Women's Primary Health Care

Protocols for Practice

Second Edition

Women's Primary Health Care

Protocols for Practice

Second Edition

Winifred L. Star, R.N., C., N.P., M.S.
Lisa L. Lommel, R.N., C., F.N.P., M.S., M.P.H.
Maureen T. Shannon, C.N.M., F.N.P., M.S.

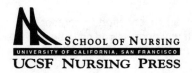

SCHOOL OF NURSING
UNIVERSITY OF CALIFORNIA, SAN FRANCISCO
UCSF NURSING PRESS

Senior Publications Coordinator: Kathleen McClung
Design/Production: Patricia Walsh Design, Monica Lacerda
Editors: Maureen Dixon, Paul Engstrom
Index: Ferreira Indexing, Inc.

For information, contact:

UCSF Nursing Press
School of Nursing
University of California, San Francisco
521 Parnassus Avenue, Room N-535C
San Francisco, CA 94143-0608 U.S.A.
Phone: (415) 476-4992
Fax: (415) 476-6042
Internet: http://nurseweb.ucsf.edu/www/books.htm

ISBN # 0-943671-21-3

Printed in U.S.A.

DISCLAIMER

The authors of *Women's Primary Health Care: Protocols for Practice* (2nd edition) and the University of California, San Francisco disavow any responsibility for the outcomes of the patients to whom any information in this publication is applied, including general assessment and treatment/ management, and in cases in which specific drug therapy has been delineated. It is the individual practicing clinician who shall remain fully responsible for the outcome of the evaluation and management of the patients to whom any clinical guidelines in this publication are applied, including instances in which specific drug therapy has been set forth. For additional information concerning specific drugs and drug therapy, health care providers should consult the drug package insert, the *Physicians' Desk Reference*, and/or a clinical pharmacist.

The contributing authors and publisher have made every effort to contact the copyright holders for borrowed material. If any permissions have been inadvertently overlooked, we will be pleased to make the necessary corrections in future printings.

To Our Mothers

Women's Primary Health Care
Protocols for Practice

Contents

Dedication .... **xiii**
Contributors .... **xv**
Medical Editors .... **xxi**
Preface to the Second Edition .... **xxiii**
Acknowledgments .... **xxv**

Section 1 — **Women's Primary Health Care—Introduction**

1-A   Women's Primary Health Care **1-2**
1-B   Scope of Practice and Medicolegal Issues **1-5**
1-C   Women's Health Across the Life Span: An Overview ... **1-8**
1-D   Lesbian Health Care **1-27**

Section 2 — **Ophthalmological Disorders**

2-A   Blepharitis **2-2**
2-B   Cataracts **2-4**
2-C   Conjunctivitis **2-6**
2-D   Dacryocystitis **2-10**
2-E   Eye Injury **2-11**
2-F   Glaucoma **2-14**
2-G   Hordeolum and Chalazion **2-17**
2-H   Keratitis **2-19**
2-I   Pinguecula and Pterygium **2-21**
2-J   Uveitis **2-22**
2-K   Bibliography **2-24**

Section 3 — **Dermatological Disorders**

3-A   Acne Rosacea **3-2**
3-B   Acne Vulgaris **3-5**
3-C   Atopic Dermatitis (Atopic Eczema) **3-8**
3-D   Burns—Minor **3-11**
3-E   Cellulitis **3-14**
3-F   Contact Dermatitis (Contact Eczema): Irritant and Allergic ... **3-16**
3-G   Dyshidrotic Eczema (Pompholyx) **3-19**
3-H   Folliculitis **3-21**

3-I Fungal Infections **3-24**
  → Tinea Versicolor (Pityriasis Versicolor) **3-24**
  → Tinea Corporis (Body Ringworm) **3-25**
  → Tinea Capitis (Scalp Ringworm) **3-26**
  → Tinea Pedis (Athlete's Foot) **3-27**
  → Tinea Cruris (Eczema Marginatum) **3-29**
  → Candidiasis (Moniliasis) **3-30**
3-J Furuncles and Carbuncles **3-32**
3-K Impetigo **3-34**
3-L Molluscum Contagiosum **3-36**
3-M Paronychia **3-38**
3-N Pediculosis **3-40**
3-O Pityriasis Rosea **3-43**
3-P Psoriasis **3-45**
3-Q Scabies **3-48**
3-R Seborrheic Dermatitis **3-51**
3-S Warts **3-53**

Section 4

Breast Disorders

4-A Breast Cancer Screening **4-2**
4-B Breast Pain and Nodularity **4-6**
4-C Duct Ectasia/Periductal Mastitis **4-10**
4-D Fat Necrosis **4-12**
4-E Fibroadenoma **4-14**
4-F Fluid Cysts **4-16**
4-G Galactocele **4-18**
4-H Galactorrhea **4-20**
4-I Intraductal Papilloma **4-23**
4-J Mastitis—Nonpuerperal **4-25**
4-K Nipple Discharge—Physiologic **4-27**
4-L Paget's Disease **4-29**
4-M Superficial Phlebitis (Mondor's Disease) **4-31**

Section 5

Respiratory/Otorhinolaryngological Disorders

5-A Asthma **5-2**
5-B Bronchiectasis **5-12**
5-C Bronchitis—Acute **5-15**
5-D Chronic Obstructive Pulmonary Disease **5-17**
5-E Epistaxis **5-23**
5-F Influenza **5-25**
5-G Otitis Externa **5-29**
5-H Otitis Media **5-31**
5-I Pharyngitis **5-33**
5-J Pneumonia **5-37**
5-K Rhinitis **5-43**
5-L Sinusitis—Acute **5-48**
5-M Sinusitis—Chronic **5-51**

Section 6

Cardiovascular Disorders

6-A Angina **6-2**
6-B Deep Vein Thrombosis **6-8**
6-C Heart Failure **6-15**

6-D	Hyperlipidemia	**6-22**
6-E	Hypertension	**6-29**
6-F	Mitral Valve Prolapse	**6-37**
6-G	Palpitations	**6-42**

Section 7

Gastrointestinal Disorders

7-A	Abdominal Pain	**7-2**
7-B	Appendicitis	**7-11**
7-C	Cholecystitis	**7-14**
7-D	Constipation	**7-18**
7-E	Diarrhea	**7-23**
7-F	Diverticular Disease	**7-29**
7-G	Gastroesophageal Reflux and Heartburn	**7-33**
7-H	Gastrointestinal Bleeding	**7-39**
7-I	Hemorrhoids and Anal Fissures	**7-43**
7-J	Hernia	**7-48**
7-K	Inflammatory Bowel Disease	**7-51**
7-L	Irritable Bowel Syndrome	**7-60**
7-M	Peptic Ulcer Disease	**7-64**

Section 8

Musculoskeletal Disorders

8-A	Common Disorders of the Musculoskeletal System—Introduction	**8-2**
8-B	Fibromyalgia	**8-3**
8-C	Osteoarthritis	**8-8**
8-D	Rheumatoid Arthritis	**8-12**
8-E	Bursitis and Tendinitis	**8-15**
8-F	Shoulder Pain	**8-18**
8-G	Elbow Pain	**8-23**
8-H	Wrist, Hand, and Finger Pain	**8-27**
	→ Carpal Tunnel Syndrome	**8-27**
	→ De Quervain's Disease	**8-30**
	→ Osteoarthritis of the Basilar Joint of the Thumb	**8-31**
	→ Trigger Fingers	**8-32**
	→ Ganglion Cysts	**8-33**
8-I	Hip Pain	**8-36**
8-J	Knee Pain	**8-39**
	→ Acute Knee Pain	**8-39**
	→ Chronic Knee Pain	**8-43**
8-K	Ankle Pain	**8-48**
8-L	Foot Pain	**8-52**
8-M	Low Back Pain	**8-58**
	→ Acute Low Back Pain	**8-59**
	→ Chronic Low Back Pain	**8-69**
8-N	Table 8N.1. Anti-inflammatory and Analgesic Medication	**8-74**

Section 9

Neurological Disorders

9-A	Bell's Palsy	**9-2**
9-B	Dizziness	**9-8**
9-C	Face Pain	**9-16**
9-D	Headache	**9-23**
	→ Migraine Headache	**9-26**
	→ Cluster Headache	**9-28**

	→ Tension-Type Headache	**9-29**
	→ Temporal or Giant Cell Arteritis	**9-30**
9-E	Seizures	**9-37**
9-F	Temporomandibular Disorder	**9-43**

Section 10

Hematological/Endocrine/Immunological Disorders

10-A	Anemia	**10-2**
10-B	Chronic Fatigue Syndrome	**10-14**
10-C	Osteoporosis	**10-18**
10-D	Systemic Lupus Erythematosus	**10-25**
10-E	Thyroid Disorders	**10-33**
10-F	Type 1 Diabetes Mellitus	**10-40**
10-G	Type 2 Diabetes Mellitus	**10-51**

Section 11

Infectious Diseases

11-A	Diarrhea—Infectious	**11-2**
11-B	Hepatitis—Viral	**11-8**
11-C	Human Immunodeficiency Virus-1 Infection	**11-20**
11-D	Lyme Disease	**11-42**
11-E	Measles (Rubeola)	**11-49**
11-F	Mononucleosis	**11-52**
11-G	Mumps	**11-55**
11-H	Rubella	**11-57**
11-I	Tuberculosis	**11-60**
11-J	Varicella Zoster Virus	**11-69**

Section 12

Genitourinary Disorders

12-A	Abnormal Uterine Bleeding	**12-3**
12-B	Abnormal Cervical Cytology	**12-13**
12-C	Amenorrhea—Secondary	**12-24**
12-D	Dysmenorrhea	**12-37**
12-E	Ectopic Pregnancy	**12-42**
12-F	Endometriosis	**12-48**
12-G	Hirsutism	**12-53**
12-H	Infertility	**12-62**
	12-HA Clomiphene Citrate	**12-76**
12-I	Pelvic Inflammatory Disease	**12-81**
12-J	Pelvic Masses	**12-87**
12-K	Pelvic Pain—Acute	**12-96**
12-L	Pelvic Pain—Chronic	**12-100**
12-M	Perimenopausal and Menopausal Symptoms and Hormone Therapy	**12-109**
12-N	Polyps—Cervical and Endometrial	**12-121**
12-O	Premenstrual Syndrome and Premenstrual Dysphoric Disorder	**12-124**
12-P	Sexual Dysfunction	**12-132**
12-Q	Toxic Shock Syndrome	**12-146**
12-R	Urinary Tract Disorders	**12-151**
	12-RA Urinary Tract Infection	**12-151**
	12-RB Female Urinary Incontinence	**12-157**
	12-RC Overactive Bladder	**12-161**
	12-RD Interstitial Cystitis	**12-164**

12-S   Vaginitis **12-167**
   12-SA   Atrophic Vaginitis **12-167**
   12-SB   Bacterial Vaginosis **12-170**
   12-SC   Candidal Vulvovaginitis **12-174**
   12-SD   Cytolytic Vaginitis **12-180**
   12-SE   *Trichomonas vaginalis* Vaginitis **12-182**
   12-SF   Table 12SF.1. Vaginal Infections **12-186**
   12-SG   Bibliography **12-187**
12-T   Vulvar Disease **12-189**
   12-TA   Red Lesions of the Vulva **12-189**
     →   Cutaneous Candidiasis **12-189**
     →   Contact Dermatitis (Reactive Vulvitis) **12-191**
     →   Paget's Disease **12-193**
   12-TB   White Lesions of the Vulva **12-195**
     →   Lichen Sclerosus **12-195**
     →   Squamous Cell Hyperplasia **12-197**
   12-TC   Dark Lesions of the Vulva **12-200**
     →   Lentigo **12-200**
     →   Nevi **12-200**
     →   Seborrheic Keratosis **12-201**
     →   Melanoma **12-202**
   12-TD   Small Lesions of the Vulva **12-205**
     →   Epidermal Cysts **12-205**
     →   Acrochordons **12-206**
     →   Hidradenitis Suppurativa **12-206**
     →   Hemangiomas **12-208**
     →   Caruncle (Urethral) **12-209**
     →   Fox-Fordyce Disease **12-209**
   12-TE   Large Lesions of the Vulva **12-211**
     →   Bartholin's Cyst/Abscess **12-211**
     →   Verrucous Carcinoma **12-214**
   12-TF   Ulcerative Lesions of the Vulva **12-216**
     →   Squamous Cell Carcinoma **12-216**
     →   Basal Cell Carcinoma **12-219**
   12-TG   Vulvar Intraepithelial Neoplasia **12-221**
   12-TH   Vulvodynia **12-224**
12-U   Vaginal Intraepithelial Neoplasia **12-233**

Section 13   **Sexually Transmitted Diseases**
13-A   Chancroid **13-2**
13-B   *Chlamydia trachomatis* **13-9**
13-C   Gonorrhea **13-17**
13-D   Granuloma Inguinale (Donovanosis) **13-25**
13-E   Genital Herpes Simplex Virus **13-29**
13-F   Human Papillomavirus **13-37**
13-G   Lymphogranuloma Venereum **13-45**
13-H   Syphilis **13-50**

Section 14   **Behavioral Disorders**
14-A   Alcohol and Other Drug Problems **14-2**
14-B   Anxiety Disorders **14-10**
14-C   Depression **14-19**

CONTENTS

14-D Domestic Violence **14-30**
14-E Eating Disorders **14-35**
14-F Sexual Abuse (Minors and Adult Survivors) **14-46**
14-G Sexual Assault **14-51**
14-H Smoking Cessation **14-64**
14-I Stress Management **14-69**

Section 15   **Occupational Health** **15-1**

Section 16   **General Nutrition Guidelines** **16-1**

Index   Index of Tables, Figures, and Appendices **I-1**
              Index **I-7**

Dedication

To my mother, Winifred V. Star, for a life well-lived. And to Dawn Isaacs, my friend and colleague, who was created in her mother Edvige's image—strong, sincere, sensitive, and full of common sense.

WLS

To my husband, Michael, and children, Liam and Tess, for letting me realize my dreams and enjoying the ride along with me. To my parents, Jerome and Rosemary, for being there every step of the way. Thank you all!

LLL

To the Shannon-Pantell Family Circus (Bob, Matt, Greg, and Megan) for their patience and humor during the preparation of this edition, to my parents with appreciation for all their support, and to my patients who continue to teach me.

MTS

Contributors

Principal Authors and Editors

Winifred L. Star, R.N., C., N.P., M.S.
Women's Health Nurse Practitioner
Coordinator, Young Mother's Clinic
Department of Obstetrics and Gynecology
Kaiser Permanente Medical Center
San Francisco, California

Associate Clinical Professor
Department of Family Health Care Nursing
University of California, San Francisco
San Francisco, California

Associate Clinical Professor
Department of Obstetrics, Gynecology, and Reproductive Sciences
University of California, San Francisco
San Francisco, California

Lisa L. Lommel, R.N., C., F.N.P., M.S., M.P.H.
Associate Clinical Professor
Family Nurse Practitioner Program
Department of Family Health Care Nursing
University of California, San Francisco
San Francisco, California

Director, Young Women's Program
University of California at Mt. Zion
San Francisco, California

Maureen T. Shannon, C.N.M., F.N.P., M.S.
Associate Clinical Professor
Department of Family Health Care Nursing
University of California, San Francisco
San Francisco, California

Certified Nurse-Midwife and Family Nurse Practitioner
Women's Specialty Clinic
Perinatal HIV Program
University of California, San Francisco
San Francisco, California

Contributing Authors

Susan L. Adams, Ph.D., R.N., N.P.
Associate Professor of Nursing
Dominican University of California
San Rafael, California

Claire L. Appelmans, R.N., C., W.H.C.N.P., M.S.
Nurse Practitioner
Santa Clara County Public Health Department
San Jose, California

Clinical Faculty
Planned Parenthood Federation of America
   Nurse Practitioner Program
Philadelphia, Pennsylvania

Toni Ayres, R.N., M.F.T., Ed.D.
Lecturer
Department of Counseling
San Francisco State University
San Francisco, California

Marriage and Family Therapist
Private Practice
Berkeley, California

Pilar Bernal de Pheils, R.N., M.S., F.N.P.
Associate Clinical Professor
Department of Family Health Care Nursing
University of California, San Francisco
San Francisco, California

Family Nurse Practitioner
Women's Clinic Faculty Practice
Mission Neighborhood Health Center
Department of Family Health Care Nursing
University of California, San Francisco
San Francisco, California

Family Nurse Practitioner
Valencia Health Services Clinic Faculty Practice
Department of Family Health Care Nursing
University of California, San Francisco
San Francisco, California

Ann M. Brennan, R.N., M.S., A.N.P., P.N.P.
Nurse Practitioner, Manager
Trauma Recovery/Rape Treatment Center
San Francisco General Hospital Emergency Department
San Francisco, California

Scott Brown, R.D., C.D.E.
Manager
Nutrition Clinics North-East Bay Area
Kaiser Permanente Medical Center
San Francisco, California

Barbara J. Burgel, R.N., M.S., C.O.H.N.S., F.A.A.N.
Clinical Professor and Adult Nurse Practitioner
Department of Community Health Systems
Occupational and Environmental Health Nursing Program
University of California, San Francisco
San Francisco, California

Geraldine M. Collins-Bride, R.N., M.S., A.N.P.
Associate Clinical Professor and Vice-Chair
Department of Community Health Systems
University of California, San Francisco
San Francisco, California

Jeanne R. Davis, R.N., F.N.P., M.P.H.
Nurse Coordinator
Glaser Pediatric Research Network
Stanford University
Palo Alto, California

Melanie Deal, R.N., C., N.P., M.S.
Clinical Program Manager
Infertility Prevention Project
California Family Health Council
Berkeley, California

Carole E. Deitrich, R.N., C., M.S., G.N.P.
Clinical Professor
Department of Physiological Nursing
University of California, San Francisco
San Francisco, California

Gerontological Nurse Practitioner
Laguna Honda Hospital and Rehabilitation Center
San Francisco, California

Sari Fredrickson, M.S., F.N.P., R.N., C.
Family Nurse Practitioner
Kaiser Permanente Medical Center
Walnut Creek, California

Jacqueline Wish Gilbert, R.N., M.S., C.F.N.P.
Family Nurse Practitioner
San Francisco Department of Public Health
Chinatown Public Health Center
San Francisco, California

St. Anthony's Free Medical Clinic in association with
The Department of Children, Youth, and Families
San Francisco Department of Public Health
Pediatric Clinic
San Francisco, California

Lynn Hanson, R.N., N.P., M.S.
Nurse Practitioner
Department of Obstetrics, Gynecology, and Reproductive
  Sciences
Department of Pediatrics, Division of Adolescent Medicine
University of California, San Francisco
San Francisco, California

Linda K. Humphrey, R.N., C., N.P., C.N.S., M.S.
Women's Health Nurse Practitioner
Department of Obstetrics and Gynecology
Kaiser Permanente Medical Center
San Rafael, California

Laura Hutkins, R.N., M.S, F.N.P., C.S.
Nurse Practitioner
Department of Internal Medicine
Kaiser Permanente Medical Center
Redwood City, California

Lecturer
Family Nurse Practitioner Program
San Jose State University
San Jose, California

Martha A. Jessup, R.N., Ph.D.
Fellow
Institute for Health Policy Studies
University of California, San Francisco
San Francisco, California

Catherine M. Kelber, R.N., M.S., A.N.P., B.C.
Associate Clinical Professor and Associate Director
Adult Nurse Practitioner Program
Department of Community Health Systems
University of California, San Francisco
San Francisco, California

Tekoa King, C.N.M., M.P.H.
Associate Clinical Professor
Department of Obstetrics, Gynecology, and Reproductive
  Sciences
University of California, San Francisco
San Francisco, California

Editor-in-Chief
Journal of Nurse Midwifery & Women's Health

Anita Levine-Goldberg, R.N., N.P., M.S.
Women's Health Nurse Practitioner
Department of Obstetrics and Gynecology
Kaiser Permanente Medical Center
Santa Rosa, California

Jenna A. Lewis, M.S.N., W.H.N.P., A.N.P.
Women's Health Nurse Practitioner
Department of Obstetrics and Gynecology
Kaiser Permanente Medical Center
San Francisco, California

Sandra L. Lindholm-Norman, R.N., M.S., N.P.
Women's Health Nurse Practitioner
Department of Obstetrics and Gynecology
Department of Urology
Kaiser Permanente Medical Center
Walnut Creek, California

Ann-Marie McNamara, R.N., C., N.P., M.S.
Clinical Instructor
Edgewood College
Madison, Wisconsin

Jane A. Newhard-Parks, R.N., M.S.N., F.N.P.
Family Nurse Practitioner
Fremont High School Tiger Clinic
Clinica Alta Vista
La Clinica de la Raza
Oakland, California

5M Women's Clinic
Department of Obstetrics and Gynecology
San Francisco General Hospital
San Francisco, California

Medical Unit
San Leandro Juvenile Justice System
Ambulatory Care Services
Alameda County, California

Loren D. Newman, R.N., F.N.P., C., B.S.N.
Employee Health Coordinator
Kaiser Permanente Medical Center
Roseville, California

Kim K. O'Hair, R.N.P., M.S.N.
Women's Health Nurse Practitioner
Women's Health Faculty Practice
University of California at Mt. Zion
San Francisco, California

Assistant Clinical Professor
Department of Family Health Care Nursing
University of California, San Francisco
San Francisco, California

Joan Y. Okasako, R.N., C.S., F.N.P., M.S.
Family Nurse Practitioner
Department of Obstetrics and Gynecology
Kaiser Permanente Medical Center
San Francisco, California

Diane C. Putney, M.N., R.N., C.F.N.P.
Nurse Practitioner
Department of Orthopedic Surgery
Kaiser Permanente Medical Center
South San Francisco, California

Julie Richards, R.N., C., W.H.N.P., F.N.P., M.S., M.S.N.
Nurse Practitioner
Nevada State Health Division
Bureau of Community Health
Carson City, Nevada

Mary M. Rubin, R.N., C., Ph.D., C.R.N.P.
Women's Health Care Specialist and Colposcopy Consultant
Associate Clinical Professor
Department of Family Health Care Nursing
University of California, San Francisco

Nurse Coordinator for Clinical Research
Department of Gynecological Oncology
University of California, San Francisco
San Francisco, California

JoAnne M. Saxe, R.N., M.S., A.N.P., B.C.
Adult Nurse Practitioner
Clinical Professor and Director
Adult Nurse Practitioner Program
Department of Community Health Systems
University of California, San Francisco
San Francisco, California

Ellen M. Scarr, R.N., C., M.S., F.N.P., W.H.N.P.
Associate Clinical Professor and Associate Director
Family Nurse Practitioner Program
Department of Family Health Care Nursing
University of California, San Francisco
San Francisco, California

Nurse Practitioner
Young Women's Program
University of California, San Francisco/Mt. Zion Medical Center
San Francisco, California

Margaret A. Scott, R.N., M.S.N., F.N.P.
Assistant Clinical Professor
Department of Family Health Care Nursing
University of California, San Francisco

Nurse Practitioner
Young Women's Program
University of California, San Francisco/Mt. Zion Medical Center
San Francisco, California

Kellie Sheehan, R.N., C., M.S.N., F.N.P.
Nurse Practitioner
General Internal Medicine
University of California, San Francisco
San Francisco, California

Jennifer L. Tagatz, R.N., C., M.S., F.N.P.
Family Nurse Practitioner
Department of Obstetrics and Gynecology
Kaiser Permanente Medical Center
San Francisco, California

Family Nurse Practitioner
Women's Options Clinic
Department of Obstetrics and Gynecology
University of California San Francisco/
    San Francisco General Hospital
San Francisco, California

Robin Taylor, R.N., M.S.N., F.N.P.
Independent Consultant
Medical/Drug Safety Writer
San Francisco, California

Kathryn Zender, R.N., M.S.N., F.N.P.
Nurse Practitioner
Department of Neurology
Kaiser Permanente Medical Center
San Francisco, California

Contributors to the First Edition

Wendy Berk, C.A.N.P.
Bell's Palsy
Face Pain
Temporomandibular Disorder

Jeanette M. Broering, R.N., M.S., C.P.N.P.
Women's Health Across the Lifespan: An Overview—
    Adolescent Health Care Issues (Women 13 to 19 Years of Age)
Human Papillomavirus

Rozane Moon Gee, R.D., M.S., C.D.E.
General Nutrition Guidelines

Michelle M. Marin, R.N., M.S., A.N.P.
Anemia

Carolyn Muir, R.N., C., N.P., M.S.
Fertility Awareness

Joan R. Murphy, R.N., C., M.S., N.P., C.N.S.
Dysmenorrhea
Genital Herpes Simplex Virus

Elisabeth O'Mara, R.N., M.S., A.N.P., C.D.E.
Type 1 Diabetes Mellitus
Type 2 Diabetes Mellitus

Jan Reddick, M.S.N., F.N.P.
Dermatological Disorders

Julie Richards, R.N., C., W.H.N.P., F.N.P., M.S., M.S.N.
Battering/Domestic Violence
Endometriosis
Sexual Assault

Diana Taylor, Ph.D., R.N., F.A.A.N.
Women's Health Across the Lifespan: An Overview—
    Health Care Issues for Women During Midlife (40 to 64 Years
    of Age)
Perimenopausal Symptoms and Hormone Therapy
Perimenstrual Symptoms and Premenstrual Syndrome

Jacqueline Wish Gilbert, R.N., M.S., C.F.N.P.
(formerly Jacqueline W. Wasserman)
Dizziness/Vertigo
Headache
Seizures

Lori M. Weseman, R.N., M.S., N.P.
Infertility
Clomiphene Citrate

Medical Editors

Amy V. Kindrick, M.D., M.P.H.
Associate Physician
San Francisco General Hospital
Department of Family and Community Medicine
University of California, San Francisco
San Francisco, California

Sarah Maria Mandel, M.S., M.D.
Senior Physician
Department of Obstetrics and Gynecology
Kaiser Permanente Medical Center
San Francisco, California

Preface to the Second Edition

The principal authors of *Women's Primary Health Care: Protocols for Practice* are pleased to bring you the second edition of this long-awaited publication. We welcome the many new contributing authors to this edition and thank the original contributors for the foundation they provided. Over the years, the first edition attracted a wide audience of practicing clinicians. It is our hope that this publication will serve as a working manual for use in many clinical practice settings, as well as a framework from which to formulate site-specific protocols and guidelines for practice. For obstetrics practitioners, our "sister book," *Ambulatory Obstetrics*,* is a helpful companion to this comprehensive volume of women's primary health care.

As in the first edition, the book is divided into several parts. Section 1 presents an overview of primary care and women's primary health care, followed by a review of standards of practice and medicolegal issues, and a discussion of health care for women across the life span.

The main body of the book contains disease- and condition-specific protocols, with each chapter utilizing the "S-O-A-P" (Subjective-Objective-Assessment-Plan) format for easy reference. These chapters address the most common entities in women's primary health care. Lastly, a general nutrition section expands upon and complements information contained in specific chapters.

Several new chapters have been added to the second edition. Original chapters have been thoroughly reviewed and revised to reflect current standards of practice. Readers are advised to consult additional literature regarding disorders/conditions for which more recent advances in research or procedures have been made.

The authors welcome your comments and suggestions. Please address all correspondence to: University of California Nursing Press
School of Nursing
521 Parnassus Avenue, Room N-535C
San Francisco, CA 94143-0608

---

*Star, W.L., Shannon, M.T., Lommel, L.L. et al. 1999. *Ambulatory obstetrics,* 3rd ed. San Francisco: University of California, San Francisco.

Acknowledgments

The publication of *Women's Primary Health Care: Protocols for Practice* (2nd edition) was facilitated by the hard work and generous support of a number of people.

The authors thank the medical editors of the book, Dr. Sarah Mandel and Dr. Amy Kindrick, for their expert review and for fine-tuning this publication to state-of-the-art standards of care.

A special thank you goes to our research assistants, Jennifer Chen and Cynthia Feakins, for organizing a multitude of literature searches and spending numerous hours in the library assembling much of the data in this second edition.

Winifred Star would like to thank her friends and colleagues for all their support during the preparation of this book, and acknowledge all her patients, who, over the years, have kept her connected in so many ways. And, to Tim Bigalke—thank you for listening.

The contributing authors thank a number of people for their support and assistance: Pilar Bernal de Pheils appreciated the support and understanding of her husband, Jon, and her two daughters, Anna Julia, and Veronica, during the many hours spent in writing her chapters. Scott Brown would like to acknowledge two nutritional science students, Caitlyn Walker and Norae Ferrara, who assisted with the development and revision of the General Nutrition Guidelines. Geraldine Collins-Bride wishes to recognize Dr. Marcus Conant for his pioneering work in the fields of herpes simplex virus and human immunodeficiency virus infections.

Jeanne Davis expresses thanks for the love and support from Eddie, her Mom and Dad, Josh, and all her friends as she worked on this project. Melanie Deal thanks Dan Fox for his unending encouragement and support. Sari Fredrickson acknowledges Wendy Berk, C.A.N.P., for her work on the first edition of the Face Pain and Bell's Palsy chapters, and thanks Carolyn Fishel, the Medical Librarian at Kaiser Permanente in Walnut Creek, California.

Jacqueline Wish Gilbert wishes to thank her husband, Clinton, for his superb computer expertise, creativity, and humorous spirit. Linda Humphrey acknowledges Gordy, who has always given her encouragement to do everything she's attempted; Diane, an incredible role model of strength and dedication; Brendan and Trevor, whose lives have enriched her more than she thought possible; and Terry, for showing her that true success lies within love and happiness.

Lynn Hanson thanks her son, Connor Martin, for his help with the computer, and her colleagues Jean Perry, R.N., N.P., M.S.; Karen Smith-McCune, M.D.; and Teresa Darragh, M.D. Laura Hutkins acknowledges Marian Brame, R.P.T.; Sari Fredrickson, F.N.P.; and Wendy Berk, N.P., for their mentoring. Kim O'Hair thanks Dick and Donna.

Marty Jessup would like to acknowledge that work on her chapter was supported by the Treatment Research Center, Department of Psychiatry, University of California, San Francisco, and the National Institute on Drug Abuse (Grant #P5ODA09253). To Joseph R. Guydish, Ph.D., James L. Sorensen, Ph.D., and Sharon M. Hall, Ph.D.—thank you for your mentoring, support, and guidance.

Sandra Lindholm-Norman wishes to thank Robert for all of his technical support. Joan Okasako acknowledges Ian, Devon, and Doug for their love and support. Diane Putney acknowledges Dr. Robert Silverstein and Dr. James Johnson for their mentoring over the past 12 years, and Geri Bodeker, M.S., C.H.E.S., who performed the literature searches for the Musculoskeletal Disorders section of the book.

JoAnne Saxe acknowledges her husband, Noel, and daughters Kelly, Jocelyn, and Lydia for their love and inspiration, and her A.N.P. colleagues and students for their words of wisdom, encouragement, and support. Ellen Scarr offers many thanks to Roberta Acker for her enthusiasm and ongoing support during the preparation of the manuscript. Meg Scott thanks her husband, Robbie Scott, whose patience and enduring support sustained her throughout this project.

Jennifer Tagatz thanks George, Susan, Kirsten, Gary, Katie, Craig, and Winnie for always believing in her and pushing her to excel. Robin Taylor is grateful to her colleagues at the Northern California Comprehensive Epilepsy Center, University of California, San Francisco with whom she worked from 1988 to 1997. Kathryn Zender wishes to thank the staff of the Department of Neurology at Kaiser Permanente, San Francisco for their support of this endeavor, Dan Rosen, M.D., for his valuable advice and support, and John Di Minno for his love, support, and ever-present sense of humor.

To Kathleen Thibadeau, Maureen Sullivan, Winifred Duggan, and Monica Lacerda—thank you for your gracious assistance and expertise with manuscript preparation of the second edition. To Michael Stadler, a thank you for the computer design work on several algorithms and figures in the book. To our editors, Maureen Dixon and Paul Engstrom, who had the immense task of getting the manuscript letter perfect, we thank you for all your efforts on this publication. And to the Walsh Design Group, thank you for putting the wonderful finishing touches on the book.

And, finally, we thank Kathleen McClung, Senior Publications Coordinator at the Nursing Press of the University of California, San Francisco for organizing the many aspects of the book's publication, and William Holzemer, Ph.D., for the generous financial support and commitment to this project.

SECTION 1

Women's Primary Health Care – Introduction

1-A Women's Primary Health Care **1-2**
1-B Scope of Practice and Medicolegal Issues **1-5**
1-C Women's Health Across the Life Span: An Overview **1-8**
1-D Lesbian Health Care **1-27**

Lisa L. Lommel, R.N., C., F.N.P., M.S., M.P.H.

1-A

Women's Primary Health Care

Women's health refers to a spectrum of research, prevention, and treatments related to maintaining and restoring the health of women. The term is used in reference to diseases, disorders, and conditions that, compared to those in men, are unique to, more prevalent among, or more serious in women or that have different risk factors or interventions (Gonen 1999).

Broadly speaking, *primary care* is a concept that describes a domain of service, a type of practitioner, or a philosophy of care (Brown et al. 1999). The latest definition of primary care, developed by the Institute of Medicine, states that "primary care is the provision of integrated, accessible health care services by clinicians who are accountable for addressing a large majority of personal health care needs, developing a sustained partnership with patients, and practicing in the context of family and community" (Donaldson et al. 1996). In addition to functioning as the initial point of contact with the health delivery system, critical features of primary health care include other systems of care:

→ *Disease prevention* (primary, secondary, tertiary)

→ *Health promotion* (maintenance and enhancement of health)

→ *Care coordination* (outreach, advocacy, referral, service coordination)

→ *Community health development* (consumer involvement, public health functions)

→ *Managed care* (cost containment, outcome evaluation) (Taylor 1993)

As the distinct health care needs of women are identified, so too are the unique primary care needs that extend beyond but include reproductive health care. The components of women's primary care include medical diseases (such as cardiology and endocrinology), reproductive care (including gynecology, obstetrics, and oncology), psychology and behavioral medicine (including depression, alcohol or drug use, eating disorders, and domestic violence), and preventive medicine (including cancer screening) (Carlson et al. 1995).

Two areas of women's primary care that have been neglected are mental and behavioral health and preventive health services. Primary care must include evaluation, diagnosis, treatment,

and referral for mental health issues to be truly comprehensive. In addition, data from the 1991 National Health Interview Survey showed that women were not engaging in preventive health behaviors to protect against serious illness, nor were they receiving screening to detect treatable disease (Gonen 1999). The study found that 46% of women over age 40 who were interviewed had not received a clinical breast exam in the past two years. Additionally, of the three in five women who reported engaging in risky behavior (smoking, alcohol, or drug use), the majority were not asked about these behaviors during the most recent check-up (Gonen 1999).

The Commonwealth Fund Survey of Women's Health indicated that the main factors positively influencing whether women received preventive services were insurance coverage and having a regular source of care. Factors negatively influencing whether women received preventive services included failure of health professionals to counsel women about prevention or refer them to screening, barriers to access such as lack of insurance, lack of transportation, or work and child care difficulties (Commonwealth Fund Commission of Women's Health 1996).

In providing women's health services, the health care provider must recognize how health risks and concerns affect certain subgroups of women—i.e., women of color, women living in poverty, substance abusers, lesbians, and immigrants. Health should be addressed and managed within the context of the individual experience. In these contexts, the value of the health norm should be evaluated and individualized. The focus of change may be on the environment rather than the individual—e.g., an emphasis on social support networks, time and role management, or stress in the workplace.

Providers of Primary Health Care for Women

The medical community has long debated what types of providers are best suited to provide primary care to women. The consensus is that women's primary care is about more than reproductive health, yet obstetrician/gynecologists (ob/gyns) historically have not been trained to deliver comprehensive non-reproductive care, and family physicians and internists have not been trained to care for more complicated disorders of the reproductive system. Primary care clinicians are supposed to care for every problem that the patient brings, no matter what type of problem or organ system; have the appropriate training to manage a large majority of these problems; and involve other practitioners for further evaluation or treatment when appropriate (Bartman 1996). Simply stated, a primary health care clinician is responsible for making decisions regarding all aspects of a woman's care. Medical education has responded to this dilemma by instituting programs and fellowships in women's health that integrate relevant issues from all specialties (Council on Graduate Medical Education 1995). Furthermore, data from the Commonwealth Fund Survey of Women's Health indicates that one-third of women regularly seek care from both a primary care physician and an ob/gyn (these women made 25% more visits than women seeing only one provider); 39% see only primary care physicians; and 16% see only ob/gyns for their primary care (Commonwealth Fund Commission of Women's Health 1996). All of this points to the need for all types of providers to become actively involved in comprehensive primary care services for women.

Nonphysician providers, including nurse practitioners, nurse midwives, and physician assistants, have long served as primary care providers for women. These clinicians also provide care to underserved women in greater numbers than do physicians. Advanced practice nursing education has always focused on health promotion and disease prevention activities and patient education as a principle goal in health care delivery. A 1986 study by the U.S. Congress, Office of Technology Assessment, found that nurse practitioners and certified nurse midwives provided primary care that was, in fact, equal in quality to the care provided by physicians, and that they outperformed physicians in the areas of communication and preventive care (U.S. Congress, Office of Technology Assessment 1986). A 1993 study by the American Nurses Association reached similar conclusions (Brown 1993).

Chronic Illness and Primary Health Care for Women

As the baby boom population ages, there will be more women over age 65 than ever before. Women, in particular, suffer from more chronic illnesses than men, live longer with more disabilities, and are more focused on the health of other family members than their own. Given this, primary health care must include continuity of care for long-term illness in addition to episodic illness care and promoting preventive health. In response to demographics, increasing numbers of programs aimed at chronic women's health problems have emerged. These programs address cardiovascular health, breast and ovarian cancer, osteoporosis, chronic pelvic pain, eating disorders, and women with disabilities (Gevirtz et al. 1999). Preventing and managing chronic illness can improve individual health and inhibit preventable skyrocketing health care costs.

Multidisciplinary Women's Primary Health Care

A multidisciplinary approach to women's health has gained momentum over the past 20 years. It is based on the concept that all of a woman's bio-psychosocial needs may be taken care of in one setting. There are many such settings throughout the world that show strong evidence of quality of care, decreased cost, and improved patient satisfaction.

The term *multidisciplinary* has two primary meanings. The first focuses on the participation of a variety of health professions in the health care of women, including physicians, nurse practitioners, nurses, psychologists, nutritionists, social workers, physical therapists, health educators, and alternative medicine practitioners (Carlson 2000). The second meaning refers to the integration of care across medical specialties, including medicine, obstetrics and gynecology, psychiatry, surgery, endocrinology, cardiology, gastroenterology, orthopedics, physiatry and gynecologic specialties such as infertility, urogynecology, and oncology (Carlson 2000).

The multidisciplinary approach to women's health care is an important model because it provides comprehensive primary care services, expands the concepts of women's health beyond its traditional focus on reproductive health (Carlson 2000), and can provide a setting for research to generate knowledge that is unique to women.

Expanding the definition of women's health to include primary health care is critical to meeting women's needs. By understanding primary care and women's health, the provider will be better able to provide optimal and appropriate care to this population. Therefore, the goal of this book is to provide assessment and management strategies for selected aspects and conditions of women's primary health care. This will assist and guide the health provider to include primary health care in the comprehensive care of women.

BIBLIOGRAPHY

Bartman, B.A. 1996. Women's access to appropriate providers within managed care: implications for the quality of primary care. *Women's Health Issues* 6(1):45–50.

Brown, C.V. 1999. Primary care role for women: the role of the obstetrician-gynecologist. *Clinical Obstetrics and Gynecology* 42(2):306–313.

Brown, S.A., and Grimes, D.E. 1993. *Nurse practitioners and certified nurse midwives: a meta-analysis of studies on nurses in primary care roles.* Washington D.C.: American Nurses Association.

Carlson, K.J. 2000. Multidisciplinary women's health care and quality of care. *Women's Health Issues* 10(5):220–225.

Carlson, K.J., Eisenstat, S.A., Frigloetto, F.D. et al. 1995. *Primary care of women.* St. Louis, Mo.: Mosby.

Commonwealth Fund Commission of Women's Health. 1996. *Prevention and women's health: a shared responsibility.* New York: The Commonwealth Fund.

Council on Graduate Medical Education. 1995. *Fifth report: women and medicine.* Chicago.

Donaldson, M.S., Yordy, K.D., Lohr, K.N. et al. eds. 1996. *Primary care: America's health in a new era.* Washington, D.C.: National Academy Press.

Gevirtz, F., Corrato, R.R., Chodoff, P., et al. 1999. Chronic disease, women's health, and "disease management": the latest trend? *Women's Health Issues* 9(1):18–29.

Gonen, J.S. 1999. Women's primary care in managed care: clinical and provider issues. *Women's Health Issues* 9(Suppl. 2): 5S–14S.

Taylor, D. 1993. Primary care and primary health care in the United States. *Primary care medicine, principles and practice.* San Francisco: University of California, San Francisco.

U.S. Congress. Office of Technology Assessment. 1986. *Nurse practitioners, physician assistants and certified nurse midwives: a policy analysis.* Washington, D.C.: U.S. Government Printing Office.

Winifred L. Star, R.N., C., N.P., M.S.
Loren D. Newman, R.N., F.N.P., C., B.S.N.

1-B

Scope of Practice and Medicolegal Issues

Standardized Procedures

The boundaries of nursing practice are delineated in statutes passed by the legislatures in individual states (Hogue 1989). These nursing practice acts, which may vary from state to state, are designed to safeguard the public interest and legally sanction the practice of nursing. The Nurse Practice Act regulates nurse practitioner (NP) practice in all 50 states. In five states, however, NPs are regulated jointly by the Boards of Medicine and Boards of Nursing (Pearson 2003). In some states, there is legislative intent to realize the existence of overlapping functions between nurses and physicians, implemented via the development of standardized procedures and protocols. In most states, the role of an advance practice nurse (APN), specifically an NP, is dependent on practice protocols. Creating appropriate practice protocols is one of the most important precursors to implementing the advanced practice role because they determine the clinician's ability to treat or manage clinical situations or disease (Paul 1999). Written protocols provide the means for expanding the practice of nursing beyond what is commonly perceived as traditional (Kauffroath 1990).

Nurse practitioners must be knowledgeable about their state nursing practice acts and guidelines for the development of standardized procedures. Copies of these documents may be obtained from each state's board of registered nursing (BRN). California requires that standardized procedures be developed through collaborative efforts among administrators, physicians, and nurses, and that these procedures must specify the scope of supervision required for their performance. Standardized procedures are not subject to prior approval by the BRN or board of medical quality assurance (BMQA). However, they must be developed according to guidelines jointly promulgated by these boards (Board of Registered Nursing 1998).

In California, standardized procedures have two components: 1) the policy component—i.e., the general intent to allow registered nurses to perform a specific clinical function or service in a particular setting; and 2) the protocols—i.e., the rules or procedures to be followed in performing the clinical function or

service authorized by the policy (California Nurses Association [CNA] 1989).

There are two types of protocols—*disease-specific* or *procedure-specific protocols* and *process protocols*. Disease-specific/procedure-specific protocols delineate steps for treating and managing a specific disease or for carrying out a specific procedure. Process protocols are function-based and describe the steps to be taken in performing a given function, such as an evaluation of chronic illness. Process protocols specify requirements for care but do not mandate medical content (CNA 1989).

The protocols in *Women's Primary Health Care: Protocols for Practice* represent disease-specific protocols. They are intended as guidelines for practice and should be adapted for use in different practice settings based on limitations and variations unique to the institution or type of practice and the needs/resources of the patient. In addition, these protocols should not be considered as *the* standard of care, as there is not one standard of care for every situation encountered in everyday practice (Gillstrap 1992).

Protocols can be used in three ways. The first is to meet the state requirement for a protocol, thereby providing a legal framework for practice. If deviation from the standard or protocol causes damage to the patient, the APN could be legally vulnerable. For that reason, protocols must reflect the minimum requirements for safe care rather than the maximum for ideal care (Paul 1999). The second use for protocols is as a guide to increasing practice excellence. Well-chosen protocols present an array of pertinent information that may enhance the outcome of a clinical situation. Finally, protocols may be used as a performance assessment tool for managers who supervise NPs. If a protocol is used as a management tool, it may be desirable that it exceeds the minimum standard for safety demanded by the state but is not as comprehensive as protocols designed to explore all avenues of excellence. Such a tool would allow for assessing current qualities in practice but would also be useful for identifying additional areas for professional growth. Hence, in order for a protocol to be optimally useful, it is important to determine the purpose for which it is intended.

Prescriptive Authority and Reimbursement

Individual states' laws concerning the furnishing of drugs and devices must be adhered to for nursing practice to be within legal bounds. In general, there has been significant advancement in NP prescribing. All 50 states and the District of Columbia have legislated some form of prescriptive authority for nurse practitioners. Forty-five states and the District of Columbia also include a provision for nurse practitioners to prescribe controlled substances (Pearson 2003). Advanced practice nurses in 38 states and the District of Columbia may apply for Drug Enforcement Agency (DEA) numbers (Pearson 2003). APNs' legal authority to practice has expanded in some states each year, and this continues to benefit health care for our nation's citizens. Twenty-five states and the District of Columbia have no specific requirement for physician supervision of nurse practitioners. Physician collaboration is required in 14 states and physician supervision in six (Pearson 2003).

With regard to reimbursement, all 50 states allow some form of Medicaid reimbursement for APNs. The majority of states reimburse at 80–100% of the amount paid for similar services provided by physicians (Pearson 2000). A major breakthrough in reimbursement came on November 2, 1999, when the Health Care Financing Administration (HCFA) published the ruling governing Medicare Part B reimbursement for nurse practitioners and clinical nurse specialists. It allows for direct billing of up to 85% of the physician fee schedule (American College of Nurse Practitioners 1999).

Restrictive barriers to nursing practice are gradually being removed. For advanced practice nursing to fulfill its mission to provide primary health care to all individuals, additional legislative reforms are needed nationwide. Political involvement by APNs is critical to changing laws governing prescriptive authority and third-party reimbursement.

Malpractice and Professional Liability Insurance

All health care providers are affected by the medical malpractice crisis in this country. With the expansion of the role of the APN comes increased responsibility and liability. Despite past surveys, which show very few malpractice cases against NPs, nurses today are increasingly being held personally accountable for their practice, and malpractice claims against nurses are continuing to increase (Feutz-Harter 1997, Nettles-Carlson et al. 1988). According to the National Practitioner Data Bank (NPDB) 2000 Annual Report (containing accumulated data since 1990), NPs have been responsible for 4.7% of all nurse malpractice payments (U.S. Department of Health and Human Services 2000).

Though medicolegal issues of health care are not routinely taught in nursing schools, nurses are responsible for knowing the law and how to comply with it (Feutz-Harter 1997). Ignorance is not defensible in a malpractice action!

Lawsuits occur when legal limits of practice have allegedly been breached and may occur despite legitimate practice. It is reported that of all medical malpractice claims filed, less than 50% result in any type of payment; less than 10% proceed to trial; and, of those that do, around 80% result in verdicts for the defendant (Feutz-Harter 1989).

Legal liability for malpractice means that an individual is accountable for acts of negligence that he or she has committed. However, liability can expand to include that individual's site manager, supervisory person, or employer (Feutz-Harter 1989). Areas of practice of particular importance with respect to liability include charting and documentation, informed consent and treatment decisions, and confidentiality and privacy issues. APNs must be especially aware of the practice implications in all these areas.

The level of conduct for which a nurse is held accountable is referred to as the *standard of care* (Feutz-Harter 1989). As discussed previously, standards of care should be flexible and individualized according to the particular situation. Nurse practitioners must keep abreast of advances in health care as they apply to clinical practice, both regionally and nationally. Competency mandates a continual process of updating knowledge and skills (Feutz-Harter 1989).

Unfortunately, protocols of care or practice standards can be used against the health care provider in a lawsuit. Failure to comply precisely with the written standard may constitute a breach of conduct and thus increase liability. Moniz (1992) suggests that to minimize malpractice risk, protocols should be realistic, represent the minimum requirements for safe care instead of the maximum for ideal care, and should be updated regularly as knowledge develops. Once adopted, Moniz warns, protocols must be *followed*—deviation can have legal implications.

Professional liability insurance offers protection for nurses in the event of patient harm when the acceptable standard of care has allegedly been breached (Feutz-Harter 1997). Nurses must be knowledgeable about which professional services are covered under their professional liability insurance policy. In securing an individual policy, the nurse should consider his or her security needs; advanced practice and professional activities in and outside the work site; personal assets; amount of coverage provided by the employer; and the individual nurse's area of nursing practice, its potential for lawsuits, and the amount of past awards (Feutz-Harter 1997).

There are many misconceptions regarding the extent to which a nurse is afforded protection under the employer's liability insurance policy. Coverage is provided for actions performed within the scope of employment and the job description. In the event of a malpractice suit, the employer may, however, seek compensation for damages awarded against the institution for acts of commission or omission by the nurse (Feutz-Harter 1997). In actual practice, this "going after" the nurse occurs rarely (if at all), as it sets up too adversarial a relationship between nurse and employer.

Actions performed outside the scope of employment may also result in malpractice claims, and the "Good Samaritan" law cannot be relied upon to provide absolute immunity. Even offering well-intentioned advice may expose a nurse to malpractice action.

For additional information on legal issues in nursing, please refer to *Nursing and the Law* by Sheryl Feutz-Harter (listed in the bibliography), to nursing professional organizations, and/or to risk management professionals at individual institutions.

BIBLIOGRAPHY

American College of Nurse Practitioners. 1999. HCFA's final rule on the notice of proposed rule making regarding the physician fee schedule/year 2000. *American College of Nurse Practitioners Bulletin November 5, 1999.* Available at: http://www.nurse.org/acnp/medicare/hcfa.991102.shtml. Accessed on August 1, 2001.

American Nurses Association. 2000. *ANA analysis and comparison chart: analysis and comparison of advanced practice recognition with Medicaid reimbursement and insurance reimbursement laws 2000 chart.* Available at: http://www.nursingworld.org/gova/charts/medicaid.htm. Accessed on September 6, 2001.

Board of Registered Nursing. 1998. *An explanation of standardized procedure requirements for nurse practitioner practice,* NPR-B-20. Available at: http://www.rn.ca.gov/policies/pdf/npr-b-20.pdf. Accessed on April 4, 2001.

_____. 1998, *Nurse practitioners,* BP2834-R. Available at: http://www.rn.ca.gov/policies/pdf/bp2834-r.pdf. Accessed on April 4, 2001.

_____. 1999. *Frequently asked questions regarding nurse practitioner practice,* NPR-I-25. Available at: http://www.rn.ca.gov/policies/pdf/npr-i-25.pdf. Accessed on April 4, 2001.

_____. 2000. *California State Board of Pharmacy rules and regulations—excerpts pertaining to nurse practitioner furnishing and certified nurse-midwife furnishing,* BP4018. Available at: http://www.rn.ca.gov/policies/pdf/bp-4018.pdf. Accessed on April 4, 2001.

_____. 2000. *Nurse practitioners new authority to provide medications,* NPR-B-26. Available at: http://www.rn.ca.gov/policies/pdf/npr-b-26.pdf. Accessed on April 4, 2001.

California Nurses Association. 1989. *Nursing practice in California: rights, responsibilities, and regulations.* San Francisco: the Author.

Feutz-Harter, S. 1989. *Nursing and the law.* Eau Claire, Wis.: Professional Education Systems.

_____. 1997. *Nursing and the law,* 6th ed. Eau Claire, Wis.: Professional Education Systems.

Gillstrap, L.C. III. 1992. Legal issues in obstetrics. Lecture presented at the Tenth National Kaiser Permanente Obstetrics and Gynecology Conference. Kamuela, Hawaii, July 1992.

Hogue, E. 1989. The importance of supporting nursing colleagues on scope of practice issues. *Pediatric Nursing* 15(1):82–83.

Kauffroath, K.A. 1990. *California statutes affecting nursing practice.* Eau Claire, Wis.: Professional Education Systems.

Mahoney, D.F. 1992. Nurse practitioners as prescribers: past research trends and future study needs. *Nurse Practitioner* 17(1):44–51.

Moniz, D.M. 1992. The danger of written protocols and standards of practice. *Nurse Practitioner* 17(9):58–60.

Nettles-Carlson, B., and Wolfe, J. 1988. Survey shows few malpracice claims against NPs. *Tar Heel Nurse* 50(1):1–11.

Paul, S. 1999. Developing practice protocols for advanced practice. *American Association of Critical-Care Nurses Clinical Issues 1999,* August 10 (3):343–355.

Pearson, L.J. 2000. Annual legislative update: how each state stands on legislative issues affecting advanced nursing practice. *Nurse Practitioner* 25(1):16–28.

_____. 2003. Fifteenth annual legislative update: how each state stands on legislative issues affecting advanced nursing practice. *Nurse Practitioner* 28(1):26–58.

U.S. Department of Health and Human Services. Health Resources and Services Administration, Bureau of Health Professions, Division of Quality Assurance. 2000. *National practitioner data bank 2000 annual report.* Available at: http://www.npdb.com/pubs/stats/00annrpt.pdf. Accessed on September 6, 2001.

Maureen T. Shannon, C.N.M., F.N.P., M.S.
Margaret A. Scott, R.N., M.S.N., F.N.P.
Carole E. Deitrich, R.N., C., M.S., G.N.P.

Jeanette M. Broering, R.N., M.S., C.P.N.P.
Diana Taylor, PH.D., R.N., F.A.A.N.

1-C

Women's Health Across the Life Span: An Overview

The purpose of this section of *Women's Primary Health Care: Protocols for Practice* is to present strategies for screening and illness prevention based on the age of a woman. It is designed to help practitioners incorporate health maintenance and illness prevention concepts into clinical practice. These strategies will eventually change as a result of the development of better methods to improve health within our society.

Overview of Women's Health Care Issues

Maureen T. Shannon, C.N.M., F.N.P., M.S.

As the concept of primary care has undergone significant changes during the past two decades, it became evident that health care for women needed to change as well. Aside from reproductive health care, the majority of health care recommendations for women have been based on studies done primarily on male research subjects. Furthermore, much of medical education and research has demonstrated a gender bias regarding health maintenance, disease prevention, and treatment of conditions for women (National Institutes of Health [NIH] 1992).

In response to this discrepancy in health care and research, NIH established the Office of Research on Women's Health (ORWH) in 1990. ORWH was established to promote women's health and to ensure that clinical research trials supported by NIH include an adequate number of women so that results extrapolated from studies would be applicable to both sexes.

During its first year of existence, ORWH convened a public hearing and a workshop to develop a research agenda on women's health. Data analyzed by ORWH during these meetings revealed the following facts about women's health in the United States (NIH 1992):

→ Women will constitute the larger part of the population and be the most *susceptible* to disease in the future.

→ Overall, women have *worse* health than men.

→ Certain health problems are more *prevalent* in women than in men.

→ Certain health problems are *unique* to women or affect women *differently* than they do men.

Although these findings apply to all women, ethnic and racial differences among women do appear to have an effect on morbidity and mortality rates associated with various diseases (NIH 1992). For example, in 1997 the average life expectancy of a white woman was five years longer than an African American woman (Hoyert et al. 2001).

Women generally live longer than men but face greater morbidity during their lifetimes. Except for injuries, categories of self-reported chronic illnesses and acute conditions are more common for women than men (Wingard 1984). Several chronic diseases have a higher reported incidence in women. These include obesity, diabetes, anemia, respiratory diseases, autoimmune diseases, gastrointestinal problems, osteoporosis, and Alzheimer's disease (NIH 1992, NIH 1999, Strickland 1988). While heart attacks are viewed as a male disease, more women die of heart disease each year than men (Halm et al. 2000, Kannel 2002, United States Department of Health and Human Services [USDHHS] Office on Women's Health 2001). Furthermore, 42% of women die within a year of myocardial infarction compared with 24% of men (USDHHS Office on Women's Health 2001).

Reproductive-age women report or seek care for acute conditions and short-term disabilities more frequently than men; and more women than men report and seek care for chronic conditions and associated disabilities during mid- to late life (Green et al. 1999, NIH 1992).

Certain health problems affect women exclusively or differently than they do men. The morbidity and mortality associated with complications of pregnancy (e.g., ectopic pregnancies, gestational diabetes, pregnancy-induced hypertension) and reproductive system cancers (e.g., ovarian, cervical, uterine) are particular to women. Breast cancer, which occurs rarely in men, is a leading cause of death of women. The incidence of this disease increased steadily from one in 20 women in the 1940s to one in nine women by 1990 (NIH 1992); since 1990 the rate has stabilized at 110 cases per 100,000 women. In 1999 breast cancer claimed the lives of 43,300 women in the United States (USDHHS Office on Women's Health 2001).

Each year, more than 6 million women acquire a sexually transmitted disease (STD); 50% of these women are between the ages of 13 and 19 (NIH 1992). STD-associated morbidity (e.g., infertility, ectopic pregnancy, chronic herpes simplex virus [HSV] infection, human papillomavirus [HPV] infection, human immunodeficiency virus [HIV] infection) and mortality also increase as a result of these infections. Although preventable, certain STDs are steadily increasing in women. Chlamydia increased from 415,051 cases in women in 1996 to 565,970 cases in 2000. As expected, the rate in women increased from 316 per 100,000 in 1996 to 400 per 100,000 in 2000 (Centers for Disease Control and Prevention [CDC] 2001a).

Behavioral factors contribute directly and indirectly to both health promotion and the development of disease. Of particular concern is the increased and sustained incidence of cigarette smoking among women compared to men. During the years between 1935 and 1965, the rate of smoking by women increased from 18% to 34%. Despite massive anti-smoking campaigns, in 2001 64% of teens had smoked—20% of them were daily cigarette smokers—and additional teens used cigars and smokeless tobacco (Grunbaum et al. 2002). As a result, an increased incidence of adverse health consequences associated with smoking is reported among women smokers that includes lung and other types of cancer, heart disease, respiratory diseases, hypertension, osteoporosis, increased pregnancy complications (e.g., preterm births), and increased perinatal and neonatal morbidity and mortality (e.g., low birthweight infants) (NIH 1992, NIH 1999).

Behavioral factors associated with the development of adverse health conditions in women include high dietary fat consumption (which may contribute to heart disease and cancers), delay in accessing medical or prenatal care, use of oral contraceptives in women over age 35 who smoke (which places them at an increased risk for cardiovascular disease), and unprotected sexual activity in women at risk for STDs.

Psychosocial issues faced by women are also different from those faced by men. Role expectations, role burdens, (e.g., traditionally the caregiver), and abilities to cope with and adapt to stressful situations have a direct impact on a woman's health (Woods 1988). Imbalances in role relationships (e.g., power, control) can also adversely affect women's health. For example, women are at greater risk of physical and sexual assault than are men (Council on Scientific Affairs, American Medical Association [AMA] 1992) and are more likely to be subjected to sexual harassment and sexual discrimination. It has been estimated that more than 4.5 million women are victims of violence each year and are six times as likely to be assaulted by someone they know than are men; often their spouse or intimate partner is the abuser (Harwell et al. 2000, USDHHS Office on Women's Health 2001).

The psychological stressors women face often require therapeutic interventions. Data indicate that approximately 12% of women have a major depressive episode during their lifetime (USDHHS Office on Women's Health 2001). However, some studies indicate that the diagnosis of psychological problems in women is often the result of gender bias on the part of the clinician, a bias resulting from a lack of knowledge about women's health care. This perspective is cited as being the reason physicians more frequently prescribe psychotropic medications for women than for men (Bernstein et al. 1981).

Socioeconomic status, ethnicity, and age play significant roles in women's access to health and health services. Recent data show that diabetes is four times more common in African American, Hispanic, and Native American women than in white women (USDHHS Office on Women's Health 2001). African American women experience the highest rate of coronary heart disease of all ethnic groups—three times higher than white women. While breast cancer has a reportedly higher incidence in white women, African American women have a higher mortality rate associated with it. The decrease in breast cancer mortality that occurred from 1990–1994 was six times greater for white women than African American women (6.1% versus 1.0%) (National Center for Health Statistics 1992, NIH 1992, USDHHS Office on Women's Health 2001). Lung and colon cancer rates are higher for African American women than white women. Disability (the inability to carry on one or more major activities of daily life) is higher among African American women compared to white women (U.S. Department of Commerce [USDC] 1991).

As a group, women are economically disadvantaged compared to men, regardless of age, race, ethnicity, education, or employment status. Although women provide a substantial contribution to the labor force, they consistently receive less pay than men for similar jobs (USDC 1991). Most low-income women of all races perceive that their health is poor, with 75% of poor minority women and 60% of poor white women reporting poor health (National Center for Health Statistics 1992, NIH 1992).

Almost 78% of the poor in the United States are women and children (USDC 1991). In 2000, 27.4% of all households were headed by a female, and 22.3% of African American and 21.2% of Hispanic women had an income below the poverty level (USDC 2001). By comparison, the poverty rate for the entire United States was 11.3% (more than 31 million people); the rate for white non-Hispanics was 7.5%, and for married-couple families it was 4.7%. The poverty rate has been falling steadily since 1993 and is half what was reported in 1959, the year statistics for poverty were initiated (Dalaker 2001). African American, Hispanic, and Native American women, particularly those who are single and heads of households, have long had high rates of poverty. They are now being joined by white, middle-class women rearing children alone, women who have recently immigrated from other countries, and older women subsisting on small fixed incomes, all of whom are at an increased risk for poor health outcomes (Rubia et al. 2002, Weitz et al. 2001).

The financial constraints women face are compounded by the lack of affordable medical insurance available to individuals today. The proportion of uninsured women under age 65 rose from 14% in 1994 to 18% in 1998. During 1998, 26% of women had no health insurance for at least part of the year (USDHHS

Office of Disease Prevention and Health Promotion 2001). Following welfare reform, a 1997 survey indicated that although a majority of women who left welfare were working, only 33% received medical coverage from their jobs, and 49% were uninsured (Garrett et al. 2000). In addition, women are the major recipients of Medicare/Medicaid and, therefore, they remain vulnerable to changes in health and social services provided by the federal government.

Improvements in women's health status are no longer likely to come solely from technological breakthroughs. Instead, improvements will have to incorporate environmental and social changes as well as behavioral changes (i.e., individual lifestyle), and will require a culturally sensitive approach to the delivery of health care (Hiatt et al. 2001). In addition, strategies to improve health outcomes should encourage the direct participation and collaboration of patients with their clinicians (O'Malley et al. 2002).

Reform at the level of health delivery systems is critical to improving women's health. The present systems of health care for women often result in overlapping services (e.g., obstetrical care, gynecological care) with duplication of some services (e.g., Pap smears) and lack of attention to issues that can have major health consequences (e.g., substance abuse, eating disorders, domestic violence).

Adolescent Health Care Issues (Women 13 to 19 Years of Age)

Margaret A. Scott, R.N., M.S.N., F.N.P.
Maureen T. Shannon, C.N.M., F.N.P., M.S.
Jeanette M. Broering, R.N., M.S., C.P.N.P.

Throughout the 1990s and into the 21st century, demographic trends for adolescents have revealed changes in population and racial composition. Although the absolute number of adolescents increased between 1990 and 2000 (from 34,868,264 to 40,847,962), it is estimated that the relative proportion of adolescents will decline from 14.5% of the total population in 2000 to 13% by the year 2020. Racial and ethnic minority shifts are also occurring. In 1998, non-Hispanic whites comprised 84% of the adolescent population; however, it is projected that by 2040 this percentage will drop below 50%. The most rapid growth will occur among Asian/Pacific Islander youth, and Hispanic youth will eclipse African American youth as the second most populous racial/ethnic group (National Adolescent Health Information Center 2000; USDC 1992, 2002).

Although adolescence is thought to be a time of optimal wellness, development, and physical growth, morbidity and mortality do occur. Cause-specific mortality by age is attributable to behavioral etiologies that include unintentional injuries such as motor vehicle accidents (MVAs) and intentional injuries such as homicide or suicide (Ozer et al. 1998). In 1999, nearly three-quarters of all deaths in 15–24 year olds were attributable to theses causes (Anderson 2002). Likewise, most morbidity

during adolescence results from risk behaviors that have outcomes such as unintentional pregnancy, sexually transmitted infections (STIs), substance abuse, injuries, and mental health problems. Some of these behaviors occur together—e.g., alcohol consumption has been highly correlated with adverse outcomes such as MVAs, suicides, and homicides; poor contraceptive and safer-sex practices can result in pregnancy and STDs. Clinicians need to be mindful of the clustering of these behaviors and ask appropriate questions regarding social behaviors when interviewing adolescents.

Health risks associated with the early onset of sexual activity have a significant effect on adolescents, and can generate

Table 1C.1.   TANNER STAGING OR SEXUAL MATURITY RATING (SMR) OF FEMALES

Breast
Breast Stage 1
  Breast-prepubertal; no glandular tissue
  Areola and papilla-areola conform to general chest line
Breast Stage 2
  Breast-breast bud; small amount of glandular tissue
  Areola and papilla-areola widen
Breast Stage 3
  Breast-larger and more elevation; extends beyond areolar parameters
  Areola and papilla-areola continue to enlarge but remain in contour with the breast
Breast Stage 4
  Breast-larger and more elevation
  Areola and papilla-areola and papilla form a mound projecting from the breast contour
Breast Stage 5
  Breast-adult (size is variable)
  Areola and papilla-areola and breast in same plane, with papilla projecting above areola

Pubic Hair
Pubic Hair Stage 1
  None
Pubic Hair Stage 2
  Small amount of long, slightly pigmented, downy hair on the labia majora
Pubic Hair Stage 3
  Moderate amount of pubic hair, more curly, coarse, and pigmented; the hair also extends more laterally
Pubic Hair Stage 4
  Hair that resembles adult hair in coarseness and curliness but does not extend down the medial aspects of the thigh
Pubic Hair Stage 5
  Adult type and quantity of hair extending down the medial aspects of the thighs

Source: Reprinted with permission from Tanner, J.M. 1982. *Growth at adolescence,* 2nd ed. Oxford: Blackwell Science.

long-term health and social problems. According to the 1999 Youth Risk Behavior Surveillance Summary, 65.8% of female students in grade 12 reported a history of sexual intercourse, compared with 32.5% of those in grade 9, demonstrating that the percentage of sexually active teenage females increases as age increases. Additionally, 4.4% of young women nationwide reported initiation of sexual intercourse prior to age 13, and 13.1% reported four or more sexual partners in their lifetime (CDC 2000). As a result, STIs are the most common and potentially destructive infectious diseases occurring among adolescents. Sexually active young women age 15–19 have consistently higher rates of chlamydia than older women, with increased prevalence rates among economically disadvantaged women. In 1997, 15–19 year old women had the highest rates of gonorrhea (USDHHS Division of STD Prevention 1998). In adolescent females, negative sequelae associated with STDs include pelvic inflammatory disease (PID) with resultant tubal scarring, ectopic pregnancy, infertility, chronic pelvic pain, exposure to viruses with oncogenic potential (e.g., human papillomavirus), and HIV infection.

Rates of pregnancy, birth, and abortion among teenage women nationally, while high relative to other developed countries, have continued to decline throughout the 1990s. In 1997, the number of total pregnancies in women younger than 20 years

Table 1C.2.   CHARACTERISTICS OF FEMALE ADOLESCENT PSYCHOSOCIAL DEVELOPMENT

Early Adolescence (11 to 13 Years)		Mid-Adolescence (14 to 17 Years)	
Cognition	1. Concrete thought dominant 2. Cannot perceive long-range implications of current decisions and acts	**Cognition**	1. Rapidly gaining competence in abstract thought 2. Capable of perceiving future implications of current acts and decisions, though capability variably applied
Psychosocial	1. Preoccupation with rapid body change 2. "Am I normal?" Concerns about appearance and attractiveness	**Psychosocial**	1. Re-establishes body image as growth decelerates and stabilizes 2. Preoccupations with fantasy and idealism in exploring expanded cognition and future options
Family	1. Defining independence/dependence boundaries 2. No major conflicts over parental control	**Family**	1. Potential conflicts over control 2. Struggle for emancipation
Peer Group	1. Peer affiliation emerging in relative importance 2. Compares own normality and acceptance with same-sex age mates	**Peer Group**	1. Strong need for identification to affirm self-image 2. Looks to peer group to define behavioral code during emancipation process
Sexuality	1. Self-exploration and evaluation 2. Limited dating 3. Limited intimacy	**Sexuality**	1. Heightened sexual activity 2. Testing abilities to attract and parameters of femininity 3. Preoccupation with romantic fantasy

Late Adolescence (17 to 21 Years)			
Cognition	1. Established abstract thought processes 2. Future-oriented 3. Capable of perceiving and acting on long-range plans	**Peer Group**	1. Recedes in importance in favor of individual friendships
Psychosocial	1. Emancipation completed 2. Intellectual and functional identity established 3. May experience crisis at age 21 years when facing societal demands for autonomy	**Sexuality**	1. Forms stable relationships 2. Capable of mutuality and reciprocity in caring for another rather than former narcissistic orientation 3. Plans for future in thinking of marriage, family 4. Intimacy involves commitment rather than exploration and romanticism
Family	1. Transition of child/parent dependency relationship to the adult/adult model		

Source: Reprinted by permission of Elsevier Science from Slap, G.B. Normal physiological and psychological growth in the adolescent. *Journal of Adolescent Health Care* 7:13S–23S. ©1986 by The Society of Adolescent Medicine.

old was 882,290, down from 1,002,650 in 1987; of these, 22,690 involved girls younger than 15 years old. Pregnancy outcomes in 1997 for women under age 20 included 493,341 live births, 263,899 induced abortions, and an estimated 125,060 miscarriages and stillbirths (Henshaw 2001). The majority (up to 90%) of these pregnancies are reported to be unintentional. Furthermore, adolescents are less likely to receive early prenatal care, thus increasing the possibility of adverse maternal and fetal outcomes. Factors that increase the risk that a mother will not seek prenatal care include being under 18 years old, unmarried, low educational attainment, and a member of a minority group (USDHHS Maternal and Child Health Bureau 1993).

A number of mental health issues have been noted to disproportionately affect adolescent females—most notably depression, suicidal ideation and attempts, eating disorders, and violence and sexual abuse. Depressive symptoms in girls increase during middle adolescence and peak between 17–18 years old (Slater et al. 2001). Young women are more likely than young men to have considered suicide (27.1% versus 15.1%), as well as to report having attempted suicide (11.6% versus 4.5%) (CDC 2000). Eating disorders are a major concern in adolescent medicine, and should be screened for at all preventive visits (Hampton 2000). Depression and eating disorders have been correlated with violence and sexual abuse in adolescents, with 12% of high school girls reporting sexual abuse compared with 5% of boys. Overall, approximately one in four young women report having experienced physical, sexual, or relationship abuse (Slater et al. 2001).

Confidentiality is a major concern of adolescents when they are seeking medical services. One survey of middle-class suburban adolescents reported that if parental knowledge were required, only 45% would seek care for severe depression, 19% for contraception, 15% for STDs, and 17% for drug abuse. If assured that medical care would be confidential, an additional 12% would seek care for depression, 45% for contraception, 50% for STDs, and 49% for drug abuse (Marks et al. 1983).

The provisions of the law regarding minors' consent for health care are not always clear. For the practicing clinician, the interpretation and implementation of existing laws concerning the reproductive health care of adolescent females can be confusing, particularly since the age of majority varies from 18 to 21 according to individual states' laws (Gans 1993). Generally, when obtaining consent for routine medical or surgical procedures for an adolescent, it is advisable for the clinician to obtain written consent from both the adolescent and his or her parent or guardian.

There are situations in which a minor can give consent for her own care. Legally emancipated minors can give consent for all forms of health care. The categories of emancipated minors include: married minors, minors serving in the armed forces, those emancipated through court declaration, mature minors, minors over a certain age, high school graduates, pregnant minors, and minor parents. Conditions for which minors may give consent independently include prescription and nonprescription contraceptive devices, pregnancy diagnosis, prenatal and postpartum care, testing for contagious diseases such as

Table 1C.3. LEADING CAUSES OF DEATH FOR WOMEN BY AGE GROUP

Cause of Death	% Total Deaths
Women 13 to 19 Years of Age	
Unintentional injuries	51.6
Homicide	8.6
Suicide	7.4
Malignant neoplasms	6.7
Heart disease	4.2
Women 20 to 24 Years of Age	
Unintentional injuries	36.6
Homicide	10.9
Malignant neoplasms	9.5
Suicide	7.2
Heart disease	5.6
Women 25 to 34 Years of Age	
Unintentional injuries	21.8
Malignant neoplasms	16.0
Heart disease	8.4
Suicide	7.1
Homicide	6.9
Women 35 to 44 Years of Age	
Malignant neoplasms	28.8
Unintentional injuries	12.4
Heart disease	12.3
HIV	4.5
Suicide	4.3
Women 45 to 54 Years of Age	
Malignant neoplasms	40.2
Heart disease	16.6
Unintentional injuries	5.3
Cerebrovascular disease	4.5
Diabetes mellitus	3.4
Women 55 to 64 Years of Age	
Malignant neoplasms	41.8
Heart disease	21.3
Chronic lower respiratory disease	5.5
Cerebrovascular disease	4.5
Diabetes mellitus	4.4
Women 65 Years of Age and Older	
Heart disease	34.1
Malignant neoplasms	19.0
Cerebrovascular disease	9.5
Chronic lower respiratory disease	5.5
Influenza and pneumonia	3.4

Source: Reprinted from Anderson, R.N. 2002. Deaths: leading causes for 1999. *National Vital Statistics Reports* 49:18–20. Hyattsville, Md.: National Center for Health Statistics.

STDs and HIV, rape and sexual assault, and, to a limited extent, drug, alcohol, and outpatient mental health counseling (English 2000). State guidelines regarding an unemancipated, unmarried minor's right to seek medical care, abortion, and other important health care services are available to the practicing clinician (Gans 1993).

Another legal issue pertaining to adolescents is the responsibility for payment, which may constitute a significant barrier to accessing medical services. Adolescents who are 18 years old or emancipated minors are financially responsible for their own care. Federally funded programs such as Title X of the Family Planning Act provide reproductive health services for adolescents in addition to other state-based programs such as Medicaid.

Essential to the assessment of an adolescent female's health is the evaluation of her physical and psychosocial maturation. Although the pubertal process in adolescent females is sequential and predictable, great variations in the intensity and duration of this event have been described (Tanner 1982). Chronological age is a poor prognosticator of pubertal status. However, classification of an adolescent female's pubertal status can be achieved through clinical assessment utilizing **Tanner Staging or Sexual Maturity Rating (SMR) of Females, Table 1C.1** (Slap 1986, Tanner 1982).

Similarly, adolescents vary in their psychological development. The major psychosocial outcomes of adolescence include cognitive and affective identity formation, emancipation from parents and family with the establishment of personal intimacy outside the primary family unit, and educational or vocational achievement as part of beginning some type of life work. Generally, this process occurs in three stages: early (11–13 years), middle (14–15 years), and late (17–21 years). Major areas for assessment include growth, body image concerns, and sexuality; cognitive development; and relationships with family, peers, and school (see **Table 1C.2, Characteristics of Female Adolescent Psychosocial Development**).

Because changes in adolescent mortality and morbidity are linked primarily to behavioral etiologies such as unintentional pregnancy, STIs, and alcohol- and drug-related consequences, current health promotion for adolescents emphasizes health guidance and prevention of behavioral and emotional disorders in addition to traditional biomedical conditions (see **Table 1C.3, Leading Causes of Death for Women by Age Group**; **Table 1C.4, Health Assessment for Women 13 to 19 Years of Age**; and **Table 1C.5, Risk Assessment, Prevention Measures, and Counseling for Women 13 to 19 Years of Age**).

Recommendations for preventive services have been promulgated by four national organizations/groups. *Guidelines for Adolescent Preventive Services (GAPS)* (AMA 1997) is a comprehensive set of recommendations by the American Medical Association providing a framework for the organization and content of preventive health services, with recommendations for health, screening, and immunizations. *GAPS* can direct clinicians regarding appropriate health maintenance and preventive aspects of the care of adolescents. Copies of *Guidelines for Adolescent Preventive Services* are available at www.ama-assn.org/ama/upload/mm/39/gapsmono.pdf or from the Department of Adoles-

cent Health, American Medical Association, 515 North State Street, Chicago, Ill. 60610 (800-621-8335).

Recommendations for adolescent preventive services have also been issued by the American Academy of Pediatrics (AAP) in *Guidelines for Health Supervision III* (1997), available through the AAP (www.aap.org); by a project initiated by the Maternal and Child Health Bureau in *Guidelines for Health Supervision of Infants, Children, and Adolescents,* 2nd edition (revised) (2000), available at www.brightfutures.org/guidelines.html; and in the U.S. Preventive Services Task Force *Guide to Clinical Preventive Services,* 2nd edition (1996), at odphp.osophs.dhhs.gov/pubs. Finally, recommendations for immunizations are updated annually by joint representatives of the AAP, the American Academy of Family Physicians (AAFP), and the CDC and are disseminated each January in an issue of *Morbidity and Mortality Weekly Report* available online at www.cdc.gov/MMWR.

Health Care Issues for Reproductive-Age Women (20 to 39 Years of Age)

Maureen T. Shannon, C.N.M., F.N.P., M.S.

In 2000, more than 40 million women in the United States were between the ages of 20 and 39 years old, constituting 28.2% of the female population, and having a median age of 36.5 years (USDC 2001). Currently, 49% of the U.S. labor force in the 20–24 year old category is made up of women, and 47% of workers between the ages of 20–54 years are women (U.S. Department of Labor 2002). Despite the increasing number of women in the workforce, child care and support for child care remains a problem. Of children younger than 5 years, an estimated 12,400,000 (63%) are in child care. Of those children in child care, only 3.8% receive any governmental support; 1.4% receive support from the women's employers (Smith 2002).

Demographic and employment data regarding reproductive-age women can be misleading. One could infer from them that women in this age category are a healthy group of individuals. In reality, personal lifestyle patterns of women between 20–39 reveal risk behaviors that contribute considerably to the mortality and morbidity observed in this population (see **Table 1C.3**).

Many of the leading causes of death for women in this age group (e.g., MVAs, homicide, and suicide) involve personal and social factors that could be altered to prevent injuries and death. The incidences of heart disease and malignant neoplasms could also be influenced by preventive measures. Of the deaths attributed to cancer in adult women, 30% are related to smoking (USDHHS 1990). Obesity increases women's risks for heart disease, stroke, diabetes, gallbladder disease, and some cancers (USDHHS Office of Disease Prevention and Health Promotion 2001). Obesity is more common in poor women and minorities. African American women and Mexican American women have more obesity than the males in their cultural groups or than white women.

Improved nutrition, cessation of smoking and substance abuse (i.e., alcohol, prescription medications, illicit drugs), regular exercise, consistent use of seat belts, personal screening for evidence of cancer (e.g., self breast examination), and early access to appropriate medical evaluation and treatment are measures that can significantly reduce mortality rates observed in women of this and older age groups (see **Table 1C.6, Health**

Assessment for Women 20 to 39 Years of Age and **Table 1C.7, Risk Assessment, Prevention Measures, and Counseling for Women 20 to 39 Years of Age**).

Reproductive health is usually the reason women in this age group seek medical care. When they do, the clinician has an opportunity to educate, screen, and intervene to prevent adverse outcomes associated with unintended pregnancies, improper

---

Table 1C.4.   HEALTH ASSESSMENT FOR WOMEN 13 TO 19 YEARS OF AGE

	Health Assessment (Every One to Three Years)
History	■ Medical history—including childhood illnesses, immunizations ■ Obstetrical/gynecological history (as indicated)—including age at the time of menarche, menstrual history, age at time of first coitus (consensual, nonconsensual), sexual and safer sex practices, contraception, sexually transmitted diseases (STDs), number of partners, sexual orientation ■ Surgical history ■ Family history ■ Current medications—prescription and over-the-counter ■ Dietary intake ■ Regular exercise practices ■ Tobacco/alcohol/drug use ■ Psychosocial history—including history of child abuse/neglect, domestic violence, emotional/physical abuse by parents or dating partner(s)
Physical Examination	■ Height, weight, basal metabolic index, and vital signs ■ Complete physical examination including: • Visual acuity • Oral cavity examination • Palpation of thyroid • Cardiovascular assessment • Skin examination • Lymph node assessment • Breast examination • Pelvic examination as indicated* • Rectal examination as indicated* • Scoliosis screening • Tanner staging or sexual maturity rating
Laboratory Tests	■ Tuberculin skin tests at least once in adolescence or as indicated in high-risk individuals* ■ Chlamydia screening annually in sexually active adolescents with urine-based ligase chain reaction (LCR) test or culture ■ STD screening as indicated* including gonorrhea and chlamydia LCR or cultures, VDRL or RPR, HIV counseling and testing ■ Pap smear as indicated* ■ Vision screening as indicated* ■ Pregnancy test as indicated* ■ Iron screening with known risk factors

*See specific chapters for indications/guidelines.

Sources: Compiled from American Academy of Pediatrics. 1997. *Guidelines for health supervision III.* Elk Grove, Ill.: the Author; United States Public Health Service (USPHS). 1998. *Clinician's handbook of preventive services,* 2nd ed. McLean, Va.: International Medical Publishing; and Centers for Disease Control and Prevention (CDC). 1998. Recommendations to prevent and control iron deficiency anemia in the United States. *Morbidity and Mortality Weekly Report* 47 (RR-3):1–36.

contraceptive method use, and STDs. It is essential that appropriate and adequate screening, testing, and treatment of STDs occur, as these infectious diseases are associated with significant morbidity (e.g., pelvic inflammatory disease, infertility, ectopic pregnancy, cancer) and mortality (e.g., HIV infection).

Counseling women about safer sex methods should be an integral component of their reproductive and primary health care. However, recommendations about contraception and safer sex must be made within the context of the individual woman's social and cultural milieu. Determining the obstacles to negoti-

Table 1C.5.   RISK ASSESSMENT, PREVENTION MEASURES, AND COUNSELING FOR WOMEN 13 TO 19 YEARS OF AGE

	Risk Assessment
Behaviors	■ Tobacco/alcohol/drug use ■ Symptoms of physical and/or emotional abuse ■ Symptoms of depression, suicide ■ Evidence of social isolation, increased stress at home or school ■ Risk factors associated with STDs, unintended pregnancy ■ Driving motor vehicles: use of seat belts, driving under the influence of alcohol/drugs ■ Lack of regular physical exercise ■ Excessive dietary intake of fat, cholesterol; inadequate intake of iron, calcium; bingeing and/or purging behaviors for weight control ■ Sun/ultraviolet light exposure ■ Evidence of social isolation, increased stress at home or school
	Prevention Measures and Counseling
Prevention Strategies	■ Use of motor vehicle seat belts; use of helmet bicycling, skateboarding ■ Prevention/cessation of tobacco/alcohol/drug use ■ Avoidance of driving/being a passenger in a vehicle driven by a person under the influence of alcohol/drugs ■ Dietary restriction of fat, cholesterol; adequate intake of iron, calcium; iron supplementation (as indicated); maintenance of balanced diet; avoidance of bingeing and purging for weight control ■ Regular exercise program ■ Teach/review breast self-examination (when appropriate) ■ Discussion of contraceptive options (when appropriate) ■ Discussion of behaviors to reduce STD exposure (when appropriate) ■ Discussion of violent behaviors and strategies to reduce exposure to violence; available resources ■ Sun/ultraviolet-light skin protection ■ Discussion of stress reduction in home and at school ■ Folic acid 0.4 mg daily for adolescents of reproductive capability (may be in the form of a multivitamin)
Immunizations	■ Tetanus/diphtheria booster once during adolescence ■ Measles/mumps/rubella once during adolescence if <2 previous immunizations ■ Hepatitis B vaccine ■ Hepatitis A vaccine in certain states, regions, and high risk individuals ■ Influenza vaccine annually in high-risk individuals* ■ Pneumococcal vaccine as indicated in high-risk individuals*
Referrals (as indicated)	■ Primary care clinician ■ Dentist ■ Obstetrician/gynecologist ■ Psychologist/psychiatrist ■ Alcohol/drug treatment programs ■ STD clinic for partner testing/treatment when indicated* ■ Community groups/resources (specific to the needs of the woman)

*See specific chapters for indications/guidelines.

Sources: Compiled from American Academy of Pediatrics. 1997. *Guidelines for health supervision II*. Elk Grove, Ill.: the Author; American Academy of Pediatrics. 2000. *Report of the Committee on Infectious Diseases*, 23rd ed., Elk Grove, Ill.: the Author; and United States Public Health Service (USPHS). 1998. *Clinician's handbook of preventive services*, 2nd ed. McLean, Va.: International Medical Publishing.

ating safer sex and the use of certain contraceptive methods are essential for these practices to be successfully incorporated into women's lives.

The majority of pregnant women are between 20–39 years old. Their health is of particular importance, as inadequate or delayed prenatal care can have an adverse impact on the health of the woman and her fetus. Infant mortality rates are a barometer of the overall health of a nation, reflecting not only infant outcomes but maternal antenatal health as well.

In the United States, 83% of women now receive prenatal care in the first trimester (Eberhardt et al. 2001). In 2000, first trimester care was obtained by 88.5% of white women, 84% of Asian or Pacific Islanders, 74.4% of Hispanics, 74.3% of blacks, and 69.3% of Native Americans (Eberhardt et al. 2001). The greatest single hazard to infant health is low birth weight, which results from lack of prenatal care, poor maternal nutrition, maternal smoking, maternal alcohol/drug use, and maternal age (increases observed in women younger than 18 and

Table 1C.6.   HEALTH ASSESSMENT FOR WOMEN 20 TO 39 YEARS OF AGE

	Health Assessment **(Every One to Three Years)**
History	▪ Medical history ▪ Review of systems—including signs/symptoms of cancer, heart disease ▪ Obstetrical/gynecological history—including menstrual history, sexual and safer sex practices, contraception, STDs, number of partners, sexual orientation ▪ Surgical history ▪ Family history—including history of breast/ovarian, cancer, cardiovascular disease, diabetes ▪ Current medications—prescription and OTC ▪ Dietary intake ▪ Regular exercise practices ▪ Travel (especially outside of the United States) ▪ Tobacco/alcohol/drug use ▪ Psychosocial history—including history of child abuse/neglect, domestic violence, emotional/physical abuse by spouse

Physical Examination	▪ Height, weight, basal metabolic index, and vital signs
	▪ Complete physical examination including:
	  • Visual acuity as indicated*
	  • Oral cavity examination
	  • Palpation of thyroid
	  • Breast examination
	  • Cardiovascular assessment
	  • Skin examination
	  • Lymph node assessment
	  • Pelvic examination
	  • Rectal examination

Laboratory Tests	▪ Pap smear as indicated* ▪ Mammogram as indicated* ▪ Chlamydia screening annually in younger, sexually active women by urine LCR or culture ▪ STD screening as indicated* including gonorrhea and chlamydia by LCR or culture, VDRL or RPR, and HIV counseling and testing ▪ Tuberculin skin tests in high-risk individuals* ▪ Rubella antibody titer as indicated* ▪ Nonfasting total blood cholesterol every five years, more frequently as indicated* ▪ Fasting plasma glucose as indicated* ▪ Urinalysis for bacteriuria as indicated* ▪ Pregnancy test as indicated*

*See specific chapters for indications/guidelines.

Sources: Compiled from USPHS. 1998. *Clinician's handbook of preventive services,* 2nd ed. McLean, Va.: International Medical Publishing; and Leitch, A.M., Dodd, G.D., Costanza, M. et al. 1997. American Cancer Society guidelines for the early detection of breast cancer: Update 1997. *CA—A Cancer Journal for Clinicians* 47:150–153.

older than 40 years) (National Center for Health Statistics 1992, USDHHS 1990).

Early and comprehensive prenatal care reduces the rates of infant mortality and number of low birth-weight infants. Recently, the low birth weight (<2,500 g) rate has fallen to 7.6%, with Hispanic women having a rate of 6.4%, non-Hispanic whites 6.6%, and black women 13.1% (Martin et al. 2002). These racial disparities are not likely due to poverty, as the black and Hispanic poverty rates are very similar at 22.1% and 21.2%, respectively (Dalaker 2001). Nor do differences in health insurance

---

Table 1C.7.   RISK ASSESSMENT, PREVENTION MEASURES, AND COUNSELING FOR WOMEN 20 TO 39 YEARS OF AGE

Risk Assessment

Behaviors	■ Tobacco/alcohol/drug use
	■ Symptoms of depression, suicide, abnormal bereavement
	■ Symptoms of physical and/or emotional abuse
	■ Risk factors associated with STDs, unintended pregnancy, high-risk pregnancy
	■ Driving motor vehicles: use of seat belts, driving under the influence of alcohol/drugs
	■ Lack of regular physical exercise
	■ Excessive dietary intake of fat, cholesterol; inadequate intake of iron, calcium
	■ Sun/ultraviolet light exposure

Prevention Measures and Counseling

Prevention Strategies	■ Use of smoke detector in home
	■ Use of motor vehicle seat belts
	■ Cessation of tobacco/alcohol/drug use
	■ Limiting alcohol consumption
	■ Avoidance of driving/being a passenger in a vehicle driven by a person under the influence of alcohol/drugs
	■ Dietary restriction of fat, cholesterol; adequate dietary intake of iron, calcium; iron, calcium supplementation (as indicated)
	■ Exercise program (appropriate to physical capabilities)
	■ Review/teach self breast examination; woman should exam breasts monthly
	■ Review/teach signs and symptoms of cancer, cardiovascular disease
	■ Discussion of contraceptive options (when appropriate)
	■ Discussion of behaviors to reduce STD exposure (when appropriate)
	■ Discussion of osteoporosis prevention
	■ Discussion of domestic violence and available resources
	■ Sun/ultraviolet-light skin protection
	■ Discussion of stress reduction in home and employment settings
	■ Folic acid 0.4 mg p.o. daily (may be in the form of a multivitamin)
Immunizations	■ Tetanus/diphtheria every 10 years
	■ Rubella vaccine as indicated*
	■ Hepatitis B vaccine as indicated in high-risk individuals*
	■ Pneumococcal vaccine as indicated in high-risk individuals*
	■ Influenza vaccine annually in high-risk individuals*
	■ Varicella vaccine vaccine if >13 years of age with no history or an unknown history of childhood chickenpox*
Referrals (as indicated)	■ Primary care clinician
	■ Dentist
	■ Obstetrician/gynecologist
	■ Psychologist/psychiatrist
	■ Alcohol/drug treatment programs
	■ STD clinic for partner testing/treatment when indicated*
	■ Community groups/resources (specific to particular needs of the woman)

*See specific chapters for indications/guidelines.

Sources: Compiled from USPHS. 1998. *Clinician's handbook of preventive services,* 2nd ed. McLean, Va.: International Medical Publishing; and Leitch, A.M., Dodd, G.D., Costanza, M. et al. 1997. American Cancer Society guidelines for the early detection of breast cancer: Update 1997. *CA–A Cancer Journal for Clinicians* 47:150–153.

explain the higher rate for black women, as they have a substantially lower uninsured rate than Hispanics (19.3% versus 33.9%, respectively) (Eberhardt et al. 2001). However, it is noteworthy that poor weight gain in pregnancy (<16 pounds) was more common in black women (21.1%) than Hispanics (11.0%) or white non-Hispanics (11.8%) (Martin et al. 2002). In addition, the rate of smoking during pregnancy by Hispanic women was only 3.5% compared with 9.9% for black women and 15.6% for white pregnant women (Martin et al. 2002). When low birth weight is adjusted by smoking status, white non-Hispanic and Hispanic smokers have low birth weight rates (10.6% and 12.3%) substantially less than black smokers (20.4%) but substantially more than nonsmokers in these respective racial groups (5.9%, 6.6%, 12.3%) (Martin et al. 2002). These data suggest that during pregnancy inadequate weight gain and smoking are both determinants of low birth weight; these are also behaviors that are somewhat amenable to control by pregnant women and possibly may be influenced by social networks that can support them. Preconception education and prevention strategies can have an important impact on perinatal outcomes, especially when these strategies target the reduction or early detection of potentially adverse conditions such as domestic violence, smoking, a lack of daily folic acid intake, and HIV/STD infections (Ahluwalia et al. 2001; Bernstein et al. 2000; CDC 1999, 2001b; Peterson et al. 2001).

Psychosocial and cultural aspects of a woman's life can have an impact on her health and her perception of illness. Conflicts regarding family, employment, and personal time commitments have been cited as major sources of stress for women between 25–34 years old (Woods 1988). In one survey, those under age 35 reported an increased incidence of physical and emotional symptoms compared to women over 35, possibly as a result of attempting to meet high expectations for professional success during those years set by themselves or others (Griffith 1983). Other studies have demonstrated increased levels of family-related (not employment-related) stress in women compared to male managers, executives, and professionals (Staats et al. 1983).

Personal relationships within the family, particularly those between the woman and her partner, also contribute to a woman's overall sense of well-being. Studies have indicated that a partner's emotional and psychological support has a protective effect on a woman's health (Woods 1988). On the other hand, a woman can suffer emotional and physical injuries as a consequence of her partner's violent behavior.

For women of reproductive age, pregnancy can be a stimulus for the emergence of violent tendencies in their partners. In one report, up to 37% of women surveyed reported having been assaulted by their partners during pregnancy (Helton et al. 1987). This situation emphasizes the need for clinicians to carefully screen and adequately educate women about domestic violence, and to be particularly vigilant in their assessment of women for partner abuse during pregnancy.

Health Care Issues for Women During Midlife (40 to 64 Years of Age)

Maureen T. Shannon, C.N.M., F.N.P., M.S.
Diana Taylor, Ph.D., R.N., F.A.A.N.

In the year 2000, more than 42 million American women were older than 50 years, compared with only 5 million women in 1900. Midlife and older women are the fastest growing segment of American society and, when combined with males of the same ages, represent more than 27% of the United States population (USDC 2002).

Midlife for women in the United States encompasses the years between 40–64, and can represent a crisis or an opportunity, based in part on the woman's perception of midlife, on how she copes with the transition, on her resources and the demands on her, and on the support she receives (Frank 1992). How a woman adjusts to midlife is likely to have an impact on her general health, reproductive status, and psychosocial well-being.

Historically, little attention has been given to women's health at midlife beyond reproductive biology. The end of reproductivity signals merely a transition from childbearing to non-childbearing capability for a woman and is a physiological process. Rather than being linear, however, a woman's life progresses with various roles, positions, and biopsychosocial states occurring in a variety of sequences and overlapping one another.

Women in their middle years are at varying points in their own life cycles. One 40-year-old woman may be a grandmother, while another may be having her first child. Multiple markers such as age, reproductive events, life events, parenting, work, menstruation, and retirement have been used to describe a woman's life in midlife. Too often, only one of these experiences has been singled out for investigation at the expense of others (e.g., menopause). However, during this phase of a woman's life, the impact of the "empty nest," entering or re-entering the job market, caring for elderly parents, perimenopausal symptoms, and daily stressors cannot be isolated from one another as separate and distinct events.

Many women in midlife have limited incomes. Compounding the stress associated with financial limitations is the lack of either private or government health coverage for 20% of American women between the ages of 44–64 (USDC 1991). In recent years the percentage of uninsured in this age group has remained relatively stable at 12% (Eberhardt 2001).

Economic disadvantage is a recognized contributing factor to increased morbidity and mortality in any age group. This is, in part, a result of poor access to necessary health screening and assessment. For example, in 1987, only 22% of low-income women age 40 or older had ever received a clinical breast examination and a mammogram compared to 36% of women in the total population (USDHHS 1990). A study of five cancer prevention screenings (breast exam, mammogram, Pap, rectal, fecal occult blood) demonstrated that having insurance resulted in significantly higher rates for all five screenings. Higher education resulted in higher screening rates for three preventive services, and higher income resulted in higher rates for two screenings. There were no racial differences after adjusting for these factors (Hegarty et al. 2000).

Because diseases that are the leading causes of death for women in this age group can be prevented in many instances, healthy behaviors and close monitoring for the emergence of diseases is especially important during midlife (see **Table 1C.3**). Malignant neoplasms—particularly lung and breast cancer, fol-

lowed by heart disease—account for the majority of deaths of women who are 40–64 years old. Cerebrovascular events, cirrhosis, accidents, and suicide are also significant causes of death observed in this population.

For many years, hormone replacement therapy had been used by nearly 40% of postmenopausal women as a preventive measure to potentially reduce menopausal symptoms, heart disease, bone density erosion (with subsequent fracture), and cancer. However, in 2002 the Women's Health Initiative Study, a

Table 1C.8.   HEALTH ASSESSMENT FOR WOMEN 40 TO 64 YEARS OF AGE

Health Assessment
(Every One to Three Years)

History	■ Medical history ■ Review of systems—including signs/symptoms of cardiovascular disease, cancer ■ Obstetrical/gynecological history—including menstrual history (when appropriate), sexual and safer sex practices, sexual orientation, number of sexual partners, contraception, STDs ■ Surgical history ■ Family history—including history of breast/ovarian/colon cancer, cardiovascular disease, diabetes ■ Current medication—prescription and over-the-counter ■ Dietary intake ■ Regular exercise practices ■ Tobacco/alcohol/drug use ■ Travel (especially outside of the United States) ■ Psychosocial history—including history of child abuse/neglect, domestic violence, emotional/physical abuse by spouse/partner(s), sexual assault

Physical Examination	■ Height, weight, basal metabolic index, and vital signs
	■ Complete physical examination including:
	  • Visual acuity (as indicated)
	  • Oral cavity examination
	  • Palpation of thyroid
	  • Breast examination
	  • Cardiovascular assessment
	  • Skin examination
	  • Lymph node assessment
	  • Pelvic examination
	  • Rectal examination

Laboratory Tests	■ Nonfasting total blood cholesterol every five years, more frequently as indicated ■ Pap smear as indicated* ■ Mammogram annually starting at age 40 years* ■ Fecal occult blood testing annually after age 50 years, earlier as indicated* ■ Sigmoidoscopy every 3–5 years after age 50 years, earlier as indicated* ■ Tuberculin skin tests in high-risk individuals* ■ STD screening as indicated—including gonorrhea and chlamydia LCR or cultures, VDRL or RPR, and HIV counseling and testing in high-risk individuals* ■ Glaucoma testing as indicated* ■ Fasting plasma glucose as indicated*

*See specific chapters for indications/guidelines.

Sources: Compiled from USPHS. 1998. *Clinician's handbook of preventive services,* 2nd ed., McLean Va.: International Medical Publishing; Leitch, A.M., Dodd, G.D., Costanza, M. et al. 1997. American Cancer Society guidelines for the early detection of breast cancer: update 1997. *CA—A Cancer Journal for Clinicians* 47:150–153; and Zoorob, R. 2001. Cancer screening guidelines. *American Family Physician* 63:1101–1112.

large study of more than 16,000 women, was halted because women on estrogen-progestin therapy had an increased rate of breast cancer, coronary artery disease, stroke, and pulmonary embolus when compared with placebo controls. The hormone replacement group had fewer cases of colon cancer, endometrial cancer, and hip fractures, however. Deaths in the two groups did not differ, but the risks were considered greater than the benefits for the population. As a result, and until further data are released, the American College of Obstetricians and Gynecologists (ACOG) recommends that women should discuss their individual circumstances with their physicians (Writing Group for the Women's Health Initiative Investigators 2002, ACOG 2002). While hormone replacement results have been disappointing as a preventive measure, such causes of mortality are

Table 1C.9.   RISK ASSESSMENT, PREVENTION MEASURES, AND COUNSELING FOR WOMEN 40 TO 64 YEARS OF AGE

Risk Assessment

Behavior	■ Tobacco/alcohol/drug use ■ Symptoms of depression, suicide, abnormal bereavement ■ Symptoms of physical and/or emotional abuse ■ Risk factors associated with STDs, unintended pregnancy ■ Driving motor vehicles: use of seat belts, driving under the influence of alcohol/drugs ■ Lack of regular physical exercise ■ Excessive dietary intake of fat, cholesterol ■ Sun/ultraviolet light exposure ■ Evidence of social isolation, increased stress at home or work

Prevention Measures and Counseling

Prevention Strategies	■ Use of smoke detector in home ■ Use of motor vehicle seat belts ■ Cessation of tobacco/alcohol/drug use ■ Limiting alcohol consumption ■ Avoidance of driving/being a passenger in a vehicle driven by a person while under the influence of alcohol/drugs ■ Dietary reduction of fat, cholesterol; adequate dietary intake of calcium ■ Exercise program (appropriate to physical capabilities) ■ Review/teach self breast examination ■ Review/teach signs and symptoms of cardiovascular disease, cancer ■ Discussion of contraceptive options (as appropriate) ■ Discussion of behaviors to reduce STD exposure ■ Sun/ultraviolet-light skin protection ■ Discussion of stress reduction in home and employment settings ■ Folic acid 0.4 mg p.o. daily with reproductive capability (may be in the form of a multivitamin)
Immunizations	■ Tetanus/diphtheria (every 10 years) ■ Hepatitis B vaccine as indicated in high-risk individuals* ■ Pneumococcal vaccine as indicated in high-risk individuals* ■ Influenza vaccine annually in high-risk individuals*
Referrals (as indicated)	■ Primary care clinician ■ Dentist ■ Ophthalmologist (for glaucoma testing) ■ Obstetrician/gynecologist ■ Psychologist/psychiatrist ■ Alcohol/drug treatment programs ■ STD clinic for partner testing/treatment (when indicated)* ■ Community groups/resources (specific to particular needs of the woman)

*See specific protocols for indications/guidelines.

Sources: Compiled from USPHS. 1998. *Clinician's handbook of preventive services,* 2nd ed., McLean Va.: International Medical Publishing; Leitch, A.M., Dodd, G.D., Costanza, M. et al. 1997. American Cancer Society guidelines for the early detection of breast cancer: update 1997. *CA—A Cancer Journal for Clinicians* 47:150–153; and Zoorob, R. 2001. Cancer screening guidelines. *American Family Physician* 63:1101–1112.

preventable only if early, comprehensive health education, health assessments, and medical interventions are integrated into the primary care of women during their midlife (see **Table 1C.8, Health Assessment for Women 40 to 64 Years of Age** and **Table 1C.9, Risk Assessment, Prevention Measures, and Counseling for Women 40 to 64 Years of Age**).

Health Care Issues for Older Women (Age 65 Years and Older)

Carole E. Deitrich, R.N., C., M.S., G.N.P.

By 2030, one in four women will be age 65 or older. A woman who reaches age 75 can expect to reach age 88, and she can expect to live longer than her male counterpart. By age 85, women outnumber men 2.5 to one (USDC 2001).

Despite living longer, women often have a poorer quality of life. They are more likely than men to be without an available caretaker, to have less money and other material resources, and are less likely to engage independently in activities that would enhance their quality of life (USDHHS Administration on Aging 2002).

The focus of health care for older women includes not only the usual early detection and treatment of disease (e.g., cardiovascular, cerebrovascular, and cancer), but also the identification of conditions associated with aging that influence morbidity, functional capacity, and quality of life, as distinct from the diagnostic and curative approaches usually considered. Screening for these conditions, aggressive teaching programs for older women, and mobilizing community resources can significantly enhance the lives of women in their later years (Goldberg et al. 1997).

The screening guidelines cited here view all people over 65 together, as if they were a homogenous group (U.S. Preventive Services Task Force 1996). The practitioner is first cautioned to evaluate each older women individually and to exercise clinical judgment, including knowledge of risks, the woman's wishes, and those of her family to determine appropriate screening. Problems such as loss of cognitive function, falling, and urinary incontinence are *not* normal consequences of aging. The presence of such symptoms indicates a need to assess an individual for an underlying pathology, which may be relieved with treatment. Undertreatment of older women can result if physiological or psychological symptoms are too quickly attributed to old age (NIH 2000).

→ Screening
  ■ Sensory losses:
    • Impaired vision and hearing are responsible for accidents and social isolation, and confound the evaluation of cognitive dysfunction. Denial of losses, especially hearing but also sight if driving ability is in question, can delay evaluation, impede the adjustment process, and decrease the likelihood of learning ways to compensate for these losses.

    – Vision: Snellen chart, referral to an ophthalmologist for glaucoma and retina exam
    – Hearing: whisper/finger rub, audiometer. Hearing aids can be helpful but require time and persistence to learn the correct usage and limitations (USDHHS Office of Disease Prevention and Health Promotion 2001).
  ■ Functional status:
    • Changes in functional status are leading indicators of medical illness, depression, and dementia (NIH 2000). There are scales to measure and track activities of daily living (e.g., bathing, dressing, toileting, eating, ambulation) and instrumental activities of daily living (e.g., paying bills, using the telephone, using public transportation) (Katz et al. 1963). A careful history can reveal an inability to carry out these activities. Start by asking the patient how she got to the clinic, who she lives with, and who does the shopping and cooking. Determine if family or other support is available and what their level of involvement is. Use of measurement scales can help track the changes.
  ■ Safety:
    • Poor physical conditioning contributes to loss of balance and impaired gait, causing falls and loss of confidence in physical capacity. A vicious cycle is established that gives rise to further loss of conditioning. Determine the factors that facilitate recovery of physical strength and confidence. Pain management, weight-bearing exercise, physical rehabilitation, and Tai Chi all contribute to improved balance and mobility (Tinetti et al. 1994).
  ■ Driving habits:
    • Include use of seat belts and whether the woman is fit to drive
  ■ Cognition:
    • The history can reveal cognitive dysfunction if practitioners are careful not to confine themselves to yes and no questions. Also, eliciting information from those who know the person and can report changes in her functional status can be helpful. Decline in functional status is a leading indicator of cognitive dysfunction, and if sudden, may herald a medical disorder. Use the mini mental status exam (MMSE), and if there is any doubt, refer for cognitive dysfunction exam with a complete dementia evaluation and the possible use of acetylcholinesterase inhibitors (e.g., Aricept®) (USDHHS Public Health Service 1996).
  ■ Depression:
    • A thorough personal and social history is a most useful screening tool, and the Geriatric Depression Scale (GDS) is standardized. The most productive information about depression may not arise when asking about depression. It is often more fruitful to inquire about what activities the patient does or used to do, whether there is a change in functional status, and what gives her pleasure, as well as questions related to appetite, sleep, and activity. Depression and dementia

often co-exist. Refer for evaluation for psychotherapy or antidepressants, as a combination of the two is often necessary to provide optimal treatment in older women, as in others (National Institute of Mental Health [NIMH] 1999).

- Urinary incontinence:
  - This problem occurs in 10–30% of ambulatory geriatric patients, with women affected twice as often as men. It is responsible for emotional distress and burden on both the woman and the caregiver. It is a leading cause

Table 1C.10.   HEALTH ASSESSMENT FOR WOMEN 65 YEARS OF AGE AND OLDER

Annual Health Assessment

History	■ Medical history ■ Review of systems—including signs/symptoms associated with cardiovascular disease, cerebrovascular disease, and cancer ■ Obstetrical/urogynecological history ■ Surgical history ■ Family history ■ Current medications—prescription, over-the-counter, herbals, polypharmacy ■ Dietary intake; who shops and cooks ■ Level of physical activity ■ Functional status ■ Tobacco/alcohol use ■ Travel (especially outside of the United States) ■ Psychosocial history—including domestic violence, physical abuse by spouse/partner, sexual assault, support systems, social involvement, recent losses, depression ■ Safety at home, driving
Physical Examination	■ Height, weight, and vital signs ■ Complete physical examination including: 　• Gait and balance 　• Visual acuity 　• Hearing assessment 　• Oral cavity examination (especially with smoking and alcohol history) 　• Palpation of thyroid 　• Cardiovascular assessment 　• Breast examination 　• Skin examination 　• Lymph node assessment 　• Neurological examination 　• Pelvic examination 　• Rectal examination
Laboratory Tests	■ Fasting fractionated blood cholesterol every five years, more frequently as indicated* ■ Fasting plasma glucose as indicated* ■ Dipstick urinalysis as indicated* ■ Fecal occult blood testing ■ Sigmoidoscopy every 3–5 years, more frequently as indicated* ■ Glaucoma testing ■ Pap smear as indicated (may be discontinued in some women >65 years of age)* ■ STD screening as indicated—VDRL or RPR, and HIV as indicated ■ Mammogram* ■ Thyroid function tests as indicated* ■ Tuberculin skin tests in high-risk individuals*

*See specific protocols for indications/guidelines.

Sources: Compiled from USPHS 1998. *Clinician's handbook of preventive services,* 2nd ed., McLean, Va.: International Medical Publishing; Leitch, A.M., Dodd, G.D., Costanza, M. et al. 1997. American Cancer Society guidelines for the early detection of breast cancer: update 1997. *CA—A Cancer Journal for Clinicians* 47:150–153; and Zoorob, R. 2001. Cancer screening guidelines. *American Family Physician* 63:1101–1112.

of admission to nursing homes and a significant barrier to discharge from them. Make it a practice to bring up the subject as many women will not. Self-report logs are useful. The patient may also be sent for urodynamic testing. This information can save having to try various

medicines or, worse, assuming that nothing can be done (USDHHS Public Health Service 1996).
- Drugs/polypharmacy:
  - This aspect of screening includes review of all medications—prescription, over-the-counter, and herbal prepa-

Table 1C.11.   RISK ASSESSMENT, PREVENTION MEASURES, AND COUNSELING FOR WOMEN 65 YEARS OF AGE AND OLDER

Risk Assessment

Behaviors	■ Changes in cognitive function
	■ Symptoms of depression, suicide, abnormal bereavement
	■ Tobacco/alcohol/drug use
	■ Driving motor vehicles: use of seat belts, driving under the influence of alcohol/drugs; no longer fit to drive
	■ Symptoms/signs of physical and/or emotional abuse
	■ Lack of physical exercise
	■ Excessive dietary intake of fat, cholesterol; unbalanced nutrient intake
	■ Evidence of social isolation
	■ Sun/ultraviolet light exposure

Prevention Measures and Counseling

Prevention Strategies	■ Prevention of falls/trauma
	■ Use of smoke detector in home
	■ Use of motor vehicle seat belts
	■ Hot water heater temperature reduction to <130°F/54°C
	■ Cessation of tobacco/alcohol/drug use
	■ Limiting alcohol consumption
	■ Avoid driving/being a passenger in a vehicle driven by a person under the influence of alcohol/drugs
	■ Dietary reduction of fat (specifically saturated fats), cholesterol
	■ Exercise program (appropriate to physical capabilities)
	■ Review/teach self breast examination
	■ Review/teach signs and symptoms of cardiovascular disease, cancer
	■ Sun/ultraviolet-light skin protection
	■ Discussion of hormone therapy, aspirin, calcium, supplements, bisphosphonates, etc.
	■ Encourage participation in social activities and contact with community resources
Immunizations	■ Influenza vaccine annually
	■ Pneumococcal vaccine
	■ Tetanus/diphtheria every 10 years
	■ Hepatitis B vaccine as indicated in high-risk individuals*
Referrals (as indicated)	■ Primary care clinician
	■ Ophthalmologist (for glaucoma testing)
	■ Dentist
	■ Geriatrician
	■ Gynecologist
	■ Psychologist/psychiatrist
	■ Physical therapist
	■ Alcohol/drug treatment programs
	■ Community groups/resources (specific to particular needs of individual)

*See specific protocols for indications/guidelines.

Sources: Compiled from USPHS. 1998. *Clinician's handbook of preventive services,* 2nd ed., McLean, Va.: International Medical Publishing; Goldberg, T.H., and Stephen, C.I. 1997. Preventive medicine and screening in older adults. *Journal of the American Geriatrics Society* 45:344–354; Leitch, A.M., Dodd, G.D., Costanza, M. et al. 1997. American Cancer Society guidelines for the early detection of breast cancer: update 1997. *CA—A Cancer Journal for Clinicians* 47:150-153; and Zoorob, R. 2001. Cancer screening guidelines. *American Family Physician* 63:1101–1112.

rations—as well as alcohol consumption. In order to discover polypharmacy and the potential for drug interactions, ask the patient to bring to her appointment a list of all medications she is currently taking. Although abuse of alcohol and nonprescription drugs is expected to increase among this age group, most substance abuse observed in older women is a result of improper use of prescription medications. Health care providers contribute to this problem if they fail to adjust dosages for older individuals, to verify renal and liver function before prescribing, or prescribe without knowledge of what has been prescribed by other providers. A thorough review of all medications and coordination of care by a designated primary-care clinician can help reduce this problem (NIH 2000).

■ Elder abuse/family violence:
  • It is estimated that only one in 14 cases of elder abuse is accurately identified. Understanding family dynamics and the circumstances in which the older woman lives, as well as exploring unexplained injuries, are useful starting points to determine if further inquiry is needed (Fullin et al. 1994).

→ See **Table 1C.10, Health Assessment for Women 65 Years of Age and Older** and **Table 1C.11, Risk Assessment, Prevention Measures, and Counseling for Women 65 Years of Age and Older.**

BIBLIOGRAPHY

Ahluwalia I.B., and Daniel, K.L. 2001. Are women with recent live births aware of the benefits of folic acid? *Morbidity and Mortality Weekly Report* 50 (RR–6):3–12.

American Academy of Pediatrics. 1997. *Guidelines for health supervision III.* Elk Grove, Ill.: the Author.

____. 2000. Report of the Committee on Infectious Diseases, 25th ed. Elk Grove Village, Ill.: the Author.

American College of Obstetricians and Gynecologists. 2002. Statement on the estrogen plus progestin trial of the Women's Health Initiative. American College of Obstetricians and Gynecologists News Release, July 9, 2002. Washington, D.C.

American Medical Association. 1997. *Guidelines for adolescent preventive services.* Chicago: the Author.

Anderson, R.N. 2002. Deaths: leading causes for 1999. *National Vital Statistics Reports* 49:18–20.

Bernstein, B., and Kane, R. 1981. Physicians' attitudes toward female patients. *Medical Care* 19:600–608.

Bernstein P.S., Sanghvi, T., and Merkatz, I.R. 2000. Improving preconception care. *Journal of Reproductive Medicine* 45:546–552.

Centers for Disease Control and Prevention (CDC). 1998. Accommodations to prevent and control iron deficiency anemia in the United States. *Morbidity and Mortality Weekly Report* 47(RR-3):1–36.

____. 1999. Cigarette smoking during the last three months of pregnancy among women who gave birth to live infants—Maine, 1988–1997. *Morbidity and Mortality Weekly Report* 48:421–423.

____. 2000. Youth risk behavior surveillance—United States, 1999. *Morbidity and Mortality Weekly Report* 49(SS-05):1–96.

____. 2001a. *Sexually transmitted disease surveillance, 2000.* Atlanta, Ga.: Centers for Disease Control.

____. 2001b. Revised recommendations for HIV screening of pregnant women. *Morbidity and Mortality Weekly Report* 50:63–85.

Coker, A.L., Sanderson, M., Fadden M.K. et al. 2000. Intimate partner violence and cervical neoplasia. *Journal of Women's Health and Gender Based Medicine* 9:1015–1023.

Council on Scientific Affairs, American Medical Association. 1992. Violence against women: relevance for medical practitioners. *Journal of the American Medical Association* 267:3184–3189.

Dalaker, J. 2001. U.S. Census Bureau current population reports. Series P 60–214. *Poverty in the United States 2000.* Washington D.C.: Government Printing Office.

Eberhardt, M.S., Ingram, D.D., and Makuc D.M. 2001. *Health in the United States 2001, with urban and rural chartbook.* Hyattsville, Md.: National Center for Health Statistics.

English, A. 1988. *Adolescent health care: a manual of California law,* 3rd ed. San Francisco: National Center for Youth Law.

____. 2000. Reproductive health services for adolescents: critical legal issues. *Obstetrics and Gynecology Clinics* 27(1): 195–211.

Frank, M.V. 1992. Transition into midlife. Clinical issues in perinatal and women's health. *Nursing* 2(4):421–428.

Fullin, K.J., Fullin, P., and Cosgrove, A. 1994. Screening patients for domestic violence in clinical practice. Proceedings of the National Conference on Family Violence. March 11–13, 1994. Washington, D.C.

Gans J.D., 1993. *Policy compendium on confidential health services for adolescents.* Chicago, Ill.: American Medical Association.

Garrett, B, and Molahan, J. 2000. Health insurance coverage after welfare. *Health Affairs* 19:175–184.

Glantz, M.D., and Backenheimer M.S. 1988. Substance abuse among elderly women. *Clinical Gerontologist* 8:3–26.

Goldberg, T.H., and Stephen, C.I. 1997. Preventive medicine and screening in older adults. *Journal of the American Geriatrics Society* 45:344–354.

Green, C.A., and Pope, C. 1999. Gender, psychosocial factors and the use of medical services: a longitudinal analysis. *Social Science and Medicine* 48:1363–1372.

Griffith, J. 1983. Women's stressors according to age groups. *Issues in the Health Care of Women* 6:311–326.

Grunbaum, J.A., Kann, L., Kinchen, S.A. et al. 2002. Youth risk behavior surveillance—United States 2001. *Morbidity and Mortality Weekly Report* 51 (SS–04):1–64.

Halm, M.A., and Penque, S. 2000. Heart failure in women. *Progress in Cardiovascular Nursing.* Fall:121–133.

Hampton, H.L. 2000. Adolescent gynecology: examination of the adolescent patient. *Obstetrics and Gynecology Clinics* 27(1):1–18.

Harwell T.S., and Spence M.R. 2000. Population surveillance for physical violence among adult men and women—Montana, 1998. *American Journal of Preventive Medicine* 19:321–324.

Hegarty, V., Burchett, B.M., Gold, G.T. et al. 2000. Racial differences in use of cancer prevention services among older Americans. *Journal of the American Geriatrics Society* 48:735–740.

Helton, A., McFarlane, J., and Anderson, E. 1987. Battered and pregnant: a prevalence study. *American Journal of Public Health* 77:1337–1339.

Henshaw, S. 2001. *U.S. teenage pregnancy statistics with comparative statistics for women aged 20–24.* New York: Alan Guttmacher Institute.

Hiatt, R.A., Pasick, R.J., Stewart, S. et al. 2001. Community-based cancer screening for underserved women: design and baseline findings from the breast and cervical cancer intervention study. *Preventive Medicine* 33:190–203.

Hoyert, D.L., Arias, E., Smith, B.L. et al. 2001. Deaths: final data for 1999. *National Vital Statistics Reports* 49(8).

Institute of Medicine. 1990. *The second 50 years.* Washington, D.C.: National Academy of Sciences.

Irwin, C.E., and Shafer, M.A. 1992. Adolescent sexuality: the problem of negative outcomes of a normative behavior. In *Adolescents at risk: medical and social perspectives,* eds., E.E. Rogers, and E. Ginzberg. Boulder, Colo.: Westview Press.

Kannel W.B. 2002. The Framingham Study: historical insight on the impact of cardiovascular risk factors in men versus women. *Journal of Gender Specific Medicine* 5:27–37.

Katz, S., Ford, A.B., Moskowitz, R.W. et al. 1963. Studies of illness and the aged: index of ADL: a standardized measure of biological and psychosocial function. *Journal of the American Medical Association* 185:914–919.

Leitch, A.M., Dodd, G.D., Costnaza, M., et al. 1997. American Cancer Society guidelines for the early detection of breast cancer: update 1997. *CA–A Cancer Journal for Clinicians* 47:150–153.

Marks, A., Malizio, J., Hoch, J. et al. 1983. Assessment of health needs and willingness to utilize health care resources of adolescents in a suburban population. *Journal of Pediatrics* 102:456–460.

National Adolescent Health Information Center. 2000. *Fact sheet on adolescent demographics.* San Francisco: the Author.

Martin, J.A., Hamilton, B.C., Ventura, S.J. et al. 2002. Births: final data for 2000. *National Vital Statistics Reports 50.* Hyattsville, Md.: U.S. Department of Health and Human Services.

National Center for Health Statistics. 1992. *Health, United States 1991.* Hyattsville, Md.: U.S. Department of Health and Human Services.

National Institutes of Health (NIH). 1992. *Report of the National Institutes of Health: opportunities for research on women's health.* Bethesda, Md.: the Author.

_____. 1999. *Report of the National Institutes of Health: opportunities for research on women's health.* Bethesda, Md.: the Author.

_____. Federal Interagency Forum on Aging Related Statistics. 2000. Older Americans 2000: key indicators of well-being. Washington, D.C.: U.S. Government Printing Office.

National Institute of Mental Health. 1999. *Older adults: depression and suicide facts.* NIH Publication No. 01–4593, pp. 1–2. Bethesda, Md.: National Institute of Mental Health.

O'Malley, A.S., and Forrest, C.B. 2002. Beyond the examination room: primary care performance and the patient-physician relationship for low income women. *Journal of General Internal Medicine* 17:66–74.

Ozer, E.M., Brindis, C.D., Millstein, S.G. et al. 1998. *America's adolescents: Are they healthy?* San Francisco: National Adolescent Health Information Center.

Peterson, R., Connelly, A., Martin, S.L. et al. 2001. Preventive counseling during prenatal care. Pregnancy risk assessment monitoring system (PRAMS). *American Journal of Preventive Medicine* 20:245–250.

Ramey, E.R. 1982. The national capacity for health in women. In *Women: a developmental perspective,* (NIH Publication No. 82-2290), eds. P.W. Berman and E.R. Ramey. Washington, D.C.: U.S. Government Printing Office.

Rubia, M., Marcos, I., and Muenning, R.A. 2002. Increased risk of heart disease and stroke among foreign-born females residing in the United States. *American Journal of Preventive Medicine* 22:30–35.

Slap, G.B. 1986. Normal physiological and psychological growth in the adolescent. *Journal of Adolescent Health Care* 7:139.

Slater, J.M., Guthrie, B.J., and Boyd, C.J. 2001. A feminist theoretical approach to understanding health of adolescent females. *Journal of Adolescent Health* 28(6):443–449.

Smith, K. 2002. Who's minding the kids? Child care arrangements: spring 1997. *Current Population Reports,* pp.70–86. Washington D.C.: United States Census Bureau.

Staats, M., and Staats, T. 1983. Differences in stress levels, stressors, and stress responses between managerial and professional males and females on the Stress Vector Analysis—research edition. *Issues in the Health Care of Women* 5:165–176.

Strickland, B.R. 1988. Sex-related differences in health and illness. *Psychology of Women Quarterly* 12:381–399.

Tanner, J.M. 1982. *Growth at adolescence,* 2nd ed. Oxford: Blackwell Scientific Publications.

Tinetti, M.E., Baker K.I., McAvay, G. et al. 1994. A multifactorial intervention to reduce the risk of falling among elderly people living in the community. *New England Journal of Medicine* 331:821–827.

U.S. Department of Commerce (USDC). 1991. *Statistical abstract of the United States 1991,* 111th ed. Washington D.C.: the Author.

____. 1992. *1990 Census of population. General population characteristics, United States.* Washington, D.C.: U.S. Government Printing Office.

____. 2001. *2000 Census of population. General population characteristics, United States.* Washington, D.C.: U.S. Government Printing Office.

____. 2002. *2000 Census of population and housing. Profiles of general demographic characteristics 2000, United States.* Washington, D.C.: U.S. Government Printing Office.

United States Department of Health and Human Services (USDHHS). 1990. *Healthy people 2000. National health promotion and disease prevention objectives.* Washington, D.C.: the Author.

____. Administration on Aging. 2002. *Profile of older Americans: 2002.* Washington, D.C.: U.S. Government Printing Office.

____. Division of STD Prevention. 1998. *Sexually transmitted disease surveillance, 1997.* Atlanta, Ga.: Centers for Disease Control and Prevention.

____. Maternal and Child Health Bureau. 1993. *Child health 1992, United States.* Washington, D.C.: U.S. Government Printing Office.

____. Office of Disease Prevention and Health Promotion 2001. *Healthy People 2010,* 2nd ed. Washington, D.C.: U.S. Government Printing Office.

____. Office on Women's Health, National Women's Health Information Center. 1999. *A report of the task force on the NIH Women's Health Research Agenda for the 21st Century, Volume 1. Executive summary.* Publication No. 99-4385. Washington, D.C.: U.S. Government Printing Office.

____. Office on Women's Health, National Women's Health Information Center. 2001. *Women's health issues: an overview.* Washington, D.C.: U.S. Government Printing Office.

____. Public Health Service, Agency for Health Care Policy and Research. 1996. *Recognition and initial assessment of Alzheimer's disease and related dementias.* AHCPR Publication No. 97–0702.

U.S. Department of Labor. Bureau of Labor Statistics. 2002. *Current population survey. Household data seasonally adjusted. Table 8-A. Employed persons by age and sex seasonally adjusted.* Bureau of Labor Statistics, August 2002. Available at: http://www.bls.gov/cps/home.htm. Accessed on September 1, 2002.

U.S. Preventive Services Task Force. 1996. *Guide to clinical preventive services*, 2nd ed. Baltimore, Md.: Lippincott Williams & Wilkins.

U.S. Public Health Service (USPHS). 1985. Report of the Public Health Service Task Force on Women's Health Issues. *Public Health Reports* 100:73.

____. 1998. *Clinician's handbook of preventive services*, 2nd ed. McLean, Va.: International Medical Publishing.

Ventura, S.J., Mosher, W.D., Curting, S.C. et al. 2001. Trends in pregnancy rates for the United States, 1976–1997: an update. *National Vital Statistics Report* 49:1–9.

Weitz, T.A., Freund, K.M., and Wright, L. 2001. Identifying and caring for underserved populations: experience of the National Centers of Excellence in Women's Health. *Journal of Women's Health and Gender-based Medicine* 10:937–952.

Wingard, D.L. 1984. The sex differential in morbidity, mortality, and lifestyle. *Annual Review of Public Health* 5:433–458.

Woods, N.F. 1988. Women's health. *Annual Review of Nursing Research* 6:210–235.

Writing Group for the Women's Health Initiative Investigators. 2002. Risks and benefits of estrogen plus progestin in healthy post-menopausal women. *Journal of the American Medical Association* 288:321–333.

Zoorob, R. 2001. Cancer screening guidelines. *American Family Physician* 63:1101–1112.

Ellen M. Scarr, R.N., C., M.S., F.N.P., W.H.N.P.

1-D

Lesbian Health Care

Defining lesbianism is difficult. This has contributed to the lack of research and understanding of the needs of the lesbian population. A broad definition is that lesbians are women who are attracted to, feel affection for, and/or have sex with women. This definition includes women who self-identify as lesbians yet have never had sex with another woman. Conversely, there are women whose behavior would suggest they are lesbian (e.g., they have had or are having sexual relationships with women), but who self-identify as bisexual or heterosexual. For clarity, the term lesbian will be used in this chapter to refer to women who self-identify as lesbians in both identity and behavior.

Studies estimate that 10% of the United States population is homosexual, with between 1.4–4.3% of women sexually active with other women (Dean et al. 2000). An estimated 2.3 million women self-identify as lesbian (Marrazzo et al. 2001). There are larger concentrations of lesbians in urban areas than in rural areas. Preliminary data from the 2000 census shows a marked increase in the number of households with same-sex couples across the country (Human Rights Campaign 2001).

Despite an increased visibility and acceptance of homosexuality in this country over the last two decades, there is still a large amount of homophobia and heterosexism, negatively impacting the civil rights of gays. Most Americans still view homosexuality as morally wrong, and there is legal as well as tacit approval for ongoing discrimination in every aspect of life. Homosexuality remains a crime in 16 states (Dean et al. 2000). Homosexuals are denied employment, housing, custody, and other rights and privileges based solely on sexual orientation.

In the past, little research has been undertaken on issues related to lesbian health, although recently this has begun to change. The Institute of Medicine released a report titled *Lesbian Health: Current Assessment and Directions for the Future* (1999). This document called for increased funding for research on health care issues significant to lesbians, and it identified numerous areas where knowledge is lacking. The report expresses concern that lesbians may be at increased risk for certain chronic illnesses due to the unique grouping of potential risks in this population, although inadequate existing data make a definitive assessment impossible. Previous small studies have identified behaviors such as lack of utilization of preventive services as increasing the risk as well. Many lesbians have felt disenfranchised from various aspects of society, including the health care system.

This chapter discusses identified areas of primary concern among the lesbian population.

Substance Use

Early studies on lesbian alcohol and tobacco use were based on convenience samples of women in gay bars (Fifield 1975, Heffernan 1998, Lewis et al. 1982). Lesbians often gather at gay bars to socialize (either women-only or mixed lesbian/gay men clientele), as these bars provide one of the few social settings outside the home where lesbians feel comfortable. Not surprisingly, these studies found a high percentage of alcohol use/abuse and cigarette smoking among the respondents.

Recent studies have undertaken to identify the prevalence of substance abuse among lesbians. Cochran et al. (2001) compared data from seven studies of lesbians (a small percentage of whom identified themselves as bisexual) against two national population-based studies. Lesbians were found to be more likely to currently smoke cigarettes and have a history of smoking than women in the general population (Cochran et al. 2001). Alcohol use was found to be similar among lesbians and women in the general population, but lesbians were more likely to have a history of current or past heavy alcohol use (five or more drinks per day for sustained periods of time) (Cochran et al. 2001). A study by Aaron et al. (2001) reported that lesbians were more likely to report cigarette and alcohol use than women in general. Work by Ryan et al. (2001) also confirmed higher tobacco use among lesbians.

Some authors have suggested that poor coping skills among lesbians are associated with an increase in substance abuse. A study by Heffernan (1998) found that increased alcohol use was not associated with increased levels of perceived stress or lack of social support but rather with reliance on bars as the primary social gathering place. In contrast to earlier studies, Heffernan also found a decrease in the number of heavy drinkers and an increase in the number of lesbians who did not drink alcohol at all (28%). Marijuana and cocaine use have been found to be no higher among lesbians than in the general population (McKirnan et al. 1989).

Obesity

Lesbian women are more likely to be overweight than heterosexual women (Aaron et al. 2001, Cochran et al. 2001). Although one-third of both groups admit to being sedentary, lesbians are more likely to engage in vigorous physical activity when active (Aaron et al. 2001). Interestingly, most lesbians have a good body image and are less likely to consider themselves overweight, perhaps reflecting the acceptance of a variety of body sizes and shapes within the lesbian community (Cochran et al. 2001). Similarly, and in contrast to the gay male population, there is less disordered eating in the lesbian population than in heterosexual women, possibly due to less attention to body appearance (Dean et al. 2000).

Mental Health

A report by the Department of Health and Human Services in 1989 identified an increased risk of suicide and depression among homosexuals (Lee 2000). The report found that 30% of completed suicides were in gay youth, and that 40% of lesbian, gay, bisexual, and transgender youth had attempted or completed suicide. Young lesbians are twice as likely to have attempted suicide as heterosexual girls are (Lee 2000). Early identification of one's own homosexuality, rejection from family and peers, isolation and lack of social support, and a history of sexual or physical abuse have been correlated with an increased risk of suicide in homosexual youth.

Homosexual adults are also at risk for suicide and depression. Social isolation, lack of support from or contact with one's family of origin, fear of discrimination and stigmatization, and the experience of discrimination and anti-gay violence create an ongoing life stress that may become overwhelming. Gilman et al. (2001) reviewed data from the National Comorbidity Survey, a nationally representative household survey, to identify the risk of psychiatric disorders among same-sex partners. Their review found that homosexuals were at increased risk for anxiety and mood disorders, as well as suicidal thoughts and plans. They postulate that the stresses associated with discrimination and stigmatization, including a sense of isolation, lack of social support, and stressful life events, increase the rates of these mental disorders in the homosexual population (Gilman et al. 2001).

Sexually Transmitted Disease

Most studies on the prevalence of sexually transmitted disease (STD) have not collected information on sexual orientation, thus little is known about the transmission of specific STDs between lesbians. Additionally, many lesbians consider themselves to be at no or minimal risk for STDs, regardless of current or past sexual behaviors. It is likely that lesbians who are exclusively sexually active with women are at low risk for the transmission of bacterial infections such as gonorrhea and chlamydia (Marrazzo et al. 2001). However, human papillomavirus (HPV) DNA has been detected in lesbians, even those who have never had sex with men. HPV can be transmitted via skin-to-skin contact, as well as by digital contact or sex toys (Marrazzo et al. 2001). In the same manner, herpes simplex virus can also be transmitted between two women (Carroll 1999).

In a study by Aaron et al (2001), 86.9% of lesbian women had sex only with women, while more than 3% had sexual contact with men to some degree. Ten percent of those who identified themselves as lesbian had not had sex with anyone in the last year. However, most lesbians have had sex with a man at some time in their lives (53–99% by some estimates), and one-third of lesbians continue to do so (Marrazzo et al. 2001). This increases the risk of STD acquisition to that of a heterosexual woman having sex with men (Marrazzo et al. 2001). Additionally, many lesbians who are sexually active with men do so without protection against pregnancy or STDs (Carroll 1999). Lesbian and bisexual women who have had sex with men in the past or continue to do so are much more likely to have had male partners who themselves were bisexual or intravenous drug users. This places not only the woman but also her partner at an increased risk for STDs, including human immunodeficiency virus (HIV).

There is little research on lesbian acquisition of HIV. In the absence of other known risk factors, whether or not HIV can be transmitted during female-to-female sexual contact is unclear, although there have been case reports in the literature (White 1997). However, if a lesbian who has had sex with a man or used intravenous drugs develops HIV, she is put in the higher risk category (Dean et al. 2000). HIV has been identified in menstrual blood, vaginal secretions, and cervical biopsy specimens (Carroll 1999). Risks for HIV transmission include sexual practices such as cunnilingus and digital/manual contact with infected fluids. Sex toys (e.g., dildos, vibrators) may be shared between partners, increasing risk. Many lesbians who attempt pregnancy via artificial insemination use donors who are known to them, often bypassing HIV and other STD testing offered by reputable sperm banks.

Gynecologic Cancers

There is concern that lesbians are at increased risk of breast, endometrial, and ovarian cancers, as the majority of them are nulliparous or conceive later in life and have not used oral contraceptives; many are obese, smoke cigarettes, and drink alcohol. These factors may also increase their risk of lung and colon cancers. While none of these known risk factors is unique to lesbian women, they may be uniquely concentrated within this population (Cochran et al. 2001). Lesbians may also be less likely than heterosexual women to utilize preventive screening, and the lack of a need for contraception eliminates a common interface with a health care provider for services.

Inadequate Utilization of Services

Overt and subtle homophobia serves to undermine the medical care provided to lesbian and bisexual women. Many lesbians have experienced discrimination due to their sexual orientation, which for many has negatively impacted their utilization of health care services. Many do not seek medical care due to prior negative experiences with providers and a perceived lack of susceptibility to disease.

Studies indicate that two-thirds of providers do not ask women their sexual orientation (Lee 2000). This places the burden of disclosure on the woman, who may be uncomfortable revealing her sexual orientation because of prior discrimination, fear of stigmatization, or fear of inferior care. There are reports in the literature of both male and female homosexuals receiving substandard care once they disclosed their sexual orientation (Dean et al. 2000). Many medical providers assume women are heterosexual, either from lack of awareness or internalized homophobia, preferring not to bring up the issue. Women are often asked what type of contraception they use, not whether or not they are sexually active and with whom. When sexual orientation is not revealed, health care risks are not appropriately identified and addressed. Lesbians may feel more comfortable discussing their sexual orientation with a provider if they have been "out" with friends and family, but even when a woman is comfortable identifying herself as lesbian or bisexual, providers often lack knowledge of sexual orientation, practices, and specific behavioral risks.

Unfortunately, many lesbians who are not sexually active with men, and many health care providers, do not believe that lesbians need annual cervical screening. However, cervical dysplasia, including high-grade squamous intraepithelial lesions, has been found in lesbians who have never had sex with men (Marrazzo et al. 2001). We know that HPV can be transmitted from female-to-female, and it is likely that intravaginal deposition occurs with digital contact. In particular, young lesbians are less likely to receive cervical screening than their heterosexual counterparts, regardless of sexual practices (Diamant et al. 2000).

In a large study by Diamant et al. (2000), 70% of lesbians age 50 or older had received mammograms in the last year. Results of a smaller study by Lauver et al. (1999) were similar and found that the reasons given by lesbians for not having mammography were no different than those given by heterosexual women (e.g., cost, fear of discomfort).

Recommendations for Providers

→ Create a nonjudgmental open atmosphere in providing care to women of all sexual orientation.
→ Take a detailed sexual history, making no assumptions. Ask every female patient, "Are you sexually active with men, women, or both?" Obtain information on the number of partners and specific practices engaged in, including oral, vaginal, and anal sex. Ask if any sex toys are used and/or shared between partners, and whether protective aids such as gloves or dental dams are used.
→ Ask about HIV risk factors in the patient and her partner(s). Ask if she has any concerns related to sexual health.
→ Providers should educate themselves about the specific risk behaviors that have been found to be more prevalent in les-

bians. Provide counseling and information on the health risks of tobacco and alcohol abuse, STD risk, the need for preventive health care, and community resources. Be prepared to teach patients about barrier methods to prevent STDs.
→ Provide annual cervical screening for all women by the age of 18 or when sexual activity begins. The frequency of cervical screening should be individualized. See specific chapters for indications and guidelines.
→ Make consistent mammography recommendations for all female patients, regardless of their sexual orientation.
→ Encourage lesbian patients to have a durable power of attorney for health care, or a health proxy, so that the woman's family of origin cannot overrule her wishes. Such documents should allow lesbian partners equal access to information and visiting privileges that are afforded heterosexual couples.

As more studies look at specific risks in the lesbian population, additional recommendations may be appropriate, and providers should maintain their awareness of the health care needs of this unique population. Optimal health care is a right of all women in this country, regardless of sexual orientation.

BIBLIOGRAPHY

Aaron, D., Markovic, N., Danielson, M. et al. 2001. *American Journal of Public Health* 91(6):972–975.

Carroll, N. 1999. Optimal gynecologic and obstetric care for lesbians. *Obstetrics and Gynecology* 93(4):611–613.

Cochran, S., Mays, V., Bowen, D. et al. 2001. Cancer-related risk indicators and preventive screening behaviors among lesbians and bisexual women. *American Journal of Public Health* 91(4):591–597.

Dean, L., Meyer, I., Robinson, K. et al. 2000. Lesbian, gay, bisexual and transgender health: findings and concerns. *Journal of the Gay and Lesbian Medical Association* 4(3):101–151.

Diamant, A., Schuster, M., and Lever, J. 2000. Receipt of preventive health care services by lesbians. *American Journal of Preventive Medicine* 19(3):141–148.

Fifield, L.G. 1975. On my way to nowhere: alienated, isolated, and drunk. Los Angeles: Gay Community Services Center.

Gilman, S., Cochran, S., Mays, V. et al. 2001. Risk of psychiatric disorders among individuals reporting same-sex sexual partners in the National Comorbidity Survey. *American Journal of Public Health* 91(6):933–939.

Heffernan, K. 1998. The nature and predictors of substance use among lesbians. *Addictive Behaviors* 23(4):517–528.

Human Rights Campaign. 2001. U.S. census figures continue to show national trend of dramatic increase in households of same-sex partners. Available at: http://www.hrc.org/newsreleases/2001/census/010627.asp. Accessed on July 30, 2002.

Institute of Medicine. 1999. *Lesbian health: current assessment and directions for the future*. Washington, D.C.: National Academy Press.

Lauver, D., Karon, S., Egan, J. et al. 1999. Understanding lesbians' mammography utilization. *Women's Health Issues* 9(5):264–274.

Lee, R. 2000. Health care problems of lesbian, gay, bisexual, and transgender patients. *Western Journal of Medicine* 172(6):403–408.

Lewis, C.E., Saghir, M.T., and Robins, E. 1982. Drinking patterns in homosexual and heterosexual women. *Journal of Clinical Psychiatry* 43:277–278.

Marrazzo, J., Koutsky, L., Kiviat, N. et al. 2001. Papanicolaou test screening and prevalence of genital human papillo-mavirus among women who have sex with women. *American Journal of Public Health* 91(6):947–952.

McKirnan, D., and Peterson, P. 1989. Alcohol and drug use among homosexual men and women: epidemiology and population characteristics. *Addictive Behaviors* 14:545–553.

Ryan, H., Wortley, P., Easton, A. et al. 2001. Smoking among lesbians, gays, and bisexuals. *American Journal of Preventive Medicine* 21(2):142–149.

White, J. 1997. HIV risk assessment and prevention in lesbians and women who have sex with women: practical information for clinicians. *Health Care for Women International* 18:127–138.

SECTION 2

Ophthalmological Disorders

2-A Blepharitis. **2-2**
2-B Cataracts **2-4**
2-C Conjunctivitis. **2-6**
2-D Dacryocystitis **2-10**
2-E Eye Injury **2-11**
2-F Glaucoma **2-14**
2-G Hordeolum and Chalazion. **2-17**
2-H Keratitis. **2-19**
2-I Pinguecula and Pterygium. **2-21**
2-J Uveitis. **2-22**
2-K Bibliography **2-24**

Lisa L. Lommel, R.N., C., F.N.P., M.S., M.P.H.
Julie Richards, R.N., C., W.H.N.P., F.N.P., M.S., M.S.N.

2-A
Blepharitis

Blepharitis is a chronic bilateral inflammation of the eyelid margins. The condition is complex and involves multiple etiologic factors, including meibomian gland dysfunction, the lipid content of meibomian secretions, and extraocular bacteria (McCulley et al. 2000). *Anterior blepharitis* is more common and involves the eyelid skin, eyelashes, and associated glands. There are two major types of anterior blepharitis—*staphylococcal blepharitis*, which may become ulcerative, and *seborrheic blepharitis*, which usually involves the scalp, brows, and ears (Sullivan et al. 1999).

Posterior blepharitis is inflammation of the eyelid secondary to dysfunction of the meibomian glands. There may be an associated staphylococcal infection. Posterior blepharitis is strongly associated with acne rosacea (Sullivan et al. 1999).

DATABASE
SUBJECTIVE

→ Symptoms may include:
- Irritation, burning, and itchy eyes
- Anterior blepharitis:
  - Staphylococcal—scaling, lesions, red lid margins, loss of lashes, crusting of lid margins
  - Seborrheic—less lid margin redness and scaling and no lesions or crusting of lid margins
  - Mixed type—red lid margin, crusting, scaling, lesions
- Posterior blepharitis:
  - Red lid margins, tearing, lid margin rolled in

OBJECTIVE

→ The patient may present with:
- Anterior blepharitis:
  - Staphylococcal—red lid margins, dry scales, broken or missing lashes, ulcerations, inflamed conjunctiva
  - Seborrheic—greasy scales, less lid redness, no ulcerations, inflamed conjunctiva
  - Mixed type—dry and greasy scales, red lid margins and ulcerations, inflamed conjunctiva

- Posterior blepharitis:
  - Lid margins hyperemic with telangiectasias
  - Inflamed meibomian gland orifice
  - Entropion
  - Frothy or greasy tears
→ Both anterior and posterior blepharitis may present with signs of:
- Hordeolum
- Chalazion
- Abnormal lid protrusion
- Conjunctivitis
- Keratitis
- Increased vascularization and thinning of inferior cornea (more common in posterior blepharitis)
→ See the **Hordeolum and Chalazion**, **Conjunctivitis**, and **Keratitis** chapters.

ASSESSMENT

→ Blepharitis
→ R/O hordeolum
→ R/O chalazion
→ R/O conjunctivitis
→ R/O acne rosacea

PLAN
DIAGNOSTIC TESTS

→ Usually not required for diagnosis and treatment.

TREATMENT/MANAGEMENT

Anterior Blepharitis

→ Responds well to lid hygiene and topical antibiotics.
- Dilute Johnson's Baby Shampoo® 1:1 with water, stabilize eyelid by gently pulling laterally, and scrub eyelids with cotton-tip applicator or clean washcloth. Rinse well with water. A commercial eyelid cleanser (e.g., Eye Scrub®, OCuSOFT®) may also be used (Shields 2000).

- Follow with application of a warm compress for 5–10 minutes to each eye. Lid margin scrubs should be done twice a day.
- For severe cases, patients may apply a thin layer of antibiotic ophthalmic ointment at bedtime to the lid margin with clean fingers or cotton-tip applicator and rub it in for 5–10 strokes:
  - Bacitracin 500–1,000 units/g ointment (Shields 2000)
    OR
  - Erythromycin 0.5% ointment (Shields 2000)
    OR
  - Sulfacetamide sodium (Sodium Sulamyd®) 10% ointment (Plewig et al. 1999).
- Treatment may continue for up to several weeks. If symptoms persist, nonurgent referral to an ophthalmologist is warranted (Shields 2000).

→ Co-existing seborrheic dermatitis is treated with low-potency topical steroids and/or shampoos for the scalp and eyebrows containing selenium sulfide, antifungals (e.g., ketoconazole), zinc pyrithione, benzoyl peroxide, salicylic acid, coal or juniper tar, or detergents (Plewig et al. 1999). (See the **Seborrheic Dermatitis** chapter in Section 3.)

Posterior Blepharitis

→ Patients with acne rosacea or seborrheic dermatitis often develop an infection or inflammation of the meibomian gland. These patients can be treated with (Shields 2000):

- Tetracycline HCL 250 mg p.o. BID–QID
  OR
- Doxycycline 50–100 mg p.o. QD–BID
- Treatment may continue for up to several weeks. If symptoms persist, nonurgent referral to an ophthalmologist is warranted (Shields 2000).

CONSULTATION

→ Referral is indicated when there is poor response to treatment or if corneal disease is present.
→ As needed for prescription(s).

PATIENT EDUCATION

→ See "Treatment/Management."
→ Explain the pathophysiology, chronicity, and treatment plan.
→ Advise the patient to avoid rubbing her eyes at all times.
→ Advise the patient to wash her hands well before and after eye treatment.
→ Advise the patient to keep eye ointment clean and not to share it with others.
→ Maintenance therapy for normal lid margins includes daily lid shampoo and warm compresses.

FOLLOW-UP

→ Document in progress notes and on problem list.

Lisa L. Lommel, R.N., C., F.N.P., M.S., M.P.H.
Julie Richards, R.N., C., W.H.N.P., F.N.P., M.S., M.S.N.

2-B
Cataracts

A *cataract* is an opacification of the crystalline lens of the eye. Most cataracts occur with aging and almost all elderly patients have some degree of opacification (Steinert 2000b.)

Aging is the most common cause of cataracts, but other associated factors include trauma, smoking, heredity, oxidative damage (from free-radical reactions), ultraviolet light damage, and malnutrition (Harper et al. 1999).

In addition, many conditions are associated with cataracts. These include uveitis, glaucoma, retinitis pigmentosa, retinal detachment, diabetes mellitus, hypoparathyroidism, myotonic dystrophy, atopic dermatitis, galactosemia, and Lowe's, Werner's, and Down's syndromes (Harper et al. 1999).

Corticosteroids and other drugs, including phenothiazines, amiodarone, and phospholine iodide, may induce cataracts (Harper et al. 1999).

DATABASE

SUBJECTIVE

→ Symptoms may include:
- Blurred vision, usually worse when viewing distant objects; progressive over months or years
- The earliest symptom may be improved near vision.
- Poor hue discrimination
- Monocular diplopia (double vision in one eye)
- Decreased visual acuity with extraneous light source (glare from sunlight), commonly disturbing the ability to drive
- No pain or redness

OBJECTIVE

→ Reduced visual acuity may be present depending on density and position of opacity on lens.
→ The pupil may be white.
→ Check for the red reflex while standing about 12 inches from the patient. Cataract formation is indicated by disruption of the red reflex.

→ Plus power (black numbers) of about 15–20 diopters will bring the lens into focus as you approach the patient. The lens is best viewed with a dilated pupil (Steinert 2000b.)
→ Senile cataracts are wedge-shaped, pointing toward the center of the pupil.
→ The ability to visualize fundus on close examination depends on the density and location of opacity.
→ Slit-lamp examination can reveal the morphology of the cataract—e.g., cataracts due to uveitis or drug use may first appear in the posterior subcapsular region.

ASSESSMENT

→ Cataract
→ R/O concomitant condition contributing to cataract formation
→ R/O other causes of decreased visual acuity

PLAN

DIAGNOSTIC TESTS

→ A complete eye examination should be performed by an ophthalmologist.
→ Examination of the eye for measurement of best eyeglass correction should be completed before a decision is made regarding surgery.
→ Additional diagnostic tests may be appropriate to rule out conditions contributing to cataract formation.

TREATMENT/MANAGEMENT

→ There is no medical treatment for cataracts.
→ Eyeglasses and/or contact lenses may provide satisfactory correction for some patients.
→ Surgery is the treatment of choice for individuals with functional visual impairment.
- Includes removing the opacity and implanting an intraocular lens, which eliminates the need for heavy cataract glasses or contact lenses.
→ Management of condition contributing to formation of cataract as indicated.

CONSULTATION

→ Referral to an ophthalmologist is indicated for comprehensive work-up and management decision.

PATIENT EDUCATION

→ Explain pathophysiology and treatment options.
→ Specifics of patient education will depend on treatment option.
→ For patients with surgical correction, advise adherence to postsurgical care.

→ Advise all individuals to protect their eyes from ultraviolet radiation with protective sunglasses and wide-brimmed hats.
→ Advise patients who smoke to stop. Referral to a smoking-cessation support group may be indicated.
→ Advise patients that steroid use should be limited to the lowest dose necessary.
→ Advise patients that a diet rich in vitamins C and E and beta carotene has been shown to lower the risk of cataract formation (Taylor 2000).

FOLLOW-UP

→ Document in progress notes and on problem list.

Lisa L. Lommel, R.N., C., F.N.P., M.S., M.P.H.
Julie Richards, R.N., C., W.H.N.P., F.N.P., M.S., M.S.N.

2-C
Conjunctivitis

Conjunctivitis is an inflammation of the conjunctiva, caused most commonly by bacteria, chlamydia, viruses, or allergies. Common bacteria that cause conjunctivitis include *Staphylococcus aureus, Streptococcus pneumoniae*, and *Haemophilus influenzae. Neisseria gonorrhoeae* and *Chlamydia trachomatis* are also important causes. The most common viral pathogens in adults are adenovirus types 8,11, and 19 (*Sanford Guide to Antimicrobial Therapy* 2001). Other causes of conjunctivitis include fungi, parasites, rickettsiae, and ocular irritants such as contact lenses. Conjunctivitis also is associated with other conditions, including rosacea, psoriasis, thyroid disease, gout, tuberculosis, syphilis, and sarcoidosis (Schwab et al. 1999).

DATABASE
SUBJECTIVE

Bacterial
→ Precipitating factors include a history of contact with a person with similar symptoms.
→ Symptoms begin in one eye and spread to the other.
→ Symptoms include:
  ■ A copious mucopurulent discharge
  ■ Crusting of eyelids in the morning
  ■ Mild discomfort and grittiness
  ■ No pain, blurred vision, or photophobia

Gonococcal
→ Precipitating factors include contact with infected genital secretions.
→ Symptoms include:
  ■ A copious purulent discharge
  ■ Associated symptoms of genital infection

Chlamydial
→ Precipitating factors include:
  ■ Contact with infected genital secretions
  ■ Young, sexually active women

→ Symptoms include:
  ■ Acute redness and irritation
  ■ Watery to mucopurulent discharge
  ■ Associated symptoms of genital infection

Viral
→ Symptoms usually involve one eye at onset with less severe involvement of the second eye after one week.
→ Symptoms include:
  ■ A copious watery discharge
  ■ Gritty, irritated eye
  ■ Photophobia
  ■ Associated symptoms of cough, malaise, fever, and sore throat

Seasonal and Perennial Allergy
→ Symptoms include:
  ■ Itching, irritation, burning, photophobia
→ History includes:
  ■ Associated allergic problems, including rhinitis, eczema, and food allergies
  ■ Seasonal allergy (hay fever conjunctivitis):
    • Most common in spring and summer
    • Related to the appearance of specific allergens or pollens
  ■ Perennial allergy:
    • Chronic and usually year-round
    • Symptoms are usually less severe than those of a seasonal allergy
    • The patient may experience seasonal exacerbation of symptoms
  ■ Watery discharge
  ■ Red conjunctiva
  ■ Mild to moderate discomfort
  ■ Commonly associated symptoms of nasal and/or pharyngeal complaints, including rhinorrhea, pharyngitis, and postnasal drip
→ Symptoms are usually bilateral.

Contact Allergy

→ A wide variety of substances—most commonly including medications, cosmetics, and contact lens solutions—may cause contact allergy.
→ Symptoms include:
- Itching, burning, and watery discharge
- Photophobia

OBJECTIVE

→ The patient may present with:

Bacterial

- A copious purulent discharge
- No keratitis or preauricular lymph nodes

Gonococcal

- A copious purulent discharge
- Red conjunctiva with edema
- Possible corneal involvement
- An enlarged preauricular lymph node

Chlamydial

- A watery to mucopurulent discharge
- Diffuse conjunctival redness
- Conjunctival follicles
- Possible corneal involvement
- A nontender, enlarged preauricular lymph node

Viral

- Pharyngitis
- Fever
- Red palpebral conjunctiva
- Watery eye discharge
- Stringy exudate
- Palpebral conjunctival follicles and central keratitis are hallmark clinical signs on slit-lamp examination
- An enlarged or palpable preauricular lymph node

Seasonal and Perennial Allergy

- Red conjunctiva with edema
- Tarsal conjunctival follicles
- Clear, stringy discharge
- Signs of perennial allergy are less severe than those of seasonal allergy or may be absent

Contact Allergy

- Red conjunctiva with edema
- Skin of eyelids reddened, edematous, scaling, and papular
- Inferior fornix presenting with a follicular response
- Severe cases that may involve cornea with infiltrates and opacities

ASSESSMENT

→ Conjunctivitis
- R/O bacterial
- R/O gonococcal
- R/O chlamydial
- R/O viral
- R/O seasonal and perennial allergy
- R/O contact allergy
→ R/O trauma
→ R/O uveitus/iritis
→ R/O keratitis
→ R/O narrow angle closure glaucoma
→ R/O concomitant sexually transmitted infection (STI)

PLAN

DIAGNOSTIC TESTS

→ Eye acuity should be measured before installation of fluorescein.
→ Slit-lamp examination may be helpful.
→ Fluorescein staining may be indicated to help rule out corneal involvement. (See the **Eye Injury** and **Keratitis** chapters.)

Bacterial

→ Severe inflammation and purulent discharge should be cultured to guide appropriate treatment.

Gonococcal

→ Suspected cases should be confirmed by culture of discharge.
→ Test for concomitant STIs—syphilis, trichomoniasis, *C. trachomatis*, HIV.

Chlamydial

→ Suspected cases should be confirmed by culture with cytologic examination of discharge.
→ Test for concomitant STIs—syphilis, *N. gonorrhoeae*, trichomoniasis, HIV.

Viral

→ No specific diagnostic tests.

Seasonal and Perennial Allergy

→ In severe cases, allergy testing may be recommended to identify specific allergens.

Contact Allergy

→ No specific diagnostic tests.
→ Skin testing can be useful in identifying specific allergens.

TREATMENT/MANAGEMENT

Bacterial

→ Usually self-limiting, lasting 10–14 days if left untreated.

→ Any conjunctivitis with severe, profuse exudates warrants immediate referral to an ophthalmologist to avoid corneal damage, loss of eye, or septicemia/meningitis (Leibowitz 2000, Schwab et al. 1999).

→ For mild cases (*Nurse Practitioners' Prescribing Reference* 2002, Steinert 2000b):

- Polymyxin B/trimethoprim ophthalmic solution, 1 drop in affected eye(s) every 3 hours for 1 week (maximum 6 doses/day)

OR

- Erythromycin 0.5% ophthalmic ointment. Instill in affected eye(s) QID for 1 week.
- Aminoglycosides and fluoroquinolones are not recommended for routine conjunctivitis.

Gonococcal

→ If gonorrhea is suspected, immediate referral to an ophthalmologist is indicated to R/O corneal involvement, which may lead to perforation.

→ If cornea is not involved (Schwab et al. 1999):

- Ceftriaxone 1 g IM for 1 dose

→ Normal saline conjunctival irrigation for 15 minutes QID.

→ Treat associated STIs.

Chlamydial (Schwab et al. 1999)

→ Tetracycline, divided doses, 1–1.5 g/day p.o. for 3–4 weeks

OR

→ Erythromycin, divided doses, 1 g/day p.o. for 3–4 weeks

OR

→ Doxycycline 100 mg p.o. BID for 3 weeks

→ Treat associated STIs.

Viral

→ Usually self-limiting, lasting approximately 2 weeks.

→ Corticosteroids are not recommended, as they might prolong course.

→ Warm compresses may relieve discomfort.

→ Often difficult to distinguish clinically from bacterial infection. A topical antibiotic often is prescribed. (See "Treatment/Management" of bacterial conjunctivitis, above.)

Seasonal and Perennial Allergy

→ Initial management is focused on identifying causative antigen(s) and eliminating them from the environment.

→ Desensitization is less effective in ocular disease than in allergic rhinitis (Schwab et al. 1999).

→ Many agents are available for treating allergic ocular conditions, including ocular decongestants, astringents, antihistamines, mast cell stabilizers, and topical nonsteroidal anti-

inflammatory drugs (NSAIDs) (Shields 2000). Many treatments are available over the counter.

- Decongestants (*Nurse Practitioners' Prescribing Reference* 2002, Shields 2000):
  - Naphazoline hydrochloride 1–2 drops in each eye up to 5 times a day

OR

  - Tetrahydrozoline hydrochloride 1–2 drops in each eye up to 5 times a day

- Decongestant/astringent combinations (*Nurse Practitioners' Prescribing Reference* 2002, Shields 2000):
  - Tetrahydrozoline plus zinc sulfate 1–2 drops in each eye up to 5 times a day

- Decongestant/antihistamine combinations (*Nurse Practitioners' Prescribing Reference* 2002, Shields 2000):
  - Naphazoline HCL 0.025%, pheniramine maleate 0.3%, 1–2 drops in each eye up to 4 times a day

- Antihistamines (*Nurse Practitioners' Prescribing Reference* 2002, Shields 2000):
  - Levocabastine HCL 0.05%, 1 drop in each eye QID. Soft contact lenses contraindicated.

OR

  - Emedastine 0.05%, 1 drop in each eye up to 4 times a day. Remove soft contact lenses. May reinsert 10 minutes after applying.

- Mast cell stabilizers (*Nurse Practitioners' Prescribing Reference* 2002, Shields 2000):
  - Lodoxamide 1–2 drops in each eye QID for up to 3 months

OR

  - Cromolyn sodium 4%, 1–2 drops in each eye 4–6 times daily at regular intervals.
    - The clinical response with mast cell stabilizers is not immediate; they must be given for about 2 weeks to prevent the release of histamine (Leibowitz 2000).

- Antihistamine/mast cell stabilizer combinations (*Nurse Practitioners' Prescribing Reference* 2002, Shields 2000):
  - Olopatadine HCL 0.1%, 1 drop in each eye BID at 6–8 hour intervals. Remove contact lenses; may reinsert them 10 minutes after applying.

- Topical NSAID (*Nurse Practitioners' Prescribing Reference* 2002, Shields 2000):
  - Ketorolac tromethamine 0.5%, 1 drop in each eye QID. Concomitant soft contact lenses are not recommended.

→ Systemic antihistamines may be effective against more severe ocular symptoms and associated nasal and pharyngeal symptoms. (See the **Rhinitis** chapter in Section 5.)

Contact Allergy

→ Eliminate contact with the offending substance.

→ Self-limiting, should subside after contact is discontinued.

→ Cool compresses may provide relief from discomfort.

→ If the cornea is involved, immediate referral to an ophthalmologist is indicated.

CONSULTATION

→ Indicated in severe cases of conjunctivitis (including gonorrhea).

→ Physician consultation is recommended if symptoms don't improve in one week or if condition worsens after beginning treatment.

→ Referral to an ophthalmologist is indicated if symptoms of bacterial conjunctivitis don't improve in one week.

→ Immediate referral to an ophthalmologist is indicated if there is corneal involvement or decreased visual acuity.

→ As needed for prescription(s).

PATIENT EDUCATION

→ Instruct the patient regarding pathophysiology, risk factors, and treatment plan.

→ Advise the patient to maintain good hygiene:
  ■ Avoid contact with towels or other fomites from an infected individual.
  ■ Wash hands well before and after touching the eyes or instilling ocular medications.
  ■ Avoid touching an infected eye with an ocular medication container.

→ Teach the patient proper instillation of ocular medications:
  ■ Tilt head back.
  ■ Place a finger on the cheek and gently pull downward, forming a pocket.
  ■ Instill drops or an approximately 0.5 inch ribbon of ointment into the pocket without touching the tip of the tube to the eye.
  ■ Look downward before closing eye.

→ For patients with gonococcal or chlamydial conjunctivitis:
  ■ Instruct the patient regarding transmission of STIs, including using condoms to avoid contracting them.
  ■ Advise the patient to avoid contact with infected genital secretions.
  ■ Advise the patient that these infections are reportable to local health departments.
  ■ Advise the patient to have sexual partners treated for infection. (See the **Gonorrhea** and *Chlamydia trachomatis* chapters in Section 13.)
  ■ Advise the patient regarding the need for additional STI testing and treatment as indicated.

→ For the patient with seasonal and perennial allergic conjunctivitis:
  ■ Instruct her to avoid allergens that precipitate symptoms.

FOLLOW-UP

→ See "Consultation," above.

→ Document in progress notes and on problem list.

Lisa L. Lommel, R.N., C., F.N.P., M.S., M.P.H.
Julie Richards, R.N., C., W.H.N.P., F.N.P., M.S., M.S.N.

2-D
Dacryocystitis

Dacryocystitis, an infection of the lacrimal sac, usually develops when the lacrimal system becomes partially or totally blocked. In acute dacryocystitis, *Staphylococcus aureus* and beta-hemolytic streptococci are the most common infectious organisms. In chronic cases, *Streptococcus pneumoniae* or, rarely, *Candida albicans* is the predominant organism.

This infection may be acute or chronic and is most common in females older than 40 years. It can be complicated by cellulitis of the surrounding skin.

DATABASE

SUBJECTIVE

→ Patients with acute cases present with:
- Pain
- Swelling
- Redness around the inner canthus of the eye
- Increased tearing
- Discharge

→ Patients with advanced cases may present with generalized facial swelling and tenderness.

→ Patients with chronic cases may present with only tearing and discharge.

OBJECTIVE

→ Patients may present with:
- Tenderness
- Swelling
- Redness around the inner canthus of the eye
- Pressure over the lacrimal sac, possibly producing mucopurulent drainage through the lacrimal puncta

→ Advanced cases may present with:
- Generalized swelling and tenderness
- Enlarged cervical lymph nodes

ASSESSMENT

→ Dacryocystitis
→ R/O orbital cellulitis

→ R/O acute conjunctivitis
→ R/O lacrimal sac neoplasm
→ R/O underlying nasolacrimal duct obstruction
→ R/O hordeolum/chalazion

PLAN

DIAGNOSTIC TESTS

→ Usually none needed for diagnosis.
→ Culture of duct drainage may assist in choice of antibiotic treatment if first-line therapy is not improving symptoms.

TREATMENT/MANAGEMENT

→ Warm compresses and massage over the lacrimal duct area 3 times a day.
→ Oral antibiotics:
- Cephalexin 500 mg QID for 10 days (Thompson 2001).

CONSULTATION

→ Referral to an ophthalmologist is indicated to R/O an underlying nasolacrimal duct obstruction.
→ Immediate emergency referral is warranted when orbital cellulitis is present.
→ As needed for prescription(s).

PATIENT EDUCATION

→ Instruct the patient regarding pathophysiology, chronicity, and treatment plan.
→ See "Treatment/Management," above.
→ Advise the patient to avoid rubbing her eyes.
→ Advise the patient to wash her hands well before and after treatment.

FOLLOW-UP

→ Document in progress notes and on problem list.

Lisa L. Lommel, R.N., C., F.N.P., M.S., M.P.H.
Julie Richards, R.N., C., W.H.N.P., F.N.P., M.S., M.S.N.

2-E
Eye Injury

Eye injuries run the gamut, from serious emergencies requiring immediate referral to an ophthalmologist to minor trauma—e.g., a foreign body lodged in an eye and extracted in an outpatient setting. The primary care provider's responsibility to a patient who presents with a serious emergency is to provide diagnosis and immediate management, and transport to an ophthalmologist and/or emergency setting. Nonemergency conditions can be managed in consultation with a physician.

DATABASE

SUBJECTIVE

Chemical, Thermal, or Radiation Burn; Penetrating Injury; Blunt Trauma

→ History should include:
  - How, when, and where the injury occurred
  - Protective eye wear, contact lens, or glasses usually worn
  - Loss of vision and presence of pain or associated manifestations
  - Presence of a foreign-body sensation
→ Identify the injurious object. Any eye injury produced by a high-velocity missile (while, e.g., mowing, hammering, or in a motor vehicle accident) should be treated as a penetrating globe injury and referred to an ophthalmologist immediately (Shields 2000).
→ In radiation burns (e.g., from sunlight, a sun lamp, or a welding arc), symptoms usually are delayed 6–12 hours, then manifest as severe pain and photophobia.
→ Tetanus immunization status should be obtained in cases of penetrating injury.

Corneal Abrasion

→ Symptoms include:
→ Pain, tearing, photosensitivity, blurring of vision, and sensation of a foreign body.
→ History includes object contact with the eye (e.g., contact lens, particulates).

→ Tetanus immunization status should be obtained.

Foreign Body

→ Symptoms include:
  - Pain, burning, and a foreign-body sensation increasing with lid movement
→ Tetanus immunization status should be obtained.

Retinal Detachment

→ Symptoms include:
  - Sudden onset of floaters, flashing lights, pain when moving the eye, headache, or peripheral field defect.
→ The patient has a history of "a curtain coming down over the eye."

OBJECTIVE

→ Signs will be influenced by the nature of the injury.
→ It is important for the clinician who isn't an ophthalmologist to keep in mind the possibility of causing further damage while attempting to do a complete eye exam (Asbury et al. 1999).
→ A physical examination may include some or all of the following, depending on the nature of the injury (Asbury et al. 1999):
  - Measurement of visual acuity
  - Evaluation of ocular motility
  - Palpation for defects in the bony orbital rim and facial structure. (Do not press on the eye with penetrating or blunt trauma.)
  - Assessment of facial sensation
  - Inspection for the presence of enophthalmos by viewing profiles of corneas over the brow.
  - Assessment of pupils for size, shape, symmetry, and reaction to light
  - Assessment of tarsal surfaces of the lids, anterior segment, corneal surface, bulbar conjunctiva, and depth and clarity of anterior chamber

- Inspection of lens, vitreous, optic disk, and retina
- A more thorough assessment of the lids, palpebral conjunctiva, and fornices if the eyeball is not damaged
- Photographic documentation for legal considerations
→ Always evaluate the apparently uninjured eye.
→ Instillation of fluorescein will reveal abnormal staining (i.e., darker green) if a corneal abrasion is present. It may also highlight a foreign body. Linear abrasion in a vertical pattern may indicate a foreign body under the eyelid.

ASSESSMENT

→ Eye injury
- R/O chemical burn
- R/O thermal burn
- R/O radiation burn
- R/O penetrating eye injury
- R/O blunt trauma
- R/O foreign body
- R/O retinal detachment

PLAN

DIAGNOSTIC TESTS

NOTE: *Any medications placed in an injured eye must be sterile. Several are available in sterile individual dosage units* (Asbury et al. 1999).

→ A slit lamp facilitates examination through magnification.
→ Fluorescein staining and ultraviolet light may be used to look for corneal epithelial defects and foreign bodies.
- May first anesthetize the eye with proparacaine 0.5%, 1–2 drops.
→ With prolonged usage, topical anesthetics are toxic to the cornea and should never be dispensed to the patient for relief of ocular discomfort. (See *Physicians' Desk Reference*.)
- Pull down the lower lid and place the edge of fluorescein paper against the conjunctiva until a small amount of dye is taken up.
- Remove the paper and rinse the eye with normal saline to remove excess dye.
- Examine with penlight or ultraviolet light.
→ Computed tomography may be indicated to assess the traumatized eye and orbit.
→ Further diagnostic testing may be indicated as per an ophthalmologist.

TREATMENT/MANAGEMENT

Chemical Burn (e.g., household cleaners, fertilizers, pesticides, and battery acid) (Shields 2000)

→ Constitutes a true emergency.
→ Briefly R/O globe perforation (chemical explosions like those involving batteries may produce a globe injury or intraocular foreign body).
→ A topical anesthetic may be instilled before irrigation and every 20 minutes. Proparacaine 0.5%, 1–2 drops. With

prolonged usage, topical anesthetics are toxic to the cornea and should never be dispensed to the patient for relief of ocular discomfort. (See *Physicians' Desk Reference*.)
→ Immediate eye irrigation—with any clean, drinkable liquid (preferably water or normal saline, if available)—using a hose, tap, or shower for at least 15 minutes before transport to an ophthalmologist or emergency setting.
→ Alkali burns are more serious and may require prolonged irrigation.
→ Remove small particles from the conjunctival sac with a wet, cotton-tip applicator.
→ Consultation with a physician may be sought before transport.

Thermal Burn (Asbury et al. 1999)

→ Consult immediately with an ophthalmologist and refer the patient.

Radiation Burn (Asbury et al. 1999)

→ Consult immediately with an ophthalmologist and refer the patient.

Perforating Eye Injury (Shields 2000)

→ Apply a nonpressure protective eye shield and refer immediately to an ophthalmologist or emergency setting.
→ Administer tetanus immunization as indicated.

Blunt Trauma (Shields 2000)

→ Refer promptly to an ophthalmologist or emergency setting.

Corneal Abrasion (Shields 2000)

→ For a small abrasion of the cornea, conjunctiva, or sclera:
- Apply a drop of a cycloplegic agent (e.g., cyclopentolate HCL 1% solution), then a small amount of antibiotic ointment (e.g., erythromycin) in the lower conjunctival sac.
- Prescribe a topical nonsteroidal anti-inflammatory agent (e.g., ketorolac tromethamine, 1 drop QID) for pain.
- Continue antibiotic prophylaxis (e.g., with erythromycin ointment) 1–2 times QD until the abrasion heals.
→ For a large abrasion or one over the pupil, or if pain persists after a local anesthetic, refer promptly to an ophthalmologist.
→ If the patient has a contact lens-associated injury, refer promptly to an ophthalmologist to rule out a corneal ulcer.
→ Refer promptly if corneal opacity is present or develops.

Foreign Body

→ The most important aspect of managing foreign bodies is to determine whether a high-velocity injury occurred. Any high-velocity injury should be treated as a penetrating injury of the globe until proven otherwise. Such patients should always be referred to an ophthalmologist (Shields 2000).
→ A topical anesthetic may be used before attempting to remove the foreign body. With prolonged usage, topical anesthetics are toxic to the cornea and should never be dispensed to the patient for relief of ocular discomfort (See *Physicians' Desk Reference*.)

■ Proparacaine 0.5%, 1–2 drops
→ A mobile foreign body may be removed with normal saline irrigation.
→ A foreign body on the conjunctiva (not the cornea) may be removed by everting the lid and gently wiping with a wet, cotton-tip applicator.
→ After removing a foreign body, instill a small amount of polymyxin-bacitracin ophthalmic ointment in the lower conjunctival sac.
→ If a foreign body is imbedded in the cornea or conjunctiva, patch the eye and refer immediately to an ophthalmologist.
→ For a small abrasion of the conjunctiva, sclera, or cornea, see "Corneal Abrasion" under "Treatment/Management," above.
→ Administer tetanus immunization as indicated.

Retinal Detachment

→ Refer immediately to an ophthalmologist.

CONSULTATION

→ See "Treatment/Management" for consultation and referral.
→ As needed for prescription(s).

PATIENT EDUCATION

→ Advise all patients to wear safety glasses when they use hazardous materials and play sports.
→ Teach the patient how to instill eye medications properly:
■ Lie down with both eyes open and look up.
■ Slightly retract the lower eyelid.

■ Instill medication into the lower eyelid cul-de-sac without touching the eye. Look down with the eyelid still retracted so the eyes do not squeeze shut.
■ Inform the patient that ointment may make vision blurry.
→ Teach the patient to apply an eye patch properly:
■ Pressure patches should be applied firmly enough to hold the lid against the cornea.
■ Nonpressure patches are laid lightly across the eye and secured at the forehead and cheek.

Corneal Abrasion

→ Instruct the patient to call a provider in case of sudden redness, pain, or tearing.

Blunt Trauma

→ Instruct the patient who has experienced a mild trauma to call a provider in case of increased pain or decreased vision.
→ Advise patients to avoid platelet-inhibiting analgesic products for pain relief (e.g., aspirin, nonsteroidal anti-inflammatory drugs).

FOLLOW-UP

Corneal Abrasion

→ Recheck daily until fluorescein staining completely resolves. Refer promptly to an ophthalmologist if the abrasion has not decreased by 50% within 24 hours or if the abrasion is not completely healed within 48–72 hours (Shields 2000).
→ Document in progress notes and on problem list.

Lisa L. Lommel, R.N., C., F.N.P., M.S., M.P.H.
Julie Richards, R.N., C., W.H.N.P., F.N.P., M.S., M.S.N.

2-F

Glaucoma

Glaucoma is an optic neuropathy in which there is damage to the optic nerve and a visual-field loss. This is usually the result of elevated intraocular pressure. The pressure in the eye is maintained by the equilibrium of aqueous humor production and outflow. Elevated intraocular pressure is caused by obstructed outflow of the aqueous humor. Elevated intraocular pressure is defined as a pressure >21 mm Hg. However, this number is not diagnostic for glaucoma, as many individuals have elevated pressures and do not develop glaucoma. Conversely, glaucoma can develop in rare instances without elevated intraocular pressure.

The two most common types of *primary glaucoma* are *acute angle-closure glaucoma* and *chronic open-angle glaucoma*. Acute angle-closure glaucoma is uncommon among Caucasians and usually presents as an acute, painful condition. It is more prevalent among Asians, especially Burmese and Vietnamese (Vaughan et al. 1999). It occurs in individuals who have a narrow anterior chamber usually resulting from an enlarging lens associated with aging. Elevated intraocular pressure is precipitated by the closure of the narrow anterior chamber, causing it to obstruct the trabecular mesh work necessary for aqueous outflow. Angle closure is also associated with pupillary dilatation secondary to being in a darkened room, stress, or mydriatic or cycloplegic drugs.

An uncontrolled, acute attack of open-angle glaucoma can lead to permanent loss of vision or chronic angle closure. Approximately one-half of patients with acute angle-closure glaucoma will develop the condition in the other eye if prophylactic surgery is not performed.

Chronic open-angle glaucoma is common, accounting for 90% of all glaucoma cases. It occurs in 0.4–0.7% of the population older than 40 years (Vaughan et al. 1999). It is four times more common and is usually more aggressive among African Americans (Vaughan et al. 1999). Elevated intraocular pressure is thought to be caused by an obstruction in aqueous outflow at the microscopic level of the trabecular mesh work. The intraocular pressure is consistently elevated and, over months or years, causes optic nerve atrophy and vision loss. This condition is insidious and often silent, causing extensive damage before the patient is aware of vision loss (Vaughan et al. 1999).

Primary glaucoma also may be due to congenital glaucoma, which is extremely rare. Secondary glaucoma may develop due to uveitis, neoplasm, lens-induced glaucoma, trauma, retinal vein thrombosis, diabetes, or prolonged steroid use (Vaughan et al. 1999).

DATABASE

SUBJECTIVE

Acute Angle-Closure Glaucoma

→ Risk groups include:
  - Individuals who are hypermetropic (far-sighted)
  - Older individuals who have larger lenses
  - Asian-Americans
→ Symptoms may include:
  - Sudden onset of reddening, pain in the eye
  - Headache, usually unilateral
  - Nausea and vomiting
  - Blurred vision, with halos around lights (like looking through frosted glass)
  - Onset associated with pupil dilatation at night, darkened rooms, stress, or mydriatic or cycloplegic drugs
  - A history of similar attacks that subsided after going to sleep (causing pupil constriction)
→ The degree of vision loss depends on extent of corneal edema.
→ If an acute episode has resolved, no signs and symptoms may be present—thus, the importance of history. Before an acute attack presents, there may be a long history of short, recurrent attacks that resolve spontaneously.

Chronic Open-Angle Glaucoma

→ Risk groups and factors include:
  - Older individuals
  - African Americans

- ■ Diabetics
- ■ Extreme myopia (short-sightedness)
- ■ Migraine
- ■ Vasospasm
- ■ Family history of glaucoma
- ■ History of ocular trauma

→ The patient is usually asymptomatic until severe damage has occurred.

→ A gradual loss of peripheral vision over years.

→ Halos around lights if intraocular pressure is markedly elevated.

→ The severity of symptoms is related to the level of intraocular pressure.

OBJECTIVE

Acute Angle-Closure Glaucoma

→ The patient presents with:
- ■ Reddened eye, hazy cornea
- ■ Semi-dilated, fixed, unreactive pupil
- ■ Ciliary injection (circumcorneal)
- ■ Affected eye is harder and tender to touch
- ■ Decreased visual acuity

Chronic Open-Angle Glaucoma

→ Possible loss of peripheral visual field and visual acuity but only with severe damage.

→ In early glaucoma, the optic disc becomes notched on the supertemporal or inferotemporal rim.

→ Later optic-disc changes include:
- ■ Increase in the depth and width of physiologic cup
- ■ Nasal displacement of central retinal vessel
- ■ Progressive pallor of the optic-disc head

→ Asymmetrical disc cupping and hemorrhages are associated signs.

→ Almost always bilateral.

→ The severity of signs is related to the level of intraocular pressure.

ASSESSMENT

→ Acute angle-closure glaucoma

→ Chronic open-angle glaucoma

→ R/O conjunctivitis

→ R/O acute uveitis

→ R/O corneal disorders

→ R/O iritis

PLAN

DIAGNOSTIC TESTS

→ The Schiotz Tonometer, for measuring intraocular pressure, should not be used in the outpatient setting when there is a suspicion of acute closed-angle glaucoma. Measurement of pressure should only be attempted by the ophthalmologist.

→ Ophthalmoscopy should be performed on all patients when there is suspicion of glaucoma.

→ Visual field testing with more-sensitive perimetry devices should be completed by the ophthalmologist.

TREATMENT/MANAGEMENT

Acute Angle-Closure Glaucoma

→ Requires urgent referral to an ophthalmologist.

→ *Immediate consultation with an ophthalmologist is indicated for treatment to lower intraocular pressure before urgent referral* (Richter 2000).

→ The treatment of choice is laser iridotomy or surgical peripheral iridectomy. Prophylactic laser iridotomy is indicated in the unaffected eye (Vaughan et al. 1999).

Chronic Open-Angle Glaucoma

→ Referral to an ophthalmologist is indicated for patients with suspected elevated intraocular pressure.

→ All primary care providers should be familiar with medications that increase intraocular pressure and use them cautiously (e.g., systemic and topical steroids, and drugs with anticholinergic effects).

→ All primary care providers should be familiar with their patient's ocular medications—specifically, their side effects and interactions with other drugs. (See *Physicians' Desk Reference*.)

Screening for Open-Angle Glaucoma

→ Mass screening efforts have been shown to be ineffective in detecting glaucoma. Current recommendations include comprehensive eye examinations (by an ophthalmologist) for the asymptomatic individual, based on the risk factors of age and race (Richter 2000):
- ■ African American patients:
  - • 20–39 years old: every 3–5 years
  - • 40–64 years old: every 2–4 years
  - • Older than 65 years: every 1–2 years
- ■ Other asymptomatic patients:
  - • 20–39 years old: every 3–5 years or less frequently
  - • 40–64 years old: every 2–4 years
  - • Older than 65 years: every 1–2 years

→ In addition, referral to an ophthalmologist is recommended for the following:
- ■ Patients who have additional risk factors should be referred to an ophthalmologist on a more frequent basis. These risk factors include:
  - • Family history
  - • Diabetes
  - • Myopia
  - • History of ocular trauma
  - • History of arterial disease
  - • Previous use of glaucoma medications
- ■ Patients with symptoms of glaucoma should be referred immediately to an ophthalmologist.

CONSULTATION

→ See "Treatment/Management," above.

→ As needed for prescription(s).

PATIENT EDUCATION

→ Explain the pathophysiology, risk factors, and management plan for glaucoma.

→ Explain to asymptomatic patients the importance of comprehensive eye examinations. (See "Screening" in "Treatment/Management," above, for recommendations.)

→ See "Treatment/Management" for special situations necessitating referral to an ophthalmologist.

→ Emphasize the importance of using ocular medications as prescribed, even if the patient is asymptomatic.

→ Patients using drops need to be educated regarding lacrimal duct occlusion in order to minimize systemic absorption through the nasal mucosa (Richter 2000). Occlude the duct either by using direct pressure while applying drops or by keeping the eyelids closed for 5 minutes after applying drops.

FOLLOW-UP

→ Emphasize the importance of follow-up examinations by the ophthalmologist.

→ Document in progress notes and on problem list.

Lisa L. Lommel, R.N., C., F.N.P., M.S., M.P.H.
Julie Richards, R.N., C., W.H.N.P., F.N.P., M.S., M.S.N.

2-G
Hordeolum and Chalazion

A *hordeolum* is an infection of the glands of the eye, usually caused by *Staphylococcus aureus*. An internal hordeolum creates a large swelling and involves the meibomian glands. The smaller and more external abscess (sty) involves Moll's or Zeis glands. Cellulitis is a complication of this condition.

A chalazion is a common sterile, granulomatous inflammation of a meibomian gland. It is differentiated from a hordeolum by the absence of acute inflammatory signs (Sullivan et al. 1999).

DATABASE

SUBJECTIVE

Hordeolum

→ Symptoms may include:
- Swelling and redness surrounding the abscess
- Possible abscess on the upper or lower conjunctival surface
- Possible abscess on the upper or lower lid margin
- Pain related to the amount of swelling
- Increased tearing
- Foreign body sensation

Chalazion

→ Symptoms may include:
- Nontender, hard mass on the upper or lower lid
- Conjunctiva possibly red and swollen
- Lesion, which, if large enough, may distort vision
- Increased tearing
- Foreign body sensation

→ Symptoms are commonly multiple and recurrent.
→ Severe hordeola and chalazia may cause corneal abrasions, especially if the patient rubs the affected eye.

OBJECTIVE

Hordeolum

→ The patient presents with:

- Red, swollen, acutely tender abscess on the upper or lower lid of the conjunctival surface or lid margin
- External abscesses usually smaller than internal abscesses
- Swelling and redness surrounding the abscess
- Usually a head of pus is present.

Chalazion

→ The patient presents with:
- Hard, nontender swelling of the upper or lower lid
  - May be tender, with abscess formation.
  - Conjunctiva may be red and swollen.

ASSESSMENT

→ Hordeolum
→ Chalazion
→ R/O sebaceous cyst
→ R/O molluscum contagiosum
→ R/O basal cell carcinoma
→ R/O cellulitis
→ R/O meibomian gland carcinoma
→ R/O blepharitis
→ R/O conjunctivitis
→ R/O corneal abrasion

PLAN

DIAGNOSTIC TESTS

→ Consider fluorescein staining to R/O corneal abrasion.

TREATMENT/MANAGEMENT

Hordeolum

→ Clean, warm compresses to the affected eye for 15 minutes QID.
→ Referral to a physician is indicated for incision if resolution does not begin within 48 hours.
→ Referral to a physician is indicated for cellulitis.

Chalazion

→ Referral to an ophthalmologist is indicated for incision and curettage of a large lesion causing vision impairment or for cosmetic reasons.

CONSULTATION

→ Referral to a physician is indicated for a hordeolum that has not resolved after 48 hours.
→ Referral to an ophthalmologist is indicated for a chalazion.
→ As needed for prescription(s).

PATIENT EDUCATION

→ Explain the pathophysiology, transmission, and treatment plan.

→ Advise the patient not to rub, scratch, or touch her eye.
→ Advise the patient to wash her hands well before and after instilling eye ointment.
→ Advise the patient not to re-use or share eye ointment.
→ Advise the patient that ointment may make vision blurry.
→ Advise the patient to apply clean, warm compresses to the affected eye QID.

FOLLOW-UP

→ If hordeolum has not improved after 48 hours of treatment, consider referral to a physician.
→ Recurrent lesions should be referred for biopsy to rule out basal cell or meibomian gland carcinoma.
→ Document in progress notes and on problem list.

Lisa L. Lommel, R.N., C., F.N.P., M.S., M.P.H.
Julie Richards, R.N., C., W.H.N.P., F.N.P., M.S., M.S.N.

2-H

Keratitis

Keratitis is an inflammation of the corneal epithelium and stroma caused by bacteria, viruses, fungi, or amoebas. The most common bacterial pathogens that invade the cornea are *Pseudomonas aeruginosa, Staphylococcus aureus, Streptococcus epidermidis, Streptococcus pneumoniae, Streptococcus pyogenes, Enterobacteriaceae,* and *Listeria.* Herpes simplex and Herpes zoster are major causes of viral keratitis. *Acanthamoeba* is a common cause of amebic keratitis, especially among contact lens wearers (*Sanford Guide to Antimicrobial Therapy* 2001).

Corneal ulcers may occur as a result of corneal infection, though there are several noninfectious causes. Because ineffective treatment of corneal ulcers and corneal infections may lead to corneal scarring and permanent vision loss, immediate referral of the patient with these conditions to an ophthalmologist is essential.

DATABASE

SUBJECTIVE

→ Symptoms include pain, photophobia, red eye, tearing, reduced vision, and conjunctival discharge.
→ If a corneal ulcer is present, the patient may have the sensation of something in the eye as a result of the lid moving over the corneal defect.

Bacterial

→ Precipitating factors may include:
  ▪ Contact lenses, especially extended wear
  ▪ Corneal trauma
  ▪ Contaminated medications or fluorescein solution
  ▪ Adjacent ocular infection—chronic bacterial conjunctivitis or dacryocystitis
  ▪ Disorders that reduce the natural antimicrobial barrier— severe dry eye, inadequate eyelid closure, severe allergic eye disease, or loss of corneal sensation

Viral

→ Herpes simplex is characterized by:
  ▪ Recurrences precipitated by stress, fever, sunlight

exposure, or menstruation. (See the **Genital Herpes Simplex Virus** chapter in Section 13.)
  ▪ A vesicular rash that becomes pustular, then crusts
→ Herpes zoster is characterized by:
  ▪ Malaise, fever, headache, burning, or itching in periorbital region
  ▪ A vesicular rash that becomes pustular, then crusts
  ▪ Ocular symptoms include conjunctivitis, anterior uveitis, and episcleritis. (See the **Conjunctivitis** and **Uveitis** chapters and the **Varicella Zoster Virus** chapter in Section 11.)

Fungal

→ Precipitating factors may include:
  ▪ Corneal injury from plant material or an agricultural setting
  ▪ Immunocompromised individuals

Amebic

→ Precipitating factors may include:
  ▪ Contact lenses
  ▪ Homemade saline solutions (for cleaning contact lenses)
→ Eye pain may be severe.

OBJECTIVE

→ The patient may present with:
  ▪ Red eye with circumcorneal injection
  ▪ Purulent or watery discharge
→ A corneal ulcer may present as a gray, necrotic area or punctate lesions that stain strongly with fluorescein dye.
→ If there is a history of trauma, the eye should be examined for the presence of a foreign body.

Bacterial

→ The patient may present with:
  ▪ A cornea hazy with a central ulcer and an adjacent stromal abscess

■ Pus in the anterior chamber in front of the iris and behind the cornea (hypopyon)

Viral

→ The patient may present with:
  ■ Herpes simplex characterized by:
    • A dendritic (branching) ulcer
    • "Geographic" ulcers if a topical steroid is used
    • A tender, preauricular node
  ■ Herpes zoster is characterized by:
    • Ocular signs such as conjunctivitis, anterior uveitis, or episcleritis. (See the **Conjunctivitis** and **Uveitis** chapters and the **Varicella Zoster Virus** chapter in Section 11.)

Fungal

→ The patient may present with multiple stromal abscesses.

Amebic

→ The patient may present with perineural and ring infiltrates in the corneal stroma.
→ Earlier changes confined to the corneal epithelium may be present.

ASSESSMENT

→ Keratitis:
  ■ R/O bacterial
  ■ R/O viral
  ■ R/O fungal
  ■ R/O amebic
  ■ R/O corneal ulcer

PLAN

DIAGNOSTIC TESTS

→ Visual acuity should be measured.
→ Slit-lamp examination may be performed with fluorescein staining, though this test is usually reserved for the ophthalmologist.
→ Further testing and cultures should be completed by an ophthalmologist.

TREATMENT/MANAGEMENT

→ Immediate referral to an ophthalmologist is indicated.

CONSULTATION

→ Immediate referral to an ophthalmologist is indicated in all cases of corneal infection or ulcer.
→ As needed for prescription(s).

PATIENT EDUCATION

→ Teach the patient about the pathophysiology of, and risk factors and management plan for, keratitis.
→ Advise the patient that a delay in or inadequate treatment of keratitis could lead to permanent vision loss.
→ Advise the patient to follow the treatment plan from the ophthalmologist carefully.
→ Advise patients with herpes simplex:
  ■ To avoid steroid medication that may increase viral activity.
  ■ That recurrences are common and to avoid activities that may precipitate a herpes outbreak.
→ See the **Genital Herpes Simplex Virus** chapter in Section 13 and the **Varicella Zoster Virus** chapter in Section 11.

FOLLOW-UP

→ Document in progress notes and on problem list.

Lisa L. Lommel, R.N., C., F.N.P., M.S., M.P.H.
Julie Richards, R.N., C., W.H.N.P., F.N.P., M.S., M.S.N.

2-1

Pinguecula and Pterygium

Pinguecula is an elevated nodule on either side of the cornea at the limbus. The nodules consist of hyaline and yellow elastic tissue, and are more common on the nasal side.

Pterygium is the encroachment of a pinguecula onto the cornea. It is a triangular, vascularized, hyperplastic process that usually occurs medially. Predisposing factors to pterygium include chronic exposure to ultraviolet radiation, wind, and dust (Schwab et al. 1999).

DATABASE
SUBJECTIVE

Pinguecula
→ The patient is usually asymptomatic.
  ■ May present with signs of inflammation: redness, tearing, and tenderness.
→ The nodule rarely increases in size.

Pterygium
→ The patient is usually asymptomatic.
  ■ She may notice a visual disturbance if a nodule is encroaching on the pupillary area.

OBJECTIVE

Pinguecula
→ The patient presents with:
  ■ A yellow, elevated nodule on either side of the cornea
  ■ Redness and tenderness

Pterygium
→ The patient presents with a pale yellow, pink, or white triangular, thin nodule on the nasal side of the cornea.
→ A recent or progressive lesion may be thick and vascular.

ASSESSMENT

→ Pinguecula
→ Pterygium

→ R/O corneal ulceration
→ R/O keratitis

PLAN
DIAGNOSTIC TESTS
→ Corneal staining to exclude ulceration may be indicated.

TREATMENT/MANAGEMENT

Pinguecula
→ Benign, doesn't require treatment.
→ In certain cases, weak topical steroids (e.g., prednisolone 0.12%) or topical anti-inflammatory medications may be given (Schwab et al. 1999). *Only ophthalmologists should prescribe ocular steroids.*
→ Excision may be desired for cosmetic purposes.

Pterygium
→ Usually doesn't require treatment.
→ A brief course of artificial tears or a topical anti-inflammatory medication may decrease symptoms (Hoffman et al. 1999).
→ Excision may be indicated if it is interfering with vision.

CONSULTATION
→ Refer the patient to an ophthalmologist for excision of a pinguecula or pterygium.

PATIENT EDUCATION
→ Explain the pathophysiology and treatment plan.
→ Explain that discomfort usually follows excision of a pterygium.
→ Advise individuals who spend lots of time outdoors to wear protective glasses and a hat.

FOLLOW-UP
→ Advise the patient that recurrence is common after a pterygium excision.
→ Document in progress notes and on problem list.

Lisa L. Lommel, R.N., C., F.N.P., M.S., M.P.H.
Julie Richards, R.N., C., W.H.N.P., F.N.P., M.S., M.S.N.

2-J

Uveitis

Uveitis is inflammation of the uveal tract, which includes the iris, ciliary body, and choroid. Uveitis occurs as *anterior* and *posterior uveitis*. The patient may also experience *panuveitis*, which includes inflammation in both areas. *Endophthalmitis* refers to a special, severe form of posterior uveitis centered within the vitreous (Kim 1997).

Anterior uveitis involves inflammation of the iris (*iritis*) or inflammation of the iris and ciliary body (*iridocyclitis*). This condition is divided into *granulomatous* or *nongranulomatous uveitis* depending on the type of keratotic precipitate seen on examination. Anterior uveitis due to a traumatic etiology, which is commonly acute, can be caused by direct, penetrating trauma to the eye (Steinert 2000a). Nontraumatic anterior uveitis can be acute, subacute, or chronic. In most patients with anterior uveitis, there is no identifiable cause.

Anterior uveitis is associated with a variety of systemic diseases, including juvenile rheumatoid arthritis, ankylosing spondylitis, psoriatic arthritis, Reiter's syndrome, Behçet's syndrome, inflammatory bowel disease, sarcoidosis, and a variety of infections, among them herpes simplex, herpes zoster, Lyme disease, syphilis, and tuberculosis (Kim 1997).

Posterior uveitis involves inflammation of the vitreous, retina, and/or choroid. Like anterior uveitis, there is often no identifiable cause. The most common cause of posterior uveitis is toxoplasmosis. There are several other systemic conditions that have been associated with posterior uveitis. These include tuberculosis, toxocariasis, ocular candidiasis, polyarteritis nodosa, herpes zoster, sarcoidosis, histoplasmosis, syphilis, Behçet's syndrome, and Vogt-Koyanagi-Harada syndrome (Kim 1997).

Complications of uveitis include glaucoma, cataracts, pupillary abnormalities, and macular dysfunction (Leibowitz 2000).

DATABASE

SUBJECTIVE

→ Patients may have signs and symptoms of uveitis either as the presenting manifestation of a systemic disease, as outlined above, or as part of a constellation of symptoms.

- If a patient presents with uveitis, consultation should be sought for evaluation of systemic disease.
→ See specific chapters as they relate to associated systemic diseases as outlined above.
→ Anterior uveitis due to trauma presents with:
  - History of trauma
  - Acute onset of pain localized to periorbital area
  - Decreased vision
→ Nontraumatic anterior uveitis may present with (George 2001):
  - Eye pain
  - Photophobia
  - Decreased vision
  - Redness
→ Posterior uveitis most often presents with blurring and/or a loss of vision.

OBJECTIVE

→ Patients may have signs and symptoms of uveitis either as the presenting manifestation of a systemic disease, as outlined above, or as a part of a constellation of symptoms. If a patient presents with uveitis, consultation should be sought for evaluation of systemic disease.
→ See specific chapters as they relate to associated systemic diseases as outlined above.
→ Traumatic anterior uveitis presents with tenderness and redness of the conjunctivae, perilimbal area, and surrounding tissues.
→ Nontraumatic anterior uveitis may present with (George 2001):
  - Red eye (typically circumcorneal)
  - Cloudy anterior chamber upon slit-lamp examination
  - Inflammatory cells (the hallmark of iritis) suspended in aqueous humor, visible with magnification
  - Flare, due to extra protein in the aqueous
  - Hypopyon. If present, it is usually highly suggestive of human leukocyte antigen B27 (HLA-B27) associated

disease (ankylosing spondylitis, Reiter's syndrome, inflammatory bowel disease, and psoriasis), Behçet's syndrome, or, less commonly, iritis due to an infection.

- White blood cells on corneal endothelium (i.e., keratic precipitates) with smaller iris nodules (nongranulomatous disease)
- Larger keratic precipitates known as "mutton fat" with larger iris nodules (granulomatous disease)

→ Posterior uveitis may present with:
- A white eye usually (not red)
- Optic-disc swelling
- Inflammatory cells in the vitreous seen on slit-lamp examination
- Retinal and choroid hemorrhages, exudates, infiltrates, and vascular sheathing

ASSESSMENT

→ Uveitis, anterior and/or posterior:
- R/O trauma
- R/O conjunctivitis
- R/O episcleritis
- R/O systemic disease
- R/O glaucoma
- R/O keratitis
- R/O scleritis
- R/O intraocular malignancy

PLAN

DIAGNOSTIC TESTS

→ The diagnosis is usually made on clinical grounds by an ophthalmologist.

→ Slit-lamp examination may be helpful to evaluate the extent of disease.
→ An initial work-up to rule out concomitant disease (after stabilization by an ophthalmologist) may include:
- Spine, chest, skull, and sinus x-rays
- CBC
- ESR
- PPD with anergy panel
- Lyme titer
- RPR and FTA-ABS
- RF and ANA
- HLA-B27 typing
→ A variety of diagnostic tests may be indicated to rule out concomitant systemic disease.

TREATMENT/MANAGEMENT

→ Immediate referral to an ophthalmologist is warranted in all cases of uveitis.

CONSULTATION

→ Consultation is warranted to rule out concomitant disease. See the introductory discussion for specific diseases.
→ Immediate referral to an ophthalmologist is warranted in all cases of uveitis.

PATIENT EDUCATION

→ Explain the pathophysiology and treatment of uveitis.
→ Explain the pathophysiology of concomitant, systemic disease as indicated.

FOLLOW-UP

→ Document in progress notes and on problem list.

Lisa L. Lommel, R.N., C., F.N.P., M.S., M.P.H.
Julie Richards, R.N., C., W.H.N.P., F.N.P., M.S., M.S.N.

2-K
Bibliography

BIBLIOGRAPHY

Asbury, T., and Sanitato, J. 1999. Ocular and orbital trauma. In *General ophthalmology*, eds. D. Vaughan, T. Asbury, and P. Riordan-Eva, pp. 347–354. Stamford, Conn.: Appleton & Lange.

Harper, R.A., and Shock, J.P. 1999. Lens. In *General ophthalmology*, eds. D. Vaughan, T. Asbury, and P. Riordan-Eva, pp. 159–166. Stamford, Conn.: Appleton & Lange.

Hoffman, R.S., and Power, W.J. 1999. Current options in pterygium management. *International Ophthalmology Clinics* 39(1):15–26.

George, R.K. 2001. Uveitis, anterior, nongranulomatous. *eMedicine Journal* 2(5):1–11.

Kim, T. 1997. Uveitis. In *Ophthalmology for the primary care physician*, eds. D.A. Palay and J.H. Krachmer, pp. 94–101. St. Louis, Mo.: Mosby.

Leibowitz, H.M. 2000. The red eye. *New England Journal of Medicine* 343(5):345–351.

McCulley, J.P., and Shine, W.E. 2000. Changing concepts in the diagnosis and management of blepharitis. *Cornea* 19(5):650–658.

Nurse practitioners' prescribing reference. 2002. Ed. J. Murphy, pp. 124, 128–130. New York: Prescribing Reference.

Plewig, G., and Jansen, T. 1999. Seborrheic dermatitis. In *Dermatology in general medicine*, eds. I.M. Freedburg, A.Z. Eisen, K. Wolff et al., pp. 1482–1489. New York: McGraw-Hill.

Richter, C.U., 2000. Management of glaucoma. In *Primary care medicine*, eds. A.H. Goroll and A.G. Mulley, pp. 1096–1098. Philadelphia: J.B. Lippincott.

Sanford guide to antimicrobial therapy. 2001. Eds. D.N. Gilbert, R.C. Moellering, and M.A. Sande, pp 8–9. Hyde Park, Vt.: Jeb C. Sanford.

Schwab, I.R., and Crawford, J.B. 1999. Conjunctiva. In *General ophthalmology*, eds. D. Vaughan, T. Asbury, and P. Riordan-Eva, pp. 92–118. Stamford, Conn.: Appleton & Lange.

Shields, S.R. 2000. Managing eye disease in primary care. Part 2. How to recognize and treat common eye problems. *Postgraduate Medicine* 108(5):83–86, 91–96.

Steinert, R.F. 2000a. Evaluation of the red eye. In *Primary care medicine*, eds. A.H. Gololl and A.G. Mulley, pp. 1076–1081. Philadelphia: J.B. Lippincott.

_____. 2000b. Management of cataracts. In *Primary care medicine*, eds. A.H. Gololl and A.G. Mulley, pp.1098–1100. Philadelphia: J.B. Lippincott.

Sullivan, J.H. , Crawford, J.B., and Whitcher, J.P. 1999. Lids, lacrimal apparatus, and tears. In *General ophthalmology*, eds. D. Vaughan, T. Asbury, and P. Riordan-Eva, pp. 74–91. Stamford, Conn.: Appleton & Lange.

Taylor, A. 2000. Nutritional influences on risk for cataract. *International Ophthalmology Clinics* 40(4):17–49.

Thompson, C.J. 2001. Review of the diagnosis and management of acquired nasolacrimal duct obstruction. *Clinical Care* 72(2):103–111.

Vaughan, D., and Riordan-Eva, P. 1999. Glaucoma. In *General ophthalmology*, eds. D. Vaughan, T. Asbury, and P. Riordan-Eva, pp. 200–215. Stamford, Conn.: Appleton & Lange.

SECTION 3

Dermatological Disorders

3-A Acne Rosacea 3-2
3-B Acne Vulgaris. 3-5
3-C Atopic Dermatitis (Atopic Eczema) 3-8
3-D Burns—Minor 3-11
3-E Cellulitis 3-14
3-F Contact Dermatitis (Contact Eczema): Irritant and Allergic 3-16
3-G Dyshidrotic Eczema (Pompholyx) 3-19
3-H Folliculitis 3-21
3-I Fungal Infections 3-24
    → Tinea Versicolor (Pityriasis Versicolor). 3-24
    → Tinea Corporis (Body Ringworm). 3-25
    → Tinea Capitis (Scalp Ringworm). 3-26
    → Tinea Pedis (Athlete's Foot) 3-27
    → Tinea Cruris (Eczema Marginatum) 3-29
    → Candidiasis (Moniliasis) 3-30
3-J Furuncles and Carbuncles. 3-32
3-K Impetigo 3-34
3-L Molluscum Contagiosum. 3-36
3-M Paronychia 3-38
3-N Pediculosis 3-40
3-O Pityriasis Rosea 3-43
3-P Psoriasis 3-45
3-Q Scabies. 3-48
3-R Seborrheic Dermatitis 3-51
3-S Warts 3-53

3-A

Acne Rosacea

Acne rosacea is a chronic inflammatory disorder of the skin on the face that is characterized by erythema, papules, pustules, and edema of the cheeks, forehead, nose, and chin (Hirsch et al. 2000, Zuber 2000). Ocular involvement can occur and result in conjunctivitis, blepharitis, and corneal abrasions (Fitzpatrick et al. 2001, Zuber 2000). It is estimated that 13 million persons in the United States have this condition. It usually affects fair-skinned persons 30–50 years old with a peak incidence between 40–50 years. Women have a higher incidence than men (Fitzpatrick et al. 2001). However, men who are affected generally have a more severe form of this condition that may include multiple facial nodules and rhinophyma (a bulbous, irregularly swollen nose with prominent pilosebaceous, dilated pores and telangiectasia) (Aloi et al. 2000, Hirsch et al. 2000). Persons affected by this condition often report a sense of low self-esteem, diminished pleasure, and frustration and perceive that their professional and social lives are negatively impacted due to acne rosacea (National Rosacea Society 1996, Zuber 2000).

The etiology of acne rosacea is unknown. There have been some reports linking this condition to *Helicobacter pylori* and *Demodex folliculorum*, a tiny mite that can be found in human hair follicles. However, other reports have not confirmed these associations (Fitzpatrick et al. 2001, Zuber 2000). Other investigations have tried to demonstrate a causal relationship between acne rosacea and immunologic, endocrine, psychologic, pharmacologic, thermal, and alimentary factors. However, none has clearly demonstrated a definite relationship. Precipitating factors include sun and wind exposure, extremes in temperature (e.g., hot or cold weather, hot baths, ingesting hot drinks, etc.), alcohol consumption, stress, exercise, and skin care products and cosmetics (Zuber 2000). Although alcohol consumption can precipitate an exacerbation, it is not a causative factor of this condition (Fitzpatrick et al. 2001). Generally, acne rosacea is considered to be a vascular disorder of the skin that occurs de novo.

Acne rosacea is recognized to have four stages that progress from mild to very severe. *Prerosacea* is characterized by episodic flushing or blushing of the skin that is often a result of irritation from cosmetics or skin cleansers. Stage I manifests as pro-

longed erythema of the skin for several hours or days, and the development of telangiectasis on the glabella, cheeks, nasolabial folds, and nose. Stage II develops when papules and tiny pustules occur in addition to the facial erythema and telangiectasis. The final stage (Stage III) is associated with the most severe manifestations, including persistent erythema, inflammatory nodules, furuncles, tissue hyperplasia, and, rarely, persistent edema of the central part of the face (Fitzpatrick et al. 2001, Zuber 2000). Spontaneous resolution of the disease occurs after a few years. However, patients with rhinophyma may require laser surgery to treat this complication if systemic therapy is not successful (Fitzpatrick et al. 2001, Zuber 2000).

DATABASE

SUBJECTIVE

The patient may report the following symptoms depending on the stage of acne rosacea (Fitzpatrick et al. 2001, Zuber 2000):
→ Prerosacea:
- Family history of acne rosacea
- Episodes of facial flushing or blushing in response to exposure to facial cleansers or cosmetics
→ Stage I:
- Flushing or blushing of the face in response to facial cleansers, cosmetics, sun exposure, extreme temperatures, ingestion of alcohol or spicy foods, exercise, or stress
- Thin, red vascular lines (telangiectases) on the glabella, cheeks, nose, chin, and eyelids
- Redness of conjunctiva or eyelids; sense of irritated eyes (similar to sense of foreign body or "dry" eyes)
- Symptoms last from several hours to several days
→ Stage II:
- Similar symptoms as noted in Stage I
- Small acne-like lesions with or without pus in the central areas of the face
- Duration of symptoms is several days to weeks or months
→ Stage III:
- Similar symptoms as noted in Stages I and II
- Large, red nodules and pustules

- Increased size and density of telangiectases
- May report edema of the central area of the face with disfigurement of the nose, eyelids, forehead, ears, and chin

OBJECTIVE

The patient will have the following clinical manifestations depending on the stage of acne rosacea (Fitzpatrick et al. 2001, Zuber 2000):

→ Vital signs will be within normal limits (WNL).
→ Prerosacea:
- Erythema of glabella, cheeks, nasolabial folds, nose, and chin
→ Stage I:
- Erythema of glabella, eyelids and eyelash areas, cheeks, nasolabial folds, nose, and chin
- Telangiectases in areas listed above
- Redness of conjunctiva
→ Stage II:
- Similar clinical manifestations as noted in Stage I
- Scattered, discrete, small (2–3 mm) papular lesions, some with very small (<1 mm) pustular apices
- Small nodules may be present.
- Lesions are characteristically in a symmetric distribution and rarely involve the scalp, neck, chest, or back.
→ Stage III:
- Similar clinical manifestations as noted in Stages I and II
- Dense areas of telangiectases
- Large nodules and furuncles
- May have edema of forehead, eyelids, nose, chin, and ears
- May have hyperplasia of the nose, forehead, eyelids, chin, or ears

ASSESSMENT

→ Acne rosacea
→ R/O acne vulgaris
→ R/O bacterial infection
→ R/O seborrheic dermatitis
→ R/O contact dermatitis
→ R/O prolonged use of topical steroids
→ R/O systemic lupus erythematosus

PLAN

DIAGNOSTIC TESTS

→ There are no specific tests to confirm the diagnosis of acne rosacea. However, the following tests may be ordered to eliminate other conditions:
- Culture of pustular lesion for bacterial or fungal organisms may reveal *D. folliculorum.*
- Skin biopsy may reveal the following depending on the patient's stage (Fitzpatrick et al. 2001):
  - Stage I: nonspecific perifollicular inflammatory infiltrates, epithelioid cells, giant cells and granulomas without caseation, lymphocytes, dilated capillaries with surrounding inflammatory infiltration
  - Stage II: neutrophils within the follicles

- Stage III: sebaceous gland hyperplasia; diffuse hypertrophy of the connective tissue; foreign-body giant cells; epithelioid granuloma without caseation
- Serology test for *H. pylori* may be positive.

TREATMENT/MANAGEMENT

→ Treatment of acne rosacea, especially prerosacea and Stage I, should involve the avoidance of aggravating factors. The use of topical steroid preparations should be avoided in most instances, as this may result in skin atrophy.
→ Once inflammatory lesions are noted, the use of systemic and topical antibiotics is indicated. Some authors recommend that topical agents be used initially for the treatment of mild disease. Of the following topical agents that are recommended, metronidazole has been shown to be the most effective (Fitzpatrick et al. 2001, Hirsch et al. 2000, Zuber 2000):
- Metronidazole cream 0.75% applied to affected areas BID
- Metronidazole cream 1% applied to affected areas QD
- Azelaic acid cream 20% applied to affected areas BID
- Sodium sulfacetamide 10% and sulfur 5% lotion applied to affected areas BID

NOTE: Therapy should continue for several weeks after the clinical manifestations resolve.
→ Systemic antibiotics are necessary for patients who have moderate to severe disease. If a patient is in need of systemic therapy, this should be started in conjunction with topical therapy. A reduction in the systemic antibiotic dose should take place when the papules and pustules significantly improve or clear (usually 3 weeks). Therapy should continue at a maintenance dose for 8 weeks (Hirsch et al. 2000). The following systemic antibiotics are recommended (Fitzpatrick et al. 2001, Hirsch et al. 2000):
- Tetracycline 1.0–1.5 g p.o. QD in divided doses. The maintenance dose is 250–500 mg p.o. QD.
- Minocycline 50–100 mg p.o. BID. The maintenance dose is 50–100 mg p.o. QD.

NOTE: A full course of systemic antibiotics is initiated when there is a recurrence of acne rosacea.
→ Patients with a severe form of this condition may require treatment with oral isotretinoin at 0.5–1.0 mg/kg/day for up to 8 months (Fitzpatrick et al. 2001, Hirsch et al. 2000). Usually patients are started on the lower dose because the increased vascularity of the rosacea may deliver more of the medication to the skin (Zuber 2000).

NOTE: This medication is contraindicated for use in pregnant women due to the risk of teratogenic effects. In premenopausal and perimenopausal women, a pregnancy test should be performed prior to initiating this treatment. Women of reproductive potential who are prescribed isotretinoin should use an effective birth control method. Any woman with reproductive potential who completes a course of this medication should avoid pregnancy until 6 months after discontinuing it.
→ Laser surgery may be required for patients with evidence of disfigurement due to this condition.

→ Patients experiencing psychosocial symptoms should be referred for appropriate counseling.

CONSULTATION

→ Physician consultation is recommended for patients with Stage II or III, or for those who may be experiencing side effects from therapy.
→ Patients with ocular involvement should have an evaluation by an ophthalmologist. Blindness, although rare, can occur as a result of acne rosacea (Zuber 2000).

PATIENT EDUCATION

→ Educate the patient about acne rosacea, including its cause, clinical course, treatment, possible side effects of treatment, and follow-up.
→ Advise the patient that the treatment for this condition requires several weeks to months of medication, and that it may recur. Patients should also be advised that this condition usually spontaneously resolves after a few years.
→ Reassure patients with facial disfigurement that laser surgery usually results in substantial improvement, especially in patients with moderate disease (Hirsch et al. 2000).
→ Educate the patient about ways to reduce the possibility of exacerbations through the avoidance of trigger factors (e.g., stress, exposure to temperature extremes, ingestion of spicy foods and alcohol, etc.).

→ Educate the patient about resources available for psychosocial support:
The National Rosacea Society
800 South Northwest Highway, Suite 200
Barrington, Ill. 60010
(888) NO-BLUSH
www.rosacea.org

FOLLOW-UP

→ Individualized according to case presentation.
→ See "Treatment/Management" and "Consultation."
→ Document in progress notes and on problem list.

BIBLIOGRAPHY

Aloi, F., Tomasini, C., Soro, E. et al. 2000. The clinicopathologic spectrum of rhinophyma. *Journal of the American Academy of Dermatology* 43(3):468–472.

Fitzpatrick, T.B., Johnson, R.A., Wolff, K. et al. 2001. *Color atlas and synopsis of clinical dermatology. Common and serious diseases*, 4th ed., pp. 8–10. New York: McGraw-Hill.

Hirsch, R.J., and Weinberg, J.M. 2000. Rosacea 2000. *Cutis* 66:125–128.

National Rosacea Society. 1996. *Coping with rosacea. Tips on lifestyle management for rosacea sufferers*. Barrington, Ill.: National Rosacea Society.

Zuber, T.J. 2000. Rosacea. *Primary Care* 27(2):309–318.

Maureen T. Shannon, C.N.M., F.N.P., M.S.

3-B

Acne Vulgaris

Acne vulgaris (acne) is the most common dermatologic disorder in the United States, affecting approximately 80% of individuals. Although it usually begins during puberty, the onset may not occur until the third or fourth decade of a person's life (Federman et al. 2000). The actual etiology of acne is unknown, but a genetic predisposition to the effects of androgens is a proposed theory. The pathophysiology of acne vulgaris is multifactorial and involves an interaction of sebum, androgens, pilosebaceous follicles, and *Propionibacterium acnes*, an anaerobic, Grampositive diptheroid bacterium (Federman et al. 2000, Johnson et al. 2000).

The inflammatory process occurs when sebum production by the sebaceous glands increases under the influence of androgens. The interaction of the sebum with fatty acids and *P. acnes* results in a sterile inflammatory response in the pilosebaceous unit (Federman et al. 2000). The collection of this material within the sebaceous glands eventually obstructs the follicular duct and results in hyperkeratinization and plugging. The visible skin lesion that occurs is known as a *closed comedone* or *whitehead*. When whiteheads mature and expand, they can provide a portal of entry at the skin that allows oxidation of the comedone, causing a black discoloration. This lesion is commonly called a *blackhead* (or an *open comedone*). If the distended follicular duct wall ruptures into the surrounding dermis, there is an inflammatory foreign body response to the irritating sebum mixture. This process results in papules, pustules, nodules, and suppurative nodules often called *cystic acne*.

Certain factors can aggravate acne, including medications (e.g., androgens, corticosteroids, oral contraceptives, antibiotics), oil-based skin products, emotional stress, and mechanical irritation (e.g., pressure on skin). Although acne is commonly associated with adolescence, if left untreated it may persist for several decades. Eventually, most untreated acne will resolve, but it may lead to scarring, cyst formation, pigment changes, and psychological problems (Berger 2002).

Classifying acne according to its various clinical manifestations helps determine effective therapeutic interventions. The presence of comedones constitutes noninflammatory acne.

Papules, pustules, nodules, or cysts are classified as inflammatory acne (Fitzpatrick et al. 2001).

DATABASE

SUBJECTIVE

The patient with acne vulgaris may report the following (Fitzpatrick et al. 2001):
→ A history of:
  ▪ Use of oily skin products
  ▪ Psychological stress
  ▪ Increased cleansing of affected areas
  ▪ Chronic antibiotic therapy
→ Papular, pustular or nodular lesions of the face, neck, back or trunk
→ Lesions may be mildly painful and pruritic.
→ Lesions may be worse in fall and winter.
→ Exposure to medications that exacerbate acne, including lithium, bromides, antibiotics, iodides, hydantoin, corticosteroids, and oral contraceptives with high androgenic activity
→ Pressure on skin (e.g., leaning on face with hands, chin straps) may aggravate lesions.

OBJECTIVE

The following physical findings may be observed (Fitzpatrick et al. 2001, Johnson et al. 2000):
→ Evidence on the face, neck, back, and/or trunk of the following types of lesions:
  ▪ Noninflammatory acne:
    • Open comedones (blackheads)
    • Closed comedones (whiteheads)
  ▪ Inflammatory acne:
    • Papules are <0.5 centimeters (cm) in diameter with or without erythema or induration.
    • Pustules are superficial.
    • Nodules are 0.5–2 cm in diameter and deep.
    • Nodulocystic scars that may be hypertrophic (keloid) or atrophic and depressed (pitted)

→ Lesions may be isolated, scattered, discrete, or coalescent.
→ Acne caused by corticosteroids usually presents as papulopustular lesions with an absence of comedones.

ASSESSMENT

→ Acne (inflammatory, noninflammatory; mild, moderate, or severe)
→ R/O chronic folliculitis
→ R/O acne rosacea
→ R/O drug eruption
→ R/O contact dermatitis
→ R/O perioral dermatitis
→ R/O adenoma sebaceum (rare)
→ R/O acne fulminans (systemic signs and symptoms, fever, arthralgia, and leukocytosis).
→ R/O polycystic ovary disease

PLAN

DIAGNOSTIC TESTS

→ No specific diagnostic tests are recommended to confirm this condition. However, the following tests may be ordered in severe pustular forms of acne:
  ▪ Gram stain to identify a possible bacterial pathogen
  ▪ Culture and sensitivity of pustular lesion drainage to confirm presence of a pathogen and any resistant strains of organisms

TREATMENT/MANAGEMENT

→ The treatment of acne is based upon the type of acne present and requires several months. Once a good response occurs, treatment should be continued for at least another 3 months.
→ Tapering of medications can begin by decreasing both the dose and strength of agents used.
  NOTE: Variations of drug strengths and dosages appear throughout this chapter. If tapering is to begin, the clinician can refer to the specific therapeutic agents listed in each "Treatment/Management" section.

Anticomedonal (Noninflammatory Lesions)

→ Various topical agents can be used for noninflammatory comedonal acne, including (Federman et al. 2000, Johnson et al. 2000, Krowchuk 2000):
  ▪ Benzoyl peroxide 2–10% gels or solutions applied to lesions QOD or daily for several weeks to months (to years) and increased to BID if needed
    NOTE: Patients can apply benzoyl peroxide to the skin of their forearm and wait 72 hours to see if contact dermatitis develops. If there is no reaction, they can apply this product to acne-affected areas of the face (Krowchuk 2000).
  ▪ Adapalene 0.1% gel or solution applied as described above
  ▪ Azelaic acid 20% is a comedolytic with some effect against *P. acnes*. In individuals with darkly pigmented

skin, this agent may reduce the hyperpigmentation associated with acne.
  ▪ Topical retinoic acid should begin with low-strength 0.025% gel or 0.025% cream QOD at bedtime. After 1 month, increase to every day. Advance to higher concentrations as tolerated (0.01% gel or 0.05–0.1% cream). Use gels for oily skin and creams for dry skin (creams are less irritating). Acne may flare after 2–3 weeks of tretinoin therapy. Resolution should occur within 6–8 weeks.
  ▪ Improvement may not be noticed for 2–5 months.
  ▪ Warn the patient of local irritation and potential photosensitivity. Recommend sunscreen (noncomedogenic, non-oily).
→ Topical therapy with antibacterial agents can have an anti-inflammatory as well as an antimicrobial effect. Agents commonly used to treat acne include (Johnson et al. 2000, Krowchuk 2000):
  ▪ Clindamycin 1% lotion or gel applied to lesions QD–BID for several weeks to months (to years)
  ▪ Erythromycin 2% topical solution applied to lesions QD–BID for several weeks to months (to years)
→ Combining topical therapy by using benzoyl peroxide and an antibiotic may be necessary in some patients. If indicated, the use of one agent during the day and one at night is recommended (Johnson et al. 2000, Krowchuk 2000).

Inflammatory Acne

→ Treatment measures combining the above therapeutic interventions with systemic antibiotic therapy are indicated in moderate to severe inflammatory acne. Oral antibiotics that may be used include one of the following (Cunliffe 2000, Johnson et al. 2000, Krowchuk 2000):
  ▪ Tetracycline 500 mg p.o. BID for 6–8 weeks, then 250 mg p.o. BID maintenance for 2–4 months
  ▪ Erythromycin 500 mg p.o. BID for 6–8 weeks, then 250 mg p.o. BID maintenance for 2–4 months
  ▪ Minocycline 50–100 mg p.o. BID for several weeks to months
  NOTE: Warn the patient about possible side effects of medications (e.g., photosensitivity reactions, vaginal candidiasis) and contraindication for use of tetracycline during pregnancy. Minocycline has rare but significant side effects, including autoimmune hepatitis, hypersensitivity reactions, and serum sickness-like reactions (Krowchuk 2000, Nietsch et al. 2000).
→ Oral contraceptives that contain progestins with low-androgenic activity have been documented to have favorable effects on acne, and can be prescribed provided there are no contraindications for their use (Federman et al. 2000, Krowchuk 2000, Williams 2000).

Severe Inflammatory Acne

→ Refer to a dermatologist for treatment. Isotretinoin may be prescribed by the physician for treatment of severe, recalcitrant, cystic acne.

NOTE: Isotretinoin is teratogenic; a woman should not become pregnant while taking this drug or for several months after discontinuing it.

→ Intralesional injections of corticosteroids, dermabrasion, laser treatments, and chemical peels may also be employed by the physician for the treatment of severe acne (Federman et al. 2000).

CONSULTATION

→ Physician referral for evaluation and treatment of severe acne
→ Physician consultation is indicated in any patient who is being prescribed oral isotretinoin preparations, who experiences adverse reactions to medications, or who has acne unresponsive to appropriate therapeutic interventions.
→ As needed for prescription(s)

PATIENT EDUCATION

→ Educate the patient about acne, including its cause, clinical course, treatment (especially length of treatment), possible side effects of treatment, and follow-up.
→ Advise patients that at least 4–8 weeks of therapy will be required to notice improvement. Encourage them not to abandon any new treatment regimen sooner than one month.
→ Educate the patient to wash the affected area(s) twice a day with a washcloth and noncreamy soap (e.g., Dial®, Neutrogena®).
→ Advise the patient to wait 10–30 minutes after washing to apply tretinoin (less irritation develops if tretinoin is applied to *dry* skin).
→ Advise the patient to avoid moisturizers (e.g., Vaseline®, baby oil, and Oil of Olay®), as these products can aggravate acne. Nutraderm® and Moisturel® lotions can be used for dryness.
→ Advise the patient that makeup should be oil-free and water-based.
→ Advise that picking of comedones and pustules should be avoided.
→ Because tetracycline may increase the skin's sensitivity to sunlight, the dosage may be lowered or the drug discontinued four days prior to travel to a sunny area. In addition, tetracycline should not be taken if a woman is pregnant because it stains fetal teeth after 20 weeks gestation.

→ Some antibiotics (e.g., tetracycline) may decrease the efficacy of oral contraceptives, so an additional form of birth control (e.g., condoms) may be indicated.
→ Advise the patient to watch for black macules at sites of acne lesions, as this may indicate Gram-negative folliculitis.
→ Educate the patient that acne is not aggravated by certain dietary practices (Federman et al. 2000).

FOLLOW-UP

→ Individualized according to case presentation.
→ See "Treatment/Management" and "Consultation."
→ Document in progress notes and on problem list.

BIBLIOGRAPHY

Berger, T.G. 2002. Skin, hair, and nails. In *2002 current medical diagnosis and treatment*, eds. L.M. Tierney, Jr., S.J. McPhee, and M.A. Papadakis, pp. 159–161. New York: Lange Medical Books/McGraw-Hill.

Cunliffe, W.J. 2000. Acne: when, where and how to treat. *Practitioner* 244:865–871.

Federman, D.G., and Kirsner, R.S. 2000. Acne vulgaris: pathogenesis and therapeutic approach. *American Journal of Managed Care* 6(1):78–87.

Fitzpatrick, T.B., Johnson, R.A., Wolff, K. et al. 2001. *Color atlas and synopsis of clinical dermatology. Common and serious diseases.* New York: McGraw-Hill.

Johnson, B.A., and Nunley, J.R. 2000. Use of systemic agents in the treatment of acne vulgaris. *American Family Physician* 62(8):1823–1832.

Krowchuk, D.P. 2000. Managing acne in adolescents. *Pediatric Clinics of North America* 47(4):841–857.

Nietsch, H.H., Libman, B.S., Pansze, T.W. et al. 2000. Minocycline-induced hepatitis. *American Journal of Gastroenterology* 95(10):2993–2994.

Williams, J.K. 2000. Noncontraceptive benefits of oral contraceptive use: an evidence-based approach. *International Journal of Fertility* 45(3):241–247.

3-C

Atopic Dermatitis (Atopic Eczema)

Atopic dermatitis is a chronic or chronically relapsing pruritic inflammation of the epidermis and dermis that affects up to 20% of individuals in the Western world. It usually occurs in patients who have a hereditary predisposition to atopic disease (Fitzpatrick et al. 2001). Other factors contributing to atopic dermatitis include environmental allergens, local infections, and psychosocial stressors (Buske-Kirschbaum et al. 2001, Helmbold et al. 2000).

Atopic dermatitis involves a complex Type I (IgE-mediated) hypersensitivity reaction that results in the release of vasoactive substances by mast cells and basophils in response to an allergen that has interacted with IgE. The actual role of IgE in this interaction is not clearly understood. However, epidermal Langerhans cells have a high affinity for IgE receptors. This association could explain the eczema-like reactions observed in atopic dermatitis patients (Fitzpatrick et al. 2001).

One of the major symptoms of atopic dermatitis is pruritus. The associated scratching is the cause of the characteristic lichenification of the skin, which is pathognomonic of atopic dermatitis (Fitzpatrick et al. 2001). Additional criteria indicating atopic dermatitis rather than other types of dermatitis include: xerosis-ichthyosis-hyperlinear palms, facial pallor, infraorbital darkening, Dennie-Morgan infraorbital fold, *keratosis pilaris* (chronic inflammation of the skin surrounding hair follicles), *pityriasis alba* (scaling and atrophy of skin), elevated serum IgE, a tendency toward recurrent skin infections, and nonspecific hand dermatitis (Fitzpatrick et al. 2001).

DATABASE

SUBJECTIVE

The following symptoms may be reported by the patient (Fitzpatrick et al. 2001, Tofte et al. 2001, Wollenberg et al. 2000):

→ Rough, red patches of skin on her face, neck, upper trunk, and at the bends of the elbows and knees. In adults, the flexural aspects of the extremities are usually involved.
→ Black individuals may report a decreased pigmentation associated with chronic irritation around the wrists and ankles.

→ Severe pruritus may be precipitated by wool, detergents, soaps, and a change in room temperature or stress.
→ Affected individuals will report history of this condition from early childhood (60% of onsets occurs by age 1 year).
→ Family history of atopy (e.g., asthma, allergic rhinitis, atopic dermatitis, nasal polyps).
→ May report a tendency toward cutaneous infections (especially *Staphylococcus aureus* and herpes simplex). These infections may trigger fresh exacerbations of the dermatitis (Leung et al. 2001).

OBJECTIVE

The following clinical manifestations may be observed (Fitzpatrick et al. 2001):

→ Xerosis
→ Facial pallor common
→ Infraorbital folds often present (Dennie-Morgan sign).
→ White *dermatographism* (i.e., with firm stroking of the skin, the area turns white) in 80% of patients
→ Orbital darkening ("allergic shiner") may be present.
→ *Keratoconus* (i.e., cone-shaped cornea) may be present.
→ Lateral eyebrow thinning (Hertoghe sign)
→ Decreased pigment in areas of lichenification may be evident in dark-skinned individuals.
→ Lesions may be present:
  - Erythema, papules, pustules, erosions, dry and wet crusts, fissures, excoriations, lichenified plaques
  - Usually confluent and ill-defined
  - Distribution may be generalized on flexor areas, neck, eyelids, lips, forehead, nipples, and dorsa of feet and hands.
  - Papillomatous lesions (if concurrent human papilloma or molluscum infection)
  - Vesiculoform lesions (if concurrent herpes virus infection)

ASSESSMENT

→ Atopic dermatitis
→ R/O contact dermatitis
→ R/O superimposed bacterial infection
→ R/O gluten-sensitive enteropathy
→ R/O hyper IgE syndrome
→ R/O selective IgA deficiency
→ R/O herpes simplex virus infection
→ R/O asthma

PLAN

DIAGNOSTIC TESTS

→ Laboratory tests are not routinely ordered but may be indicated in some cases (e.g., significant bacterial infection). The following tests may be ordered as indicated (Fitzpatrick et al. 2001):
  ▪ Serum IgE (may be increased)
  ▪ Culture and sensitivity for bacteria and culture for herpes
  ▪ Complete blood count (CBC) (may reveal eosinophilia)

TREATMENT/MANAGEMENT

→ General measures include reducing irritation by (Berger 2002, Fitzpatrick et al. 2001):
  ▪ Bathing with soap, only once a day and only in the axillary region, groin, and feet. Brushes and washcloths should not be used.
  ▪ Use of nondrying soap (e.g., Dove®, Aveeno®, Alpha Keri®, or Basis®)
  ▪ After bathing, patting dry (do not rub) using a soft towel. Application of a thin emollient film of Eucerin®, mineral oil, Nivea®, or Vaseline® on the body (except for the face) is recommended within 3 minutes after bathing.
  ▪ Wearing clothing made of nonirritating fabrics (i.e., avoid wool, acrylics) and fabrics that can breathe (e.g., cotton)
→ Initial treatment (for acute inflammation):
  ▪ Weeping lesions should be treated by applying astringent compresses of Burow's solution or colloidal oatmeal to the lesions for 10–30 minutes BID–QID.
  ▪ High-potency topical steroid lotion or cream (not ointment) should be applied to the lesions after the astringent compress/bath treatment.
  ▪ Recommended fluorinated steroid preparations include:
    • Fluocinonide 0.05% cream—thin coating applied to lesion(s) BID until acute inflammation resolves.
    • Halcinonide 0.1% cream—thin coating applied to lesion(s) BID until acute inflammation resolves.
    NOTE: Avoid use of fluorinated topical steroids on the face.
  ▪ Systemic antihistamines will reduce associated pruritus:
    • Hydroxyzine 10–50 mg p.o. every 6 hours prn
    • Diphenhydramine 25–50 mg p.o. every 6 hours prn
    NOTE: Advise the patient about associated drowsiness and the need to avoid activities that require concentration (e.g., driving).

▪ Secondary bacterial infection can be treated with either local or systemic antimicrobials, depending upon extent and severity of symptoms.
  • Topical treatment:
    – Mupirocin 2% ointment applied to infected lesions TID for 10 days
  • Systemic treatment:
    – Dicloxacillin 250–500 mg p.o. QID for 7–10 days
→ Subsequent therapy (subacute or chronic stages):
  ▪ Continue systemic antihistamines as needed.
  ▪ Compresses are no longer needed but daily colloidal oatmeal baths may promote hydration.
  ▪ Reduce topical corticosteroid agent from high-potency to mid-potency agents in ointment form, such as:
    • Triamcinolone acetonide 0.1% applied BID to affected area(s)
    • Betamethasone dipropionate 0.05% applied BID to affected areas
  ▪ Therapy should continue until pruritus, scaling, and elevated skin lesions resolve. Patients should then begin to taper from BID to daily, then to alternate day use over the next 2–4 weeks to avoid recurrence or tachyphylaxis.

CONSULTATION

→ Physician consultation is indicated for any patient with extensive involvement (as systemic corticosteroids may be needed), resistant episodes, or with severe secondary infection.
→ As needed for prescription(s).

PATIENT EDUCATION

→ Educate the patient about atopic dermatitis, including the cause, clinical course, treatment, possible complications, side effects of medications, and indicated follow-up.
→ Advise the patient to avoid known irritants (e.g., wool and acrylic clothing).
→ Warn the patient about the sedating effects of antihistamines and the need to avoid activities that require concentration (e.g., driving).
→ Advise the patient to avoid rubbing and scratching the affected areas.
→ Advise the patient to trim her nails to avoid excoriation.
→ Advise the patient to use soaps that are nondrying (e.g., Dove®, Aveeno®, or Eucerin®). The patient should only use soap on her axilla, groin, and feet.
→ Advise the patient to avoid frequent baths due to their drying effect on skin. The patient should apply a moisturizing cream within 3 minutes after bathing.
→ Advise the patient to avoid lotions and creams that can exacerbate underlying dry skin conditions.
→ Recommend a cool-air humidifier, which can be especially helpful during the winter.
→ Discuss methods to reduce stress.

FOLLOW-UP

→ Individualized according to case presentation.
→ See "Consultation."
→ Document in progress notes and on problem list.

BIBLIOGRAPHY

Berger, T.G. 2002. Skin, hair, and nails. In *2002 current medical diagnosis and treatment*, eds. L.M. Tierney, Jr., S.J. McPhee, and M.A. Papadakis, pp. 138–140. New York: Lange Medical Books/McGraw-Hill.

Buske-Kirschbaum, A., Geiben, A., and Hellhammer, D. 2001. Psychobiological aspects of atopic dermatitis: an overview. *Psychotherapy and Psychosomatics* 70:6–16.

Fitzpatrick, T.B., Johnson, R.A., Wolff, K. et al. 2001. *Color atlas and synopsis of clinical dermatology. Common and serious diseases*, pp. 30–35. New York: McGraw-Hill.

Helmbold, P., Gaisbauer, G, Kupfer, J. et al. 2000. Longitudinal case analysis in atopic dermatitis. *Acta of Dermatology and Venereology* 80:348–352.

Leung, D.Y.M., and Soter, N.A. 2001. Cellular and immunologic mechanisms in atopic dermatitis. *Journal of the American Academy of Dermatology* 44:S1–S12.

Tofte, S.J., and Hanifin, J.M. 2001. Current management and therapy of atopic dermatitis. *Journal of the American Academy of Dermatology*, S13–S16.

Wollenberg, A., and Bieber, T. 2000. Atopic dermatitis: from the genes to skin lesions. *Allergy 2000* 55:205–213.

3-D

Burns—Minor

Burn injuries occur as a result of exposure to heat. They are classified according to the etiology of the exposure (e.g., thermal, electrical, chemical, or radiation) and by the severity of tissue damage (e.g., first, second, or third degree). In the United States, the incidence and severity of burns has been declining (Cohen et al. 2002). Approximately 2 million burn injuries occur annually, with the majority of these considered to be minor and involving less than 10% of the body (Brandt et al. 2000, Cohen et al. 2002). First- and second-degree thermal burns will be covered in this section.

First-degree burns are the result of damage to the epidermis. The release of histamines, kinins, prostaglandins, and other mediators leading to vasodilation and edema are responsible for the clinical manifestations associated with first-degree burns. A first-degree burn does not blister and has excellent capillary refill; recovery from the injury is usually quick (Pearson et al. 2000).

Second-degree burns result from damage to the epidermis and variable levels of the dermis, with blistering common. The tissue damage correlates with the depth of the burn. Re-epithelialization is dependent upon vascularization of the damaged area(s), with rapid healing and minimal or no scarring in areas with good circulation. Recovery usually takes 1–3 weeks. Deep second-degree burns often require treatment similar to third-degree burns. In addition, secondary bacterial infections may convert a partial-thickness second-degree burn to a full-thickness burn resulting in a longer period of time for recovery (Cohen et al. 2002, Pearson et al. 2000).

When assessing burns, it is essential to determine the amount of body surface affected by the burn as well as the level of skin traumatized. For adults, the *rule of nines* can be used to rapidly assess the extent of the burn. This is done to determine the need for fluid and electrolyte replacement. Generally, this assessment should be done after cleansing of areas that contain soot or other debris that would interfere with the estimate. A score of nine is given to the entire head and neck, each upper and lower extremity, the anterior upper torso, the posterior upper torso, the anterior lower torso, and the posterior lower torso. The perineum is given a score of one. Minor burns are defined as those that involve less than 15% of the total burn surface area in adults up to age 50 or a full-thickness burn of less than 2% in adults of any age (Pearson et al. 2000).

DATABASE

SUBJECTIVE

The patient may report one or more of the following depending on the type of burn (Pearson et al. 2000):
→ Pain is often present.
   NOTE: Absence of pain in a severe burn is more indicative of third-degree burn.
→ Redness at the site of exposure or trauma
→ Blistering at the site of exposure or trauma (if a second-degree burn)
→ History of exposure to sun, heat, flame, chemicals, or hot equipment (e.g., iron, pan)
→ History of taking medication that is associated with phototoxicity (e.g., doxycycline)

OBJECTIVE

The following may be evident depending on the type of burn (Pearson et al. 2000):
→ Vital signs are usually within normal limits, but the pulse rate may be increased if the patient has significant pain or anxiety.

First-Degree Burn

→ Blanches with pressure
→ Erythematous, smooth skin
→ No blisters
→ Tenderness to palpation may or may not be present.

Second-Degree Burn

→ Red, pink, or white thickened skin
→ Presence of single, multiple, or coalescent vesicular lesions

ASSESSMENT

→ First-degree burn
→ Second-degree burn
→ R/O third-degree burn
→ Evaluate percentage of body affected
→ R/O secondary bacterial infection
→ R/O electrical trauma

PLAN

DIAGNOSTIC TESTS

→ No specific diagnostic tests are indicated for the diagnosis or management of uncomplicated minor burns covering ≤10% of the body.

TREATMENT/MANAGEMENT

First- and Second-Degree Burns

→ Immediate management:
- Immediately after the burn has occurred, immerse the area in cool or room-temperature water or saline solution for up to 20 minutes to reduce further damage. Avoid prolonged application of cold water or ice packs to large surfaces (possible causes of hypothermia or arrhythmias).
- Remove clothing in contact with the affected area.
- If melted synthetics, tar, or molten metal are in contact with the area, cool this/these substance(s) as rapidly as possible and do not remove immediately after the injury due to the possibility of increasing tissue damage and depth of injury.

First-Degree Burn

→ Will usually resolve within 7 days after the skin peels and requires minimal treatment.
→ Application of an occlusive dressing that is waterproof and allows visualization of the site may be beneficial in reducing further trauma to the site. If the burn covers a pressure point, then application of a more pliable dressing (e.g., hydrocolloid) may provide additional protection (Pearson et al. 2000).
→ Aspirin, acetaminophen, or nonsteroidal anti-inflammatory drugs (NSAIDs) can be used for analgesia.

Second-Degree Burn

→ Apply a topical antibacterial cream (e.g., 1% silver sulfadiazine) to the area and cover with a sterile dressing TID–QID. **NOTE:** Sulfa preparations are contraindicated in patients who are pregnant, have G6PD deficiency, or a history of hypersensitivity to the particular drug.
→ Prophylactic systemic antibiotics are not usually recommended for uncomplicated minor second-degree burns. However, systemic prophylactic antibiotics for deep or extensive second-degree burns may be indicated. Patients

with these injuries require consultation with a physician or an outpatient burn unit.
→ Administer tetanus/diphtheria (Td) booster to patients who have completed the initial immunization series and whose last Td injection was more than 5 years ago.
→ In patients with unknown tetanus immunization status or incomplete initial immunization series, human tetanus immune globulin (TIG) is indicated for passive immunization. These patients should also receive Td to initiate the active immunization series.
→ Aspirin, acetaminophen, or NSAIDs can be used for analgesia.
→ Deep second-degree burns may require excision and autograft. Refer patients with these injuries to a physician.

CONSULTATION

→ Physician consultation is warranted in patients with any of the following (Pearson et al. 2000):
- Nonminor burns
- More than 5% of her body is affected.
- The injuries involve the face, hands, feet, or perineum.
- Chemical or electrical burns, or burns complicated by inhalation
- Burns suspected to be associated with abuse or trauma
- Circumferential limb burns or burns crossing a major joint
- Partial-thickness or full-thickness burns and diabetes or chronic vascular insufficiency
→ Occupational medical consult is indicated if the burn is work-related.
→ As needed for prescription(s)

PATIENT EDUCATION

→ Instruct the patient how to care for the burn.
→ Discuss the signs of infection and instruct the patient to return for follow-up if infection occurs.
→ Educate the patient about the risks associated with exposure to sources of heat trauma (e.g., overexposure to sun and associated skin cancer or melanoma) and ways to minimize these risks (e.g., by using sun block).
→ If the patient experienced a thermal burn due to accidental exposure (e.g., a cooking accident or accidental spill), educate her about the ways to prevent similar accidents, especially when small children are around.
→ If the burn was work-related, safety training and/or modification of workplace procedures may be necessary.

FOLLOW-UP

→ See "Consultation."
→ For individuals with second-degree burns, follow-up evaluation in 24–48 hours.
→ Document in progress notes and on problem list.

BIBLIOGRAPHY

Brandt, C.P., Coffee, T., Yurko, L. et al. 2000. Triage of minor burn wounds: avoiding the emergency department. *Journal of Burn Care and Rehabilitation* 21:26–28.

Cohen, R., and Moelleken, B.R.W. 2002. Disorders due to physical agents. In *2002 current medical diagnosis and treatment*, 41st ed., eds. L.M. Tierney, Jr., S.J. McPhee, and M.A. Papadakis, pp. 1596–1600. New York: Lange Medical Books/McGraw-Hill.

Pearson, A.S., and Wolford, R.W. 2000. Management of skin trauma. *Primary Care* 27(2):475–492.

3-E
Cellulitis

Cellulitis is a diffuse, spreading infection of the dermis and subcutaneous tissue (Fitzpatrick et al. 2001). It can occur either as a primary condition or as a complication to a pre-existing dermatosis (e.g., tinea pedis, atopic dermatitis, trauma) (Baddour 2000, Rhoudy 2000).

An increased risk of cellulitis is seen among injection drug users, alcoholics, and persons with diabetes mellitus, hematologic malignancies, chronic lymphedema, and immunosuppression. (Baddour 2000, Biswanger et al. 2000). Group A beta-hemolytic streptococci and *Staphylococcus aureus* are the most common etiologic agents. However, other organisms, including Gram-negative rods or anaerobes, may be responsible for cellulitis in diabetics or immunocompromised individuals (Baddour 2000, Rhoudy 2000).

Lymphangitis and lymphadenitis may arise as common manifestations of cellulitis at the site of an infected wound. Lymphatic involvement may progress rapidly and can lead to septicemia and death (Baddour 2000, Rhoudy 2000).

DATABASE

SUBJECTIVE

→ History may include:
- Recent break in the skin (e.g., puncture wound, laceration, abrasion, insect bite, or surgical incision)
- Prior episode of cellulitis
- Injection drug use (IDU) or alcohol abuse
- Immunosuppression
- Diabetes mellitus

→ Symptoms may include (Fitzpatrick et al. 2001):
- Fever
- Chills
- Malaise
- Anorexia
- Tenderness at site of infection
- Red, swollen area with or without purulent discharge
- Warmth at infection site and surrounding tissue

OBJECTIVE

→ Vital signs may include:
- Elevated temperature
- Increased heart rate

→ Patient may present with (Fitzpatrick et al. 2001):
- Diffuse, sharply defined, erythema or plaque-like areas of skin of varying size
- Edema
- Vesicles, bullae, erosions, abscesses, hemorrhage, or necrosis
- Red streaks (toxic striations) from area of cellulitis toward regional lymph node with tender, enlarged lymph node if lymphangitis/lymphadenitis exists
- Break in or trauma to the skin (surgical or nonsurgical)

ASSESSMENT

→ Cellulitis
→ R/O lymphangitis/lymphadenitis
→ R/O superficial/deep-vein thrombophlebitis
→ R/O soft-tissue infection
→ R/O necrotizing fasciitis
→ R/O gangrene
→ R/O contact dermatitis
→ R/O fixed drug eruptions
→ R/O erythema migrans
→ R/O prevesicular herpes zoster
→ R/O erysipelas
→ R/O cat scratch disease
→ R/O IDU
→ R/O underlying disease processes, if indicated (e.g., diabetes)

PLAN

DIAGNOSTIC TESTS

The following tests are not required for diagnosis but may be ordered as indicated (Fitzpatrick et al. 2001):

→ Cultures may identify a specific pathogen, but often specimens for these tests are not obtained unless primary treatment has failed or an atypical microorganism is suspected.

→ Gram stain may demonstrate a Gram-positive or Gram-negative pathogen.

→ Microscopic evaluation of a specimen from skin biopsy after application of potassium hydroxide may reveal hyphae (for fungal pathogens).

→ Erythrocyte sedimentation rate (ESR) may be elevated but is a nonspecific finding.

→ CBC will usually reveal an increased leukocyte count with a shift to the left.

TREATMENT/MANAGEMENT

→ During the febrile stage of illness, the patient should rest, increase fluid intake, and take antipyretic medications (e.g., acetaminophen).

→ Immobilize the affected area(s).

→ Elevate the affected extremity or extremities.

→ Apply moist heat to the affected area(s) for 20–30 minutes BID–TID.

→ The patient may require prescription analgesia to decrease the discomfort depending on the severity or extent of the area involved.

→ Incision and drainage of fluctuant abscesses should be performed. Patients undergoing incision and drainage of abscesses may require local anesthetic and/or prescription analgesics to help with pain relief.

→ For mild early cellulitis, antibiotic therapy with one of the following medications should be initiated (Fitzpatrick et al. 2001):
  ▪ Dicloxacillin 250–500 mg p.o. every 6 hours for 10 days
  ▪ Cephalexin 250–500 mg p.o. every 6 hours for 10 days
  ▪ Clindamycin 150–300 mg p.o. every 6 hours for 10 days
  ▪ Erythromycin 500 mg p.o. every 6 hours for 10 days for penicillin-allergic individuals

→ If there is underlying dermatosis (e.g., tinea pedis), institute appropriate therapy. See appropriate chapters.

→ Patients with moderate to severe symptoms or associated complications should be referred to a physician immediately.
  ▪ Hospitalization may be required.

CONSULTATION

→ Physician consultation is warranted for any patient with systemic or rapidly progressive symptoms, lymphangitis/lymphadenitis, cellulitis of the face, suspected necrotizing cellulitis, history of immune suppression (e.g., HIV infection) or other immunosuppressive medical conditions (e.g., diabetes mellitus, hematologic malignancies), or patients not demonstrating significant improvement after 48 hours of antibiotic therapy.
  ▪ Hospitalization and parenteral therapy may be indicated in some of these circumstances.

→ As needed for prescription(s)

PATIENT EDUCATION

→ Educate the patient regarding the cause of cellulitis, signs/symptoms of complications, and indicated follow-up.

→ If the patient has a history of IDU or alcohol abuse, provide information about available treatment programs. Educate regarding adverse effects of drug use and the need to consider HIV testing.

FOLLOW-UP

→ Have the patient return for a follow-up evaluation in 24–48 hours. If there is no improvement, consult with/refer patient to a physician.

→ Refer patients with IDU or alcohol abuse to appropriate treatment programs and social services.

→ See "Consultation."

→ Document in progress notes and on problem list.

BIBLIOGRAPHY

Baddour, L.M. 2000. Cellulitis syndromes: an update. *International Journal of Antimicrobial Agents* 14:113–116.

Biswanger, I.A., Kral, A.H., Bluthenthal, R.N. et al. 2000. High prevalence of abscesses and cellulitis among community-recruited injection drug users in San Francisco. *Clinical Infectious Diseases* 30:579–581.

Fitzpatrick, T.B., Johnson, R.A., Wolff, K. et al. 2001. *Color atlas and synopsis of clinical dermatology*, pp. 606–613. New York: McGraw-Hill.

Rhoudy, C. 2000. Bacterial infections of the skin. *Primary Care* 27(2):459–473.

3-F

Contact Dermatitis (Contact Eczema): Irritant and Allergic

Contact dermatitis is an acute or chronic inflammation of the epidermis and dermis caused by direct skin contact with irritants. It is characterized by itching, burning, and erythema. The skin manifestations are concentration-dependent reactions to exposure to chemical or physical agents, or allergens. These responses are characterized by itching, burning, and erythema (Fitzpatrick et al. 2001). Most episodes of contact dermatitis are self-limited and resolve in 2–3 weeks unless the individual is re-exposed or experiences a superimposed bacterial or fungal infection.

Eighty percent of contact dermatitis in the United States is due to occupational exposure to a chemical irritant, with the remaining 20% associated with allergens (Lushniak 2000). Common irritants and allergens responsible for contact dermatitis include soaps, detergents, organic solvents, hair dye, topical medications (e.g., antibiotics [especially neomycin], antihistamines, corticosteroids, anesthetics [e.g., benzocaine]), perfumes, certain metals (especially nickel), rubber products, and poison ivy or poison oak. In recent years, latex allergy is increasingly a problem. Individuals at greatest risk for latex allergy include those with spina bifida, health care professionals, and patients who have frequent contact with health care settings (Korniewicz et al. 1995, Lopes et al. 2000).

DATABASE

SUBJECTIVE

The patient may report the following (Berger 2002, Fitzpatrick et al. 2001):
→ History of a similar dermatitis
→ History of work involving exposure to:
- Water, detergents, cleaning products (e.g., cleaning, dishwashing)
- Nickel products (e.g., costume jewelry)
  - Individuals at high risk for development of nickel allergy include:
    - Hairdressers, restaurant workers, nurses, cashiers
    - Workers in metal industries

- Chromates (e.g., cement, leather products tanned with chromates)
- Rubber products (e.g., latex gloves)
- Topical drugs or cosmetics (e.g., lanolin, neomycin, local anesthetics, formaldehyde, and preservatives such as the parabens and benzoisothiozides)
- Perfumes and fragrances
- Epoxy resin
- Pesticides (e.g., agriculture)
- Plants (e.g., poison oak and poison ivy)
→ One or more of the following symptoms:
- Acute:
  - Rash that may be red, papular, blister-like with or without swelling
  - Pruritis or burning sensation (or pain) at site of contact with irritant or allergen
  - Fever in severe cases (e.g., poison ivy)
- Chronic:
  - Reddened, plaque-like areas of skin with scaling

OBJECTIVE

The following physical findings may be evident (Berger 2002, Fitzpatrick et al. 2001):
→ Lesions vary in appearance depending on the stage of response and type of dermatitis (allergic or chemical), with a distribution pattern that may be localized (to the site of contact) or generalized.
NOTE: The site of the reaction will often suggest the cause (e.g., facial involvement may be due to soap or cosmetics; scalp involvement may be due to hair products).
→ Acute inflammation:
- Allergic:
  - Erythema with macules, papules, tiny vesicles, edema, and oozing, crusted lesions
- Chemical:
  - Well-marginated erythema, vesicles, erosions, crusting and scaling

→ Subacute inflammation:
  ▪ Patches of mild erythema with small, dry scales or superficial desquamation
→ Chronic inflammatory reaction:
  ▪ Allergic:
    • Excoriation, scaling, erythema, and lichenification
  ▪ Chemical:
    • Scaling and fissures with poorly defined borders

ASSESSMENT

→ Contact dermatitis (physical, chemical, allergen reaction)
→ R/O secondary bacterial infection
→ R/O atopic dermatitis
→ R/O seborrheic dermatitis
→ R/O psoriasis
→ R/O viral infection (e.g., herpes simplex, herpes zoster)
→ R/O dermatophytosis (fungal infections)
→ R/O nummular eczema
→ R/O dyshidrotic eruptions
→ R/O lichen planus
→ R/O drug eruptions
→ R/O scabies

PLAN

DIAGNOSTIC TESTS

The following tests may be ordered if indicated:
→ Patch testing to identify a specific allergen cannot be done during the acute episode if the individual's back is involved, because a false-positive reaction can result. Patch testing can be done after the contact dermatitis has resolved, though not all potential allergens are available for testing (Elston et al. 2000, Fitzpatrick et al. 2001).
→ Potassium hydroxide 10% (KOH) may reveal the presence of hyphae if there is a coexistent fungal infection.
→ Culture and sensitivity may reveal a bacterial or viral pathogen if primary or secondary infection.

TREATMENT/MANAGEMENT

→ Identify and avoid contact with etiological agents.
  NOTE: Animals and clothing can cause re-exposure to some types of allergens (e.g., poison oak).
→ Avoid scrubbing the lesions with soap and water.
→ Topical therapy usually is effective for most individuals with mild, uncomplicated dermatitis and involves (Berger 2002):
  ▪ Compresses of Burow's solution can be applied to weeping areas for 15–20 minutes TID. The astringent effect of the solution will help dry the lesion(s).
  ▪ Potent topical corticosteroids in a drying vehicle can be used as follows:
    • Fluocinonide gel 0.5% applied to affected areas BID
  ▪ Nonfluorinated topical corticosteroid agents should be used for lesions of the face or intertriginous areas.
    • Hydrocortisone 2.5% cream applied to affected area BID
    • Dexamethasone 0.1% gel applied to affected area BID

→ Systemic corticosteroid therapy is indicated for severe episodes (e.g., significant skin involvement, swelling of the face or genitalia, or large areas of bullae). The course of treatment should be 12–21 days; otherwise, a rebound flaring of symptoms can occur. The following regimen is one example of recommended dosing (Berger 2002, Fitzpatrick et al. 2001):
  ▪ Prednisone 60 mg p.o. QD with a reduction in dose by 5 mg p.o. daily over a 2-week course
                    OR
  ▪ Prednisone 60 mg p.o. for 4–7 days, then 40 mg p.o. for 4–7 days, then 20 mg p.o. for 4–7 days
→ Oral antihistamine therapy may be helpful in relieving pruritus:
  ▪ Diphenhydramine 25–50 mg p.o. every 6 hours prn
  ▪ Hydroxyzine 10–25 mg p.o. every 6 hours prn
  NOTE: Warn the patient about drowsiness associated with these agents and the need to avoid activities that require concentration (e.g., driving).

CONSULTATION

→ Physician consultation is warranted for any patient with severe manifestation (e.g., generalized distribution), evidence of secondary bacterial infection, and/or in cases where systemic corticosteroid therapy is being considered.
→ As needed for prescription(s)

PATIENT EDUCATION

→ Educate the patient about contact dermatitis—the probable cause, clinical course, diagnostic tests, treatment options, possible complications, adverse effects of medications, and indicated follow-up.
→ Advise the patient to avoid additional exposure to known allergens or irritants.
→ Patients using systemic corticosteroids should be educated about the possible side effects, including emotional lability and gastrointestinal upset. See the *Physicians' Desk Reference*.
→ Prevention strategies may include the use of barrier creams (e.g., Stokogard®, Ivy Shield®) to decrease the risk of allergic reaction to plants (e.g., poison ivy or oak), and Iodoquinol cream (Vioform®) for individuals with nickel allergies (Berger 2002).

FOLLOW-UP

→ Individualized according to case presentation
→ See "Consultation."
→ Document in progress notes and on problem list.

BIBLIOGRAPHY

Berger, T.G. 2002. Skin, hair, and nails. In *2002 current medical diagnosis and treatment,* eds. L.M. Tierney, Jr., S.J. McPhee, and M.A. Papadakis, pp. 157–159. New York: Lange Medical Books/McGraw-Hill.

Elston, D., Licata, A., Rudner, E. et al. 2000. Pitfalls in patch testing. *American Journal of Contact Dermatitis* 11(3):184–188.

Fitzpatrick, T.B., Johnson, R.A., Wolff, K. et al. 2001. *Color atlas of clinical dermatology. Common and serious diseases,* pp. 18–23. New York: McGraw-Hill.

Korniewicz, D.M., and Kelly, K.J. 1995. Barrier protection and latex allergy associated with surgical gloves. *Association of Operating Registered Nurses Journal* 61:1037–1044.

Lopes, M.H.B., and Lopes, R.A. 2000. Latex allergy in health care personnel. *Association of Operating Registered Nurses Journal* 72:42–46.

Lushniak, B.D. 2000. Occupational skin diseases. *Primary Care* 27(4):895–915.

3-G
Dyshidrotic Eczema (Pompholyx)

Dyshidrotic eczema (pompholyx) is a chronic, recurrent, self-limited dermatitis of the finger, palms of the hands, and soles of the feet (Lehucher-Michel et al. 2000). It is a very common type of hand dermatitis. Acute episodes are characterized by pruritic, "tapioca-like" vesicular lesions, and secondary infection of the lesions may occur (Fitzpatrick et al. 2001). Spontaneous remission usually takes place 2–3 weeks after development of the initial lesions. However, recurrences can occur several weeks to months later. After the acute episode, fissures, scaling, and lichenification of the involved area are commonly observed (Berger 2002).

Usually, the condition does not occur until a patient's second or third decade of life. Although the name of this condition implies a relationship between the vesicular lesions and eccrine and sweat gland dysfunction, this is not accurate. It has been postulated that this condition may be an allergic or hypersensitivity condition, especially to nickel. Up to 50% of individuals with dyshidrotic eczema have a history of atopic reactions. Exacerbations of the condition are often associated with stressful events (Berger 2002, Fitzpatrick et al. 2001).

DATABASE

SUBJECTIVE

The patient may report the following (Berger 2002, Fitzpatrick et al. 2001):
→ Atopic history
→ Allergy to nickel
→ Symptoms absent prior to the second decade of life
→ Symptoms may include:
  ▪ Pruritus
  ▪ Blister-like eruptions on sides of fingers, palms, and soles of the feet
  ▪ Fissures, scaling after the initial blister-like lesions dry
  ▪ Pain if fissures develop
  ▪ Redness and pustules if secondary infection

OBJECTIVE

→ Vesicles are:
  ▪ Usually about 1–2 mm in diameter
  ▪ Deep-seated
  ▪ May coalesce to form tapioca-like clusters
→ Scaling, lichenification, fissures, and erosions may be present.
→ Lesions usually observed on sides of fingers, palms of the hands, and soles of the feet. Approximately 80% of the affected area is on the hands.
→ Nails may be ridged, pitted, or thickened.
→ Erythema and pustules may be evident if secondary infection.

ASSESSMENT

→ Dyshidrotic eczema (pompholyx)
→ R/O acute contact dermatitis
→ R/O vesicular tinea
→ R/O herpes simplex viral infection
→ R/O bacterial superinfection
→ R/O dermatitis herpetiformis
→ R/O nonsteroidal anti-inflammatory drug reaction

PLAN

DIAGNOSTIC TESTS

→ No specific diagnostic tests are required, as the clinical presentation and history are characteristic of the condition. However, if the patient has a vesicular eruption, the following tests may be ordered if indicated:
  ▪ Potassium hydroxide (KOH) 10% preparation of scraping from a vesicle to rule out the presence of dermatophytosis (i.e., evidence of hyphae would indicate a fungal infection) (Berger 2002).
  ▪ Bacterial culture may reveal a pathogen (e.g., *Staphylococcus aureus*) if coexistent infection (Fitzpatrick et al. 2001).
  ▪ A viral culture may be sent to rule out herpes simplex infection.

TREATMENT/MANAGEMENT

→ Lesions often spontaneously resolve within 2–3 weeks.

→ Vesicular stage (early) treatment may include:

■ Burow's solution compresses applied to affected areas for 15–20 minutes BID–TID to help dry the vesicles

→ Eczematous stage treatment may include:

■ High-potency topical steroids, which are beneficial in treating the scaling and fissuring that occur after the vesicular stage.

• Fluocinonide 0.05% ointment or cream applied to affected areas BID until resolution

• Betamethasone dipropionate 0.05% ointment applied to affected areas BID until resolution

→ Systemic steroid therapy is not indicated because the risks associated with this treatment outweigh the benefits.

→ The patient should avoid contact with any irritating substance(s), use gloves (cotton gloves covered by vinyl gloves) when exposure to water is necessary, and apply hand cream to prevent a recurrence.

→ In patients with a history of nickel allergy along with several recurrences, a nickel-free diet may be necessary. Referral to a nutritionist for proper instruction is indicated.

CONSULTATION

→ Referral to a nutritionist for proper evaluation and instruction regarding a nickel-free diet.

→ As needed for prescription(s)

PATIENT EDUCATION

→ Educate the patient about dyshidrotic eczema (pompholyx)—the possible cause(s), clinical course, treatment, prevention, and indicated follow-up.

→ Reassure the patient that the symptoms will usually resolve in 2–3 weeks.

FOLLOW-UP

→ Individualized according to case presentation

→ See "Consultation."

→ Document in progress notes and on problem list.

BIBLIOGRAPHY

Berger, T.G. 2002. Skin, hair, and nails. In *2002 current medical diagnosis and treatment*, eds. L.M. Tierney, Jr., S J. McPhee, and M.A. Papadakis, pp. 154–155. New York: Lange Medical Books/McGraw-Hill.

Fitzpatrick, T.B., Johnson, R.A., Wolff, K. et al. 2001. *Color atlas of clinical dermatology. Common and serious diseases*, pp. 39–41. New York: McGraw-Hill.

Lehucher-Michel, M.P., Koeppel, M.C., Lanteaume, S. et al. 2000. Dyshidrotic eczema and occupation: a descriptive study. *Contact Dermatitis* 43:200–205.

3-H
Folliculitis

Folliculitis is a superficial inflammation or infection of hair follicles without involvement of the surrounding skin. Typically, this inflammation involves the face, extensor surface of the extremities, and the buttocks, although any skin area can be involved. Bacterial and nonpathogen-associated forms of folliculitis can occur (Berger 2002). *Bacterial folliculitis* is usually caused by penicillin-resistant strains of *Staphylococcus aureus*, although *Pseudomonas aeruginosa* (responsible for "hot-tub" folliculitis) and a range of Gram-negative organisms (more prevalent in individuals taking antibiotics) have also been implicated. Recurrent folliculitis may be a result of chronic nasal carriage of *S. aureus* (Berger 2002).

Nonbacterial folliculitis can result from follicle occlusion by oil or oil-based cosmetics, or by friction and sweating that occur with tight clothing. Chronic, recalcitrant folliculitis of the head and neck is called *sycosis* and is caused by the trauma and autoinoculation associated with shaving (Berger 2002). Folliculitis associated with systemic steroid use *(steroid acne)* usually occurs during the first week of steroid therapy and often resolves as the dose is tapered. In HIV-infected individuals with advanced immunosuppression, a nonbacterial form of folliculitis demonstrating eosinophilic infiltrations is common and may be caused by fungal or parasitic pathogens (Berger 2002).

Systemic antibiotic therapy is usually not required to treat this condition. Local treatment includes cleansing and drying of the affected areas and avoiding irritants (Wilhelm et al. 2001). *Furunculosis* (e.g., abscess formation) is a major complication that can occur. Cavernous sinus thrombosis, although rare, is also a serious, life-threatening complication that may result from folliculitis that involves the upper lip, nose, or eyes (Berger 2002).

DATABASE

SUBJECTIVE

The patient may report the following (Berger 2002, Wilhelm et al. 2001):
→ History of:
- Exposure to tar, mineral oil, oil-based cosmetics, adhesive tape, or plastic occlusive dressing
- Recent hot tub or public pool use (1–4 days prior to symptoms)
- Diabetes mellitus
- HIV infection
- Shaving
- Recent use of systemic antibiotics or topical/systemic steroids
→ Symptoms:
- Red, slightly raised lesions on the face or extremities
- Itching and/or burning that is usually mild
- Itching and burning associated with lesions may be aggravated by shaving and other sorts of friction against the skin (e.g., clothing, scratching).

OBJECTIVE

→ Vital signs may be within normal limits (WNL) or the temperature may be elevated.
→ Patient may present with small, erythematous pustules at the hair follicle(s).
→ Lesions may be isolated, scattered, discrete, or grouped.
→ Scalp and extremities are affected the most, but this condition may also involve the face and neck (sycosis) (Berger 2002).
→ Sycosis lesions often involve the area(s) surrounding the hair follicle; lesions may have crusting in addition to erythema.
→ HIV-associated eosinophilic folliculitis is often associated with urticarial papules. Approximately 90% of the lesions are observed on the patient's head, neck, proximal extremities, and upper back and chest (Sande et al. 2001).

ASSESSMENT

→ Folliculitis
→ R/O acne vulgaris
→ R/O warts
→ R/O molluscum contagiosum
→ R/O tinea corporis
→ R/O impetigo

→ R/O urticaria

→ R/O furunculosis

→ R/O staphylococcal carriage (if frequent recurrences of bacterial folliculitis)

→ R/O diabetes mellitus (if frequent recurrences of bacterial folliculitis)

→ R/O eosinophilic folliculitis (in HIV-infected patients)

PLAN

DIAGNOSTIC TESTS

→ Though diagnostic tests usually are not necessary in uncomplicated, localized episodes of folliculitis, the following tests may be ordered as indicated by history and physical findings (Berger 2002, Wilhelm et al. 2001):

- Gram stain to identify the infecting organism
- Culture and sensitivity on specimen from inflamed follicle for confirmation of the infecting organism and antibiotic susceptibility
- Nasal swab for culture for *S. aureus* in patients suspected of nasal carriage of this bacteria. Results will be positive in patients who are chronic carriers.

TREATMENT/MANAGEMENT

→ General measures (Berger 2002, Wilhelm et al. 2001):

- Avoid friction or irritating the affected area(s).
- Cleanse the affected area(s) with a topical antibacterial solution (e.g., chlorhexidine) BID.
- If exudative, apply saline compresses to the affected areas for 15 minutes BID.
- Make sure that hot tubs, pools, and spas have proper disinfectant (e.g., chlorine).
- Application to the affected area(s) of anhydrous ethyl chloride containing 6.25% aluminum chloride QD–BID will aid in drying the lesions.

→ Bacterial folliculitis (Berger 2002, Wilhelm et al. 2001):

- After cleansing the affected area, localized, uncomplicated folliculitis can be treated with topical antimicrobials:
  - Mupirocin ointment applied to affected area(s) BID for 5 days
- If folliculitis is resistant to topical therapy or there is evidence of severe, extensive involvement, systemic antibiotic therapy should be prescribed using:
  - Dicloxacillin 250–500 mg p.o. QID for 7–10 days
  - Cephalexin 250–500 mg p.o. QID for 7–10 days
- Most hot-tub folliculitis resolves without the need for antibiotic therapy. However, in patients with persistent symptoms, consider systemic antibiotic therapy with:
  - Ciprofloxacin 500 mg p.o. BID for 5 days

→ Irritant folliculitis:

- See "General Measures," above, for instructions about the use of drying agents.
- Avoid irritants.

→ Steroid (culture-negative) folliculitis:

- Usually resolves as the steroid dose is tapered. The use of isotretinoin is recommended for severe cases. See the **Acne Vulgaris** chapter and *Physicians' Desk Reference*. **NOTE:** This medication is teratogenic if use occurs prior to or during pregnancy.

→ Eosinophilic folliculitis (Berger 2002, Sande et al. 2001):

- Severe cases may require treatment with one of the following if it is associated with an opportunistic fungal or parasitic pathogen:
  - Permethrin application every 12 hours every other day for 6 weeks
  - Itraconazole 200–400 mg p.o. QD for 14–21 days
  - Metronidazole 250 mg p.o. TID for 21–28 days
  - Isotretinoin 0.5 mg/kg/day for several weeks up to 5 months

→ In patients with recurrent furunculosis, evaluation and possible concomitant antimicrobial therapy for family members/intimate contacts who are chronic staphylococcal carriers may be indicated. Topical therapy with mupirocin applied to the individual's nares, axillae, and anogenital area BID for 5 days usually resolves the carrier state in otherwise healthy individuals. Eradication may be more difficult in individuals with a chronic illness or immunosuppression. **NOTE:** Mupirocin may be irritating when applied intranasally (Berger 2002).

CONSULTATION

→ Physician consultation is indicated for any patient with recurring episodes of folliculitis for further work-up, for complications associated with folliculitis, or if there is an underlying medical condition such as diabetes mellitus or HIV infection (Berger 2002).

→ As needed for prescription(s)

PATIENT EDUCATION

→ Educate the patient about folliculitis—causes, treatment options, possible complications of the condition, possible side effects of medication, prevention, and indicated follow-up.

→ Instruct the patient to avoid tight-fitting clothing, moisture, and potential irritants that may aggravate the condition. Wearing cotton underwear should be recommended.

→ Patients with hot-tub, spa, or pool folliculitis should be instructed about proper treatment of the water (i.e., with chlorine).

→ Instruct patients about the importance of handwashing to reduce infection(s); demonstrate proper handwashing techniques.

→ Instruct the patient to return if complications develop or if symptoms persist despite therapy.

FOLLOW-UP

→ Individualized according to case presentation

→ See "Consultation" and "Patient Education."

→ Document in progress notes and on problem list.

BIBLIOGRAPHY

Berger, T.G. 2002. Skin, hair, and nails. In *2002 current medical diagnosis and treatment*, eds. L.M. Tierney, Jr., S.J. McPhee, and M.A. Papadakis, pp. 163–164. New York: Lange Medical Books/McGraw-Hill.

Hirschmann, J.V. 2000. Antimicrobial prophylaxis in dermatology. *Seminars in Cutaneous Medicine and Surgery* 19(1):2–9.

Sande, M.A., Gilbert, D.N., and Moellering, R.C., Jr. 2001. *The Sanford guide to HIV/AIDS therapy*, 10th ed. Hyde Park, Vt.: Antimicrobial Therapy.

Wilhelm, M.P., and Edson, R.S. 2001. Skin and soft-tissue infections. In *Current diagnosis and treatment in infectious diseases*, eds. W.R. Wilson and M.A. Sande, pp. 180–183. New York: Lange Medical Books/McGraw-Hill.

3-1

Fungal Infections

Dermatophytes, or parasitic skin fungi, have an affinity for keratin and therefore affect the keratinized tissues of the body: the nails, hair, and stratum corneum of the skin. This chapter covers the common dermatomycoses, or superficial, noninvasive dermatophytosis. Tinea refers to all noninvasive cutaneous mycoses, except those caused by *Candida*, which are called *candidiasis* or *moniliasis*. The following discussion of fungal infections includes: *Tinea versicolor* (pityriasis versicolor), *Tinea corporis* (body ringworm), *Tinea capitis* (scalp ringworm), *Tinea pedis*, *Tinea cruris* (eczema marginatum), and *mucocutaneous candidiasis* (moniliasis)

Tinea Versicolor (Pityriasis Versicolor)

Tinea versicolor is caused by a lipophilic fungus, *Malassezia furfur* (also known as *Pityrosporum orbiculare* and *P. ovale*), which affects the superficial layer of skin. *M. furfur* is normally present in the skin flora, but can proliferate under certain conditions, such as excessive heat, pregnancy, use of some medications (e.g., oral contraceptives, oral corticosteroids), and immunosuppression. Infected individuals usually become symptomatic during hot, humid weather. Overgrowth of the organism results in an asymptomatic dermatosis characterized by areas of well-demarcated scaling with variable changes in pigmentation (Fitzpatrick et al. 2001, Smith et al. 2001). This condition is not contagious.

DATABASE

SUBJECTIVE

→ Patient may report a history of this condition.
→ Symptoms may include:
  ▪ Changes in skin pigmentation, especially hypopigmentation; may also include tan, pink, whitish, or brown macules varying in size usually noted on the trunk.
  ▪ Mild itching aggravated by bathing or sweating.

OBJECTIVE

→ Lesions are (Fitzpatrick et al. 2001, Smith et al. 2001):
  ▪ Initially oval or circular, sharply marginated macules varying in color from white or pink to brown
  ▪ Fine scaling
  ▪ Lesion(s) expand and cover wider area(s) of the body.
  ▪ Hypo- or hyperpigmented area(s) are evident. In untanned skin, the affected areas become light brown; in tanned skin, the areas become whitish; and in darkly pigmented skin, the areas become dark brown.
→ Involvement may be anywhere from a small area (a few millimeters) to a large, confluent distribution.
→ The trunk, neck, and upper extremities are most often affected. However, lesions may appear on the face, neck, and groin in individuals applying topical glucocorticosteroids to these areas (Fitzpatrick et al. 2001).
→ The palms of the hands, soles of the feet, and mucous membranes are never affected.

ASSESSMENT

→ Tinea versicolor
→ R/O vitiligo (no scaling)
→ R/O café-au-lait spots (no scaling)
→ R/O seborrheic dermatitis
→ R/O pityriasis rosea
→ R/O allergic contact dermatitis
→ R/O erythrasma
→ R/O psoriasis

PLAN

DIAGNOSTIC TESTS

→ The following tests may be performed as needed:
  ▪ Potassium hydroxide (KOH) 10–20% microscopic exam of skin scrapings reveals "spaghetti and meatballs" pattern (i.e., large blunt hyphae with clusters of budding spores).

- Scales will fluoresce bright blue-green with a Wood's lamp. If the individual showered recently, the Wood's lamp examination may be negative because the fluorescent chemical in the organism is water soluble (Fitzpatrick et al. 2001).
- Mycologic cultures are not helpful because the causative organisms are common skin colonizers in unaffected as well as affected individuals.

TREATMENT/MANAGEMENT

→ Topical therapy includes application of one of the following solutions (Fitzpatrick et al. 2001, Smith et al. 2001):
- Selenium sulfide shampoo (Selsun®, Exsel®), which is the most economical therapy. Apply the shampoo daily for 1 week from the base of the scalp to the knees; leave on for 10–15 minutes and then shower.
- Zinc parathion, sulfur, and salicylic acid shampoos (e.g., Sebulex®) may be effective in preventing exacerbations (Berger 2002).
  - The shampoo is applied to affected areas; leave on for 24 hours and then shower. This process should be repeated once a week for 4 weeks (Smith et al. 2001).
  - For maintenance therapy, shampooing the same areas described above once a month is recommended.
→ Systemic therapy may be necessary for the treatment of widespread or recalcitrant infections. Current recommendations include:
- Ketoconazole 400–800 mg p.o. once
  OR
- Ketoconazole 200 mg p.o. every day for 7 days
  NOTE: The patient should be instructed not to shower for 12–18 hours after taking oral ketoconazole because it is delivered via sweat to the skin (Berger 2002).
- Itraconazole 200 mg p.o. QD for 5–7 days
  NOTE: Ketoconazole and itraconazole therapy has been associated with hepatotoxicity and drug reactions. Refer to the *Physicians' Desk Reference (PDR)*.

CONSULTATION

→ Physician consultation is indicated in widespread or recalcitrant infection.
→ As needed for prescription(s)

PATIENT EDUCATION

→ Educate the patient about tinea versicolor—the cause, clinical course, treatment options, recurrence, possible complications, side effects of medications, and indicated follow-up.
→ Inform the patient that return of pigmentation may lag behind completion of therapy by several months and is influenced by skin color and exposure to the sun.
→ Inform the patient that discarding or laundering frequently worn clothing in hot water may help prevent the infection.

FOLLOW-UP

→ As indicated by case presentation.

→ See "Consultation."
→ Document in progress notes and on problem list.

Tinea Corporis (Body Ringworm)

Tinea corporis affects the smooth, nonhairy portions of skin (i.e., glabrous skin) (Smith et al. 2001). Typically, it manifests as erythematous, scaling lesions with central clearing, but it also can appear as vesicles, pustules, and psoriatic-like lesions (Fitzpatrick et al. 2001, Goldstein et al. 2000). *Trichophyton rubrum* is the most common dermatophyte causing tinea corporis and is often a result of autoinoculation from tinea pedis (Fitzpatrick et al. 2001).

Tinea corporis is more frequently reported among adults and is more common in hot, humid climates. Occasionally, individuals report exposure to an infected cat. Complications are rare, but include extension of the infection to scalp, hair, or nails, secondary bacterial infection, and dermatophytid (i.e., an allergy or sensitivity to fungus) (Berger 2002).

DATABASE

SUBJECTIVE

→ Patient may report annular, erythematous skin eruption(s) on exposed areas of body (e.g., face, arms).
→ Patient may report a history of or concurrent tinea pedis infection.
→ Mild pruritus is commonly reported.
→ Patient may report exposure to an infected cat.

OBJECTIVE

→ Erythematous, papular, well-circumscribed, and scaling lesion(s) with central clearing are most commonly observed. The lesions may fuse and cover a large area.
→ Concentric, red, scaly rings may be observed.
→ Vesicles and/or pustules may be present with secondary bacterial infection or zoophilic infection (i.e., tinea corporis resulting from contact with an infected animal) (Fitzpatrick et al. 2001).

ASSESSMENT

→ Tinea corporis
→ R/O annular lesions of psoriasis
→ R/O seborrheic dermatitis
→ R/O contact dermatitis
→ R/O pityriasis rosea
→ R/O erythema multiforme
→ R/O furunculosis
→ R/O erythema chronica migrans
→ R/O dermatitis herpetiformis

PLAN

DIAGNOSTIC TESTS

→ Potassium hydroxide (KOH) 10–20% microscopic exam of scraping of scaly lesion will reveal hyphae.
→ Fungal cultures can be ordered if confirmation of diagnosis is needed; however, this is usually not necessary.

TREATMENT/MANAGEMENT

→ Skin should be kept dry and clean.
→ Topical antifungal agents are effective when applied BID to lesion(s) until 1–2 weeks after the lesions disappear. Commonly used agents include:
- Miconazole 2% cream or lotion
- Clotrimazole 1% cream or lotion
- Ketoconazole 2% cream
- Sulconazole 1% cream
- Terbinafine 1% cream
- Butenafine 1% cream

NOTE: Treatment with terbinafine and butenafine usually results in a clinical response in a shorter time than with other topical agents (Berger 2002).
→ Use of systemic agents for the treatment of cutaneous dermatophyte infections associated with significant inflammation requires consultation with a physician prior to initiation of treatment. Agents that may be used include (Berger 2002):
- Terbinafine 250 mg p.o. QD for 3–4 weeks (or longer depending on the severity of the clinical presentation)
- Griseofulvin 250–500 mg p.o. BID for 2–4 weeks
- Itraconazole 200 mg p.o. QD for 7 days
→ A short course of oral prednisone may be necessary in some patients with severe inflammatory manifestations, but this should be prescribed after consultation with a physician.

CONSULTATION

→ Seek dermatology consultation for chronic, scaly ringworm or if the patient is experiencing moderate to severe inflammation. Treatment in these patients may require long-term oral antifungal agents and possibly systemic steroids. In addition, this may be a manifestation of a severe underlying medical problem such as lymphoma and immunological deficiencies (Smith et al. 2001).
→ As needed for prescription(s)

PATIENT EDUCATION

→ Educate the patient about the cause and indicated treatment, emphasizing the need to continue therapy for 1–2 weeks after lesions have disappeared.
→ Advise the patient to avoid contact with infected animals. Household pets should be evaluated and treated for tinea microorganisms by a veterinarian (Berger 2002).
→ Discuss proper laundering of clothing (e.g., in hot water) to prevent re-exposure.

FOLLOW-UP

→ Individualized according to case presentation
→ See "Consultation."
→ Document in progress notes and on problem list.

Tinea Capitis (Scalp Ringworm)

Tinea capitis, or ringworm of the scalp and hair, is the most common fungal infection in children. It is rarely reported in adults due to the fungistatic effects of triglycerides found in the sebum produced after puberty (Fitzpatrick et al. 2001). Two dermatophyte species are primarily responsible for this infection, *Microsporum* species and *Trichophyton tonsurans*. *T. tonsurans* is the most common etiological pathogen in the United States and is responsible for resistant infections that may persist into adulthood. Other dermatophytes that can cause tinea capitis include *Microsporum audouinii*, *Microsporum canis*, *Trichophyton schoenleinii*, and *Trichophyton mentagrophytes*. The type of dermatophyte that is responsible for tinea capitis varies depending on geographic regions and migratory patterns of populations (Gupta et al. 2000).

Tinea capitis inoculation results from contact with an infected individual, animal, or fomite. However, other factors contribute to the establishment of infection after exposure, including trauma (e.g., haircuts, tight braiding of hair) and application of oil to the hair, which promotes adherence of the organisms to the scalp (Gupta et al. 2000). The resulting infections are classified as ectothrix, endothrix, or favus. Ectothrix infection is usually caused by *M. audouinii*, endothrix by *T. tonsurans*, and favus by *T. schoenleinii*. Usually ectothrix and endothrix infections are noninflammatory and characterized by gray, annular, scaly patches of alopecia. Favus infections are associated with inflammation and yellow crusting around the hair shafts (Elewski 2000).

DATABASE

SUBJECTIVE

→ The patient may report the following symptoms, depending on the type of microorganism and associated infection (Berger 2002, Elewski 2000, Fitzpatrick et al. 2001, Gupta et al. 2000):
- Noninflammatory:
  • Patient may report:
    – Persistent dandruff unrelieved by proper use of dandruff shampoos
    – Exposure to infected farm animals or pets
    – Focal hair loss
    – A history of tinea capitis prior to or during adolescence
  • Symptoms may include:
    – Mild to moderate pruritus of affected areas
    – Areas of baldness
    – Enlarged lymph nodes
- Inflammatory:
  • Symptoms as noted above and:
    – Tender, oozing lesions in affected areas

OBJECTIVE

→ Vital signs are usually within normal limits, but an elevated temperature may be noted with inflammatory tinea.
→ Patient may present with the following physical findings depending on the type of tinea infection (Berger 2002, Elewski 2000, Fitzpatrick et al. 2001, Gupta et al. 2000):

- Erythematous papules at the hair shaft with dry scaling extending outwards
- Patches of partial or complete alopecia (noninflammatory type)
- Acutely inflamed exudative lesions, with or without pustules that may be boggy to palpation (inflammatory type)
- Hair looks dry, lusterless, grayish
- Broken hairs at or just above the scalp. This variety of tinea capitis is known as "black dot" because broken hairs may be seen as black or blond dots on the scalp.
- Occipital or posterior auricular lymphadenopathy (especially with inflammatory reaction)

ASSESSMENT

→ Tinea capitis
→ R/O seborrheic dermatitis
→ R/O psoriasis
→ R/O atopic dermatitis
→ R/O bacterial infection
→ R/O alopecia from other causes
→ R/O syphilis
→ R/O lupus erythematosus
→ R/O eczema

PLAN

DIAGNOSTIC TESTS

→ Diagnostic tests are usually not required; however, in some patients the following tests may be ordered as needed:
- Potassium hydroxide (KOH) 10% microscopic examination of the scalp scales and black dystrophic hairs should be done. Evidence of spores on or in the hair shafts indicates tinea capitis infection (Fitzpatrick et al. 2001).
- Hair shaft may be pulled from its follicle and sent for fungal culture to identify species (Gupta et al. 2000).
- Wood's lamp examination can be done but is not helpful in diagnosing *T. tonsurans*, as this species does not fluoresce. However, it may be helpful in diagnosing *M. canis* or *M. audouinii*. If these are present, the specimen will appear bright green under Wood's lamp illumination (Fitzpatrick et al. 2001, Gupta et al. 2000).
- Bacterial culture can be sent if secondary infection is suspected, although the results can be difficult to interpret if normal skin-colonizing organisms are recovered.

TREATMENT/MANAGEMENT

→ Selenium sulfide shampoo (Selsun®, Excel®) can be used to reduce the shedding and help with the eradication of spores.
→ Topical antifungal agents are not effective in the treatment of adult tinea capitis.
→ Systemic therapy is indicated in adults and should continue until culture results are negative. Some authorities recommend the continuation of therapy for 1–2 weeks after culture results are negative. The following agents can be used (Berger 2002, Fitzpatrick et al. 2001, Elewski 2000, Friedlander 2000):

- Microcrystalline griseofulvin 500 mg p.o. QD for 4–6 weeks or until culture is negative
- Ketoconazole 200 mg p.o. QD for 4–6 weeks or until culture is negative
- Fluconazole 200 mg p.o. QD for 4–8 weeks or until culture is negative
- Itraconazole 200 mg p.o. QD for 4–8 weeks or until culture is negative
- Terbinafine, an allylamine, is a potent antifungal that requires a shorter duration of therapy. For *T. tonsurans* infection, use 250 mg p.o. QD for 2–3 weeks. *M. canis* infection requires 4–8 weeks of treatment.

NOTE: Side effects, toxicities (e.g., hepatotoxicities, neutropenia) and drug interactions can occur with these agents. Consult the *PDR* and monitor the patient as indicated.
→ If kerion is present, additional therapy includes:
- Hot compresses to the lesions BID–TID
→ If the patient has a secondary bacterial infection, antibiotics should be prescribed to cover staphylococcal and/or group A streptococcal organisms.

CONSULTATION

→ Physician consultation is indicated in patients undergoing systemic therapy.
→ Consultation with a dermatologist is indicated for patients with kerion celsi. Oral steroids may be indicated to prevent scarring and resultant permanent hair loss (Smith et al. 2001).
→ As needed for prescription(s)

PATIENT EDUCATION

→ Educate the patient about tinea capitis—the cause, treatment options, and indicated follow-up.
→ Educate the patient about possible side effects and drug interactions associated with systemic treatments.
→ Advise the patient against sharing her hats, combs, or brushes with others (Fitzpatrick et al. 2001).

FOLLOW-UP

→ As indicated by case presentation
→ See "Consultation.".
→ Document in progress notes and on problem list.

Tinea Pedis (Athlete's Foot)

Tinea pedis, commonly known as *athlete's foot*, is the most prevalent acute or chronic fungal infection. Transmission of the infecting organism occurs when individuals walk barefoot on contaminated floors. Several different dermatophytes colonize the skin, including *Trichophyton rubrum* and *T. mentagrophytes*. Once colonization occurs, the dermatophyte penetrates the stratum corneum, the outermost layer of the epidermis. Variable and complex host/parasite reactions follow, resulting in different forms of infection, including interdigital (the most common type), vesicular, and dry, scaly moccasin (Fitzpatrick et al. 2001, Robbins 2000). The breaks in the skin associated with this condition provide a portal of entry for such pathogens as *Staphylococcus aureus* or group A streptococcus, resulting in localized infection or spreading infections such as ascending lymphangitis, cellulitis, or lymphadenitis (Fitzpatrick et al. 2001).

DATABASE

SUBJECTIVE

→ The patient may report a history of tinea pedis.
→ Symptoms may include (Fitzpatrick et al. 2001, Robbins 2000):
  ▪ Pruritus, which may be intense
  ▪ Burning, stinging at site of infection
  ▪ Pain associated with blisters, cracks, or fissures
  ▪ Erythema, edema, purulent drainage if secondary bacterial infection
  ▪ Enlarged, tender, local and regional lymph nodes if concomitant lymphadenitis

OBJECTIVE

→ Interdigital (Fitzpatrick et al. 2001, Robbins 2000):
  ▪ Typically does not spread beyond intertriginous areas
  ▪ Patient presents with:
    • Scaling, maceration, fissuring
    • Fourth interspace most commonly affected
  ▪ Ulcerations may be observed that indicate an extension of the interdigital infection into the dermis due to maceration and secondary bacterial infection.
→ Vesicular (Fitzpatrick et al. 2001, Robbins 2000):
  ▪ Patient presents with:
    • Intense inflammation
    • Lesions occurring anywhere on the foot, but most often observed in the webspaces, soles, or instep of the foot
    • Lesions are usually clustered and may resemble an allergic contact dermatitis.
→ Dry, scaly moccasin (Fitzpatrick et al. 2001, Robbins 2000):
  ▪ Patient presents with:
    • Well-demarcated area(s)
    • Dull erythema, powdery-white to pinkish-red hue of plantar surface, dryness, scaling, and hyperkeratosis
    • Involvement confined to the soles, heels, and lateral aspects of the foot
    • May be unilateral or bilateral

ASSESSMENT

→ Tinea pedis
→ R/O interdigital intertrigo
→ R/O candidiasis
→ R/O psoriasis
→ R/O contact dermatitis
→ R/O atopic dermatitis
→ R/O cellulitis
→ R/O lichen planus
→ R/O ichthyosis

PLAN

DIAGNOSTIC TESTS

→ Potassium hydroxide (KOH) 10–20% microscopic exam of affected skin scrapings may reveal hyphae.
→ Fungal cultures may be positive and confirm the diagnosis.
→ Bacterial culture may be positive if there is secondary infection.

TREATMENT/MANAGEMENT

→ Topical therapeutic interventions are divided into remedies for the treatment of macerated lesions and for dry, scaly lesions.
  ▪ Macerated lesions (Fitzpatrick et al. 2001, Robbins 2000):
    • Apply aluminum subacetate (Domeboro®) solution soaks for 20 minutes BID–TID to help dry lesions.
    • Apply topical antifungal agents after completely washing and drying affected area(s). The following antifungal preparations can be used and should continue to be applied for 2 weeks after the lesions resolve:
      – Terbinafine 1% cream applied BID
      – Clotrimazole 1% cream or lotion applied BID
      – Miconazole 2% cream or lotion applied BID
      – Tolnaftate preparations can be used BID but are less effective than miconazole or clotrimazole preparations.
  ▪ Dry, scaly lesions (Berger 2002, Fitzpatrick et al. 2001, Smith et al. 2001):
    • Can be treated with the topical antifungal agents listed above.
→ Systemic therapy may be necessary in patients with recurrent, severe, or persistent symptoms, and includes use of the following agents:
  ▪ Terbinafine 250 mg p.o. QD for 14 days
  ▪ Itraconazole 200 mg p.o. BID for 7 days or QD for 14 days
  ▪ Ketoconazole 200 mg p.o. QD for 3–6 weeks
  NOTE: Significant side effects, toxicities (e.g., hepatotoxicity, neutropenia) and drug interactions can occur with these agents. Consult the *PDR*.

CONSULTATION

→ Physician consultation is indicated for severe inflammation, bullae, or if secondary bacterial infections.
→ As needed for prescription(s)

PATIENT EDUCATION

→ Educate the patient about tinea pedis—the cause, treatment options, possible complications, preventive measures, and indicated follow-up.
→ Teach the patient that moisture will promote fungal infections. Whenever possible, shoes should be removed to reduce moisture. Encourage the use of cotton socks. Advise the patient to wear rubber thongs or sandals in showers, pools, and spa areas, and to completely dry toes and feet after bathing/swimming.

→ Educate the patient about the need for twice-daily application of antifungals, as improvement is unlikely if the medication is used less frequently.
→ Educate the patient about the possibility of autoinoculation and the need to use proper handwashing after foot care and treatment.

FOLLOW-UP

→ As indicated by case presentation
→ See "Consultation."
→ Document in progress notes and on problem list.

Tinea Cruris (Eczema Marginatum)

Tinea cruris is an infection caused by dermatophytes (specifically *T. rubrum* and *T. mentagrophytes*) that affects the groin, perineum, and perianal regions (Fitzpatrick et al. 2001, Smith et al. 2001). The pathology of tinea cruris is similar to that of tinea pedis, with moisture, maceration, carbon dioxide tension, friction, and chronic use of topical steroids thought to be promoting factors. Tinea cruris is more common in hot, humid climates, and in males, obese individuals, athletes, and individuals who report increased perspiring tendencies (Fitzpatrick et al. 2001).

DATABASE

SUBJECTIVE

→ Patient may be asymptomatic.
→ Patient may report (Fitzpatrick et al. 2001, Smith et al. 2001):
- History of increased perspiring
- Moderate to severe itching and/or burning in intertriginous areas
- Erythema and/or macular lesions in affected areas, usually bilaterally
- Concomitant fungal infection of feet

OBJECTIVE

→ Lesions are confined to the groin, perineum, and gluteal fold. Characteristics include (Fitzpatrick et al. 2001, Smith et al. 2001):
- Sharply marginated borders with thin scales, erythema, and central clearing observed bilaterally
- Vesicles and pustules at borders of lesion (rare)
- Usually dry

ASSESSMENT

→ Tinea cruris
→ R/O candidiasis
→ R/O erythrasma (erythrasma fluoresces red with Wood's light)
→ R/O seborrheic dermatitis
→ R/O intertrigo
→ R/O psoriasis
→ R/O contact dermatitis
→ R/O neurodermatitis (indistinct borders)
→ R/O Bowen's disease (asymmetrical)
→ R/O extramammary Paget's disease (asymmetrical distribution)

PLAN

DIAGNOSTIC TESTS

→ Potassium hydroxide (KOH) 10–20% microscopic exam of skin scrapings from the lesions' borders will reveal hyphae.
→ Fungal culture will differentiate tinea cruris from *Candida albicans*.
→ Bacterial culture can be obtained if secondary bacterial infection is suspected.

TREATMENT/MANAGEMENT

→ The affected area should be kept clean and dry, and excessive bathing avoided.
→ Clothing should be loose-fitting and made of absorbent material (e.g., cotton). Avoid irritating and rough materials.
→ Topical antifungal therapy is effective when recommended regimens are followed. Using any of the following agents in solution or lotion form (for increased penetration of skin folds) is acceptable, but therapy must continue for up to 2 weeks after resolution of the lesion(s) (Berger 2002, Fitzpatrick et al. 2001):
- Terbinafine 1% applied to affected area BID
- Miconazole 2% applied to affected area BID
- Clotrimazole 1% applied to affected area BID
- Ketoconazole 2% applied to affected area every day
- Sulconazole 1% applied to affected area every day
→ Systemic antifungal therapy is not routinely indicated unless the patient is experiencing severe symptoms. If systemic therapy is being considered, consultation with a physician is indicated.

CONSULTATION

→ Physician consultation is warranted with severe or recurrent tinea cruris or if secondary bacterial infection is suspected (because lymphangitis can occur).
→ As needed for prescription(s)

PATIENT EDUCATION

→ Educate the patient about tinea cruris—the cause, treatment options, possible complications, preventive measures, and indicated follow-up.
→ Advise the patient to avoid tight clothing, thereby decreasing moisture and friction.
→ Advise the patient to keep the affected areas dry.
→ Advise the patient to apply medication as instructed to promote resolution of infection.
→ Educate the patient about the possibility of autoinoculation and the need for proper handwashing after applying treatment to affected areas.

FOLLOW-UP

→ Individualized according to case presentation
→ See "Consultation."
→ Document in progress notes and on problem list.

Candidiasis (Moniliasis)

Cutaneous candidiasis is an infection that occurs in moist, occluded areas of the body. It is most often caused by *Candida albicans*, although other candida species can cause the classic beefy-red, intertriginous fungal infection. A complex complement reaction of the host is activated by the invading candida organism, resulting in pustule formation. Precipitating factors include moisture, obesity, diabetes mellitus, antibiotic therapy, immune deficiency, oral contraceptive use, and pendulous breasts (Fitzpatrick et al. 2001, Fox et al. 2001).

Cutaneous candidiasis can have a prolonged course, especially in patients with a depressed immune function. Superficial cutaneous lesions may be manifestations of systemic infections (e.g., disseminated candidiasis, candidemia). *Chronic mucocutaneous candidiasis* is a recurrent infection of the skin and mucous membranes that can progress to granulomatous lesions even after the completion of antifungal therapy. It is a result of an abnormality of cell-mediated immunity and may be associated with autoimmune endocrine dysfunction (e.g., hypoparathyroidism, adrenal insufficiency) (Fox et al. 2001).

DATABASE

SUBJECTIVE

→ Patient may report:
- A history of diabetes, obesity, systemic antibiotic use, oral contraceptive use, or immunological deficiency
- Episodes of vulvar/vaginal burning, itching, or discharge (see the **Vaginitis** chapters in Section 12).

→ Symptoms may include burning, stinging, itching, and tenderness of the affected areas.

OBJECTIVE

→ Lesions are:
- Beefy-red, with scalded-looking skin
- Irregular, with sharp margins
- Occasionally scaly

→ Lesions have satellite pustules.

→ Paronychia may be evident.

→ Lesions usually occur in intertriginous areas of the groin, axilla, inframammary areas, and between the third and fourth fingers (Berger 2002, Fitzpatrick et al. 2001, Fox et al. 2001).

ASSESSMENT

→ Candidiasis (cutaneous)
→ R/O seborrheic dermatitis
→ R/O intertrigo (nonspecific and psoriatic)
→ R/O tinea corporis
→ R/O erythrasma
→ R/O folliculitis
→ R/O contact dermatitis
→ R/O tinea cruris (usually less red)
→ R/O pediculosis
→ R/O underlying medical condition (e.g., diabetes mellitus, HIV infection)

PLAN

DIAGNOSTIC TESTS

→ Potassium hydroxide (KOH) 10–20% microscopic exam of the contents of a vesicle or pustule reveals budding cells or short hyphae (scraping of the beefy-red area will not demonstrate hyphae) (Berger 2002).

→ Fungal cultures may be useful in situations where symptoms are refractory to standard treatment (Fitzpatrick et al. 2001).

→ Bacterial culture can be obtained if a secondary infection is suspected.

TREATMENT/MANAGEMENT

→ Affected areas should be kept dry. Whenever possible, expose the affected areas to air.

→ Topical antifungal therapy for cutaneous lesions includes (Berger 2002, Fitzpatrick et al. 2001):
- Miconazole 2% cream or lotion applied TID–QID to affected area(s) until complete resolution
- Clotrimazole 1% applied TID–QID to affected area(s) until complete resolution
- Ketoconazole 2% applied TID to affected area(s) until complete resolution

→ Topical anti-inflammatory therapy may help reduce severe symptoms:
- Hydrocortisone 1% cream applied BID to affected area(s) for a limited time (3–5 days)

→ Disseminated candidiasis requires systemic antifungal therapy. Affected patients typically are critically ill and often have compromised immune function. Hospitalization and consultation with a physician in these situations is necessary prior to initiating treatment.

CONSULTATION

→ Physician consultation for evaluation of potential underlying conditions is indicated in patients with recurrent, persistent, severe cutaneous candidiasis infections or if disseminated candidiasis is suspected.

→ As needed for prescription(s)

PATIENT EDUCATION

→ Educate the patient about cutaneous candidiasis infection— the cause, treatment options, possible side effects of medications, and indicated follow-up.

→ Advise the patient to minimize moisture and occlusion to promote resolution and diminish the chance of recurrence.

→ For individuals with diabetes, stricter surveillance and control of blood sugar levels should be considered.

→ In severe or recurrent cutaneous infection or disseminated disease, the patient should be counseled about and offered HIV testing.

FOLLOW-UP

→ Individualized according to case presentation
→ See "Consultation."
→ Document in progress notes and on problem list.

BIBLIOGRAPHY

Berger, T.G. 2002. Skin, hair, and nails. In *2002 current medical diagnosis and treatment*, eds. L.M. Tierney, Jr., S.J. McPhee, and M.A. Papadakis, pp. 144–146. New York: Lange Medical Books/McGraw-Hill.

Elewski, B.E. 2000. Tinea capitis: a current perspective. *Journal of the Academy of Dermatology* 42(1):1–20.

Fitzpatrick, T.B., Johnson, R.A., Wolff, K. et al. 2001. *Color atlas and synopsis of clinical dermatology. Common and serious diseases*. New York: McGraw-Hill.

Fox, C.R., and Sande, M.A. 2001. Candida species. *Current diagnosis and treatment in infectious diseases*, eds. W.R. Wilson and M.A. Sande, pp. 734–744. New York: Lange Medical Books/McGraw-Hill.

Friedlander, S.F. 2000. The optimal therapy for tinea capitis. *Pediatric Dermatology* 17(4):325–326.

Goldstein, A.O., Smith, K.M., Ives, T.J. et al. 2000. Mycotic infections. Effective management of conditions involving the skin, hair, and nails. *Geriatrics* 55(5):40–52.

Gupta, A.K., and Summerbell, R.C. 2000. Tinea capitis. *Medical Mycology* 38:255–287.

Robbins, J.M. 2000. Recognizing, treating, and preventing common foot problems. *Cleveland Clinic Journal of Medicine* 67(1):45–57.

Smith, D.S., and Relman, D.A. 2001. Dermatophytes. In *Current diagnosis and treatment in infectious diseases*, eds. W.R. Wilson and M.A. Sande, pp. 777–784. New York: Lange Medical Books/McGraw-Hill.

3-J

Furuncles and Carbuncles

A *furuncle* is a deep-seated infection of a hair follicle involving the surrounding subcutaneous tissue that appears as an erythematous nodule or abscess (Wilhelm et al. 2001). A *carbuncle* is a group of multiple, coalescing furuncles with multiple drainage points that are usually located in areas of thick subcutaneous tissue. The usual infecting organism is coagulase-positive *Staphylococcus aureus* (Fitzpatrick et al. 2001, Wilhelm et al. 2001).

The most frequent sites on the body for furuncle/carbuncle formation are hairy portions exposed to friction, irritation, moisture, or the obstructive effect of petrolatum products (Wilhelm et al. 2001). The development of furuncles/carbuncles occurs more commonly in obese individuals with oily skin and in staphylococcal carrier states (Fitzpatrick et al. 2001, Von Eiff et al. 2001). Rare complications associated with manipulation of furuncles include osteomyelitis, perinephric abscess, endocarditis, and cavernous sinus thrombosis (secondary to manipulation of a nasolabial fold or central upper-lip furuncles) (Wilhelm et al. 2001).

DATABASE

SUBJECTIVE

→ The patient may report the following (Fitzpatrick et al. 2001, Wilhelm et al. 2001):
  ▪ History of previous furuncle, carbuncle, or hidradenitis suppurativa
  ▪ Symptoms may include:
    • Redness and swelling at site of the affected follicle
    • Lesion is usually extremely painful
    • Fever and/or malaise

OBJECTIVE

→ Vital signs are usually within normal limits but may reveal a low-grade temperature.
→ Lesions are initially hard, indurated nodules with a surrounding erythematous flame.
→ The nodule develops into a pustule or becomes a fluctuant abscess.

→ Usually a spontaneous rupture with discharge of pus occurs after a few days to 1–2 weeks.
→ Most frequent sites for furuncles are the face, neck, upper back, axillae, buttocks, and groin. Carbuncles are most frequently noted at the nape of the neck, back, and thighs (Wilhelm et al. 2001).

ASSESSMENT

→ Furuncle
→ Carbuncle
→ R/O inflamed epidermal inclusion cyst
→ R/O pustular acne
→ R/O erysipelas
→ R/O cellulitis
→ R/O necrotic herpes simplex virus infection
→ R/O hidradenitis suppurativa
→ R/O ecthyma (deep form of impetigo)
→ R/O staphylococcal carrier state
→ R/O immunosuppression (if recurrent, severe furuncle/carbuncle)

PLAN

DIAGNOSTIC TESTS

→ The following diagnostic tests may be ordered if indicated (Wilhelm et al. 2001):
  ▪ Culture and sensitivity after incision and drainage (I&D) should be considered in certain patients (e.g., immunocompromised) to rule out methicillin-resistant *S. aureus*.
  ▪ Nasal swab for culture for *S. aureus* in patients suspected of nasal carriage of this bacterium. This will be positive in patients who are chronic carriers (Wilhelm et al. 2001).
  ▪ CBC is rarely indicated but, if done, may reveal a slight leukocytosis.

TREATMENT/MANAGEMENT

→ Immobilization of the affected part is indicated to prevent over-manipulation.

→ Apply moist heat for 15–30 minutes BID to help localize the lesion (Fitzpatrick et al. 2001).

→ Systemic antibiotics are indicated for the treatment of carbuncles and for the treatment of furuncles in immunosuppressed individuals and to assist resolution in healthy individuals. The antibiotic regimen chosen should provide antimcrobial activity against coagulase-positive *S. aureus.* The following antibiotics may be used (Wilhelm et al. 2001):

- Dicloxacillin 250–500 mg p.o. QID for 10 days
- Cephalexin 500 mg p.o. QID for 10 days
- Clindamycin 150–300 mg p.o. QID for 10 days
- Ciprofloxacin 500 mg p.o. BID for 10 days
- Erythromycin 250–500 mg p.o. QID for 10 days can be used in penicillin-allergic patients if the isolate is sensitive to it.

NOTE: Carbuncle therapy may require parenteral antibiotics.

→ After lesions are "mature," I&D may be performed.

→ Recurrent furunculosis may require combination antimicrobial therapy. Consultation with a physician is indicated in such instances.

→ In patients with recurrent furunculosis, evaluation and possible concomitant antimicrobial therapy for family members/intimate contacts who are chronic staphylococcal carriers may be indicated. Topical therapy with mupirocin applied to the individual's nares, axillae, and anogenital area BID for 5 days usually resolves the carrier state.

NOTE: Mupirocin may be irritating when applied intranasally (Berger 2002, Hirschmann 2000, Kaye 2000).

CONSULTATION

→ Consultation with a physician is indicated in a patient with a nasolabial fold or central upper-lip furuncle who has recurrent furunculosis, who has carbuncles, who is immunosuppressed, or who does not respond to therapy (Wilhelm et al. 2001).

→ As needed for prescription(s)

PATIENT EDUCATION

→ Educate the patient regarding furuncles/carbuncles—the cause, clinical course, treatment, possible complications, possible side effects of medications, and indicated follow-up.

→ Advise the patient to wear loose-fitting clothing and cotton underwear and to avoid using oil-based body lotions and make-up.

→ Advise the patient to avoid manipulating lesions.

→ After I&D, advise the patient to apply an antibacterial ointment and keep the area loosely bandaged.

FOLLOW-UP

→ The patient should return for evaluation and I&D of a mature furuncle. If packing is inserted into the wound site, advise the patient to return for advancement/removal of the packing material.

→ If the patient develops signs or symptoms of complications, she should return for immediate evaluation.

→ See "Consultation."

→ Document in progress notes and on problem list.

BIBLIOGRAPHY

Berger, T.G. 2002. Skin, hair, and nails. In *2002 current medical diagnosis and treatment,* eds. L.M. Tierney, Jr., S.J. McPhee, and M.A. Papadakis, pp. 163–164. New York: Lange Medical Books/McGraw-Hill.

Fitzpatrick, T.B., Johnson, R.A., Wolff, K. et al. 2001. *Color atlas and synopsis of clinical dermatology. Common and serious diseases,* pp. 600–601. New York: McGraw-Hill.

Hirschmann, J.V. 2000. Antimicrobial prophylaxis in dermatology. *Seminars in Cutaneous Medicine and Surgery* 19(1):2–9.

Kaye, E.T. 2000. Topical antibacterial agents: role in prophylaxis and treatment of bacterial infections. *Current Clinical Topics in Infectious Diseases* 20:43–62.

Von Eiff, C., Becker, K., Machka, K. et al. 2001. Nasal carriage as a source of *Staphylococcus aureus* bacteremia. *New England Journal of Medicine* 344(1):11–16.

Wilhelm, M.P., and Edson, R.S. 2001. Skin and soft-tissue infections. In *Current diagnosis and treatment in infectious diseases,* eds. W.R. Wilson and M.A. Sande, pp. 182–183. New York: Lange Medical Books/McGraw-Hill.

3-K

Impetigo

Impetigo is a superficial bacterial infection of the skin caused by group A streptococcus and/or *Staphylococcus aureus*. It is common in childhood as a primary disease but often occurs secondary to other dermatologic conditions such as eczema or in immunocompromised patients. Typically, the skin becomes colonized by group A streptococcus, usually transmitted from another person (American Academy of Pediatrics [AAP] 2000). Impetigo may begin following a break in the skin from an insect bite or some other minor trauma. Generally it is confined to the epidermis but may progress to the dermal layer of skin, becoming known as *ecthyma*. The lesions are characteristically vesicular; following a weeping phase, they appear as honey-colored crusts. Itching is quite prominent and scratching frequently leads to secondary infection with *S. aureus*. *Bullous impetigo* is another disorder caused by an exfoliative toxin produced by phage group 2 *S. aureus*; it is not the result of progressive impetigo infection (Wilhelm 2001).

Impetigo is common in young children and quite contagious; following skin infection, the throat often becomes colonized. Certain M serotypes of group A streptococci (2, 49, 52, 55, 57, 59-61) are likely to cause impetigo (Swartz 2000). Group A streptococci responsible for impetigo are also capable of causing acute glomerulonephritis within 7–10 days of the onset of infection. Unfortunately, antibiotics have not been demonstrated to prevent acute glomerulonephritis in patients with impetigo but can prevent further colonization and spread to other individuals (AAP 2000).

DATABASE

SUBJECTIVE

→ Symptoms may include:
  ▪ Itching rash
  ▪ Ongoing outcropping of lesions
→ History may include:
  ▪ Contact with individuals having similar rash
  ▪ Recent history of insect bites or break in skin

OBJECTIVE

→ Vital signs:
  ▪ Temperature should be normal; elevation suggests cellulitis.
  ▪ Blood pressure should be normal; elevation suggests glomerulonephritis.
→ Lesions begin as pinpoint papules, progress to fluid-filled lesions that erupt into a clear, honey-colored, dew-drop appearance, and eventually dry and scab. Lesions may appear on any part of body. They may leave pits in the skin or hypopigmentation.
→ The presence of periorbital or peripheral edema suggests an onset of acute glomerulonephritis.

ASSESSMENT

→ Impetigo
→ R/O folliculitis
→ R/O varicella
→ R/O viral exanthem
→ R/O contact dermatitis
→ R/O scabies
→ R/O insect bites
→ R/O herpes zoster
→ R/O ecthyma
→ R/O pediculosis corporis

PLAN

DIAGNOSTIC TESTS

→ Diagnostic tests are generally not necessary in uncomplicated impetigo; however, both Gram stain and culture can be done on lesions to confirm group A streptococci.
→ Suspicion of lesions due to infestation (scabies, pediculosis) requires skin scraping to look for scabies mites, or examination of hair follicles for nits (egg sacs of lice); rarely, lice may be seen on the skin.

TREATMENT/MANAGEMENT

→ Topical 2% mupirocin ointment (Bactroban®) may be applied to affected areas TID for 7 days if only few superficial lesions are present. Mupirocin cream is also effective (Gisby et al. 2000).

→ Systemic therapy may be initiated with one of the following:

- Dicloxacillin (Dynapen®) 500 mg QID for 7 days
  OR
- Cephalexin (Keflex®) 500 mg QID for 7 days
  OR
- Erythromycin (E-Mycin®) 500 mg QID for 7 days for penicillin-allergic patients

CONSULTATION

→ Physician consultation is indicated for a febrile, sick-appearing, immunodeficient, or immunosuppressed patient.

→ Consultation is also required for any signs of glomerulonephritis, including hypertension, edema, and/or blood in urine.

→ As needed for prescription(s)

PATIENT EDUCATION

→ Advise the patient about the highly transmissible nature of the disease.

→ Advise the patient about handwashing if there are children for whom they are providing care.

→ Educate the patient about the natural course of the disease and the importance of following the prescribed therapeutic regimen.

→ Inform patients about potentially developing symptoms that should prompt a re-visit (fever, skin erythema, edema).

FOLLOW-UP

→ Individualized according to case presentation

BIBLIOGRAPHY

American Academy of Pediatrics (AAP). 2000. Group A strep-tococcal infections. In *2000 red book report of the Committee on Infectious Diseases*, 25th ed., ed. L.K. Pickering, pp. 526–536. Elk Grove Village, Ill.: American Academy of Pediatrics.

Gisby, J., and Bryant, J. 2000. Efficacy of a new cream formulation of mupirocin: comparison with oral and topical agents in experimental skin infections. *Antimicrobial Agents and Chemotherapy* 44: 255–259.

Swartz, M. 2000. Cellulitis and subcutaneous tissue infections. In *Mandell, Douglas and Bennett's principles and practice of infectious diseases*, 5th ed., eds. G.L. Mandell, J.E. Bennett, and R. Dolin, pp. 1037–1040. New York: Churchill Livingstone.

Wilhelm, M.P. 2001. Skin and soft tissue infections. In *Current diagnosis and treatment in infectious diseases*, eds. W.R. Wilson and M.A. Sande, pp. 177–190. New York: Lange Medical Books/McGraw-Hill.

3-L

Molluscum Contagiosum

Molluscum contagiosum is a contagious, self-limited, and relatively common skin disorder (especially in children and sexually active adults) with a higher incidence observed in men than women. It is caused by *Molluscipoxvirus*, a member of the poxvirus family (Drew 2001, Fitzpatrick et al. 2001). Infection usually results in the development of flesh-colored, waxy, smooth, spherical, centrally umbilicated lesions ranging in size from 2–10 mm in diameter, though giant molluscum papules larger than 15 mm in diameter have occurred. Usually, molluscum appears in clusters of 5–20 lesions.

In immunocompetent adults, lesions are usually found on the lower abdomen, pubic region, and inner thighs. Facial or neck lesions, or a generalized distribution, are often are seen in immunocompromised individuals (e.g., HIV-infected). Complications associated with molluscum contagiosum include bacterial superinfection and cosmetic disfigurement (Fitzpatrick et al. 2001).

Molluscum contagiosum is transmitted through close physical contact, including sexual contact. Autoinoculation is another means. The incubation period is 1–8 weeks. The period of communicability is unknown but probably lasts as long as lesions are present. If left untreated in immune-competent hosts, lesions may persist for 2–12 months and then resolve spontaneously (Berger 2002, Fitzpatrick et al. 2001).

DATABASE

SUBJECTIVE

→ The patient may report the following (Berger 2002, Fitzpatrick et al. 2001):
  ▪ Small, flesh-colored lesions in clusters; distribution may be disseminated or localized
  ▪ Lesions may be painful if there is secondary infection.
  ▪ History of exposure to someone with molluscum
  ▪ History of immunosuppression (e.g., HIV infection)
  ▪ Symptoms of other sexually transmitted diseases (STDs)

OBJECTIVE

→ The following physical examination findings may be evident (Berger 2002, Fitzpatrick et al. 2001):
  ▪ Discrete, umbilicated, pearly white, smooth papules
    • Usually 2–10 mm, but lesions may be as large as 1.5–2.0 cm in diameter.
  ▪ Pubic and genital areas are most commonly affected. Lesions also may appear on the trunk, inner thighs, and proximal extremities. In HIV-infected individuals, the eruption may include the face or neck, or have a generalized distribution (Berger 2002, Drew 2001).
  ▪ Eyelid lesions may be associated with a unilateral conjunctivitis.
  ▪ Molluscum dermatitis presents with a sharply bordered eczematoid reaction 3–10 cm in diameter, may involve only a portion of a molluscum lesion, and usually disappears as the lesion resolves.

ASSESSMENT

→ Molluscum contagiosum
→ R/O warts (especially condyloma acuminata)
→ R/O keratoacanthoma
→ R/O lichen planus
→ R/O epithelial/intradermal nevi
→ R/O intradermal dermatitis
→ R/O human papillomavirus infection
→ R/O basal cell epithelioma
→ R/O secondary infection
→ R/O coexistent STDs
→ R/O HIV infection (if evidence of widely distributed and/or persistent infection)
→ R/O disseminated invasive fungal infection (e.g., cryptococcosis) in HIV-infected individual

PLAN

DIAGNOSTIC TESTS

→ The diagnosis is usually made on the basis of physical findings. However, in patients for whom confirming the diagnosis is desired, the following tests may be performed:

- Wright's or Giemsa stain of the lesion's central core will demonstrate large cytoplasmic inclusion bodies.
- Biopsy for confirmation of diagnosis can be done, although it is rarely indicated (Fitzpatrick et al. 2001).

→ Screen for other STDs as indicated.

TREATMENT/MANAGEMENT

→ In immunocompetent patients, the lesions usually resolve spontaneously and do not require treatment. However, when treatment is indicated (e.g., persistent infection), the following options are available (Berger 2002, Fitzpatrick et al. 2001):

- Application of liquid nitrogen for 1–15 seconds. Molluscum lesions require a shorter application time than HPV lesions (see the **Human Papillomavirus** chapter in Section 13).
- Removal of the lesion and its core through curettage.
- Lesions refractory to freezing with liquid nitrogen, or large lesions, may require electrodessication or laser treatment.

→ If bacterial superinfection or molluscum dermatitis exists, the patient may require systemic antibiotics or topical corticosteroids. (See the **Furuncles and Carbuncles** and **Atopic Dermatitis [Atopic Eczema]** chapters.)

→ Treatment of coexisting STDs as indicated.

→ For patients with disseminated or persistent molluscum, counseling and testing for HIV should be offered.

CONSULTATION

→ Physician consultation is indicated for a patient with diffuse or persistent molluscum, and/or in cases of significant bacterial superinfection or molluscum dermatitis.

→ Refer patients requiring electrodessication or laser treatments to a physician with experience in these therapies.

PATIENT EDUCATION

→ Educate the patient about molluscum contagiosum—the cause, communicability, clinical course, treatment options, length of treatment, possible complications, and indicated follow-up.

→ Advise the patient that as long as lesions are present, they are infectious and to avoid close, intimate contact with others, as well as autoinoculation. Individuals should avoid shaving in areas where lesions are present.

→ Discuss the need for additional STD testing (including HIV, especially if the patient has disseminated infection) and treatment as indicated.

→ Inform patients that people with whom they have intimate contact should be evaluated for molluscum contagiosum or other STDs as indicated.

FOLLOW-UP

→ The patient should return every two weeks for additional treatment until no lesions are present.

→ See "Consultation."

→ Document in progress notes and on problem list.

BIBLIOGRAPHY

Berger, T.G. 2002. Skin, hair, and nails. In *2002 current medical diagnosis and treatment*, eds. L.M. Tierney, Jr., S.J. McPhee, and M.A. Papadakis, p. 174. New York: Lange Medical Books/McGraw-Hill.

Drew, W.L. 2001. Poxviruses. In *Current diagnosis and treatment in infectious diseases*, eds. R. Wilson and M.A. Sande, p. 215. New York: Lange Medical Books/McGraw-Hill.

Fitzpatrick, T.B., Johnson, R.A., Wolff, K. et al. 2001. *Color atlas and synopsis of clinical dermatology. Common and serious diseases*, pp. 754–757. New York: McGraw-Hill.

3-M
Paronychia

Paronychia is an inflammation of the lateral or proximal tissue fold surrounding the nail. In general, the patient's fingernail folds are more commonly affected than the toenail folds.

The initial inflammatory response is caused by exposure to an allergen or irritant. Secondary bacterial infection due to *Staphylococcus aureus, Streptococcus pyogenes*, or *Pseudomonas* results in symptoms and signs associated with acute infection. Chronic inflammation results from infection with a fungal pathogen, usually *Candida albicans* (Fitzpatrick et al. 2001, Fox et al. 2001, Mayeaux 2000, Tosti et al. 2000).

DATABASE

SUBJECTIVE

→ Patient may have a history of frequent water exposure (e.g., daily dishwashing for restaurants) (Fitzpatrick et al. 2001).
→ Symptoms include pain, redness, swelling, and tenderness of the affected area.

OBJECTIVE

→ Patient presents with:
  ■ Edema surrounding the nail fold
  ■ Erythema of the nail fold
  ■ Affected area is warm to the touch.
  ■ Pustular formation may be evident.

ASSESSMENT

→ Paronychia (bacterial or candidal)
→ R/O cellulitis
→ R/O herpetic whitlow

PLAN

DIAGNOSTIC TESTS

→ Potassium hydroxide (KOH) 10% preparation and microscopic evaluation of purulent material will reveal hyphae if *Candida* are present.

→ Culture and sensitivity of purulent material may be ordered if there is evidence of significant infection or when there is a history of recurrence (Fox et al. 2001).

TREATMENT/MANAGEMENT

→ General measures:
  ■ Avoid exposure to irritants, allergens, moisture, and microtrauma.
→ Bacterial paronychia:
  ■ Incision and drainage are indicated when there is pustule formation.
  ■ For deep pustular lesions, systemic antibiotic therapy should be initiated with:
    • Dicloxacillin 250 mg p.o. QID for 7–10 days
                OR
    • Erythromycin 250–500 mg p.o. QID for 7–10 days in penicillin-allergic patients
→ *Candida* paronychia:
  ■ Incise and drain the lesion if fluctuant.
  ■ Topical antifungal therapy includes:
    • Miconazole 2% cream applied TID for 1–2 weeks after resolution of lesion
    • Clotrimazole 1% cream applied TID for 1–2 weeks after resolution of lesion
  ■ Oral antifungals may be prescribed in severe instances of chronic paronychia, but this is rarely needed. If oral antifungals are being considered, consultation with a physician is advised.
  ■ If there is evidence of superimposed bacterial infection, initiation of systemic antibiotics is indicated. See the "Bacterial Paronychia" section above and the **Furuncle and Carbuncle** chapter.
  ■ With chronic paronychia in the absence of water exposure, consider an evaluation for diabetes mellitus.

CONSULTATION

→ Refer the patient to a dermatologist if paronychia is progressing, if it is associated with cellulites, or if it persists after appropriate treatment.

→ As needed for prescription(s)

PATIENT EDUCATION

→ Educate the patient about paronychia—the causes, treatment, possible complications, and any indicated follow-up.

→ Advise the patient to keep her hands dry and warm. If rubber gloves are worn to keep hands dry, they should be placed over cotton gloves.

FOLLOW-UP

→ Individualized according to case presentation

→ See "Consultation."

→ Document in progress notes and on problem list.

BIBLIOGRAPHY

Fitzpatrick, T.B., Johnson, R.A., Wolff, K. et al. 2001. *Color atlas and synopsis of clinical dermatology. Common and serious diseases*, pp. 958–959. New York: McGraw-Hill.

Fox, C.R., and Sande, M.A. 2001. *Candida* species. In *Current diagnosis and treatment in infectious diseases*, eds. W.R. Wilson and M.A. Sande, p. 735. New York: Lange Medical Books/McGraw-Hill.

Mayeaux, E.J., Jr. 2000. Nail disorders. *Primary Care* 27(2): 333–351.

Tosti, A., and Piraccini, B.M. 2000. Treatment of common nail disorders. *Dermatologic Clinics* 18(2):339–348.

3-N
Pediculosis

Pediculosis is a parasitic infestation caused by three species of lice: *Pediculus humanus capitis* (the head louse, infesting the scalp), *Pediculus humanus corporis* (the body or clothing louse, infesting the trunk), and *Pthirus pubis* (the crab louse, infesting pubic and other hair-bearing areas of the body) (Fitzpatrick et al. 2001).

Transmission of pediculosis capitis usually occurs through the use of contaminated hats and/or hair grooming articles, pediculosis corporis as a result of overcrowded living conditions or poor hygiene, and pediculosis pubis through sexual contact. However, close, nonsexual, physical contact can also result in transmission (Fitzpatrick et al. 2001). Head and body lice are highly mobile (i.e., can migrate 23 cm/minute), while pubic lice are very slow (10 cm/day). Pubic lice are able to survive off the human host for 12–48 hours, head lice for up to 55 hours, and body lice for 1–7 days. The manifestations of pediculosis are a result of the host's reaction to saliva or anticoagulant injected by the louse into the dermis while feeding.

Lice eggs are deposited at the base of hair shafts. They are opalescent when viable and less than 0.5–1 mm in diameter. When the nits hatch (6–10 days after laying), the empty egg cases remain on the hair shaft (Fitzpatrick et al. 2001).

DATABASE
SUBJECTIVE

→ The following may be reported by the patient:
  - A history of exposure to pediculosis
  - Symptoms include mild to intense pruritus, worsening at night

Pediculosis Capitis
→ More common in children, but also occurs in adults
→ History of shared caps/hats, combs/brushes
→ History of outbreak in an institution (e.g., school)

Pediculosis Corporis
→ Patient may have a history of poor hygiene.
→ More common among people living in overcrowded conditions (e.g., shelters)

Pediculosis Pubis
→ More common in young adults
→ May coexist with other sexually transmitted diseases (STDs)

OBJECTIVE
The following physical examination findings may be evident (Berger 2002, Fitzpatrick et al. 2001):

Pediculosis Capitis
→ Typically confined to the postauricular and occipital regions (Fitzpatrick et al. 2001)
→ Patient may present with:
  - Erythema and scaling
  - Linear excoriations at hairline from scratching
  - Urticarial eruption over neck and shoulders
  - Variable maculopapular rash on trunk
  - Excoriations, crusts, and secondary impetiginized lesions involving the neck, forehead, face, and ears. In extreme secondary infections, the scalp becomes a confluent mass of matted hair, lice, mites, crusts, and purulent discharge called plica polonica.
  - Cervical lymphadenopathy, especially if secondary bacterial infection
  - Examination of hair shaft may reveal the presence of a louse (which appears to be between 1–4 mm long with a translucent or grayish-white body and six legs); or nits (which appear to be between 0.5–1 mm and whitish in color if they are viable or translucent if the casing is empty).
→ Unlike dandruff, the egg casings cannot be separated from the hair shafts.

Pediculosis Corporis

→ Patient may present with the following:
- Erythematous macules, papules, or urticarial papules with central areas of hemorrhage
- Numerous excoriations caused by intense itching
- Postinflammatory pigmentation of lesions
- Few or no adult organisms evident on body (they attach to host only to feed, then return to the seams of clothing or bedding)
- Louse or nit found in seams of clothing

Pediculosis Pubis

→ Usually affects the pubic area, but can affect any hairy area (e.g., axillae, thighs, periumbilical area, eyelashes).
→ Often there are characteristic maculae ceruleae (bluish-gray macules up to 1 cm in diameter, nonblanching) at feeding sites. The blue color is thought to be a breakdown product of heme caused by louse saliva.
→ Adult organisms can be seen with the naked eye or with the aid of a magnifying lens. Adults are 1–2 mm long, brownish-gray in color, and attached to the hair shaft. Nits are whitish-gray in appearance, 0.5 mm long, and round.

ASSESSMENT

Pediculosis Capitis

→ R/O hair casts, hair gels
→ R/O seborrheic dermatitis
→ R/O contact dermatitis
→ R/O eczema
→ R/O impetigo
→ R/O psoriasis
→ R/O lichen simplex chronicus
→ R/O tinea capitis
→ R/O Candida

Pediculosis Corporis

→ R/O seborrheic dermatitis
→ R/O pyoderma
→ R/O impetigo
→ R/O psoriasis
→ R/O pruritus vulvae
→ R/O folliculitis
→ R/O contact dermatitis
→ R/O tinea cruris
→ R/O Candida

Pediculosis Pubis

→ R/O anogenital eczema/pruritus
→ R/O seborrheic dermatitis
→ R/O tinea cruris
→ R/O folliculitis
→ R/O blepharitis (if eyelash involvement)
→ R/O scabies
→ R/O concomitant STDs

PLAN

DIAGNOSTIC TESTS

→ On microscopic examination in patients with pediculosis capitis and pubis, a plucked hair will show oval nits (eggs) cemented to it.

TREATMENT/MANAGEMENT

Pediculosis Capitis

→ Permethrin (1%) cream rinse applied to the head and scalp and washed off after 30 minutes. Reapplication of treatment is recommended 7–14 days after the first treatment to destroy incubating/hatching nits (Berger 2002, Fitzpatrick et al. 2001).

Pediculosis Corporis

→ Permethrin (1%) cream rinse applied to body and washed off after 10 minutes or permethrin cream 5% applied to the body for 8 hours are effective treatments (Berger 2002). Reapplication of treatment is recommended 7–14 days after the first treatment to destroy incubating/hatching nits (Berger 2002, Fitzpatrick et al. 2001).
→ Lindane lotion 1% in a thin layer applied to the entire skin surface from the patient's neck down, and washed off after 8–12 hours. Retreatment 7–10 days after initial application is necessary to destroy eggs. Not recommended for pregnant or lactating women (Berger 2002, Fitzpatrick et al. 2001). **NOTE:** Overtreatment may be associated with neurotoxicity.
→ Proper hygiene practices are essential.

Pediculosis Pubis

→ Permethrin 1% cream applied to areas of body hair, then completely washed off after 10 minutes. **NOTE:** Permethrin has less potential for toxicity than Lindane in the event of inappropriate use.
→ Lindane 1% shampoo applied to areas of body hair for 4 minutes and then thoroughly washed off. Not recommended for pregnant or lactating women. This agent is used in persons who have not responded to other therapies or who are intolerant of other agents. It has low ovicidal activity. Repeat treatment 7–10 days after the initial treatment is recommended (American Academy of Pediatrics [AAP] 2000).
→ Patients with this condition need counseling and possible testing for other STDs as indicated.
→ Additional considerations:
- Systemic treatment for secondary bacterial infection may be necessary, including:
  - Dicloxacillin 250–500 mg p.o. QID for 10 days
    OR
  - Erythromycin 250–500 mg p.o. QID for 10 days
- If the bacterial infection is minimal and confined to a small area, consider topical antibiotic therapy with mupirocin 2% applied to affected area(s) TID for 10 days. The recommended regimens should not be applied to the eyes.

■ Infestation of eyelashes can be treated with a thick application of petrolatum BID for 8 days with removal of nits after therapy (Berger 2002, Fitzpatrick et al. 2001).

CONSULTATION

→ Physician consultation is indicated in persistent or recurrent infestations, or if there is evidence of significant superimposed bacterial infection.
→ As needed for prescription(s)

PATIENT EDUCATION

→ To prevent future infestations, advise the patient not to share her towels, combs, clothing, or bedding with others and to avoid exposure to known contaminated persons/areas.
→ Advise the patient to treat combs/brushes by soaking them in pediculicidal solution for 15 minutes, or alcohol or Lysol 2% for one hour, and then rinsing them completely.
→ To remove nits from the hair, patients should use a fine-toothed comb. Nit removal is best attempted the day after treatment with a pediculicidal agent. To loosen the glue by which nits attach to the hair shaft, soak the hair with white vinegar (3–5% acetic acid) and apply a towel soaked in the same solution for 30–60 minutes (AAP 2000).
→ Bedding, clothing, and head gear should be machine-washed and dried using the hot cycle of the dryer, or removed from body contact for at least 72 hours.
→ Advise the patient to vacuum floors and furniture completely.

→ Household and close contacts of the infested individual should be examined and treated accordingly.
→ See "Patient Education" in the **Scabies** chapter for management of clothing and bed linens.

FOLLOW-UP

→ Retreatment may be necessary if lice or eggs are seen. **NOTE:** New viable eggs are a creamy-yellow color; empty egg casings are translucent. Empty egg casings are not indicative of active infestation (Fitzpatrick et al. 2001).
→ Alternative treatment regimens may be tried if patient is not responding to the primary regimen(s).
→ See "Consultation."
→ Document in progress notes and on problem list.

BIBLIOGRAPHY

American Academy of Pediatrics (AAP). Committee on Infectious Diseases. 2000. *2000 red book report of the Committee on Infectious Diseases,* 25th ed., ed. L.K. Pickering, pp. 427–431. Elk Grove Village, Ill.: American Academy of Pediatrics.

Berger, T.G. 2002. Skin, hair, and nails. In *2002 current medical diagnosis and treatment,* eds. L.M. Tierney, Jr., S.J. McPhee, and M.A. Papadakis, pp. 179–180. New York: Lange Medical Books/McGraw-Hill.

Fitzpatrick, T.B., Johnson, R.A., Wolff, K. et al. 2001. *Color atlas and synopsis of clinical dermatology. Common and serious diseases,* pp. 826–833. New York: McGraw-Hill.

3-0

Pityriasis Rosea

Pityriasis rosea is a common, mild, self-limited inflammatory skin eruption that is believed to be caused by human herpes virus type 7 (HHV-7) (Berger 2002, Fitzpatrick et al. 2001). The lesions that develop in this condition have a characteristic pattern and will spontaneously resolve within 4–8 weeks (Berger 2002). Pityriasis rosea most often affects young adults, especially women, with an increased incidence during spring and fall. Although infections may be reported in household members, pityriasis rosea is not highly infectious (Berger 2002).

DATABASE

SUBJECTIVE

→ A "herald patch," a single plaque, precedes the generalized rash by 1–2 weeks.
→ Pruritus is usually present but is mild (Berger 2002).
→ Patient may report an oval, pale-brown macular eruption on trunk, back, and extremities, preceded by a bright-red, scaly patch.
→ Patient may report a household contact who has a similar rash.

OBJECTIVE

→ Patient presents with:
  ▪ Herald patch (80% of patients) that is 2–5 cm in diameter, slightly raised, bright-red oval plaque with scaling at the periphery (Berger 2002, Fitzpatrick et al. 2001).
  ▪ Generalized, discrete, maculopapular oval lesions 4–5 mm in diameter with fine scaling, typically distributed symmetrically over the trunk, along cleavage lines, over the back in a "Christmas tree" pattern, and along proximal portions of the extremities.
    • The central portion of lesions may have a crinkled appearance (so-called "cigarette paper" appearance) (Berger 2002).

ASSESSMENT

→ Pityriasis rosea
→ R/O secondary syphilis (feet and hands usually have palmar erythema)
→ R/O drug eruption
→ R/O tinea corporis
→ R/O tinea versicolor
→ R/O seborrheic dermatitis
→ R/O psoriasis (especially guttate psoriasis)
→ R/O erythema migrans
→ R/O viral exanthem

PLAN

DIAGNOSTIC TESTS

→ Though specific diagnostic tests to confirm diagnosis are not necessary, the following tests may be done:
  ▪ VDRL or RPR to rule out secondary syphilis (Berger 2002).
  ▪ A scraping of the eruption can be examined microscopically using potassium hydroxide (KOH) 10% to rule out a fungal infection (Berger 2002).
  ▪ Skin biopsy should be considered if the rash/lesions persist for more than eight weeks (Fitzpatrick et al. 2001).

TREATMENT/MANAGEMENT

→ Usually no treatment is required other than symptomatic relief measures.
→ In patients with pruritus, the following antipruritic solutions can be applied to the affected areas as needed (varying results reported):
  ▪ Camphor 5%, menthol 5%, phenol 5% (Sarna®) lotion (an over-the-counter product)
  ▪ Pramoxine hydrochloride 1% cream or lotion
→ Medium-strength topical corticosteroids may be prescribed for darker pigmented patients as a means of reducing hyperpigmentation (Berger 2002). These include:

- Triamcinolone acetonide 0.1% cream or lotion applied to affected areas BID–TID
- Alclometasone dipropionate 0.5% cream or ointment applied to affected areas BID–TID

→ Antihistamines may be prescribed if the patient is experiencing severe pruritus:
- Hydroxyzine 25 mg every 6 hours as needed
  NOTE: Warn patient regarding associated drowsiness. It may be beneficial for the patient to take 50 mg at bedtime.

CONSULTATION

→ Refer patients whose lesions do not clear up after eight weeks to a dermatologist.
→ As necessary for prescription(s)

PATIENT EDUCATION

→ Reassure the patient that spontaneous clearing will occur, usually within 6–8 weeks.

→ Although pityriasis rosea is infectious, it is not highly contagious, so affected individuals do not need to isolate themselves from others.
→ Educate the patient regarding possible side effects associated with recommended medications.

FOLLOW-UP

→ Individualized according to case presentation
→ See "Consultation."
→ Document in progress notes and on problem list.

BIBLIOGRAPHY

Berger, T.G. 2002. Skin, hair, and nails. In *2002 current medical diagnosis and treatment*, eds. L.M. Tierney, Jr., S.J. McPhee, and M.A. Papadakis, p. 143. New York: Lange Medical Books/McGraw-Hill.

Fitzpatrick, T.B., Johnson, R.A., Wolff, K. et al. 2001. *Color atlas and synopsis of clinical dermatology. Common and serious diseases*, pp. 106–108. New York: McGraw-Hill.

3-P

Psoriasis

Psoriasis is a common skin condition that affects 3–5 million people in the United States. It is characterized by scaling papules or plaques appearing acutely or chronically on elbows, knees, or the scalp (Berger 2002, Fitzpatrick et al. 2001). The cause of psoriasis is not known, but its association with specific HLA types, including HLA-B13, HLA-B17, HLA-Bw57, and HLA-Cw6, suggests a genetic predisposition (Fitzpatrick et al. 2001). If an individual has a parent with psoriasis, her risk of developing the condition is 8%; if both parents have psoriasis, the risk is 41% (Fitzpatrick et al. 2001).

The pathogenesis of psoriasis involves an abnormality in the function of keratinocytes that results in a shortening of the cell lifecycle with increased production of epidermal cells at 28 times the normal rate (Fitzpatrick et al. 2001). This pathophysiologic activity is the basis for the clinical manifestations associated with this condition. Factors associated with an acute exacerbation of psoriasis include stress, trauma (e.g., irritation, injury), alcohol consumption, infection (e.g., human immunodeficiency virus [HIV], streptococcal infection), or exposure to certain medications (e.g., lithium, oral glucocorticosteroids) (Berger 2002, Fitzpatrick et al. 2001).

There are various types of psoriasis, including the plaque-like form, *guttate psoriasis* (which often follows streptococcal pharyngitis), and a generalized erythrodermic pustule form (von Zumbusch syndrome), which is rare but may be life-threatening. In addition, arthritis occurs in 5–8% of individuals with psoriasis, with approximately 10% of these patients not manifesting other signs or symptoms of psoriasis. However, there is usually a family history of psoriasis in this group (Fitzpatrick et al. 2001).

DATABASE

SUBJECTIVE

→ The patient may report the following (Berger 2002, Fitzpatrick et al. 2001):
  ■ History may include:
    • Minor trauma of affected area (Koebner phenomenon)
    • Use of systemic corticosteroids, lithium, alcohol, or chloroquine

  • Exposure to sunlight
  • Pharyngitis
  • Stress
  • Family history of psoriasis
  ■ Symptoms include:
    • Localized or generalized eruption(s) of pink lesions with scaling lasting for a few days (acute exacerbation) to several months (chronic form)
    • Pruritus (common)
    • Brownish-yellow, thick, pitted nails
    • Pain and swelling of finger joints
    • Obesity
    • Generalized pustules, fever, weakness, and chills (von Zumbusch syndrome)

OBJECTIVE

The following findings may be evident upon physical examination:

→ Vital signs are usually within normal limits but there may be an increased temperature if coexistent streptococcal infection or von Zumbusch syndrome.

→ Lesions:
  ■ May reveal sharply marginated, erythematous papules and plaques covered with silver-white scales, usually on the scalp, palms, soles, and the extensor surfaces of the elbows and knees. In addition, the sacrum, perineum, and genitalia may be involved.
  ■ May erupt on the face, but are rare
  ■ May be round, oval, or annular
  ■ Are usually bilateral, often symmetric
  ■ Hands are usually less erythematous than other sites.

→ Auspitz's sign (pinpoint bleeding) may occur if scale(s) are removed.

→ Nails may be stippled or pitted, yellow, thick, or distorted with swelling, redness, and scaling of the paronychial margin and arthritis of the distal interphalangeal joint. Salmon patches, a localized reddish discoloration in the central por-

tion of the nail, are pathognomonic. Oil drop sign is onycholysis localized at the nailbed, which appears like a "drop of oil on a piece of paper" (Mayeaux 2000).
NOTE: Nail involvement is noted in 10–50% of patients with psoriasis, but in some persons nail manifestations may occur without other signs and symptoms of psoriasis.
→ Edema, tenderness of interphalangeal joints
→ Guttate psoriasis (rare) presents as 2.0–1.0 cm, salmon-pink, "drop-like" lesions distributed diffusely over the trunk, face, and scalp. Palms and soles are unaffected.

ASSESSMENT

→ Psoriasis
→ R/O seborrheic dermatitis
→ R/O lichen simplex chronicus
→ R/O candidiasis (confused with intertriginous psoriasis)
→ R/O psoriasiform drug eruptions (especially beta-blockers, gold, and methyldopa)
→ R/O eczema
→ R/O glucagonoma syndrome (malignant tumor of pancreatic islet cells)
→ R/O guttate psoriasis
→ R/O von Zumbusch syndrome
→ R/O pityriasis rosea
→ R/O secondary syphilis
→ R/O tinea
→ R/O onychomycosis
→ R/O Reiter's syndrome
→ R/O HIV infection (especially when symptoms are severe)

PLAN

DIAGNOSTIC TESTS

→ Usually, the skin eruption and distribution are diagnostic. However, the following tests may be ordered as indicated:
  ▪ VDRL or RPR to rule out syphilis
  ▪ Skin scrapings of lesions for potassium hydroxide 10% microscopic evaluation to rule out fungal infections
  ▪ Throat culture—may be positive for group A beta-hemolytic streptococcus in guttate psoriasis.
  ▪ Uric acid may be elevated.
  ▪ Rheumatoid factor will be negative.
  ▪ HIV antibody test may or may not be positive.

TREATMENT/MANAGEMENT

→ In individuals with mild disease involving less than 5% of the body surface, treatment can be initiated by the primary care clinician. In other individuals with psoriasis, referral to a dermatologist is advised. The following therapeutic strategies can be initiated depending on the amount and severity of disease (Berger 2002, Chu 2000, Drew 2000, Fitzpatrick et al. 2001):
  ▪ Mild, limited disease can be managed with the following therapeutic interventions:

  • After soaking the lesion and removing the scaling skin, application of a mid- to high-potency topical corticosteroid such as:
    – Fluocinonide 0.05% cream or gel applied BID for 14–21 days
    – Fluocinolone acetonide 0.2% cream or 0.025% ointment applied BID for 14–21 days
    NOTE: After 14–21 days of daily topical corticosteroid therapy, pulse therapy consisting of TID–QID on weekends thereafter (Berger 2002). It often is beneficial to apply an occlusive, plastic-wrap covering over the area after using the topical steroid, especially if the covering can be left in place overnight. Avoid using mid- to high-potency topical corticosteroids on the face, breasts, genitalia, or body folds, or for extended periods of time to avoid tachyphylaxis and atrophy of the skin.
  • Vitamin D analogues (calcipotriene 0.001% cream or ointment) are nonsteroidal agents that can be combined with high-potency topical corticosteroid agents. By using calcipotriene daily during the week, topical steroids can be used on the weekends.
    NOTE: Calcipotriene should not be used on ≥40% of the body surface and not >100 g per week. Do not use on the face or groin due to irritation.
  • In patients with mild, isolated lesions, occlusive dressings using Duoderm® (applied to lesion and left in place for 5–7 days) may be beneficial without topical corticosteroids.
  • Retinoid analogues (e.g., Tazarotene® 0.5–1% gel or cream) can be used QD–BID. They can be used in conjunction with other treatments such as topical steroids to treat plaques.
  • Scalp involvement can be treated initially with a tar shampoo used daily. If thick scales are present, the application of salicylic acid gel 6% to the scalp and then covering the scalp with a shower cap may be beneficial.
▪ If moderate to severe pruritus is reported by the patient, consider prescribing an antihistamine such as:
  • Hydroxyzine 10–50 mg p.o. at bedtime prn
  NOTE: Advise the patient regarding drowsiness associated with these medications and to avoid driving or other potentially dangerous activities while taking them.
▪ Psoriasis that covers more than 30% of the body surface is difficult to treat with topical corticosteroids and usually requires outpatient UVB-light exposure 3 times a week for several weeks. Refer to a dermatologist for evaluation and treatment.
▪ If the patient has a positive throat culture for group A beta-hemolytic streptococcal infection, then treatment with the appropriate antibiotic (e.g., penicillin VK) should be initiated.

CONSULTATION

→ Consultation with a dermatologist is indicated if guttate psoriasis is suspected.

→ Consult with a physician as needed for prescription(s) and when using high-potency topical corticosteroids.

→ Refer patients with psoriasis that covers more than 5% of the body to a dermatologist for evaluation and treatment (Fitzpatrick et al. 2001).

PATIENT EDUCATION

→ Educate the patient regarding psoriasis—the cause(s), possible therapeutic interventions, length of treatment, possible complications/side effects of medications, and indicated follow-up.

→ Advise the patient to avoid factors that can aggravate psoriasis (e.g., sunlight exposure, alcohol consumption, stress, and trauma to the area).

→ Review hygiene and advise the patient to avoid rubbing or scratching the lesions to prevent the Koebner phenomenon and the possibility of a secondary bacterial infection.

FOLLOW-UP

→ Individualized according to case presentation

→ See "Consultation."

→ Document in progress notes and on problem list.

BIBLIOGRAPHY

Berger T.G. 2002. Skin, hair, and nails. In *2002 current medical diagnosis and treatment,* eds. L.M. Tierney, Jr., S.J. McPhee, and M.A. Papadakis, pp. 141–143. New York: Lange Medical Books/McGraw-Hill.

Chu, T. 2000. Better patient compliance in psoriasis. *Practitioner* 244:238–244.

Drew, G.S. 2000. Psoriasis. *Primary Care* 27(2):385–406.

Fitzpatrick, T.B., Johnson, R.A., Wolff, K. et al. 2001. *Color atlas and synopsis of clinical dermatology. Common and serious diseases,* pp. 50–65. New York: McGraw-Hill.

Mayeaux, E.J. 2000. Nail disorders. *Primary Care* 27(2): 333–351.

3-Q

Scabies

Scabies is a skin infestation caused by a mite, *Sarcoptes scabiei*. It is often described as a sexually transmitted disease. However, because the mite can remain alive off the host for more than two days, transmission can occur through close personal contact or shared clothing or bedding (Fitzpatrick et al. 2001). In a primary scabies infection, there is an incubation period of 2–6 weeks between the time of infection and the onset of itching. With subsequent infestation, symptoms may begin within 1–3 days after reinfestation because the person is sensitized to the mite (Fitzpatrick et al. 2001).

In immunocompromised individuals and debilitated or senile patients, scabies infection may present with a generalized dermatitis characterized by scaling, vesicles, and crusting of the eruption. Pruritus may be absent or minimal. These clinical manifestations are associated with a type of scabies called *Norwegian scabies*, which is highly transmissible due to the high concentration of mites in the exfoliating scales (Berger 2002).

DATABASE

SUBJECTIVE

→ Patient may report exposure to a close contact with scabies.
→ Symptoms may include:
  ■ Moderate to severe generalized itching, worsening at night
  ■ Papulovesicular lesions

OBJECTIVE

→ Patient may present with:
  ■ Evidence of "burrows" or "runs" that are 2–3 mm long with a papule or vesicle at the end of the tunnel (Fitzpatrick et al. 2001). Burrows are usually found in/on digital webs, palms, wrists, vulva, nipples, gluteal folds, buttock, axillae, or toes, with a minute vesicle or papule at the end. Infestation of the face, neck, and soles of the feet is rare but may occur in the elderly or immunocompromised (e.g., human immunodeficiency virus [HIV] infection).
  ■ Vesicles in isolation, often on sides of fingers

  ■ Nodules that are indurated, brownish-red, 0.5–2.0 cm in diameter, often on axillary folds, upper back, groin, buttocks
  ■ Papules on abdomen, buttocks, or inner thighs
  ■ Eczematous plaques and/or excoriations often on the hands and axillae; if on the breasts, may resemble Paget's disease
  ■ Excoriation or lichenification if chronic rubbing or scratching
  ■ Crusting of lesions, suggesting secondary bacterial infection
  ■ Erythema, tenderness, crusting, pustules if secondary bacterial infection
  ■ Lymphadenopathy may be noted.
  ■ Diffuse, urticarial, edematous papules on the forearms, anterior trunk, thighs, and buttocks if autosensitization type ("Id") reaction
  ■ Norwegian or "crusted" scabies presents as psoriasiform or eczematous lesions often observed on the face, scalp, palms, and soles (Fitzpatrick et al. 2001).
→ Atypical crusted or "exaggerated" scabies may occur in HIV-infected patients.

ASSESSMENT

→ Scabies
→ R/O atopic dermatitis
→ R/O papular urticaria
→ R/O pyoderma
→ R/O impetigo
→ R/O insect bites
→ R/O dermatitis herpetiformis

PLAN

DIAGNOSTIC TESTS

→ For microscopic detection of mites:
  ■ Locate a burrow in typical sites for burrows (as described above) and isolate a "dark point" (the mite) at the end of the burrow (a magnifying lens may aid this process). The

best areas in which to attempt to isolate a mite are on the finger webs or flexor aspects of the wrists.

- Slowly open burrow at the dark point, using a needle or thin surgical blade (e.g., #15 scalpel blade). The mite will stick to the point of the needle/blade.
- It can then be transferred to a slide containing immersion oil or mineral oil and viewed microscopically (Fitzpatrick et al. 2001).
- Visualization of the mite, egg, or mite feces (scybole) is diagnostic.

→ Bacterial culture can be performed if secondary infection is suspected.

TREATMENT/MANAGEMENT

→ Topical treatment is usually successful in treating scabies. Topical agents include:

- Permethrin 5% cream is the drug of choice because many scabies infestations are resistant to other antiscabies medications. Topical application should occur after the patient has bathed. The cream is applied to the entire skin surface from the neck down (with special attention to hands, feet, and intertriginous area), left on for 8–14 hours, then washed off (shower or bath). Generally, 1 application is curative; however, a repeat treatment can be done 1 week after the initial treatment if severe pruritus continues (Berger 2002, Fitzpatrick et al. 2001).
- Other agents that have been used include lindane 1% and crotamiton applied from the neck down overnight for 4 consecutive nights. See the *Physicians' Desk Reference* for details on use and contraindications.
  NOTE: Lindane has been associated with neurotoxicity and should be avoided in infants, pregnant women, and patients with open skin or widespread excoriations (Berger 2002).

→ Topical treatment failures, especially in patients with crusted scabies, may require systemic therapy using ivermectin 200 µg/kg p.o. single dose with a second dose administered 1 week later (Berger 2002, Fitzpatrick et al. 2001).
NOTE: Ivermectin should not be used in children or pregnant women.

→ Because scabicidal therapy is antibacterial, most patients with secondary bacterial infection do not require antibiotic therapy. However, in certain cases, antibiotic therapy may be indicated.

- Topical therapy—if a few small areas are involved—using:
  • Mupirocin 2% ointment applied to affected area(s) TID for 10 days
- Systemic therapy should be instituted in cases of extensive secondary bacterial infection, with one of the following:
  • Dicloxacillin 500 mg p.o. every 6 hours for 10 days
  OR
  • Erythromycin 500 mg p.o. every 6 hours for 10 days

→ Post-scabietic pruritus can persist for up to 2 weeks after successful eradication of mites. Systemic antipruritic therapy for this may include the use of an antihistamine such as hydroxyzine 25 mg p.o. every 6 hours prn.
NOTE: Advise the patient that drowsiness is associated with this medication and to avoid activities that require concentration (e.g., driving).

→ Systemic glucocorticosteroids may be needed in patients with severe hypersensitivity reaction to scabies.

CONSULTATION

→ Refer a patient with hypersensitivity reaction to scabies, with recalcitrant scabies, or with persistent nodules to a dermatologist. These may require systemic treatment and/or intralesional corticosteroids (Berger 2002, Fitzpatrick et al. 2001).

→ For cases in which there is severe secondary bacterial infection

→ As necessary for prescription(s)

PATIENT EDUCATION

→ Educate the patient about scabies—the cause, infectivity, clinical course, treatment, and prevention.

→ Advise the patient:

- Not to wash her hands after applying the medication due to the need to treat any infestation involving hands
- Not to overtreat the condition, as this may lead to irritant dermatitis
- That 24 hours after completing therapy, she is no longer able to transmit the disease. However, symptoms may persist for weeks as a result of a hypersensitivity reaction to the mite.

→ Sexual and close personal or household contacts of the patient should be treated prophylactically (Orkin et al. 1990).

→ Clothing and bed linen should be changed before treatment to avoid reinfestation. Towels, bedding, and clothing used within four days prior to treatment should be machine washed in hot, soapy water. Nonwashable clothing or bedding should be stored in plastic for two weeks (American Academy of Pediatrics [AAP] 2000).

→ Infested individuals may return to work or school after completing a single recommended treatment (AAP 2000).

→ Prophylactic treatment of sexual contacts or close personal household contacts within the past month is recommended. All members of a household should be treated at the same time to prevent re-exposure and re-infection (AAP 2000, Fitzpatrick et al. 2001).

→ Vacuuming environmental surfaces is recommended in households where a patient has been diagnosed with Norwegian ("crusted") scabies (AAP 2000).

FOLLOW-UP

→ If itching or lesions persist for more than two weeks, or new lesions appear more than one week after treatment, a second application of antiscabies medication may be indicated (Berger 2002, Fitzpatrick et al. 2001).

→ See "Consultation."

→ Document in progress notes and on problem list.

BIBLIOGRAPHY

American Academy of Pediatrics (AAP). Committee on Infectious Diseases. 2000. In *2000 red book report of the Committee on Infectious Diseases*, 25th ed., ed. L.K. Pickering, pp. 506–508. Elk Grove Village, Ill.: American Academy of Pediatrics.

Berger, T.G. 2002. Skin, hair, and nails. In *2002 current medical diagnosis and treatment*, eds. L.M. Tierney, Jr., S.J. McPhee, and M.A. Papadakis, pp. 178–179. New York, NY: Lange Medical Books/McGraw-Hill.

Fitzpatrick, T.B., Johnson, R.A., Wolff, K. et al. 2001. *Color atlas and synopsis of clinical dermatology. Common and serious diseases*, pp. 834–842. New York: McGraw-Hill.

Orkin, M., and Maibach, H. 1990. Scabies. In *Sexually transmitted diseases*, 2nd ed., eds. K.K. Holmes, P.-A. Mårdh, P.F. Sparling et al., pp. 473-479. New York: McGraw-Hill.

3-R
Seborrheic Dermatitis

Seborrheic dermatitis is an acute or chronic inflammatory condition of the skin characterized by erythema; dry, scaling skin; and yellow, crusted patches usually occurring on the scalp, central face, body folds, umbilicus, and presternal and interscapular areas of the body (Berger 2002, Fitzpatrick et al. 2001, Johnson et al. 2000).

Though the etiology is unknown, causal relationships have been postulated. These include a genetic predisposition to the condition and an inflammatory response to *Pityrosporum ovale* (also known as *Malassezia furfur*), a yeast organism found on the scalp of all humans (Berger 2002, Fitzpatrick et al. 2001). Additional factors that may aggravate seborrheic dermatitis include certain medications (e.g., methyldopa [Aldomet®]), emotional stress, alcohol intake, hormones, and some infections, such as human immunodeficiency virus (HIV) infection (Berger 2002, Fitzpatrick et al. 2001).

Seborrheic dermatitis often exists with other dermatologic conditions, such as psoriasis, acne rosacea, and acne vulgaris. The majority of individuals affected are adults 20–50 years old. Exacerbations are frequently noted during winter months or when the individual is exposed to high temperatures (e.g., from heaters) or increased humidity (Berger 2002, Fitzpatrick et al. 2001).

DATABASE

SUBJECTIVE

→ Symptoms may include (Berger 2002, Fitzpatrick et al. 2001, Johnson et al. 2000):
- Pruritus
- Dry scaling and erythema of eyelid margins
- Erythematous, dry scaling of skin on scalp, face, chest, back, skin folds

→ Patient may report:
- A family history of seborrheic dermatitis
- Coexisting dermatological conditions
- Medical conditions associated with increased incidence of seborrheic dermatitis (e.g., HIV infection, Parkinson's disease)

- Use of medications that may aggravate the condition (e.g., Aldomet®)

OBJECTIVE

→ Characteristics of lesions include (Berger 2002, Fitzpatrick et al. 2001, Johnson et al. 2000):
- Erythema
- May have a yellow or orange hue
- Vary in size from 5–20 mm
- Sharp margins
- May be psoriaform and plaque-like
- Dry, moist, or greasy scaling (Berger 2002, Fitzpatrick et al. 2001)
- Sticky or weeping crusts

→ Lesions are most often located in/on:
- Perinasal areas
- Ears
- Scalp
- Supraorbital areas
- Eyelids
- Genitalia
- Perianal area and gluteal folds
- Chest, submammary areas
- Umbilicus
- Back
- Axillae

ASSESSMENT

→ Seborrheic dermatitis
→ R/O pityriasis rosea
→ R/O tinea versicolor
→ R/O psoriasis
→ R/O candidiasis
→ R/O zinc deficiency
→ R/O impetigo
→ R/O lupus erythematosus
→ R/O pemphigus foliaceous

PLAN

DIAGNOSTIC TESTS

→ Usually, no specific diagnostic tests are required to confirm the diagnosis in the majority of patients. However, the following tests may be ordered as indicated to eliminate the possibility of other conditions:

- Scraping of lesion for microscopic examination with potassium hydroxide (KOH) 10% to evaluate for presence of fungal organisms
- Fungal culture if a particular fungal organism is suspected and a definitive diagnosis is desired

TREATMENT/MANAGEMENT

→ Underlying conditions (e.g., Parkinson's disease, emotional stress) that may aggravate seborrheic dermatitis should be treated.

→ Seborrhea of the scalp (mild to moderate) (Berger 2002, Johnson et al. 2000):

- May be treated with over-the-counter shampoos that contain tar, zinc, pyrithione, or selenium (e.g., Neutrogena T/Gel®, Selsun®). The patient should shampoo daily with one of these products.
- Ketoconazole 2% shampoo can be used twice a week.
- Topical corticosteroid solutions or lotions can be added if symptoms persist. To prevent tachyphylaxis, use these agents intermittently and only when the symptoms persist. The patient should apply a small amount of one of the following agents to the affected areas at bedtime:
  - Triamcinolone acetonide 0.1%
  - Betamethasone dipropionate 0.05%
  - Fluocinonide 0.05%

→ Seborrhea of the face (Berger 2002, Johnson et al. 2000):

- Use mild soaps to cleanse the face as a means of avoiding further irritation.
- Scalp treatment usually reduces facial involvement.
- Low-potency topical corticosteroids can be used intermittently (avoid area surrounding the eyes), including:
  - Hydrocortisone 1% applied to affected area(s) BID
  - Alclometasone dipropionate 0.5% applied to affected area BID
- Use of fluorinated topical corticosteroids on the face is not recommended due to the possibility of atrophy, telangiectasia, or steroid rosacea.
- If symptoms persist after scalp therapy and use of mild soaps, ketoconazole 2% cream can be applied to the affected areas BID for 4 weeks.

→ Seborrhea of the body (Berger 2002, Johnson et al. 2000):

- Use of mild soaps in axillary and groin areas only with daily bathing
- Low-potency topical steroids can be effective in non-hairy areas, including:
  - Hydrocortisone 1.0–2.5% cream BID–TID to affected areas until resolution

  - Desonide 0.05% cream BID–TID to affected areas until resolution
  - Alclometasone dipropionate 0.5% cream BID–TID until resolution
- Ketoconazole 2% cream BID to affected areas can be used as an alternate therapy to topical steroids but is reportedly less effective (Fitzpatrick et al. 2001).

→ Seborrhea of intertriginous areas (Berger 2002, Johnson et al. 2000):

- Apply low-potency topical steroids (under "Treatment/Management," see "Seborrhea of the body") BID for 5–7 days and then once or twice a week.
- Avoid the use of oil-based ointments in these areas.

→ Seborrhea of the eyelids:

- Gentle cleansing of the eyelid margins with undiluted Johnson & Johnson Baby Shampoo® using a soft, cotton-tip swab at bedtime is usually effective (Berger 2002).

CONSULTATION

→ Refer severe or persistent cases to a dermatologist for further evaluation and treatment.

→ As needed for prescription(s)

PATIENT EDUCATION

→ Educate the patient about seborrheic dermatitis, including the cause(s), aggravating factors, treatment options and length of treatment, possible side effects of medications, and indicated follow-up.

→ Advise the patient to avoid the use of fluorinated corticosteroids on the face and prolonged use elsewhere to prevent telangiectasia and erythema.

→ If tar shampoos dry hair, advise the patient to use hair conditioners.

→ If severe, intractable seborrheic dermatitis, consider HIV counseling and testing.

FOLLOW-UP

→ Individualized according to case presentation

→ See "Consultation."

→ Document in progress notes and on problem list.

BIBLIOGRAPHY

Berger T.G. 2002. Skin, hair, and nails. In *2002 current medical diagnosis and treatment*, eds. L.M. Tierney, Jr., S.J. McPhee, and M.A. Papadakis, pp. 143–144. New York: Lange Medical Books/McGraw-Hill.

Fitzpatrick, T.B., Johnson, R.A., Wolff, K. et al. 2001. *Color atlas and synopsis of clinical dermatology. Common and serious diseases*, pp. 45–48. New York: McGraw-Hill.

Johnson, B.A., and Nunley, J.R. 2000. Treatment of seborrheic dermatitis. *American Family Physician* 61(9):2703–2712.

3-S

Warts

Warts are caused by various types of *human papillomaviruses (HPV)*, each manifesting as a different form of wart. There are four types of warts: *flat warts* (verruca plana), *common warts* (verruca vulgaris), *plantar warts* (verruca plantaris), and *genital warts* (condyloma acuminata). There is an increased incidence of warts in younger individuals, with a reduction in common warts noted after age 25. Flat warts and plantar warts are more common in women. (Genital warts are discussed in the **Sexually Transmitted Diseases** chapters in Section 13.)

Warts may be spread by personal contact, by fomites, and autoinoculation from one part of the body to another through minor trauma to the skin (Fitzpatrick et al. 2001). The average incubation period is approximately three months, with a range of 2–18 months (Berger 2002). In 50% of individuals, warts spontaneously resolve; however, recurrences are frequent (Berger 2002, Drew 2001). Twenty-three of more than 150 HPV subtypes are associated with malignant neoplasms. HPV types 5, 8, and 19 are associated with squamous cell carcinoma, especially in patients with epidermodysplasia verruciformis (an autosomal recessive condition) or immunosuppression (Fitzpatrick et al. 2001). However, the majority of nongenital warts are benign (Fitzpatrick et al. 2001).

DATABASE

SUBJECTIVE

→ The majority of patients are asymptomatic.
→ Symptoms may include:
- In plantar warts, occasional pain with pressure
- Occasionally mild pruritus
- Mechanical obstruction, which may be reported if the wart is located in nostril or ear canal
- Plantar warts may appear at sites of trauma or pressure.

OBJECTIVE

Verruca Plana ("Flat Wart")
(Fitzpatrick et al. 2001)

→ Mesa-like, flat-topped, round, oval, polygonal, or linear papules, usually 1–2 mm thick
→ Skin-colored or light brown
→ Numerous, discrete, and closely set
→ Favor face, dorsa of hands, and shins

Verruca Vulgaris (Common Wart)

→ Firm papules 1–10 mm in diameter
→ Hyperkeratotic, cleft, with multiple conical projections (vegetations)
→ Skin-colored, "reddish-brown dots" (thrombosed capillary loops) may be seen.
→ Isolated or scattered discrete lesions
→ Usually occur on hands, fingers, and knees

Verruca Plantaris (Plantar Wart)

→ Shiny, sharply marginated papule or plaque with hyperkeratotic surface
→ Skin-colored; may need to pierce wart with a scalpel to see reddish-brown dots diagnostic of warts.
→ Usually appear as an isolated lesion but more may be present in a mosaic pattern (Fitzpatrick et al. 2001)

ASSESSMENT

→ Verruca vulgaris
→ Verruca plantaris
→ Verruca plana
→ R/O basal cell carcinoma
→ R/O squamous cell carcinoma
→ R/O actinic keratosis
→ R/O molluscum contagiosum

→ R/O condyloma acuminata
→ R/O inflammatory dermatoses
→ R/O callus
→ R/O foreign body

PLAN

DIAGNOSTIC TESTS

→ Though the physical findings usually are adequate to make the diagnosis of warts, a biopsy of a wart-like lesion may be indicated in the following situations to rule out squamous cell carcinoma:
  - Large, chronic warts in an older individual
  - Wart-like lesions in sun-damaged skin areas

TREATMENT/MANAGEMENT

Verruca Plana

- Usually involve spontaneously over months to years without scarring, so avoid destructive treatments (Berger 2002, Fitzpatrick et al. 2001).
- Retinoic acid 0.1% cream or 0.25% gel applied BID for 4–6 weeks may be effective in the treatment of facial warts (Berger 2002, Fitzpatrick et al. 2001).
- Imiquimod 5% cream applied at HS 3 times a week to affected areas that are not thickly keratinized may be effective (Fitzpatrick et al. 2001).

Verruca Vulgaris

→ Keratolytic agents are safe and effective, with minimal or no side effects when used properly (Berger 2002).
→ Small lesions: salicylic acid/lactic acid collodion 10–20% gel or liquid applied to affected area under occlusion at bedtime, then washed off in the morning (Berger 2002). **NOTE:** Patient should hydrate the area by soaking the affected area(s) for 5 minutes in warm water prior to the application of the keratolytic agent.
→ Large lesions: 40% salicylic-acid plaster for 1 week, followed by salicylic acid/lactic acid collodion or liquid nitrogen for 10–30 seconds to flat lesions. The area of freezing should extend 1–2 mm beyond the lesion and thaw time should be 30–45 seconds. A second freezing is done as above. A blister will appear in 12–24 hours. This should be left intact. The patient should be seen again in 2–3 weeks and assessed for retreatment (Berger 2002, Fitzpatrick et al. 2001).

Verruca Plantaris

- If asymptomatic, do not treat because 50% will involute in 6 months.
- Surgical removal is not recommended, as painful scarring can result (Berger 2002).
- Salicylic-acid 40% plaster applied after soaking the warts in warm water and scraping off dead tissue and leaving on for 4–6 days can be effective. This is continued until normal skin lines return (Berger 2002, Fitzpatrick et al. 2001).
- Soaking the warts in hot water for ½–¾ hour, 2–3 times a week for 16 treatments can be effective because warts are thermolabile (Berger 2002, Fitzpatrick et al. 2001).

CONSULTATION

→ Refer to a dermatologist those patients with periungual warts, facial warts, unresponsive warts, suspicious wart-like lesions, and individuals with peripheral vascular diseases or diabetes mellitus who have warts on their extremities.
→ Refer to a dermatologist for laser, injection, electrocautery, or surgical treatment of warts.

PATIENT EDUCATION

→ Educate the patient regarding warts—the cause, clinical course, treatment options, possible side effects or complications associated with treatment(s), and indicated follow-up.
→ Teach patients to avoid shaving flat warts, as this may spread lesions.

FOLLOW-UP

→ See "Treatment/Management" and "Consultation."
→ Document in progress notes and on problem list.

BIBLIOGRAPHY

Berger, T.G. 2002. Skin, hair, and nails. In *2002 current medical diagnosis and treatment*, eds. L.M. Tierney, Jr., S.J. McPhee, and M.A. Papadakis, pp. 171–172. New York: Lange Medical Books/McGraw-Hill.

Drew, W.L. 2001. Papoviruses. In *Current diagnosis and treatment in infectious diseases*, eds. W.R. Wilson and M.A. Sande, pp. 471–474. New York: Lange Medical Books/ McGraw-Hill.

Fitzpatrick, T.B., Johnson, R.A., Wolff, K. et al. 2001. *Color atlas and synopsis of clinical dermatology. Common and serious diseases*, pp. 761–765. New York: McGraw-Hill.

SECTION 4

Breast Disorders

4-A Breast Cancer Screening 4-2
4-B Breast Pain and Nodularity 4-6
4-C Duct Ectasia/Periductal Mastitis. 4-10
4-D Fat Necrosis 4-12
4-E Fibroadenoma 4-14
4-F Fluid Cysts 4-16
4-G Galactocele 4-18
4-H Galactorrhea 4-20
4-I Intraductal Papilloma 4-23
4-J Mastitis—Nonpuerperal. 4-25
4-K Nipple Discharge—Physiologic 4-27
4-L Paget's Disease 4-29
4-M Superficial Phlebitis (Mondor's Disease) 4-31

4-A

Breast Cancer Screening

One out of every nine American women will develop breast cancer during her lifetime. Breast cancer is the second leading cause of cancer death in women (lung cancer ranks first), accounting for 30% of all female cancers (Leitch 2001). Recent studies show that the mortality rate from breast cancer has decreased substantially over the last decade at a rate of 1.8% per year (Leitch 2001). The primary reason for this change is the increasing incidence of in situ breast cancer (early stage) found through increasing use of screening mammography. The proportion of in situ breast cancer has increased from 3.6% in 1983 to 18% in 1999 (Leitch 2001).

Although some of the risk factors that increase a woman's risk of developing breast cancer are understood, researchers do not know what causes most breast cancers. Scientists are looking at how changes (mutations) in the DNA can cause normal breast cells to become cancerous. Most breast cancers have several gene mutations that are not inherited but instead develop over a woman's lifetime. Recent studies show that approximately 10% of breast cancer cases are due to inherited mutations in breast cancer genes. The most common mutations are in the genes BRCA1 and BRCA2. About 50–60% of women with an inherited mutation will develop breast cancer by age 70. Women with these inherited mutations also have an increased risk of developing ovarian cancer. Inherited mutations of the p53 tumor suppressor gene can also increase a woman's risk of developing breast cancer as well as other cancers. This is known as the *Li-Fraumeni syndrome*.

Breast cancer greatly concerns women, especially those who have significant risk factors. Since only 25% of cancers of the breast occur in defined risk groups, breast cancer screening should be done for all asymptomatic women. It should be emphasized that screening guidelines only apply to asymptomatic women. Women with significant risk factors or those with a history or current breast symptoms may need more frequent screening and diagnostic evaluation.

DATABASE

SUBJECTIVE

→ Risk factors include (American Cancer Society 2001a, Apantaku 2000):
- Gender
  - Breast cancer is about 100 times more common in women than in men.
- Increasing age
  - There is a progressive rise in incidence with age.
  - Women under 30 years account for only 0.3% of cases.
- Genetic risk factors
  - Women with inherited mutations of BRCA1, BRCA2, or the p53 tumor suppressor gene have an increased risk of developing breast cancer. (See **Table 4A.1, Characteristics of BRCA1 and BRCA2 Mutations**.)
- Family history
  - First-degree relative (mother, sister, or daughter) from either the mother's or father's side of the family with breast cancer doubles a woman's risk. Women with premenopausal first-degree relatives with breast cancer have a three- to fourfold increase in risk. Having two first-degree relatives increases the risk fivefold.
- Personal history of breast cancer
  - Women with a history of primary breast cancer have a three- to fourfold increase in risk for primary cancer in the contralateral or same breast.
- Menstrual periods
  - Women who started menstruating at an early age (before age 12) or who went through menopause late (after age 50) have a slightly higher risk (American Cancer Society 2001a).
- Pregnancy
  - Risk is higher in women who have never had a child or whose first full-term pregnancy occurred after age 30.
  - Aborted pregnancy does not affect breast cancer risk.

- Alcohol
  - There is a positive, dose-dependent association between alcohol consumption and risk for breast cancer. One alcoholic drink per day confers a slightly higher risk for breast cancer. Two to five drinks per day confers a 1.5% increase in risk over nondrinkers.
- Irradiation
  - Women who have had chest area radiation as a child or young woman have a significantly higher risk of breast cancer.
- Biopsy-proven breast changes
  - Risk for breast cancer is increased in women with certain types of breast tissue changes. (See **Table 4A.2, Benign Breast Disease and Relative Risk for Subsequent Invasive Breast Cancer**.)
- Oral contraceptive (OC) use
  - The relationship between OC use and breast cancer risk is unclear. Recently, one large study found that women currently using OCs are at slightly higher risk for developing breast cancer than are nonusers. Women who stopped using OCs for more than 10 years appear to have no increased risk (American Cancer Society 2001a).
- Hormone therapy
  - Most studies suggest that current or recent long-term use of hormone replacement therapy (HRT) after menopause may slightly increase the risk for breast cancer. A woman's breast cancer risk returns to that of the general population within five years of stopping HRT. These studies are controversial (American Cancer Society 2001a).
- Obesity and high-fat diets
  - Obesity is associated with an increased risk of developing breast cancer, especially in women after menopause. This risk appears to be increased for women who gained weight as an adult but not among those who were overweight as a child. Excess fat in the waist area affects risk more than the same amount in the hips and thighs. More research is needed on the impact of fat intake and breast cancer, but there is clear evidence of a relationship between fat intake and other types of cancer (American Cancer Society 2001a).
- Physical activity
  - Additional research is needed to confirm the relationship between vigorous activity and protection against breast cancer.
- Environmental pollution
  - Currently, research does not show a clear link between cancer risk and exposure to environmental pollutants.
→ Patient may have one or more risk factor(s) for breast cancer. Most women with breast cancer have no identifiable risk factors.
→ Symptoms may include:
  - Usually painless, hard mass with irregular edges. Some rare cancers may be tender, soft, and rounded.

Table 4A.1. CHARACTERISTICS OF BRCA1 AND BRCA2 MUTATIONS

High-Risk Patient for BRCA1, BRCA2 Mutation

Family history of onset of cancer at young age

Bilaterality of breast cancer

More than three relatives on same side of family

Family history of ovarian cancer

BRCA1	BRCA2
80% lifetime risk of breast cancer	80% lifetime risk of breast cancer
65% risk of contralateral breast cancer	Breast cancer expressed in males
20–50% risk of ovarian cancer	Small increase in risk of ovarian cancer
Possible increase in risk of cancer and prostate cancer	

Source: Reprinted by permission from Hansen, N., and Morrow, M. 1998. Breast disease. *Medical Clinics of North America* 82(2):203–222.

Table 4A.2. BENIGN BREAST DISEASE AND RELATIVE RISK FOR SUBSEQUENT INVASIVE BREAST CANCER

Classification	Relative Risk

Nonproliferative lesions
  Cyst, micro or macro
  Duct ectasia
  Fibroadenoma
  Papillary apocrine changes
  Mild sclerosing adenosis
  Fibrosis
  Mastitis
  Metaplasia, squamous or
    apocrine
  Mild epithelial hyperplasia
	1
	(no increase in risk)

Proliferative lesions
  Moderate or florid hyperplasia
  Intraductal papilloma
  Florid sclerosing adenosis
	1.5–2.0
	(slight increase in risk)

Proliferative lesions with atypia
  Atypical hyperplasia,
    lobular or ductal
	4.0–5.0
	(moderate increase in risk)

Carcinoma in situ
  Ductal carcinoma in situ
  Lobular carcinoma in situ
	8.0–10.0
	(high risk)

Source: Reprinted by permission from Hansen, N., and Morrow, M. 1998. Breast disease. *Medical Clinics of North America* 82(2):203–222.

- Spontaneous, unilateral, serous, or bloody nipple discharge in nonlactating breast
- Itching, burning, dimpling, swelling, or erythema of the skin
- Change in contour of the breast
- Nipple retraction
- Axillary swelling

OBJECTIVE

→ Inspection and palpation of the breasts—supraclavicular and axillary regions (supine and sitting)—may reveal a breast mass, nipple retraction, skin dimpling (*peau d'orange*), erythema, edema, induration, and/or change in breast contour.

→ Patient may present with:
- Breast mass
- Unilateral, serous, or bloody discharge or crusting on nipple
- Supra/infraclavicular or axillary adenopathy
- Screening mammogram suspicious for breast cancer

→ Carefully document findings using descriptive terms.
- Mass(es) should be described assuming a clock position, locating the mass by distance from the base of the nipple, the dimensions measured with a centimeter tape or ruler.
- Consistency, shape, presence of tenderness, mobility, and associated skin changes should be described. Diagrams are helpful.

ASSESSMENT

→ Breast mass (with or without adenopathy, nipple discharge or skin changes)

→ R/O breast cancer

→ R/O benign breast disease

→ R/O cervical/dorsal radiculitis

→ R/O Tietze's syndrome (costochondritis)

PLAN

DIAGNOSTIC TESTS

→ Technologies for evaluating breast findings include:
- Mammography—effective in diagnosing early-stage cancers
  - Most effective in women over 30 years old, whose breasts are less dense
  - Not recommended in pregnancy
  - Screening mammography usually involves two views of each breast. Additional views may be needed in some women to include as much breast tissue as possible.
  - Diagnostic mammography, performed when there is a breast complaint or an abnormal screening mammogram, may include additional views and cone views with magnification.
  - Digital mammography is similar to standard mammography with the advantage of images being stored digitally so modifying the brightness or contrast can enhance them.

- The Breast Imaging Reporting and Data System (BIRADS) is a standard way of reporting mammography results that allows consistent use of language and ensures better follow-up on suspicious findings (American Cancer Society 2001c).
  - Category 0: Assessment is incomplete and additional imaging evaluation is needed.
  - Category 1: Negative. There is no significant abnormality to report.
  - Category 2: Benign finding. Negative mammogram but ensures documentation to use in future mammogram assessments.
  - Category 3: Probably benign finding. Follow-up in a short time frame is suggested.
  - Category 4: Suspicious abnormality. Biopsy should be considered.
  - Category 5: Highly suggestive of malignancy. Biopsy is strongly recommended.
- Mammography after breast augmentation with implants—x-rays cannot penetrate silicone or saline implants well enough to image under- and overlying breast tissue. Four additional images (implant displacement views), in addition to the standard four images, should be taken. The implant is pushed forward against the chest wall and the breast is pulled forward over it. These views are not successful in women who have contractures around the implants. They are easiest to obtain when implants have been placed underneath the chest muscle. Screening guidelines are otherwise the same as for women without implants (American Cancer Society 2001c, Schumann 1994).
- Sonography—primary use is for differentiating between a solid versus cystic mass and to guide needles during biopsy.
  - Some studies suggest ultrasound be considered in screening women with dense breasts, but ultrasound cannot reliably detect microcalcifications (earliest signs of cancer) or lesions smaller than 1 cm, thus it should not be recommended (American Cancer Society 2001c).
- Ductography—used to evaluate nipple discharge in non-lactating breast. This involves cannulating the involved duct, injecting radiopaque dye, and evaluating by x-ray.
- Biopsy
  - Fine-needle aspiration biopsy (FNAB) utilizes a 20-gauge needle to aspirate fluid or small tissue fragments from a mass. Usually performed with ultrasound or stereotactic guidance. Stereotactic guidance is used when a lesion cannot be palpated. A small electric motor controlled by a computer guides needle placement.
  - Core needle biopsy (CNB) utilizes a larger needle (14-gauge) to remove a cylindrical core of tissue. Usually requires a small skin incision and local anesthesia. Usually performed with ultrasound or stereotactic guidance.
  - Excisional biopsy is used to remove the entire lesion and surrounding margin. Done when needle biopsies

are negative but the mass is clinically suspicious for malignancy. May be done without initial needle biopsy if lesion is very suspicious. May be performed with wire localization. Requires local anesthesia with intravenous sedation for outpatients.

- Serum DNA analysis to assess for inherited mutated BRCA1 or BRCA2 has become part of cancer genetic testing. Testing for the p53 tumor suppressor gene is not part of the usual breast cancer genetic testing but may be done by specialized cancer genetic centers if the family history raises the possibility of Li-Fraumeni syndrome.

TREATMENT/MANAGEMENT

→ Second examiner to corroborate breast findings.
→ Refer patient to a breast specialist if a dominant mass or any suspicious findings are present.
→ Discussion of treatment of breast cancer is beyond the scope of this chapter. Refer to a current publication on breast cancer management.

CONSULTATION

→ For suspicious mass or findings
→ Women considering genetic testing should be referred to a qualified genetic counselor, nurse, or physician. Testing is expensive, often not covered by health insurance, and abnormal genetic test results may preclude women from getting life insurance (Ang et al. 2001).
→ If a mutated BRCA or p53 gene is found, referral to a qualified health care team is recommended to develop a plan of care that includes more frequent screening to monitor for early signs of cancer and to review risk reduction strategies (i.e., tamoxifen or surgery). **NOTE:** Women positive for these inherited genes are also at higher risk for ovarian cancer and should be managed appropriately.
→ Patients with diagnosed breast cancer are managed by a surgeon and oncologist.

PATIENT EDUCATION

→ Allay patient's concerns regarding breast findings.
→ Advise risk modification: decrease fat and alcohol intake, avoid excessive radiation exposure (mammography not included).
→ Patients undergoing mammography should obtain prior mammogram results for comparison if done at a different facility, have their mammograms scheduled one week after their menses, and not wear deodorant during the exam.

FOLLOW-UP

→ Patients undergoing screening mammography should receive their results in a timely manner.

→ Follow-up appointment with a breast specialist as indicated.
→ Teach the American Cancer Society's recommendation for routine breast screening (Zoorob et al. 2001):
  - Breast self-examination monthly starting at age 20.
  - Clinical breast examination (CBE) every three years at ages 20–39 and every year after age 40.
  - Mammography every year starting at age 40. CBE should take place at a short interval prior to mammography because if a mass is identified it can be brought to the attention of the radiologist (Smith et al. 2000).
→ Women with a personal or family history of breast cancer may need earlier and/or more frequent clinical breast examinations and/or mammograms. Physician consultation should be sought (Zoorob et al. 2001).
→ Women at higher risk for breast cancer have options that can be suggested for cancer prevention. They include prophylactic mastectomy, tamoxifen therapy, clinical trial participation, and diet and lifestyle modification. Physician referral should be sought when surgery or pharmacological therapy is being considered.
→ Call the American Cancer Society at (800) ACS-2345 for mammogram facilities in the patient's area.
→ Document in progress notes and on problem list.

BIBLIOGRAPHY

American Cancer Society. 2001a. *What are the risks for breast cancer?* Available at: http://www.cancer.org. Accessed on September 1, 2002.

American Cancer Society. 2001b. *Breast cancer: detection and symptoms.* Available at: http://www.cancer.org. Accessed on September 1, 2002.

American Cancer Society. 2001c. *Mammography and other breast imaging procedures.* Available at: http://www.cancer.org. Accessed on September 1, 2002.

Ang, P., and Garber, J.E. 2001. Genetic susceptibility for breast cancer—risk assessment and counseling. *Seminars in Oncology* 28(4):419–433.

Apantaku, L.M. 2000. Breast cancer diagnosis and screening. *American Family Physician* 62(3):596–602.

Hansen, N., and Morrow, M. 1998. Breast disease. *Medical Clinics of North America* 82(2):203–222.

Leitch, A.M. 2001. Breast cancer: screening and early detection. *Texas Medicine* 97(2):74–78.

Schumann, D. 1994. Health risks for women with breast implants. *Nurse Practitioner* 19(7):19–30.

Smith, R.A., Mettlin, C.J., Davis, K.J. et al. 2000. American Cancer Society guidelines for the early detection of cancer. *Cancer Journal for Clinicians* 50(1):34–49.

Zoorob, R., Anderson, R., Cefalu, C. et al. 2001. Cancer screening guidelines. *American Family Physician* 63(6):1101–1112.

Lisa L. Lommel, R.N., C., F.N.P., M.S., M.P.H.

4-B
Breast Pain and Nodularity

Breast pain (*mastalgia*) is the most common breast complaint for women. It is reported to occur in as many as 66% of adolescent and adult women (Neinstein 1999). Three discrete patterns of breast pain have been recognized: *cyclical mastalgia, noncyclical mastalgia,* and *chest wall pain* (Steinbrunn et al. 1997).

Cyclical breast pain is pain that begins the week preceding menses and resolves with menstruation, though pain of varying degrees may persist throughout the menstrual cycle. It is most common in women 20–40 years old with resolution in the perimenopausal years. Though the exact etiology of cyclical breast pain is unclear, it is thought to be related to gonadotrophic and ovarian hormonal fluctuations during the menstrual cycle (Hansen et al. 1998, Zylstra 1999). Other studies have shown a decrease in essential fatty acids in patients with mastalgia, suggesting an increase in the prolactin effect on the breast due to decreased progesterone production that normally inhibits prolactin (BeLieu 1994). There have been no reported changes in the histology of breast tissue in women with mastalgia (Neinstein 1999). Cyclical mastalgia often coexists with cyclical nodularity, but each may occur independently.

Since mastalgia is not considered a pathologic condition, there is a new consensus relating to the correct terminology for this condition. *Benign breast changes* is now used in lieu of fibrocystic changes and mastitis.

Cyclical breast nodularity and swelling are also due to the effects of estrogen and progesterone on breast tissue. Prior to menses, breast lobules, alveoli, and ducts become engorged, causing swelling and nodularity. With the onset of menses, the ducts regress and epithelial cells desquamate and are maintained until the second week of the cycle, when proliferation begins again. Over time, alveoli enlargement can lead to cyst formation. Although this condition is usually associated with tenderness, it is not necessarily painful.

Noncyclical mastalgia occurs in pre- and postmenopausal women and does not coincide with events in the menstrual cycle. It presents most commonly in women over age 40. Pain may begin and resolve at any time, often without a defined pattern. While the etiology of noncyclical pain is poorly understood,

radiological abnormalities consistent with coarse calcification and ductal dilation are commonly seen. There is no histological evidence, however, that noncyclical pain results from the pathological changes of duct ectasia. Nodularity is much less prominent than in the cyclical pain pattern.

Noncyclical breast pain may also present as postbiopsy mastalgia (trauma-related), fat necrosis, sclerosing adenosis, stretching of Cooper's ligaments and possibly, although uncommonly, breast cancer (Drukker 1997).

Chest wall pain may be felt as breast pain but may be caused by a painful costochondral junction syndrome (*Tietze's syndrome*). This pain is a chronic condition, often unilateral, increases with activity, and can occur at any age. The pain emanates from the area of the breast that overlies the tender costocartilage (Drukker 1997).

DATABASE

SUBJECTIVE

→ Elicit duration, site, periodicity, and characteristic of the pain.

→ Elicit what impact pain has on the patient's lifestyle (e.g., sex, sleep, touching, hugging, general activity).

→ Elicit any personal or family history of benign or malignant breast problems.

→ Symptoms include:

- Cyclical pain—heaviness, achiness, tenderness, unilaterally or bilaterally, beginning approximately one week (but may be as long as four weeks) prior to menses and resolving with onset of menses.

- Usually not well-localized, occurring most typically in upper outer quadrants.

- May radiate to axilla and down medial aspect of upper arm.
  - Some women report mastalgia for the first time with initiation or change in estrogen replacement therapy or oral contraceptive use.

- May report diffuse lumpiness or nodularity without a dominant mass.
  - Nodularity is more common in upper outer quadrants.

- ■ May have breast swelling, causing change in breast contour and size; bra may feel tighter.
  - • Symptom severity may fluctuate from cycle to cycle.
- ■ Noncyclical pain of duct ectasia:
  - • Unilateral, sharp, burning, drawing pain, exacerbated by cold
  - • Site precisely located most often subareolar or upper inner quadrant, tender to touch (see the **Duct Ectasia/ Periductal Mastitis** chapter).
- ■ Noncyclical pain of sclerosing adenosis:
  - • Spontaneous onset of well-localized pain.
- ■ Noncyclical pain of fat necrosis:
  - • History of trauma by injury, compression by an abscess, or incision for biopsy, localized to area of trauma. Pain may occur months to years after trauma (see the **Fat Necrosis** chapter).
- ■ Chest wall pain (Tietze's syndrome):
  - • Unilateral chronic, sharp, or aching pain in the medial quadrants of the breast over the costocartilages. Pain occurs with pressure over the affected cartilage.

OBJECTIVE

→ Carefully document findings using descriptive terms.
- ■ Mass(es) should be described by using a clock position, locating the mass by distance from the base of the nipple, the dimensions measured with a centimeter ruler or tape.
- ■ The consistency, shape, presence of tenderness, mobility, and associated skin changes should be described. Diagrams are helpful.

Cyclical Pain

→ Inspection and palpation of the breasts—supraclavicular and axillary regions (supine and sitting)—may not reveal a definite mass. If premenstrual, breasts may feel fuller and tense and demonstrate a prominent venous pattern.
- ■ Finely granular to grossly lumpy nodularity may be palpated particularly in upper outer quadrants.

Noncyclical Pain

→ No discrete palpable masses may be felt at the site of pain. Nodularity is less prominent. Scar tissue may be felt over the site of pain with postbiopsy trauma. A small, firm, fixed mass may be felt in fat necrosis.

Chest Wall Pain

→ No discrete palpable mass at the site of pain, but the involved costal cartilage may be enlarged. Palpation may elicit pain.
→ Examine the patient in the left lateral decubitus position, which allows the breast to fall away from the chest wall.

ASSESSMENT

→ Mastalgia—cyclical
→ Mastalgia—noncyclical
- ■ R/O duct ectasia
- ■ R/O fat necrosis

- ■ R/O sclerosing adenosis
- ■ R/O postbiopsy trauma
- ■ R/O breast cancer
→ Chest wall pain
- ■ R/O Tietze's syndrome
- ■ R/O degenerative disorders
- ■ R/O hiatal hernia
- ■ R/O angina
- ■ R/O cholelithiasis
- ■ R/O pulmonary disorders
→ Cyclical nodularity

PLAN

DIAGNOSTIC TESTS

→ In absence of a dominant mass, no specific diagnostic test is recommended.
→ Mammography may be recommended in women over 30 years old for reassurance or because of suspicion of mass.
→ Consider pregnancy test, as appropriate.

TREATMENT/MANAGEMENT

→ Ask a second examiner to corroborate findings.
→ Refer to a breast specialist if a dominant mass is present.
→ Pain chart (kept for a minimum of 3 months) is helpful to define the pain pattern severity and to give a baseline measurement of the number of days of pain per cycle. This alone may provide reassurance if the pain is hormonally related. For patients receiving pharmacologic therapy, a pain chart should be part of the treatment plan to assess for a change in symptoms.
→ Breast pain should be treated when it is severe enough to interfere with a patient's lifestyle and occurs more than a few days each month (Morrow 2000).
→ Generalized nodularity alone does not usually require treatment. Reassurance that the condition is benign and normal should be offered.

Cyclical Pain

First-line Therapy: Mild to Moderate Symptoms

→ Combined oral contraceptives (OCs) may be of benefit to women with a history of mild to moderate cyclical mastalgia. Breast pain improvement is evident after 6 months in 70–90% women (Neinstein 1999). Risk factors for OCs should be considered before initiating therapy.
- ■ Routine cycling of a low-dose pill containing 30–35 μg of estrogen and a low-dose/potency progestin is recommended, although studies have shown that a greater benefit was achieved with higher doses of progesterone (Drukker 1997).
→ For women who experience mastalgia or nodularity after starting OCs, withdrawal of the pill may decrease symptoms.
- ■ If the patient wants to continue OC use, a change to a higher progestin pill may be of benefit.
→ For women on estrogen replacement therapy, complete withdrawal or substitution with a low-dose combined prepa-

ration may be of benefit. (See also the **Perimenopausal and Menopausal Symptoms and Hormone Therapy** chapter in Section 12.)

→ Evening primrose oil is a rich source of essential fatty acids (EFAs). Studies suggest that patients with mastalgia have abnormally low levels of EFAs.

- Studies suggest a 44% improvement rate in mild to moderate cases of mastalgia with no change in nodularity (Neinstein 1999, Steinbrunn et al. 1997).

- Younger patients who are likely to need treatment of long duration, women who want to continue on OCs, or women with less severe symptoms may initially have evening primrose oil (EPO) recommended to them (Steinbrunn et al. 1997).

- Dosing recommendation: Three 500 mg tablets BID. Because EPO is a dietary supplement, the effect is slow, and at least 4 months of treatment are required (BeLieu 1994, Holland et al. 1994). If there is no improvement of symptoms after 4 months, consider alternative therapy. If symptoms improve, continue treatment for 2 more months, then discontinue. Some patients report long-lasting effects after discontinuing EPO. May restart regimen if symptoms return (Mansel 1994, Steinbrunn et al. 1997). Side effects include mild nausea.

Second-Line Therapy: Severe Symptoms and/or Second-Line Treatment

→ Danazol was found to be 70–80% effective in relieving severe breast mastalgia by inhibiting pituitary gonadotropins. Nodularity also decreased, although more slowly (Morrow 2000, Steinbrunn et al. 1997). Danazol is the only drug labeled by the U.S. Food and Drug Administration for the treatment of breast pain.

- Symptoms recur in 30–65% of patients following discontinuation.

- Dosage recommendations: 100–300 mg daily for 1 month, then reduce to maintenance doses of 25 mg–50 g/day. For some women, a dose of 100 mg a day for 5 days a month during the luteal phase is therapeutic (Holland et al. 1994). Adjust therapy in accordance with symptoms and side effects (Steinbrunn et al. 1997). Danazol should be stopped every 12 months to assess whether treatment is still required.

- Common side effects include amenorrhea, irregular menses, mild androgenic effects such as weight gain, acne and hirsutism, voice change, reduction in breast size, leg cramps, and decreased libido. These are generally dose-dependent. See *Physicians' Desk Reference (PDR).*

- Contraindications: Pregnancy, lactation, abnormal vaginal bleeding, markedly impaired renal and/or cardiac function, or liver dysfunction.

→ Bromocriptine, a dopamine antagonist, is effective in lowering prolactin levels, thereby reducing mastalgia and nodularity in 65% of patients (Steinbrunn et al. 1997).

- Dosing recommendations (Steinbrunn et al. 1997):

Day of Menstrual Cycle	Dose
1–3	1.25 mg at night with food
4–8	2.5 mg at night with food
9–14	1.25 mg in morning with food and 2.5 mg at night with food
15 onward	2.5 mg in morning with food and 2.5 mg at night with food

- Common side effects may be mild to severe and include nausea, vomiting, dizziness, irritability, and headache. (See *PDR.*) Side effects can be minimized by gradually introducing the dosage regimen, by taking the drug with meals, and by using the smallest amount to obtain the desired results. Bromocriptine should not be used in patients on diuretic or hypotensive drug therapy.

→ Tamoxifen binds to estrogen receptors and has both agonistic and antagonistic actions. It has a response rate of approximately 80–90% in the treatment of cyclic mastalgia (Steinbrunn et al. 1997). Response rates for nodularity are not available.

→ Studies of tamoxifen use in breast cancer patients have shown an increased risk of a second primary tumor of the endometrium. However, studies have shown no increase in tumor incidence with short-term use (less than 6 months)(Steinbrunn et al. 1997). Use should be limited to patients who fail to respond to oral contraceptives, EPO, danazol, or bromocriptine.

→ Studies have shown a similar response rate at 3 months of therapy as at 6 months of therapy. Relapse rate after discontinuation is approximately 30% (Steinbrunn et al. 1997).

- Dosage recommendations (BeLieu 1994): 20 mg/day p.o. on cycle Days 5–25 or 15–25, or daily for 1–4 cycles.

- Side effects: menstrual irregularity, bleeding secondary to endometrial hyperplasia, vaginal atrophy, menopausal symptoms (hot flashes), and leukorrhea. (See *PDR.*)

- Contraindications: pregnancy

→ GnRH agonists have had some success in treating mastalgia and to a lesser extent nodularity. Limited studies have shown a response rate of 50–81% depending on route of delivery (Steinbrunn et al. 1997).

- GnRH agonists work by increasing the body's secretion of luteinizing hormone (LH) and follicle-stimulating hormone (FSH). Eventually there is a depletion of stores of these hormones, which decreases the amount of estrogen. The decreased amounts of estrogen then limit the breast symptoms.

- Side effects include those of the perimenopause: menstrual irregularity, vasomotor symptoms, vaginal dryness, theoretical loss of bone density beginning after 6 months of therapy, and effects on lipoprotein chemistry. (See *PDR.*)

- Contraindications: pregnancy

  NOTE: A pregnancy test should be done before initiating treatment with danazol, tamoxifen, bromocriptine, or GnRH agonists.

→ Patients at risk for pregnancy who are taking bromocriptine, danazol, or tamoxifen should use a barrier contraceptive method because these agents are potentially teratogenic and may reduce effectiveness of oral contraceptives. Women using oral contraception may take evening primrose oil.

→ An association between methylxanthine (caffeine, theophylline, theobromine) consumption and mastalgia/nodularity has not been substantiated; however, as many as 60–65% of patients will report a reduction in premenstrual mastalgia after several months of decaffeination (Drukker 1997).

→ Closely controlled studies of vitamin E have found no evidence of specific improvement, although anecdotally, many patients using 400 mg BID have noted a benefit (Drukker 1997).

Noncyclical Pain

→ Danazol appears to be effective, with 75% of patients responding to treatment (Morrow 2000). Recommended dosages for noncyclical mastalgia are similar to those for cyclical mastalgia treatment.

Chest Wall Pain

→ Chest wall pain from Tietze's syndrome may be treated with lidocaine/steroid injection for intense, localized, persistent pain. For less severe pain, a trial of nonsteroidal anti-inflammatory drugs (NSAIDs) is recommended.

CONSULTATION

→ For suspicion of mass
→ Advised for management of noncyclical and chest wall pain
→ Consultation and/or referral to physician for management with danazol, bromocriptine, tamoxifen, or GnRH agonists
→ Physician management is warranted for injection treatment of chest wall pain
→ As needed for prescription(s)

PATIENT EDUCATION

→ Nonpharmaceutical modalities that might help some women include:
  ▪ Lower salt intake, especially prior to and during mastalgia symptoms
  ▪ Heat to breasts; wearing a well-fitting supportive bra, especially with exercise
  ▪ Wearing a bra at night
  ▪ Analgesics
→ Teach/review breast self-examination.
→ Allay patient's concerns regarding breast findings.
→ Teach/review use of pain chart.
→ Advise correct use of OC, danazol, bromocriptine, or EPO therapy including dose, regimen, side effects, and treatment plan.
→ Although an association between methylxanthine and mastalgia/nodularity has not been substantiated, a reduction in caffeine intake is safe.

FOLLOW-UP

→ In two or three months, re-examine breasts during the first half of the menstrual cycle, when pain and nodularity are minimal, to re-evaluate for discrete masses.
→ Continue breast pain chart throughout treatment to provide a quantitative means of measuring response to treatment.
→ Teach the American Cancer Society's recommendation for routine breast screening (Zoorob et al. 2001):
  ▪ Breast self-examination monthly starting at age 20.
  ▪ Clinical breast examination (CBE) every three years at ages 20–39 and every year after age 40.
  ▪ Mammography every year starting at age 40. CBE should take place at a short interval prior to mammography because if a mass is identified it can be brought to the attention of the radiologist (Smith et al. 2000).
→ Women with a personal or family history of breast cancer may need earlier and/or more frequent clinical breast examinations and/or mammograms. Physician consultation should be sought (Zoorob et al. 2001).
→ Women at higher risk for breast cancer have options that can be suggested for cancer prevention. They include prophylactic mastectomy, tamoxifen therapy, clinical trial participation, and diet and lifestyle modification. Physician referral should be sought when surgery or pharmacological therapy is being considered.
→ Call the American Cancer Society at (800) ACS-2345 for mammogram facilities in the patient's area.
→ Document in progress notes and on problem list.

BIBLIOGRAPHY

BeLieu, R.M. 1994. Mastodynia. *Obstetrics and Gynecology Clinics of North America* 21(3):461–477.

Drukker, B.H. 1997. Breast disease: a primer in diagnosis and management. *International Journal of Fertility* 42(5):278–287.

Hansen, N., and Morrow, M. 1998. Breast disease. *Medical Clinics of North America* 82(2):203–222.

Holland, P.A., and Gateley, C.A. 1994. Drug therapy in mastalgia. *Drugs* 48(5):709–716.

Mansel, R.E. 1994. Breast pain. *British Medical Journal* 309:866–868.

Morrow, M. 2000. The evaluation of common breast problems. *American Family Physician* 61(8):2371–2378.

Neinstein, L.S. 1999. Breast disease in adolescents and young women. *Pediatric Clinics of North America* 46(3):607–629.

Smith, R.A., Mettlin, C.J., Davis, K.J. et al. 2000. American Cancer Society guidelines for the early detection of cancer. *Cancer Journal for Clinicians* 50(1):34–49.

Steinbrunn, B.S., Zera, R.T., and Rodriguez, J.L. 1997. Mastalgia. *Postgraduate Medicine* 102(5):183–198.

Zoorob, R., Anderson, R., Cefalu, C. et al. 2001. Cancer screening guidelines. *American Family Physician* 63(6):1101–1112.

Zylstra, S. 1999. Office management of benign breast disease. *Clinical Obstetrics and Gynecology* 42(2):234–248.

Lisa L. Lommel, R.N., C., F.N.P., M.S., M.P.H.

4-C

Duct Ectasia/Periductal Mastitis

Mammary *duct ectasia/periductal mastitis* is the result of inflammation and enlargement of the ducts behind the nipple. The sequence and pathogenesis of events are not clear, but certain histological changes have been found to predominate with age.

Severe inflammation with lack of duct dilation is seen more often in younger women. "Scanty" inflammatory changes but more multiple duct dilation are seen in older women. From these findings, it has been postulated that duct ectasia begins as periductal inflammation. As the inflammation resolves, the involved ducts become fibrotic and dilated.

Duct ectasia does not increase a women's risk for breast cancer. However, this condition can be complicated by severe inflammation, which can cause significant morbidity. Duct ectasia is considered a primary cause of noncyclical breast mastalgia (see the **Breast Pain and Nodularity** chapter).

DATABASE

SUBJECTIVE

→ Duct ectasia/periductal mastitis is more common in women ages 45–55, those who have borne children, and those with a history of nipple manipulation (Zylstra 1999).
→ Periareolar or subareolar mass may be palpable.
→ Nipple inversion with areolar thickening may be present.
→ Pain of varying intensity may be felt depending on the degree of inflammation.
  ▪ Burning in nature
  ▪ Exacerbated by cold
  ▪ Located in subareolar area or in the upper inner quadrant
  ▪ Usually noncyclical
  ▪ Tends to affect younger patients
→ Discharge symptoms include spontaneous, intermittent, unilateral, or bilateral nipple discharge usually from multiple ducts.
  ▪ More commonly thin and watery in the younger patient, and thick, sticky, or toothpaste-like in the older patient
  ▪ Multicolored discharge (yellow, white, brown, gray, or reddish brown) but most commonly greenish or blackish

  ▪ With more advanced inflammation, discharge may change and present as bloody

OBJECTIVE

→ Inspection and palpation of the breasts—supraclavicular and axillary regions (supine and sitting)—may reveal a 1–2 cm worm-like or tubular, firm, and tender mass in the subareolar region, not attached to surrounding tissue.
  ▪ Mass may appear rapidly and subside spontaneously within a week.
  ▪ May recur at the same site, at intervals of a few months to 10 years or more. With each recurrence, the condition tends to be more severe than the last.
  ▪ Bilateral masses may develop or the original mass may subside and a new mass begin in the opposite breast.
  ▪ Mass may also persist and become chronic in nature.
  ▪ Any of these masses may form abscesses.
→ Areola may be red and swollen.
→ Mild degrees of nipple retraction may occur in early inflammation. Retraction is present in 75% of patients with periareolar inflammation.
→ Young patients commonly present with pain and/or an inflammatory mass. Older patients more likely have nipple retraction or a nontender mass. This correlates with the suggested pathogenesis of this condition.
→ Findings should be carefully documented using descriptive terms.
  ▪ Masse(s) should be described assuming a clock position, locating the mass by distance from the base of the nipple, the dimensions measured with a centimeter ruler or tape.
  ▪ Consistency, shape, presence of tenderness, mobility, and associated changes should be described. Diagrams are helpful.
→ Attempt to elicit nipple discharge.
  ▪ Apply mild pressure over each quadrant of the periareolar region.
  ▪ Note the location of discharge, and the consistency and color of the discharge.

ASSESSMENT

→ Duct ectasia/periductal mastitis
→ R/O breast cancer

PLAN

DIAGNOSTIC TESTS

→ Nipple discharge should be examined for occult blood with hemostick (urine dipstick can be substituted) or hemoccult testing.
→ Cytology is generally not recommended because the absence of malignant cells does not exclude cancer and a positive result does not distinguish intraductal cancer from invasive cancer (Morrow 2000).
→ Diagnostic mammography with magnification of the retroareolar region is recommended in women over 35 years old to evaluate for breast cancer (Morrow 2000).

TREATMENT/MANAGEMENT

→ Ask a second examiner to corroborate findings.
→ Refer patient to a breast specialist if mass is present.
→ In early stages of inflammation, no intervention may be necessary. Advise patient to keep nipples clean, apply heat locally, and use nonsteroidal anti-inflammatory agents as needed.
→ When nipple discharge resembles galactorrhea, a serum prolactin should be done to rule out prolactinemia (see the **Galactorrhea** chapter).
→ Development of moderate to severe inflammation and/or periareolar mass or abscess warrants antibiotic therapy and incision and drainage by a physician.
→ Local excision of involved ducts may be effective in controlling symptoms (McCool et al. 1998).

CONSULTATION

→ For confirmation of diagnosis.
→ All patients with dominant mass; moderate to severe inflammation or abscess; or bloody, spontaneous, and/or unilateral nipple discharge should be referred for physician evaluation.

PATIENT EDUCATION

→ Allay patient's concerns regarding breast findings.
→ Advise patient to keep nipples clean with mild soap and water and to refrain from nipple manipulation.

FOLLOW-UP

→ For patients with only mild inflammation, re-examine at routine visits.
→ Follow-up appointment with a breast specialist for patients with moderate to severe inflammation or abscess.
→ Teach the American Cancer Society's recommendation for routine breast screening (Zoorob et al. 2001):
  ■ Breast self-examination monthly starting at age 20.
  ■ Clinical breast examination (CBE) every three years at ages 20–39 and every year after age 40.
  ■ Mammography every year starting at age 40. CBE should take place at a short interval prior to mammography because if a mass is identified it can be brought to the attention of the radiologist (Smith et al. 2000).
→ Women with a personal or family history of breast cancer may need earlier and/or more frequent clinical breast examinations and/or mammograms. Physician consultation should be sought (Zoorob et al. 2001).
→ Women at higher risk for breast cancer have options that can be suggested for cancer prevention. They include prophylactic mastectomy, tamoxifen therapy, clinical trial participation, and diet and lifestyle modification. Physician referral should be sought when surgery or pharmacological therapy is being considered.
→ Call the American Cancer Society at (800) ACS-2345 for mammogram facilities in the patient's area.

BIBLIOGRAPHY

McCool, W.F., Stone-Condry, M., and Bradford, H.M. 1998. Breast health care. *Journal of Nurse-Midwifery* 43(6):406–430.

Morrow, M. 2000. The evaluation of common breast problems. *American Family Physician* 61(8):2371–2378.

Smith, R.A., Mettlin, C.J., Davis, K.J. et al. 2000. American Cancer Society guidelines for the early detection of cancer. *Cancer Journal for Clinicians* 50(1):34–49.

Zoorob, R., Anderson, R., Cefalu, C. et al. 2001. Cancer screening guidelines. *American Family Physician* 63(6):1101–1112.

Zylstra, S. 1999. Office management of benign breast disease. *Clinical Obstetrics and Gynecology* 42(2):234–249.

4-D

Fat Necrosis

Fat necrosis of the breast refers to the death of fat tissue that is surrounded by healthy tissue. Necrosis of adipose (fatty) tissue within the breast is a benign condition. It can be linked to direct trauma of the breast in approximately 50% of patients (Drukker 1997). Fat necrosis often arises secondary to breast biopsy, cyst aspiration, reduction mammoplasty, breast reconstruction, lumpectomy, radiotherapy, implant removal, anticoagulant therapy, and malignant neoplasms (Hogge et al. 1995).

As the area affected by the trauma attempts to heal, scar tissue develops. Some areas of fat necrosis respond by releasing greasy fluid, forming a sac-like collection called an *oil cyst*. Oil cysts can be diagnosed by fine needle aspiration, which also serves as a treatment (American Cancer Society 2001).

This condition may simulate cancer on physical examination and mammography. Since breast cancer is more common than fat necrosis, a history of trauma should not rule out the possibility of carcinoma. Fat necrosis does not increase a woman's risk for breast cancer.

DATABASE

SUBJECTIVE

→ Fat necrosis is more common in overweight, perimenopausal, large-breasted women.
→ Patient has history of:
  ■ Trauma to the breasts (50% of patients)
  ■ Breast biopsy, reduction mammoplasty, lumpectomy, radiotherapy, implant removal, anticoagulant therapy, cyst aspiration, breast reconstruction, or malignant neoplasm
  ■ Ecchymosis (20–30% of patients)
  ■ Noncyclical breast pain, though more commonly painless
→ Single or multiple breast mass may be felt.
→ Retraction of the skin may be present.
→ A mass associated with trauma and ecchymosis may exhibit an initial increase in size followed by regression or the mass may remain unchanged for years.

OBJECTIVE

→ Inspection and palpation of the breasts—supraclavicular and axillary regions (supine and sitting)—may reveal a firm, rounded, and smooth or irregular, single, or multiple mass(es) fixed to surrounding breast tissue and sometimes associated with skin retraction.
→ Ecchymosis may be present or there may be evidence—in the form of pigmentation—of recent hemorrhage.
→ Mammography appearance may mimic carcinoma; cannot reliably distinguish between the two.
→ Carefully document findings using descriptive terms.
  ■ Mass(es) should be described assuming a clock position, locating the mass by distance from the base of the nipple, the dimensions measured with a centimeter ruler.
  ■ Consistency, shape, presence of tenderness, mobility, and associated skin changes should be described. Diagrams are helpful.

ASSESSMENT

→ Fat necrosis
→ R/O breast cancer
→ R/O benign breast disease

PLAN

DIAGNOSTIC TESTS

→ Although needle biopsy may be adequate, excisional biopsy irrespective of mammographic finding is warranted to rule out carcinoma (Drukker 1997, Giuliano 2001).

TREATMENT/MANAGEMENT

→ Second examiner to corroborate breast findings.
→ Refer to a breast specialist if dominant mass or any suspicious findings are present.
→ When major trauma to the breast has occurred, accompanied by ecchymosis and a palpable mass, expectant management may be employed.

→ In the absence of clear evidence of trauma and presence of mass, biopsy is warranted.

CONSULTATION

→ Consultation is recommended if the patient has a history and evidence of trauma and palpable mass.
→ Referral is warranted when there is a palpable mass but an absence of history and evidence of trauma.

PATIENT EDUCATION

→ Allay patient's concerns regarding breast findings.
→ Advise ways to avoid trauma to the breasts—e.g., by wearing supportive bra, placing seat belt strap below breast, avoiding sports-related injuries.

FOLLOW-UP

→ Follow-up appointment with a breast specialist as indicated.
→ If breast trauma is diagnosed, assess for possibility of violence. Refer to social services, safe shelter, and/or appropriate violence prevention program as indicated.
→ Teach the American Cancer Society's recommendation for routine breast screening (Zoorob et al. 2001):
  ▪ Breast self-examination monthly starting at age 20.
  ▪ Clinical breast examination (CBE) every three years at ages 20–39 and every year after age 40.
  ▪ Mammography every year starting at age 40. CBE should take place at a short interval prior to mammography because if a mass is identified it can be brought to the attention of the radiologist (Smith et al. 2000).
→ Women with a personal or family history of breast cancer may need earlier and/or more frequent clinical breast examinations and/or mammograms. Physician consultation should be sought (Zoorob et al. 2001).
→ Women at higher risk for breast cancer have options that can be suggested for cancer prevention. They include prophylactic mastectomy, tamoxifen therapy, clinical trial participation, and diet and lifestyle modification. Physician referral should be sought when surgery or pharmacological therapy is being considered.
→ Call the American Cancer Society at (800) ACS-2345 for mammogram facilities in the patient's area.
→ Document in progress notes and on problem list.

BIBLIOGRAPHY

American Cancer Society 2001. *Benign breast conditions.* Available at: http://www.cancer.org. Accessed on September 1, 2002.

Drukker, B.H. 1997. Breast disease: a primer on diagnosis and management. *International Journal of Fertility* 42(5): 278–287.

Giuliano, A.E. 2001. Breast. In *Current medical diagnosis and treatment,* eds. L.M. Tierney, Jr., S.J. McPhee, and M.A. Papadakis. New York: McGraw-Hill.

Hogge, J.P., Robinson, R.E., Magnant, C.M. et al. 1995. The mammographic spectrum of fat necrosis of the breast. *Radiographics* 15:1347–1356.

Smith, R.A., Mettlin, C.J., Davis, K.J. et al. 2000. American Cancer Society guidelines for the early detection of cancer. *Cancer Journal for Clinicians* 50(1):34–49.

Zoorob, R., Anderson, R., Cefalu, C. et al. 2001. Cancer screening guidelines. *American Family Physician* 63(6):1101–1112.

Lisa L. Lommel, R.N., C., F.N.P., M.S., M.P.H.

4-E

Fibroadenoma

Fibroadenomas are the most common benign solid tumor of the female breast. A fibroadenoma is a benign tumor made up of both glandular breast tissue and stromal (fibroconnective) tissue. Under hormonal influence, these two tissues proliferate and grow in size, becoming large enough to be palpable. Recent studies have shown the presence of estrogen receptors in fibroadenomas. Since these tumors are hormonally responsive, they may increase in size toward the end of the menstrual cycle and during pregnancy (Hansen et al. 1998, Isaacs 1994).

A fibroadenoma may grow progressively, remain the same size, or regress. The average fibroadenoma will grow to 2–3 cm in size. Fibroadenomas may grow rapidly, reaching a size larger than 4 cm. Such tumors are called *giant fibroadenomas* and occur most commonly in adolescents (Hansen et al. 1998). Fibroadenomas may be present in postmenopausal women, but this is most likely due to the tumor developing before menopause and becoming apparent with involution of the surrounding breast tissue (Zylstra 1999).

Fibroadenomas are most common in African American women who are in their 20s and early 30s. Twenty percent of women with a fibroadenoma will have bilateral lesions and 10–15% of women will have multiple lesions (Zylstra 1999). Historically, fibroadenomas have not been considered a risk factor for breast cancer, but several large studies have shown that there is an increased risk for cancer if the fibroadenoma has a complex histology, proliferates quickly, or contains chromosomal abnormalities (Alderman 1999).

DATABASE

SUBJECTIVE

→ Breast mass may be palpable during breast self-exam.
  ▪ Unless very large, almost always painless
  ▪ More commonly singular but may be multiple
  ▪ May increase in size at end of each menstrual cycle

OBJECTIVE

→ Inspection and palpation of breasts—supraclavicular and axillary regions (supine and sitting)—may reveal a mass

that is firm, rubbery, smooth, well-circumscribed, freely mobile, nontender and rounded, and lobulated or discoid in configuration.
  ▪ After menopause, mass may regress—becoming stony, hard, discrete, and moderately mobile—but it usually will not disappear totally.
  ▪ Single mass is more common, though there may be multiple and/or bilateral masses.
    • Multiple masses occur in 20% of women (Isaacs 1994).
  ▪ Majority of masses located in upper outer quadrants.
  ▪ Mass may be found incidentally on mammography.
  ▪ Masses may grow rapidly during pregnancy.
→ Findings should be carefully documented using descriptive terms.
  ▪ Masses should be described assuming a clock position, locating the mass by distance from the base of the nipple, the dimensions measured with a centimeter tape or ruler.
  ▪ Consistency, shape, presence of tenderness, mobility, and associated skin changes should be described. Diagrams are helpful.

ASSESSMENT

→ Fibroadenoma
→ R/O fluid cyst
→ R/O benign mass
→ R/O breast cancer

PLAN

DIAGNOSTIC TESTS

→ Sonography may be employed to differentiate a solid from a cystic mass.
  ▪ For women under age 25, sonography, together with clinical examination and fine needle aspiration (FNA) cytology, will confirm diagnosis.
  ▪ Sonography is not an effective assessment tool for women older than 25–30 whose breasts are less dense.
  ▪ Other limitations to sonography include:

- Cannot detect microcalcifications
- Difficulty in imaging fatty breast
- Unreliably depicts solid masses smaller than 1 cm

→ Mammography is recommended in women over age 30 who have a breast mass.

→ FNA should be considered to confirm diagnosis in women under age 25 with a palpable mass (Drukker 1997).

- Cytological testing should be completed on all solid tumor aspirates for specific diagnosis.

TREATMENT/MANAGEMENT

→ Ask a second reviewer to corroborate breast findings.

→ Refer to a breast specialist if dominant mass is present.

→ Excision is recommended for women older than 25 or those with large fibroadenomas. Since the risk of cancer is low in women younger than 25, these women can be given a choice regarding excision of a fibroadenoma (Drukker 1997).

CONSULTATION

→ For suspicion of a mass

→ Physician management is warranted if a dominant mass is present.

PATIENT EDUCATION

→ Teach/review breast self-examination.

→ Allay patient's concerns regarding breast findings.

FOLLOW-UP

→ Follow-up appointment with a breast specialist as indicated.

→ Teach the American Cancer Society's recommendation for routine breast screening (Zoorob et al. 2001):

- Breast self-examination monthly starting at age 20.
- Clinical breast examination (CBE) every three years at ages 20–39 and every year after age 40.

■ Mammography every year starting at age 40. CBE should take place at a short interval prior to mammography because if a mass is identified it can be brought to the attention of the radiologist (Smith et al. 2000).

→ Women with a personal or family history of breast cancer may need earlier and/or more frequent clinical breast examinations and/or mammograms. Physician consultation should be sought (Zoorob et al. 2001).

→ Women at higher risk for breast cancer have options that can be suggested for cancer prevention. They include prophylactic mastectomy, tamoxifen therapy, clinical trial participation, and diet and lifestyle modification. Physician referral should be sought when surgery or pharmacological therapy is being considered.

→ Call the American Cancer Society at (800) ACS-2345 for mammogram facilities in the patient's area.

→ Document in progress notes and on problem list.

BIBLIOGRAPHY

Alderman, E.M. 1999. Breast problems in the adolescent. *Contemporary Pediatrics* 16(9):99–120.

Drukker, B.H. 1997. Breast disease: a primer on diagnosis and management. *International Journal of Fertility* 42(5):278–287.

Hansen, N., and Morrow, M. 1998. Breast disease. *Medical Clinics of North America* 82(2):203–222.

Isaacs, J.H. 1994. Benign tumors of the breast. *Obstetrics and Gynecology Clinics of North America* 21(3):487–497.

Smith, R.A., Mettlin, C.J., Davis, K.J. et al. 2000. American Cancer Society guidelines for the early detection of cancer. *Cancer Journal for Clinicians* 50(1):34–49.

Zoorob, R., Anderson, R., Cefalu, C. et al. 2001. Cancer screening guidelines. *American Family Physician* 63(6): 1101–1112.

Zylstra, S. 1999. Office management of benign breast disease. *Clinical Obstetrics and Gynecology* 42(2):234–248.

4-F

Fluid Cysts

Cysts are fluid-filled sacs that can occur within the breast tissue. Cysts are often solitary, but they may be multiple. A simple cyst is defined sonographically as one with smooth margins, a well-defined posterior wall, enhanced distal sound transmission, and an echo-free interior. It is the most common dominant mass in women ages 35–50 (Hansen et al. 1998, Isaacs 1994).

Fluid-filled cysts usually cease with menopause, except for women on hormone therapy. There is no evidence that simple cysts increase a woman's risk for breast cancer (McCool et al. 1998).

DATABASE

SUBJECTIVE

→ Symptoms include:
- Single or multiple palpable mass(es)
  - Mass may have developed as rapidly as overnight.
  - Mass may be visible when patient is lying down.
- Possible nipple discharge, evident when a duct is involved
→ Pain:
- May or may not be associated with the menstrual cycle
- May be associated with a mass that develops rapidly, with a large mass, or with rapid disappearance of a mass (due to rupture or discharge of contents into a duct)
- May radiate to axilla of affected side

OBJECTIVE

→ Inspection and palpation of breasts—supraclavicular areas and axillary regions (supine and sitting)—may reveal a single or multiple mass(es) that is/are firm, mobile, partially attached to the breast tissue, well-delineated, and tense and tender if fully filled, or soft, fluctuant, and tender if partially filled.
- Two-thirds of fluid-filled cysts occur in upper outer quadrant.
- It is difficult to distinguish a cystic lesion from a solid mass on physical examination.

→ A cyst may be found incidentally on mammography for breast cancer screening.
→ Carefully document findings using descriptive terms.
- Masses should be described assuming a clock position, locating the mass by distance from the base of the nipple, the dimensions measured with a centimeter tape or ruler.
- Consistency, shape, presence of tenderness, mobility, and associated skin changes should be described. Diagrams are helpful.

ASSESSMENT

→ Fluid cyst
→ R/O fibroadenoma
→ R/O other benign mass
→ R/O breast cancer

PLAN

DIAGNOSTIC TESTS

→ Sonography is recommended as the primary imaging technique for women under 30–35 years old to differentiate between a cystic and a solid mass.
- If fine needle aspiration (FNA) is done, sonography may be used to aid in directed aspiration.
→ Mammography is recommended for women over 30–35 years old to assist in the diagnosis of a cyst and to exclude an incidental cancer.
→ FNA is both diagnostic and therapeutic for a simple cyst, and it is recommended for a palpable mass in women older than 25.
- Routine cytologic testing of cyst fluid is not indicated because of low likelihood of cancer in the absence of clinical findings of bloody fluid or a residual mass after aspiration.
- Cytological testing should be completed on aspirates that are bloodstained.
- Normal cyst fluid ranges in color from pale yellow to dark green to brown (Morrow 2000).

TREATMENT/MANAGEMENT

→ Ask a second examiner to corroborate breast findings.

→ Refer to a breast specialist if a dominant mass is present.

→ FNA is therapeutic. Re-aspiration may be necessary if cyst recurs.

→ Further evaluation in consultation with a breast specialist is necessary if:

- The palpable mass does not disappear with aspiration
- The fluid in the cyst is bloody
- The same cyst recurs multiple times in a short time interval

→ If the mass is not seen by ultrasound, mammography may be indicated, primarily to look for microcalcifications.

CONSULTATION

→ For suspicion of a mass

→ Physician management is warranted if a dominant mass is present.

PATIENT EDUCATION

→ Teach/review breast self-examination.

→ Allay patient's concern regarding breast finding.

FOLLOW-UP

→ Follow-up appointment with a breast specialist as indicated.

→ Re-examine in three to four weeks to confirm that cyst has not refilled.

→ Teach the American Cancer Society's recommendation for routine breast screening (Zoorob et al. 2001):

- Breast self-examination monthly starting at age 20.
- Clinical breast examination (CBE) every three years at ages 20–39 and every year after age 40.

- Mammography every year starting at age 40. CBE should take place at a short interval prior to mammography because if a mass is identified it can be brought to the attention of the radiologist (Smith et al. 2000).

→ Women with a personal or family history of breast cancer may need earlier and/or more frequent clinical breast examinations and/or mammograms. Physician consultation should be sought (Zoorob et al. 2001).

→ Women at higher risk for breast cancer have options that can be suggested for cancer prevention. They include prophylactic mastectomy, tamoxifen therapy, clinical trial participation, and diet and lifestyle modification. Physician referral should be sought when surgery or pharmacological therapy is being considered.

→ Call the American Cancer Society at (800) ACS-2345 for mammogram facilities in the patient's area.

→ Document in progress notes and on problem list.

BIBLIOGRAPHY

Hansen, N., and Morrow, M. 1998. Breast disease. *Medical Clinics of North America* 82(2):203–222.

Isaacs, J.H. 1994. Benign tumors of the breast. *Obstetrics and Gynecology Clinics of North America* 21(3):487–497.

McCool, W.F., Stone-Condry, M., and Bradford, H.M. 1998. Breast health care. *Journal of Nurse Midwifery* 43(6):406–430.

Morrow, M. 2000. The evaluation of common breast problems. *American Family Physician* 61(8):2371–2378.

Smith, R.A., Mettlin, C.J., Davis, K.J. et al. 2000. American Cancer Society guidelines for the early detection of cancer. *Cancer Journal for Clinicians* 50(1):34–49.

Zoorob, R., Anderson, R., Cefalu, C. et al. 2001. Cancer screening guidelines. *American Family Physician* 63(6):1101–1112.

Lisa L. Lommel, R.N., C., F.N.P., M.S., M.P.H.

4-G

Galactocele

A *galactocele* is an uncommon, milk-filled mass caused by over-distention and/or obstruction of a lactiferous duct (Isaacs 1994). Most galactoceles develop after cessation of lactation. Galactoceles do not put a woman at increased risk for breast cancer.

DATABASE

SUBJECTIVE

→ Symptoms may include:
  ▪ Milky-white nipple discharge may occur, and in later stages the discharge may be green or yellow
  ▪ Firm, nontender mass, commonly in upper outer quadrants beyond the areolar border
→ Typical history includes:
  ▪ Abrupt or gradual cessation of lactation
  ▪ History of galactorrhea
  ▪ Current oral contraceptive use

OBJECTIVE

→ Inspection and palpation of breasts—supraclavicular and axillary regions (supine and sitting)—may reveal a mass that is smooth, mobile, well-delineated, and firm or soft and fluctuant.
→ Patient may present with:
  ▪ Single or multiple masses
  ▪ Milky-white, green, or yellow discharge
→ Findings should be carefully documented using descriptive terms.
  ▪ Mass(es) should be described assuming a clock position, locating the mass by distance from the base of the nipple, the dimensions measured with a centimeter tape or ruler.
  ▪ Consistency, shape, presence of tenderness, mobility, and associated skin changes should be described. Diagrams are helpful.

ASSESSMENT

→ Galactocele
→ R/O galactorrhea
→ R/O fibroadenoma
→ R/O other benign mass
→ R/O breast cancer

PLAN

DIAGNOSTIC TESTS

→ Fine needle aspiration (FNA) is advised in any woman over age 25 who has a breast mass or in any woman with suspicious findings.
  ▪ Withdrawal of milky discharge is diagnostic for galactocele.
  ▪ Evidence of fat lobules can be identified with microscopy.

TREATMENT/MANAGEMENT

→ Ask a second examiner to corroborate breast findings.
→ Refer to a breast specialist if a dominant mass is present.
→ FNA is often curative, although multiple aspirations may be needed.
→ Galactocele may be self-limiting and may subside in a few weeks.

CONSULTATION

→ For suspicion of a mass
→ Physician management is warranted if a dominant mass is present.

PATIENT EDUCATION

→ Allay patient's concerns regarding breast findings.
→ Advise patient to taper weaning rather than abruptly discontinue breast-feeding to decrease the risk of recurrence.

FOLLOW-UP

→ Re-examine in 3–4 weeks to confirm that cyst has not refilled.

→ Follow-up appointment with a breast specialist as indicated.

→ Teach the American Cancer Society's recommendation for routine breast screening (Zoorob et al. 2001):

- Breast self-examination monthly starting at age 20.
- Clinical breast examination (CBE) every three years at ages 20–39 and every year after age 40.

→ Mammography every year starting at age 40. CBE should take place at a short interval prior to mammography because if a mass is identified it can be brought to the attention of the radiologist (Smith et al. 2000).

→ Women with a personal or family history of breast cancer may need earlier and/or more frequent clinical breast examinations and/or mammograms. Physician consultation should be sought (Zoorob et al. 2001).

→ Women at higher risk for breast cancer have options that can be suggested for cancer prevention. They include prophylactic mastectomy, tamoxifen therapy, clinical trial participation, and diet and lifestyle modification. Physician referral should be sought when surgery or pharmacological therapy is being considered.

→ Call the American Cancer Society at (800) ACS-2345 for mammogram facilities in the patient's area.

→ Document in progress notes and on problem list.

BIBLIOGRAPHY

Isaacs, J.H. 1994. Benign tumors of the breast. *Obstetrics and Gynecology Clinics of North America* 21(3):487–497.

Smith, R.A., Mettlin, C.J., Davis, K.J. et al. 2000. American Cancer Society guidelines for the early detection of cancer. *Cancer Journal for Clinicians* 50(1):34–49.

Zoorob, R., Anderson, R., Cefalu, C. et al. 2001. Cancer screening guidelines. *American Family Physician* 63(6): 1101–1112.

4-H

Galactorrhea

Galactorrhea is a spontaneous, multiple-duct, milky, nipple discharge most commonly seen in nonpregnant, nonlactating women of childbearing age. It is most often caused by an increased production of prolactin (hyperprolactinemia), either directly by pituitary gland activity or indirectly by inadequate hypothalamic inhibition of the pituitary gland.

Physiologic galactorrhea may present at menarche, early in menopause, for 1–2 years following cessation of lactation, or as a result of physical and emotional stress, coitus, mechanical and sexual stimulation of the nipples, or traumatic stimulation of the anterior thoracic nerves (Arnold et al. 1997).

There are many drugs associated with elevated prolactin levels. These drugs either deplete dopamine levels or block dopamine receptors, subsequently suppressing the prolactin-inhibiting factor. Drugs that are commonly associated with galactorrhea are oral contraceptives, antihypertensives, marijuana, opiates, tricyclic antidepressants, and phenothiazines (McCool et al. 1998, Speroff et al. 1999). (See **Table 4H.1, Causes of Chronic Hyperprolactinemia in the Nonpregnant Female**.)

Pathologic causes of hyperprolactinemia are hypothyroidism, diseases affecting the hypothalamic-pituitary axis, and nonpituitary sources. In hypothyroidism, with lowered levels of thyroid hormone, the thyroid-releasing hormone is produced in excess and acts as a prolactin-releasing factor causing release of pituitary prolactin. Hypothalamic disorders include tumors, infections, and vascular, degenerative, or granulomatous lesions. Pituitary disorders include tumors, Cushing's disease, or Nelson syndrome. Nonaxis causes include disorders affecting the clearance of serum prolactin (i.e., renal failure and liver failure). Although rare, elevated levels of prolactin may be the result of ectopic production of prolactin by bronchogenic or renal carcinomas, or stalk lesions or compression (Arnold et al. 1997). (See **Table 4H. 1**.)

DATABASE

SUBJECTIVE

→ Symptoms may include:
- Milky discharge—spontaneous and intermittent or persistent, unilateral or bilateral

- Hypoestrogenic symptoms (e.g., vasomotor symptoms, decreased breast size, vaginal atrophy) in patients with moderate to severe hyperprolactinemia
→ Patient may experience menstrual irregularities varying from polymenorrhea to amenorrhea.
- Oligomenorrhea and amenorrhea are the most common.
- Approximately one-third of women with galactorrhea will have normal menses.
→ Mild hirsutism may accompany ovulatory dysfunction (see the **Hirsutism** chapter in Section 12).
→ Patient may have history or signs and symptoms of:
- Any of the causes of hyperprolactinemia (see **Table 4H.1**).
  - For example, neoplastic lesions may produce headaches and visual changes (Jardines 1996).
- Endocrine anovulatory disorders including Chiari-Frommel, Forbes-Albright, and Ahumada-Del Castillo syndromes
→ A careful drug history, including illicit drug use, is important to assess for medications associated with galactorrhea.

OBJECTIVE

→ Inspection and palpation of the breasts—supraclavicular and axillary regions (supine and sitting) and compression of the breast, areola, or nipple—may reveal a milky nipple discharge. A mass is usually not present.
→ Physical examination should include thyroid exam, fundoscopic exam, and complete neurological exam, including visual field determination.
→ Patients with a history or symptoms of any of the causes of hyperprolactinemia may elicit manifestations of the condition (see **Table 4H.1**).
→ Clinical symptoms of galactorrhea or menstrual irregularities do not always correlate with prolactin levels.
→ See the **Amenorrhea—Secondary** chapter in Section 12.

ASSESSMENT

→ Galactorrhea
→ R/O hyperprolactinemia

→ R/O any of the possible causes of hyperprolactinemia (see **Table 4H.1**)

PLAN

DIAGNOSTIC TESTS

→ Observation of fat globules on microscopic exam will confirm galactorrhea.

→ Pregnancy test should be obtained to rule out pregnancy.

→ A serum prolactin level should be obtained in all cases of spontaneous discharge and in cases of elicited discharge when physiological causes cannot be ruled out (see the **Nipple Discharge—Physiologic** chapter).

■ Serum prolactin exceeding 20 ng/mL (varies by lab) is suggestive of hyperprolactinemia.

■ The optimal sampling time is between 8:00 a.m. and 12:00 noon.

■ Avoid sampling during and after events that may result in transient physiological hyperprolactinemia: excessive breast stimulation, stress, pelvic examination, coitus, surgical procedures, during midcycle, after an extended sleep, and following a protein-rich meal.

NOTE: The half-life for prolactin is 50–60 minutes.

→ Computerized axial (assisted) tomographic (CAT, CT) scanning or magnetic resonance imaging (MRI) is indicated with a prolactin ≥100 ng/mL, for lesser values in consultation with a physician, or in patients who have CNS symptoms such as headache or focal neurological signs (Alderman 1999).

■ CT scan with cone-down views of the sella turcica is more useful in the diagnosis of small pituitary tumors that do not distort or alter the size of the gland.

■ Magnetic resonance imaging (MRI), although more expensive and not as widely available, is an improvement over CT scanning for the visualization of structures adjacent to the pituitary, which may be affected by tumoral growth, and to diagnose empty-sella syndrome (Speroff et al. 1999).

→ Thyroid-stimulating hormone (TSH) should be obtained to rule out thyroid disease.

→ A variety of diagnostic tests to rule out underlying disorders may be obtained, depending on the history and physical examination.

→ See the **Amenorrhea—Secondary** chapter in Section 12.

Table 4H.1.   CAUSES OF CHRONIC HYPERPROLACTINEMIA IN THE NONPREGNANT FEMALE

Physiological	Excessive breast manipulation		Stress, surgery, venipuncture, etc.
Pharmacological	Estrogens Progestins Phenothiazines • Prochlorperazine • Chlorpromazine • Trifluoperazine • Thioridazine • Fluphenazine • Perphenazine • Acetophenazine • Mesoridazine • Methotrimeprazine • Pericyazine • Pipotiazine • Promazine • Thiopropazate • Thioproperazine • Triflupromazine	Butyrophenones • Haloperidol • Droperidol • Pimozide Thioxanthenes • Thiothixene • Chlorprothixene • Flupenthixol Tricyclic antidepressants • Amitriptyline • Amoxapine • Imipramine • Clomipramine • Desipramine • Doxepin • Nortriptyline • Protriptyline • Trimipramine	Miscellaneous antidepressants • Maprotiline • Fluoxetine • Paroxetine • Fluvoxamine Atypical antipsychotics • Clozapine • Loxapine • Molindone Antihypertensives • Methyldopa • Reserpine • Verapamil • Flunarizine Miscellaneous antidopaminergics • Metoclopramide	Others • Cimetidine • Danazol • Isoniazid • Arginine

Pathological	Primary hypothyroidism
	Hypothalamic disorders
	   Neoplastic, infectious, vascular, degenerative, or
	   granulomatous hypothalamic lesions
	Pituitary stalk section
	Pituitary disorders
	   Prolactin-secreting adenoma
	   Acromegaly, Cushing's disease, Nelson syndrome
			Ectopic production of prolactin
			   Bronchogenic carcinoma, hypernephroma
			Chronic renal failure
			Chest wall lesions
			Surgical scars, herpes zoster	

Functional	Idiopathic (no demonstrable tumor)			

Source: Compiled from Arnold, G.J., and Neiheisel, M.D. 1997. A comprehensive approach to evaluating nipple discharge. *Nurse Practitioner* 22(7):96–111; Katz, E., and Adashi, E.Y. 1990. Hyperprolactinemic disorders. *Clinical Obstetrics and Gynecology* 33(3):622–639.

TREATMENT/MANAGEMENT

→ Hyperprolactinemia due to physiological causes should be managed by discontinuing or reducing the precipitating events (e.g., a decrease in breast manipulation).

→ Hyperprolactinemia of pharmacological origin is managed by eliminating the causative drug.

■ In cases where the drug is necessary or when an alternative drug is not available, the presence of galactorrhea and associated symptoms should be weighed against the consequences of discontinuing the drug.

→ Management of hyperprolactinemia due to pathology other than pituitary tumors or idiopathic hyperprolactinemia should include treatment of the underlying condition (e.g., treatment of hypothyroidism).

→ Hyperprolactinemia due to prolactin-secreting pituitary tumors should be managed by a physician with dopaminergic agents (e.g., bromocriptine or, rarely, surgery).

→ Women with moderate to severe hyperprolactinemia due to idiopathic causes who have normal radiologic studies and regular menses may be managed expectantly and/or with bromocriptine.

→ Women with a normal prolactin and regular menses have a low risk of pituitary tumor and can be managed expectantly.

■ Periodic prolactin levels should be done to confirm the stability of the underlying process.

■ If the presence or amount of galactorrhea is unsatisfactory to the patient, bromocriptine may be used to reduce the occurrence.

CONSULTATION

→ Physician management is indicated for management with bromocriptine or when surgery is indicated.

PATIENT EDUCATION

→ Teach/review breast self-examination.

→ Allay patient's concerns regarding breast findings.

→ Patient should be advised before withdrawal of pharmacological agents that may be causing hyperprolactinemia.

→ For women with physiological causes of hyperprolactinemia, advise ways of omitting the offending event.

■ For example, to reduce breast stimulation, if sexually related, teach alternative means of stimulation.

■ For example, if stress-induced, provide suggestion for stress reduction.

NOTE: Advise women using bromocriptine to use an effective form of contraception because of the medication's teratogenic potential.

■ Review common side effects of this drug:

• Nausea
• Vomiting
• Headaches
• Faintness
• Dizziness
• Nasal congestion
• Fatigue

• Abdominal cramps
• (Rarely) neuropsychiatric symptoms (Speroff et al. 1999). (See *Physicians' Desk Reference*.)

→ See the **Amenorrhea—Secondary** chapter in Section 12.

FOLLOW-UP

→ Women with galactorrhea, normal prolactin levels, and normal menses can be followed with periodic prolactin levels every year.

■ If prolactin levels increase, a CT scan or MRI can be ordered.

→ Teach the American Cancer Society's recommendation for routine breast screening (Zoorob et al. 2001):

■ Breast self-examination monthly starting at age 20.

■ Clinical breast examination (CBE) every three years at ages 20–39 and every year after age 40.

■ Mammography every year starting at age 40. CBE should take place at a short interval prior to mammography because if a mass is identified it can be brought to the attention of the radiologist (Smith et al. 2000).

→ Women with a personal or family history of breast cancer may need earlier and/or more frequent clinical breast examinations and/or mammograms. Physician consultation should be sought (Zoorob et al. 2001).

→ Women at higher risk for breast cancer have options that can be suggested for cancer prevention. They include prophylactic mastectomy, tamoxifen therapy, clinical trial participation, and diet and lifestyle modification. Physician referral should be sought when surgery or pharmacological therapy is being considered.

→ Call the American Cancer Society at (800) ACS-2345 for mammogram facilities in the patient's area.

→ Document in progress notes and on problem list.

BIBLIOGRAPHY

Alderman, E.M. 1999. Breast problems in the adolescent. *Contemporary Pediatrics* 16(9):99–120.

Arnold, G.J., and Neiheisel, M.B. 1997. A comprehensive approach to nipple discharge. *Nurse Practitioner* 22(7):96–111.

Jardines, L. 1996. Management of nipple discharge. *American Surgeon* 62(2):119–122.

Katz, E., and Adashi, E.Y. 1990. Hyperprolactinemic disorders. *Clinical Obstetrics and Gynecology* 33(3):622–639.

McCool, W.F., Stone-Condry, M., and Bradford, H.M. 1998. Breast health review. *Journal of Nurse Midwifery* 43(6): 406–430.

Smith, R.A., Mettlin, C.J., Davis, K.J. et al. 2000. American Cancer Society guidelines for the early detection of cancer. *Cancer Journal for Clinicians* 50(1):34–49.

Speroff, L., Glass, R.H., and Kase, N.G. 1999. The breast. In *Clinical gynecologic endocrinology and infertility*, 6th ed. Baltimore, Md.: Lippincott Williams & Wilkins.

Zoorob, R., Anderson, R., Cefalu, C. et al. 2001. Cancer screening guidelines. *American Family Physician* 63(6): 1101–1112.

Lisa L. Lommel, R.N., C., F.N.P., M.S., M.P.H.

4-1

Intraductal Papilloma

Intraductal papillomas are finger-like projections that invade the lumen of the breast duct and are attached by a single stalk to the duct wall. The papilloma is a delicate villous structure caused by proliferation of the ductal epithelium, which creates a small dilation of the duct. The lesions most commonly develop adjacent to the areola and are usually less than 0.5 cm in size. Trauma to the ducts that contain papillomas will cause bleeding into the duct lumen and subsequent spontaneous serous, serosanguineous, or sanguineous nipple discharge. Pain at the point of location of the papilloma is uncommon (Drukker 1997).

Intraductal papillomas are the most common cause of benign pathologic nipple discharge in women who are not pregnant or lactating and are more common in the perimenopausal and menopausal woman. Solitary forms of intraductal papilloma (i.e., only one duct involved) are the most common type and do not increase a woman's risk for breast cancer. Multiple forms of this condition (intraductal papillomatosis), involving multiple ducts, have been shown to be linked with malignant transformation (Drukker 1997). Intraductal papillomatosis, usually affecting younger women, is more likely to present with a mass in the periphery of the breast and less often with nipple discharge.

DATABASE

SUBJECTIVE

→ Symptoms may include:
- Spontaneous, serous, serosanguineous, or sanguineous nipple discharge
- More commonly unilateral, though may be bilateral
- Palpable mass—if present, most commonly in the periphery of breast
- Tenderness with pressure over the involved duct

OBJECTIVE

→ Inspection and palpation of the breasts—supraclavicular and axillary regions (supine and sitting)—may reveal a subareolar mass, but this is very uncommon.

- With multiple forms of intraductal papilloma, the mass is more commonly in the periphery of the breast.
→ For women with a history of nipple discharge, the involved duct can be located by exerting gentle pressure at the areolar margin in a circular path around the nipple.
- When a discharge is seen, document location and whether it emanates from a single duct or multiple ducts, as well as its consistency and color.
→ Carefully document findings using descriptive terms.
- Mass(es) should be described assuming a clock position, locating the mass by distance from the base of the nipple, the dimensions measured with a centimeter ruler or tape.
- Consistency, shape, presence of tenderness, mobility, and associated skin changes should be described. Diagrams are helpful.

ASSESSMENT

→ Solitary intraductal papilloma
→ R/O multiple intraductal papilloma
→ R/O duct ectasia
→ R/O physiological nipple discharge
→ R/O breast cancer

PLAN

DIAGNOSTIC TESTS

→ Mammography is recommended in women over age 30 to rule out breast cancer. Magnification of the retroareolar region may be helpful.
→ Hemocult testing of nipple discharge for presence of blood should be performed.
→ Cytological analysis of the discharge is not reliable because the absence of malignant cells does not exclude cancer (Morrow 2000).

TREATMENT/MANAGEMENT

→ Ask a second examiner to corroborate breast finding.
→ Refer to a breast specialist for management.

→ Surgical excision with biopsy of the involved duct is the usual treatment.

CONSULTATION

→ For suspicion of a mass
→ Physician referral is recommended for diagnosis.

PATIENT EDUCATION

→ Teach/review breast self-examination.
→ Allay patient's concerns regarding breast finding.

FOLLOW-UP

→ Encourage follow-up appointment with a breast specialist.
→ Teach the American Cancer Society's recommendation for routine breast screening (Zoorob et al. 2001):
  - Breast self-examination monthly starting at age 20.
  - Clinical breast examination (CBE) every three years at ages 20–39 and every year after age 40.
  - Mammography every year starting at age 40. CBE should take place at a short interval prior to mammography because if a mass is identified it can be brought to the attention of the radiologist (Smith et al. 2000).

→ Women with a personal or family history of breast cancer may need earlier and/or more frequent clinical breast examinations and/or mammograms. Physician consultation should be sought (Zoorob et al. 2001).
→ Women at higher risk for breast cancer have options that can be suggested for cancer prevention. They include prophylactic mastectomy, tamoxifen therapy, clinical trial participation, and diet and lifestyle modification. Physician referral should be sought when surgery or pharmacological therapy is being considered.
→ Call the American Cancer Society at (800) ACS-2345 for mammogram facilities in the patient's area.
→ Document in progress notes and on problem list.

BIBLIOGRAPHY

Drukker, B.H. 1997. Breast disease: a primer on diagnosis and management. *International Journal of Fertility* 42(5): 278–287.

Morrow, M. 2000. The evaluation of common breast problems. *American Family Physician* 61(8):2371–2378.

Smith, R.A., Mettlin, C.J., Davis, K.J. et al. 2000. American Cancer Society guidelines for the early detection of cancer. *Cancer Journal for Clinicians* 50(1):34–49.

Zoorob, R., Anderson, R., Cefalu, C. et al. 2001. Cancer screening guidelines. *American Family Physician* 63(6): 1101–1112.

Lisa L. Lommel, R.N., C., F.N.P., M.S., M.P.H.

4-J

Mastitis—Nonpuerperal

Nonpuerperal mastitis, or squamous metaplasia, is described as the benign transformation of glandular or mucosal epithelium into stratified squamous epithelium. The origin of the condition is unknown. It has been postulated to occur as a result of a congenital anomaly of the ductal system, cigarette smoking, or vitamin A deficiency (Marchant 1998). It is not known whether inflammation occurs first followed by squamous metaplasia or if squamous metaplasia causes an obstruction and subsequent inflammation in the ductal system (Marchant 1998).

The diagnosis of squamous metaplasia is made by histologic evaluation. A careful evaluation is required, as squamous metaplasia occasionally appears with fibrous breast tissue, which results in an atypical cellular appearance (Marchant 1998).

Nonpuerperal mastitis is often misdiagnosed and improperly treated. Antibiotics are not helpful. Total excision of the involved duct system is the only complete cure.

DATABASE

SUBJECTIVE

→ More common in premenopausal women
→ Multicolored nipple discharge from nipple or nipple-areolar complex near a Montgomery's follicle
→ May have nipple retraction
→ May have palpable peri- or subareolar mass
→ History of multiple visits to health provider that may include multiple attempts to incise and drain mass and repeated antibiotic treatments without relief
→ History of duct ectasia, intraductal papilloma, or trauma (see the **Duct Ectasia/Periductal Mastitis** and **Intraductal Papilloma** chapters)

OBJECTIVE

→ Inspection and palpation of the breasts—supraclavicular and axillary regions (supine and sitting)—may reveal a tender peri- or subareolar mass. May have axillary lymphadenopathy.
→ Multicolored nipple discharge

→ Nipple retraction may be present.
→ Findings should be carefully documented using descriptive terms.
  ■ Mass(es) should be described assuming a clock position, locating the mass by distance from the base of the nipple, the dimensions measured with a centimeter ruler or tape.
  ■ Consistency, shape, presence of tenderness, mobility, and associated skin changes should be described. Diagrams are helpful.

ASSESSMENT

→ Nonpuerperal mastitis (squamous metaplasia)
→ R/O duct ectasia
→ R/O intraductal papilloma
→ R/O carcinoma of the breast

PLAN

DIAGNOSTIC TESTS

→ Fine needle aspiration for diagnostic culture may be indicated, though it usually does not alter the management plan.

TREATMENT/MANAGEMENT

→ Ask a second examiner to corroborate breast findings.
→ Successful treatment requires complete excision of involved duct system. Cultures should be taken during surgery, but they are usually negative.
→ Tissue should also be sent to pathology to rule out carcinoma. Recurrence is rare.

CONSULTATION

→ For suspicious mass or finding
→ Referral to a physician is indicated for diagnosis and treatment

PATIENT EDUCATION

→ Allay patient's concerns regarding breast findings.

FOLLOW-UP

→ Follow-up appointment with a breast specialist as indicated.

→ Teach the American Cancer Society's recommendation for routine breast screening (Zoorob et al. 2001):

■ Breast self examination monthly starting at age 20.

■ Clinical breast examination (CBE) every three years at ages 20–39 and every year after age 40.

■ Mammography every year starting at age 40. CBE should take place at a short interval prior to mammography because if a mass is identified it can be brought to the attention of the radiologist (Smith et al. 2000).

→ Women with a personal or family history of breast cancer may need earlier and/or more frequent clinical breast examinations and/or mammograms. Physician consultation should be sought (Zoorob et al. 2001).

→ Women at higher risk for breast cancer have options that can be suggested for cancer prevention. They include prophylactic mastectomy, tamoxifen therapy, clinical trial participation, and diet and lifestyle modification. Physician referral should be sought when surgery or pharmacological therapy is being considered.

→ Call the American Cancer Society at (800) ACS-2345 for mammogram facilities in the patient's area.

→ Document in progress notes and on problem list.

BIBLIOGRAPHY

Marchant, D.J. 1998. Controversies in benign breast disease. *Surgical Oncology Clinics of North America* 7(2):285–289.

Smith, R.A., Mettlin, C.J., Davis, K.J. et al. 2000. American Cancer Society guidelines for the early detection of cancer. *Cancer Journal for Clinicians* 50(1):34–49.

Zoorob, R., Anderson, R., Cefalu, C. et al. 2001. Cancer screening guidelines. *American Family Physician* 63(6): 1101–1112.

4-K

Nipple Discharge—Physiologic

Physiologic nipple discharge is a normal finding and can be elicited manually from the breasts of the majority of nonpregnant, nonlactating women. It begins in the early neonatal period as "witches milk" when neonates experience a few weeks of physiologic nipple discharge. Neonatal discharge is caused by a rapid decrease in neonatal estrogen in the presence of a high neonatal prolactin level, which stimulates the rudimentary breast tissue. After menarche, the cyclical rise and fall of estrogen and progesterone is responsible for secretory activity in the tubulo-alveolar units of the breast. After menopause, with the absence of hormone activity, the secretory activity ceases. Ductal elements remain, however, and are capable of producing pathologic secretions (Arnold et al. 1997).

The incidence and/or volume of physiologic discharge can increase under specific conditions. Certain medications can increase physiologic discharge, with combined oral contraceptives being the most common (see the **Galactorrhea** chapter). Chest wall surgery or trauma can cause a discharge through activation of afferent thoracic nerves and reflex stimulation of the breast through the hypothalamic-pituitary axis (Arnold et al. 1997). Vigorous sexual activity may also cause physiologic discharge. Recent or early pregnancy events are associated with physiologic discharge although they are categorized as lactational discharge.

Although not true nipple discharge, *pseudo-discharge* may present as physiologic discharge. Pseudo-discharge is caused by dermatological conditions affecting the nipple, areola, and/or breast. They include eczema, atopic dermatitis, viral lesions, infection of Montgomery's glands, traumatic nipple erosions (jogger's nipples), nipple trauma (piercing), or Paget's disease (see the **Paget's Disease** chapter) (Arnold et al. 1997).

DATABASE

SUBJECTIVE

→ Patient may notice nipple discharge either unilaterally or, more frequently, bilaterally during compression of the breast, areola, or nipple during breast self-exam or sexual stimulation. Physiologic discharge is usually not spontaneous.

→ Nipple discharge may be noted on bra, nightclothes, or sheets.

→ Physiologic discharge is most often milky white, multicolored (yellow, green, or gray), or bloody. By contrast, pathologic discharge is more often multicolored, purulent, or bloody.

→ History may include:
- Use of medications that can cause nipple discharge (see the **Galactorrhea** chapter)
- Recent chest wall surgery
- Recent or early pregnancy event
- Evidence of current dermatological breast lesions

OBJECTIVE

→ Inspection and palpation of the breasts—supraclavicular and axillary regions (supine and sitting)—may reveal a few drops of nipple discharge that are milky-white, multicolored (yellow, green, or gray), or serous.

→ Each quadrant of the areolar complex should be milked separately to assess for single or multiple duct discharge. Physiologic discharge is usually multiductal.

→ Presence of nipple, areolar, or breast lesions may indicate pseudo-discharge.

→ A magnifying glass will aid in differentiating single-duct from multiple-duct discharges. It will also differentiate true nipple discharge from pseudo-discharge (i.e., skin lesions).

→ With physiologic nipple discharge, usually no mass or lymphadenopathy is found.

→ There may be evidence of dermatological breast lesion.

ASSESSMENT

→ Physiologic nipple discharge
→ R/O galactorrhea
→ R/O dermatologic lesion
→ R/O mastitis
→ R/O duct ectasia
→ R/O intraductal papilloma
→ R/O breast cancer

PLAN

DIAGNOSTIC TESTS

→ Occult blood testing of the nipple discharge is advised to rule out presence of blood.

→ The practitioner may consider pregnancy test to rule out lactational discharge.

→ Microscopic evaluation of milky discharge can be performed to assess for evidence of fat globules, confirming the presence of milk.

→ Mammography is recommended for women over 35 years old (Morrow 2000).

TREATMENT/MANAGEMENT

→ Ask a second examiner to corroborate breast findings.

→ With milky discharge, see the **Galactorrhea** chapter.

→ Appropriate topical dermatological medications for women with topical breast lesions.

→ With serous or bloody discharge, refer to a breast specialist.

→ For women with physiologic nipple discharge, no treatment is necessary.

CONSULTATION

→ As appropriate for milky discharge (see the **Galactorrhea** chapter)

→ For serous discharge

→ For abnormal mammogram

→ For suspicion of a mass

PATIENT EDUCATION

→ Teach/review breast self-examination.

→ Allay patient's concerns regarding breast findings.

→ For women with milky discharge, see the **Galactorrhea** chapter.

→ Encourage proper nipple hygiene (i.e., washing with mild soap and water and keeping nipples dry).

→ Patient may use breast pads (commercially bought or clean cotton pads) if she finds discharge embarrassing.

→ Discourage manual or oral breast stimulation to decrease amount of discharge.

→ Review with health care provider medications that may be causing physiologic discharge.

FOLLOW-UP

→ Encourage follow-up appointment with a breast specialist.

→ Teach the American Cancer Society's recommendation for routine breast screening (Zoorob et al. 2001):

- Breast self-examination monthly starting at age 20.
- Clinical breast examination (CBE) every three years at ages 20–39 and every year after age 40.
- Mammography every year starting at age 40. CBE should take place at a short interval prior to mammography because if a mass is identified it can be brought to the attention of the radiologist (Smith et al. 2000).

→ Women with a personal or family history of breast cancer may need earlier and/or more frequent clinical breast examinations and/or mammograms. Physician consultation should be sought (Zoorob et al. 2001).

→ Women at higher risk for breast cancer have options that can be suggested for cancer prevention. They include prophylactic mastectomy, tamoxifen therapy, clinical trial participation, and diet and lifestyle modification. Physician referral should be sought when surgery or pharmacological therapy is being considered.

→ Call the American Cancer Society at (800) ACS-2345 for mammogram facilities in the patient's area.

→ Document in progress notes and on problem list.

BIBLIOGRAPHY

Arnold, G.J., and Neiheisel, M.B. 1997. A comprehensive approach to nipple discharge. *Nurse Practitioner* 22(7): 96–111.

Morrow, M. 2000. The evaluation of common breast problems. *American Family Physician* 61(8):2371–2378.

Smith, R.A., Mettlin, C.J., Davis, K.J. et al. 2000. American Cancer Society guidelines for the early detection of cancer. *Cancer Journal for Clinicians* 50(1):34–49.

Zoorob, R., Anderson, R., Cefalu, C. et al. 2001. Cancer screening guidelines. *American Family Physician* 63(6): 1101–1112.

Lisa L. Lommel, R.N., C., F.N.P., M.S., M.P.H.

4-L

Paget's Disease

Paget's disease is characterized by an infiltration of breast carcinoma cells into the epidermis of the nipple along the mammary ducts, without direct invasion. Paget's disease includes cancer lesions such as infiltrating ductal carcinoma, which are usually well-differentiated, or a ductal carcinoma in situ. This infiltration can be microscopic or present with erosion, scaling, or ulceration of the areola and/or nipple. When a palpable tumor is also present, it is easier to identify the nipple lesion as Paget's disease. If no palpable tumor is present, nipple lesions may be diagnosed as dermatitis, which can delay correct diagnosis and treatment (Giuliano 2001). Paget's disease of the breast is rare, constituting only about 1% of all breast cancers (Giuliano 2001).

DATABASE

SUBJECTIVE

→ Symptoms include:
  ■ Nipple and/or areolar itching, burning, or pain
  ■ Nipple and/or areolar scaling, erythema, erosion, or ulceration
  ■ Subareolar mass may be palpable

OBJECTIVE

→ Inspection and palpation of the breasts
  ■ Supraclavicular and axillary regions (supine and sitting) may reveal nipple and/or areolar scaling, erythema, erosion, or ulceration.
  ■ Subareolar mass may be palpable.
  ■ Axillary or clavicular lymph nodes are possibly enlarged.

ASSESSMENT

→ Paget's disease
→ R/O dermatitis
→ R/O fluid cyst
→ R/O fibroadenoma

PLAN

DIAGNOSTIC TESTS

→ Mammography is indicated in cases of discrete mass and in patients with nipple/areolar involvement without palpable mass (Giuliano 2001).
→ Physician referral is indicated for biopsy.

TREATMENT/MANAGEMENT

→ Refer to a physician for mammography follow-up if abnormal.
→ Physician management is indicated if the diagnosis is Paget's disease.

CONSULTATION

→ Referral is indicated for mammography follow-up and management if the diagnosis is Paget's disease.

PATIENT EDUCATION

→ Explain need for diagnostic mammography and biopsy.
→ When providing breast self-exam, stress to the patient the importance of alerting her health care provider about any nipple/areolar skin changes.

FOLLOW-UP

→ Encourage follow-up appointment with a breast specialist.
→ Teach the American Cancer Society's recommendation for routine breast screening (Zoorob et al. 2001):
  ■ Breast self-examination monthly starting at age 20.
  ■ Clinical breast examination (CBE) every three years at ages 20–39 and every year after age 40.
  ■ Mammography every year starting at age 40. CBE should take place at a short interval prior to mammography because if a mass is identified it can be brought to the attention of the radiologist (Smith et al. 2000).

→ Women with a personal or family history of breast cancer may need earlier and/or more frequent clinical breast examinations and/or mammograms. Physician consultation should be sought (Zoorob et al. 2001).

→ Women at higher risk for breast cancer have options that can be suggested for cancer prevention. They include prophylactic mastectomy, tamoxifen therapy, clinical trial participation, and diet and lifestyle modification. Physician referral should be sought when surgery or pharmacological therapy is being considered.

→ Call the American Cancer Society at (800) ACS-2345 for mammogram facilities in the patient's area.

→ Document in progress notes and on problem list.

BIBLIOGRAPHY

Giuliano, A.E. 2001. Breast. In *Current medical diagnosis and treatment,* eds. L.M. Tierney, Jr., S.J. McPhee, and M.A. Papadakis. New York: McGraw-Hill.

Smith, R.A., Mettlin, C.J., Davis, K.J. et al. 2000. American Cancer Society guidelines for the early detection of cancer. *Cancer Journal for Clinicians* 50(1):34–49.

Zoorob, R., Anderson, R., Cefalu, C. et al. 2001. Cancer screening guidelines. *American Family Physician* 63(6): 1101–1112.

Lisa L. Lommel, R.N., C., F.N.P., M.S., M.P.H.

4-M

Superficial Phlebitis (Mondor's Disease)

Superficial phlebitis of the breast *(Mondor's disease)* is an inflammation of a subcutaneous vein most commonly located on the lateral surface of the breast and chest wall. It begins as a painful thrombosed vein that develops into a fixed fibrous cord (Fiorica 1994). Although any vein may be involved, the vein usually affected is the thoraco-epigastric vein, which runs from the hypochondrium up across the lateral aspect of the breast to the anterior axillary fold (Zylstra 1999). It is a rare condition that occurs more commonly in women 21–55 years old. The etiology is unknown. Mondor's disease is benign and does not increase a woman's risk for breast cancer.

DATABASE

SUBJECTIVE

→ Symptoms may include:
- Acute onset of pain in lateral half of involved breast or anterior chest wall
- Progressing to dull aching tenderness in the breast
- Slight elevation in temperature over the affected area
- An elongated, firm cord (string phlebitis) in area of tenderness
- More commonly presents in women with heavy, poorly supported, pendulous breasts and/or with history of (Drukker 1997):
  - Parturition
  - Augmentation or reduction mammoplasty
  - Breast biopsy
  - Muscular strain
  - Traumatic injury to the breast

OBJECTIVE

→ Inspection and palpation of the breasts—supraclavicular and axillary regions (supine and sitting)—may reveal acute, tender, thickened cord typical of a thrombosed vein.
- With the arm and breast elevated, the cord-like or tubular vein may be taut and raised above the level of the skin.
- Dimpling of the skin may occur over the affected area.

- The affected vein may be v-shaped, and if there is branching the vein may have an inverted v-shape.
→ No adenopathy should be present.
→ No mass should be palpable.
→ Both breasts are rarely involved.
→ Findings should be carefully documented using descriptive terms.
- Mass(es) should be described assuming a clock position, locating the mass by distance from the base of the nipple, the dimensions measured with a centimeter tape or ruler.
- Consistency, shape, presence of tenderness, mobility, and associated skin changes should be described. Diagrams are helpful.

ASSESSMENT

→ Superficial thrombophlebitis (Mondor's disease)
→ R/O breast cancer

PLAN

DIAGNOSTIC TESTS

→ Mammography should be obtained in all patients with a palpable cord, even without an associated mass (Fiorica 1994).
→ Biopsy is indicated if:
- There is uncertainty of diagnosis
- There is a contiguous mass
- There is a suspicion of malignancy
- The condition does not resolve in 2–3 weeks with conservative treatment

TREATMENT/MANAGEMENT

→ Ask a second examiner to corroborate breast findings.
→ Treat conservatively with analgesics and local application of heat.
→ Advise rest for the affected arm and support for the affected breast.
→ This condition is self-limiting and usually lasts 2–3 weeks.

→ Refer to a breast specialist if a dominant breast mass is present.

CONSULTATION

→ Recommended for diagnosis
→ Refer to a breast specialist if a dominant mass is present.

PATIENT EDUCATION

→ Allay patient's concern regarding breast findings.

FOLLOW-UP

→ Encourage a follow-up appointment with a breast specialist.
→ Teach the American Cancer Society's recommendation for routine breast screening (Zoorob et al. 2001):
  - Breast self-examination monthly starting at age 20.
  - Clinical breast examination (CBE) every three years at ages 20–39 and every year after age 40.
  - Mammography every year starting at age 40. CBE should take place at a short interval prior to mammography because if a mass is identified it can be brought to the attention of the radiologist (Smith et al. 2000).
→ Women with a personal or family history of breast cancer may need earlier and/or more frequent clinical breast examinations and/or mammograms. Physician consultation should be sought (Zoorob et al. 2001).

→ Women at higher risk for breast cancer have options that can be suggested for cancer prevention. They include prophylactic mastectomy, tamoxifen therapy, clinical trial participation, and diet and lifestyle modification. Physician referral should be sought when surgery or pharmacological therapy is being considered.
→ Call the American Cancer Society at (800) ACS-2345 for mammogram facilities in the patient's area.
→ Document in progress notes and on problem list.

BIBLIOGRAPHY

Drukker, B.H. 1997. Breast Disease: a primer on diagnosis and management. *International Journal of Fertility* 42(5):278–287.

Fiorica, J.V. 1994. Special problems: Mondor's disease, macrocysts, trauma, squamous metaplasia, miscellaneous disorders of the nipple. *Obstetrics and Gynecology Clinics of North America* 21(3):479–485.

Smith, R.A., Mettlin, C.J., Davis, K.J. et al. 2000. American Cancer Society guidelines for the early detection of cancer. *Cancer Journal for Clinicians* 50(1):34–49.

Zoorob, R., Anderson, R., Cefalu, C. et al. 2001. Cancer screening guidelines. *American Family Physician* 63(6): 1101–1112.

Zylstra, S. 1999. Office management of benign breast disease. *Clinical Obstetrics and Gynecology* 42(2):234–249.

SECTION 5

Respiratory/ Otorhinolaryngological Disorders

5-A Asthma **5-2**
5-B Bronchiectasis **5-12**
5-C Bronchitis—Acute **5-15**
5-D Chronic Obstructive Pulmonary Disease **5-17**
5-E Epistaxis **5-23**
5-F Influenza **5-25**
5-G Otitis Externa **5-29**
5-H Otitis Media **5-31**
5-I Pharyngitis **5-33**
5-J Pneumonia **5-37**
5-K Rhinitis **5-43**
5-L Sinusitis—Acute **5-48**
5-M Sinusitis—Chronic **5-51**

5-A
Asthma

Asthma has long been regarded as a lung disease resulting from airway hyperresponsiveness and inflammation characterized by intermittent reversible airway obstruction. Recent advances have led to a new definition of asthma as:

"…a chronic inflammatory disorder of the airways in which many cells and cellular elements play a role, in particular, mast cells, eosinophils, T lymphocytes, neutrophils and epithelial cells. In susceptible individuals, this inflammation causes recurrent episodes of wheezing, breathlessness, chest tightness and cough. These episodes are usually associated with widespread but variable air flow obstruction that is often reversible. The inflammation also causes an associated increase in the existing bronchial hyperresponsiveness" (National Institutes of Health [NIH] 1997).

The airways of patients with asthma are hyperresponsive to a variety of inhaled irritants, including allergens, pollens (Busse et al. 2001), dust mites, cockroaches (Arruda et al. 2001), occupational irritants (Toren et al. 1999), viruses, or cold air. Some individuals experience symptoms principally following exercise (i.e., *exercise-induced bronchospasm*) (Anderson et al. 2000). Asthma occurs in individuals with a genetic predisposition (Larj et al. 2002). Many individuals have family members with asthma or other atopic disorders, such as allergic rhinitis or eczema.

When the individual's airway is exposed to a triggering event or antigen, there is immediate bronchoconstriction of smooth muscle and degeneration of mast cells that leads to release of inflammatory mediators. These, in turn, cause an inflammatory response involving a variety of cells and other mediators (Busse et al. 2001). The physiological response to this inflammatory sequence is smooth muscle contraction (i.e., *bronchospasm*), edema, and excess mucus production and plugging. The narrowing of small airways can lead to air trapping, hypoxemia, carbon dioxide retention, increasing pulmonary vascular resistance, and negative pleural pressure. These physiological processes are responsible for the common clinical symptoms of wheezing, shortness of breath, and cough, and can lead to progressive use of accessory muscles, pulsus paradoxicus, and respiratory failure.

Asthma is classified as either intermittent or chronic and as mild, moderate, or severe. Clinical characteristics and lung function measurement are used to determine an individual's classification, which in turn determines a specific level of therapy. The current classification system is described in **Table 5A.1, Stepwise Approach to Asthma Classification Clinical Features**. Additionally, some patients have special conditions—such as *cough variant asthma*, with most of their symptoms occurring during sleep—while others experience exercise-induced bronchospasm.

Asthma now affects more than 15 million Americans; estimated costs in 2000 reached $14.5 billion (Centers for Disease Control and Prevention [CDC] 2001). In 1998, 39 people per 1,000 had experienced an asthma episode or attack in the previous 12 months. In 1991, with more than 8.8 million visits to physician offices, asthma ranked 10th among medical diagnoses in the United States (Schappert 1993); however, by 1998 there were 13.9 million visits to physician offices or hospital clinics for asthma (CDC 2001). Although mortality and hospitalization rates for asthma increased in the 1980s, deaths are uncommon. In 1998, there were 423,000 hospitalizations and 5,438 deaths (CDC 2001).

Because asthma is such a widespread chronic disease with acute exacerbations causing considerable patient dysfunction and extensive use of health care services, the National Heart, Lung, and Blood Institute of NIH created a National Asthma Education and Prevention Program (NAEPP) that has developed *Guidelines for the Diagnosis and Management of Asthma* (NIH 1997). The guidelines still have to be tested to document their effectiveness, but they should nevertheless be considered for incorporation into clinical practice.

Many components of the guidelines are included in this chapter, which presents the care plan for individuals with mild to moderate asthma. The care of an individual with severe asthma or asthma that is unresponsive to appropriate therapy is beyond the scope of this chapter. An individual with these conditions should be referred to a physician or pulmonary clinic for evaluation and treatment.

DATABASE

SUBJECTIVE

→ History may include:
- Other allergic disorders (e.g., allergic rhinitis, sinusitis, eczema, nasal polyps)
- Lower respiratory infections in childhood (e.g., bronchitis, pneumonia)
- Passive exposure to smoke
- Smoking
- Environmental/occupational exposure to allergens, pets
- Environmental/occupational exposure to chemicals/pollutants/irritants (e.g., aerosols, perfumes, detergents, construction materials, fumigants)
- Medications (especially aspirin, nonsteroidal anti-inflammatory medications, beta-blockers)
- Exposure to weather (temperature) change
- Exacerbation of symptoms with exercise
- Endocrine factors (e.g., pregnancy, menses, thyroid disease)
- Family history of asthma, allergic rhinitis, eczema

→ Note age of initial diagnosis of asthma.

→ The patient may report one or more of the following symptoms:
- Wheezing
- Chest tightness
- Shortness of breath
- Daytime cough
- Nighttime cough
- Sputum production (adults)
- Activity limitation
- Fever
- Chest pain
- Lethargy
- Anxiety
- Confusion
- Palpitations

NOTE: When assessing the patient's symptoms, it is important to determine the following: onset, duration, pattern (e.g., episodic, continuous symptoms with intermittent exacerbations), course of disease, treatment(s) that relieve symptoms, aggravating factors or seasonal variations, and any use of medical services (e.g., hospital, emergency room, or urgent-care clinic).

OBJECTIVE

→ Physical examination may reveal the following:
- Vital signs:
  - Elevation in temperature, along with increasing pulse and respirations. Blood pressure may reveal pulse paradoxicus in severe cases. These measurements, in part, determine therapeutic interventions.
- The patient appears fatigued, lethargic, or disoriented, or coughs persistently when attempting to talk.
- Cyanosis
- Evidence of eczema
- Rhinitis
- Nasal flaring
- Nasal polyps
- Neck vein distention
- Use of accessory muscles of respiration—i.e., neck, chest, abdomen
- Hunched posture while breathing
- Pigeon chest
- Hollow sound upon chest wall percussion

→ Auscultation of the chest may reveal:
- Decreased intensity of breath sounds
- Prolonged expiration
- Wheezing
- Crackles
- Rhonchi

→ Auscultation of the heart may reveal a cardiac gallop or increased P_2.

Table 5A.1.   STEPWISE APPROACH TO ASTHMA CLASSIFICATION CLINICAL FEATURES

	Days with Symptoms	**Nights with Symptoms**	**Pulmonary Function**
Step 4 **Severe Persistent**	Continual	Frequent	$FEV_1/PEF \leq 60\%$ PEFR variability $>30\%$
Step 3 **Moderate Persistent**	Daily	>1/week	$FEV_1/PEF >60\%-<80\%$ PEFR variability $>30\%$
Step 2 **Mild Persistent**	3–6/week	>2/month	$FEV_1/PEF \geq 80\%$ PEFR variability 20–30%
Step 1 **Mild Intermittent**	≤2/week	≤2/month	$FEV_1/PEF \geq 80\%$ PEFR variability <20%

Source: National Institutes of Health (NIH). 2002. National Asthma Education and Prevention Program. *Expert panel report. Guidelines for the diagnosis and management of asthma. Update on selected topics 2002.* Publication No. 02-5075. Bethesda, Md.: the Author.

ASSESSMENT

$\rightarrow$ Asthma

$\rightarrow$ R/O chronic bronchitis (chronic obstructive pulmonary disease [COPD Type B])

$\rightarrow$ R/O emphysema (COPD Type A)

$\rightarrow$ R/O congestive heart failure

$\rightarrow$ R/O drug reaction (e.g., to beta-blockers, aspirin, angiotensin-converting enzyme inhibitors, antibiotics)

$\rightarrow$ R/O acute inhalation of irritating substance

$\rightarrow$ R/O mechanical obstruction (especially a mediastinal mass)

$\rightarrow$ R/O pulmonary embolism

$\rightarrow$ R/O pulmonary infection (e.g., pneumonia, acute bronchitis)

$\rightarrow$ R/O gastroesophageal reflux disorder

$\rightarrow$ R/O pulmonary eosinophilia syndrome

PLAN

DIAGNOSTIC TESTS

$\rightarrow$ It is recommended that all patients have objective measures of lung function performed to establish a diagnosis, monitor progress, and judge severity during acute exacerbations of asthma. It is important to use objective measures of lung function because a patient's history and physical examination findings may not correlate with the severity of airflow obstruction.

$\rightarrow$ The following tests usually are ordered (see **Table 5D.2, Pulmonary Function Tests (PFTs)—Definitions and Results in Obstructive and Restrictive Pulmonary Disease** in the **Chronic Obstructive Pulmonary Disease** chapter):

- Spirometry:
  - Airway obstruction will impact flow rates and produce changes in the forced vital capacity (FVC), forced expiratory volume in one second (FEV$_1$), and the maximum midexpiratory flow rate (MMEF). An obstructive pattern will be demonstrated.
  - Spirometry equipment is not frequently found in most primary care offices; therefore, the patient may need to be referred to a pulmonologist.
- Peak expiratory flow rate (PEFR) meters:
  - PEFR correlates well with FEV$_1$. Asthma reduces PEFR and FEV$_1$.
  - PEFR meters are widely available as small office equipment or inexpensive plastic portable models.

$\rightarrow$ Depending on clinical history and physical examination, the following additional tests may be ordered after consultation with a physician:

- Chest x-ray:
  - To rule out pneumonia in febrile patients, to assess other cardiopulmonary disease if other obstructive phenomena are suspected, and to assess pneumothorax or atelectasis in acutely ill patients
- Sputum for Gram stain and/or culture-and-sensitivity:
  - To rule out a co-existing pulmonary infection

- Complete blood count (CBC):
  - May reveal eosinophilia
- Skin testing:
  - To determine hypersensitivity to specific allergens
- Nasal secretions smear:
  - To evaluate for the presence of eosinophilia
- Serum theophylline level (evaluate baseline and/or therapeutic levels in patients using theophylline for symptom relief)

$\rightarrow$ In *acute* exacerbations of asthma with moderate to severe symptoms, the following tests can be ordered after consultation with a physician:

- Oxygen saturation
- Blood gasses:
  - pO$_2$ will be decreased.
  - pCO$_2$ will be increased in severe asthma episodes, and normal or low in mild to moderate asthma (because of hyperventilation).

NOTE: Although some sources had recommended arterial blood gas measurement (NIH 1991), this test is technically difficult and potentially has more complications than other sampling methods. Oxygenation is adequately assessed by measuring transcutaneous oxygen saturation with a digital pulse oximeter (Elborn et al. 1991, Holmgren et al. 1992), and elevations in pCO$_2$ and reductions in pH are obtainable with capillary or venous blood. The NAEPP guidelines use pCO$_2$ values that are based on arterial blood; pCO$_2$ measured on capillary or venous blood, or measured transcutaneously, will be slightly higher. Transcutaneous pO$_2$ also will be lower than corresponding arterial values (Holmgren et al. 1992).

TREATMENT/MANAGEMENT

$\rightarrow$ A wide variety of treatment strategies are available to control asthma.

- A number of different symptom patterns can be classified as mild, moderate, or severe persistent. The more severe or frequent the symptoms, the greater the dosages of medications.
- Tailoring the medication regimen to allow maximum patient functioning with minimum symptoms and side effects is the goal of individualized management.

$\rightarrow$ The following are general guidelines for environmental control and medication management for asthma therapy:

- Environmental control should be based on the patient's history of allergic/irritant exposure.
  - Outdoor measures:
    - Patients do not have to avoid the outdoors but should avoid activities that may increase symptoms (e.g., mowing the lawn) or involve unnecessarily heavy exposure to outdoor allergens (e.g., pollens, ragweed, molds).
  - Indoor measures:
    - Keeping the house as clean as possible, especially the patient's bedroom

- Wearing a mask when vacuuming and using special vacuums with high efficiency particulate air (HEPA) filters
- Having pets sleep outdoors or, if that is not possible, in areas where there is limited exposure of the patient to animal hair, fur, and dander
- Maintaining low humidity to discourage mold growth
- Encasing mattresses and pillows in plastic covers
- Washing bedding every week in water with a temperature of at least 54° C/130° F
- Having a minimum of rugs, upholstered furniture, and stuffed animals, and keeping these out of the bedroom if possible
- Removing carpets on concrete slabs and from other types of floors if possible.
- Pharmacological interventions: Refer to **Table 5A.2, Medications for the Treatment of Asthma** and **Table 5A.3, Daily Dosages for Inhaled Steroids** for the medications recommended for each asthma classification by the NAEPP guidelines for treating asthma, and to

Table 5A.4, Types of Medication Used in Asthma for a summary of available medications.
- Patients exhibiting severe symptoms or symptoms that persist after therapy, or patients classified as severe persistent, need an immediate evaluation by a physician.
- If control is not maintained, the NAEPP guidelines recommend "stepping up" to the regimen for the next level of severity (i.e., from the mild to moderate regimen) after reviewing the patient's medication technique, compliance, and control of environmental triggers.
- Patient treatments also can be stepped down if a review of status suggests that reducing pharmacologic treatment is possible.

NOTE: There are special precautions when treating patients older than 65 years. High-dose inhaled steroids may increase the risk of open angle glaucoma and decreased bone mineral density. However, the latter can be reduced by vitamin D and calcium supplementation (NIH 1997). Theophylline clearance is hampered by other medications, such as propranolol and cimetidine. Finally, the use of

Table 5A.2. MEDICATIONS FOR THE TREATMENT OF ASTHMA

	Daily Medication for Long-Term Control	Medication for Quick Relief
Step 4 **Severe Persistent**	Preferred: inhaled steroid, high dose AND long-acting inhaled β_2-agonist AND, IF NEEDED oral steroid (attempt to reduce)	Short-acting inhaled β_2-agonist 2–4 puffs as needed for symptoms. Up to 3 treatments at 20-minute intervals. Daily use or increasing use indicates need for additional long-term therapy.
Step 3 **Moderate**	Preferred: inhaled steroid, low dose AND long-acting inhaled β_2-agonist AND, IF NEEDED increase inhaled steroid to medium dose OR low to medium inhaled steroid with leukotriene modifier or theophylline	Short-acting inhaled β_2-agonist 2–4 puffs as needed for symptoms. Up to 3 treatments at 20-minute intervals for acute exacerbation. Daily use or increasing use indicates need for additional long-term therapy.
Step 2 **Mild Persistent**	Preferred: inhaled steroid, low dose OR cromolyn 2–4 puffs TID-QID OR nedocromil 2–4 puffs BID-QID OR sustained-release theophylline OR leukotriene modifiers	Short-acting inhaled β_2-agonist 2–4 puffs as needed for symptoms. Up to 3 treatments at 20-minute intervals for acute exacerbation. Daily use or increasing use indicates need for additional long-term therapy.
Step 1 **Mild Intermittent**	No daily medication	Short-acting inhaled β_2-agonist 2–4 puffs as needed for symptoms. Up to 3 treatments at 20-minute intervals for an acute exacerbation. Use more than twice weekly may indicate need to initiate long-term therapy.

Source: National Institutes of Health (NIH). 2002. National Asthma Education and Prevention Program. *Expert panel report. Guidelines for the diagnosis and management of asthma. Update on selected topics 2002.* Publication No. 02-5075. Bethesda, Md.: the Author.

Table 5A.3.   DAILY DOSAGES FOR INHALED STEROIDS

Inhaled Steroid	Low Dose	Medium Dose	High Dose
Beclomethasone 42 mcg/puff 84 mcg/puff	168–504 mcg 4–12 puffs 2–6 puffs	504–840 mcg 12–20 puffs 6–10 puffs	>840 mcg >20 puffs >10 puffs
Budesonide Dry powder inhaler (DPI): 200 mcg/dose	200–400 mcg 1–2 inhalations	400–600 mcg 2–3 inhalations	>600 mcg >3 inhalations
Flunisolide 250 mcg/puff	500–1,000 mcg 2–4 puffs	1,000–2,000 mcg 4–8 puffs	>2,000 mcg >8 puffs
Fluticasone Metered dose inhaler: 44, 110, 220 mcg/puff DPI: 50, 100, 250 mcg/dose	88–264 mcg 2–6 puffs, 44 mcg 2 puffs, 110 mcg 2–6 inhalations, 50 mcg	264–660 mcg 2–6 puffs, 110 mcg 3–6 inhalations, 100 mcg	>660 mcg >6 puffs, 110 mcg >3 puffs, 220 mcg >6 inhalations, 100 mcg >2 inhalations, 250 mcg
Triamcinolone acetonide 100 mcg/puff	400–1,000 mcg 4–10 puffs	1,000–2,000 mcg 10–20 puffs	>2,000 mcg >20 puffs

Source: National Institutes of Health (NIH). 1999. *Practical guide to the diagnosis and management of asthma.* Publication No. 99-4055. Bethesda, Md.: the Author.

Table 5A.4.   TYPES OF MEDICATION USED IN ASTHMA

Medication	Other Drug Label	Preparations Available	Mechanism of Action	Uses/Advantages	Disadvantages
Quick Relief					
Short-Acting β₂-Adrenergic Agonists					
Albuterol	Ventolin®, Proventil®	Inhaled, nebulized, oral	Relaxes smooth muscles and produces bronchodilation.	Efficacious and first choice for acute bronchospasm. Inhaled route fastest. Can be delivered with metered dose inhaler.	Can produce cardiovascular and muscle stimulation. Minimized by avoiding oral route and less ß₂-selective medicines (isoproterenol, metaproterenol, isoetharine, and epinephrine).
Bitolterol	Tornalate®	Inhaled			
Pirbuterol	Maxair®	Inhaled, oral			
Terbutaline	Brethaire®, Brethine®	Inhaled, oral, subQ			
Ipratropium	Atrovent®	Inhaled	Reduces vagal tone to airways.	Effective in status asthmaticus in conjunction with β₂-agonists.	Limited use outside of emergencies. Causes drying of mouth and respiratory secretions.
Systemic Corticosteroids					
Prednisone	Prednisone, Solu-Medrol®, SoluCortef®	Oral IV IV	Anti-inflammatory: interrupts the development of and terminates ongoing inflammatory response.	For moderate to severe exacerbations to avoid progression and reduce chance of relapse.	Fluid retention, gastric irritation, weight gain, mood alteration, increased blood pressure. May be fatal if varicella develops.
Prednisolone	Prelone®	Oral			
Methylprednisolone	Medrol®	Oral			
Hydrocortisone					

(continued)

Table 5A.4.   TYPES OF MEDICATION USED IN ASTHMA (continued)

Medication	Other Drug Label	Preparations Available	Mechanism of Action	Uses/Advantages	Disadvantages
Long-Term Control					
Inhaled Corticosteroids					
Beclomethasone	Vanceril®	Inhaled	Anti-inflammatory: interrupts responses to allergens, reduces airway hyperresponsiveness.	Long-term control of mild, moderate, and severe persistent asthma.	Thrush, cough, dysphonia. Potential for systemic effects.
Dipropionate	Beclovent®	Inhaled			
Budesonide		Inhaled			
Flunisolide	AeroBid®	Inhaled			
Fluticasone propionate	Flovent®	Inhaled			
Triamcinolone acetonide	Pulmicort®, Azmacort®	Inhaled			
Cromolyn Sodium	Intal®	Inhaled (MDI, nebulizer)	Stabilize mast cells, prevent mediator release. Inhibit response to exercise and cold air.	Long-term prevention of symptoms of persistent asthma, to prevent exercise-induced bronchospasm (EIB).	Unpleasant taste.
Nedocromil Sodium	Tilade®				
Long-Acting β₂-Agonists					
Salmeterol	Serevent®	Inhaled, oral	Bronchodilation; slower onset and longer duration than short-acting agents.	Long-term prevention of symptoms of persistent asthma, preventing EIB and nighttime symptoms.	Tachycardia, hypokalemia, muscle tremors; use with caution in elderly.
Formoterol	Foradil®	Aerosolized			
Albuterol	Proventil®, Repetabs®, Volmax® extended-release tablets	Oral			
Methylxanthines					
Theophylline sustained-release capsules and tablets	Elixophyllin®, Slo-Bid™, Gyrocaps®, Slo-Phyllin®, Theo-Dur®, Theolair®, Uniphyl®	Oral	Smooth muscle relaxation produces bronchodilation.	Mainstay for decades, but many side effects. Long-term control of persistent asthma (added to β-agonists) can be monitored for therapeutic level; helpful for nocturnal symptoms.	Narrow therapeutic range, GI upset and muscle tremors at low doses, cardiovascular and CNS toxicities at higher levels.
Leukotriene Modifiers					
Montelukast	Singulaire®	Oral	Inhibit or modify leukotriene and leukotriene receptors.	May be considered as an alternative in mild persistent asthma.	Elevation of liver enzymes with zileuton.
Zafirlukast	Accolate®	Oral			
Zileuton	Zyflo®	Oral			
Systemic Corticosteroids					
Prednisone	Prednisone, Deltasone®	Oral	Anti-inflammatory	Given by short bursts of 5–10 days to control acute exacerbations. Long-term control in persistent severe asthmatics.	Short-term use has reversible side effects of fluid retention, mood swings, hypertension. Long-term use associated with adrenal axis suppression.
Prednisolone	Prelone®	Oral			
Methylprednisolone	Medrol®	Oral			

Source: National Institutes of Health (NIH). 1999. *Practical guide to the diagnosis and management of asthma*. Publication No. 99-4055. Bethesda, Md.: the Author.

metered dose inhalers (MDIs) can be challenging for many elderly women (Kitch et al. 2000).

- Exercise-induced bronchospasm: Use of the following medication(s) 5–60 minutes before exercise is often beneficial:
  - Inhaled cromolyn: 2 inhalations. Duration of effect is usually 1–2 hours.
  - An inhaled, short-acting, β_2-adrenergic agent such as albuterol: 2 inhalations. Duration of effect is usually 2–3 hours.
  - An inhaled, long-acting, β_2-adrenergic agent such as salmeterol taken at least 30 minutes before exercise will last 10–12 hours.
  NOTE: If moderate to severe symptoms characteristically accompany exercise, then inhaled cromolyn and an inhaled β_2-adrenergic agent can be combined 15 minutes before exercise.

- Cough variant asthma: Treatment can follow the typical treatment of asthma, except inhaled medications may worsen the symptoms (Irwin et al. 1998). Use of the following medications may be beneficial:
  - An inhaled β_2-adrenergic agent such as albuterol at bedtime (Jenne 1984)
  - Sustained-release theophylline 200 mg p.o. taken between 6:00 p.m. and 8:00 p.m. (Arkinstall 1988)
  - Zafirlukast 20 mg p.o. BID (Dicpinigaitis et al. 2002)
  NOTE: In patients with nocturnal asthma symptoms, a work-up should be considered to rule out the possibility of gastroesophageal reflux.

- Mild intermittent asthma: Use of β_2-agonists is recommended because these agents act faster, have fewer adverse side effects, and achieve the desired results at lower doses than do oral medications. The following medications can be prescribed:
  - Albuterol: Patients can take 1–2 puffs every 3–4 hours as needed during the acute exacerbation of the asthma episode. Up to 3 treatments of 2–4 puffs at least 20 minutes apart can be used during an acute attack (NIH 1997).
  NOTE: The need to use an inhaler daily or 3–4 times a day indicates the need for additional therapy (NIH 2002).

- Mild persistent asthma: Use of inhaled anti-inflammatory agents is indicated. Mild persistent asthma is characterized by exacerbations that occur more than twice a week or that affect the patient's sleep and/or daily living activities, or by pulmonary function as documented in **Table 5A.1** (NIH 2002). One of the following agents can be prescribed:
  - Preferred treatment:
    ➤ Inhaled steroids, low dose. (See **Table 5A.3**.)
  - Alternative treatment:
    ➤ Cromolyn sodium 2–4 puffs TID-QID
    NOTE: A 4- to 6-week trial of this agent is necessary before its effectiveness can be determined.
    ➤ Nedocromil 2–4 puffs BID-QID

➤ Zafirlukast 20 mg p.o. BID or montelukast 10 mg p.o. qHS

- Moderate persistent asthma: Use of inhaled anti-inflammatory agents is indicated. Moderate persistent asthma is characterized by daytime symptoms that occur daily, affect the patient's sleep more than once weekly, and/or interfere with daily living activities, or by pulmonary function as indicated in **Table 5A.1** (NIH 2002). The following agents can be prescribed:
  - Preferred treatments:
    ➤ Inhaled steroid, medium dose (see **Table 5A.3**)
    OR
    ➤ Inhaled steroid, low dose (see **Table 5A.3**) in combination with a long-acting, inhaled, β_2-agonist such as salmeterol
  - Alternative treatment:
    ➤ Inhaled steroid, low dose in combination with a leukotriene antagonist or theophylline
    ➤ In patients with severe recurring exacerbations, medium-dose steroids can be substituted for the low-dose, inhaled steroids listed above.
    ➤ Since release of the NAEPP guidelines in 1999, information has become available indicating the efficacy of formoterol (Bensch et al. 2002) and the efficacy of a fluticasone/salmeterol combination (Kavuru et al. 2000).
  NOTE: Attaining maximum benefit from the above medications may require 2–4 weeks of therapy. Side effects of these agents include occasional coughing, dysphonia, and oral candidiasis. Use of a spacer device or having the patient rinse her mouth after inhaling medication will reduce the incidence of side effects.

- If a patient's symptoms persist after the use of inhaled steroids at the above doses, consultation with a physician is indicated.

- Therapeutic options at this point include increasing the dose of the inhaled steroid or using a longer-acting bronchodilator or sustained-release theophylline preparations.

- If theophylline is prescribed, the usual initial dose is 200 mg p.o. BID with adjustments in the dose based on clinical symptoms and serum theophylline levels. (Obtaining serum theophylline levels after increasing therapy is indicated to determine if a therapeutic level of 5–15 µg/mL has been attained.) Toxicity occurs when the level is 20 µg/mL or greater but also may occur in some patients with levels of at least 15 µg/mL. Symptoms and physical findings associated with theophylline toxicity include nausea, vomiting, tachycardia, tachypnea, arrhythmias, hyperglycemia, hypokalemia, and seizures (NIH 1997).

- Persistence of symptoms after initiating maximum doses of inhaled steroids, bronchodilators, cromolyn sodium, and leukotriene modifiers may require oral steroids. In these situations, refer the patient to a physician for further evaluation and treatment.

Figure 5A.1.   STEPS FOR USING YOUR INHALER

1. Remove the cap and hold inhaler upright.

2. Shake the inhaler.

3. Tilt your head back slightly and breathe out slowly.

4. Position the inhaler in one of the following ways (A or B is optimal, but C is acceptable for those who have difficulty with A or B. C is required for breath-activated inhalers):

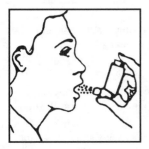 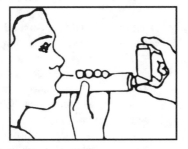 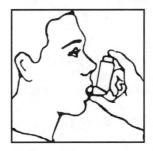 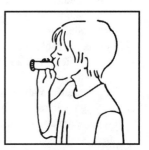

A. Open mouth with inhaler 1–2 inches away.

B. Use spacer/holding chamber (that is recommended especially for young children and for people using corticosteroids).

C. In the mouth. Do not use for corticosteroids.

D. **NOTE:** Inhaled dry powder capsules require a different inhalation technique. To use a dry powder inhaler, it is important to close the mouth tightly around the mouthpiece of the inhaler and to inhale rapidly.

5. Press down on the inhaler to release medication as you start to breathe in slowly.

6. Breathe in slowly (3–5 seconds).

7. Hold your breath for 10 seconds to allow the medicine to reach deeply into your lungs.

8. Repeat puff as directed. Waiting 1 minute between puffs may permit the second puff to penetrate your lungs better.

9. Spacers/holding chambers are useful for all patients. They are particularly recommended for young children and older adults and for use with inhaled corticosteroids.

Avoid common inhaler mistakes. Follow these inhaler tips:

- Breathe out *before* pressing your inhaler.

- Inhale *slowly*.

- Breathe in through your mouth, not your nose.

- Press down on your inhaler at the *start* of inhalation (or within the first second of inhalation).

- Keep inhaling as you press down on the inhaler.

- Press your inhaler only *once* while you are inhaling (one breath for each puff).

- Make sure you breathe in evenly and deeply.

NOTE: Other inhalers are becoming available in addition to those illustrated above. Different types of inhalers may require different techniques.

Source: National Institutes of Health (NIH). 1997. National Asthma Education and Prevention Program. *Expert panel report 2. Guidelines for the diagnosis and management of asthma.* Publication No. 97-4051. Bethesda, Md.: the Author.

- If the patient smokes, she should be advised to stop and be referred to a smoking cessation program.
- Psychological evaluation and/or counseling may be indicated for patients exhibiting significant signs or symptoms of depression, anxiety, or other psychological sequelae associated with chronic disease.

CONSULTATION

→ Consultation with a physician is indicated for a patient who exhibits moderate to severe asthma symptoms or for a patient who is having significant side effects associated with medications.

→ Physician consultation is indicated:
  - For a patient with a history of multiple emergency room visits, hospital stays, and symptoms that are atypical and raise questions about other diagnostic possibilities.
  - If diagnostic testing for allergens is indicated.
  - If there are complicating factors requiring special care (e.g., concomitant cardiac disease, nasal polyps) or other significant complications (e.g., pneumonia, suspected tension pneumothorax).

→ Any patient with severe persistent asthma should be referred to an asthma specialist.

→ As needed for prescription(s).

PATIENT EDUCATION

→ Educate the patient about asthma—the cause(s), clinical course, preventive measures, treatment options, possible complications, side effects of medications, and when to seek immediate medical care.

→ Educate the patient about the need to avoid triggering agents and to prevent exacerbations.

→ If the patient smokes, discuss the need to stop smoking and refer her to community programs.

→ Instruct the patient about the proper use of MDIs and spacer devices for inhaled medications. (See **Figure 5A.1, Steps for Using Your Inhaler**.) The following steps should be emphasized:
  - Make sure there is enough medicine in the canister. An easy way to determine this is to place the canister in a container of water: If it sinks to the bottom, it is full; if it floats on the surface (tipped sideways), it is empty.
  - Hold the canister upright, remove the cap, and shake.
  - Tilt head back slightly and breathe out.
  - Open mouth, holding the inhaler 1–2 inches away.
  - Press down on the top of the canister and breathe in slowly. Continue to breathe in slowly for 3–5 seconds.
  - After breathing in, hold breath for 10 seconds, allowing the medicine to reach the lungs.
  - If repeat puffs are necessary, wait one minute between puffs so the medication can reach the lungs.

→ Educate the patient about medications, their proper use, possible side effects, and when to notify health care providers after initiating therapy (e.g., if the expected response does not occur or if there are significant side effects).

→ Reinforce the use of peak flow meters for additional monitoring of pulmonary functions, as recommended by physician consultants.

→ Educate the patient and her family regarding emergency measures (e.g., contacting emergency care providers if the patient does not respond to therapy).

→ Educate the patient about signs and symptoms of depression, anxiety, or other emotional/psychological sequelae associated with chronic disease.

FOLLOW-UP

→ The patient with stable, mild persistent asthma should be seen at least every six months for evaluation.
  - The patient should return more frequently if she experiences any exacerbation of symptoms.

→ If the patient experiences severe, acute symptoms, she should be seen immediately by a physician for evaluation and treatment.

→ If the patient is taking theophylline, she should return for serum theophylline levels as recommended by the consulting physician (usually every six months when stable). She should also do so if she begins taking another medication (e.g., erythromycin) that can alter theophylline serum levels or if she experiences any signs or symptoms associated with theophylline toxicity.

→ Document in progress notes and on problem list.

BIBLIOGRAPHY

Anderson, S.D., and Daviskas, E. 2000. The mechanism of exercise induced asthma is... *Journal of Allergy and Clinical Immunology* 106:453–459.

Arkinstall, W.W. 1988. Review of the North American experience with evening administration of Uniphyl tablets, a once daily regimen for nocturnal asthma. *American Journal of Medicine* 85:60–63.

Arruda, L.K., Vailes, L.D., Ferriani, V.P. et al. 2001. Cockroach allergens and asthma. *Journal of Clinical Allergy and Immunology* 107:419–428.

Bensch, G., Gerger, W.E., Blokhin, B.M. et al. 2002. One-year efficacy and safety of inhaled formoterol dry powder in children with persistent asthma. *Annals of Allergy and Asthma Immunology* 89:180–190.

Busse, W.W., and Lemanske, R.F. 2001. Asthma. *New England Journal of Medicine* 344:350–362.

Centers for Disease Control and Prevention (CDC). 2001. National Center for Health Statistics. *New asthma estimates: tracking prevalence, health care, and mortality.* Available at: http://www.cdc.gov/nchs/products/pubs/pubd/hestats/hestats.htm. Accessed on October 5, 2001.

Dicpinigaitis, P.V., Dobkin, J.B., and Reichel, J. 2002. Antitussive effect of the leukotriene receptor antagonist zafirlukast in subjects with cough variant asthma. *Journal of Asthma* 39:291–297.

Elborn, J.S., Finch, M.B., and Stanford, C.F. 1991. Non-arterial assessment of blood gas status in patients with chronic pulmonary disease. *Ulster Medical Journal* 60:164–167.

Holmgren, D., and Sixt, R. 1992. Transcutaneous and arterial blood gas monitoring during acute asthmatic symptoms in older children. *Pediatric Pulmonology* 14:80–84.

Irwin, R.S., Boulet, L.-P., Cloutier, M.M. et al. 1998. Managing cough as a defense mechanism and as a symptom. A consensus panel report of the American College of Chest Physicians. *Chest* 114:133S–181S.

Jenne, J.W. 1984. Theophylline use in asthma. Some current issues. *Clinics in Chest Medicine* 84:645–648.

Kavuru, M., Melamed, J., Gross, G. et al. 2000. Salmeterol and fluticasone combining in a new powder inhalation device for the treatment of asthma: a randomized, double blind, placebo-controlled trial. *Journal of Allergy and Clinical Immunology* 105:1108–1116.

Kitch, B.T., Levy, B.D., and Fanta, C.H. 2000. Late onset asthma: epidemiology, diagnosis, and treatment. *Drugs and Aging* 17:385–397.

Larj, M.J., Meyers, D.A., and Bleecker, E.R. 2002. Genetics of asthma. *Immunology and Allergy Clinics of North America* 20:129–136.

National Institutes of Health (NIH). 1991. National Asthma Education and Prevention Program (NAEPP). *Expert panel report. Guidelines for the diagnosis and management of asthma.* Publication No. 91-3042. Bethesda, Md.: the Author.

_____. 1997. National Asthma Education and Prevention Program. *Expert panel report 2. Guidelines for the diagnosis and management of asthma.* Publication No. 97-4051. Bethesda, Md.: the Author.

_____. 1999. *Practical guide to the diagnosis and management of asthma.* Publication No. 99-4055. Bethesda, Md.: the Author.

_____. 2002. National Asthma Education and Prevention Program. *Expert panel report. Guidelines for the diagnosis and management of asthma. Update on selected topics 2002.* Publication No. 02-5075. Bethesda, Md.: the Author.

Schappert, S.M. 1993. *National ambulatory medical care survey: 1991 summary. Advance data from vital and health statistics.* No. 230. Hyattsville, Md.: National Center for Health Statistics.

Toren, K., Balder, B., Brisman, J. et al. 1999. The risk of asthma in relation to occupational exposures: a case-control study from a Swedish city. *European Respiratory Journal* 13:496–501.

5-B
Bronchiectasis

Bronchiectasis is a condition characterized by permanent dilation and bacterial colonization with inflammation of the bronchi that results in the destruction of bronchial wall tissue (Chesnutt et al. 2002). The pulmonary changes resulting in bronchiectasis can be a consequence of congenital or acquired conditions, including lung infections, cystic fibrosis, immunodeficiency states, and localized pulmonary obstruction (Chesnutt et al. 2002, Pasteur et al. 2000). Patients usually present with a history of persistent or intermittent productive cough in the absence of contributing factors such as smoking or asthma (although these factors also may be reported by patients).

The actual incidence of bronchiectasis is unknown because in many patients the symptoms are often mild and intermittent, unless an exacerbation of pulmonary symptoms occurs secondary to bacterial infection. A decreased incidence of acquired bronchiectasis has been reported in the United States, probably as a result of more effective treatment of bronchopulmonary infections (Chesnutt et al. 2002).

The symptoms associated with bronchiectasis vary from mild to severe and are related to the pulmonary damage that has occurred. The pathophysiology of bronchiectasis involves minor to severe epithelial damage, hyperplasia of goblet cells, reduced connective tissue, bronchial dilation, and inflammatory changes.

Such pulmonary damage, in turn, results in reduced mucociliary clearance with increased mucus retention and bacterial colonization (most commonly with *Haemophilus influenzae* or *Pseudomonas aeruginosa*, which may be intermittent or continuous [Pasteur et al. 2000]). Bacterial colonization stimulates an increase in neutrophils in the pulmonary secretions, which then contributes to further pulmonary damage and repair, and which is often responsible for an exacerbation of symptoms. Complications associated with bronchiectasis include right ventricular hypertrophy, heart failure, amyloidosis, and the development of secondary abscesses at extrapulmonary sites (e.g., the brain).

DATABASE

SUBJECTIVE

→ Predisposing factors may include (Chesnutt et al. 2002, Pasteur et al. 2000):
  ■ Congenital conditions:
    • Cystic fibrosis
    • Immune defect (e.g., immunoglobulin deficiency, neutrophil adhesion defect)
    • Immotile cilia syndrome
    • Allergic bronchopulmonary aspergillosis
    • Alpha-1 antitrypsin deficiency
  ■ Acquired conditions:
    • History of:
      – Pulmonary infections (e.g., tuberculosis, pneumonia, fungal infections, lung abscess)
      – Inflammatory disease (e.g., rheumatoid arthritis, inflammatory bowel disease)
      – Pulmonary fibrosis
      – Acquired immunodeficiency (e.g., human immunodeficiency virus [HIV] infection, chemotherapy)

→ The patient may report one or more of the following symptoms, which can vary in intensity from mild to severe (Chesnutt et al. 2002, Irwin et al. 2000, Pasteur et al. 2000):
  ■ Chronic cough producing copious amounts of mucus (often foul-smelling)
  ■ Hemoptysis
  ■ Dyspnea (increasing with exertion)
  ■ Wheezing
  ■ Fever (if co-existent with bacterial infection)
  ■ Malaise
  ■ Weight loss

OBJECTIVE

→ Physical findings are often nonspecific but may include the following (Chesnutt et al. 2002):

- Elevated temperature if there is a superimposed bacterial infection
- Increased respiratory rate and pulse if there is significant pulmonary or cardiac disease
- Auscultation of the patient's lungs reveals persistent bibasilar crackles
- Collection of sputum in a specimen cup reveals copious amounts of purulent mucus (often foul-smelling) that will separate into three distinct layers.

ASSESSMENT

→ Bronchiectasis
→ R/O acute pulmonary infection (e.g., bronchitis, pneumonia, tuberculosis)
→ R/O chronic obstructive pulmonary disease
→ R/O cor pulmonale
→ R/O congestive heart failure
→ R/O immune defect
→ R/O immotile cilia syndrome (rare)

PLAN

DIAGNOSTIC TESTS

→ Complete blood count (CBC) may be within normal limits or may demonstrate leukocytosis if secondary pulmonary infection co-exists.
→ Gram stain of sputum may reveal an organism requiring antimicrobial treatment. (See the **Pneumonia** chapter.)
→ Sputum culture may reveal a pathogenic organism requiring antimicrobial treatment. (See the **Pneumonia** chapter.)
→ In moderate to severe bronchiectasis, pulmonary function tests will reveal obstructive dysfunction (see **Table 5D.2, Pulmonary Function Tests (PFTs)—Definitions and Results in Obstructive and Restrictive Pulmonary Disease** in the **Chronic Obstructive Pulmonary Disease** chapter for definitions of PFT tests):
- Spirometry testing will demonstrate a normal or decreased FVC and a decreased FEV_1, FEV_1/FVC, FEF_{25-75}, PEFR, and maximum voluntary ventilation (MVV).
- Lung volume testing will demonstrate an increased total lung capacity (TLC), functional residual capacity (FRC), and residual volume (RV)/TLC.
→ Arterial blood gases will reveal hypoxemia in patients with severe bronchiectasis.
→ Chest x-ray will demonstrate peribronchial fibrosis and cystic spaces at the lung bases.
→ High-resolution computerized tomography (HRCT) is the preferred diagnostic study and may reveal bronchial dilatation with lack of bronchial tapering as well as peribronchial fibrosis and cystic spaces at the lung bases (Chesnutt et al. 2002, Pasteur et al. 2000).
→ A tuberculosis skin test will be negative.
→ Bronchoscopy may be indicated to:
- Evaluate the etiology of hemoptysis
- Rule out the possibility of a malignancy or an obstructive airway lesion, and/or to remove retained secretions

→ Consultation with a physician is indicated for the initial evaluation.

TREATMENT/MANAGEMENT

→ If there is evidence of pulmonary infection (based on Gram stain or sputum culture results), initiation of a specific antibiotic therapy is indicated. When a patient exhibits an acute exacerbation of symptoms without evidence of a specific pathogen, empiric antibiotic therapy may be initiated with one of the following agents for 10–14 days (Chesnutt et al. 2002):
- Amoxicillin 500 mg p.o. TID
- Amoxicillin-clavulanic acid 500 mg p.o. TID or 875 mg p.o. BID
- Trimethoprim/sulfamethoxazole 160 mg/800 mg p.o. every 12 hours
→ In patients with severe bronchiectasis and copious amounts of purulent sputum, alternating 2 or 3 of the above antibiotics with one another for up to 4 weeks may be necessary to resolve symptoms of an exacerbation.
→ Pulmonary toilet (including chest physiotherapy, chest percussion, postural drainage) may be instituted; however, the efficacy of this is inconclusive. Some studies have found a beneficial effect of pulmonary toilet in reducing sputum production but not in improving pulmonary function tests (Jones et al. 2000).
→ If moderate to severe symptoms are evident, bronchodilators should be prescribed. (See the **Chronic Obstructive Pulmonary Disease** chapter.)
→ Avoidance of situations that may aggravate bronchiectasis (e.g., smoking, exposure to air pollutants) should be recommended.
→ Immunization with pneumococcal vaccine and influenza vaccine should be advised. (See the **Pneumonia** and **Influenza** chapters.)
→ Occasionally, surgical resection is indicated in patients with localized bronchiectasis and adequate PFTs who are not responding to conservative management. Decisions and referrals would be the responsibility of the consulting physician.

CONSULTATION

→ Consultation is indicated for any patient, especially those with moderate to severe symptoms (e.g., hypoxemia), significant hemoptysis, or symptoms persisting after appropriate conservative treatment.
→ Patient referral to a respiratory physical therapist—so she can be properly instructed about pulmonary toilet techniques—may be beneficial.
→ As needed for prescription(s).

PATIENT EDUCATION

→ Educate the patient about bronchiectasis—the possible cause(s), clinical manifestations, ways to prevent exacerbation, signs and symptoms of complications, possible diagnostic tests required, and any indicated follow-up.

→ Discuss with the patient prophylactic measures (e.g., pneumococcal and influenza vaccinations) that are indicated and why such measures can be beneficial.

→ When appropriate, educate the patient about the possible psychological sequelae (e.g., depression) of an obstructive pulmonary disorder and provide her with referrals and resources.

→ Review the potential side effects of medications (see *Physicians' Desk Reference* as needed). In women using long-term antibiotic therapy, education about possible vaginal candidiasis infections—signs, symptoms, preventative measures, treatment options—is essential. (See the **Vaginitis** chapters in Section 12.) Some antibiotics decrease the effectiveness of oral contraceptive pills.

FOLLOW-UP

→ Patients with evidence of acute pulmonary infection who are treated as outpatients should have a follow-up visit scheduled after completion of their antibiotic therapy. If symptoms persist or worsen during the course of antibiotic therapy, the patient should return for re-evaluation before finishing the antibiotics.

→ If there has been consultation/management with a physician, follow-up visits should be upon recommendation of the physician.

→ Document in progress notes and on problem list.

BIBLIOGRAPHY

Chesnutt, M.S., and Prendergast, T.J. 2002. Lung. In *2002 current medical diagnosis & treatment*, 41st ed., eds. L.M. Tierney, Jr., S.J. McPhee, and M.A. Papadakis, pp. 295–296. New York: Lange Medical Books/McGraw-Hill.

Irwin, R.S., and Madison, J.M. 2000. The diagnosis and treatment of cough. *New England Journal of Medicine* 343(23):1715–1721.

Jones, A., and Rowe, B.H. 2000. Bronchopulmonary hygiene physical therapy in bronchiectasis and chronic obstructive pulmonary disease: a systematic review. *Heart & Lung* 29(2):125–135.

Pasteur, M.C., Halliwell, S.M., Houghton, S.J. et al. 2000. An investigation into the causative factors in patients with bronchiectasis. *American Journal of Respiratory and Critical Care Medicine* 162:1277–1284.

5-C

Bronchitis—Acute

Acute bronchitis is an acute or subacute infection of the upper respiratory tract characterized by fever and cough. It usually occurs during the winter months. In 50% of adult patients, the etiology is unknown; however, in approximately 40% of adults, a viral pathogen is responsible for the infection. Bacterial pathogens (e.g., *Haemophilus influenzae, Streptococcus pneumoniae, Bordetella pertussis, Mycoplasma pneumoniae,* and *Chlamydia pneumoniae*) are responsible for acute bronchitis in a minority of adults (Gonzales et al. 2000a, 2000b). Pertussis has been documented in 10–20% of adults with a coughing illness that persists beyond 2–3 weeks (Gonzales et al. 2000a, 2000b).

In most patients, the episode is self-limited, lasts 1–2 weeks, and requires only symptomatic treatment. However, in patients with a history of chronic obstructive pulmonary disease (COPD), acute bronchitis may require pharmacological interventions, especially if the patient has an increased volume and purulence of sputum with dyspnea (Niederman 2000). Use of antibiotics for acute bronchitis in healthy patients without a history of COPD has not demonstrated significant benefit and is associated with an increase in bacterial resistance to antimicrobials. Therefore, antibiotic therapy in this group of adults is not recommended (Bent et al. 1999, Gonzales et al. 2000a, Smucny et al. 1998).

DATABASE

SUBJECTIVE

→ Predisposing factors may include a history of (Gonzales et al. 2000a):
- Recent upper respiratory infection (URI)
- Smoking or exposure to an environment with secondhand smoke
- Recent influenza or exposure to influenza or respiratory syncytial virus
→ The patient may report one or more of the following symptoms (Gonzales et al. 2000a, Hueston et al. 2000):
- URI symptoms—headache, malaise, pharyngitis, nasal congestion
- Low-grade fever
- Cough that may produce a clear to purulent discharge
- Substernal chest discomfort
- Wheezing

OBJECTIVE

→ Physical examination may reveal (Gonzales et al. 2000a, Hueston et al. 2000):
- Mild temperature elevation (usually <38° C)
- Blood pressure, pulse, and respiratory rate are usually within normal limits (WNL).
- Pharyngeal erythema
- Rhonchi or crackles without focal consolidation upon auscultation of the lungs

ASSESSMENT

→ Acute bronchitis
→ R/O URI
→ R/O asthmatic bronchitis
→ R/O cough-variant asthma
→ R/O postnasal drip syndrome
→ R/O pneumonia
→ R/O influenza
→ R/O pertussis

PLAN

DIAGNOSTIC TESTS

→ The diagnosis of acute bronchitis is usually made based on the clinical presentation and physical examination findings. However, in patients with a history of COPD or severe or persistent symptoms, the following diagnostic tests can be ordered (Gonzales et al. 2000a, 2000b):
- Chest x-ray: usually WNL.
- Sputum cultures: may reveal a pathogen such as *M. pneumoniae.* However, common oropharyngeal contaminants usually are recovered and are of unknown significance in the presence of acute bronchitis symptoms.

- Serum C-reactive protein: usually WNL in most viral illnesses; will be elevated in serious bacterial infections, adenovirus or Epstein-Barr viral illnesses, or certain inflammatory diseases (e.g., rheumatoid arthritis). Elevated levels must be evaluated on an individual basis (Gonzales et al. 2000a).
- Pulmonary function tests: may have an FEV_1 <80% (an obstructive pattern), but this is transient and will return to WNL after the acute illness.
- Methacholine test: will be negative unless the patient has asthma.

TREATMENT/MANAGEMENT

→ Symptomatic treatment for acute bronchitis in patients without COPD includes rest, increased fluid intake, and the use of antipyretics (e.g., acetaminophen) as needed.
→ Cough suppression can be attempted through the use of over-the-counter medications containing dextromethorphan. The usual dose of dextromethorphan is 15 mg p.o. every 6 hours. In patients with severe cough, a codeine preparation may be necessary.
→ If the patient is suspected of having co-existent influenza A, use of neuraminidase inhibitors (e.g., Zanamivir) can be considered. (See the **Influenza** chapter.)
→ Patients with wheezing or significant/persistent cough often benefit from the use of inhaled β-agonists (via metered dose inhalers), such as:
  - Albuterol 90 μg/puff, 2 puffs every 4–6 hours prn
  - Bitolterol 370 μg/puff, 2–3 puffs every 6–8 hours prn
  - Terbutaline 200 μg/puff, 2 puffs every 4–6 hours prn
→ Antimicrobial therapy is not indicated in healthy adults with uncomplicated disease because most acute bronchitis in this population is caused by viruses.
  - In elderly patients, patients with COPD who develop dyspnea and increased sputum purulence and volume, patients with persistent symptoms, or patients with significant medical problems (e.g., those who are immunocompromised), antimicrobial therapy may be indicated and may include (Niederman 2000):
    - Erythromycin 500 mg p.o. QID for 10–14 days
      NOTE: Erythromycin provides a wide spectrum of coverage with limited cost and side effects. For pertussis therapy, 14 days of erythromycin are necessary.
    - Tetracycline 250 mg p.o. QID for 7–10 days
    - Clarithromycin 500 mg p.o. BID for 10 days
    - Azithromycin 500 mg p.o. on the first day, then 250 mg p.o. QD for 5 days

CONSULTATION

→ Consultation with a physician may be indicated in patients with COPD, severe or persistent symptoms, or significant underlying medical conditions.
→ As needed for prescription(s).

PATIENT EDUCATION

→ Educate the patient about acute bronchitis—the most common cause(s), usual symptomatic treatments, signs and/or symptoms of complications, and any follow-up that may be indicated.
→ If the patient requires antibiotic therapy, educate her about the need to take the medications as prescribed and discuss any potential side effects.
→ If the patient smokes or lives/works in an environment where she is exposed to secondhand smoke, educate her about the adverse effects of smoking (e.g., lung disease, cancer, heart disease) and possible ways to reduce or stop smoking (e.g., smoking cessation programs). (See the **Smoking Cessation** chapter in Section 14.)

FOLLOW-UP

→ If physician consultation is indicated, follow-up per physician recommendation.
→ Document in progress notes and on problem list.

BIBLIOGRAPHY

Bent, S., Saint, S., Vittinghoff, E. et al. 1999. Antibiotics in acute bronchitis: a meta-analysis. *American Journal of Medicine* 107:62–67.

Gonzales, R., and Sande, M.A. 2000a. Uncomplicated acute bronchitis. *Annals of Internal Medicine* 133:981–991.

_____. 2000b. Acute bronchitis in the healthy adult. *Current Topics in Infectious Diseases* 20(4):158–173.

Hueston, W.J., Mainous, A.G., Dacus, E.N. et al. 2000. Does acute bronchitis really exist? *Journal of Family Practice* 49(5):401–406.

Niederman, M.S. 2000. Antibiotic therapy of exacerbations of chronic bronchitis. *Seminars in Respiratory Infections* 15(1):59–70.

Smucny, J.J., Becker, L.A., Glazier, R.H. et al. 1998. Are antibiotics effective treatment for acute bronchitis? A meta-analysis. *Journal of Family Practice* 47(6):453–460.

5-D
Chronic Obstructive Pulmonary Disease

Chronic obstructive pulmonary disease (COPD) is a condition characterized by expiratory airway obstruction. COPD is comprises two diseases: *emphysema* and *chronic bronchitis*. In most patients, elements of both these diseases co-exist.

It is estimated that 14 million people in the United States have COPD (Flaherty et al. 2000). It is the fourth leading cause of death in the United States, with a higher death rate noted among elderly men (Chesnutt et al. 2002). Additionally, there is significant morbidity associated with this condition, including frequent pulmonary infections, cor pulmonale, and psychosocial sequelae associated with chronic disease (e.g., depression).

The most important factor associated with COPD is cigarette smoke; up to 90% of patients with COPD have had significant exposure to it (Sethi et al. 2000b). There is a direct correlation between the amount and duration of cigarette use and the acceleration of decline in lung function in patients with COPD (Sethi et al. 2000b). Other factors that contribute to COPD include the genetic predisposition of patients (e.g., the alpha-1-antitrypsin deficiency), exposure to environmental and occupational pollutants (e.g., air pollution or bacterial or viral infections), and host factors (e.g., atopy or bronchial hyperresponsiveness) (Hogg 2000, Kunzli et al. 2000, Murphy 2000, Sethi et al. 2000a, 2000b).

Emphysema

Emphysema is characterized by permanent enlargement of lung parenchyma distal to the terminal bronchioles, resulting in destruction and coalescence of alveolar walls without obvious fibrosis (Hogg 2001). Emphysematous changes are thought to occur in response to excessive lysis of elastin by elastase and other enzymes produced by lung neutrophils, mononuclear cells, and macrophages (Chesnutt et al. 2002).

There are two types of emphysema: *panlobular* or *panacinar*, which is characterized by destructive changes in the alveoli and alveolar sacs, and is associated with alpha-1 antitrypsin deficiency or idiopathic causes; and *centrilobular* or *centriacinar*, which is characterized by pathology in the respiratory bronchioles and is the result of chronic bronchitis (Hogg 2001).

Chronic Bronchitis

Chronic bronchitis is characterized by a recurrent, chronic, productive cough that is present for at least three months, annually for two consecutive years, in the absence of other causes for the symptoms (Flaherty et al. 2000). It involves airway obstruction and inflammation. Although not an active infection, chronic bronchitis is associated with an increased incidence of acute respiratory infections (e.g., acute bronchitis or pneumonia) (Chesnutt et al. 2002).

DATABASE

SUBJECTIVE

→ The patient may report one or more of the following predisposing factors associated with COPD (Chesnutt et al. 2002, Sethi et al. 2000b):
- History of cigarette smoking
- Exposure to air pollution
- History of recurrent respiratory infections
- History of a hereditary disorder associated with COPD (e.g., alpha-1 antitrypsin deficiency, immotile cilia syndrome, or cystic fibrosis)

Emphysema

→ Patients with emphysema usually report the onset of the following symptoms after age 50 years (Chesnutt et al. 2002, Sethi et al. 2000b):
- Shortness of breath that becomes more severe and constant
- Weight loss (usually noted in advanced disease)
- Minimal or no cough
- If a cough is present, it is associated with little or no mucous production. If mucous is reported, it is usually clear or mucoid, not purulent.

Chronic Bronchitis

→ Patients with chronic bronchitis usually report the onset of symptoms when they are in their fourth or fifth decade of life. Symptoms include (Chesnutt et al. 2002):

- A persistent, severe cough producing copious amounts of purulent, often foul-smelling sputum. The cough is usually most intense in the morning.
- Mild, intermittent shortness of breath and dyspnea associated with increased exertion. As the disease progresses, moderate to severe shortness of breath and dyspnea are noted, even at rest.
- Hemoptysis (may be reported in associated with aspirin intake)
- Patients often report weight gain.
- Patients may report a swelling of extremities.

OBJECTIVE

→ See **Table 5D.1, Patterns of Disease in Advanced COPD.**

Emphysema

→ The following physical findings may be evident, depending on disease severity (Chesnutt et al. 2002, Flaherty et al. 2000):

- Vital signs: Blood pressure and temperature will be within normal limits (WNL) unless there is a co-existing condition (e.g., hypertension or infection). The respiratory rate and pulse may be WNL or increased, depending on the level of respiratory distress the patient is experiencing.
- The patient may appear thin and wasted in advanced disease.
- Examination of the chest will reveal an increased anteroposterior diameter ("barrel chest") and hypertrophied accessory respiratory muscles.
- Palpation of the chest will reveal normal to decreased tactile fremitus.
- Percussion of the chest will reveal hyperresonance.
- Auscultation of the lungs may reveal diminished breath sounds usually without adventitious sounds.
- Clubbing of the fingers may be evident.

Table 5D.1.   PATTERNS OF DISEASE IN ADVANCED COPD

	Type A: Pink Puffer (Emphysema Predominant)	Type B: Blue Bloater (Bronchitis Predominant)
History and Physical Examination	Major complaint is dyspnea, often severe, usually presenting after age 50 years. Cough is rare, with scant, clear, mucoid sputum. Patients are thin, with recent weight loss common. They appear uncomfortable, with evident use of accessory muscles of respiration. Chest is very quiet without adventitious sounds. No peripheral edema.	Major complaint is chronic cough, productive of mucopurulent sputum, with frequent exacerbations due to chest infections. Patient often presents in late 30s and 40s. Dyspnea usually mild, though patients may note limitations to exercise. Patients frequently overweight and cyanotic but seem comfortable at rest. Peripheral edema is common. Chest is noisy, with rhonchi invariably present; wheezes are common.
Laboratory Studies	Hemoglobin usually normal (12–15 g/dL). PaO_2 normal to slightly reduced (65–75 mm Hg), but SaO_2 normal at rest. $PaCO_2$ normal to slightly reduced (35–40mm Hg). Chest radiograph shows hyperinflation with flattened diaphragms. Vascular markings are diminished, particularly at the apices.	Hemoglobin usually elevated (15–18 g/dL). PaO_2 reduced 45–60 mm Hg and $PaCO_2$ slightly to markedly elevated (50–60 mm Hg). Chest radiograph shows increased interstitial markings ("dirty lungs"), especially at bases. Diaphragms are not flattened.
Pulmonary Function Tests	Airflow obstruction ubiquitous. Total lung capacity increased, sometimes markedly so. D_LCO reduced. Static lung compliance increased.	Airflow obstruction ubiquitous. Total lung capacity normal but may be slightly increased. D_LCO normal. Static lung compliance normal.
Special Evaluations V/Q Matching	Increased ventilation to high V/Q area—i.e., high dead space ventilation.	Increased perfusion to low V/Q areas.
Hemodynamics	Cardiac output normal to slightly low. Pulmonary artery pressures mildly elevated and increased with exercise.	Cardiac output normal. Pulmonary artery pressures elevated, sometimes markedly so, and worsen with exercise.
Nocturnal Ventilation	Mild to moderate degree of oxygen desaturation not usually associated with obstructive sleep apnea.	Severe oxygen desaturation, frequently associated with obstructive sleep apnea.
Exercise Ventilation	Increased minute ventilation for level of oxygen consumption. PaO_2 tends to fall, $PaCO_2$ rises slightly.	Decreased minute ventilation for level of oxygen consumption. PaO_2 may rise; $PaCO_2$ may rise significantly.

Source: Chesnutt, M.S., and Prendergast, T.J. 2002. Lung. In *2002 current medical diagnosis & treatment*, 41st ed., eds. L.M. Tierney, Jr., S.J. McPhee, and M.A. Papadakis, p. 292. New York: Lange Medical Books/McGraw-Hill. © The McGraw-Hill Companies Inc. Reproduced with permission.

Chronic Bronchitis

→ Physical examination may reveal the following findings depending on disease severity (Chesnutt et al. 2002, Flaherty et al. 2000):

- Vital signs: Blood pressure and temperature will be WNL unless there is a co-existing condition (e.g., hypertension or infection). The patient's respiratory rate and pulse may be WNL or increased, depending on the severity of the condition.
- Skin: Plethora and, in advanced disease, central cyanosis may be present.
- Examination of the chest will reveal a normal anteroposterior diameter.
- Palpation of the chest may reveal decreased tactile fremitus.
- Percussion of the chest may be normal to dull.
- Auscultation of the lungs may reveal normal to decreased breath sounds with diffuse wheezes and rhonchi.
- Examination will reveal copious amounts of mucopurulent or purulent sputum.
- Clubbing of the fingers and/or edema of the extremities may be evident.

ASSESSMENT

→ COPD
→ Emphysema
→ Chronic bronchitis
→ R/O acute infection (e.g., pneumonia)
→ R/O asthmatic bronchitis

Table 5D.2.   PULMONARY FUNCTION TESTS (PFTS)—DEFINITIONS AND RESULTS IN OBSTRUCTIVE AND RESTRICTIVE PULMONARY DISEASE

Test	Definition	Results in Obstructive Pulmonary Disease*	Results in Restrictive Pulmonary Disease*
Tests Derived from Spirometry			
Forced vital capacity (FVC) in liters	The volume of gas that can be forcefully expelled from the lungs after maximal inspiration.	N or ↓	↓
Forced expiratory volume in 1 second (FEV$_1$)	The volume of gas expelled in the first second of the FVC maneuver.	↓	N or ↓
Forced expiratory flow from 25–75% of the vital capacity (FEF$_{25-75}$) in liters per second (L/s)	The maximal midexpiratory airflow rate.	↓	N or ↓
Peak expiratory flow rate (PEFR) in L/s	The maximal airflow rate achieved in the FVC maneuver.	↓	N or ↑
Maximum voluntary ventilation (MVV) in liters per minute (L/min)	The maximum volume of gas that can be breathed in 1 minute (usually measured for 15 seconds and multiplied by 4).	↓	N or ↓
FEV$_1$/FVC percentage	N/A	↓	N or ↑
Lung Volumes			
Slow vital capacity (SVC) in liters	The volume of gas that can be slowly exhaled after maximal inspiration.	N or ↓	↓
Total lung capacity (TLC) in liters	The volume of gas in the lungs after a maximal inspiration.	N or ↑	↓
Functional residual capacity (FRC) in liters	The volume of gas in the lungs at the end of a normal tidal expiration.	↑	N or ↓
Expiratory reserve volume (ERV) in liters	The volume of gas representing the difference between functional residual capacity and residual volume.	N or ↓	N or ↓
Residual volume (RV) in liters	The volume of gas remaining in the lungs after maximal expiration.	↑	N, ↑, or ↓
RV/TLC ratio	N/A	↑	N or ↑

*N = normal
↓ = less than predicted
↑ = greater than predicted

Source: Reprinted with permission from Stauffer, J.L. 1993. Pulmonary diseases. In *Current medical diagnosis & treatment*, 32nd ed., eds. L.M. Tierney, Jr., S.J. McPhee, M.A. Papadakis et al., pp. 183–262. Norwalk, Conn.: Appleton & Lange. © The McGraw-Hill Companies Inc. Reproduced with permission.

→ R/O bronchiectasis
→ R/O cor pulmonale
→ R/O central airway obstruction
→ R/O congestive heart failure

PLAN

DIAGNOSTIC TESTS

→ See **Table 5D.1** and **Table 5D.2, Pulmonary Function Tests (PFTs)—Definitions and Results in Obstructive and Restrictive Pulmonary Disease**.
→ CBC may reveal an increased hemoglobin (15–18 g/dL) secondary to polycythemia in advanced COPD due to chronic hypoxemia (Chesnutt et al. 2002).
→ Chest x-ray findings (Chesnutt et al. 2002):

Emphysema

- Hyperinflation of the lungs with decreased bronchovascular markings. Retrosternal air may be visible on lateral view.
- Bullae (parenchymal) and blebs (subpleural) will be evident and are pathognomonic.
- The diaphragm will be low and flat.
- The heart will be a normal size.

Chronic Bronchitis

- May reveal increased peribronchial and perivascular markings.
- Enlargement of central pulmonary arteries may be evident if there is advanced disease.
- The diaphragm will be normal.
- Heart size may be increased.

→ An electrocardiogram can be ordered if heart disease is suspected. It will demonstrate right axis deviation, right ventricular hypertrophy, and "p" pulmonale secondary to cor pulmonale in patients with severe COPD (Chesnutt et al. 2002).
→ A computerized tomography (CT) scan is not usually done but, if performed, may reveal the following:
- Chronic bronchitis: bronchial wall thickening (nonspecific)
- Emphysema: areas of "low attenuation without definable walls" (Flaherty et al. 2000, p. 215)
→ Pulmonary function tests will demonstrate the following (also see **Table 5D.2**) (American Thoracic Society 1991, Chesnutt et al. 2002):

Emphysema

- Spirometry will reveal an obstructive pattern.
- Total lung capacity (TLC) will be increased.
- Residual volume (RV) will be increased.
- The RV/TLC ratio will be increased (indicating air trapping).
- Forced expiratory volume in the first second (FEV_1) will be decreased.
- The FEV_1 to forced vital capacity (FVC) ratio will be decreased.
- Diffusing capacity for carbon dioxide (D_LCO_2) will be decreased.

- Alveolar volume (V_A) will be decreased.
- The D_LCO/V_A ratio will be low.

Chronic Bronchitis

- Spirometry will reveal an obstructive pattern.
- TLC will be normal to decreased.
- RV will be normal to decreased.
- FEV_1 will be decreased.
- The FEV_1 to FVC ratio will be decreased.
- The alveolar-arterial oxygen difference (A-a DO_2) will be increased.
- D_LCO_2 will be decreased.
- V_A will be decreased.
- D_LCO_2/V_A ratio will be low.

→ Blood gases are not routinely done unless indicated. If performed, the following results may be noted, depending on the severity of the patient's disease (Chesnutt et al. 2002, Flaherty et al. 2000):

Emphysema

- Resting arterial oxygen pressure (PaO_2): slight decrease
- Exercise PaO_2: decreased
- $PaCO_2$: normal to increased
- Exercise $PaCO_2$: slight decrease to increase (advanced disease is associated with CO_2 retention)

Chronic Bronchitis

- Resting PaO_2: moderate to severe decrease (especially at night)
- Exercise PaO_2: may increase
- $PaCO_2$: increased
- Exercise $PaCO_2$: significantly increased

→ Gram stain of sputum may reveal increased white blood cells and a pathogen (e.g., *Streptococcus pneumoniae*, *Haemophilus influenzae*, or *Moraxella catarrhalis*) if there is a co-existing active infection.
→ Culture of sputum may identify a pathogen if there is a co-existing active infection.

TREATMENT/MANAGEMENT

→ For patients with evidence of significant symptoms or disease (e.g., respiratory distress or pneumonia), hospitalization may be required for effective treatment. Physician consultation and management are indicated.
→ For patients with mild to moderate symptoms, outpatient management is possible as long as their symptoms respond to conservative therapy.
→ An essential component of treatment is improving ventilation by reducing respiratory secretions (e.g., pulmonary toilet, deep breathing, and coughing).
- Some patients may require referral to a respiratory therapist for instruction in proper pulmonary toilet techniques.
→ Patients need to maintain adequate hydration and nutritional intake.

- For those patients exhibiting weight loss, supplemental caloric intake is indicated.
- Referral to a nutritionist for specific recommendations may be necessary.

→ If the patient smokes cigarettes, she must be advised to stop.
  - Referral to community programs or support groups may be necessary.
  - Nicotine chewing gum (a 2 mg piece chewed slowly for 30 minutes) or a nicotine patch may be helpful during her withdrawal from cigarettes. (See the **Smoking Cessation** chapter in Section 14.)

→ Reducing exposure to potential respiratory irritants and allergens (e.g., air pollution, secondary smoke, and toxic inhalants) is essential. Specific recommendations for each patient should be based on individual circumstances.

→ Improving the patient's airway diameter—by reducing edema and inflammation, and relieving bronchospasm—may require pharmacological therapies, including beta-agonists, theophylline compounds, inhaled anticholinergic agents, and corticosteroid agents.
  - Individualized therapeutic regimens may include one or more of the following agents (Chesnutt et al. 2002):
    • Bronchodilators are indicated to partially reverse airway obstruction in patients with exacerbation of disease, wheezing, or asthmatic bronchitis. Medications include:
      – Ipratropium bromide spray, an anticholinergic bronchodilator, 2–4 inhalations every 6 hours
      – Albuterol, a sympathomimetic bronchodilator, 1–4 inhalations every 4–6 hours
      NOTE: Ipratropium bromide combined with albuterol is slightly more effective than either agent alone (Chesnutt et al. 2002).
      – Theophylline 400–1,000 mg/24 hours p.o. in 2 divided doses
      NOTE: Theophylline use in COPD generally is reserved for those patients who fail to respond to or are intolerant of inhaled bronchodilators, or who have sleep-related respiratory symptoms. Its value in COPD treatment may be due to improved respiratory muscle performance (Chesnutt et al. 2002). Careful monitoring of theophylline levels is recommended when initiating therapy and adjusting doses. A baseline serum theophylline level should be obtained when initiating therapy. Additional theophylline levels should be obtained 3–5 days after initiating therapy.
    • Corticosteroid therapy may reduce inflammation. Agents that may be prescribed include:
      – Inhaled corticosteroids. Studies have demonstrated improvement in patients' airway reactivity and respiratory symptoms, especially those of patients with chronic bronchitis. However, corticosteroid therapy does not affect the decline in lung function associated with COPD (Lung Health Study Research Group 2000).
        ➤ Beclomethasone 2 inhalations TID-QID
        ➤ Triamcinolone 2 inhalations TID-QID (maximum dose not to exceed 16 inhalations/24 hours)
        ➤ Flunisolide 2–4 inhalations BID (maximum dose not to exceed 4 inhalations BID)
        NOTE: Instruct the patient to rinse her mouth after use to prevent oral candidiasis.
      – Oral corticosteroid therapy may be necessary in patients with exacerbation of symptoms after conventional therapy (Chesnutt et al. 2002). The following dosages may be prescribed:
        ➤ Prednisone 5–40 mg p.o. every day or every other day.
        NOTE: Discontinue oral corticosteroids if there is no evidence of spirometric improvement after 2–4 weeks of therapy. Tapering the dose by increments of 5–10 mg every 2–3 days can be done when oral corticosteroid therapy has continued beyond 2–3 weeks.

→ Antibiotic therapy should be initiated in patients with evidence of acute infection.
  - Ideally, such therapy should be based on the results of sputum Gram stain or culture results.
  - If acute exacerbation of symptoms is evident (especially in chronic bronchitis patients), empiric antibiotic therapy may be initiated with one of the following agents for 7–10 days (Chesnutt et al. 2002):
    • Amoxicillin 500 mg p.o. TID
    • Amoxicillin/clavulanic acid 500 mg p.o. TID or 875 mg p.o. BID
    • Doxycycline 100 mg p.o. BID
    • Trimethoprim/sulfamethoxazole 160 mg/800 mg p.o. BID
    NOTE: Clinicians should be aware of local antibiotic resistance patterns when selecting empiric antibiotic therapy. Beta-lactamase and sulfa resistance is increasingly common in organisms associated with COPD exacerbations.

→ Prophylactic immunizations (e.g., yearly influenza vaccination and pneumococcal immunization) should be administered to COPD patients and household members in close contact with them. (See the **Pneumonia** and **Influenza** chapters.)

→ Home oxygen therapy may be necessary for certain patients with significant hypoxemia. If home oxygen therapy is being considered, consultation with a physician is indicated.

→ Patients should be carefully monitored for the development of any signs and symptoms of complications, including cor pulmonale, respiratory infections, and psychosocial problems (e.g., depression).

→ In patients exhibiting signs or symptoms of depression, psychological evaluation and therapy should be recommended.

CONSULTATION

→ Consultation with a physician is warranted for any patient with moderate to severe symptoms or signs of COPD, if

there is evidence of complications associated with COPD, or for patients who do not respond to conservative therapy.
→ As needed for prescription(s).

PATIENT EDUCATION

→ Educate the patient about COPD—the cause(s), clinical manifestations, recommended diagnostic tests, therapeutic interventions, prognosis, possible complications, and indicated follow-up.
→ Discuss ways the patient can prevent further lung damage and complications (e.g., by not smoking cigarettes, not inhaling toxic substances and pollutants, and receiving recommended immunizations).
   ▪ If the patient smokes cigarettes, referral to community resources and support groups for cessation may be beneficial. (See the **Smoking Cessation** chapter in Section 14.)
   ▪ When appropriate, educate the patient about the possible psychological sequelae she may experience as a result of COPD (e.g., depression) and provide her with referrals and resources.
   ▪ Educate the patient about any potential side effects of the medications that are prescribed (see the *Physicians' Desk Reference* as needed), the need to monitor for these, and the importance of reporting them to her clinician.

FOLLOW-UP

→ Patients requiring hospitalization, consultation, or management of care by a physician should have follow-up evaluations per a physician's recommendation.
→ Follow-up evaluations of patients receiving outpatient care should be based on the severity of their symptoms before, during, and after therapeutic interventions. Patients without evidence of improvement in their symptoms should return as soon as possible for further evaluation.
→ Document in progress notes and on problem list.

BIBLIOGRAPHY

American Thoracic Society. 1991. Lung function testing: selection of reference values and interpretative strategies. *American Review of Respiratory Diseases* 144:1202–1218.

Chesnutt, M.S., and Prendergast, T.J. 2002. Lung. In *2002 current medical diagnosis & treatment*, 41st ed., eds. L.M. Tierney, Jr., S.J. McPhee, and M.A. Papadakis, pp. 290–295. New York: Lange Medical Books/McGraw-Hill.

Flaherty, K.R., Kazerooni, E.A., and Martinez, F.J. 2000. Differential diagnosis of chronic airflow obstruction. *Journal of Asthma* 37(3):201–223.

Hogg, J.C. 2000. Chronic bronchitis: the role of viruses. *Seminars in Respiratory Infections* 15(1):32–40.

_____. 2001. Chronic obstructive pulmonary disease: an overview of pathology and pathogenesis. *Novartis Foundation Symposium* 234(1):4–26.

Kunzli, N., Kaiser, R., Medina, S. et al. 2000. Public-health impact of outdoor and traffic-related air pollution: a European assessment. *Lancet* 356:795–801.

Lung Health Study Research Group. 2000. Effect of inhaled triamcinolone on the decline in pulmonary function in chronic obstructive pulmonary disease. *New England Journal of Medicine* 343:1902–1909.

Murphy, T.F. 2000. *Haemophilus influenzae* in chronic bronchitis. *Seminars in Respiratory Infections* 15(1):41–50.

Sethi, J.M., Muscarella, K., Evans, N. et al. 2000a. Airway inflammation and etiology of acute exacerbations of chronic bronchitis. *Chest* 118(6):1557–1565.

Sethi, J.M., and Rochester, C.L. 2000b. Smoking and chronic obstructive pulmonary disease. *Clinics in Chest Medicine* 21(1):67–86.

Stauffer, J.L. 1993. Pulmonary diseases. In *Current medical diagnosis & treatment*, 32nd ed., eds. L.M. Tierney, Jr., S.J. McPhee, M.A. Papadakis et al., pp. 183–262. Norwalk, Conn.: Appleton & Lange.

5-E

Epistaxis

Epistaxis (nosebleed) is a common problem. Most epistaxis episodes are self-limited and associated with minimal blood loss. However, in approximately 5% of patients, the bleeding persists and requires medical evaluation and interventions (Jackler et al. 2002). Most cases of epistaxis requiring medical evaluation are successfully managed by conservative treatments (e.g. nasal packing, local chemical cautery, or electrocautery) (Frazee et al. 2000, Koh et al. 2000).

In patients unresponsive to such treatments, a diagnosis of *intractable epistaxis* is made. Intractable epistaxis, although uncommon, can be life-threatening if the bleeding cannot be controlled. Hospitalization is necessary to stop the bleeding, determine and treat the underlying cause, and stabilize patients who have lost a significant amount of blood (Koh et al. 2000, Shellenberger 2000). Complications associated with intractable epistaxis include anemia, infection, hemorrhage, and, in severe cases, death.

There are two anatomic sites associated with epistaxis episodes. Anterior nasal bleeding occurs in the anterior portion of the nasal septum where a thin nasal mucous membrane covers a plexus of blood vessels. When exposed to dry air or minor trauma (e.g., finger picking), bleeding can occur. The most frequent type of epistaxis, anterior nasal bleeding, is responsible for most epistaxis occurring in children and young adults. Usually, anterior epistaxis is self-limited and does not require medical evaluation (Frazee et al. 2000, Jackler et al. 2002, Koh et al. 2000, Shellenberger 2000).

Posterior nasal bleeding originates in the area posterior to the middle turbinate, an area that is difficult to assess for treatment. This type of epistaxis often is associated with older patients and patients with certain medical conditions (e.g. hypertension, bleeding disorders). Medical evaluation and interventions are usually necessary to treat this epistaxis episode and minimize blood loss (Frazee et al. 2000, Jackler et al. 2002, Koh et al. 2000, Srinivasan et al. 2000).

DATABASE

SUBJECTIVE

→ Predisposing factors may include:
- Decreased ambient humidity
- Trauma
- Nasal infection
- Anatomic deviations (deviated nasal septum, septal spur)
- Allergic rhinitis
- Hypertension
- Bleeding disorders
- Chronic, excessive alcohol intake
- Overuse of a platelet-inhibiting medication (e.g., aspirin, nonsteroidal anti-inflammatory drug)
- Severe liver disease
- Neoplasm (especially hematologic malignancies)
- Use of decongestants, nasal steroids
- Recreational intranasal drug use
- Systemic vasculitis

→ Symptoms may include:
- Nasal bleeding, unilateral or bilateral
- Symptoms associated with upper respiratory infection or allergic rhinitis
- Dizziness (if there is increased blood loss)
- Lightheadedness (if there is increased blood loss)
- Bleeding from other sites (with overuse of platelet-inhibiting medication, coagulopathy, or severe liver disease)
- Symptoms associated with severe liver disease (e.g., anorexia, jaundice)

OBJECTIVE

→ The patient may present with the following changes in vital signs:
- Blood pressure. Postural change in blood pressure may be observed if there is significant blood loss.
- Pulse may be increased if there is significant blood loss.
- Skin pallor may be observed if there is significant blood loss.

→ Direct observation with a nasal speculum may reveal a localized bleeding site in the anterior portion of the nasal vestibule. The bleeding site may not be visible if it is located posterior to the middle turbinate.

→ Crusting, inflammation, and ulceration may be observed if nasal mucosa has been traumatized.

ASSESSMENT

→ Epistaxis
→ R/O nasal trauma
→ R/O allergic rhinitis
→ R/O infection
→ R/O anatomic deviations
→ R/O hypertension
→ R/O bleeding disorders
→ R/O overuse of platelet-inhibiting medications
→ R/O chronic alcohol use
→ R/O liver disease
→ R/O neoplasm
→ R/O intranasal drug use
→ R/O systemic vasculitis

PLAN

DIAGNOSTIC TESTS

→ If significant blood loss is suspected, the following tests may be ordered in consultation with a physician:

- Complete blood count (CBC): A decreased hemoglobin and hematocrit may be noted with significant blood loss.
- Platelet count: may be decreased in patients with idiopathic thrombocytopenia, severe liver disease.
- Prothrombin time (PT), partial thromboplastin time (PTT), bleeding time: may be increased in patients with severe liver disease, anticoagulation therapy (e.g., warfarin sodium), or clotting disorder
- Bone marrow biopsy

TREATMENT/MANAGEMENT

→ If the patient does not have a history of prolonged epistaxis and there is no evidence of excessive blood loss (e.g., postural changes), she should apply direct digital pressure—tightly compressing the soft nasal tip of the nose (not the bony portions of the nose) between the index finger and thumb—for at least 5 minutes and for as long as 30 minutes (Shellenberger 2000).

- During this time, the patient should be sitting with her head bent *slightly* forward to reduce the swallowing of blood (Shellenberger 2000).

→ After application of digital pressure, evaluate the patient for cessation of bleeding.

- If bleeding has stopped, attempt to view and identify the site of the epistaxis to rule out specific pathology.
- Observe the patient for several minutes to ensure that bleeding will not resume.

→ If the bleeding recurs or continues despite application of digital pressure, the patient should be evaluated immediate-

ly by a physician for additional diagnostic and therapeutic interventions. Epistaxis can lead to severe blood loss and death if inadequately evaluated and treated, though this is a rare occurrence.

→ Treatment of underlying pathology (e.g., rhinitis, infection, hypertension, liver disease, bleeding disorder) is essential to reduce the likelihood of recurrence.

→ Patients with epistaxis caused by decreased ambient humidity should be educated about ways to increase ambient humidity (e.g., by using a vaporizer) to maintain adequate hydration, and about avoiding nasal mucosa trauma (e.g., finger picking). Nasal saline spray can be used to help loosen and remove crusting as a means of reducing nose blowing or picking (Shellenberger 2000). Application of a small (less than pea size) lubricating cream (e.g., petroleum jelly) with a cotton-tip swab to just inside the nares at night can further reduce dryness (Shellenberger 2000).

CONSULTATION

→ Consultation with a physician is warranted in all instances of suspected intractable epistaxis, if the bleeding site cannot be seen, or when significant underlying medical conditions are suspected.

→ As needed for prescription(s).

PATIENT EDUCATION

→ Educate the patient about epistaxis—the most common cause, treatment, signs and symptoms of complications, preventive measures, and, if epistaxis recurs, the proper technique to use when applying direct pressure to the nostrils.

→ Educate the patient about avoiding hot and spicy foods and tobacco, as vasodilation may result from their ingestion/use (Jackler et al. 2002).

FOLLOW-UP

→ If there has been physician consultation, follow up per physician recommendation.

→ Document in progress notes and on problem list.

BIBLIOGRAPHY

Frazee, T.A., and Hauser, M.S. 2000. Nonsurgical management of epistaxis. *Journal of Oral and Maxillofacial Surgery* 58:419–424.

Jackler, R.K., and Kaplan, M.J. 2002. Ear, nose, and throat. In *2002 current medical diagnosis & treatment*, 41st ed., eds. L.M. Tierney, Jr., S.J. McPhee, and M.A. Papadakis, pp. 246–247. New York: Lange Medical Books/McGraw-Hill.

Koh, E., Frazzini, V.I., and Kagetsu, N.J. 2000. Epistaxis: vascular anatomy, origins, and endovascular treatment. *American Journal of Roentgenology* 174(3):845–851.

Shellenberger, T. 2000. Nosebleeds: not just kids' stuff. *RN* 63(2):50–54.

Srinivasan, V., Sherman, I.W., and O'Sullivan, G. 2000. Surgical management of intractable epistaxis: audit of results. Journal of Laryngology & Otology 114:697–700.

Maureen T. Shannon, C.N.M., F.N.P., M.S.

5-F

Influenza

Influenza is a respiratory illness caused by one of three types of orthomyxoviruses: type A, B, or C. Influenza epidemics that occur in the fall or winter months are caused by types A and B; the viral infections are similar in their clinical presentations. Type C influenza virus does not cause epidemics and is associated with either no symptoms or a milder respiratory illness than types A and B (Centers for Disease Control and Prevention [CDC] 2001, Danzig et al. 2001).

The influenza viruses are capable of changing their envelope proteins in response to the development of immunity by populations exposed to the viruses. After such a change in the envelope proteins, persons previously immunized or infected with a type of influenza virus may again be susceptible to infection by the same virus type (CDC 2001, Chien et al. 2000, Danzig et al. 2001).

Viral shedding from nasal secretions is the method of transmission, with an individual most infectious 24 hours before the onset of symptoms (Chien et al. 2000). Cessation of viral shedding occurs by seven days after the onset of symptoms. The incubation period after exposure is 1–4 days, with clinical illness usually lasting 1–2 weeks. The malaise and cough associated with influenza infection may persist for two or more weeks after other symptoms subside (CDC 2001).

The annual mortality rate associated with influenza is estimated to be 10,000–40,000 persons in the United States annually, with the highest rates observed in persons 65 years old or older, very young children, and persons of any age with certain underlying medical conditions (e.g., pulmonary disease, cardiovascular disease, immunodeficiency) (CDC 2001, Mossad 2001). Deaths are usually a result of pneumonia but also can be due to exacerbations of cardiopulmonary or other medical conditions during the influenza infection (CDC 2001).

Complications associated with influenza include otitis media, sinusitis, myositis, bronchitis, secondary bacterial pneumonia, and, rarely, pericarditis, myocarditis, and thrombophlebitis (Danzig et al. 2001). Reye's syndrome is a rare but serious complication of influenza, occurring 2–3 weeks after symptom onset. It is usually reported in school-age children.

Although the exact pathogenesis is unknown, the incidence of Reye's syndrome is associated with the ingestion of aspirin (Danzig et al. 2001).

The most effective way to reduce the morbidity and mortality, as well as work and school absenteeism, associated with influenza is to prevent outbreaks. Annually, vaccines are developed to target the viral strains of type A and B influenza that are predicted to erupt during the fall and winter months. In healthy individuals younger than 65 years, the efficacy of influenza immunizations in preventing illness or complications associated with the infection is 70–90%. In elderly populations, the development of antibodies after influenza immunization is less than that observed in younger, healthier populations. However, there is a significant reduction in influenza complications and mortality rates reported in elderly vaccinated populations (CDC 2001).

DATABASE

SUBJECTIVE

→ The patient may report exposure to an individual with similar symptoms.

→ The patient may report one or more of the following symptoms, ranging from mild to severe (CDC 2001, Danzig et al. 2001, Montalto et al. 2000, Monto et al. 2000):

- Sudden onset of high-grade fever
- Cough—initially nonproductive but may become productive
- Malaise
- Chills and/or rigors
- Generalized myalgia
- Arthralgia
- Headache
- Nasal congestion
- Sore throat
- Substernal chest discomfort
- Conjunctivitis
- Abdominal pain
- Anorexia
- Nausea
- Vomiting

OBJECTIVE

→ Physical examination may reveal the following (Danzig et al. 2001):
- Elevated temperature (however, in elderly patients there may be no increase in temperature noted)
- Weight loss and/or orthostasis if there is severe nausea and vomiting
- Mild pharyngeal injection
- Anterior cervical lymph nodes may be enlarged and tender to palpation
- Conjunctival erythema and/or discharge
- Auscultation of the lungs may reveal basilar crackles or rhonchi if there is bronchitis or pneumonia
- Auscultation of the heart may reveal a rub if there is pericarditis
- A change in mental status may be observed in patients with central nervous system complications or Reye's syndrome (such signs and symptoms usually occur 2–3 weeks after the onset of illness if Reye's syndrome complicates influenza)

ASSESSMENT

→ Influenza (type A, B, or C)
→ R/O upper respiratory infection
→ R/O otitis media
→ R/O sinusitis
→ R/O bronchitis
→ R/O pneumonia
→ R/O other viral infections (e.g., mononucleosis)
→ R/O West Nile virus infection

PLAN

DIAGNOSTIC TESTS

→ Diagnostic testing is not necessary for most patients who exhibit signs and symptoms associated with influenza. However, some diagnostic tests may be helpful when patients are severely ill, when prophylaxis is necessary or treatment decisions need to be made (e.g., whether or not to initiate anti-influenza medications), or to determine whether or not an influenza outbreak is occurring in a community. If diagnostic testing is indicated, one or more of the following tests may be ordered after consultation with a physician (Danzig et al. 2001):
- CBC:
  - May demonstrate leukopenia.
- Cultures of nasopharyngeal swabs or aspirates may be positive.
  - Cultures should be obtained within 72 hours of illness secondary to the rapid decline in quantity of virus after 72 hours.
  - Culture requires 5–10 days before results are available (CDC 2003).
- Viral antigen testing (e.g., immunofluorescence, enzyme immunoassay, time-resolved fluoroimmunoassay) of nasopharyngeal specimens for influenza A or B may be

positive. Most of these tests can provide results to clinicians within two hours after specimen collection. These tests have a sensitivity of approximately 70% and a specificity of 90% for detection of influenza (CDC 2003). However, not all available assays detect both type A and B influenza. Therefore, clinicians should confirm with their laboratories the type of assay(s) available before obtaining the specimens.
- Reverse transcriptase polymerase chain reaction (RT-PCR) of nasopharyngeal swabs or sputum specimens may be positive for type A or B influenza, with results available within 1–2 days (CDC 2003).
- Acute and convalescent titers of serum may reveal a significant increase in influenza virus titer for type A or B. The acute serum sample must be obtained within the first week of illness and the convalescent sample collected 2–4 weeks later (CDC 2003). Getting results from these tests requires 2–4 weeks after sample collection.
- Chest x-ray:
  - May reveal evidence of bronchitis or pneumonia in patients with these complications (Chien et al. 2000).
- If Reye's syndrome is suspected, the following will be noted (Danzig et al. 2001):
  - Decreased blood glucose
  - Increased serum transaminase levels
  - Increased blood ammonia levels
  - Increased prothrombin time

TREATMENT/MANAGEMENT

→ During the symptomatic phase of influenza, the patient should rest, increase fluid intake, and use acetaminophen for fever and myalgia (Chien et al. 2000, Danzig et al. 2001).
- The patient should avoid contact with others, especially those most susceptible to possible complications from influenza (e.g., patients 65 years old or older and immunocompromised patients).
→ For severely ill patients or patients at high risk for the development of complications, the use of anti-influenza medications should be considered. There are currently four medications available for use to decrease the severity and duration of symptoms, and the complications associated with influenza. However, all of these medications must be initiated within 48 hours of symptom development to maximize their efficacy. The medications, dosages, and side effects are presented in **Table 5F.1, Anti-Influenza Medications**.
→ Immunization with a polyvalent influenza virus vaccine (1, 0.5 mL IM injection for adults) during the fall or winter months provides partial immunity for up to 1 year. A patient will develop antibodies against the viral types approximately 2 weeks after being immunized. Therefore, the optimum time to administer the vaccine is between October and November, the months before peak influenza season. However, health care providers should continue to offer immunization throughout the influenza season to unvaccinated patients, as influenza activity may persist through early

Table 5F.1.   ANTI-INFLUENZA MEDICATIONS

Characteristic(s)	Amantadine (Symmetrel®)*	Rimantadine (Flumadine®)**¶	Zanamivir (Relenza®)	Oseltamivir*** (Tamiflu®)
Mechanism of Action	Inhibits M_2 ion channel (only present on influenza type A)	Inhibits M_2 ion channel (only present on influenza type A)	Neuraminidase inhibitor	Neuraminidase inhibitor
Indication(s)	Prevention and treatment of influenza type A	Prevention and treatment of influenza type A	Treatment of influenza type A and B	Prevention and treatment of influenza type A and B
FDA-Approved Age Categories for Use	For treatment and prophylaxis in patients ≥1 year old	For prophylaxis in patients ≥1 year old; for treatment in patients ≥13 years old	For treatment in patients >7 years old	For prophylaxis in patients ≥13 years old; for treatment in patients >1 year old
Pregnancy Category	C	C	C	C
Route of Administration	Oral	Oral	Inhalation	Oral
Dosage: Prophylaxis	Ages 13–64: 100 mg BID§ Ages ≥65: ≤100 mg QD (duration = 10 days)	Ages 13–64: 100 mg BID Ages ≥65: 100 or 200 mg QD§§ (duration = 10 days)	Not FDA-approved for prophylaxis	Ages 13–64: 75 mg QD Ages ≥65: 75 mg QD (duration = 7 days after exposure)
Dosage: Treatment	Ages 13–64: 100 mg BID§ Ages ≥65: ≤100 mg QD (duration = 5–7 days or 1–2 days after symptoms resolve)	Ages 13–64: 100 mg BID§ Ages ≥65: 100 or 200 mg QD§§ (duration = 5–7 days or 1–2 days after symptoms resolve)	Ages 13–64: 10 mg BID Ages ≥65: 10 mg BID (duration = 5 days)	Ages 13–64: 75 mg BID Ages ≥65: 75 mg BID (duration = 5 days)
Side Effects	Nausea, anorexia, nervousness, anxiety, difficulty concentrating, lightheadedness	Similar to amantadine but less severe	Nasal and throat discomfort; possible bronchospasm in asthmatics and patients with COPD	Nausea, vomiting (↓ if drug is taken with food)
Drug Interactions	↓ renal clearance with septra, hydrochlorothiazide, quinidine, quinine; ↑ CNS toxicity if concurrent use of CNS stimulants, antihistamines, anticholinergic drugs	↓ peak levels with acetaminophen and aspirin; ↓ renal clearance with cimetidine	Limited data, but no drug interactions reported	Possible ↓ renal clearance if concurrent administration of drugs excreted via anionic pathway of renal tubular system (e.g., probenecid)

*Consult package insert for dosage recommendations for administering amantadine to patients with creatinine clearance ≤50 mL/min/1.73 m².

**Only approved for treatment in adults; approved for prophylaxis in children and adults.

¶The dosage of rimantadine for patients with severe hepatic dysfunction or a creatinine clearance ≤10 mL/min is 100 mg/day. Patients with less hepatic or renal disease taking 100 mg rimantadine/day should be observed closely; the dose should be reduced or discontinued, if necessary.

***The dose of oseltamivir should be reduced in patients with creatinine clearances <30 mL/min.

§ Children >10 years old who weigh <40 kg should be administered amantadine or rimantadine in a dosage of 5 mg/kg/day.

§§ A reduction in rimantadine dose to 100 mg/day should be considered for all patients ≥65 years old who experience side effects at 200 mg/day. In addition, elderly patients in nursing homes should only receive 100 mg/day.

Source: Adapted from Centers for Disease Control and Prevention (CDC). 2001. Prevention and control of influenza. Recommendations of the Advisory Committee on Immunization Practices (ACIP). *Morbidity and Mortality Weekly Report* 50(RR-4):1–63; Mossad, S.B. 2001. Prophylactic and symptomatic treatment of influenza. Current and developing opinions. *Postgraduate Medicine* 109(1):97–105; Sandhu, S.K., and Mossad, S.B. 2001. Influenza in the older adult. Indications for the use of vaccine and antiviral therapy. *Geriatrics* 56(1):43–51.

March (CDC 2001). For information about immunization doses and schedules for children, refer to the CDC Web site at www.cdc.gov/nip/flu or to the *Morbidity and Mortality Weekly Report*.

- Annual immunization is necessary because the antigenic configuration of the virus changes yearly.
- Annual immunization is recommended for individuals at greatest risk of having serious complications associated with influenza or individuals who can transmit influenza to high-risk groups, such as:
  - Persons 50 years old or older
    NOTE: Persons 65 years old or older are considered at high risk for complications associated with influenza infection and should be targeted for immunization as soon as vaccine is available. In addition, adults 50–64 years old have an increased prevalence of high-risk conditions but may not be aware of the condition or perceive a need for influenza vaccination. The CDC recommends vaccinating all individuals in this age group to ensure adequate vaccination coverage for those with medical conditions that place them at risk for serious complications associated with influenza infection (CDC 2001). However, if there is a shortage of vaccine, individuals 65 years old or older should be targeted for immunization first, followed by the 50–64 year age group (unless an individual in this age group has an identified high-risk medical condition such as cardiovascular disease).
  - Persons with chronic heart or lung disease (including asthma)
  - Residents of nursing homes or other chronic care facilities
  - Persons who required ongoing medical care or hospitalization during the previous year because of chronic medical diseases (e.g., diabetes mellitus), hemoglobinopathies, renal dysfunction, or immunosuppression (including pharmacologically induced immunosuppression)
  - Children and adolescents (6 months to 18 years old) receiving long-term aspirin therapy (and therefore at risk of developing Reye's syndrome after influenza infection)
  - Persons who are HIV-positive
  - Pregnant women who will be in the second or third trimester of pregnancy during the influenza season
    NOTE: Whenever possible, influenza vaccine should be administered after the first trimester.
  - Persons preparing to travel to foreign countries. The risk of exposure depends on the destination, the season during which the arrival is planned, and whether or not the person received an influenza vaccination during the previous fall or winter months. In the tropics, influenza can occur throughout the entire year; in the southern hemisphere, the peak influenza season is between April and September.
  - Health care workers, nursing-home/chronic-care facility employees, providers of home care, or household members who have contact with high-risk persons
    NOTE: Influenza vaccinations should not be administered

to patients with a known anaphylactic hypersensitivity to eggs or other components of the influenza vaccine without first consulting a physician. Persons with an acute febrile illness should not be vaccinated until the symptoms subside (CDC 2001).

CONSULTATION

→ Consultation with a physician is warranted for any patient with suspected or diagnosed complications associated with influenza, or before prescribing anti-influenza medications.
→ As otherwise indicated.
→ As necessary for prescription(s).

PATIENT EDUCATION

→ Educate the patient about influenza—the cause, clinical course, diagnostic tests that may be necessary, treatment options, possible complications, and any indicated follow-up.
→ Educate high-risk patients about preventive measures (e.g., influenza vaccination) to avoid influenza infection.

FOLLOW-UP

→ If a consultation with a physician was necessary, follow up as recommended by the physician.
→ If symptoms of complications develop, the patient should return for re-evaluation.
→ Document in progress notes and on problem list.

BIBLIOGRAPHY

Centers for Disease Control and Prevention (CDC). 2001. Prevention and control of influenza. Recommendations of the Advisory Committee on Immunization Practices (ACIP). *Morbidity and Mortality Weekly Report* 50(RR-4):1–63.

_____. 2003. Laboratory and diagnostic procedures for influenza. Available at: http://www.cdc.gov/ncidod/hip/INFECT/flu_acute.htm#table. Accessed on February 15, 2003.

Chien, J.W., and Johnson, J.L. 2000. Viral pneumonias. *Postgraduate Medicine* 107(3):41–52.

Couch, R.B. 2000. Prevention and treatment of influenza. *New England Journal of Medicine* 343(24):1778–1787.

Danzig, L., and Fukuda, K. 2001. Influenza. In *Current diagnosis & treatment in infectious diseases*, eds. W.R. Wilson and M.A. Sande, pp. 380–388. New York: Lange Medical Books/McGraw-Hill.

Montalto, N.J., Gum, K.D., and Ashley, J.V. 2000. Updated treatment for influenza A and B. *American Family Physician* 62(11):2467–2476.

Monto, A.S., Gravenstein, S., Elliott, M. et al. 2000. Clinical signs and symptoms predicting influenza infection. *Archives of Internal Medicine* 160:3243–3247.

Mossad, S.B. 2001. Prophylactic and symptomatic treatment of influenza. Current and developing opinions. *Postgraduate Medicine* 109(1):97–105.

Sandhu, S.K., and Mossad, S.B. 2001. Influenza in the older adult. Indications for the use of vaccine and antiviral therapy. *Geriatrics* 56(1):43–51.

5-G

Otitis Externa

Otitis externa is an inflammation of the external auditory canal caused by pathogens that grow readily in moist environments (e.g., *Pseudomonas aeruginosa*, *Staphylococcus aureus*, group A *Streptococcus*, or fungi such as *Candida* species and *aspergillus*). Usually, exposure to water followed by some type of trauma to the auditory canal (e.g., insertion of a cotton-tip swab or hairpin) precedes the onset of symptoms (Jackler et al. 2002, Virk et al. 2001).

Necrotizing (malignant) external otitis is a rare but potentially lethal infection that can occur in immunocompromised patients (e.g., those with cancer or diabetes). It is caused by *P. aeruginosa* and occasionally by *aspergillus*. This infection is characterized by severe otalgia and persistent, foul aural discharge (Jackler et al. 2002, Virk et al. 2001).

DATABASE

SUBJECTIVE

→ The patient may report the following (Jackler et al. 2002, Virk et al. 2001):
- A history of exposure to water
- A history of diabetes mellitus, immunosuppression (especially in malignant otitis externa)
- Pain in the affected ear
- Pruritis in the affected ear
- Discharge from the affected ear

OBJECTIVE

→ A scant amount of discharge from the affected ear may be observed.
→ Manipulation of the auricle of the affected ear will cause/increase pain.
→ Otoscopic examination of the auditory canal will reveal edema, erythema, and possible discharge (purulent, bloody, serous). Insufflation of the tympanic membrane (TM) will be within normal limits; however, the canal may be too edematous or full of exudate to allow visualization of the TM.
→ Pre- and postauricular lymph node enlargement, with or without tenderness to palpation, may be noted.

→ If necrotizing otitis externa is suspected, examination of the cranial nerves (VI, VII, IX, X, XI, and/or XII) may reveal palsies.
→ Facial erythema, tenderness, and/or warmth adjacent to the affected ear (in malignant otitis externa)

ASSESSMENT

→ Acute otitis externa
→ R/O otitis media
→ R/O foreign body in external auditory canal
→ R/O necrotizing external otitis
→ R/O perforated TM

PLAN

DIAGNOSTIC TESTS

→ Culture of discharge is rarely necessary, as most cases readily respond to topical therapy.
→ Potassium hydroxide (KOH) 10% wet prep of discharge may reveal elements of hyphae and/or yeast buds in suspected cases of fungal infection.

TREATMENT/MANAGEMENT

→ Rinsing of the canal using gentle suction is recommended before beginning treatment.
- This also may result in better visualization of the TM if visualization has been a problem (Virk et al. 2001).
- Instillation of cerumenolytics and/or irrigation of the canal is not recommended.
→ Direct instillation of topical medications into the affected ear is the standard treatment. Occasionally, a wick may need to be inserted into the ear to help facilitate topical therapy if the canal has evidence of substantial edema (Jackler et al. 2002, Virk et al. 2001).
- Otic preparations available for therapy include acid/alcohol solutions or antibiotic/steroid solutions/suspensions.
  • Acid/alcohol otic preparations reduce inflammation and

have a drying and an antifungal effect. Available preparations include:

– Acetic acid 2% solution. Instill 4 gtt in affected ear TID-QID for 7–10 days.
– Hydrocortisone 1% and acetic acid 2% solution. Instill 5 gtt in affected ear TID-QID for 7–10 days.

• Antibiotic/steroid otic preparations have an antimicrobial effect and reduce inflammation. Available preparations include:

– Hydrocortisone 1%, 5 mg neomycin sulfate, 10,000 units polymyxin B per mL suspension/solution. Instill 5 gtt in affected ear TID-QID for 7–10 days.
– Hydrocortisone 1%, 3.3 mg neomycin sulfate, 3 mg colistin sulfate per mL suspension. Instill 4 gtt in affected ear TID-QID for 7–10 days.

NOTE: Neomycin-containing solutions/suspensions may be locally irritating. They also may sensitize the patient to neomycin and result in a more pronounced reaction if neomycin-containing preparations are used in the future.

→ The affected ear canal should be protected from water exposure for at least 2 weeks.
→ For recurrent episodes of otitis externa, prophylactic treatment with boric acid 2.75% in isopropyl alcohol solution may be an option before swimming or bathing.
→ A systemic analgesic (e.g., a nonsteroidal anti-inflammatory drug) may be necessary if the patient is experiencing severe discomfort.
→ If periauricular cellulitis or recalcitrant infection occurs, systemic antibiotic therapy with an agent effective against *P. aeruginosa* species should be prescribed, such as (Jackler et al. 2002):

■ Ciprofloxacin 500 mg p.o. BID for 10 days

CONSULTATION

→ If necrotizing (malignant) external otitis is suspected, physician consultation is warranted.
→ For resistant, recurrent episodes.
→ As needed for prescription(s).

PATIENT EDUCATION

→ Educate the patient about otitis externa—the cause(s), treatment, and the importance of avoiding future trauma as a means of preventing future episodes.
→ If episodes occur after exposure to water (e.g., swimming), discuss the possibility of using an otic preparation before swimming to reduce the possibility of recurrence. The patient should also use a hand-held hair dryer to facilitate drying of the canal after water exposure.

FOLLOW-UP

→ If the condition is resistant to treatment or as recommended by a physician after consultation.
→ Document in progress notes and on problem list.

BIBLIOGRAPHY

Jackler, R.K., and Kaplan, M.J. 2002. Ear, nose, and throat. In *2002 current medical diagnosis & treatment*, 41st ed., eds. L.M. Tierney, Jr., S.J. McPhee, and M.A. Papadakis, pp. 229, 232. New York: Lange Medical Books/McGraw-Hill.

Virk, A., and Henry, N.K. 2001. Upper respiratory tract infections. In *Current diagnosis & treatment in infectious diseases*, eds. W.R. Wilson and M.A. Sande, pp. 112–113. New York: Lange Medical Books/McGraw-Hill.

5-H

Otitis Media

Otitis media is an inflammation of the mucous membrane of the middle ear, the tympanic membrane (TM), and the mastoid air cells. It is observed frequently in children, but its incidence in adults is less common. The pathophysiology of otitis media involves a combination of factors, including Eustachian tube dysfunction (secondary to mucous membrane edema, obstruction, or anatomic deformity), impaired ciliary function of the mucosa, barotrauma, and/or infection with a specific pathogen (Jackler et al. 2002, Virk et al. 2001).

Complications associated with otitis media include diminished hearing, mastoiditis, meningitis, brain abscess, subdural empyema, facial paralysis, cavernous sinus thrombosis, sinus vein thrombosis, petrous apicitis (infection of the petrous bone), and chronic perforation of the TM (Jackler et al. 2002).

The most common pathogens isolated in adult otitis media are *Streptococcus pneumoniae*, *Haemophilus influenzae*, *Branhamella catarrhalis*, and, less frequently, *Staphylococcus aureus*, group A *streptococci*, and *Pseudomonas aeruginosa* (Virk et al. 2001). Penicillin-resistant *S. pneumoniae* is becoming more prevalent and is believed to contribute to some cases of recalcitrant acute otitis media (Virk et al. 2001).

DATABASE

SUBJECTIVE

→ Predisposing factors may include a history of:
- Recent upper respiratory infection (URI)
- Allergies
- Otitis media

→ The patient may report one or more of the following symptoms:
- Otalgia
- Fever
- Diminished hearing
- Tinnitus
- Otorrhea
- Sore throat (may be unilateral)
- Temporomandibular joint (TMJ) pain
- Vertigo
- Anorexia
- Nausea
- Vomiting

OBJECTIVE

→ Temperature may be elevated but often is normal in adults.

→ The external auditory canal may contain a purulent discharge if TM perforation has occurred.

→ The TM may be bulging or retracted, opaque, erythematous, bullous, or hyperemic. Air-fluid level or purulent fluid may be observed behind the TM. There may be distorted or absent TM landmarks and light reflex. The TM may be immobile when insufflation is attempted.

→ Enlarged and tender pre- and postauricular lymph nodes may be palpated.

→ Tenderness to palpation of mastoid prominence may be noted.

→ Diminished gross hearing tests (e.g., wristwatch ticking, whispering) of affected ear may be evident.

ASSESSMENT

→ Otitis media
→ R/O middle ear effusion
→ R/O URI
→ R/O otitis externa
→ R/O TM perforation
→ R/O barotrauma
→ R/O anatomic deformity
→ R/O foreign body in external auditory canal
→ R/O cerumen impaction
→ R/O TMJ syndrome
→ R/O facial pain syndrome

PLAN

DIAGNOSTIC TESTS

→ Usually otitis media is a clinical diagnosis and does not require additional testing; however, in some patients the following diagnostic tests may be indicated:

- Audiometry testing may demonstrate diminished hearing in affected ear(s).
- Tympanocentesis may reveal purulent discharge. Bacterial and/or fungal cultures of this discharge may be performed if indicated (e.g., if a penicillin-resistant organism is suspected). If tympanocentesis is being considered, the patient should be referred to an otolaryngologist.

TREATMENT/MANAGEMENT

→ Initiate antibiotic treatment with amoxicillin 500 mg p.o. TID for 10 days (Virk et al. 2001).

→ Patients who are not responding to amoxicillin after 3–5 days of treatment or who experience a recurrence of symptoms should be treated with one of the following (Virk et al. 2001):

- Amoxicillin-clavulanic acid 500 mg p.o. BID or 875 mg p.o BID for 10 days
- Cefpodoxime 100–400 mg p.o. BID for 10 days
- Cefaclor 250 mg p.o. BID for 10 days
- Trimethoprim/sulfamethoxazole 1 tablet p.o. BID for 10 days (if the patient is penicillin-allergic)
- Erythromycin 250 mg p.o. QID for 10 days (if the patient is penicillin-allergic)

→ If penicillin-resistant *S. pneumoniae* is suspected (e.g., the patient fails to respond to appropriate therapy with standard medications), consultation with an otolaryngologist is indicated to determine the need for further diagnostic testing and treatment.

→ Decongestants, air humidification, and nasal steroids for severe cases may be beneficial. (See the **Rhinitis** chapter.)

→ Analgesics (e.g., aspirin, acetaminophen) may help diminish the otalgia associated with otitis media.

CONSULTATION

→ As indicated in otitis media that is unresponsive to therapy or associated with significant hearing loss, or if complications are suspected.

→ As needed for prescriptions.

PATIENT EDUCATION

→ Educate the patient about otitis media—the cause, treatment options and possible side effects, and signs and symptoms of complications.

→ Educate the patient about nonpharmacological management of common side effects associated with antibiotic therapy (e.g., vaginal candidiasis, diarrhea).

→ Advise the patient to avoid activities that can aggravate the condition (e.g., traveling to high altitudes, scuba diving) until resolution of symptoms and completion of therapy.

→ Educate the patient about the importance of completing all antibiotics as prescribed to reduce the possibility of developing resistant organisms or a recurrence of the infection.

FOLLOW-UP

→ If otitis media has been associated with hearing loss, consider repeating audiometry testing 4–6 weeks after completion of therapy to determine if this problem was resolved.

→ If consultation with a physician was required, follow up as recommended by the physician.

→ Document in progress notes and on problem list.

BIBLIOGRAPHY

Jackler, R.K., and Kaplan, M.J. 2002. Ear, nose, and throat. In *2002 current medical diagnosis & treatment*, 41st ed., eds. L.M. Tierney, Jr., S.J. McPhee, and M.A. Papadakis, pp. 230–233. New York: Lange Medical Books/McGraw-Hill.

Virk, A., and Henry, N.K. 2001. Upper respiratory tract infections. In *Current diagnosis & treatment in infectious diseases*, eds. W.R. Wilson and M.A. Sande, pp. 108–111. New York: Lange Medical Books/McGraw-Hill.

5-1

Pharyngitis

Pharyngitis is an inflammation of the pharynx that can result from several etiological factors. In 50% of cases, the cause is a virus, such as adenovirus, respiratory syncytial virus, Epstein-Barr virus (EBV), coxsackievirus, influenza, or parainfluenza virus, associated with an upper respiratory infection (URI) (Bisno 2001, Virk et al. 2001).

Of the bacterial pathogens associated with pharyngitis, *group A beta-hemolytic streptococcus* (GABHS) is the most common etiologic agent and accounts for 10–40% of infections. Other less-frequent bacterial pathogens responsible for pharyngitis include nongroup A *Streptococci, Neisseria gonorrhoeae, Haemophilus influenzae, Corynebacterium diphtheriae, Mycoplasma pneumoniae,* and *Chlamydia trachomatis* (Virk et al. 2001). Pharyngitis also is associated with other conditions, such as the acute retroviral syndrome that may occur when an individual is seroconverting to human immunodeficiency virus (HIV) infection. However, in approximately 40% of patients with pharyngitis, an exact etiology is not determined (Virk et al. 2001). Environmental factors such as exposure to cigarette smoke, dry air, postnasal drip, and air pollution also may be responsible for pharyngitis symptoms.

Possible serious sequelae (e.g., acute rheumatic fever, peritonsillar abscesses, glomerulonephritis, jugular vein thrombophlebitis) associated with GABHS are a major concern when evaluating and considering treatment of a patient with pharyngitis.

DATABASE

SUBJECTIVE

Viral

→ Symptoms may include:
- Sore throat
- Dysphagia
- Fever (can be high)
- Anorexia (often associated with coxsackievirus)
- Rhinorrhea
- Cough
- Hoarseness
- Malaise

→ The patient may report exposure to HIV via unprotected sex, use of an unclean needle, or occupation. The symptoms may be mild to severe and include (Zavasky et al. 2001):
- Fever
- Sore throat
- Rash
- Myalgia
- Headache
- Stiff neck
- Nausea, vomiting
- Altered mental status

GABHS

→ The patient may report exposure to a person with GABHS within the previous two weeks.
→ Patients may present with minimal symptoms or experience all of the following:
- Severe dysphagia
- High fever
- Cervical lymphadenopathy
- Headache
- Lethargy
- Anorexia
- Abdominal pain
- Scarlatiniform (e.g., sunburn-like) rash with generalized distribution
  NOTE: URI symptoms are less commonly associated with GABHS than with viral pathogens that cause pharyngitis.

Gonococcal

→ The patient is usually asymptomatic but can present with symptoms associated with pharyngitis.
→ The patient has a history of orogenital sexual contact.
→ See the **Gonorrhea** chapter in Section 13 for other symptoms.

Diphtheria

→ Rarely observed today in the United States because of immunizations (Committee on Infectious Diseases 2000).

→ The patient has a history of no or incomplete immunizations.

→ Symptoms may include:
- Low-grade fever
- Sore throat
- Dysphagia
- Hoarseness
- Malaise
- Swollen neck ("bull neck" appearance)
- Shortness of breath, if there is associated myocarditis
- Stridor
- Double vision, slurred speech if there is associated neuropathy
- Skin lesions similar to insect bites

OBJECTIVE

Viral

→ The patient may present with:
- Elevated temperature
- Mild erythema, edema of mucosa of pharynx
- Exudate on tonsils
- Small vesicles on tonsils, uvula, and palate, and on palms and soles of the feet (coxsackievirus)
- Generalized and tender or nontender adenopathy
- Inflammation, erythema of conjunctiva; whitish-yellow discharge from the eyes

→ See the **Rhinitis** chapter for additional physical findings.

→ See the **Human Immunodeficiency Virus-1 Infection** chapter in Section 11 for additional physical findings associated with acute retroviral syndrome.

GABHS

→ The patient may present with:
- Elevated temperature (often >38.3° C)
- Erythematous (flushed) face with circumoral pallor if there is scarlet fever (Chambers 2001)
- Erythema, edema of tonsils and pharynx
- Tongue with enlarged red papillae ("strawberry" tongue) if there is scarlet fever (Chambers 2001)
- Exudate on tonsils and pharynx
- Palatal petechiae
- Enlarged, tender, anterior cervical lymph nodes
- Scarlatiniform rash (diffuse, erythematous, sunburn-like rash with fine papules; blanches with pressure; most intense in axillae and groin)

Gonococcal

→ Occasionally may observe exudative pharyngitis.

→ Cervical adenitis may be present.

→ See the **Gonorrhea** chapter in Section 13 for other physical findings.

Diphtheria

→ The patient may present with:
- Elevated temperature
- Gray, tenacious, tonsillar/pharyngeal pseudomembrane
- Tachycardia (disproportionate to temperature elevation)

→ Cranial nerve testing of the 9th and 10th nerves may be abnormal (if there is neuropathy).

→ Cutaneous pustules and/or ulcers with a grayish-brown membrane at the base

ASSESSMENT

→ Pharyngitis
→ R/O GABHS pharyngitis
→ R/O URI
→ R/O mononucleosis
→ R/O peritonsillar abscess
→ R/O coxsackievirus infection
→ R/O diphtheria (rare)
→ R/O HIV acute retroviral syndrome

PLAN

DIAGNOSTIC TESTS

Viral

→ Complete blood count (CBC) with differential may reveal atypical lymphocytosis if there is an EBV infection.

→ Heterophile test: positive if there is an EBV infection.

→ Throat cultures: negative for bacteria.

→ HIV antibody test is usually negative or indeterminate in patients with acute retroviral syndrome. However, viral tests for HIV (e.g., viral load) will demonstrate positive results. (See also the **Human Immunodeficiency Virus-1 Infection** chapter in Section 11.)

GABHS

→ Because it is not possible to distinguish GABHS pharyngitis from other types of pharyngitis on clinical presentation, certain diagnostic tests are indicated to confirm the diagnosis.

→ Strategies vary regarding when certain tests should be done and are based on such factors as cost(s) of the test(s), sensitivity/specificity of the test(s), and time required to perform the test(s), as well as the incidence in the geographic area of pharyngitis *not* due to GABHS and the likelihood of patient follow-up.

→ Throat culture:
- Considered the gold standard. Has a sensitivity of 90–95% and a specificity of 100%.
- A cotton-tip swab is used to obtain the specimen from the posterior pharynx and tonsillar fossae. This specimen is plated on sheep's-blood agar medium with a bacitracin disc. Results are available 24–48 hours later.
- Positive culture indicates the presence of beta-hemolytic streptococcus. However, it will not distinguish between serologically infected patients versus GABHS carriers or

group C and G streptococci infection (beta-hemolytic strains that may cause pharyngitis) (Virk et al. 2001).

→ Rapid tests:

- Rapid antigen detection test (RADT) for group A beta-hemolytic strep is less costly than the throat culture and results are available within 1–2 hours. Sensitivity is 80–95% and specificity is 90–95% (Jackler et al. 2002, Virk et al. 2001, Webb et al. 2000).
- A positive RADT result indicates hemolytic streptococcus infection.
- Some authors recommend confirming a negative RADT result with a throat culture (Chambers 2001, Virk et al. 2001).

→ CBC: Leukocytosis may or may not be observed; usually not done for work-up of GABHS pharyngitis.

→ Lateral neck x-ray should be obtained in patients with stridor to rule out laryngeal obstruction (Virk et al. 2001).

Gonococcal

→ Throat culture:

- Two or three swabs rubbed over the posterior pharynx and tonsils for 10–20 seconds and plated on Thayer-Martin medium.
- Positive result indicates gonococcal infection.

→ Obtain other tests (e.g., cervical, rectal cultures) to rule out the presence of gonococcus at other sites, and tests such as chlamydia culture and VDRL to rule out co-existent sexually transmitted diseases (STDs). (See the **Gonorrhea** and *Chlamydia trachomatis* chapters in Section 13.)

Diphtheria

→ Diagnosis is usually made by clinical findings.

→ Throat culture:

- Swab the posterior pharynx and tonsils beneath the pseudomembrane and plate on Loeffler's or tellurite selective medium to confirm the diagnosis.
- Because of the special medium that is necessary, laboratory staff should be notified in advance that diagnostic testing for diphtheria is being requested.

TREATMENT/MANAGEMENT

→ Recommended for all episodes of pharyngitis are rest, increased fluids, use of analgesics (e.g., acetaminophen) as needed, and warm saline gargles (¼ tsp. of salt in 8 oz. of warm water) TID to help alleviate symptoms.

- Viral pharyngitis is usually a self-limited, benign condition and requires no additional therapy.

→ GABHS antibiotic therapy is recommended to prevent serious sequelae. The following agents may be prescribed (Chambers 2001, Jackler et al. 2002):

- Penicillin V 250–500 mg p.o. every 6–8 hours for 7–10 days

OR

- Amoxicillin 500 mg p.o. TID for 10 days

→ In beta-lactamase-resistant cases of GABHS, alternative antibiotic therapy is necessary and may include:

- Cefuroxime axetil 250 mg p.o. every 12 hours for 10 days

OR

- Dicloxacillin 250 mg p.o QID for 10 days

OR

- Amoxicillin with clavulanate acid 500 mg p.o TID for 10 days
- For penicillin-allergic patients, the following medications can be prescribed:
  - Erythromycin 500 mg p.o. QID for 10 days

OR

  - Clarithromycin 250 mg p.o. every 12 hours for 10 days

OR

  - Azithromycin 500 mg p.o for 3 days

OR

  - Cefuroxime axetil 250 mg p.o. BID for 10 days (if the patient does not have a history of cephalosporin allergy)
- If compliance with oral therapy is of concern, benzathine penicillin G 1.2 million units IM can be administered.

→ Treatment of gonococcal pharyngitis consists of ceftriaxone 125 mg IM or ciprofloxacin 500 mg p.o. in a single dose. (See the **Gonorrhea** chapter in Section 13.)

- Treatment of any suspected or co-existent STDs also is indicated. (See the appropriate chapters.)

→ If diphtheria is suspected, the patient should be hospitalized and isolated. Treatment includes administering antitoxin, the dose of which depends on the severity/duration of disease. Before administering antitoxin, the patient should undergo a scratch test to make sure there is no allergy to equine antitoxin (Committee on Infectious Diseases 2000).

- Antitoxin is available through the Drug Service, Centers for Disease Control and Prevention, (404) 639-3670 (during business hours, Monday through Friday), (404) 639-2888 (nights, weekends, and holidays), www.cdc.gov/ncidod/srp/drugservice
- Antibiotic therapy also is indicated and includes (Loutit et al. 2001):
  - Penicillin 500 mg QID p.o. for 14 days

OR

  - Erythromycin 500 mg p.o. QID for 14 days

→ For patients with severe odynophagia, hospitalization for hydration and parenteral antibiotic therapy may be necessary.

→ Surgical intervention (i.e., tonsillectomy) is rarely indicated and should be considered only for patients with documented recurrent GABHS pharyngitis.

→ Symptomatic contacts of patients with GABHS should have throat cultures done and receive appropriate treatment as indicated.

→ Sexual contacts of patients with gonococcal pharyngitis should be evaluated and treated as indicated. (See the **Gonorrhea** chapter in Section 13.)

→ If HIV infection is diagnosed, initiation of antiretroviral agents may be indicated and should be prescribed in consultation with an infectious disease specialist. Sexual contacts of the patient should be evaluated.

CONSULTATION

→ As indicated in recurrent pharyngitis, suspected peritonsillar abscess, or HIV infection, or for patients with severe symptoms that may require hospitalization for treatment.
→ As needed for prescription(s).

PATIENT EDUCATION

→ Educate the patient about the cause of pharyngitis, the clinical course, treatment, possible complications, and any required follow-up.
→ Discuss the need for evaluation of symptomatic contacts (in nongonococcal pharyngitis) and for evaluation and treatment of all sexual contacts of patients with gonococcal pharyngitis.
→ Advise the patient to call or return for evaluation of any signs/symptoms of complications (including antibiotic reactions).

FOLLOW-UP

→ Test of cure usually is not necessary in GABHS pharyngitis but should be obtained in patients with gonococcal pharyngitis.
→ Because gonococcal infections and diphtheria are state-mandated reportable diseases, a morbidity report must be filed with the local department of public health. In some states, HIV infection is also a state-mandated reportable disease.
→ Document in progress notes and on problem list.

BIBLIOGRAPHY

Bisno, A.L. 2001. Acute pharyngitis. *New England Journal of Medicine* 344(3):205–211.

Chambers, H.F. 2001. Infectious diseases: bacterial and chlamydial. In *2002 current medical diagnosis & treatment*, 41st ed., eds. L.M. Tierney, Jr., S.J. McPhee, and M.A. Papadakis, pp. 1348–1351. New York: Lange Medical Books/McGraw-Hill.

Committee on Infectious Diseases. 2000. *Red book 2000. Report of the Committee on Infectious Diseases*, 25th ed. Elk Grove Village, Ill.: American Academy of Pediatrics.

Jackler, R.K., and Kaplan, M.J. 2002. Ear, nose, and throat. In *2002 current medical diagnosis & treatment*, 41st ed., eds. L.M. Tierney, Jr., S.J. McPhee, and M.A. Papadakis, pp. 246–249. New York: Lange Medical Books/McGraw-Hill.

Loutit, J., and Relman, D. 2001. Gram-positive aerobic bacilli. In *Current diagnosis & treatment in infectious diseases*, eds. W.R. Wilson and M.A. Sande, pp. 533–536. New York: Lange Medical Books/McGraw-Hill.

Virk, A., and Henry, N.K. 2001. Upper respiratory tract infections. In *Current diagnosis & treatment in infectious diseases*, eds. W.R. Wilson and M.A. Sande, pp. 100–103. New York: Lange Medical Books/McGraw-Hill.

Webb, K.H., Needham, C.A., and Kurtz, S.R. 2000. Use of high-sensitivity rapid strep test without culture confirmation of negative results: 2 years' experience. *Journal of Family Practice* 49(1):34–38.

Zavasky, D.M., Gerberding, J.L., and Sande, M.A. 2001. Patients with AIDS. In *Current diagnosis & treatment in infectious diseases*, eds. W.R. Wilson and M.A. Sande, pp. 315–327. New York: Lange Medical Books/McGraw-Hill.

5-J

Pneumonia

Pneumonia is an infection of the lung caused by various pathogens, including bacteria, viruses, and fungi. Pneumonia accounts for approximately 10 million clinician visits and 500,000 hospitalizations annually in the United States (Bartlett et al. 2000). It is the sixth leading cause of death in the United States, with a mortality rate of 1% for outpatient cases compared to 14% for hospitalized patients (Chesnutt et al. 2002).

Community-acquired pneumonia (CAP) is defined as pneumonia that "begins outside of the hospital or is diagnosed within 48 hours after admission to the hospital in a patient who has not resided in a long-term care facility for 14 days or more before the onset of symptoms" (Chesnutt et al. 2002, p. 295). Risk factors associated with an increased risk of morbidity and mortality include advanced age (older than 65 years), co-existing lung disease (e.g., chronic obstructive pulmonary disease [COPD]), immunosuppression, alcoholism, and other comorbid medical conditions (e.g., renal disease and cardiac disease) (Bartlett et al. 2000, Chesnutt et al. 2002, Cunha 2001a).

Individuals who develop pneumonia are exposed to the infecting organism by transmission from colonization in the upper respiratory tract, through hematogenous spread, or by inhaling infected droplets. The bacterial organisms commonly responsible for CAP include *Streptococcus pneumoniae*, *Haemophilus influenzae*, *Moraxella catarrhalis*, *Mycoplasma pneumoniae*, *Chlamydia pneumoniae*, and *Legionella pneumophila* (Bartlett et al. 2000, Cunha 2001a). Of these pathogens, *S. pneumoniae*, *H. influenzae*, and *M. catarrhalis* are responsible for approximately 85% of CAP cases, with the remaining 15% attributed to the more "atypical" pathogens (Cunha 2001a). In approximately 40–60% of CAP cases, an etiologic pathogen is not identified.

The most common viral pathogens that cause pneumonia in adults include influenza viruses Type A and B (responsible for 50% of viral pneumonias), respiratory syncytial virus, adenovirus, parainfluenza viruses, and viruses associated with exanthems (e.g., measles) (Chien et al. 2000a, 2000b). In immunocompromised individuals, the herpes viruses (e.g., herpes simplex virus, varicella zoster virus, and cytomegalovirus [CMV]) are the most common cause of viral pneumonias (Chien et al. 2000a).

Pneumonia resulting from fungi (e.g., *Pneumocystis carinii*, *Cryptococcus neoformans*, *Aspergillus fumigatus*, *Histoplasma capsulatum*, and *Coccidioides immitis*) is rarely seen in individuals with competent immune systems but is of concern in immunocompromised patients (e.g., HIV-positive patients and patients undergoing cytotoxic therapy) who are in advanced stages of immune dysfunction (Bartlett et al. 2000).

Nosocomial (i.e., hospital-acquired) pneumonias also can occur and usually are present 48 hours after admission to the hospital in individuals without an incubating infection at the time of admission (Chesnutt et al. 2002). These pneumonias have a mortality rate of 20–50%, with the highest risk among patients in intensive care units or among patients using mechanical ventilation (Chesnutt et al. 2002). Pathogens frequently—though not exclusively—associated with nosocomial infection include *Staphylococcus aureus*, *Klebsiella pneumoniae*, *Escherichia coli*, and *Pseudomonas aeruginosa*, along with influenza viruses Type A and B (Chesnutt et al. 2002).

Complications associated with pneumonia are related directly to the infecting organism and the immune status of the patient. In most healthy adults, CAP usually can be treated effectively with oral antibiotics on an outpatient basis, without serious sequelae developing. However, in patients with diminished immune responses (e.g., the elderly, alcoholics, malnourished patients, and immune-deficient patients) or those with a history of pre-existing pulmonary disease, there is an increased risk of complications, which can include pleural effusion, bacteremia, lung abscesses, meningitis, or death (Bartlett et al. 2000, Cunha 2001a). In patients who are at increased risk of such complications, hospitalization often is indicated. The Pneumonia Patient Outcomes Research Team (PORT) developed and validated a prediction schema to help clinicians identify patients' risk of CAP-associated mortality within 30 days of diagnosis. (See **Table 5J.1, PORT Criteria and Scoring**.) This system uses 19 variables to place patients in one of five risk classes. Individuals in the PORT Risk Class I have <1% risk of mortality; however, individuals in the other categories have incremental increases in mortality risk up to 29% in Class V.

This system can be useful in initially determining whether or not a patient with CAP should be hospitalized for treatment (Bartlett et al. 2000, Chesnutt et al. 2002).

An in-depth presentation that includes all pathogens, clinical manifestations, and treatment modalities for the various types of pneumonia is beyond the scope of this chapter, which will present information about the clinical manifestations, diagnostic testing, and current treatment recommendations for uncomplicated CAP.

DATABASE

SUBJECTIVE

→ The patient may be elderly.
→ The patient may have a history of:
  ▪ Cigarette smoking
  ▪ COPD
  ▪ Splenectomy

▪ Chronic illness(es): diabetes mellitus, chronic liver or kidney disease, neoplasm, cardiac disease
▪ Substance abuse (e.g., alcohol or injection drug use)
▪ Immune deficiency
▪ Malnutrition
▪ Recent upper respiratory infection, influenza, or viral exanthem (e.g., measles or varicella)
▪ Recent hospitalization
→ The symptoms and their intensity will vary depending on the pathogen causing the pneumonia and on the patient's baseline health status.

Bacterial Pneumonia (Chesnutt et al. 2002)

→ Symptoms may include:
  ▪ Fever often >38° C/100.4° F (especially in patients with pneumococcal pneumonia)

Table 5J.1.   PORT* CRITERIA AND SCORING

Patient Predictor Criteria/Condition	PORT Points
Age	Men = 1 per year of age Women = 1 per year of age minus 10
Nursing home resident	10 points
Renal disease Congestive heart failure Cerebral vascular disease Pleural effusion Pulse >125 beats/minute Hematocrit <30% Arterial partial pressure of oxygen <60 mm Hg Glucose >250 mg/dL	Each condition = 10 points
Temperature >40° C or <35° C	15 points
Liver disease (e.g., cirrhosis, chronic active hepatitis) Altered mental status (e.g., coma, stupor, or disorientation to time, place, person) Systolic blood pressure <90 mm Hg Respiratory rate ≥30/minute BUN ≥30 mg/dL Serum sodium <130 mEq/L	Each condition = 20 points
Neoplastic disease (other than basal or squamous cell cancer of the skin diagnosed within 1 year of presentation with pneumonia) Arterial pH <7.35	Each condition = 30 points

Risk Class, Number of PORT Points, and 30-Day Mortality Rate (MR)			Recommended Site of Care
Risk Class I:	no predictors	MR = 0.1%	Outpatient
Risk Class II:	≤70 points	MR = 0.6%	Outpatient
Risk Class III:	71–90 points	MR = 2.8%	Outpatient or brief hospitalization
Risk Class IV:	91–130 points	MR = 8.2%	Hospitalize
Risk Class V:	>130 points	MR = 29.2%	Hospitalize

* The Pneumonia Patient Outcomes Research Team

Source: Adapted with permission from Bartlett, J.G., Dowell, S.F., Mandell, L.A. et al. 2000. Practice guidelines for the management of community-acquired pneumonia in adults. *Clinical Infectious Diseases* 31:352; Chesnutt, M.S., and Prendergast, T.J. 2002. Lung. In *2002 current medical diagnosis & treatment*, 41st ed., eds. L.M. Tierney, Jr., S.J. McPhee, and M.A. Papadakis, p. 292. New York: Lange Medical Books/McGraw-Hill.

- Hypothermia, especially in elderly patients (Virk et al. 2001)
- Cough may or may not be productive of copious amounts of thick, purulent, and/or blood-tinged mucus
- Chills and/or rigors
- Dyspnea
- Chest pain
- Malaise
- Headache (rare)
- Myalgia
- Change in mental status (often noted in *L. pneumophila*)
- Nausea, vomiting, diarrhea (usually associated with *L. pneumophila*)

→ Patients with COPD may report less significant symptoms and note only a gradually increasing intensity of shortness of breath, increased cough, and possibly a low-grade temperature.

→ Elderly patients often present with a minimal cough (usually nonproductive), dehydration, mental status changes, and no fever.

Viral Pneumonia

→ The symptoms associated with viral pneumonia are similar to those of bacterial pneumonias. However, the following symptoms may be reported as a result of the patient's underlying viral illness (Chien et al. 2000a, 2000b):

- History of a viral exanthem that may include recent measles or varicella zoster virus infection. (See the **Measles [Rubeola]** and **Varicella Zoster Virus** chapters in Section 11.)
- History of symptoms that may indicate recent influenza infection, including:
  - Fever
  - Nausea
  - Vomiting
  - Myalgias
  - Malaise
  - Arthralgias
  - Headache

Atypical Pneumonia

→ The patient with *M. pneumoniae*, *C. pneumoniae*, or *L. pneumophila* pneumonia may report the onset of the following symptoms:

- Headache
- Malaise
- Low-grade fever
- Sore throat
- Enlarged cervical glands (if *M. pneumoniae*)
- Persistent, nonproductive cough (especially if *M. pneumoniae*)
- Chest muscle discomfort (not pleuritic pain)
- Symptoms associated with sinusitis. (See the **Sinusitis— Acute** chapter.)

- Dry cough, earache, aural discharge, and altered mental status can be associated with *M. pneumoniae* (Virk et al. 2001).
- Nausea, vomiting, and diarrhea can be associated with *L. pneumophila* (Virk et al. 2001).

OBJECTIVE

→ The following physical findings may be noted in patients with pneumonia (Bartlett et al. 2000, Chesnutt et al. 2002, Chien et al. 2000a, 2000b):

- They may appear anxious, apprehensive, or confused, depending on the level of hypoxia.
- Vital signs:
  - Temperature may be elevated, normal, or decreased (usually noted in elderly patients).
  - Blood pressure may be normal or decreased in patients with shock (secondary to bacteremia/sepsis) or dehydration.
    - Pulse may be elevated (>90 beats/minute).
  - Respiratory rate may be normal or the patient may be tachypneic.
- Skin:
  - Color may be normal or grayish to cyanotic, depending on the patient's oxygen perfusion.
  - Poor tissue turgor may be evident if the patient is dehydrated.
  - A rash of viral exanthem may be evident in patients with a concomitant viral infection (e.g., measles or varicella zoster).
  - Erythema nodosum may be observed in association with *C. pneumoniae* or fungal infections.
- Examination of the ears may reveal bullous myringitis in association with *M. pneumoniae*.
- Examination of the chest may reveal diminished excursion of the thorax secondary to pain.
- Palpation of the chest wall may reveal tenderness to palpation of intercostal muscles. Increased tactile fremitus may be noted in area(s) of consolidation.
- Percussion of the chest may reveal:
  - Decreased diaphragmatic excursion on the affected side if there is pleural fluid accumulation at the lung bases
  - Dullness in area(s) of consolidation
- Auscultation of the lungs may reveal:
  - Crepitation
  - Bronchial or tubular breath sounds (if there is consolidation)
  - A pleural friction rub if there is pleural effusion
  - Diminished or absent vesicular breath sounds if there is pleural effusion
  - Increased bronchophony, egophony, and whispered pectoriloquy if there is consolidation or pleural effusion
- Auscultation of the heart may reveal a systolic murmur if endocarditis is present.
- Neurological examination may reveal nuchal rigidity and/or altered mentation if there is CNS involvement.

ASSESSMENT

→ Pneumonia (bacterial, viral, atypical)
→ R/O bacteremia
→ R/O meningitis
→ R/O cardiac disease (e.g., congestive heart failure)
→ R/O COPD
→ R/O influenza infection
→ R/O tuberculosis
→ R/O adult respiratory distress syndrome
→ R/O pulmonary embolism and infarction
→ R/O neoplasm
→ R/O reactive airway disease
→ R/O immune deficiency

PLAN

DIAGNOSTIC TESTS

→ Multiple diagnostic tests, other than a chest x-ray, to confirm mild CAP in a patient are not necessary (Bartlett 2000). However, a number of the following diagnostic tests may be ordered to determine the etiology of the illness in patients with comorbid conditions or clinical manifestations that may indicate more severe pulmonary disease. These tests include:

- Chest x-rays. They are essential in making the differential diagnosis (e.g., pneumonia versus acute bronchitis) and evaluating the patient for underlying pulmonary disease (e.g., COPD). In addition, a baseline chest x-ray can be helpful for comparison purposes in situations where the response to therapy is lacking or protracted (Bartlett 2000, Bartlett et al. 2000, Chesnutt et al. 2002, Virk et al. 2001). Chest x-ray findings may demonstrate local or diffuse changes, including infiltration, consolidation, pleural effusion, and, rarely, abscess formation (Bartlett et al. 2000, Chesnutt et al. 2002, Chien et al. 2000a, 2000b).
- CBC:
  - Bacterial pneumonias usually will result in leukocytosis (WBC count >13,000 cells/mm³) with a left shift present. However, up to 25% of patients may have a WBC count within normal limits or suppressed (e.g., in severe pneumococcal infection).
  - Hematocrit/hemoglobin (Hct/Hgb) may be decreased if there is hemolytic anemia associated with severe infections or other medical conditions (e.g., significant malnutrition or chronic alcohol abuse).
  - Decreased platelets may be noted in severe infection associated with disseminated intravascular coagulation (Virk et al. 2001).
- Serum chemistry panel may reveal elevated transaminases (alanine aminotransferase, aspartate aminotransferase) and decreased serum sodium (<130 mEq/L) in severe infections.
- Increased serum bilirubin (>3–4 mg/dL) and lactose dehydrogenase (>250 U/L) are often noted in severe infections.
- Gram stain of sputum may reveal the organism if an adequate specimen is obtained.

- A reliable sputum specimen must contain >25 polymorphonuclear cells/field and <10 squamous epithelial cells on low magnification (i.e., x 100) to minimize the possibility of contamination from upper airway organisms (Virk et al. 2001).
- Specimens for culture:
  - Sputum culture to identify a specific organism may be obtained but is not as sensitive or specific as Gram stain and in approximately 50% of cases is not diagnostic of a pathogen. Anaerobic cultures are of no diagnostic assistance due to oropharyngeal contamination (Virk et al. 2001).
    - If the patient is unable to produce an adequate specimen, sputum induction may be necessary.
  - For patients presenting with significant symptoms, blood or pleural fluid specimens should be obtained for culture.
    - A positive culture result is considered diagnostic for the causative organism (e.g., *S. pneumoniae*, *H. influenzae*, or influenza virus Type A) (Virk et al. 2001).
  - Rarely, cultures from urine and stool specimens may be obtained to identify possible pathogens (e.g., CMV).
- Antigen detection (e.g., counterimmunoelectrophoresis, bacterial antigen testing, and radioimmunoassays) may be used to rapidly detect *L. pneumophila* (serotype I), *S. pneumoniae*, *H. influenzae*, respiratory syncytial virus, influenza virus, and parainfluenza viruses. The sensitivity of these antigen tests is >80% and depends on the specimen source, type of test used, and type of pathogen being identified (Virk et al. 2001).
- Serum antibody titer(s):
  - Acute and convalescent serum antibody titers for a viral pathogen, when suspected, may demonstrate a fourfold rise, indicating recent infection (e.g., CMV, herpes simplex virus, or measles. See specific viral infection chapters.). However, these tests are not helpful if rapid identification of the etiologic pathogen is desired.
  - IgM titer rise may indicate acute infection with a viral pathogen. (See specific viral infection chapters.)
  - Serum cold agglutinins is a nonspecific test for *M. pneumoniae* with a sensitivity of 30–60% (Virk et al. 2001).

TREATMENT/MANAGEMENT

→ Patients with moderate to severe symptoms, with underlying medical conditions that may impair immune response (e.g., the elderly or patients with chronic medical conditions, neutropenia, or immune deficiency), or in whom a particularly virulent organism is suspected, should be hospitalized for parenteral therapy. (See **Table 5J.1**.)

→ In a *healthy* adult patient with uncomplicated CAP, outpatient therapy is possible. Empiric antibiotic treatment for suspected bacterial pneumonia includes the following agents, which provide coverage for the most common pathogens (Bartlett 2000, Virk et al. 2001):

- Levofloxacin 500 mg p.o. QD for 10–14 days
  OR

- Azithromycin 500 mg p.o. on the first day, then 250 mg p.o. QD for 4 days

OR

- Doxycycline 100 mg p.o. BID for 10–14 days

OR

- Amoxicillin/clavulanic acid: 875/125 mg p.o. BID for 10–14 days

OR

- Erythromycin 500 mg p.o. QID for 10 days

→ If influenza virus Type A infection is suspected because of evidence of an epidemic in the community, consider amantadine HCl or rimantadine HCl therapy. (See the **Influenza** chapter.)

→ Symptomatic treatment includes rest, increased fluid intake, adequate nutrition, and antipyretics (e.g., acetaminophen) as needed.

→ If the patient smokes, advise her to stop to prevent exacerbation of symptoms and further damage to her lung tissue.
  - If the patient does not smoke but lives in an environment in which she is exposed to secondary smoke, she should be advised to limit her exposure as much as possible.

→ Prevention strategies include immunization of individuals for whom pneumococcal and influenza vaccinations are recommended.
  - Pneumococcal vaccination is recommended for individuals at risk of pneumococcal disease and its complications. These patients include:
    - Immune-competent individuals with chronic illness (e.g., diabetes mellitus, cardiovascular disease, pulmonary disease, alcoholism, cirrhosis, or cerebrospinal fluid leaks)
    - Individuals 65 years old or older
    - Immunocompromised adults (e.g., individuals with chronic renal failure, nephrotic syndrome, splenic dysfunction or anatomic asplenia, Hodgkin's disease, lymphoma, multiple myeloma, or a transplanted organ)
    - Adults with HIV infection (both asymptomatic and symptomatic)
    - Individuals living in environments or social settings where there is an identified increased risk of pneumococcal disease and its complications
  - Administering pneumococcal vaccine will afford protection against 23 strains of *S. pneumoniae* that reportedly are responsible for most clinical pneumococcal diseases.
    - The duration of immunity is unknown but has been documented to last for 5–7 years in healthy adults.
    - The efficacy of the vaccine in preventing bacteremic pneumococcal infection is approximately 60% (Bartlett et al. 2000).
  - Immunizing before discharge hospitalized patients who are considered at risk of pneumococcal disease and its complications should be considered.
  - Influenza vaccination should be administered annually to individuals at risk of complications associated with this infection, as well as to individuals who are caregivers or have close household contact with persons at risk of complications of influenza infection. (See the **Influenza** chapter.)

CONSULTATION

→ Physician consultation is warranted for any patient with:
  - A history of complications of pneumonia (e.g., respiratory distress, CNS involvement, or abscess)
  - An underlying medical condition that may impair immune response or response to therapy
  - A poor response to initial therapy

→ As needed for prescription(s).

PATIENT EDUCATION

→ If the patient's condition requires hospitalization for treatment, the physician responsible for her care should discuss with her the treatment options and need for hospitalization.

→ Educate the patient about pneumonia—the causes, clinical course, indicated diagnostic tests, treatment options, possible complications, and the need for follow-up.

→ Educate the patient regarding signs and symptoms of possible complications associated with pneumonia, and the need for medical evaluation if any occur.

→ Educate the patient about the need to comply with treatment regimens to facilitate resolution of the pneumonia.

→ If the patient smokes, advise her to stop and provide her with information regarding smoking cessation programs and available community resources. (See the **Smoking Cessation** chapter in Section 14.)

→ Educate the patient about the need for any immunizations as indicated (e.g. influenza or pneumococcal).

FOLLOW-UP

→ If the patient is hospitalized, follow-up visits should be as recommended by the physician responsible for her care.

→ Follow-up evaluation of any patient is indicated when there are persistent symptoms after initiation of appropriate therapy, when patients may not comply with treatment regimens, or when patients develop symptoms of complications.

→ Document in progress notes and on problem list.

BIBLIOGRAPHY

Bartlett, J.G. 2000. Treatment of community-acquired pneumonia. *Chemotherapy* 46(Suppl. 1):24–31.

Bartlett, J.G., Dowell, S.F., Mandell, L.A. et al. 2000. Practice guidelines for the management of community-acquired pneumonia in adults. *Clinical Infectious Diseases* 31:347–382.

Chesnutt, M.S., and Prendergast, T.J. 2002. Lung. In *2002 current medical diagnosis & treatment*, 41st ed., eds. L.M. Tierney, Jr., S.J. McPhee, and M.A. Papadakis, pp. 299–307. New York: Lange Medical Books/McGraw-Hill.

Chien, J.W., and Johnson, J.L. 2000a. Viral pneumonias. Infection in the immunocompromised host. *Postgraduate Medicine* 107(2):67–80.

Chien, J.W., and Johnson, J.L. 2000b. Viral pneumonias. Epidemic respiratory viruses. *Postgraduate Medicine* 107(3):41–52.

Cunha, B.A. 2001a. Community-acquired pneumonia. Diagnostic and therapeutic approach. *Medical Clinics of North America* 85(1):43–77.

Cunha, B.A. 2001b. Nosocomial pneumonia. Diagnostic and therapeutic considerations. *Medical Clinics of North America* 85(1):79–114.

Virk, A., and Wilson, W.R. 2001. Tracheobronchitis and lower respiratory tract infections. In *2001 current diagnosis & treatment in infectious diseases*, eds. W.R. Wilson and M.A. Sande, pp. 118–154. New York: Lange Medical Books/ McGraw-Hill.

5-K
Rhinitis

Rhinitis is an inflammation of the nasal mucosa resulting in congestion and rhinorrhea. There are several causes of rhinitis, including viral infection, allergic and vasomotor responses, intranasal recreational drug use, and/or nasal decongestant overuse. Although many of the clinical manifestations of the various types of rhinitis are similar, there are differences in the clinical presentations that can help determine the type and indicated therapy for each.

Viral Rhinitis (Common Cold)

Viral rhinitis is an infection of the upper respiratory tract that can be caused by more than 200 different serological types of viruses. The most common types of viruses associated with rhinitis include rhinovirus (cause of 30–50% of colds), coronavirus, adenovirus, parainfluenza virus, respiratory syncytial virus, and influenza types A, B, and C (Drew 2001).

These viruses are transmitted by direct or close contact, entering the body via the ciliated epithelium of the nose. Exposure of ciliated epithelium to the virus causes edema and hyperemia of the nasal mucosa, resulting in increased secretion of the glands responsible for the production of both serous and mucinous fluid.

The nasal obstructive symptoms associated with viral rhinitis are caused by the narrowing of the nasal passages, which, in turn, results from the edema of the mucous membranes (Jackler et al. 2002).

Susceptibility to viruses associated with the common cold varies, though there is an increased incidence during the fall, winter, and spring. The incubation period for most of the causative viruses is 1–6 days. The course of the infection is usually self-limited, with acute symptoms lasting up to seven days.

Complications associated with viral rhinitis are uncommon, with most resulting from secondary bacterial infections. These include acute otitis media, acute sinusitis, bronchitis (usually in patients with chronic obstructive pulmonary disease), and, rarely, pneumonia (usually in high-risk populations, such as immunocompromised individuals) (Drew 2001, Jackler et al. 2002).

Allergic Rhinitis

Allergic rhinitis is a chronic, recurrent inflammation of the mucous membranes of the nose, resulting in nasal congestion and discharge. It is the most common chronic condition in the United States, affecting 5–22% of Americans (Bellanti et al. 2000). Allergic rhinitis often occurs seasonally or perennially and is the result of an antigen-specific IgE response by the nasal mucosa, usually to an inhaled allergen (Bellanti et al. 2000, Kishiyama et al. 2001).

The seasonal variation of symptoms can provide information about the type of allergen causing an individual's symptoms. Common allergens responsible for allergic rhinitis symptoms include grass (symptoms usually noted during summer), pollens (symptoms usually noted during spring), ragweed (symptoms usually noted during fall), and animal dander and dust (symptoms usually noted throughout the year) (Bellanti et al. 2000, Jackler et al. 2002, Kishiyama et al. 2001).

Vasomotor Rhinitis

Vasomotor rhinitis is a nasal mucous membrane inflammation not associated with infection or allergy. Though its etiology is unknown, an autonomic imbalance resulting in vasodilation, nasal congestion, and increased mucous secretion is one theory (Jackler et al. 2002).

Precipitating factors associated with vasomotor rhinitis include emotional stress, environmental factors (e.g. toxins, smoke), exercise, and recumbency. Rhinitis observed during pregnancy and in hypothyroid patients also is thought to be due to this vasomotor response.

DATABASE
SUBJECTIVE

Viral Rhinitis

→ The patient may report recent exposure to a person with viral rhinitis symptoms.

→ The patient may report one or more of the following symptoms:
- Nasal congestion
- Sneezing
- Rhinorrhea, usually watery but may be purulent if there is secondary bacterial infection
- "Scratchy" sore throat
- Nonproductive cough
- Headaches
- Low-grade fever
- Malaise
- Myalgia
- Hoarseness
- Lymphadenopathy

Allergic Rhinitis

→ The patient may report a history of one or more of the following:
- Asthma
- Eczema
- Other allergic reactions (e.g., urticaria)
- Nasal polyps

→ The patient may report one or more of the following symptoms, usually in a seasonal or perennial pattern:
- Rhinorrhea:
  - Usually watery
- Sneezing:
  - Usually in the morning
- Recurrent nasal obstruction
- Lacrimation
- Itching of the eyes, nose, and oropharynx
- Frequent sore throats:
  - Usually secondary to nasopharyngeal dryness from mouth breathing or postnasal drip
- Recurrent/persistent, nonproductive cough
- Frequent clearing of throat
- Halitosis
- Snorting (to attempt to clear nasal passages)

Vasomotor Rhinitis

→ Recent history may include:
- Emotional stress
- Exercise
- Exposure to smoke, odors, noxious fumes, and other environmental toxins
- Recumbency

→ The patient may report one or more of the following symptoms:
- Nasal congestion:
  - May be unilateral or bilateral, may be in alternate sides of the nose
- Rhinorrhea may or may not be reported.

OBJECTIVE

(Bellanti et al. 2000, Drew 2001, Kishiyama et al. 2001)

Viral Rhinitis

→ Physical examination will reveal one or more of the following:
- Vital signs usually within normal limits (WNL), although a low-grade temperature may be observed.
- Erythema, edema of nasal mucosa
- Nasal discharge:
  - May be thin and watery or thick and purulent
- Mild erythema, edema of pharyngeal mucous membranes
- Enlarged tonsillar and/or cervical lymph nodes may be palpated.
- Auscultation of lungs WNL.

Allergic Rhinitis

→ Physical examination may reveal one or more of the following:
- Vital signs usually WNL
- Transverse crease of the nose
- Pale, bluish discoloration of the nasal turbinates
- Edema of nasal mucosa
- Nasal discharge:
  - Usually clear, thin, and watery
  - May be yellow (due to increased eosinophils)
- Nasal polyps
- Gingival hypertrophy, halitosis, and/or enlarged adenoid or tonsillar lymphoid tissue (signs of chronic mouth breathing)
- Edema of eyelids
- Conjunctival erythema
- Lacrimation
- Bluish discoloration of the infraorbital area

Vasomotor Rhinitis

→ Physical examination may reveal one or more of the following:
- Nasal turbinate edema
- Nasal mucosa bluish to dark red
- Thin, clear nasal discharge

ASSESSMENT

→ Rhinitis—viral, allergic, vasomotor
→ R/O influenza
→ R/O sinusitis
→ R/O otitis media, serous otitis
→ R/O nasal polyposis
→ R/O drug-induced rhinitis
→ R/O asthma
→ R/O pneumonia
→ R/O eosinophilic nonallergic rhinitis
→ R/O intranasal recreational drug use
→ R/O nasal decongestant overuse

PLAN

DIAGNOSTIC TESTS

Viral Rhinitis

→ No specific diagnostic tests are indicated in cases of viral rhinitis.

■ If secondary bacterial complications are suspected, then tests indicated for the diagnosis of such conditions may be ordered. (See the **Sinusitis—Acute, Sinusitis— Chronic**, and **Pneumonia** chapters.)

Allergic Rhinitis

→ Specific diagnostic tests for allergic rhinitis should be ordered only as clinically indicated by the frequency and severity of a patient's symptoms.

■ Tests may include:

• White blood cell (WBC) count and differential

– An increase in eosinophils may be noted. However, absence of absolute eosinophilia does not rule out rhinitis.

• Serum IgE levels may be elevated but are of limited use-fulness because of a lack of sensitivity and specificity.

• A smear of nasal secretions can be air dried and prepared with Giemsa or Hansel's stain to demonstrate eosinophilia.

– In acute allergic rhinitis, 10–100% eosinophils may be observed.

• Allergy testing:

– Various types of allergy tests are available, including the prick test, the scratch test, intradermal testing, and in vitro tests.

– These tests are done to determine the presence or absence of allergen-specific IgE antibodies.

– These tests are not routinely done on all patients with rhinitis. They must be used only according to a patient's severity of symptoms and history of allergy.

– Patient referral to an allergist is indicated when such testing is being considered because of the cost, indicated treatment and follow-up, and possibility of anaphylaxis in some patients.

Vasomotor Rhinitis

→ No specific diagnostic testing is indicated for vasomotor rhinitis. (If allergy testing is done, the results will be nega-tive.)

TREATMENT/MANAGEMENT

Viral Rhinitis

→ No specific treatment has been found effective in shortening or eliminating symptoms of the common cold.

■ Prescribing antibiotics is unnecessary, as they are ineffective in treating the condition and will not prevent the development of associated complications.

■ Antibiotics should be prescribed for patients who develop secondary bacterial infections (e.g., sinusitis, pneumonia).

→ Symptomatic treatment with simple home remedies should be recommended and includes:

■ Increased rest (especially if the patient is febrile)

■ Increased fluid intake (especially warm liquids)

■ Use of a steam vaporizer to help liquefy secretions

NOTE: Warn patients about placing steam vaporizers in hazardous areas where small children or other household members could be harmed if the steaming liquid is spilled. Instruct patients to clean the vaporizer regularly to prevent overgrowth of bacteria and molds.

■ Acetaminophen every 4–6 hours as needed to reduce fever and alleviate generalized discomfort.

NOTE: Aspirin should not be used because it may increase viral shedding, and in children and adolescents should be avoided because of the risk of Reye's syndrome.

→ Systemic antihistamines may relieve some nasal congestion and sneezing. They include (Bellanti et al. 2000, Drew 2001, Scadding et al. 2000):

■ Chlorpheniramine 4–8 mg p.o. BID or TID (maximum daily dose ≤24 mg) or sustained-release chlorpheniramine 8–12 mg p.o. once at bedtime or every 8 hours (maximum daily dose ≤24 mg)

■ Clemastine 1.34–2.68 mg p.o. BID

NOTE: Warn the patient about CNS effects associated with systemic antihistamines (e.g., drowsiness, dizziness).

→ Systemic decongestants also may reduce nasal congestion and sneezing (Bellanti et al. 2000, Drew 2001, Scadding et al. 2000).

■ Several over-the-counter (OTC) preparations, containing pseudoephedrine as their active ingredient, are available.

• The dose of short-acting pseudoephedrine is 30–60 mg p.o. every 4–6 hours (maximum daily dose ≤240 mg).

• The dose of sustained-released pseudoephedrine is 120 mg every 12 hours (maximum daily dose ≤240 mg).

NOTE: Patients with severe hypertension, heart disease, seizure disorders, or hyperthyroidism, or those taking monoamine oxidase (MAO) inhibitor medications, should not be given preparations containing pseudoephedrine. Consult *Physicians' Desk Reference* and a clinical pharmacist as indicated for additional information.

→ In elderly patients, use short-acting, systemic antihistamine or decongestant preparations before recommending sustained-release products. An increased sensitivity to CNS side effects has been noted in elderly patients.

→ Antitussive preparations containing dextromethorphan may help reduce the frequency of coughing episodes.

■ The usual dose for dextromethorphan is 10–20 mg p.o. every 3–4 hours prn (maximum daily dose ≤120 mg).

→ Although expectorants (e.g., guaifenesin) often are recommended for treating cold symptoms, they have not been shown to be any more effective than a placebo.

→ Although topical decongestant sprays often provide patients with a sense of improved nasal patency, their use must be monitored carefully and limited to 3–5 days to prevent rebound nasal hyperemia and tachyphylaxis (Jackler et al. 2002).

- Common OTC topical nasal decongestants include:
  - Phenylephrine 0.125–1.0% solutions. Apply 1–2 intranasal sprays every 4 hours prn (begin with ≤0.25% solutions).

  NOTE: Precautions and contraindications similar to those regarding the use of pseudoephedrine products also apply to phenylephrine. (See "Viral Rhinitis" under "Treatment/Management," above.)
  - Oxymetazoline 0.025% solution. Apply 2–3 intranasal sprays BID prn or 0.05% solution 2–3 drops BID prn.

→ If influenza type A is suspected because of a community epidemic and the patient is being seen within 48 hours of symptom onset, consider initiating antiviral therapy to shorten the symptomatic phase of the illness. (See the **Influenza** chapter for indications for antiviral therapy.)

Allergic Rhinitis

→ Maintaining an allergen-free environment is essential. The following steps may help reduce symptoms (Jackler et al. 2002, Scadding et al. 2000):

- Removing dust-collecting household fixtures (e.g., drapes, carpets)
- Substituting synthetic materials for animal products (e.g., wool)
- Covering mattresses, pillows, and cushions with plastic or anti-allergenic covers

→ An air purifier may help decrease allergen exposure.

→ Systemic antihistamines and decongestants may help reduce symptoms. Because they reduce allergic mechanisms, antihistamines usually are more effective than decongestants in relieving symptoms. See "Viral Rhinitis," above, for dosages and possible side effects.

→ Nonsedating antihistamines are preferable for patients unable to tolerate the CNS side effects associated with OTC antihistamine products. However, the former are available only by prescription and are more costly than OTC preparations.

- Antihistamine products that have minimal or no sedating side effects include (Jackler et al. 2002):
  - Cetirizine 10 mg p.o. QD
  - Fexofenadine 60 mg p.o. BID or 120 mg p.o. QD
  - Ebastine 10–20 mg p.o. QD
  - Mizolastine 10 mg p.o. QD

→ Intranasal steroid sprays often are helpful. But patients need to be advised that symptoms may not improve until after 2 weeks of proper use (Jackler et al. 2002).

- Intranasal steroid sprays include:
  - Beclomethasone intranasal spray per nostril BID
  - Flunisolide intranasal spray per nostril BID.
  NOTE: Potential side effects include nasal dryness, irritation, or stinging.
  - Intranasal cromolyn 4% spray, 2 intranasal sprays BID before exposure to allergen.

→ Systemic corticosteroids for allergic rhinitis are rarely necessary and, if indicated, should be prescribed in consultation with a physician.

→ When indicated, immunotherapy (e.g., desensitization or hyposensitization) of patients with severe symptoms should be managed by an allergist.

Vasomotor Rhinitis

→ Whenever possible, avoiding precipitating factors will help reduce the symptoms associated with vasomotor rhinitis.

→ Symptomatic treatment of this condition may include the use of oral antihistamines and/or decongestants. (See "Viral Rhinitis," above.)

→ Intranasal saline drops may relieve symptoms in patients with nasal congestion. The usual dose is 2 drops in each nostril TID-QID.

CONSULTATION

→ As necessary, depending on the severity of the patient's symptoms, evidence of complications (e.g., sinusitis, pneumonia with viral rhinitis), or the need for referral to a specialist (e.g., an allergist) for additional diagnostic testing and/or treatment.

→ As needed for prescription(s).

PATIENT EDUCATION

→ Educate the patient about rhinitis (viral, allergic, vasomotor)—the cause(s), clinical course, treatment options, any potential side effects associated with medications, possible complications, preventive measures, and any indicated follow-up. (See specific sections of this chapter for all of these educational components.)

FOLLOW-UP

→ Follow-up evaluations usually are not indicated in most patients unless severe symptoms or complications develop. If a patient was referred to a physician for further diagnostic testing and/or treatment, then follow-up is per recommendation of the consulting physician.

→ Document in progress notes and on problem list.

BIBLIOGRAPHY

Bellanti, J.A., and Wellerstedt, D.B. 2000. Allergic rhinitis update: epidemiology and natural history. *Allergy and Asthma Proceedings* 21(6):367–370.

Drew, W.L. 2001. Rhinoviruses. In *Current diagnosis & treatment in infectious diseases*, eds. W.R. Wilson and M.A. Sande, pp. 377–379. New York: Lange Medical Books/McGraw-Hill.

Jackler, R.K., and Kaplan, M.J. 2002. Ear, nose, and throat. In *2002 current medical diagnosis & treatment*, 41st ed., eds. L.M. Tierney, Jr., S.J. McPhee, and M.A. Papadakis, pp. 241, 244–245. New York: Lange Medical Books/McGraw-Hill.

Kishiyama, J.L., and Adelman, D.C. 2001. Allergic and immunologic disorders. In *2002 current medical diagnosis & treatment*, 41st ed., eds. L.M. Tierney, Jr., S.J. McPhee, and M.A. Papadakis, pp. 791–795. New York: Lange Medical Books/McGraw-Hill.

Scadding, G.K., Richards, D.H., and Price, M.J. 2000. Patient and physician perspectives on the impact and management of perennial and seasonal allergic rhinitis. *Clinical Otolaryngology* 25:551–557.

5-L

Sinusitis—Acute

Acute sinusitis is an infection of the mucosa of the paranasal sinuses that results from a combination of factors, including edema of the nasal mucosa, which causes a narrowing of the sinus ostia; decreased (sinus) ciliary transport of mucous secretions; overproduction of mucous secretions; and a reduction in oxygen tension, which, in turn, promotes the growth of certain pathogens (Jackler et al. 2002, Virk et al. 2001). Because the paranasal sinuses directly communicate with a nonsterile cavity, infection often is a component of acute sinusitis.

In adults, the most common organisms associated with acute sinusitis are *Streptococcus pneumoniae, Haemophilus influenzae, Staphylococcus aureus,* and *Branhamella catarrhalis.* Viral pathogens such as rhinovirus, influenza, and parainfluenza viruses have been observed in 15–30% of studies investigating sinusitis, and fungi such as *Aspergillus* and *Candida albicans* also have been identified as etiologic pathogens, particularly in immunocompromised individuals (Jackler et al. 2002, Kahn et al. 2000).

Cellulitis, meningitis, abscess formation, osteomyelitis, and cavernous sinus thrombosis are possible complications associated with untreated or inadequately treated acute sinusitis (Jackler et al. 2002).

DATABASE

SUBJECTIVE

→ Predisposing factors may include (Jackler et al. 2002, Virk et al. 2001):
  - Allergic rhinitis
  - Upper respiratory infection (URI)
  - Asthma
  - Deviated nasal septum
  - Environmental irritants
  - Excessive topical decongestant use
  - Nasal polyps, tumors, or foreign bodies
  - Hypertrophied adenoids
  - Swimming/diving
  - Barotrauma
  - Dental infection
  - Nasal surgical packing
  - Cystic fibrosis
  - Bronchiectasis
  - Immobile cilia syndrome
  - Immune deficiency

→ Symptoms may include (Corey et al. 2000, Jackler et al. 2002):
  - Fever (may not be documented in up to 65% of patients)
  - Chills (may not be documented in up to 65% of patients)
  - Headache
  - Facial pain or facial fullness, which is aggravated by coughing, straining, a head-down position, or an acute change in barometric pressure
  - Malaise
  - Nasal discharge (may be clear, mucoid, or purulent)
  - Postnasal discharge
  - Photophobia
  - Anorexia
  - Symptoms of a URI persisting beyond 10 days
  - Morning cough
  - Halitosis

OBJECTIVE

→ The patient may present with (Corey et al. 2000, Jackler et al. 2002):
  - Temperature of 39° C/102.2° F or above (may not be documented in up to 65% of patients)
  - Discharge in the nasal meatus, which may be thin or thick, clear, mucoid, or purulent
  - Discharge observed in the posterior pharynx
  - Tenderness to palpation over the frontal, periorbital, maxillary, or subzygomatic regions of the head
  - Conjunctivitis
  - Edema of eyelid(s) and/or medial canthus.

→ Transillumination for frontal and maxillary opacification can be performed but generally is not reliable.

ASSESSMENT

→ Acute sinusitis
→ R/O chronic sinusitis
→ R/O allergy (allergic rhinitis, asthma)
→ R/O nasal obstruction (tumor, polyp, deviated septum, foreign body)
→ R/O dental infection
→ R/O overuse of topical nasal decongestants
→ R/O immotile cilia syndrome (rare)

PLAN

DIAGNOSTIC TESTS

→ Diagnostic tests usually are not required in uncomplicated presentations; however, the following tests may be ordered if indicated:
  ▪ A sinus x-ray series may demonstrate air-fluid levels, mucosal thickening ≥5 mm, or opacification of an infected sinus, and will confirm the diagnosis of acute sinusitis.
  ▪ Computerized tomography (CT) scan findings of thickened mucosa within the sinuses and stenosis of anatomic structures. CT scans are more sensitive and specific than x-rays.
    • CT scans are recommended for patients who are not responding appropriately to antibiotic therapy for acute sinusitis, to rule out the spread of infection to the brain.
    • If possible, the patient should be on antibiotics for three weeks before the scan.
      – This will help reduce tissue edema and facilitate better visualization of the area during the scan.
    • Maxillary antrum aspiration for culture and sensitivity should be reserved only for patients failing antibiotic therapy, for patients with immunodeficiency (e.g., HIV-positive patients, patients with diabetes mellitus), or for patients with nosocomial infections.

TREATMENT/MANAGEMENT

→ Initiate antibiotic therapy (in patients without a history of penicillin allergy) with one of the following (Jackler et al. 2002, Virk et al. 2001):
  ▪ Amoxicillin 500 mg p.o. TID for 10 days. It is the first choice because amoxicillin provides better sinus penetration than ampicillin does.
  ▪ Amoxicillin-clavulanate potassium 500 mg p.o. TID or 875 mg p.o. BID for 10 days (if beta-lactamase-positive organisms are suspected).
→ If the patient is allergic to penicillin or is unresponsive to the above antibiotic therapy after 72 hours, treatment can be initiated with one of the following (Jackler et al. 2002, Virk et al. 2001):
  ▪ Trimethoprim/sulfamethoxazole 1 double-strength tablet p.o. every 12 hours for 10 days
  ▪ Cephalexin 250–500 mg. p.o. QID for 10 days
  ▪ Cefixime 400 mg p.o. QD for 10 days
  ▪ Ciprofloxacin 500 mg p.o. BID for 10 days

  ▪ Clarithromycin 500 mg p.o. BID for 14 days
  ▪ Azithromycin 500 mg p.o. QD for 3 days
→ Oral decongestants may provide some symptom relief in uncomplicated sinusitis.
  ▪ If appropriate, the patient could initiate therapy with pseudoephedrine 30–60 mg p.o. every 4–6 hours as needed (maximum daily dose not to exceed 240 mg). **NOTE:** Pseudoephedrine is contraindicated in severe hypertension and/or coronary artery disease.
→ In simple sinusitis, limited use of topical decongestant can be initiated with one of the following:
  ▪ Oxymetazoline 0.05% spray 1–2 sprays in each nostril every 8 hours prn for up to 3 days
  ▪ Xylometazoline 0.05–0.1% spray 1–2 sprays in each nostril every 8 hours prn for up to 3 days
→ Nasal saline spray may be useful in maintaining moist nasal mucosa and avoiding desiccation.
→ Humidification with warm, moist air helps clear sinus congestion and avoid desiccation.

CONSULTATION

→ Physician consultation is indicated for patients who are unresponsive to antibiotic therapy after 72 hours or when resistant organisms are suspected. Further evaluation, treatment, and/or possible referral to an otolaryngologist may be indicated.
→ As needed for prescription(s).

PATIENT EDUCATION

→ Educate the patient about sinusitis—the cause(s), clinical course, treatment options, possible complications and side effects of medications, and any indicated follow-up.
→ Educate the patient about the adverse effects on nasal mucosa of antihistamines and the overuse of topical decongestants.
  ▪ Antihistamines can cause desiccation of the mucosa, resulting in an increase in viscous secretions. They should be avoided.
  ▪ Topical nasal decongestants can cause ciliastasis and a decreased blood flow to the nasal mucosa, resulting in an inhibited clearance of nasal secretions and a reduced amount of antibiotics delivered to the sinuses.

FOLLOW-UP

→ See "Consultation," above.
→ Document in progress notes and on problem list.

BIBLIOGRAPHY

Corey, J.P., Houser, S.M., and Ng, B.A. 2000. Nasal congestion: a review of its etiology, evaluation, and treatment. *Ear, Nose, & Throat Journal* 79(9):690–693, 696, 698.

Jackler, R.K., and Kaplan, M.J. 2002. Ear, nose, & throat. In *2002 current medical diagnosis & treatment*, 41st ed., eds. L.M. Tierney, Jr., S.J. McPhee, and M.A. Papadakis, pp. 232–325. New York: Lange Medical Books/McGraw-Hill.

Kahn, D.A., Cody, D.T., George, T.J. et al. 2000. Allergic fungal sinusitis: an immunohistologic analysis. *Journal of Allergy and Clinical Immunology* 106(6):1096–1101.

Virk, A., and Henry, N.K. 2001. Upper respiratory tract infections. In *Current diagnosis & treatment in infectious diseases*, eds. W.R. Wilson and M.A. Sande, pp. 113–117. New York: Lange Medical Books/McGraw-Hill.

5-M
Sinusitis—Chronic

Chronic sinusitis is a prolonged infection of the paranasal sinuses resulting from interference with the normal transport and clearance of nasal mucous secretions. It is usually caused by a mechanical obstruction (anatomical or pathophysiological) of the osteomeatal unit, resulting in diminished mucociliary movement and an increased accumulation of mucous secretions. When mucous secretions continue to accumulate, there is a reduction in the oxygenation of the nasal mucosa, resulting in a proliferation of pathogens.

Pathogens most commonly associated with chronic sinusitis are *Streptococcus pneumoniae, Staphylococcus aureus, Bacteroides fragilis* group, *Peptostreptococcus* species, and beta-lactamase-producing *Haemophilus influenzae* or *Branhamella catarrhalis*. More recently, allergic sinusitis due to fungal organisms of the *Dematiaceae* family have been associated with chronic sinusitis symptoms (Jackler et al. 2002, Kahn et al. 2000, Virk et al. 2001).

DATABASE

SUBJECTIVE

→ Predisposing factors may include (Jackler et al. 2002, Virk et al. 2001):
  ▪ History of recent sinus infection, allergic rhinitis, asthma
  ▪ Anatomic deviations of the nose (e.g., obstructed osteomeatal unit, deviated septum)
  ▪ Nasal polyps, tumor, foreign body
  ▪ Immune deficiency.
→ Symptoms may include (Corey et al. 2000, Jackler et al. 2002, Virk et al. 2001):
  ▪ Dull ache or pressure of the midface
  ▪ Pressure between the eyes
  ▪ Morning headache aggravated by head movement
  ▪ Nasal congestion
  ▪ Postnasal drip
  ▪ Otalgia
  ▪ Epistaxis
  ▪ Dental pain

  ▪ Halitosis
  ▪ Chronic cough:
    • Usually most noticeable in the morning
  ▪ Bronchitis
  ▪ Fatigue
  ▪ Lightheadedness
  ▪ Dizziness
  ▪ Recurrent laryngitis
  ▪ Nausea (from swallowing postnasal discharge)

OBJECTIVE

→ The patient may present with:
  ▪ Purulent nasal discharge
  ▪ Nasal polyp
  ▪ Deviated septum
  ▪ Tenderness to palpation over involved sinuses

ASSESSMENT

→ Chronic sinusitis
→ R/O failed therapy for acute sinusitis
→ R/O chronic rhinitis
→ R/O nasal polyposis
→ R/O dental infection
→ R/O migraine or tension headache
→ R/O temporal arteritis
→ R/O temporal mandibular joint disorder
→ R/O asthma

PLAN

DIAGNOSTIC TESTS

→ In consultation with a physician, the following tests may be ordered to confirm the diagnosis of chronic sinusitis and to rule out other significant conditions (e.g., abscess, neoplasm) (Jackler et al. 2002):
  ▪ Nasal smear:
    • May reveal eosinophils or neutrophils, differentiating allergic from bacterial sinusitis

- Sinus series x-rays:
  - May reveal findings consistent with sinusitis (e.g., air fluid levels, opacification of an infected sinus) and eliminate the presence of an abscess
- Computerized tomography (CT) scan:
  - May identify osteomeatal unit disease
  - Three weeks of antibiotic therapy should be completed before a CT scan to reduce tissue edema, allowing better visualization of anatomic structures during the scan.
- Magnetic resonance imaging (MRI) is useful only in identifying soft-tissue masses, mucosal diseases, and fungus balls.
- Nasal cultures, if done, correlate poorly with bacteria causing infection of the sinuses because normal nasal flora often grow in such cultures.
- Maxillary antrum aspiration may be necessary in resistant cases. If so, referral to an otolaryngologist is warranted.

TREATMENT/MANAGEMENT

→ When chronic sinusitis is suspected, antibiotic therapy should be initiated with an antimicrobial agent effective against beta-lactamase-producing organisms. These agents include (Jackler et al. 2002, Virk et al. 2001):
- Amoxicillin-clavulanate potassium 500 mg p.o. TID for 4–6 weeks

OR

- Trimethoprim/sulfamethoxazole 1 double-strength tablet p.o. BID for 4–6 weeks

OR

- Cefaclor 500 mg p.o. QID for 4–6 weeks
→ When using prolonged antibiotic therapy in women or immune-deficient patients, consider prophylaxis (e.g., vaginal antifungal agents, oral candidiasis therapies) for yeast infections and review nonpharmacological methods to diminish the likelihood of a yeast infection.
→ Humidification with warm, moist air may help prevent desiccation.
- Other helpful measures include forcing fluids orally, use of a nasal saline spray, and avoidance of physical or chemical irritants.
→ Oral decongestants (e.g., pseudoephedrine) may help reduce the edema of the nasal mucosa. (See the **Sinusitis—Acute** chapter for doses.)
- Because sleeplessness is a common side effect of such medications, they should be used in the morning and avoided in the late afternoon or evening.

→ Topical steroid nasal sprays should be avoided during the initial acute phase of therapy because of the potential suppression of local immune response to the organism.
- However, their use to decrease the tissue edema observed in association with allergic or vasomotor rhinitis may be beneficial. (See "Allergic Rhinitis" or "Vasomotor Rhinitis" in the **Rhinitis** chapter.)

CONSULTATION

→ Consultation with a physician is indicated in patients who do not respond to therapy within 72 hours, who may require maxillary antrum aspiration, or who have an underlying immunodeficiency.
→ As needed for prescription(s).

PATIENT EDUCATION

→ Educate the patient about chronic sinusitis—the cause(s), the therapeutic interventions (including possible side effects of medications), possible complications, and indicated follow-up. Discuss ways to prevent further episodes.

FOLLOW-UP

→ If symptoms do not improve within 72 hours, the patient should return for further evaluation or per recommendation of a physician if consultation was required.
→ Document in progress notes and on problem list.

BIBLIOGRAPHY

Corey, J.P., Houser, S.M., and Ng, B.A. 2000. Nasal congestion: a review of its etiology, evaluation, and treatment. *Ear, Nose, & Throat Journal* 79(9):690–693, 696, 698.

Jackler, R.K., and Kaplan, M.J. 2002. Ear, nose, & throat. In *2002 current medical diagnosis & treatment*, 41st ed., eds. L.M. Tierney, Jr., S.J. McPhee, and M.A. Papadakis, pp. 232–325. New York: Lange Medical Books/McGraw-Hill.

Kahn, D.A., Cody, D.T., George, T.J. et al. 2000. Allergic fungal sinusitis: an immunohistologic analysis. *Journal of Allergy and Clinical Immunology* 106(6):1096–1101.

Virk, A., and Henry, N.K. 2001. Upper respiratory tract infections. In *Current diagnosis & treatment in infectious diseases*, eds. W.R. Wilson and M.A. Sande, pp. 113–117. New York: Lange Medical Books/McGraw-Hill.

SECTION 6

Cardiovascular Disorders

6-A Angina 6-2
6-B Deep Vein Thrombosis 6-8
6-C Heart Failure 6-15
6-D Hyperlipidemia 6-22
6-E Hypertension 6-29
6-F Mitral Valve Prolapse 6-37
6-G Palpitations 6-42

Ellen M. Scarr, R.N., C., M.S., F.N.P., W.H.N.P.

6-A
Angina

Angina pectoris, commonly known as chest pain, is most often caused by atherosclerosis, or *coronary heart disease* (CHD), the result of localized deposits of fat and fibrous tissue (plaque) in the subintimal layer of the coronary arteries (Brashers 2002). The precipitating factor for the development of arterial plaque is thought to be endothelial injury caused by conditions such as hypertension, hyperlipidemia, and cigarette smoking. Recent data suggest that inflammation may also play a role: lipoprotein(a) has been shown to have inflammatory, as well as atherogenic and thrombogenic, properties (Albert 2000, Drown 2000). Increased levels of lipoprotein(a) have been found to increase the risk of CHD in men, although the effect in women is less clear (Bedinghaus et al. 2001). There is current speculation that infectious agents, such as *Chlamydia pneumoniae* and cytomegalovirus, also may play a role in plaque development and progression, as well as in thrombogenesis (Albert 2000), although more study is needed.

Angina is the symptomatic manifestation of a lack of oxygen to the myocardium, or the mismatch between supply and demand, and is often classified as *stable* or *unstable*. Stable angina occurs predictably: a secure, stenotic plaque that has developed in the lumen of a coronary artery impedes adequate blood flow and oxygen delivery to the heart muscle during times of increased demand (e.g., exertion or emotional or mental stress). Symptoms typically are relieved with rest. Unstable angina, an acute coronary syndrome, can occur at any time, even at rest or during sleep. Unstable angina can be initiated by the rupture of a plaque, resulting in intraluminal clot formation. The clot and its associated ischemia are responsible for the symptoms of unstable angina or myocardial infarction (MI) (Schoenhagen et al. 2000). The pain is unpredictable, unrelieved with rest, and often unrelieved with nitroglycerin.

Angina also can develop from coronary artery spasm. Vasoconstriction of the artery leads to decreased blood flow, ischemia, and then chest pain. Usually seen with atherosclerosis, spasm also can occur in normal coronary arteries. *Prinzmetal's (variant) angina*, typically found in women younger than 50 years, develops at rest without precipitating factors, often waking the woman from sleep. In Prinzmetal's angina, the coronary arteries may demonstrate no occlusion (Massie et al. 2002).

It is estimated that 4 million women in the United States experience angina. The age-adjusted prevalence of angina is higher in women than men (American Heart Association [AHA] 2001). Cardiovascular disease, which includes CHD, remains the leading cause of death for women in the United States, accounting for more than 225,000 deaths in 1998 (AHA 2001). One-third of all deaths in women can be attributed to CHD (Rosenfeld 2000). Twice as many women die of cardiovascular disease as die from cancer. In particular, the number of deaths from CHD is 4–6 times higher than deaths from breast cancer, although women are more aware of and more afraid of breast cancer than CHD (Andrews et al. 2000, Bedinghaus et al. 2001).

In the third and fourth decade of life, men have three times more cardiovascular disease than women do. Women develop CHD approximately 10 years later than men do, usually beginning after menopause, and suffer more severe manifestations of CHD (e.g., MI, heart failure, sudden death) approximately 20 years after the onset of CHD (AHA 2001). By the seventh decade, women have the same prevalence of CHD as men. The later onset of CHD in women is generally attributed to the cardioprotective effects of endogenous estrogen (Penckofer et al. 2001). It is postulated that the effect of estrogen on lipid metabolism, particularly its ability to lower low-density lipoprotein (LDL) cholesterol—the main atherogenic lipoprotein—reduces women's risk for developing CHD. Estrogen also raises high-density lipoprotein (HDL), the lipoprotein that transports free cholesterol to the liver for excretion, thereby lowering serum cholesterol. This effect is important because having low HDL levels has been shown to be associated with increased cardiovascular risk in women (Rosenfeld 2000). Estrogen also exerts vasodilatory effects on the coronary vasculature by stimulating production and release of nitric oxide, a potent vasodilator.

Years of observational studies led researchers to believe that exogenous estrogen would provide similar protective effects for postmenopausal women, preventing—or at least delaying—the onset of CHD. The objective of one arm of the Women's

Health Initiative, a randomized, controlled trial of more than 16,000 healthy, ethnically diverse women, was to evaluate the risks and benefits of combination hormone replacement therapy. In July 2002, after 5.2 years of the eight-year study, this arm of the study was stopped because the risks were found to outweigh the benefits. Women receiving estrogen and progesterone supplementation had a 29% higher incidence of coronary events than did women receiving a placebo (Rossouw et al. 2002).

Many questions still need to be addressed, such as what length of therapy is safe and whether different hormone formulations will alter risk. However, as of late 2002, the U.S. Preventive Services Task Force (USPSTF) was recommending that hormone replacement therapy should not be initiated or continued to prevent CHD (USPSTF 2002).

There are other gender differences regarding CHD. Women are more likely to be incorrectly diagnosed with CHD, in part because they are less likely to present with the "typical" symptoms of angina. Pain may be localized to the shoulder or neck, and the absence of classic substernal chest pain is not associated with a negative predictive value as it is in men (Deaton et al. 2000). Additionally, fatigue and dyspnea commonly are associated with CHD in women. Studies concerning access to care and utilization of health care resources have shown that women are less likely than men to be referred for noninvasive diagnostic testing, less likely to be referred for invasive testing (even when initial studies are abnormal), and less likely to be treated aggressively with pharmacologic modalities, even though there is substantial evidence as to their benefit in the literature (Bedinghaus et al. 2001, Deaton et al. 2000).

Management includes both primary and secondary prevention strategies. Primary prevention (prevention of the development of CHD or first MI) is aimed at risk-factor identification and reduction. Clinical trials are in place to assess the effectiveness of primary prevention strategies in women. Secondary prevention (prevention of subsequent cardiovascular events or death) involves ongoing risk reduction and aggressive treatment of comorbid conditions such as hypertension and hyperlipidemia.

Many of the following risk factors for CHD (Bedinghaus et al. 2001, Massie et al. 2002) are amenable to lifestyle changes:
→ Age (postmenopausal)
→ Hypertension
→ Hyperlipidemia
→ Hypertriglyceridemia
→ Diabetes mellitus
→ Insulin resistance (Syndrome X)
→ Increased lipoprotein(a) (possibly)
→ Sedentary lifestyle
→ Obesity
   ■ Central obesity (waist:hip ratio >0.8)
   ■ Generalized obesity (body mass index [BMI] >30)
→ Cigarette smoking
→ Family history of premature cardiac death
   ■ First-degree male relative younger than 45 years
   ■ First-degree female relative younger than 55 years

DATABASE

SUBJECTIVE

→ Symptoms may include:
   ■ Chest discomfort, usually described as burning, squeezing, tightness, pressure or "indigestion"
   ■ Nausea, dizziness, diaphoresis
      • Localization of discomfort:
         – Typically behind or slightly to the left of mid-sternum
         – May radiate to the left shoulder, left arm
         – May radiate to the jaw, neck, back, or right anterior chest
         – May occur only in the shoulder, arm, or jaw ("atypical" presentation)
      • Timing of chest pain:
         – Usually begins with exertion, after meals, or with stress.
         – As disease progresses or if the patient has spasm, it can occur at rest, even during sleep.
      • Duration of chest pain:
         – Usually lasts several minutes, often resolves after the patient stops the precipitating activity; resolves without residual pain.
         – Persistent pain may be a precursor to MI.
      • Relieving factors:
         – Decreases with rest
         – Decreases with nitroglycerin (NTG)
→ Past medical history may include:
   ■ Risk factors for cardiovascular disease, including:
      • Diabetes
      • Hypertension
      • Coronary artery spasm
      • Hyperlipidemia
      • Hypertriglyceridemia
      • Insulin resistance
         – Polycystic ovary syndrome
   ■ Conditions related to cardiovascular disease, including:
      • Cerebrovascular accident
      • Peripheral vascular disease
      • Thyroid disease. Patients with hyperthyroidism may present with chest pain.
      • Obesity. BMI >30 is a risk factor for all-cause mortality and is associated with diabetes, hyperlipidemia, and hypertension.
→ Social history:
   ■ May include the use of:
      • Cigarettes. As few as three cigarettes per day increase coronary risk. More than 60% of MIs in women younger than 50 years are attributable to smoking (Bedinghaus et al. 2001).
      • Alcohol. Low or moderate consumption (14 or fewer drinks per week) has been associated with favorable lipid profiles and a reduction in CHD (Nanchahal et al. 2000).
      • Caffeine

- Drugs (including recreational drugs, especially stimulants such as cocaine or amphetamines)
  - Activity level. Sedentary patients are at higher risk for coronary disease.
→ Family history may include:
  - Hypertension
  - Coronary disease (especially sudden death or MI in a first-degree male relative before age 45 years and a female relative before age 55 years)
  - Hyperlipidemia
  - Hypertriglyceridemia
  - Diabetes
  - Cerebrovascular accident
  - Peripheral vascular disease

OBJECTIVE

→ If the patient is asymptomatic at the time of her visit, a physical assessment should include:
  - Vital signs
  - Weight, height, BMI
  - General appearance
  - Fundoscopic examination to assess for hypertensive changes, diabetic retinopathy
  - Neck examination to assess for carotid bruits, jugular vein distention, thyroid abnormalities
  - Cardiac examination to assess for murmurs, clicks, gallops, rubs, cardiomegaly, arrhythmia
  - Lung examination
  - Extremity examination to assess for neuropathy, clubbing, edema, cyanosis
→ If the patient is having chest pain at the time of examination, an initial brief assessment is indicated to determine the need for emergency intervention. There may be changes in:
  - Vital signs (hypertension, irregular pulse, bradycardia, tachycardia are often noted)
  - General appearance (anxiety, discomfort, pallor, or diaphoresis may be noted)
  - Cardiac examination (gallop or murmur that is absent when the patient is asymptomatic, or a sustained or intermittently irregular heartbeat, may be heard)

ASSESSMENT

→ Angina: stable versus unstable:
  - R/O coronary heart disease
  - R/O coronary spasm
  - R/O other cardiovascular etiologies:
    - Mitral valve prolapse
    - Cardiomyopathy
    - Myocarditis
    - Pericarditis
    - Aortic valve disease
    - Aortic dissection
  - R/O metabolic etiologies:
    - Thyroid disease
  - R/O anemia

- R/O musculoskeletal etiologies:
  - Costochondritis
  - Intercostal neuritis
  - Cervical spine disease
  - Degenerative joint disease
- R/O gastrointestinal etiologies:
  - Peptic ulcer disease
  - Esophageal spasm
  - Esophageal reflux
- R/O pulmonary etiologies:
  - Pneumonia
  - Pneumothorax
  - Pulmonary embolism
- R/O anxiety/panic attack

PLAN

DIAGNOSTIC TESTS

→ Electrocardiogram (EKG):
  - May be normal in a patient who is asymptomatic at the time of examination. Common abnormalities include:
    - Old Q waves
    - Nonspecific ST-T wave changes
    - Intraventricular conduction defects (e.g., bundle branch block)
    - Atrioventricular conduction defects (e.g., 1°, 2°, or 3° block)
    - Left ventricular hypertrophy
    - Rhythm disturbances
    - Ectopy
  - If the patient is having angina at the time an EKG is performed, may note:
    - ST segment depression (horizontal or downsloping)
    - ST segment elevation (with coronary artery spasm or infarction)
→ Laboratory data:
  - Fasting lipid panel (total cholesterol, LDL, HDL, triglycerides)
  - Electrolytes, blood urea nitrogen (BUN), creatinine
  - Thyroid tests if indicated by history or exam: thyroid stimulating hormone (TSH), free T_4, T_3
  - Hematocrit if clinically indicated
  - Fasting blood sugar if clinically indicated
  - Troponin-I and/or creatine kinase [CK] to rule out infarction if clinically indicated
→ Exercise stress test:
  - The initial diagnostic test of choice.
    - The patient must be ambulatory.
    - Contraindicated if angina is unstable.
  - Looks for ischemia precipitated by exercise.
  - Confirms the diagnosis of angina.
  - Determines activity level/limitation.
    - Noninvasive tests may be less accurate in women (Deaton et al. 2000):
      - Less able to achieve maximal heart rate due to age or physical disability.

- Estrogen (both endogenous and exogenous) can interfere with ST depression due to vasodilatory effects.
■ Testing of asymptomatic patients is indicated only if they are high-risk:
  • Patients with a strong family history of CHD, especially early-onset
  • Patients with hyperlipidemia
  • Older patients beginning an exercise program
  • Individuals in occupations involving potential risk to other people (e.g., airline pilots)
■ Positive test: ≥1 mm horizontal or downsloping ST depression
  • 60–80% of those with CHD will have positive tests.
  • 10–30% false positives (fewer if 2 mm is a criterion for ST depression) (Massie et al. 2002)
■ Duration of exercise is a strong prognostic indicator of long-term survival (Zanger et al. 1999).
→ Stress cardiac imaging:
  ■ Pharmacologic stress takes the place of exercise.
    • Useful if the patient is physically impaired.
  ■ Stress echocardiography or nuclear single-photon emission computed tomography (SPECT)
  ■ Pharmacologic agents: vasodilator (e.g., adenosine or dipyridamole) or inotrope (e.g., dobutamine)
→ Cardiac catheterization:
  ■ Localizes coronary atherosclerosis
  ■ Determines the need for revascularization or angioplasty
  ■ May demonstrate coronary artery spasm
  ■ Determines valvular and myocardial function

TREATMENT/MANAGEMENT

→ For patients with acute angina or a history suggesting unstable angina, emergent monitored transport to the nearest acute-care facility is indicated.
→ For patients with a history suggesting stable angina, begin risk-factor modification. (See "Patient Education," below.)
→ In consultation with a physician, medication should be started for symptoms suggesting stable angina (Gibbons et al. 1999, Massie et al. 2002, Zanger et al. 2000):
  ■ Nitrate therapy:
    • Nitric oxide is a potent vasodilator and exhibits antiplatelet effects. Nitrate therapy provides an exogenous source of nitric oxide.
    • Short-acting nitrate (all patients with suspected angina should be given NTG):
      – NTG 0.3–0.6 mg: 1 tablet sublingually at the onset of chest pain, may repeat 2 more times at 5-minute intervals. If chest pain persists after 15 minutes, advise the patient to call 911 or initiate emergency care. Can be used prophylactically 5 minutes before a known precipitant.
  • Beta blockers:
    – Propranolol, nadolol, atenolol, and metoprolol are approved for treating angina; it is likely that all beta blockers are effective. A first-line therapy for most

patients with chronic angina, they act by decreasing heart rate and contractility, thereby decreasing myocardial oxygen demand and increasing coronary perfusion. Use caution with higher doses when left ventricular dysfunction is present. (See **Table 5D.1, Pharmacologic Therapy for Hypertension [Selected Agents]** in the **Hypertension** chapter.)
• Calcium channel blockers:
  – Act by decreasing heart rate, contractility, and afterload (peripheral vascular resistance), resulting in decreased myocardial oxygen demand and increased perfusion. May be used as initial therapy if beta blockers are contraindicated. Diltiazem or verapamil are preferred agents. Use caution in cases of left ventricular dysfunction. Avoid short-acting dihydropyridines. (See **Table 5D.1** in the **Hypertension** chapter.)
• Antiplatelet therapy:
  – Acetylsalicylic acid: 81–325 mg p.o. every day or 325 mg QOD
    ➤ Inhibits prostaglandins, especially thromboxane A_2, a potent vasoconstrictor and platelet activator.
• Lipid-lowering agents:
  – Reduce CHD mortality in men; benefit is less clear in women. Can slow the progression of plaque and possibly lead to plaque regression. Initiate lipid-lowering therapy with documented or suspected CHD and LDL cholesterol >130mg/dL; the goal is LDL <100 mg/dL. (See the **Hyperlipidemia** chapter.)
• Long-acting nitrates:
  – Indicated as initial therapy (solely or in conjunction with a calcium channel blocker) when beta blockers are contraindicated. May also be used if unacceptable side effects occur with beta blockers.
    ➤ Isosorbide dinitrate: begin 5 mg p.o. QID. Gradually increase dosage over 1–2 weeks to a maximum of 10–40 mg TID.
    ➤ Isosorbide mononitrate: 10–40 mg p.o. BID or 60–120 mg p.o. sustained-release tablets
    ➤ NTG ointment (2%): 6.25–25 mg BID–QID
    ➤ NTG transdermal patch: 5–20 mg/24 hours
      ✱ Continuous nitrate blood levels are associated with the development of nitrate tolerance. The patient needs 8–10 nitrate-free hours/day.

NOTE: Recently released findings from the Heart and Estrogen/Progestin Replacement Study (HERS II) confirmed earlier reports that the use of hormones does not reduce the risk of coronary events in older women with CHD. Estrogen should not be prescribed for secondary prevention of heart disease (Grady et al. 2002, Hulley et al. 1998).

CONSULTATION

→ Consult with a physician about new symptoms requiring medication.
→ Consult with a physician about persistent or worsening symptoms requiring modification of the medication regime

(increased dosage of a single agent or addition of a second agent).

→ Refer to a cardiologist for cardiac catheterization when a diagnosis of CHD is suspected, given the results of exercise or stress testing.

→ Refer to a cardiologist for percutaneous revascularization (e.g., stents, percutaneous transluminal coronary angioplasty) or to a surgeon for bypass grafting, depending on the anatomical lesion and location, and the patient's age, symptoms, comorbid conditions (e.g., diabetes, hypertension, hyperlipidemia, obesity), and preference.

→ As needed for prescription(s).

PATIENT EDUCATION

→ Advise the patient to reduce aggravating factors, including strenuous exercise, large meals, and emotional stressors.

→ Advise the patient to premedicate with NTG before activities known to precipitate angina (e.g., overexertion, large meals, stress, or exposure to cold temperatures).

→ Advise the patient to eliminate or modify risk factors:
- Smoking cessation:
  - Three years after quitting, risks decrease to those for women who have never smoked (Rosenfeld 2000).
  - In women, concerns about weight gain and increased levels of stress interfere with successful nicotine cessation. A combination of nicotine patch and buproprion is most effective (Bedinghaus et al. 2001).
- Reduce elevated total cholesterol, LDL, and triglyceride levels:
  - Although the benefits are less clear in women, it is prudent to recommend lipid lowering.
  - Advise the patient to reduce saturated fats and carbohydrates in her diet. (See Section 16, **General Nutrition Guidelines**.)
  - The goal is to lower LDL cholesterol to <160 (primary prevention), <130 (two or more CHD risk factors present but no known CHD), or <100 (known CHD).
  - See the **Hyperlipidemia** chapter.
- Increase exercise:
  - A sedentary lifestyle is an independent risk factor for MI and also contributes to obesity (Bedinghaus et al. 2001).
  - Encourage at least 30 minutes of exercise three times per week.
- Weight loss (if the patient is obese):
  - Dietary modification to achieve ideal weight and BMI <25 (Giardina 2000).
  - Exercise is less effective in reducing obesity in women than in men (Bedinghaus et al. 2001).

→ Educate the patient about medications she uses:
- NTG must be stored in a dark bottle and discarded after six months.
- NTG ointment and patches should be applied over hairless skin, rotating the site to minimize local irritation.
- Long-acting nitrates must not be discontinued abruptly.
- Antianginal medication reduces symptoms but has not been shown to improve mortality (Zanger et al. 2000).

→ Discuss the safety of sexual activity, giving individual guidelines to the patient based on her activity level and test results. Initiate open and direct discussion because many patients may be hesitant to do so.

→ Encourage the patient to participate in a cardiac exercise class if angina is stable.

FOLLOW-UP

→ Maintain weekly contact with the patient while initiating and maximizing medication therapy.

→ Once the patient has stabilized, visits 3–4 times per year are appropriate to discuss ongoing risk reduction, exercise tolerance, symptom control, medication side effects, and the possible need for intervention.

→ Document in progress notes and on problem list.

BIBLIOGRAPHY

Albert, N. 2000, Inflammation and infection in acute coronary syndromes. *Journal of Cardiovascular Nursing* 15(1):13–26.

American Heart Association (AHA). 2001. Statistics on heart disease. Available at: http://www.americanheart.org. Accessed on July 20, 2002.

Andrews, J., Graham-Garcia, J., and Raines, T. 2000. Heart disease mortality in women: racial, ethnic, and geographic disparities. *Journal of Cardiovascular Nursing* 15(3):83–87.

Bedinghaus, J., Leshan, L., and Diehr, S. 2001. Coronary artery disease prevention: What's different for women? *American Family Physician* 63(7):1393–1400, 1405–1406.

Brashers, V. 2002. Alterations in cardiovascular function. In *Pathophysiology: the biologic basis for disease in adults and children*, 4th ed., eds. K. McCance and S. Huether. St. Louis, Mo.: Mosby.

Deaton, C., Kunik, C., Hachamovitch, R. et al. 2000. Diagnostic strategies for women with suspected coronary artery disease. *Journal of Cardiovascular Nursing* 15(3):39–53.

Drown, D. 2000. High sensitivity C-reactive protein: Can it predict cardiovascular risk in postmenopausal women? *Progress in Cardiovascular Nursing* 15(4):152–153.

Giardina, E. 2000. Heart disease in women. *International Journal of Fertility and Women's Medicine* 45(6):350–357.

Gibbons, R., Chatterjee, K., Daley, J. et al. 1999. ACC/AHA/ACP-ASIM guidelines for the management of patients with chronic stable angina. A report of the American College of Cardiology/American Heart Association Task Force on Practice Guidelines (Committee on Management of Patients with Chronic Stable Angina). *Journal of the American College of Cardiology* 33(7):2092–2197.

Grady, D., Herrington, D., Bitner, V. et al. 2002. Cardiovascular disease outcome during 6.8 years of hormone therapy: Heart and Estrogen/Progestin Replacement Study (HERS II). *Journal of the American Medical Association* 288(1):49–57.

Hulley, S., Grady, D., Bush, T. et al. 1998. Randomized trial of estrogen plus progestin for secondary prevention of coronary heart disease in postmenopausal women. *Journal of the American Medical Association* 280(7):605–613.

Massie, B., and Amidon, T. 2002. Heart. In *Current medical diagnosis and treatment*, 41st ed., eds. L. Tierney, S. McPhee, and M. Papadakis, pp. 363–457. New York: Lange Medical Books/McGraw-Hill.

Nanchahal, K., Aston, W., and Wood, D. 2000. Alcohol consumption, metabolic cardiovascular risk factors, and hypertension in women. *International Journal of Epidemiology* 29(1):57–64.

Penckofer, S., and Schwertz, D. 2001. Hormone replacement therapy: primary and secondary prevention. *Journal of Cardiovascular Nursing* 15(3):1–25.

Rosenfeld, J. 2000. Heart disease in women: gender-specific statistics and prevention strategies for a population at risk. *Postgraduate Medicine* 107(6):111–116.

Rossouw, J., Anderson, G. Prentice, R. et al. 2002. Risks and benefits of estrogen plus progesterone in healthy postmenopausal women. Principal results from the Women's Health Initiative randomized controlled trial. *Journal of the American Medical Association* 288(3):321–333.

Schoenhagen, P., McErlean, E., and Nissen, S. 2000. The vulnerable coronary plaque. *Journal of Cardiovascular Nursing* 15(1):1–12.

U.S. Preventive Services Task Force (USPSTF). 2002. Hormone replacement therapy. Available at: http://www.ahrq.gov/clinic/3rduspstf/hrt. Accessed on December 13, 2002.

Zanger, D., Solomon, A., and Gersh, B. 1999. Contemporary management of angina. Part I: risk assessment. *American Family Physician* 60(9):2543–2552.

_____. 2000. Contemporary management of angina. Part II: medical management of chronic stable angina. *American Family Physician* 61(1):129–138.

6-B
Deep Vein Thrombosis

Deep vein thrombosis (DVT) involves the partial or complete blockage of a vein by a clot (thrombus) accompanied by inflammatory changes in the vessel wall (Messina et al. 2002). DVT is the cause of significant morbidity and mortality worldwide. Each year in the United States, more than 800,000 DVTs are diagnosed, accounting for more than 250,000 hospitalizations and 50,000 deaths (Kim et al. 2001). However, it is postulated that because the diagnosis is often unsuspected or missed, the actual incidence is twice that high (American Thoracic Society [ATS] 1999).

Three factors (*Virchow's triad*) predispose to the development of DVT: venous stasis, hypercoagulability, and vascular wall injury. Of these, stasis is thought to be the most important, as it triggers coagulation by means of thrombin activation, platelet aggregation, and fibrin formation (Kennedy et al. 2001).

Many patients with DVT have no *known* risk factors, with half of DVTs thought to be "idiopathic." However, there is increased recognition of the role of an underlying chronic hypercoagulability, either inherited or acquired; once present, there is heightened susceptibility to external events (e.g., risk factors) that may trigger venous stasis, vascular endothelial injury, and/or coagulation, with subsequent DVT (Brewster 2000). A number of risk factors have been identified. They include:

→ History of a previous DVT, which confers a fivefold risk for recurrence (Kennedy et al. 2001, Lee et al. 2001). For this reason, it is suggested that DVT should be viewed as a chronic disease.

→ Surgery is a major risk factor, particularly orthopedic (total hip replacement, total knee replacement) and major abdominal and pelvic procedures with general anesthesia. Mechanisms include direct endothelial injury and postoperative immobilization.

→ Immobility caused by any condition, including surgery or other illness, paralysis after stroke or spinal cord injury, casting or traction of an extremity, prolonged travel (e.g., by air, train, or car for longer than four hours), or a sedentary lifestyle.

→ Aging, which naturally results in changes in blood flow and increased blood viscosity. Generally, risk increases proportionately after the age of 40 years. An exception is women of childbearing age, who have a higher incidence of DVT when compared to age-matched males, likely due to estrogen (see below) (Kim et al. 2001).

→ Inherited coagulation defects may be responsible for up to 20% of DVTs (Kennedy et al. 2001). Affected persons often present with DVT at an early age, especially when exposed to other risk factors (e.g., surgery, pregnancy, oral contraceptives). Half will have recurrent DVTs unless they receive lifelong anticoagulation therapy. Inherited defects include:

■ Antithrombin III deficiency, a direct inhibitor of thrombin

■ Protein S deficiency, a vitamin K-dependent plasma protein that inhibits clotting factors V and VIII

■ Protein C deficiency, which inhibits clotting factors Va and VIIIa. Deficiency of Protein C increases the risk of DVT by 8–10 times (Kim et al. 2001). Heterozygosity for this defect (as well as for Antithrombin III and Protein S deficiencies) carries more risk than homozygosity (Brewster 2000).

■ Factor V Leiden, a common inherited disorder that prevents activated Protein C from inhibiting clotting. Uncommon in Asians and blacks, Factor V Leiden may be found in 5% of those with Northern European ancestry (Kim et al. 2001). While conferring low risk by itself, it increases the risk of DVT when coupled with other risk factors.

■ Prothrombin gene mutation is an inherited disorder that increases the risk of DVT.

■ Hyperhomocysteinemia leads to vascular injury, early atherosclerosis, and increased risk of DVT.

→ Antiphospholipid antibodies directly damage vascular walls or interact with other abnormal clotting factors, leading to hypercoagulability. These acquired antibodies are produced after infection, during pregnancy, and with systemic lupus erythematosus and other autoimmune disorders, and also may be found in normal persons. The antibodies, which include anticardiolipin and lupus anticoagulant, greatly increase DVT risk (Brewster 2000).

→ Estrogen use has long been implicated in thrombogenesis. The high doses of estrogen (50 µg) in early oral contraceptives were thought to be responsible. However, decreasing the estrogen dose has not resulted in a parallel decrease in the incidence of DVT in women using lower-dose oral contraceptives. It has been postulated that while the overall risk of DVT while taking oral contraceptives is low, women with inherited coagulation deficiencies, particularly Factor V Leiden or exposure to other known risk factors (e.g., surgery, cigarette smoking), demonstrate an increased incidence of DVT. Additionally, elevated estrogen levels during pregnancy and postpartum (including after spontaneous or therapeutic abortion) are known to increase the risk of DVT.

■ Women taking estrogen for hormone replacement therapy, particularly women with coronary heart disease, have a two- to threefold increased risk of DVT compared to nonusers, similar to the risk with oral contraceptives despite the lower dose of estrogen (Farrell 2001, Grady et al. 2000, Mayo 1997).

→ The role of progestins in thrombus formation also has been recognized. In the mid-1990s, the third-generation progestins (gestodene, desogestrel) were implicated in a twofold increased risk of DVT in young women (although perhaps as a result of poorly designed studies). These agents were taken off the market in several European countries. Subsequent study has shown that third-generation progestins carry no more risk than second-generation progestins (Farmer et al. 1998).

→ Cigarette smoking places women at risk for DVT. Although the mechanism is unclear, it is thought to be related to smoking's role in the development of atherosclerosis.

→ Malignancy is known to cause accelerated coagulation early in disease, even before symptoms develop. Up to 10% of all patients diagnosed with a new DVT are subsequently diagnosed with cancer within six months (usually lung cancer). Although this is an area of controversy, currently there are no recommendations for cancer screening in those diagnosed with a DVT (Kennedy et al. 2001, Kim et al. 2001).

→ Obesity has been implicated as an independent risk factor in women (but not men), separate from any associated immobility. Obesity predisposes to venous stasis and hypercoagulation (Lee et al. 2001).

→ Medical conditions also confer an increased risk of DVT. These conditions include cardiac disease (myocardial infarction, heart failure), nephrotic syndrome, and systemic lupus erythematosus (Brewster 2000).

The spectrum of venous thromboembolic disease encompasses localized deep vein thromboses to massive, life-threatening pulmonary emboli. While any large vein may develop a venous thromboembolism, DVT occurs most often in a lower extremity and is the major cause of pulmonary embolism. Thrombosis in a jugular, sinus, upper extremity, mesenteric, or pelvic vein is uncommon and beyond the scope of this chapter (Volturo et al. 2001).

DVT is most commonly a clot that forms in the lower extremity, usually the calf. If untreated, there may be progression proximally into the thigh, with a risk of subsequent embolization. A proximal DVT (involving the popliteal vein or higher) is associated with a 50% incidence of pulmonary embolism (PE) if untreated; distal DVTs (e.g., those localized to the calf) carry less than a 20% risk of PE (Ofri 2000).

Superficial thrombophlebitis is a common, localized condition wherein a superficial vein (often the long saphenous vein) becomes inflamed. Risks include venipuncture (including intravenous drug use), trauma, and, most commonly, varicosities (causing venous stasis). Septic thrombophlebitis may present with systemic symptoms of infection. While usually benign, there is some risk of propagation to a deep vein, including a 10% risk of PE. Additionally, an occult DVT may coexist with superficial thrombophlebitis (Messina et al. 2002, Volturo et al. 2001).

Pulmonary embolism is a thrombus that lodges in the pulmonary venous system, most often the result of embolization from a clot in the deep veins of a lower extremity, proximal to and involving the popliteal veins (ATS 1999). Responsible for an estimated 50,000 deaths per year in the United States, PE often presents acutely, although increasingly it is thought that many persons with PE are asymptomatic or present with vague symptoms (e.g., tachypnea, tachycardia), making diagnosis difficult (Chesnutt et al. 2002). The true incidence of PE is now thought to be higher than previously recognized (Volturo et al. 2001).

DATABASE

SUBJECTIVE

→ The patient may report:
■ General:
  • Feeling apprehensive
  • Chills and/or fever
■ Respiratory:
  • Dyspnea, at rest or with exertion
  • Chest pain
    – Pleuritic
    – Nonpleuritic
  • Cough
    – Hemoptysis
■ Musculoskeletal:
  • Lower extremity pain
    – Unilateral
    – Usually gradual in onset, increasing over days
      ➤ Sudden onset is more likely to be associated with musculoskeletal trauma than DVT.
    – Pain is worse with ambulation or dependency, better with rest and elevation.
  • Lower extremity swelling
    – Feeling of fullness may increase with standing or walking.
→ Past medical history may reveal:
■ History of DVT

- A known coagulation defect:
  - Factor V Leiden deficiency
  - Protein C deficiency
  - Protein S deficiency
  - Antithrombin III deficiency
  - Anticardiolipin antibody
- Recent surgery, especially with general anesthesia:
  - Orthopedic surgery:
    - Total hip replacement
    - Total knee replacement
  - Major abdominal surgery
  - Pelvic surgery
- Recent or ongoing immobility for any reason:
  - Prolonged bed rest
  - Paralysis, paresthesia of an extremity/extremities
    - Stroke
    - Spinal cord injury
  - Casting or traction of an extremity
  - Sedentary lifestyle
  - Obesity
  - Recent travel (by air, plane, or car) for more than four hours
- Malignancy
→ Family history may reveal:
  - History of DVT
    - May suggest inherited coagulation defect
  - History of specific coagulation defect
→ Medications may include:
  - Oral contraceptive
  - Estrogen replacement therapy

OBJECTIVE

→ The physical examination is important but often inconclusive for DVT. Even in the presence of PE or lower-extremity DVT, the physical examination may be unremarkable.
→ The presentation of DVT in younger adults may be more subtle than in older adults (Lee et al. 2001).
→ Patients with suspected PE should have a thorough examination, including of the extremities, to assess for DVT.
→ Patients with suspected lower-extremity DVT should have a thorough cardiorespiratory examination; 50% of patients with DVT may have an asymptomatic PE at the time of presentation (Lee et al. 2001).
→ General appearance may reveal apprehension, diaphoresis with PE.
→ Vital signs may be altered with PE:
  - Tachypnea
    - Most patients with PE will have a respiratory rate ≥16 breaths/minute.
  - Tachycardia (heart rate >100 beats per minute)
  - Low-grade fever (<38.3° C)
  - Hypotension
    - Systolic blood pressure <90 mmHg with massive PE
→ Cardiac examination may be altered in cases of PE:
  - May hear murmur and/or gallop.

- May note increased intensity of pulmonic S_2.
- May note jugular venous distention.
NOTE: Normal cardiac examination does not rule out PE.
→ Respiratory examination may be altered in cases of PE:
  - May hear rales or crackles with PE.
  - May note cyanosis with massive PE.
NOTE: Normal respiratory examination does not rule out PE.
→ Musculoskeletal examination may reveal:
  - Unilateral leg swelling:
    - Measure the calf circumference of each leg 10 cm below the tibial tuberosity.
    - Unilateral leg edema is a sensitive marker of DVT (Brewster 2000).
    - A calf circumference discrepancy of >1 cm in the affected leg is clinically significant. No discrepancy in calf circumference does not rule out DVT (Kennedy et al. 2001).
  - Lower-extremity warmth and/or erythema
    - Cyanosis if a marked venous obstruction is present.
  - Tenderness along the involved vein
    - Rarely, there is a palpable clot with DVT.
    - A tender, warm, discolored, subcutaneous cord or knot is suggestive of superficial thrombophlebitis.
  - Distention of superficial veins
  - Homan's sign (pain in the calf with dorsiflexion of the foot) is neither sensitive nor specific for DVT; its presence or absence neither rules in nor rules out DVT (Kennedy et al. 2001).
NOTE: A thorough extremity examination should be done, from ankle to thigh, to assess for proximal extension of DVT. A normal musculoskeletal examination does not rule out DVT.

ASSESSMENT

→ R/O DVT
→ R/O pulmonary embolism
→ R/O lower-extremity deep vein thromboembolism
→ R/O superficial thrombophlebitis

PLAN

DIAGNOSTIC TESTS

→ The diagnosis of DVT or PE cannot (and should not) be made on the basis of history and/or physical examination alone. Imaging studies are required to confirm the diagnosis.
→ For suspected PE, consider:
  - V/Q scan (ventilation/perfusion scan):
    - First-line diagnostic test
    - Low risk
    - Many pulmonary conditions can interfere with test interpretations, decreasing the specificity of a scan (ATS 1999).
  - Pulmonary angiogram:
    - The gold standard
    - Useful when a V/Q scan is abnormal but nondiagnostic
    - Invasive (requires contrast dye) and expensive (ATS 1999)

- Safe but not without risks: contrast dye reaction, transient renal dysfunction (Chesnutt et al. 2002)
- Chest x-ray:
  - Abnormal, although nonspecific, in most patients with PE.
  - May show pulmonary infiltrate, infarction, atelectasis, effusion, pulmonary edema, or vascular redistribution (Weiner et al. 2001).
- Arterial blood gases (ABG):
  - May reveal hypoxia, although patients with PE may have normal ABG.
- Electrocardiogram (EKG):
  - May demonstrate right heart strain and other nonspecific abnormalities; a normal EKG does not rule out PE.
- D-dimer assay (enzyme-linked immunosorbent assay [ELISA]):
  - A recently available screening test for DVT. D-dimers are specific products of fibrin degradation that are released into the blood. The test is highly sensitive, so a negative test can rule out PE. But it has poor specificity, as many conditions (e.g., malignancy, liver failure, sepsis, recent surgery) may result in a positive test (Weiner et al. 2001).
- Lower-extremity ultrasound (see below):
  - Most PEs originate in a lower extremity; some authors suggest that patients with suspected PE also should be evaluated for DVT.
→ For suspected lower-extremity DVT:
- Compression ultrasound:
  - Excellent sensitivity and specificity for proximal DVTs
  - May include duplex or color flow
  - Noninvasive, inexpensive, widely available
  - First-line test
    - A negative test does not rule out DVT; need to consider clinical presentation and patient risk. (See **Table 6B.1, Clinical Model for Predicting Pretest Probability for DVT** and **Figure 6B.1, Diagnostic Algorithm for Evaluation of Proximal DVT Using Ultrasonography and Venography Based on Pretest Probability.**)
- Contrast venogram:
  - The gold standard; nearly 100% sensitivity and specificity
  - Detects DVT in the calf, iliac vein, and inferior vena cava that may be missed on ultrasound
  - Not appropriate as a first-line test (ATS 1999)
  - Invasive, uncomfortable, and may cause phlebitis or contrast-dye reaction
  - More expensive, not available in all settings
  - Useful with negative or equivocal ultrasound in the patient with a high likelihood of DVT or in the patient with prior DVT on nondiagnostic ultrasound (Rosen et al. 2001).
- Magnetic resonance imaging (MRI):
  - Nearly 100% sensitivity and specificity

- More accurate than ultrasound for calf or pelvic DVT; also can determine old versus new DVT
- Expensive, not available in all settings
- Use when other tests are inconclusive (Rosen et al. 2001)
- Impedance plethysmography:
  - A noninvasive test that measures changes in venous outflow
  - Less sensitive than Doppler ultrasound, especially in asymptomatic patients
- D-dimer assay (see above)

NOTE: In a number of studies, 40–60% of patients with DVT were found to have an asymptomatic PE. Controversy exists as to whether all patients with DVT should be routinely evaluated for PE with a baseline V/Q scan or pulmonary angiography (Lee et al. 2001).

→ For superficial thrombophlebitis:
- In most patients, no diagnostic testing is indicated.
- Superficial thrombophlebitis in the greater saphenous vein carries some risk of propagation to a deep vein; if there is evidence that the saphenous vein may be involved, ultrasound may be ordered (Brown 2001).

TREATMENT/MANAGEMENT

PE

→ Patients with PE should be hospitalized promptly for anticoagulation therapy with intravenous heparin, oxygenation, and possibly venous filter devices.

Table 6B.1. CLINICAL MODEL FOR PREDICTING PRETEST PROBABILITY FOR DVT

Clinical Feature	Score*
Active cancer within 6 months	1
Paralysis, paresis, or cast of lower extremity	1
Recently bedridden >3 days or Major surgery within 4 weeks	1
Localized tenderness along distribution of deep vein system	1
Calf diameter >3 cm larger than opposite leg[1]	1
Pitting edema	1
Collateral superficial veins (nonvaricose)	1
Alternative diagnosis as likely or greater than that of DVT	-2

*Interpretation: 0 = low probability = 3% frequency of DVT; 1–2 = medium probability = 17% frequency of DVT; ≥3 = high probability = 75% frequency of DVT.
[1] Measured 10 cm below tibial tuberosity.

Source: Ofri, D. 2000. Diagnosis and treatment of deep vein thrombosis. *Western Journal of Medicine* 173(3):194–197. Reprinted with permission from the BMJ Publishing Group.

Lower-Extremity DVT

→ The primary goal of treatment is to stop ongoing thrombus progression and prevent embolization (e.g., PE). While an established clot is unaffected by heparin, clot dissolution will occur by natural fibrinolysis (Messina et al. 2002). Patients with a proximal DVT should be treated immediately with anticoagulation therapy, given the high incidence of PE if this condition is left untreated.

→ Proximal DVT:

■ Anticoagulation therapy:

• Hospitalization for intravenous anticoagulation therapy with unfractionated heparin (UFH) has been the mainstay of treatment for years. Oral anticoagulation with warfarin also is initiated at admission and the dose of UFH gradually decreased. Patients are discharged on warfarin when adequate anticoagulation has been achieved.

• Low molecular weight heparins (LMWHs) recently have been approved for use in venous thromboembolic disease. While similar in action to UFH and equally efficacious, these agents have less interaction with platelets and thrombin, cause less bleeding, have a longer half-life, have a more predictable anticoagulant effect, carry less risk of heparin-induced thrombocy-

topenia, and overall cause less mortality (Ofri 2000). LMWHs can be used on an outpatient basis for selected patients, avoiding costly hospitalization. There is no need to monitor the partial thromboplastin time with LMWHs, even in the outpatient setting (Brown 2001). The two agents used most widely for outpatient anticoagulation are enoxaparin and dalteparin, which is less expensive.

– Use of LMWH:

➤ Dosage: dalteparin 100 units/kg or enoxaparin 1 mg/kg by SQ injection every 12 hours. Additionally, an oral anticoagulant (e.g., warfarin) is begun within 1–3 days of initiating heparin. No loading dose of warfarin is needed; 5 mg/day p.o. is the starting dose (Brown 2001).

➤ Check prothrombin time (to assess coagulation) and platelet count (to assess for heparin-induced thrombocytopenia) on Day 3 and Day 7 (Brewster 2000).

➤ LMWH is continued for 4–7 days until the prothrombin time is elevated and the international normalized ratio (INR) is >2.0 on 2 consecutive days. Maintain an INR of 2.0–3.0 with warfarin; the usual dosage is 2–15 mg/day.

Figure 6B.1.   DIAGNOSTIC ALGORITHM FOR EVALUATION OF PROXIMAL DVT USING ULTRASONOGRAPHY AND VENOGRAPHY BASED ON PRETEST PROBABILITY

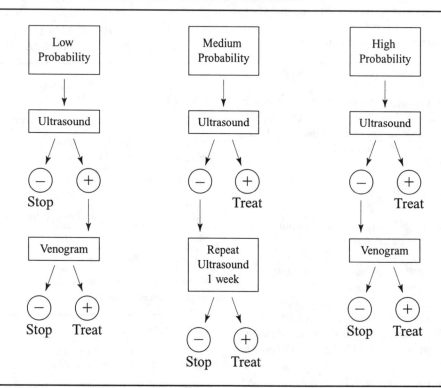

Source: Ofri, D. 2000. Diagnosis and treatment of deep vein thrombosis. *Western Journal of Medicine* 173(3):194–197. Reprinted with permission from the BMJ Publishing Group.

➤ The patient (or a family member) must be able to administer SQ LMWH.

➤ Daily contact with the patient (e.g., with a public health nurse) is appropriate.

– Length of anticoagulation therapy:

➤ Once the patient has a DVT, she is at increased risk of recurrence. The optimal duration of treatment is unknown. See suggested guidelines (**Table 6B.2, Length of Anticoagulation Therapy for DVT**).

• Candidates for outpatient therapy should be medically and hemodynamically stable. Contraindications to outpatient therapy include:

– Older than 75 years or younger than 18 years
– Suspected PE
– Known heparin allergy or history of heparin-induced thrombocytopenia
– Known bleeding disorder or active bleeding
– Concurrent illness with increased risk of bleeding
– Pregnancy
– Recent surgery
– Malignancy
– Noncompliance

■ Pain relief with a nonsteroidal anti-inflammatory drug (NSAID) as needed.

→ Distal DVT: Treatment is controversial. If a distal DVT remains localized to the calf, there is <1% risk of PE and approximately 2% risk of recurrent DVT (Ofri 2000). Thus, a distal DVT may be managed more conservatively with observation and serial diagnostic studies.

■ Anticoagulation therapy:

• Initiate anticoagulation as for proximal DVT if thrombus progression (e.g., extension into or above the popliteal veins) is noted on serial ultrasound.

■ Analgesics:

• A NSAID as needed for pain relief

NOTE: While many patients resolve spontaneously, up to 25% with an untreated calf DVT will develop chronic venous insufficiency within 1 year, so some authors recommend full anticoagulation for all patients with calf DVT (Brown 2001).

→ Superficial thrombophlebitis:

■ A NSAID as needed for discomfort
■ An antibiotic as needed if there is evidence of infection

CONSULTATION

→ Any patient with suspected PE should be urgently referred to an emergency setting for further diagnosis and treatment.

→ Refer to a vascular specialist any patient with proximal DVT who requires hospitalization for anticoagulation therapy.

→ Some patients with proximal DVT (e.g., involving iliofemoral veins) may be candidates for thrombolytic therapy (with streptokinase or tissue plasminogen activator [TPA]). Consult with or refer to a vascular specialist.

→ Some patients with proximal DVT may be candidates for saphenous vein ligation. Consult with or refer to a vascular surgeon.

→ Consultation as needed for suspected diagnosis and selection of appropriate diagnostic testing.

→ Consult with a physician regarding the appropriateness of home therapy with LMWH for selected patients, and as needed for ongoing management of anticoagulation.

→ If superficial thrombophlebitis is located above the knee and is progressing proximally, consult regarding the need for anticoagulation therapy or surgical referral.

→ As needed for prescriptions.

PATIENT EDUCATION

→ Explain the pathophysiology of DVT as appropriate for diagnosis.

→ For appropriate candidates for home LMWH use, instruct the patient or family about the SQ injection technique and about the possible symptoms and signs of excessive anticoagulation.

→ For lower extremity DVT, elevate the involved leg 15–20° with the knee slightly flexed. The patient should avoid sitting upright with legs in a dependent position.

→ For superficial thrombophlebitis, local heat and compression on the affected extremity is advised. Encourage ambulation.

→ Advise the woman of her risk of recurrence as appropriate for the diagnosis, reinforcing possible symptoms and signs that should be reported.

Table 6B.2.   LENGTH OF ANTICOAGULATION THERAPY FOR DVT

Type of DVT	Length of Anticoagulation
First DVT with identified, reversible risk factors (e.g., surgery, temporary immobility, estrogen therapy)	3–6 months
First DVT with heterozygous Factor V Leiden	3–6 months
First DVT, unknown etiology	6 months or longer (optimal duration unknown, 6 month minimum)
First DVT with malignancy; other known coagulation disorders; persistent antiphospholipid antibodies; recurrent DVT	Lifelong

Source: Compiled from Brewster, D. 2000. Management of peripheral venous disease. In *Primary care medicine: office evaluation and management of the adult patient*, 4th ed., eds. A. Goroll and A. Mulley, pp. 242–249. Philadelphia: Lippincott Williams & Wilkins; Brown, D. 2001. Treatment options for deep vein thrombosis. *Emergency Medicine Clinics of North America* 19(4):913–923; Ofri, D. 2000. Diagnosis and treatment of deep vein thrombosis. *Western Journal of Medicine* 173(3):194–197.

→ Advise the woman regarding risk factors for DVT, emphasizing those that are amenable to intervention (e.g., weight management, avoidance of immobility, smoking cessation).

→ Educate the woman about her risk of DVT related to estrogen use. Discontinue estrogen (oral contraceptives or estrogen replacement) in a woman with documented DVT or PE.

→ Discuss the relationship of cigarette smoking to increased risk of DVT. Encourage smoking cessation and assist the patient in developing a plan to accomplish this goal.

→ Advise the woman that if she needs surgery in the future, she should inform her surgeon of her history of DVT. Prophylactic preoperative and postoperative anticoagulation therapy may be necessary. Aspirin is inadequate prophylaxis for high-risk patients (Pineo 2001).

FOLLOW-UP

→ For ongoing care of a patient requiring anticoagulation therapy, monitor prothrombin time/international normalized ratio (PT/INR) as needed, decreasing frequency once the patient is stable. Adjust warfarin dosage as needed in consultation.

→ For patients with documented DVT, consider testing for inherited coagulation defects. It may be appropriate for women who present with DVT at young age (e.g., younger than 50 years), no known risk factors, a family history of DVT, or DVT of unusual location or severity (Ofri 2000).

→ Heparin-induced osteoporosis may occur in women who are anticoagulated for seven weeks or longer (Ressel 2001). Monitor as appropriate. Short-term or prophylactic heparin use poses no risk of osteoporosis.

→ Work-up for malignancy in a woman with documented DVT is not warranted in the absence of other suggestive symptoms and/or signs, other than a careful history and physical, and a routine, age-appropriate cancer screening (e.g., mammography, Pap smear, stool for occult blood, and sigmoidoscopy).

→ Document in progress notes and on problem list.

BIBLIOGRAPHY

American Thoracic Society (ATS). 1999. The diagnostic approach to acute venous thromboembolism. *American Journal of Respiratory and Critical Care Medicine* 160: 1043–1066.

Brewster, D. 2000. Management of peripheral venous disease. In *Primary care medicine: office evaluation and management of the adult patient*, 4th ed., eds. A. Goroll and A. Mulley, pp. 242–249. Philadelphia: Lippincott Williams & Wilkins.

Brown, D. 2001. Treatment options for deep vein thrombosis. *Emergency Medicine Clinics of North America* 19(4): 913–923.

Chesnutt, M., and Prendergast, T. 2002. Lung. In *Current medical diagnosis and treatment*, 41st ed., eds. L. Tierney, S. McPhee, and M. Papadakis, pp. 269–362. New York: Lange Medical Books/McGraw-Hill.

Farmer, R., and Lawrenson, R. 1998. Oral contraceptives and venous thromboembolic disease: the findings from database studies in the United Kingdom and Germany. *American Journal of Obstetrics and Gynecology* 179:578–586.

Farrell, S. 2001. Special situations: pediatric, pregnant, and geriatric patients. *Emergency Medicine Clinics of North America* 19(4):1013–1023.

Grady, D., Wenger, N., Herrington, D. et al. 2000. Postmenopausal hormone therapy increases risk for venous thromboembolic disease. The Heart and Estrogen/Progestin Replacement Study. *Annals of Internal Medicine* 132(9):689–696.

Kennedy, D., Setnik, G., and Li, J. 2001. Physical examination findings in deep vein thrombosis. *Emergency Medicine Clinics of North America* 19(4):869–876.

Kim, V., and Spandorfer, J. 2001. Epidemiology of venous thromboembolic disease. *Emergency Medicine Clinics of North America* 19(4):839–859.

Lee, L., and Shah, K. 2001. Clinical manifestations of pulmonary embolism. *Emergency Medicine Clinics of North America* 19(4):925–942.

Mayo, D. 1997. Thrombosis and hemostasis in women throughout the lifespan. *Critical Care Nursing Clinics of North America* 9(4):535–543.

Messina, L., and Tierney, L. 2002. Blood vessel and lymphatics. In *Current medical diagnosis and treatment*, 41st ed., eds. L. Tierney, S. McPhee, and M. Papadakis, pp. 485–516. New York: Lange Medical Books/McGraw-Hill.

Ofri, D. 2000. Diagnosis and treatment of deep vein thrombosis. *Western Journal of Medicine* 173(3):194–197.

Pineo, G. 2001. New developments in the prevention and treatment of venous thromboembolism. *Pharmacotherapy* 21(6 Part 2):51S–55S.

Ressel, G. 2001. ACOG practice bulletin on preventing deep venous thrombosis and pulmonary embolism. *American Family Physician* 63(11):2279–2280.

Rosen, C., and Tracy, J. 2001. The diagnosis of lower extremity deep venous thrombosis. *Emergency Medicine Clinics of North America* 19(4):895–912.

Volturo, G., and Repeta, R. 2001. Non-lower extremity deep vein thrombosis. *Emergency Medicine Clinics of North America* 19(4):877–893.

Weiner, S., and Burstein, J. 2001. Nonspecific tests for pulmonary embolism. *Emergency Medicine Clinics of North America* 19(4):943–955.

6-C

Heart Failure

Heart failure is a complex condition with characteristic clinical symptomatology and physical findings. Heart failure develops when the heart is unable to maintain adequate cardiac output to meet cellular metabolic needs or is able to do so only with markedly increased ventricular filling pressures (Shamsham et al. 2000). A wide variety of cardiac and noncardiac diseases can lead to heart failure.

Despite an increase in our understanding of the mechanisms of heart failure over the last decade and improvements in diagnostic and treatment strategies, the incidence and prevalence of heart failure continue to increase. Five million Americans have heart failure and 400,000–700,000 new diagnoses are made each year (Heart Failure Society of America [HFSA] 2001). Heart failure is associated with a high morbidity and mortality. Deaths from heart failure currently average 250,000 per year and have more than doubled in the last 20 years. Fewer than 50% of patients survive more than five years after initial diagnosis (Chavey et al. 2001a, HFSA 2001).

Nearly half of the patients with heart failure in this country are women, and among patients older than 70 years, more women than men are affected (Richardson 2001). Women are diagnosed with heart failure later than men are and suffer more quality of life impairment than men do, including poorer physical and social function (Riedinger et al. 2001).

Multiple etiologies contribute to the development of heart failure (see "Database," below). The most common causes include coronary heart disease, hypertension (HTN), and valvular heart disease (Shamsham et al. 2000). However, any condition that impairs cardiac structure and/or function can result in heart failure, and once heart failure is present, dysfunction is usually progressive (Adams et al. 1999).

In the healthy heart, systolic function (measured as cardiac output) is determined by myocardial contractility, ventricular preload (the end-diastolic volume and resulting fiber length of the ventricles before contraction), ventricular afterload (the amount of resistance to left ventricular ejection), and heart rate (Massie et al. 2002). Diastolic function is determined by ventricular relaxation, which allows for optimal filling during diastole.

The pathophysiology of heart failure includes the concepts of *systolic dysfunction* and *diastolic dysfunction*. It is important to understand the distinction between these, as treatment differs, although many patients may have components of both types of heart failure and symptom presentation is similar. In systolic dysfunction (the "big, boggy heart"), the left ventricle markedly dilates, becoming hypertrophic and more spherical in shape (Diller et al. 2000). This structural remodeling allows for ventricular filling but impairs ventricular wall motion, which decreases cardiac output. An ejection fraction (the amount of blood pumped by the left ventricle during systole) of <40% is characteristic of systolic dysfunction (Chavey et al. 2001a, Hunt et al. 2001).

Falling cardiac output leads to activation of the neurohormonal system. Initially, the increased adrenergic effects of the sympathetic nervous system stimulate the failing heart, increasing heart rate and contractility in an effort to boost cardiac output. At the same time, decreased renal perfusion activates the renin-angiotensin system, which results in fluid retention and a subsequent increase in intravascular volume to compensate for the falling cardiac output. Elevated levels of angiotensin II increase aldosterone secretion, promoting sodium and water retention. The resulting increase in preload, ventricular filling pressures, and afterload further accelerates structural (e.g., ventricular) remodeling. Elevated levels of neurohormones, including norepinephrine, endothelin, vasopressin, and other cytokines, act both independently and synergistically to impair cardiac function. Chronic neurohormonal stimulation leads to myocardial fibrosis and cellular death (*apoptosis*), ongoing ventricular remodeling, and worsening heart failure (Brashers 2002).

Approximately 20–40% of patients with heart failure have diastolic dysfunction (Hunt et al. 2001). In diastolic dysfunction (the "stiff heart"), the left-ventricle chamber size remains normal or becomes smaller, but muscle abnormalities lead to increasing ventricular wall stiffness and thickness, diastolic filling is impaired, and ventricular pressures increase as ventricular relaxation is inhibited. In the absence of advanced diastolic dysfunction, systolic contractility is preserved and the ejection fraction is usually normal/near normal (Halm et al. 2000).

Diastolic dysfunction is more common in women than men, particularly in elderly women. Diastolic dysfunction is less well understood than systolic dysfunction. It is postulated that some, but not all, of the changes associated with diastolic dysfunction are related to normal aging (Hunt et al. 2001, Richardson 2001).

Despite the difference in physiological mechanisms, both systolic dysfunction and diastolic dysfunction impair blood flow out of the left ventricle, resulting in increased filling pressures. Eventually, this pressure increase is transmitted back to the pulmonary circulation, resulting in pulmonary congestion and the classic heart-failure symptoms of dyspnea and exercise intolerance. Because not all patients with heart failure demonstrate symptoms of pulmonary or peripheral congestion in the earlier stages of disease, however, the term *heart failure* is increasingly used rather than the older term *congestive heart failure*.

Patient symptoms often are characterized as either being characteristic of *left heart failure* or *right heart failure*. Symptoms common in left heart failure include those related to pulmonary congestion and cardiomegaly. Right heart failure is associated with jugular venous distention, hepatomegaly, and peripheral edema. The most common cause of right heart failure is left heart failure; many patients with left heart failure eventually will develop symptoms of right heart failure as well. Pulmonary disease is the other major cause of right heart failure; in such cases, the right heart failure is referred to as "primary" (Brashers 2002).

Information about optimal pharmacologic treatment of heart failure in women has been limited by their underrepresentation in clinical trials, despite a nearly equal prevalence of heart failure in women and men. Women have averaged only 20% of study populations in the last 10 years (Riedinger et al. 2001). Because more women than men have diastolic dysfunction, women may be excluded from heart failure studies for which systolic dysfunction is an entry criterion. In addition, trials focusing on diastolic dysfunction have been less common than those for systolic dysfunction, further limiting women's access to trial participation. Studies that include large numbers of women and examine gender differences in response to treatment need to be undertaken.

DATABASE

SUBJECTIVE

→ Patients may present with vague symptoms that often are attributed to aging or physical disability, making the diagnosis of heart failure difficult. Heart failure is correctly diagnosed on initial presentation in only 50% of cases (Shamsham et al. 2000).
→ Symptoms may include:
   ▪ Initial presentation in mild cases:
      • Easily fatigued
      • Exercise intolerance
         − Limitation of routine and/or pleasurable activities
      • Dyspnea on exertion

   • Unexplained weight gain
   • Mild peripheral edema
▪ Progressive symptoms:
   • Worsening fatigue, decreased exercise tolerance
   • Dyspnea on exertion or at rest
   • Cough
      − Nocturnal, with activity, nonproductive
   • Orthopnea
   • Paroxysmal nocturnal dyspnea
   • Chest pains (exertional and/or at rest)
      − Compensatory tachycardia jeopardizes coronary artery perfusion during diastole
   • Palpitations (intermittent or sustained)
   • Gastrointestinal disturbances
      − Anorexia, nausea, vomiting, right upper quadrant (RUQ) pain, bloating, early satiety
   • Edema
      − Dependent edema is most common (e.g., in the legs)
      − May note upper-extremity and periorbital edema
→ Past medical history may include:
   ▪ Cardiac conditions associated with the development of heart failure:
      • Coronary heart disease (CHD)
         − Angina
         − Myocardial infarction (MI)
      • HTN
         − Systolic and/or diastolic
      • Valvular heart disease
         − Aortic stenosis or regurgitation
         − Mitral stenosis or regurgitation
         − Infective endocarditis
      • Rheumatic fever
      • Congenital heart disease
      • Constrictive pericarditis
      • Cardiomyopathy
         − Dilated
         − Hypertrophic
         − Restrictive
   ▪ Other conditions associated with heart failure:
      • Diabetes
      • Arrhythmias
      • Hyperlipidemia
      • Peripheral vascular disease
      • Connective tissue disease
      • Neuromuscular disease
         − Muscular dystrophy
      • Infiltrative disease
         − Sarcoidosis, amyloidosis, hemochromatosis
      • Thyroid disease
         − Hyperthyroidism
         − Hypothyroidism
      • Anemia
      • Malignancy, treated with chemotherapeutic drugs and/or radiation
      • Pheochromocytoma

- Pregnancy
- Infections
  - Bacterial
  - Viral (e.g., human immunodeficiency virus [HIV])
  - Parasitic (e.g., Chagas' disease)
→ Medication history may include the use of:
  - Antiarrhythmics
  - Antihypertensives
  - Antianginals
  - Steroids
  - Nonsteroidal anti-inflammatory drugs (NSAIDs)
  - Diet pills (e.g., fenfluramine)
→ Family history may include:
  - Cardiovascular disease
    - CHD
    - HTN
    - Valvular heart disease
    - Cardiomyopathy
    - Sudden death
    - Arrhythmias
  - Connective tissue disease
→ Social history:
  - May include the use of:
    - Tobacco
    - Alcohol
    - Illicit drugs
      - Cocaine
      - Amphetamines
  - Dietary habits: excess salt, highly processed foods
  - Exercise
  - Risk factors for HIV

OBJECTIVE

→ Vital signs may include:
  - Elevated temperature
    - Infection may precipitate heart failure.
  - Alterations in pulse
    - Tachycardia related to compensatory adrenergic stimulation
    - Pulsus alternans (alternating strong and weak pulse) related to impaired left ventricular function
    - Weak, thready pulse related to impaired left ventricular function
  - Increase or decrease in blood pressure
    - Initially elevated or maintained as a result of fluid retention and increased heart rate, but subsequently falls
  - Increased respiratory rate
    - Tachypnea results from pulmonary congestion and hypoxia.
  - Increased weight
    - Is a parameter for measuring the efficacy of treatment or worsening of symptoms.
  - Decreased weight
    - Over time, the patient loses muscle mass and body fat ("cardiac cachexia") (Hunt et al. 2001).

→ Physical examination to include:
  - Mental-status examination to assess for decreased cerebral blood flow
  - Ophthalmic examination to assess for retinal changes
  - Pulmonary examination to assess for:
    - Rales, usually bibasilar
    - Bronchospasm/wheezing
    - Tachypnea
    - Decreased oxygen saturation; assess SAO_2 with pulse oximetry
    - Pleural effusion
  - Cardiac examination to assess for:
    - Rhythm/rate
    - Heaves, lifts, point of maximal impulse (PMI)
      - PMI displaced laterally/inferiorly with cardiomegaly
    - Murmurs, especially systolic (mitral regurgitation or aortic stenosis)
    - Gallops
      - S_3: indicative of decreased ejection fraction, left ventricular dilatation, and increasing left atrial pressure
      - S_4: indicative of left ventricular stiffness
      - Decreased heart sounds (may indicate pericardial effusion)
  - Jugular venous distention
    - >4 cm elevation above sternal angle (with patient at 45° angle)
    - Reliable indicator of fluid overload
  - Abdominal examination to assess for:
    - Ascites
    - Hepatojugular reflex
      - Elevation of neck veins by >3 cm with sustained pressure on liver
    - Hepatomegaly
    - RUQ tenderness
  - Extremity examination to assess for:
    - Edema
      - Legs, presacral area
    - Stasis dermatitis
      - Edema, hyperpigmentation, ulceration
    - Cyanosis
    - Coldness

ASSESSMENT

→ Heart failure
  - R/O valvular heart disease
  - R/O CHD
  - R/O pericarditis
  - R/O arrhythmias
  - R/O hypertensive heart disease
  - R/O hypertrophic cardiomyopathy
  - R/O pulmonary embolism
  - R/O alcoholic or postviral cardiomyopathy
  - R/O chronic obstructive pulmonary disease
  - R/O pulmonary hypertension
  - R/O infection (endocarditis, pneumonia)

- R/O liver disease
- R/O renal disease
- R/O venous insufficiency

PLAN

DIAGNOSTIC TESTS

→ Identification of an underlying cause is an important component of the management of heart failure.

→ Initial diagnostic work-up:
  - Chest x-ray to assess for:
    - Prominent pulmonary vasculature
    - Pleural effusions
    - Increased interstitial markings
      - Kerley B lines or perihilar haziness
    - Presence/degree of cardiomegaly
  - EKG to assess for:
    - Left ventricular hypertrophy (LVH)
    - "p" mitrale
    - Cor pulmonale
    - Left atrial hypertrophy (LAH)
    - Arrhythmias
    - ST-T wave changes suggestive of ischemia
    - Prior MI
  - Labs may include:
    - Complete blood count (CBC)
    - Electrolytes
      - Including potassium, sodium, calcium, magnesium, glucose
    - Renal function tests
      - Blood urea nitrogen (BUN), creatinine
    - Liver function tests
      - Bilirubin, alanine aminotransferase (ALT), aspartate aminotransferase (AST), alkaline phosphatase
    - Thyroid function tests
      - Thyroid stimulating hormone (TSH)
    - Complete lipid panel
      - Total cholesterol, high-density lipoprotein (HDL), low-density lipoprotein (LDL), triglycerides
    - Arterial blood gases or pulse oximetry
    - HIV testing if indicated (although heart failure due to HIV cardiomyopathy usually develops after other manifestations of HIV disease [Hunt et al. 2001])

→ Other diagnostic tests (in consultation):
  - 2-D echocardiogram with Doppler flow studies. Assess:
    - Left ventricular mass and chamber size
    - Systolic function, measure ejection fraction
    - Diastolic function
    - Wall motion abnormalities
    - For primary etiology of heart failure:
      - Valvular disease
      - Pericardial disease
      - Myocardial disease
      - Presence/severity of systolic dysfunction
      - Presence/severity of diastolic dysfunction
  - Radionuclide ventriculography:
    - Assess systolic and diastolic function.

- Computerized tomography (CT) or magnetic resonance imaging (MRI):
  - Assess ejection fraction, wall motion, ventricular mass, pericardial disease
- Cardiac catheterization:
  - Left and right heart hemodynamics
  - Assess cardiac function
  - Indicated to rule out or evaluate ischemic CHD
  - Assess hemodynamics in pericarditis
- Exercise stress testing:
  - Assess concomitant CHD
- Ambulatory rhythm monitoring:
  - Assess for arrhythmias, a major cause of mortality in patients with heart failure (Chavey et al. 2001a).

→ Future diagnostic tests may include:
  - Measurement of the following peptides, which have been found in patients with heart failure and are thought to confer a worse prognosis. These are investigational and not recommended for routine use in primary care at present (Chavey et al. 2001a, Shamsham et al. 2000):
    - Atrial natriuretic peptide (ANP)
      - Secreted in response to an increase in atrial pressure
    - Brain natriuretic peptide (BNP)
      - Secreted in response to ventricular failure

TREATMENT/MANAGEMENT

→ Establish the patient's status using the New York Heart Association classification.
  - This is a measure of functional capacity in the patient with heart failure, based on exercise ability. The higher the class, the worse the prognosis. It is useful for monitoring status over time (Chavey et al. 2001a, Massie et al. 2002):
    - Class I: asymptomatic
    - Class II: symptomatic with moderate exertion
    - Class III: symptomatic with minimal exertion
    - Class IV: symptomatic at rest

→ Acute onset heart failure:
  - May require hospitalization (in consultation) for:
    - Oxygen
    - Diuretics
    - Vasoactive drugs
    - Treatment of identified underlying primary etiology
    - Correction of identified precipitating factors:
      - Infection/high fever
      - Severe anemia
      - Tachycardia

→ Mild or chronic/stable heart failure caused by *systolic dysfunction*. (See **Table 6C.1, Drugs Commonly Used for Treatment of Chronic Heart Failure**):
  - Low-dose diuretics:
    - Reduce preload (by eliminating excess fluid).
    - Lower the right- and left-heart filling pressures.
    - Improve dyspnea, orthopnea, edema.
    - Loop diuretics are commonly used, although thiazide diuretics may be adequate for mild heart failure.

- Allow the patient to change the dose as needed based on daily weight.
- Angiotensin converting enzyme (ACE) inhibitors:
  - Interfere with the renin-angiotensin system, preventing conversion of angiotensin I → II and associated secretion of aldosterone.
  - Improve cardiac output, decrease peripheral vascular resistance, increase sodium excretion, reduce fluid retention, and lead to regression of ventricular remodeling.
  - All ACE inhibitors effectively reduce symptoms and improve mortality.
  - Initiate for all patients (asymptomatic or symptomatic) with systolic dysfunction unless contraindicated.
  - Initiate at a low dose, then gradually increase as tolerated. The ideal dose is controversial, with some authors advocating higher doses than those in **Table 6C.1** (Chavey et al. 2001b).
  - Monitor renal function and potassium level within 1–2 weeks after initiation of therapy and periodically thereafter.
- Beta blockers:
  - Once considered contraindicated in heart failure, they are now known to interfere with the adverse effects that neurohormones have on cardiac structure and function.
  - Recommended for clinically stable patients (Class II and III), unless contraindicated (Chavey 2000). Their use in Class I patients has not been studied; however, many Class I patients have a history of MI or HTN and might be expected to benefit from beta blockers (Chavey 2000).
  - Improve symptoms, increase cardiac output, and reduce mortality.
  - Initiate at a low dose, then gradually increase as tolerated, not more often than every 2–4 weeks (Adams et al. 1999).

Table 6C.1. DRUGS COMMONLY USED FOR TREATMENT OF CHRONIC HEART FAILURE

Drug	Initial Dose	Maximum Dose
Loop Diuretics*		
Bumetanide	0.5–1.0 mg once or twice daily	Titrate to achieve dry weight (up to 10 mg daily)
Furosemide	20–40 mg once or twice daily	Titrate to achieve dry weight (up to 400 mg daily)
Torsemide	10–20 mg once or twice daily	Titrate to achieve dry weight (up to 200 mg daily)
ACE† Inhibitors		
Captopril	6.25 mg 3 times daily	50 mg 3 times daily
Enalapril	2.5 mg twice daily	10–20 mg twice daily
Fosinopril	5–10 mg once daily	40 mg once daily
Lisinopril	2.5–5 mg once daily	20–40 mg once daily
Quinapril	10 mg twice daily	40 mg twice daily
Ramipril	1.25–2.5 mg once daily	10 mg once daily
Beta Blockers		
Bisoprolol	1.25 mg once daily	10 mg once daily
Carvedilol	3.125 mg twice daily	25 mg twice daily (50 mg twice daily for patients >85 kg)
Metoprolol tartrate	6.25 mg twice daily	75 mg twice daily
Metoprolol succinate extended release+	12.5–25 mg daily	200 mg once daily
Digitalis Glycosides		
Digoxin	0.125–0.25 mg once daily	0.125–0.25 mg once daily

* Thiazide diuretics are not listed in this table but may be appropriate for patients with mild heart failure or associated hypertension or as a second diuretic in patients refractory to loop diuretics alone.

† Angiotensin converting enzyme

+ Referred to in some publications as metoprolol CR/XL

Source: Reprinted with permission from Hunt, S.A., Baker, D.W., Chin, M.H. et al. 2001. ACC/AHA guidelines for the evaluation and management of chronic heart failure in the adult: a report of the American College of Cardiology/American Heart Association Task Force on Practice Guidelines (Committee to Revise the 1995 Guidelines for the Evaluation and Management of Heart Failure). © 2001 by the American College of Cardiology and American Heart Association Inc. Available at: http://www.acc.org/clinical/guidelines/failure/hf_index.htm. Accessed on August 10, 2002.

- No clinical differences exist among those beta blockers shown to be of benefit in heart failure (Chavey et al. 2001b). Carvedilol was the first beta blocker labeled by the Food and Drug Administration for use in slowing the progression of heart failure (Ramahi 2000). Recently, metoprolol also was approved.
- Digitalis:
  - Has been a mainstay of therapy for years. It inhibits Na^+-K^+ adenosine triphosphatase (ATPase), which blocks sympathetic nervous system effects (Hunt et al. 2001).
  - Many digitalis preparations are available. Digoxin is the most widely studied and is preferred (Hunt et al. 2001).
  - No effect on mortality, but it decreases symptoms and improves exercise tolerance.
  - Useful in atrial fibrillation. Its use in patients with sinus rhythm is controversial, although the benefits noted above were seen in patients regardless of whether they were in atrial fibrillation or sinus rhythm. Recent guidelines recommend using it as part of a long-term management plan (Haji et al. 2000, Hunt et al. 2001).
- Other pharmacologic considerations (Hunt et al. 2001, Kayser 2000):
  - Spironolactone:
    - An aldosterone antagonist. Consider using it for those with recent or recurrent Class IV symptoms as an adjunct to ACE inhibitors, beta blockers, digoxin, and diuretics.
  - Angiotensin II receptor blockers:
    - Consider them as an alternative in patients intolerant of ACE inhibitors.
    - Studies are evaluating the concomitant use of angiotensin II receptor blockers and ACE inhibitors (Cohn 2000).
  - Hydralazine and isosorbide dinitrate:
    - May be an adjunct to ACE inhibition or useful in those intolerant of ACE inhibitors or angiotensin II receptor blockers.
  - Calcium channel blockers have no proven benefit in treating heart failure and may be detrimental.
→ Mild or chronic/stable heart failure caused by *diastolic dysfunction* (Hunt et al. 2001, Richardson 2001):
  - There is a lack of consensus about treating diastolic dysfunction, as there have been few clinical trials assessing effective interventions.
  - Current recommendations suggest that beta blockers, diuretics, and coronary revascularization be used as appropriate to achieve adequate control of heart rate, blood pressure, fluid status, and ischemia.
  - There are no clinical trials to support the use of ACE inhibitors, angiotensin II receptor blockers, calcium channel blockers, or digoxin for diastolic dysfunction. Use of these agents remains controversial.

CONSULTATION

→ For patients with acute-onset heart failure, consult a physician regarding initial work-up, treatment, and possible hospitalization.
→ For patients with progressive heart failure refractory to medical therapy, refer to a cardiologist or an internist for stabilization.
→ For treatment of the underlying etiology of heart failure (if possible):
  - Valvular heart disease/CHD/arrhythmias:
    - Initiate medication per consultation.
    - Refer for cardiology/cardiothoracic surgery.
  - Hypertension:
    - Initiate medication. (See the **Hypertension** chapter.)
    - Consider the underlying etiologies of hypertension.
  - Thyroid disease:
    - Initiate medication per consultation. (See the **Thyroid Disorders** chapter in Section 10.)
  - Pulmonary disease:
    - Refer for pulmonary evaluation.
  - Infection:
    - Treat the underlying etiology as appropriate.
→ For patients with end-stage heart failure, referral to a cardiologist is indicated.
  - Cardiac transplantation may be considered.
→ As needed for prescription(s).

PATIENT EDUCATION

→ Educate the patient and her family regarding the pathophysiology and treatment plan.
  - Provide medication instructions, including the:
    - Possibility of multiple medications
    - Timing of diuretic dosing (avoid evenings)
    - Symptoms of drug toxicity
→ Advise patients with symptoms of worsening heart failure to:
  - Record their daily weight before eating breakfast.
  - Call if they gain more than 2–3 pounds in one week.
→ Advise the patient regarding dietary management, including:
  - Avoiding salting foods at the table or while cooking.
  - Avoiding foods with high sodium content.
  - Increasing dietary potassium, especially if she is on diuretic therapy, with:
    - 10 ounces of orange, pineapple, or grapefruit juice
    - One medium banana
    - Two oranges
    - A medium-size baked potato
    - All of the above include 15 mEq of potassium. If the patient is taking potassium supplements, they may be mixed with any of the above juices.
  - Weight reduction if necessary.
  - Free water restriction if the patient is hyponatremic or in severe heart failure.
→ Advise the patient to schedule daily rest but avoid prolonged bed rest.

→ Advise the patient about preventing and managing chronic venous stasis.

→ Educate the patient regarding stress-reduction activities.

FOLLOW-UP

→ For patients on diuretic therapy:
  - Monitor serum potassium, BUN, and creatinine weekly until stabilized, then every 2–3 months as indicated.
  - Monitor postural vital signs to assess for hypovolemia.
  - Assess the need for potassium supplementation (usually necessary when the patient is on furosemide).
  - If hypokalemia occurs, begin potassium chloride elixir, 20 mEq in 1 tablespoon (15 cc) QD–TID until repleted.

→ For patients on ACE-inhibitor therapy, monitor blood pressure, BUN, creatinine, and potassium weekly, then every 2–3 months.

→ For patients on beta blocker therapy:
  - Monitor pulse rate and check for symptoms/signs of hypoperfusion or congestion.

→ For patients on digitalis therapy:
  - Monitor pulse rate, rhythm, BUN, creatinine, potassium, and serum digitalis level 1 week after initiation, adjusting the dose as necessary.
  - Digitalis levels should be monitored at least every 3–4 months.

→ Monitor exercise tolerance via patient report. The patient may note decreased symptoms at rest but not with activity.

→ Adjust/maximize medications as indicated.

→ Document in progress notes and on problem list.

BIBLIOGRAPHY

Adams, K., Baughman, K., Dec, W. et al. 1999. HFSA guidelines for management of patients with heart failure caused by left ventricular systolic dysfunction: pharmacological approaches. Heart Failure Society of America (HFSA) Practice Guidelines. Available at: http://www.hfsa.org. Accessed on August 10, 2002.

Brashers, V. 2002. Alterations in cardiovascular function. In *Pathophysiology: the biologic basis for disease in adults and children*, 4th ed., eds. K. McCance and S. Huether, pp. 980–1047. St. Louis, Mo.: Mosby.

Chavey, W. 2000. The importance of beta blockers in the treatment of heart failure. *American Family Physician* 62(11): 2453–2462.

Chavey, W., Blaum, C., Bleske, B. et al. 2001a. Guidelines for the management of heart failure caused by systolic dysfunction. Part I: Guideline development, etiology, and diagnosis. *American Family Physician* 64(5):769–774.

_____. 2001b. Guidelines for the management of heart failure caused by systolic dysfunction. Part II: Treatment. *American Family Physician* 64(6):1045–1054.

Cohn, J. 2000. Heart failure: future treatment approaches. *American Journal of Hypertension* 13(5 Part 2):74S–78S.

Diller, P., and Smucker, D. 2000. Management of heart failure. *Primary Care* 27(3):651–675.

Haji, S., and Movahed, A. 2000. Update on digoxin therapy in congestive heart failure. *American Family Physician* 62(2): 409–416.

Halm, M., and Penque, S. 2000. Heart failure in women. *Progress in Cardiovascular Nursing* 15:121–135.

Heart Failure Society of America (HFSA). 2001. Statistics on heart failure. Available at: http://www.hfsa.org/pdf/ lvsd_heart_failure.pdf. Accessed on August 12, 2002.

Hunt, S., Baker, D., Chin, M. et al. 2001. ACC/AHA guidelines for the evaluation and management of chronic heart failure in the adult. A report of the American College of Cardiology/American Heart Association Task Force on Practice Guidelines. Available at: http://www.acc.org/ clinical/guidelines/failure/hf_index.htm. Accessed on August 10, 2002.

Kayser, S. 2000. Spironolactone in the management of congestive heart failure. *Progress in Cardiovascular Nursing* 15(4): 145–148.

Massie, B., and Amidon, T. 2002. Heart. In *Current medical diagnosis and treatment*, 41st ed., eds. L. Tierney, S. McPhee, and M. Papadakis, pp. 363–457. New York: Lange Medical Books/McGraw-Hill.

Ramahi, T. 2000. Beta blocker therapy for chronic heart failure. *American Family Physician* 62(10):2267–2274.

Richardson, L. 2001. Women and heart failure. *Heart and Lung* 30(2):87–97.

Riedinger, M., Dracup, K., Brecht, M. et al. 2001. Quality of life in patients with heart failure: Do gender differences exist? *Heart and Lung* 30(2):105–116.

Shamsham, F., and Mitchell, J. 2000. Essentials of the diagnosis of heart failure. *American Family Physician* 61(5): 1319–1328.

6-D

Hyperlipidemia

Hyperlipidemia refers to the elevation of plasma lipids, primarily cholesterol and triglyceride. In the liver, cholesterol and triglycerides are incorporated into lipoproteins, which transport lipids from the gastrointestinal tract into the plasma. There are three major types of lipoproteins, which are characterized by their protein and lipid content: high-density lipoprotein (HDL), low-density lipoprotein (LDL), and very low-density lipoprotein (VLDL).

Total cholesterol is the sum of HDL cholesterol, LDL cholesterol, and VLDL cholesterol levels. The classification of lipids is summarized in **Table 6D.1, Lipid Classification**. Most cholesterol is carried in LDL and most triglycerides in VLDL cholesterol. VLDL is computed by dividing the triglyceride level by 5.

Cholesterol is a necessary component of bile acid and steroid hormone production, and is essential for cell membrane formation. However, hyperlipidemia is a significant risk factor for atherosclerosis and coronary heart disease (CHD). While all cholesterols contribute to the development of atherosclerosis, LDL cholesterol is thought to be especially atherogenic due to the damage that elevated LDL levels can do to the vascular endothelium. Once cellular injury occurs, these cells stop producing prostaglandins and nitric oxide, which are necessary for vasodilation. LDL is ingested by macrophages; elevated LDL results in an increased number of macrophages, further contributing to narrowing of the vessel lumen. Macrophages that have ingested LDL become foam cells, forming a fatty streak within the vascular lumen that progresses to plaque (Brashers 2002). Cytokine release attracts additional inflammatory cells that weaken the fibrous cap of the plaque; plaque rupture results in an acute coronary event (e.g., myocardial infarction [MI]). Lowering LDL cholesterol levels slows plaque formation and, in some patients, induces plaque regression (Pradka 2000).

Conversely, HDL cholesterol is anti-atherogenic, conferring protection against the development of CHD. HDL levels are higher in women (by approximately 10 mg/dL) than in men across the lifespan (Yu et al. 2000), offering cardioprotection even in the presence of elevated LDL levels. Low HDL levels are a more significant predictor of CHD in women than are high LDL levels (Bales 2000). In addition, low HDL levels have been associated with hypertriglyceridemia, obesity, sedentary lifestyle, cigarette smoking, Type 2 diabetes, and certain medications (National Cholesterol Education Program [NCEP] Expert Panel 2001).

The effect of hyperlipidemia treatment on CHD risk in women is less well understood than in men because of a lack of

Table 6D.1. LIPID CLASSIFICATION

Classification of LDL Cholesterol		Classification of HDL Cholesterol		Classification of Total Cholesterol		Classification of Triglycerides	
<100 mg/dL	Optimal	<40 mg/dL	Low	<200 mg/dL	Desirable	<150 mg/dL	Normal
100–129	Near/above optimal	≥60	High (optimal)	200–239	Borderline high	150–199	Borderline high
130–159	Borderline high			≥240	High	200–499	High
160–189	High					≥500	Very high
≥190	Very high						

Source: National Heart, Lung, and Blood Institute. National Cholesterol Education Program Expert Panel. 2001. *Detection, evaluation, and treatment of high blood cholesterol in adults (Adult Treatment Panel III)*. National Institutes of Health Publication No. 01-3670.

long-term cohort studies that have included women (Rosenfeld 2000). In numerous studies of men, treatment of hyperlipidemia has been shown to decrease the incidence of MI, cerebrovascular accident (CVA), sudden death, and overall mortality. There is sufficient evidence that lipid-lowering therapy for secondary prevention (the reduction of cardiovascular events in patients with established CHD) is beneficial for women (Amsterdam et al. 1998, Bedinghaus et al. 2001, Sorrentino 2000). The efficacy of pharmacologic treatment in primary prevention, or risk reduction in women without known CHD, has yet to be definitively established. The Air Force/Texas Coronary Atherosclerosis Prevention Study did show some reduction in CHD risk in women who received lipid-lowering therapy, although no change in overall mortality was demonstrated (Farnier et al. 1998). The most recent NCEP Expert Panel recommends the same treatment for women and men for both primary and secondary prevention, although it suggests that providers, when making decisions about primary prevention, consider that women generally develop CHD later in life than men do (NCEP 2001).

The Postmenopausal Estrogen/Progestin Intervention (PEPI) Trial found that estrogen, with or without progestin, reduced LDL cholesterol levels and increased HDL cholesterol levels in women (Bales 2000). Unopposed estrogen was most effective, while the use of a progestin, especially medroxyprogesterone acetate, reduced (but did not eliminate) the favorable impact of estrogen on HDL levels. Cyclic micronized progestin used with estrogen provided a more desirable effect on HDL levels. However, recent studies (including the Heart and Estrogen/Progestin Replacement Study [HERS] and early data from the Women's Health Initiative) have failed to demonstrate the efficacy of hormone replacement therapy (HRT) in lowering CHD risk in postmenopausal women (Bales 2000, Grady et al. 2002, Hulley et al. 1998, Rossouw et al. 2002). Without more compelling evidence to support its use, HRT should not be initiated with the sole purpose of primary or secondary prevention of CHD.

The PEPI trial found that estrogen, with or without progestin, reduced LDL cholesterol levels and increased HDL cholesterol levels in women (Bales 2000). Unopposed estrogen was most effective, while the use of a progestin, especially medroxyprogesterone acetate, reduced (but did not eliminate) the favorable impact of estrogen on HDL levels. Cyclic micronized progestin used with estrogen provided a more desirable effect on HDL levels. However, recent studies (including the HERS and the Women's Health Initiative) have failed to demonstrate the efficacy of HRT in reducing CHD risk in postmenopausal women (Bales 2000, Grady et al. 2002, Hulley et al. 1998, Rossouw et al. 2002). Of note, the Women's Health Initiative study participants taking HRT experienced a 29% higher rate of CHD that did those taking a placebo (Rossouw et al. 2002). Without more compelling evidence to support its use, HRT should not be initiated with the sole purpose of primary or secondary prevention of CHD.

Hypertriglyceridemia is an independent risk factor for CHD in women as well as men. Hypertriglyceridemia is associated with obesity and overweight, sedentary lifestyle, cigarette smoking, excessive alcohol use, high carbohydrate diets, diseases such as Type 2 diabetes and metabolic syndrome (Syndrome X), specific medications (including steroids, estrogens, retinoids, and high doses of beta blockers), and inherited disorders (e.g., familial hypertriglyceridemia, familial hyperlipidemia) (NCEP 2001). Treatment begins with lifestyle changes, including exercise and dietary modification, and may include treatment of underlying causes as well as triglyceride and LDL cholesterol-lowering therapy (NCEP 2001).

DATABASE

SUBJECTIVE

→ Past medical history may include a history of hyperlipidemia:
- Elevated cholesterol levels:
  - Increased total cholesterol
  - Increased LDL
  - Increased triglycerides
→ Past medical history may include other conditions associated with hyperlipidemia:
- CHD
- Cerebrovascular disease
- CVA
- Transient ischemic attacks
- Diabetes mellitus
- Hypertension
- Obesity
- Hypothyroidism
- Renal disease:
  - Chronic renal failure
  - Nephrotic syndrome
- Peripheral vascular disease
- Anorexia nervosa
- Obstructive liver disease
- Cushing's syndrome
→ Medication history may include:
- Steroids (anabolic, glucocorticoid)
- Oral contraceptives/progestins
- Isotretinoin
- Cyclosporin
- Disulfiram
- Diuretics (short-term elevation of cholesterol)
- Beta blockers (short-term elevation of cholesterol; nonintrinsic sympathomimetic activity [non-ISA] agents only)
- Human immunodeficiency virus antiretrovirals
→ Family history may include:
- Hyperlipidemia:
  - Familial hypercholesterolemia
  - Familial hypertriglyceridemia
- Atherosclerotic vascular disease:
  - CHD (especially early onset)
  - Cerebrovascular disease
  - Peripheral vascular disease
→ Social history may include:
- Cigarette smoking
- Alcohol use
- Sedentary lifestyle
→ Dietary history may include:

- Excessive intake of high fat and/or high cholesterol foods:
  - By preference
  - Due to budgetary restrictions

OBJECTIVE

→ Most patients with hyperlipidemia exhibit no physical manifestations of this disorder.
→ Physical examination to include:
- Weight and height
- Blood pressure
- Skin examination to assess for:
  - Eruptive xanthomas (yellowish red papules)
  - Tendinous xanthomas (located on tendons)
- Eye examination to assess for:
  - Lipemia retinalis (yellowish blood vessels on fundoscopy)
- Cardiovascular examination to assess for:
  - Bruits
  - Signs of arterial insufficiency:
    - Absent or decreased pulses
    - Pale color on extremity elevation; dusky red color when extremity is dependent
    - Cool skin temperature
    - Extremities with thin, shiny skin; absent hair
    - Thick, ridged finger nails

ASSESSMENT

→ Hyperlipidemia:
- R/O genetic hypercholesterolemia
- R/O genetic hypertriglyceridemia

PLAN

DIAGNOSTIC TESTS

→ Lipid testing should be done after a 9–12 hour fast (preferably overnight).

Patients Without CHD

→ Screening guidelines for healthy women remain controversial. The guidelines recently released by the Adult Treatment Panel III [ATP III] (NCEP 2001) recommend that a complete fasting lipid profile (total cholesterol, HDL cho-

lesterol, LDL cholesterol, and triglycerides) be obtained once every five years in all adults 20 years old or older. Other sources (e.g., the American College of Physicians and the U.S. Preventive Services Task Force) do not recommend screening in healthy women until age 45 years, unless a strong family history suggests increased risk.
→ Some providers screen low-risk women by obtaining a total cholesterol level only or a total cholesterol and HDL level. A complete fasting lipid panel is obtained if total cholesterol is >200mg/dL or HDL is ≤40.
→ Some providers discontinue screening women without CHD for hyperlipidemia after age 75 years.

Patients With CHD

→ All patients with cardiovascular disease should be screened with a complete fasting lipid profile.

Diagnostic Follow-up

→ Once hyperlipidemia is established, additional testing for secondary causes should be undertaken if clinically indicated (e.g., testing for diabetes or thyroid disease).

TREATMENT/MANAGEMENT

Treatment and management are based on the recommendations of the NCEP Expert Panel (2001). Treatment is stepwise and is guided by the presence of known risk factors for CHD. (See **Table 6D.2, Risk Factors for CHD in Women with Hyperlipidemia.**) Current guidelines recommend that, before initiating treatment, 10-year absolute CHD risk (i.e., the probability that a woman will develop CHD within 10 years) be calculated using the Framingham table. (See **Table 6D.3, Estimate of 10-Year Risk for Women [Framingham Point Scores].**) Assessing 10-year absolute CHD risk identifies those patients who would benefit from more aggressive intervention (NCEP 2001). The guidelines also recommend that certain other conditions (summarized in **Table 6D.4, CHD Risk Equivalents**) be considered as CHD risk equivalents (i.e., equivalent to CHD in predicting clinical complications).

After the 10-year absolute CHD risk (including risk equivalents) is determined, a stepwise management program is initiated.

Table 6D.2. RISK FACTORS FOR CHD IN WOMEN WITH HYPERLIPIDEMIA

Age ≥55 years (or early menopause)
Hypertension (≥140/90 or on antihypertensive medication)
HDL <40 mg/dL (HDL ≥60 is considered a "negative" risk factor; when present, subtract 1 risk factor from total)
Family history of premature CHD: parent or first-degree relative, male <55 years old, female <65 years old
Cigarette smoking

Source: National Heart, Lung, and Blood Institute. National Cholesterol Education Program Expert Panel. 2001. *Detection, evaluation, and treatment of high blood cholesterol in adults (Adult Treatment Panel III)*. National Institutes of Health Publication No. 01-3670.

Step One

→ Determine the patient's lipid profile. Treatment strategies are determined by the patient's LDL.
→ Goals of therapy include:
  ▪ LDL to <160 mg/dL in patients with 0–1 risk factor for CHD
  ▪ LDL to <130 mg/dL in patients with 2 or more risk factors
  ▪ LDL to <100 mg/dL in patients with CHD or a CHD risk-equivalent

Step Two

→ If LDL is ≥160 mg/dL in patients with 0–1 risk factor, ≥130 in patients with 2 or more risk factors, or ≥100 in patients with CHD or a CHD risk equivalent, initiate therapeutic lifestyle changes:
  ▪ Dietary therapy
  ▪ Weight management
  ▪ More physical activity

Table 6D.3.   ESTIMATE OF 10-YEAR RISK FOR WOMEN (FRAMINGHAM POINT SCORES)

Age	Points
20–34	-7
35–39	-3
40–44	0
45–49	3
50–54	6
55–59	8
60–64	10
65–69	12
70–74	14
75–79	16

Total Cholesterol	Points				
	Age 20–39	40–49	50–59	60–69	70–79
<160	0	0	0	0	0
160–199	4	3	2	1	1
200–239	8	6	4	2	1
240–279	11	8	5	3	2
≥280	13	10	7	4	2

	Points				
	Age 20–39	40–49	50–59	60–69	70–79
Nonsmoker	0	0	0	0	0
Smoker	9	7	4	2	1

HDL (mg/dL)	Points
≥60	-1
50–59	0
40–49	1
<40	2

Systolic BP (mmHg)	If Untreated	If Treated
<120	0	0
120–129	1	3
130–139	2	4
140–159	3	5
≥160	4	6

Point Total	10-Year Risk %
<9	<1
9	1
10	1
11	1
12	1
13	2
14	2
15	3
16	4
17	5
18	6
19	8
20	11
21	14
22	17
23	22
24	27
≥25	≥30

Source: National Heart, Lung, and Blood Institute. National Cholesterol Education Program Expert Panel. 2001. *Detection, evaluation, and treatment of high blood cholesterol in adults (Adult Treatment Panel III)*. National Institutes of Health Publication No. 01-3670.

Table 6D.4.   CHD RISK EQUIVALENTS

Diabetes mellitus

Atherosclerosis
  Carotid artery disease (symptomatic)
  Peripheral arterial disease
  Abdominal aortic aneurysm

Multiple risk factors that confer >20% 10-year risk for CHD: See **Table 6D.3**, which includes age, total cholesterol, HDL, blood pressure, and cigarette smoking.

Source: National Heart, Lung, and Blood Institute. National Cholesterol Education Program Expert Panel. 2001. *Detection, evaluation, and treatment of high blood cholesterol in adults (Adult Treatment Panel III)*. National Institutes of Health Publication No. 01-3670.

→ The goal of dietary therapy is to decrease the intake of saturated fats and cholesterol. Dietary therapy is difficult for patients to follow for any length of time, and long-term effects are usually modest (0–17% LDL reduction in a variety of studies [Yu et al. 2000]). Results can vary greatly among patients. In considering dietary modification, it is important to balance the need for osteoporosis prevention with the need for fat and cholesterol reduction. (See **Table 6D.5, Dietary Recommendations for Hyperlipidemia**.)

  ▪ Very-low-fat diets can lower HDL cholesterol as well as LDL; the net effect on CHD risk is unclear.

→ Re-evaluation after six weeks of dietary therapy:

  ▪ If LDL cholesterol is decreased to the desired level, continue therapeutic lifestyle changes and assess every 4–6 months for adherence.

  ▪ If the desired LDL cholesterol level is not achieved, reinforce the need to decrease saturated fat and cholesterol intake and increase fiber. Consider referral to a dietician. Recheck LDL in six weeks.

  ▪ If the desired LDL level still is not achieved, consider drug therapy and referring the patient to a dietician. Evaluate the patient for other causes of hyperlipidemia. Stress exercise and weight management.

Step Three

→ Consult drug therapy guidelines. (See **Table 6D.6, Drug Therapy for Hyperlipidemia**.)

→ Drug therapy is an adjunct to ongoing therapeutic lifestyle changes, which should be continually encouraged and reinforced.

→ Medications available include HMG-CoA reductase inhibitors ("statins"), nicotinic acid, fibric acid derivatives ("fibrates"), and bile acid sequestrants. (See **Table 6D.6**.)

  ▪ Numerous studies have demonstrated the efficacy of statins, which decrease LDL by 15–25%. These drugs should be the first choice for isolated hypercholesterolemia. Statins have been shown to be as efficacious in women as in men and prevent coronary events in women with and without CHD. (Bales 2000). Some statins also are beneficial for treating hypertriglyceridemia. Statins are expensive, although newer agents on the market are less so

(Yu et al. 2000). Applications are pending to make some agents available over-the-counter.

  ▪ Initiation of drug therapy for elevated LDL cholesterol:

  • If LDL is ≥130 mg/dL in the presence of CHD or a CHD risk equivalent, begin drug therapy.

  • If LDL is 100–129 mg/dL, consider drug therapy in the presence of CHD or a CHD risk equivalent.

  • If LDL is ≥130 mg/dL (with a 10–20% 10-year risk) or ≥160 mg/dL (with a <10% 10-year risk) in the presence of 2 or more CHD risk factors, begin drug therapy.

  • If LDL is ≥190 mg/dL in the absence of CHD risk factors, begin drug therapy.

  • If LDL is 160–189 mg/dL in the absence of CHD risk factors, consider drug therapy.

  ▪ Initiation of drug therapy for elevated triglycerides:

  • The first step is reducing LDL to an optimal level, as above, in conjunction with exercise and weight management.

  • If triglyceride level is <200 mg/dL, no treatment is indicated.

  • If triglyceride level is 200–400 mg/dL, begin therapeutic lifestyle changes (including alcohol restriction) and consider drug treatment in high-risk patients.

  • If triglyceride level is 400–1,000 mg/dL, begin treatment.

  • If triglyceride level is >1,000 mg/dL, begin vigorous treatment, including medication, a very-low-fat diet, avoidance of alcohol, and treatment of underlying conditions.

CONSULTATION

→ A registered dietician can facilitate dietary instruction and planning of meals.

→ Patients with severe hyperlipidemia should be referred to a lipid specialist, as hyperlipidemia frequently is associated with inherited conditions and is likely to require complex pharmacologic management.

→ See additional consultation/referral under "Treatment/ Management" and "Follow-up."

→ As needed for prescription(s).

Table 6D.5.   DIETARY RECOMMENDATIONS FOR HYPERLIPIDEMIA

Saturated fat	<7% of calories
Monounsaturated fat	≤20% of calories
Polyunsaturated fat	≤10% of calories
Total fat	25–30% of calories
Dietary cholesterol	<200 mg/day
Fiber	20–30 g/day
Total calories	As necessary to achieve and maintain ideal body weight

Source: National Heart, Lung, and Blood Institute. National Cholesterol Education Program Expert Panel. 2001. *Detection, evaluation, and treatment of high blood cholesterol in adults (Adult Treatment Panel III)*. National Institutes of Health Publication No. 01-3670.

Table 6D.6.   DRUG THERAPY FOR HYPERLIPIDEMIA

Drug Class	Mechanism of Action	Lipid Effects	Drugs and Doses	Adverse Effects	Monitoring/Comments

HMG-CoA Reductase Inhibitors (Statins)	Inhibits HMG-CoA reductase, a rate-limiting step in cholesterol synthesis	↓ total cholesterol
		↓ LDL
		↓ TG
		Minimal ↑ HDL
			1) Atorvastatin
			   Start: 10 mg @ HS
			   Max: 80 mg @ HS
			2) Cerivastatin
			   Start: 0.2 mg @ HS
			   Max: 0.4 mg @ HS
			3) Fluvastatin
			   Start: 20 mg @ HS
			   Max: 40 mg @ HS
			4) Lovastatin
			   Start: 20 mg @ HS
			   Max: 40 mg BID
			5) Pravastatin
			   Start: 10 mg @ HS
			   Max: 40 mg @ HS
			6) Simvastatin
			   Start: 10 mg @ HS
			   Max: 40 mg @ HS
				CNS: headaches
				GI: nausea, vomiting, abdominal pain, bowel alterations
				MSK: myalgias
				Skin: rash
				Lab: ↑ LFTs, ↑ CK (especially when co-administered with fibrate).
				Numerous drug interactions. Some statins metabolized by cytochrome p450 system.
					Obtain baseline LFTs. Recheck at 6 and 12 weeks, then every 6 months. Recheck after dosage adjustment. Discontinue drug if LFTs ≥3x normal. Recheck fasting lipids 4 weeks after start. Best-tolerated agents, considered first-line. Avoid with active liver disease. Use with fibrates with extreme caution.

Nicotinic Acid	Unknown.
	↓ VLDL synthesis in liver
	↓ LDL synthesis
		↓ total cholesterol
		↓ LDL
		↓ HDL
		↓ TG
			1) Niacin (OTC)
			   Start: 50–100 mg x 1 week; double dose every week to 1,000–1,500 mg in 2–3 divided doses.
			   If inadequate response, increase dose to max of 3 g/day.
			2) Extended-release nicotinic acid
			   Start: 500 mg @ HS
			   Max: 2 g @ HS
			   Increase by no more than 500 mg/month.
				GI: nausea, vomiting, diarrhea, peptic ulcer exacerbation
				Skin: flushing
				Lab: ↑ LFTs,
				   ↑ glucose,
				   ↑ uric acid
					Obtain baseline LFTs. Recheck every 6 weeks until optimal dose achieved, then every 3–6 months. Discontinue drug if LFTs ≥3x normal. Flushing may be minimized by premedication with ASA or ibuprofen 30 minutes before dose. Avoid with active liver disease and peptic ulcer disease.

Fibric Acid Derivatives (Fibrates)	↑ activity of lipoprotein lipase
	↓ VLDL synthesis
	
	↑ catabolism of LDL
		↓ VLDL
		↓ TG
		↑ HDL
			1) Gemfibrozil
			   Start: 600 mg BID
			   Max: 1,600 mg in divided doses.
			   Take 30 minutes before meals.
			
			2) Fenofibrate
			   Start: 67 mg daily at main meal
			   Max: 201 mg daily at main meal
			   Increase dose at 1-month intervals as tolerated.
				CNS: vertigo, headache
				GI: gallstones, nausea, vomiting, dyspepsia, abdominal pain
				MSK: myalgias, arthralgias
				Skin: rash
				Lab: ↑ LFTs,
				   ↑ CK (especially when given with statin),
				   ↓ WBC, ↓ Hgb/Hct
					Obtain baseline LFTs and CK.
					Periodic monitoring of LFTs.
					Avoid in severe liver or renal disease and pre-existing gallbladder disease.
					Co-administer with statins with extreme caution.

Bile Acid Resins	Combine with bile in the intestine, forming insoluble complexes excreted in stool	↓ total cholesterol
		↓ LDL
			1) Cholestyramine
			   Start: 4 g/day in divided doses.
			   Increase dose at 1-month intervals as tolerated.
			   Max: 24 g/day
			2) Colestipol
			   Start: 10 g/day
			   Max: 30 g/day
				GI: constipation, bloating, gas
				Lab: ↑ LFTs (rarely)
					Check lipid levels at 2–4 weeks.
					Interferes with absorption of various vitamins and minerals.
					Decreases absorption of numerous medications.
					May require laxatives for constipation.
					Not well-tolerated.

Medications are listed in order of compliance (e.g., statins with best compliance, bile acids with least compliance).

ASA = aspirin
BID = twice daily
CK = creatine kinase
CNS = central nervous system

GI = gastrointestinal
HDL = high-density lipoprotein
HMG-CoA = hydroxymethylglutaryl CoA
HS = at bedtime

LDL = low-density lipoprotein
LFTs = liver function tests
MSK = musculoskeletal
OTC = over the counter

TC = total cholesterol
TG = triglycerides
VLDL = very low-density lipoprotein
WBC = white blood count

Source: Compiled from Miller, J. 2002. Disorders of lipid metabolism. In *Integrated pharmacology*, 2nd ed., eds. C. Page, M. Curtis, M. Sutter et al., pp. 300–304. New York: Mosby; Safeer, R., and Lacivita, C. 2000. Choosing drug therapy for patients with hyperlipidemia. *American Family Physician* 61(11):3371–3382.

PATIENT EDUCATION

→ Educate the patient regarding the correlation between hyperlipidemia and CHD. Advise the patient that hyperlipidemia is a risk factor that she can modify. This requires a life-long commitment.

→ Advise the patient that many dietary aids are available to help plan low-cholesterol meals, including cookbooks from the American Heart Association and other sources, cholesterol counters, and the cholesterol and fat information on most food labels.

→ Educate the patient regarding specific dietary planning, taking into consideration individual food preferences and budgetary restrictions. (See Section 16, **General Nutrition Guidelines.**)

→ Advise the patient that regular aerobic exercise, quitting smoking (if applicable), and weight loss (if she is obese) can raise desirable HDL.

→ If drug therapy is initiated, advise the patient that maximal dietary modification still is necessary.

→ If drug therapy is initiated, provide detailed information regarding side effects and specific measures to monitor and manage them. (See **Table 6D.6.**)

FOLLOW-UP

→ Maintain contact with the patient to encourage treatment adherence, as compliance with therapy is often difficult (Safeer et al. 2000). At every visit, encourage patients to continue with diet and pharmacologic therapy as indicated.

→ Schedule frequent visits for those women who have trouble meeting dietary, weight, and LDL goals.

→ Obtain serum cholesterol from all healthy women once every five years.

→ For women on dietary modification, recheck lipid levels every 4–6 months to assess compliance.

→ For women on pharmacologic therapy, lipid reassessment depends on the specific agent used. (See **Table 6D.6.**)

→ Document in progress notes and on problem list.

BIBLIOGRAPHY

Amsterdam, E. and Deedwania, P. 1998. A perspective on hyperlipidemia: concepts of management in the prevention of coronary artery disease. *American Journal of Medicine* 105(1A):69S–74S.

Bales, A. 2000. In search of lipid balance in older women. *Postgraduate Medicine* 108(7):57–71.

Bedinghaus, J., Leshan, L., and Diehr, S. 2001. Coronary artery disease prevention: What's different for women? *American Family Physician* 63(7):1393–1400, 1405–1406.

Brashers, V. 2002. Alterations in cardiovascular function. In *Pathophysiology: the biologic basis for disease in adults and children*, 4th ed., eds. K. McCance and S. Huether. St. Louis, Mo.: Mosby.

Farnier, M., and Davignon, J. 1998. Current and future treatment of hyperlipidemia: the role of statins. *American Journal of Cardiology* 82(4B):3J–10J.

Grady, D., Herrington, D., Bitner, V. et al. 2002. Cardiovascular disease outcome during 6.8 years of hormone therapy: Heart and Estrogen/Progestin Replacement Study (HERS II). *Journal of the American Medical Association* 288(1):49–57.

Hulley, S., Grady, D., Bush, T. et al. 1998. Randomized trial of estrogen plus progestin for secondary prevention of coronary heart disease in postmenopausal women. *Journal of the American Medical Association* 280(7):605–613.

Miller, J. 2002. Disorders of lipid metabolism. In *Integrated pharmacology*, 2nd ed., eds. C. Page, M. Curtis, M. Sutter et al., pp. 300–304. New York: Mosby.

National Heart, Lung, and Blood Institute. National Cholesterol Education Program Expert Panel. 2001. *Detection, evaluation, and treatment of high blood cholesterol in adults (Adult Treatment Panel III)*. National Institutes of Health Publication No. 01-3670.

Pradka, L. 2000. Lipids—how low do you go: plaque regression and passivation. *Journal of Cardiovascular Nursing* 15(1):43–53.

Rosenfeld, J. 2000. Heart disease in women: gender-specific statistics and prevention strategies for a population at risk. *Postgraduate Medicine* 107(6):111–116.

Rossouw, J., Anderson, G., Prentice, R. et al. 2002. Risks and benefits of estrogen plus progestin in healthy postmenopausal women: principal results from the Women's Health Initiative randomized controlled trial. *Journal of the American Medical Association* 288(3):321–333.

Safeer, R., and Lacivita, C. 2000. Choosing drug therapy for patients with hyperlipidemia. *American Family Physician* 61(11):3371–3382.

Sorrentino, M. 2000. Cholesterol reduction to prevent CAD. *Postgraduate Medicine* 108(7):40–52.

Yu, J., Cunningham, J., Thouin, S. et al. 2000. Hyperlipidemia. *Primary Care* 27(3):541–587.

6-E

Hypertension

High blood pressure, or *hypertension* (HTN), is defined as a systolic blood pressure (SBP) of ≥140 mmHg or a diastolic blood pressure (DBP) ≥90 mmHg (Joint National Committee [JNC] [JNC VI] 1997). Blood pressure is determined by cardiac output (CO) and peripheral vascular resistance (PVR). Any condition that raises CO, which is controlled by heart rate and stroke volume, or PVR will result in elevated blood pressure. In nonhypertensive patients, blood pressure homeostasis is appropriately regulated by the renin-angiotensin-aldosterone system and the sympathetic nervous system. Renin, secreted by the renal cortex, is released when the kidney senses a decrease in renal blood flow (as a marker for decreased CO and blood pressure). Renin splits angiotensinogen to form angiotensin I, which is catalyzed by angiotensin-converting enzyme (ACE) to angiotensin II. Angiotensin II stimulates the adrenal glands to release aldosterone, which acts directly on the renal tubules to increase sodium reabsorption (Brashers 2002). These mechanisms increase plasma volume, which in turn raises stroke volume and cardiac output, and subsequently blood pressure. Angiotensin II, a potent vasoconstrictor, also raises blood pressure by increasing PVR.

The sympathetic nervous system also regulates blood pressure. Heightened sympathetic activity results in an increase in cardiac output, elevating blood pressure. An increase in blood flow also leads to increased vascular resistance.

HTN is classified as either *essential* (or *primary*) or *secondary*. In essential HTN (95% of cases), no specific cause can be determined. While our understanding of the multifactorial nature of essential HTN has broadened in the last decade, the exact mechanisms remain elusive. A number of genetic and environmental factors likely contribute to the development of essential HTN. These factors include:

→ Family history: A family history of one or both parents with HTN increases the likelihood of developing HTN. There may be genetic inheritance of defects in *natriuresis* (renal sodium excretion), intracellular sodium and/or calcium transport, or sympathetic nervous system response to stimuli (Massie 2002).

→ Aging: The risk of HTN increases as women age. HTN typically develops 5–20 years after menopause, making it likely that other factors in addition to lack of estrogen are responsible (Reckelhoff 2001).

→ Sodium sensitivity: Long debated, the role of "salt sensitivity" remains unclear. Studies do show an association between sodium intake and level of blood pressure (JNC 1997, Peters et al. 2000). Women and those who are elderly, African Americans, and diabetics seem most sensitive to the fluid retention resulting from excess sodium. The typical American diet averages >150 mmol/day of sodium (nearly 4 g); in cultures where sodium intake is <100 mmol/day, HTN is rare (Peters et al. 2000).

→ Increased sympathetic nervous system activity: Hyperactivity of the sympathetic nervous system has been implicated in the pathogenesis of HTN (Smith et al. 2002). Overstimulation of both α-adrenergic and β-adrenergic receptors leads to vasoconstriction, increased CO, and increased blood pressure. While excess levels of plasma norepinephrine are found in essential HTN, the correlation with blood pressure is poor (Massie 2002).

→ Excessive alcohol intake: Drinking three or more alcoholic drinks per day is associated with an increase in blood pressure as well as stroke. While the exact mechanism is unknown, the effect may be a result of increased catecholamine release (Massie 2002). Women typically weigh less than men, absorb more alcohol than their male counterparts, and are more susceptible to the effects of alcohol. The association between excessive alcohol intake and HTN is most pronounced in women older than 49 years (Frazier 2000).

→ Obesity: Obesity raises blood pressure by increasing vascular volume and cardiac output (Massie 2002). A body mass index (BMI) ≥27 correlates with blood pressure elevation (JNC 1997). Additionally, a waist circumference ≥34 inches in women is associated with HTN, as well as with insulin resistance and dyslipidemia.

→ Sedentary lifestyle: Lack of exercise predisposes women to obesity and HTN. Women who are sedentary have a 20–50% higher risk of developing HTN than do active women (JNC 1997). Exercise enhances weight loss, decreases all-cause mortality, and lowers blood pressure, perhaps by depressing sympathetic activity (Frazier 2000).

→ Cigarette smoking: Nicotine acutely raises both SBP and DBP, but the effect is transient. However, it is well-established that smoking increases the risk of cardiovascular disease.

In the remaining cases (approximately 5%), there is an identifiable cause of hypertension. While uncommon, women younger than 35 years who develop HTN are more likely to have *secondary hypertension* than essential HTN (Dumas 1999). Causes of secondary HTN include:

→ Renal disorders:
  - Most common cause of secondary hypertension (Massie 2002)
  - Disorders of the renal parenchyma:
    - Glomerular disease
    - Tubal interstitial disease
    - Polycystic kidney disease
    - Diabetic nephropathy
  - Stenosis of the renal arteries:
    - Atherosclerotic vascular disease

→ Endocrine disorders:
  - Hyper/hypothyroidism
  - Hypercalcemia
  - Adrenal disease:
    - Adrenal adenoma
    - Congenital adrenal hyperplasia
    - Glucocorticoid excess (e.g., Cushing's syndrome)
  - Pheochromocytoma

→ Drug use:
  - Estrogen
  - Steroids
  - Stimulants
  - Nonsteroidal anti-inflammatory drugs (NSAIDs)

→ Pregnancy-induced hypertension

→ Coarctation of the aorta:
  - Congenital aortic narrowing, usually discovered in childhood or adolescence

→ Neurological disorders

Isolated systolic HTN, defined as a SBP ≥140 mmHg and a DBP <90 mmHg, is a common finding in the elderly (Hall 1999). Affecting nearly 20% of those 80 years old or older, an elevated SBP results from an increase in PVR, CO, or both. Commonly, vascular stiffness (poor compliance) from atherosclerosis leads to an increased PVR, elevating blood pressure. Aortic valve calcification often develops as part of the normal aging process, requiring an increased CO to maintain forward flow through the narrowing valve. Previously thought to be a benign reflection of "aging" blood vessels, isolated systolic HTN is a known risk factor for cardiovascular disease and stroke (Moser 1999).

An elevated blood pressure detected only in the office setting is often referred to as *white coat HTN*. As many as 30% of patients with office blood pressure readings >140/90 have normal readings outside of the office setting (Kaplan 1998). Traditionally, white coat HTN has been considered a transient phenomenon, with no treatment deemed necessary. However, recent evidence suggests that white coat HTN may not be entirely benign. Central sympathetic hyperactivity does occur, which may lead to target organ damage and may represent a prehypertensive state (Smith et al. 2002).

HTN is a preventable and treatable cause of cardiovascular morbidity and mortality. Complications of HTN include the development of target organ damage (TOD), such as left ventricular hypertrophy (LVH); coronary heart disease (CHD); nephrosclerosis; and hypertensive retinopathy. Angina, myocardial infarction (MI), and stroke are all directly related to HTN and account for the high mortality associated with HTN.

HTN is the most common problem encountered in primary care, affecting 50 million Americans (Dumas 1999). Data from the third National Health and Nutrition Examination Survey (NHANES III) indicate that only 70% of hypertensives are aware of the diagnosis; half of these are receiving treatment but only one-quarter have blood pressure that is adequately controlled (<140/90) (Julius 2000). Increased public awareness and adoption of lifestyle changes in recent years have reduced the prevalence of HTN as well as the age-adjusted mortality rates from stroke and CHD. However, the age-adjusted incidence of stroke, end-stage renal disease, and heart failure continues to rise (Barker 2003).

Nearly 20% of women have HTN (Frazier 2000). Women of color are disproportionately afflicted: 32% of African American women and 21% of Mexican American women have HTN versus 18.3% of Caucasian women. African American women (and men) suffer an earlier onset of HTN, more severe HTN, more rapid progression to complications, and more TOD than do Caucasians (Peters et al. 2000).

Studies have shown that blood pressure is higher in younger men than age-matched females, likely due to the influence of testosterone. Yet after menopause, women's blood pressure continues to increase; approximately half of postmenopausal women in the United States are hypertensive (Affinito et al. 2001). By the age of 70–79 years, women have higher blood pressure than men do (Reckelhoff 2001). This contributes significantly to the age-related increase in MI, heart failure, and stroke seen in women (Rosenthal et al. 2000).

HTN in women has received less attention than has HTN in men. Most clinical trials published to date have enrolled mostly men, and studies have typically focused on outcomes as they relate to men (Rosenthal et al. 2000). Fortunately, more women are now being enrolled in clinical trials; results obtained in the coming years should highlight gender differences affecting the management of HTN.

DATABASE

SUBJECTIVE

→ Most patients are asymptomatic but may complain of headaches, blurred vision, dizziness, tinnitus, chest pain, shortness of breath, nausea, edema, and/or anxiety.

→ Medical history may include:

- Elevated blood pressure. Elicit information regarding:
  - Level of elevation
  - Duration of elevation
- Hypertension. Elicit information regarding:
  - Type of therapy
  - Length of therapy
  - Efficacy of treatment
  - Side effects of pharmacological therapy
- Diabetes
- Hyperlipidemia
- CHD
- Heart failure
- Cerebrovascular disease
- Peripheral vascular disease
- Renal disease
- Obesity
- Menopause

→ Medication history may include the following:
- Estrogen:
  - Oral contraceptives
  - Hormone replacement therapy
- Steroids
- NSAIDs
- Decongestants
- Appetite suppressants
- Tricyclic antidepressants
- Monoamine oxidase inhibitors
- Cocaine
- Amphetamines
- Cyclosporine
- Erythropoietin

→ Family history may include:
- Hypertension
- Premature CHD
- Hyperlipidemia
- Stroke
- Diabetes
- Renal disease

→ Social history:
- May include the use of:
  - Tobacco products
  - Alcohol
  - Caffeine
  - Recreational drugs
- Obtain information about:
  - Activity level
    - Quantify the amount of aerobic exercise per week.
  - Ethnicity, food habits
    - Obtain a description of usual diet, noting sodium intake, highly processed and fast food intake, and total calories.
  - Emotional stressors
    - Obtain a description of stressors and coping mechanisms.
  - Economic situation, occupation
    - Include information about job stress and the ability to pay for health care and medicines.

OBJECTIVE

→ Physical examination to include:
- Vital signs:
  - Blood pressure in both arms, sitting and standing
    - An appropriate size cuff should be used; the cuff bladder should encircle at least 80% of the upper arm.
    - The average of two or more readings, separated by two or more minutes.
    - The patient should avoid smoking or drinking caffeine for 30 minutes before blood pressure is taken, and should rest for five minutes before blood pressure is taken (Massie 2002).
    - Measure blood pressure in the legs if lower extremity pulses are decreased.
  - Heart rate, respiratory rate
  - Obtain height and weight, waist circumference
    - Calculate BMI (weight in kg divided by height in meters squared); ≥27 is associated with elevated blood pressure.
- Fundoscopic examination to assess for spasm or thickening of arteriolar walls, silver wire arterioles, copper wire arterioles, and arteriovenous (AV) nicking
- Neck examination to assess for jugular vein distention, carotid bruits, and an enlarged thyroid
- Chest examination to assess for rales, rhonchi, and wheezes
- Heart examination to assess rate, rhythm, murmurs, gallops, rubs, thrills, heaves, and increased or displaced point of maximal impulse (PMI)
- Abdomen examination to assess for aortic bruit, renal artery bruit, iliac bruit, hepatomegaly, increased kidney size, abnormal aortic pulsations, and hepatojugular reflex
- Extremity examination to assess for edema, clubbing, and cyanosis; bilateral comparison of peripheral pulses
- Neurological examination if there is any evidence of encephalopathy

ASSESSMENT

→ HTN
- Essential (primary) HTN
- R/O secondary HTN

PLAN

DIAGNOSTIC TESTS

→ Laboratory data:
- Before initiating pharmacological therapy, obtain baseline laboratory tests to rule out treatable causes of hypertension (as clinically indicated) and evaluate other cardiovascular risks. Laboratory tests are usually normal in uncomplicated cases of essential HTN.
- CBC, urinalysis, renal function tests (BUN, creatinine), electrolytes (potassium, sodium), fasting blood glucose,

fasting lipid panel (total cholesterol, high-density lipo-protein [HDL] cholesterol)

→ EKG:

- May show LVH or nonspecific ST-T wave abnormalities.

→ Chest x-ray:

- Usually normal, although it may show cardiomegaly, aortic dilatation or calcification, congestive heart failure; rarely, rib notching in coarctation of the aorta.
- May defer in uncomplicated HTN.

→ Echocardiography:

- Not routinely indicated. Consider it if there is clinical evidence of LVH, heart failure, or valvular disease.

→ Further studies:

- Intravenous pyelogram, renal sonogram, and thyroid tests are warranted only if symptoms suggest secondary hypertension. Consult with a physician.

TREATMENT/MANAGEMENT

→ HTN should be managed in a stepwise approach (JNC 1997):

- Determine the blood pressure stage:

	Systolic BP (mmHg)		Diastolic BP (mmHg)
Optimal	<120	and	<80
Normal	<130	and	<85
High Normal	130–139	or	85–89
Hypertension			
Stage 1	140–159	or	90–99
Stage 2	160–179	or	100–109
Stage 3	≥180	or	≥110

Source: Joint National Committee (JNC). 1997. *The sixth report of the Joint National Committee on the prevention, detection, evaluation, and treatment of high blood pressure (JNC VI).* National Institutes of Health Publication No. 98-4080.

- If a woman's systolic and diastolic blood pressures fall into different stages, the higher category is used to classify the blood pressure. The diagnosis of HTN is based on the average of two or more readings taken at each of two or more visits after the initial screening.
- Determine the risk group by major risk factors and target organ damage (TOD)/clinical cardiovascular disease (CCD):
  - Major risk factors:
    - Smoking
    - Dyslipidemia
    - Diabetes mellitus
    - Older than 60 years
    - Gender: postmenopausal women
    - Family history: women younger than 65 years, men younger than 55 years

- TOD/CCD:
  - Heart disease:
    - LVH
    - Angina or prior MI
    - Prior coronary artery bypass grafting
    - Heart failure
  - Stroke or transient ischemic attack
  - Nephropathy
  - Peripheral arterial disease
  - Hypertensive retinopathy

Risk Group A	No major risk factors No TOC/CCD
Risk Group B	At least one major risk factor (not including diabetes) No TOC/CCD
Risk Group C	TOC/CCD and/or diabetes with or without other risk factors

Source: Joint National Committee (JNC). 1997. *The sixth report of the Joint National Committee on the prevention, detection, evaluation, and treatment of high blood pressure (JNC VI).* National Institutes of Health Publication No. 98-4080.

- Determine treatment recommendations:

Blood Pressure (mmHg)	Risk Group A	Risk Group B	Risk Group C
High–Normal (130–139/ 85–89)	Lifestyle modification	Lifestyle modification	Drug therapy for those with heart failure, renal insufficiency or diabetes Lifestyle modification
Stage 1 (140–159/ 90–99)	Lifestyle modification (up to 12 months)	Lifestyle modification (up to 6 months) For patients with multiple risk factors, consider drugs as initial therapy plus lifestyle modification	Drug therapy Lifestyle modification
Stages 2 and 3 (≥160/≥100)	Drug therapy Lifestyle modification	Drug therapy Lifestyle modification	Drug therapy Lifestyle modification

Source: Joint National Committee (JNC). 1997. *The sixth report of the Joint National Committee on the prevention, detection, evaluation, and treatment of high blood pressure (JNC VI).* National Institutes of Health Publication No. 98-4080.

- Determine goal blood pressure:

Goal Blood Pressure	
<140/90 mmHg	Uncomplicated HTN, Risk Group A, Risk Group B, Risk Group C except for the following:
<130/85 mmHg	Diabetes, renal failure, heart failure
<125/75 mmHg	Renal failure with proteinuria >1 g/24 hours

Source: Joint National Committee (JNC). 1997. *The sixth report of the Joint National Committee on the prevention, detection, evaluation, and treatment of high blood pressure (JNC VI)*. National Institutes of Health Publication No. 98-4080.

- Refer to specific treatment recommendations as detailed below.

Lifestyle Modification

→ Lifestyle modifications should be initiated for all patients with HTN. For some patients, lifestyle changes will be definitive therapy; for others, they will be an adjunct to pharmacologic therapy. Recommendations include (JNC 1997):

- Smoking cessation to reduce cardiovascular risk
- Weight reduction, if indicated:
  - Even modest decreases in weight can lower blood pressure and improve the efficacy of antihypertensive medications (Niedfeldt 2002).
  - Increase vegetables and fruits, minimize saturated fats.
- Sodium restriction:
  - Restrict sodium intake to ≤100 mmol/day (2.4 gm/Na⁺, equivalent to 6 gm NaCl/day).
  - No salt added to cooking.
  - No salt added at the table.
  - Most sodium comes from processed foods; encourage the patient to read labels.
- Decrease alcohol consumption:
  - Limit alcohol to no more than 1 ounce (30 ml) of ethanol per day. One ounce ethanol = 2 ounces (60 ml) of 100-proof whiskey, 10 ounces (300 ml) of wine, and 24 ounces (720 ml) of beer.
  - Lighter weight women should limit alcohol intake to 0.5 ounces (15 ml) daily.
- Increase exercise:
  - Begin with 30 minutes 2–3 times per week and increase as tolerated.
  - Goal: at least 30–45 minutes of aerobic activity on most days of the week.
- Maintain adequate potassium intake:
  - 90 mmol/day
  - Vegetables and fruits provide adequate potassium for most patients.
- Increase calcium intake:
  - At least 800 mg/day
- Increase dietary potassium:
  - Fresh fruits, vegetables
- Maintain adequate intake of calcium and magnesium.
- Stress reduction techniques:
  - Breathing, deep muscle relaxation, meditation
  - The relationship between stress and the development of HTN is unclear. However, psychosocial stress and social isolation may increase the risk of HTN, especially in women (Levenstein et al. 2001). Stress reduction may improve a woman's sense of well-being and enhance her ability to make other lifestyle changes.

Pharmacologic Therapy

→ Pharmacologic therapy should be initiated immediately as indicated for Stages 2 and 3 HTN, as well as for those in Risk Group C (see above). After an appropriate trial of lifestyle modification (e.g., up to 12 months for Risk Group A/Stage 1 HTN, and up to 6 months for Risk Group B/Stage 1 HTN), pharmacologic therapy should be added if blood pressure remains below the goal.

- For uncomplicated HTN, begin with a diuretic or beta blocker unless there are compelling reasons to use other agents. Diuretics and beta blockers have been extensively studied and shown to reduce morbidity and mortality (JNC 1997). (See **Table 6E.1, Pharmacologic Therapy for Hypertension [Selected Agents]** and **Table 6E.2, Considerations for Individualizing Antihypertensive Drug Therapy**.)
- Begin with low dose of a long-acting, once-daily drug.
  - Once-daily dosing increases compliance and provides more consistent blood pressure control (Julius 2000).
- If an adequate response is not achieved:
  - Increase the dose of the current medication
    OR
  - Try a drug from another class
    OR
  - Add a second agent from a different class
    – Add a diuretic if one is not already being used.

NOTE: The Seventh Report of the Joint National Committee on the Prevention, Detection, Evaluation, and Treatment of High Blood Pressure (JNC VII) was originally scheduled for release in 2001. However, publication was suspended until the evaluation of the Antihypertensive and Lipid Lowering Treatment to Prevent Heart Attack Trial (ALLHAT), the largest randomized, double-blind, active-controlled HTN trial ever performed, which was completed in 2002. (This study has enrolled a large number of women.) It has been suggested that JNC VII will revise recommendations for initial drug therapy to include ACE-inhibitors, even in the absence of diabetes, as many clinicians currently consider them appropriate for first-line use (Basile 2001, Massie 2002). As this publication goes to press, the full JNC VII report is scheduled for release in Fall 2003.

CONSULTATION

→ Immediate referral is warranted in hypertensive emergencies:
- SBP >240 mmHg and/or DBP >130 mmHg (asymptomatic)

Table 6E.1.   PHARMACOLOGIC THERAPY FOR HYPERTENSION (SELECTED AGENTS)

Drug	Dosage (Initial/Maximum/ Frequency per Day)	Side Effects	Comments
Diuretics			
Thiazide			
Chlorthalidone	12.5 mg/50 mg (1)	$\downarrow$ K$^+$, Na$^+$, Mg$^+$; $\uparrow$ Ca$^+$ (may benefit postmenopausal women), uric acid, glucose, LDL (not indapamide), triglycerides (not indapamide); rash; erectile dysfunction in men	Act by interfering with Na$^+$ reabsorption in the distal tubule, $\downarrow$ blood volume; low doses well–tolerated without significant lab abnormalities; may need K$^+$ supplementation; inexpensive
Hydrochlorothiazide	12.5–25 mg/50 mg (1)		
Indapamide	1.25 mg/5 mg (1)		
Metolazone	2.5 mg/10 mg (1) (as Zaroxolyn®; dosing of other formulations varies)		
Loop			
Bumetanide	0.5 mg/4mg (2–3)	Same as thiazide diuretics, but higher risk of electrolyte abnormalities; hypotension; hearing loss (at high doses)	Act at Loop of Henle, enhance free water clearance; reserve furosemide for renal insufficiency
Ethacrynic acid	25 mg/100 mg (2–3)		
Furosemide	40 mg/320 mg (2–3)		
Torsemide	5 mg/100 mg (1–2)		
Potassium-Sparing			
Amiloride	5 mg/10 mg (1)	Risk of hyperkalemia, otherwise similar to thiazides; gynecomastia in men	Act on distal tubule
Spironolactone	25 mg/100 mg (1)		
Triamterene	25 mg/100 mg (1)		
Combination Products			
Amiloride 5 mg/ Hydrochlorothiazide 50 mg	(1–2)	Risk of hyperkalemia, otherwise similar to thiazides; GI disturbances; triamterene–renal dysfunction, stones; spirinolactone-gynecomastia in men	Multiple combinations available; limit use to women with need for potassium-sparing
Triamterene 50 mg/ Hydrochlorothiazide 25 mg	(1–2)		
Hydrochlorothiazide 25 mg/ Spirinolactone 25 mg	(1–2)		
Beta Blockers			
Acebutolol#*	200 mg /800 mg (1)	Fatigue, weakness, dizziness, bradycardia, heart block, hypotension; $\downarrow$ HDL, $\uparrow$ TG; avoid in bradycardia, advanced heart block, reactive airway disease; relatively contraindicated in diabetes (can mask symptoms of hypoglycemia)	Block β-adrenergic receptors in heart and lung; act by decreasing myocardial oxygen demand, lowering heart rate and cardiac output #Agents with intrinsic sympathomimetic activity (less bradycardia, fewer lipid changes) *Cardioselective agents (affect β$_1$ only)
Atenolol*	25 mg/100 mg (1–2)		
Betaxolol*	5 mg/20 mg (1)		
Bisoprolol*	2.5 mg/10 mg (1)		
Carteolol#	2.5 mg/10 mg (1)		
Metoprolol tartrate*	50 mg/300 mg (2)		
Metoprolol succinate*	50 mg/300 mg (1)		
Nadolol	40 mg/320 mg (1)		
Penbutolol#	10 mg/20 mg (1)		
Pindolol#	10 mg/60 mg (2)		
Propranolol	40 mg/480 mg (2)		
Propranolol LA	40 mg/480 mg (1)		
Timolol	20 mg/60 mg (2)		
ACE Inhibitors			
Benazepril	5 mg/40 mg (1–2)	Cough, dizziness, hyperkalemia, hypotension, impaired renal function Rare: angioedema, rash, hyperkalemia, altered taste, blood dyscrasias (leukopenia)	Block conversion of angiotensin I to angiotensin II Preferred for patients with diabetes and/or heart failure; cough is class side effect
Captopril	25 mg/150 mg (2–3)		
Enalapril	5 mg/40 mg (1–2)		
Fosinopril	10 mg/40 mg (1–2)		
Lisinopril	5 mg/40 mg (1)		
Moexipril	7.5 mg/15 mg (2)		
Quinapril	5 mg/80 mg (1–2)		
Ramipril	1.25 mg/20 mg (1–2)		
Trandolapril	1 mg/4 mg (1)		
Calcium Channel Blockers			
Nondihydropyridines			
Diltiazem	120 mg/360 mg (2)	Edema, headache, GI disturbances (nausea, constipation), conduction defects, heart failure (worsens systolic dysfunction), urinary frequency, gingival hypertrophy	Block calcium transport; relax smooth muscle, leading to peripheral vasodilation
Diltiazem LA	120 mg/360 mg (1)		
Mibefradil	50 mg/100 mg (1)		
Verapamil	90 mg/480 mg (2)		
Verapamil LA	120 mg/480 mg (1)		
Dihydropyridines			
Amlodipine	2.5 mg/10 mg (1)	Ankle edema, flushing, headache, gingival hypertrophy	As above
Felodipine	2.5 mg/20 mg (1)		
Isradipine	5 mg/20 mg (2)		
Nicardipine	60 mg/90 mg (2)		
Nifedipine	30 mg/120 mg (1)		
Nisoldipine	20 mg/60 mg (1)		

Source: Adapted from Joint National Committee (JNC). 1997. *The sixth report of the Joint National Committee on the prevention, detection, evaluation, and treatment of high blood pressure (JNC VI)*. National Institutes of Health Publication No. 98-4080.

Table 6E.2.   CONSIDERATIONS FOR INDIVIDUALIZING ANTIHYPERTENSIVE DRUG THERAPY

Indication	Drug Therapy
Compelling Indications Unless Contraindicated	
Diabetes mellitus (Type I) with proteinuria	ACE-I
Heart failure	ACE-I, diuretics
Isolated systolic hypertension (older women)	Diuretics (preferred), CCB (long-acting DHP)
Myocardial infarction	β-blocker (non-ISA), ACE-I (with systolic dysfunction)
May Have Favorable Effects on Comorbid Conditions	
Angina	β-blockers, CCB
Atrial tachycardia and fibrillation	β-blockers, CCB (non-DHP)
Cyclosporine-induced hypertension (caution with dose of cyclosporine)	CCB
Diabetes mellitus (Type I and II) with proteinuria	ACE-I (preferred), CCB
Diabetes mellitus (Type II)	Low-dose diuretics
Dyslipidemia	α-blockers
Essential tremor	β-blockers (noncardioselective)
Heart failure	Carvedilol, losartan potassium
Hyperthyroidism	β-blockers
Migraine	β-blockers (noncardioselective)
Myocardial infarction	Diltiazem, verapamil
Osteoporosis	Thiazides
Preoperative hypertension	β-blockers
Prostatism (benign prostatic hyperplasia)	α-blockers
Renal insufficiency (caution with renovascular hypertension and creatinine ≥3 mg/dL)	ACE-I
May Have Unfavorable Effects on Comorbid Condition (may be used with special monitoring unless contraindicated)	
Bronchospastic disease	β-blockers (contraindicated)
Depression	β-blockers, central α-agonists, reserpine (contraindicated)
Diabetes mellitus (Type I and II)	β-blockers, high-dose diuretics
Dyslipidemia	β-blockers (non-ISA), diuretics (high dose)
Gout	Diuretics
2° or 3° heart block	β-blockers (contraindicated), CCB (non-DHP contraindicated)
Heart failure	β-blockers (except carvedilol), CCB (except amlodipine, felodipine)
Liver disease	Labetalol, methyldopa (contraindicated)
Peripheral vascular disease	β-blockers
Pregnancy	ACE-I (contraindicated), angiotensin II receptor blockers (contraindicated)
Renal insufficiency	Potassium-sparing agents
Renovascular disease	ACE-I, angiotensin II receptor blockers

ACE-I = ACE inhibitor   CCB = calcium channel blocker   DHP = dihydropyridine   ISA = intrinsic sympathomimetic activity

Source: Adapted from Joint National Committee (JNC). 1997. *The sixth report of the Joint National Committee on the prevention, detection, evaluation, and treatment of high blood pressure (JNC VI)*. National Institutes of Health Publication No. 98-4080.

- SBP >200 mmHg and/or DBP >120 mmHg (symptomatic)
  - Associated with angina, CHF, headaches
- Hypertensive encephalopathy:
  - Headache, irritability, confusion, altered mental status, ± papilledema
- Hypertensive nephropathy:
  - Hematuria, proteinuria, renal dysfunction
→ Consultation or referral is recommended for refractory hypertension.
→ Consultation is recommended in suspected cases of secondary HTN.
→ As needed for prescription(s).

PATIENT EDUCATION

→ Educate the patient and family about the pathophysiology of hypertension.
→ Encourage the patient to monitor her blood pressure on a regular basis, involving the family as appropriate.
→ Encourage lifestyle modifications, sharing the rationale for each with the patient.
→ Support achievements, however small, at every visit.
→ Educate the patient regarding medication side effects and the importance of compliance.
  - Sexual dysfunction in women taking antihypertensives is not well-studied, despite the large numbers of women involved. One study by Duncan et al. (2000) found that hypertensive women suffered decreased vaginal lubrication, less frequent orgasm, and more pain, irrespective of the menopausal state or medication used. Discuss sexual dysfunction openly and provide alternate ways to deal with problems should they develop.
  - Many women with HTN are asymptomatic and unconvinced of the need for medication. After beginning treatment, they may develop side effects that prompt discontinuation of medication. Encourage medication compliance and be willing to adjust medications as needed.

FOLLOW-UP

→ Reassess blood pressure control and medication side effects within a time period—usually 1–8 weeks—to be determined by patient reliability, compliance, severity of HTN, and other medical problems.
→ If blood pressure control is inadequate, assess possible causes before changing the drug therapy:
  - Patient noncompliance
  - Subtherapeutic dosage of the medication
  - Use of other medications interfering with the efficacy of an antihypertensive
  - Unrecognized secondary hypertension
→ In patients with good response to medication, consider a trial of decreased dosage after six months to one year.
→ Document in progress notes and on problem list.

BIBLIOGRAPHY

Affinito, P., Palomba, S., Bonifacio, M. et al. 2001. Effects of hormonal replacement therapy in postmenopausal hypertensive patients. *Maturitas* 40:75–83.

Barker, L. 2003. Hypertension. In *Principles of ambulatory medicine*, 6th ed., eds. L. Barker, J. Burton, and P. Zieve, pp. 980–1018. Philadelphia: Lippincott Williams & Wilkins.

Basile, J. 2001. Hypertension 2001: pearls for the clinician. *Southern Medical Journal* 94(11):1054–1057.

Brashers, V. 2002. Alterations of cardiovascular function. In *Pathophysiology: the biologic basis for disease in adults and children*, 4th ed., eds. K. McCance and S. Huether, pp. 980–1047. St. Louis, Mo.: Mosby.

Dumas, M. 1999. Hypertension in primary care. *American Journal for Nurse Practitioners* 3(2):7–32.

Duncan, L., Lewis, C., Jenkins, P. et al. 2000. Does hypertension and its pharmacotherapy affect the quality of sexual function in women? *American Journal of Hypertension* 13(6):640–647.

Frazier, L. 2000. Factors influencing blood pressure: development of a risk model. *Journal of Cardiovascular Nursing* 15(1):62–79.

Hall, W. 1999. A rational approach to the treatment of hypertension in special populations. *American Family Physician* 60:156–162.

Joint National Committee (JNC). 1997. *The sixth report of the Joint National Committee on the prevention, detection, evaluation, and treatment of high blood pressure (JNC VI)*. National Institutes of Health Publication No. 98-4080.

Julius, L. 2000. Worldwide trends and shortcomings in the treatment of hypertension. *American Journal of Hypertension* 13(5 Part 2):57S–61S.

Kaplan, N. 1998. Treatment of hypertension: insights from the JNC VI report. *American Family Physician* 58(6):1323–1330.

Levenstein, S., Smith, M., and Kaplan, G. 2001. Psychosocial predictors of hypertension in men and women. *Archives of Internal Medicine* 161(10):1341–1346.

Massie, B. 2002. Systemic hypertension. In *Current medical diagnosis and treatment*, 41st ed., eds. L. Tierney, S. McPhee, and M. Papadakis, pp. 459–484. New York: Lange Medical Books/McGraw-Hill.

Moser, M. 1999. Hypertension treatment and the prevention of coronary heart disease in the elderly. *American Family Physician* 59(5):1248–1256.

Niedfeldt, M. 2002. Managing hypertension in athletes and physically active adults. *American Family Physician* 66(3):445–452, 457–458.

Peters, R., and Flack, J. 2000. Salt sensitivity and hypertension in African Americans: implications for cardiovascular nurses. *Progress in Cardiovascular Nursing* 15(4):138–144.

Reckelhoff, J. 2001. Gender differences in the regulation of blood pressure. *Hypertension* 37:1199–1208.

Rosenthal, T., and Oparil, S. 2000. Hypertension in women. *Journal of Human Hypertension* 14(10–11):691–704.

Smith, P., Graham, L., Mackintose, A. et al. 2002. Sympathetic neural mechanisms in white-coat hypertension. *Journal of the American College of Cardiology* 40(1):126–132.

6-F

Mitral Valve Prolapse

Mitral valve prolapse (MVP) is the abnormal displacement of one or both mitral valve leaflets into the left atrium during systole. Often asymptomatic and benign, MVP is the one of the most common valvular heart diseases. In the early 1980s, the Framingham study found a prevalence of 7.6% in women (as high as 17% in young women) and 2.5% in men (Savage et al. 1983). However, recently revised echocardiographic criteria for the diagnosis of MVP suggest the prevalence of MVP is approximately 3% (Freed et al. 1999, Singh et al. 2000). In the past, patients with normal mitral leaflets that appeared bowed or saddle-shaped on certain echocardiographic views were incorrectly identified as having MVP; only the presence on 2-D echocardiogram of systolic displacement of mitral leaflets beyond the plane of the mitral apparatus into the left atrium in the parasternal long-axis view meets diagnostic criteria for MVP. Some minor degree of displacement can be normal. Leaflets that are thickened and redundant are additional features of MVP, although they may not always be present (Liberthson 2000).

MVP may be classified as *primary* or *secondary*. Primary MVP, the most common form, may be inherited. It may also be associated with Marfan's syndrome and other connective tissue diseases. Secondary MVP may result from damage to the mitral valve apparatus (e.g., chordae tendineae) associated with myocardial infarction, rheumatic heart disease, or cardiomyopathy (Bonow et al. 1998).

The symptoms of MVP vary considerably. In most cases, MVP is an incidental finding not associated with other cardiac anomalies, and the patient remains asymptomatic with a normal life expectancy. However, a number of patients with MVP suffer from autonomic dysfunction, with palpitations being the most common complaint (Bouknight et al. 2000). The palpitations may be due to premature ventricular contractions, although often no arrhythmias are found on continuous ambulatory monitoring. Another frequent symptom is atypical chest pain, the exact cause of which is unclear. Dyspnea also may be noted, even when mitral regurgitation is absent and exercise testing reveals no evidence of exercise impairment (Bonow et al. 1998).

Neuropsychiatric symptoms, including manic depression and panic attacks, occur in a small number of patients with MVP. Although such symptoms previously were thought to be associated with MVP, recent studies suggest no correlation between the two (Shipton et al. 2001). Additionally, previous studies had reported an increased incidence of embolic stroke in patients with MVP. But according to revised criteria for MVP, the disorder is no more common in young stroke patients than in healthy individuals (Gillon et al. 1999).

Studies suggest a MVP complication rate of <2% per year (Bouknight et al. 2000). Although MVP represents a benign finding in most cases and has an excellent prognosis, patients with this disorder are at an increased risk for bacterial endocarditis, arrhythmias, and the development of mitral regurgitation (Singh et al. 2000). The risk of mitral regurgitation may be associated with the presence of obesity and hypertension, both of which place a hemodynamic burden on an already defective valve. Patients without mitral regurgitation are most likely at no increased risk for complications.

DATABASE

SUBJECTIVE

→ Symptoms may include:
  - Palpitations
  - Atypical chest pain unrelieved by rest or nitroglycerin and poorly correlated with exercise
  - Dyspnea on exertion
  - Shortness of breath
  - Dizziness/lightheadness
  - Fatigue
  - Hyperventilation
→ Past medical history may include:
  - Cardiac disease (e.g., rheumatic heart disease, endocarditis, pericarditis, arrhythmias)
  - Syncopal episodes
  - Endocrine disorders (e.g., thyroid disorders)
  - Anemia

- Connective tissue disorders
→ Family history may include:
  - Valvular heart disease
  - History of sudden death
  - Connective tissue disorders
→ Social history may include the use of:
  - Caffeine
  - Tobacco
  - Recreational drugs
→ Inquire about recent weight change.

OBJECTIVE

→ Physical examination to include:
  - Vital signs
  - Height and weight
→ Cardiac examination may include midsystolic click and late systolic murmur (*click/murmur syndrome*):
  - Midsystolic click (soft or loud, high-pitched, short duration) occurs with sudden tensing of the mitral valve apparatus as leaflets prolapse into the left atrium.
  - Late systolic murmur (medium- to high-pitched, loudest at apex, intensity varies)

- Maneuvers to elicit these findings:
  - The click moves toward S_1 and the murmur is accentuated with standing or Valsalva maneuvers that decrease left ventricular volume and increase mitral prolapse.
  - Conversely, the click/murmur moves toward S_2 and may even disappear with squatting or isometric exercises. These maneuvers enhance left ventricular volume by increasing venous return; the increased left ventricular volume helps maintain tension on the chordae tendineae and decreases prolapse.
→ If mitral regurgitation is present, the cardiac exam may include (Massie et al. 2002):
  - Prominent and hyperdynamic apical impulse to left of the midclavicular line
  - Forceful, brisk point of maximal impulse (PMI); systolic thrill over PMI
  - Midsystolic click; prominent S_3
  - Blowing, high-pitched pansystolic murmur heard maximally at the apex; radiates into left axilla, infrascapular area, and occasionally the base
→ Musculoskeletal exam to assess for:

Table 6F.1. CARDIAC CONDITIONS FOR WHICH ENDOCARDITIS PROPHYLAXIS IS RECOMMENDED

High Risk	Prosthetic cardiac valves, including bioprosthetic and homograft valves Previous bacterial endocarditis Complex cyanotic congenital heart disease (e.g., single ventricle states, transposition of the great arteries, tetralogy of Fallot) Surgically constructed, systemic-pulmonary shunts or conduits
Moderate Risk	Most other congenital cardiac malformations (other than those above and below) Acquired valvular dysfunction (e.g., rheumatic heart disease) Hypertrophic cardiomyopathy* Mitral valve prolapse with valvular regurgitation and/or thickened leaflets

*The American College of Cardiology/American Heart Association Task Force on Practice Guidelines (Committee on Management of Patients with Valvular Heart Disease) recommends prophylaxis in hypertrophic cardiomyopathy only when there is latent or resting obstruction.

Source: Adapted with permission from Taubert, K., and Dajani, A. 2001. Optimisation of the prevention and treatment of bacterial endocarditis. *Drugs and Aging* 18(6):415–424.

Table 6F.2. CARDIAC CONDITIONS FOR WHICH ENDOCARDITIS PROPHYLAXIS IS NOT RECOMMENDED

Negligible Risk*	Isolated secundum atrial septal defect Surgical repair of atrial septal defect, ventricular septal defect, or patent ductus arteriosus (without residua beyond 6 months) Previous coronary artery bypass graft surgery Mitral valve prolapse without valvular regurgitation Physiologic, functional, or innocent heart murmurs Previous Kawasaki disease without valvular dysfunction Previous rheumatic fever without valvular dysfunction Cardiac pacemakers (intravascular and epicardial) and implanted defibrillators Coronary stents

*No greater risk than the general population.

Source: Adapted with permission from Taubert, K., and Dajani, A. 2001. Optimisation of the prevention and treatment of bacterial endocarditis. *Drugs and Aging* 18(6):415–424.

- ■ Thoracic skeletal abnormalities:
  - ● Scoliosis
  - ● Narrow anterior-posterior (A-P) chest diameter
  - ● Signs of Marfan's syndrome
    - – Tall stature, with long arms and legs
    - – Pectus excavatum
    - – Joint laxity

ASSESSMENT

- → Mitral valve prolapse
- → R/O arrhythmias
- → R/O mitral regurgitation
- → R/O ischemia

PLAN

DIAGNOSTIC TESTS

- → Laboratory studies:
  - ■ Consider a complete blood count (CBC) to assess for anemia.
  - ■ Consider thyroid function studies to assess for hyperthyroidism. (See the **Thyroid Disorders** chapter in Section 10.)
- → EKG:
  - ■ Usually is normal in patients with MVP.
    - ● May see ST-T wave depression (inferior leads), T wave inversion, prolonged QT interval, prominent U waves (Bonow et al. 1998).
  - ■ Probably not necessary if the patient has asymptomatic click/murmur syndrome.

- → 2-D echocardiogram with Doppler flow study:
  - ■ Highly sensitive and specific
  - ■ The most useful noninvasive diagnostic test for MVP (Bonow et al. 1998)
  - ■ Useful in symptomatic patients for diagnosis and to determine the need for therapy
  - ■ Useful if the diagnosis is in question; consider for patients diagnosed with MVP before criteria revision (Freed et al. 1999) and who have no physical findings of MVP, to rule out the disorder.
  - ■ Not indicated if there are no physical findings of MVP, unless there is other evidence of structural heart disease or a strong family history of myxomatous valvular disease (Cheitlin et al. 1997).

TREATMENT/MANAGEMENT

Asymptomatic Patients

- → Reassurance
  - ■ Most patients are asymptomatic with an excellent prognosis.
- → Patients with MVP and valvular regurgitation and/or thickened leaflets should receive prophylaxis when undergoing certain procedures to prevent bacterial endocarditis. (See **Table 6F.1, Cardiac Conditions for Which Endocarditis Prophylaxis is Recommended**; **Table 6F.3, Procedures for Which Endocarditis Prophylaxis is Recommended**; and **Table 6F.4, Procedures for Which Endocarditis Prophylaxis is Not Recommended**.) Prophylaxis for

Table 6F.3.   PROCEDURES FOR WHICH ENDOCARDITIS PROPHYLAXIS IS RECOMMENDED

Dental Procedures[1]	Dental extractions Periodontal procedures including surgery, scaling and root planing, probing, recall maintenance Dental implant placement and reimplantation of avulsed teeth Endodontic (root canal) instrumentation or surgery only beyond the apex Subgingival placement of antibacterial fibers/strips Initial placement of orthodontic bands but not brackets Intraligamentary local anesthetic injections Prophylactic cleaning of teeth or implants where bleeding is anticipated
Respiratory Tract	Tonsillectomy and/or adenoidectomy Surgical operations that involve respiratory mucosa Bronchoscopy with a rigid bronchoscope
Gastrointestinal Tract[2]	Sclerotherapy for esophageal varices Esophageal stricture dilation Endoscopic retrograde cholangiography with biliary obstruction Biliary tract surgery Surgical operations that involve intestinal mucosa
Genitourinary Tract	Prostatic surgery Cystoscopy Urethral dilation

[1]Prophylaxis is recommended for high- and moderate-risk cardiac conditions.
[2]Prophylaxis is recommended for high-risk patients; optional for moderate-risk patients.

Source: Adapted with permission from Taubert, K., and Dajani, A. 2001. Optimisation of the prevention and treatment of bacterial endocarditis. *Drugs and Aging* 18(6):415–424.

patients with MVP and no valvular regurgitation is not recommended. (See **Table 6F.2, Cardiac Conditions for Which Endocarditis Prophylaxis is Not Recommended**.)
→ If indicated, provide bacterial endocarditis prophylaxis (Taubert et al. 2001):
- For dental, respiratory tract, or esophageal procedures:
  - Amoxicillin 2 g p.o. 1 hour before the procedure
  - If the patient is allergic to penicillins, clindamycin 600 mg p.o. 1 hour before the procedure, azithromycin 500 mg 1 hour before the procedure, or clarithromycin 500 mg 1 hour before the procedure
- For genitourinary or gastrointestinal (excluding esophageal) procedures:
  - Amoxicillin 2 g 1 hour before the procedure
  - If the patient is allergic to penicillins, vancomycin 1 g IV over 1–2 hours is recommended

Symptomatic Patients

→ Patients with palpitations, chest pain, and/or anxiety often respond to beta blocker therapy. (See the **Palpitations** chapter.)
→ Patients with dizziness and/or orthostatic symptoms:
- Increase fluids and dietary sodium.
- Recommend support stockings.
→ Bacterial endocarditis prophylaxis as above.

CONSULTATION

→ Symptomatic patients with click/murmur syndrome should be referred to a cardiologist for evaluation and/or managed in consultation with an internist.
→ Patients with physical findings of mitral regurgitation should be referred to a cardiologist or managed in consultation with an internist.
→ As needed for prescription(s).

Table 6F.4.   PROCEDURES FOR WHICH ENDOCARDITIS PROPHYLAXIS IS NOT RECOMMENDED

Dental Procedures	Restorative dentistry[1] (operative and prosthodontic) with or without retraction cord[2] Local anesthetic injections (nonintraligamentary) Intracanal endodontic treatment, postplacement and build-up Placement of rubber dams Postoperative suture removal Placement of removable prosthodontic/orthodontic appliances Taking of oral impressions Fluoride treatments Taking of oral radiographs Orthodontic appliance adjustment Shedding of primary teeth
Respiratory Tract	Endotracheal intubation Bronchoscopy with a flexible bronchoscope, with or without biopsy[3] Tympanostomy tube insertion
Gastrointestinal Tract	Transesophageal echocardiography[3] Endoscopy with or without gastrointestinal biopsy[3]
Genitourinary Tract	Vaginal hysterectomy[3] Vaginal delivery[3] Cesarean section
Genitourinary Tract (Uninfected Tissue)	Urethral catheterization Uterine dilatation and curettage Therapeutic abortion Sterilization procedures Insertion or removal of intrauterine devices
Other	Cardiac catheterization, including balloon angioplasty Implanted cardiac pacemakers, implanted defibrillators, and coronary stents Incision or biopsy of surgically scrubbed skin Circumcision

[1]Includes restoration of decayed teeth (filling cavities) and replacement of missing teeth.
[2]Clinical judgment may indicate antibacterial use in selected circumstances that may create significant bleeding.
[3]Prophylaxis is optional for high-risk patients.

Source: Adapted with permission from Taubert, K., and Dajani, A. 2001. Optimisation of the prevention and treatment of bacterial endocarditis. *Drugs and Aging* 18(6):415–424.

PATIENT EDUCATION

→ Reassure asymptomatic patients that this is a common condition that most often remains benign.

→ Advise asymptomatic patients that there is no need for medication, diet restriction, or limitation of activities.

FOLLOW-UP

→ Asymptomatic patients with absent or mild mitral regurgitation:

- Clinical evaluation every 3–5 years to assess for change in symptoms and the need for further studies. Serial echocardiograms are not necessary unless there is clinical evidence of development or worsening of mitral regurgitation (Cheitlin et al. 1997).

→ High-risk patients:

- A physical exam every year

→ Document in progress notes and on problem list.

BIBLIOGRAPHY

Bonow, R., Carabello, B., De Leon, A. et al. 1998. ACC/AHA guidelines for the management of patients with valvular heart disease. A report of the American College of Cardiology/American Heart Association Task Force on Practice Guidelines (Committee on Management of Patients with Valvular Heart Disease). *Journal of the American College of Cardiology* 32(5):1486–1588.

Bouknight, D., and O'Rourke, R. 2000. Current management of mitral valve prolapse. *American Family Physician* 61 (11):3343–3350, 3353–3354.

Cheitlin, M., Alpert, T., Armstrong, W. et al. 1997. ACC/AHA guidelines for the clinical application of echocardiography. A report of the American College of Cardiology/American Heart Association Task Force on Practice Guidelines (Committee on Clinical Application of Echocardiography). *Circulation* 95(6):1686–1744.

Freed, L., Levy, D., Levine, R. et al. 1999. Prevalence and clinical outcome of mitral valve prolapse. *New England Journal of Medicine* 341(1):1–7.

Gillon, D., Buonanno, F., Joffe, M. et al. 1999. Lack of evidence of an association between mitral valve prolapse and stroke in young patients. *New England Journal of Medicine* 341(1):8–13.

Liberthson, R. 2000. Management of valvular heart disease. In *Primary care medicine: office evaluation and management of the adult patient*, 4th ed., eds. A. Goroll and A. Mulley, pp. 227–236. Philadelphia: Lippincott Williams & Wilkins.

Massie, B., and Amidon, T. 2002. Heart. In *Current medical diagnosis and treatment*, 41st ed., eds. L. Tierney, S. McPhee, and M. Papadakis, pp. 363–457. New York: Lange Medical Books/McGraw-Hill.

Savage, D., Garrison, R., Devereus, R. et al. 1983. Mitral valve prolapse in the general population: epidemiologic features. The Framingham Study. *American Heart Journal* 106(3): 571–576.

Shipton, B., and Wahba, H. 2001. Valvular heart disease: review and update. *American Family Physician* 63(11): 2201–2208.

Singh, R., Cappucci, R., Kramer-Fox, R. et al. 2000. Severe mitral regurgitation due to mitral valve prolapse: risk factors for development, progression, and need for mitral valve surgery. *American Journal of Cardiology* 85(2):193–198.

Taubert, K., and Dajani, A. 2001. Optimisation of the prevention and treatment of bacterial endocarditis. *Drugs and Aging* 18(6):415–424.

6-G

Palpitations

Palpitations are one of the most common complaints in primary care practice, reported by as many as 16% of patients (Summerton et al. 2001). Often described as the disturbing awareness of one's own heartbeat, palpitations may be worrisome and even frightening to a patient. In most cases, palpitations are benign and not indicative of cardiovascular disease, although in some patients palpitations may be associated with clinically significant arrhythmias related to underlying disease (Zimetbaum et al. 1998). The challenge facing clinicians is to distinguish between palpitations that are benign and require only reassurance, and palpitations that signal cardiovascular pathology.

It can be difficult for clinicians to determine whether palpitations are benign or pathologic. Several studies have attempted to predict, based on clinical features, which patients with palpitations will have benign versus more serious outcomes. A study by Barsky (2001) found that those who somatize and have more health-related anxieties were less likely to have demonstrable arrhythmias associated with palpitations. In research by Ehlers et al. (2000), patients who were female, had higher heart rates, were less active, and suffered from panic attacks or depression were more aware of normal sinus rhythm than other patients were, suggesting that clinicians should include screening for mood disorders in patients who present with palpitations.

A careful history and physical examination are essential components in determining the appropriate work-up. In taking the history, the clinician should be mindful of the numerous causes of palpitations and elicit as detailed a description as possible from the patient. The following characteristics of palpitations may be useful in determining the etiology:
→ Isolated palpitations:
  ■ Premature atrial, junctional, or ventricular contraction (PAC, PJC, or PVC)
    • The premature beat may be felt, or the subsequent beat (with or without a compensatory pause) may be more perceptible, because of an increase in stroke volume and contractility.
  ■ 2° AV block, type 1 (Wenckebach)

→ Palpitations characterized by rapid rate and regular rhythm:
  ■ Catecholamine excess
    • Anxiety
    • Exercise
    • Fever
    • Stress
    • Sympathomimetic medications
    • Stimulant drug use
  ■ Hypovolemia
  ■ Hyperthyroidism
  ■ Pheochromocytoma
  ■ Marked anemia
  ■ Certain medications
  ■ Arrhythmias with constant block or 1:1 conduction:
    • Atrial flutter
    • Paroxysmal atrial tachycardia
    • Supraventricular tachycardia
    • Wolff-Parkinson-White syndrome
    • *Torsade de pointes* tachycardia
→ Palpitations characterized by rapid rate and irregular rhythm:
  ■ Arrhythmias
    • Atrial fibrillation
    • Multifocal atrial tachycardia
    • Atrial flutter with variable block
    • Paroxysmal atrial tachycardia with variable block
    • Supraventricular tachycardia with variable block
    • Multiple PACs, PJCs, or PVCs

DATABASE

SUBJECTIVE

→ The patient presents with a complaint of palpitations. While many patients have difficulty being specific about their symptoms, an accurate history of the palpitations, including descriptors, may indicate the underlying etiology or narrow the differential diagnosis.
  ■ When did the symptoms begin?

- How often do the palpitations occur?
- How long do the episodes last?
- How fast is the pulse?
- Is the pulse regular or irregular?
- Is the heart "pounding," "fluttering," "flopping," "racing," or "skipping"?
- Do the episodes occur with exercise, after medication or drug use, with stress, or at random?
- How does the episode resolve?
- Are there any other associated symptoms with the palpitations?

→ Associated symptoms may include:
- Tremor
- Nervousness
- Syncope/near fainting
- Dizziness/lightheadedness
- Perioral and/or peripheral paresthesias
- Chest pain
- Shortness of breath
- Dyspnea on exertion
- Perspiration

→ Precipitating events, if known, may include:
- Anxiety/panic attack
- Emotional upset
- Exercise
- Dehydration
- Medication or recreational drug use

→ Past medical history may include:
- Anemia
- Heart murmur
- Heart disease:
  - Valvular heart disease
  - Coronary heart disease
  - Arrhythmias/conduction disorders
- Risk factors for heart disease:
  - Diabetes
  - Hypertension
  - Hyperlipidemia
  - Smoking
  - Family history of heart disease
- Insulin-dependent diabetes
- Mood disorders:
  - Anxiety
  - Depression
  - Panic disorder
- Pheochromocytoma
- Thyroid disease

→ Medications may include:
- Antiarrhythmics
- Anticholinergics
- Antihistamines (long-acting)
- Appetite suppressants
- Decongestants
- Digoxin
- Insulin/oral hypoglycemic agents
- Theophylline compounds

- Sympathomimetics
- Psychoactive drugs

→ Social history may include the use of:
- Caffeine
- Alcohol
- Tobacco
- Recreational drugs:
  - Amphetamines
  - Cocaine
  - Ecstasy
  - Marijuana

→ Family history may include:
- Coronary artery disease
- Valvular heart disease
- Sudden death
- Early cardiac death:
  - Female death younger than 55 years
  - Male death younger than 45 years

OBJECTIVE

→ The patient's general appearance may exhibit:
- Anxiousness
- Tremulousness
- Depressed mood
- Sad affect
- Pallor
- Exophthalmus

→ Vital signs should be assessed for:
- Temperature, which may be elevated with infection
- Apical heart rate: regularity, character; comparison with radial pulse for pulse deficit
- Blood pressure, including orthostatic measurements:
  - May be hypotensive if the patient is hypovolemic or has low cardiac output.
  - Widened pulse pressure may be present.

→ Neck examination should assess for:
- Thyroid:
  - Goiter
  - Nodules
  - Tenderness
- Jugular venous distention
- Bruits

→ Lung examination should assess for:
- Adventitious sounds
- Respiratory rate and pattern

→ Heart examination should assess for:
- Rhythm characteristics:
  - Regular
  - Bounding
  - Thready
  - Occasionally irregular (i.e., PACs, PVCs)
  - Irregularly irregular (i.e., atrial fibrillation, multifocal atrial tachycardia, atrial flutter with variable block)
  - Regularly irregular (i.e., bigeminy, trigeminy, quadrigeminy, Wenckebach)

- Murmurs:
  - Location
  - Grade
  - Systolic and/or diastolic
  - Radiation
- Rubs
- Gallops:
  - S_3
  - S_4
- Heaves
- Thrills
- Point of maximal impulse
→ Extremity examination should assess for:
- Pulses
- Color
- Warmth
- Capillary refill
- Cyanosis
- Clubbing
- Edema
- Calf tenderness

ASSESSMENT

→ Palpitations
→ R/O arrhythmias/heart disease
→ R/O systemic etiologies:
- Anemia
- Thyroid disease
- Pheochromocytoma
- Medication side effect
- Stimulant side effect
→ R/O mood disorders:
- Anxiety
- Depression
- Panic disorder
- Somatization disorder

PLAN

DIAGNOSTIC TESTS

→ 12-lead EKG:
- Assess for rate, rhythm, ectopy, ischemia.
  - Indicated for most patients, even those with a normal exam.
→ Ambulatory monitoring:
- Continuous-loop event recorder:
  - Indicated for those with evidence of underlying heart disease.
  - Two-week monitoring period. The patient activates the device when palpitations occur.
  - The device saves a rhythm strip for several minutes before and after an event, which may be transmitted by telephone for interpretation.
  - More cost-effective and more useful than Holter monitoring in establishing the diagnosis (Goroll 2000).

→ Holter monitor:
- Most useful for the patient complaining of daily symptoms.
- Requires a diary to correlate symptoms with arrhythmia.
- Can repeat if the 48-hour rhythm strip is negative but yield is low.
- Questionably helpful for a healthy patient with a normal EKG.
→ Thyroid function tests (see the **Thyroid Disorders** chapter in Section 10):
- If symptoms suggest thyroid disease
→ CBC:
- To rule out anemia
→ Electrolytes:
- To rule out hypoglycemia in diabetic patients
- To rule out abnormalities in patients with underlying heart disease
→ Exercise treadmill test (ETT):
- If symptoms occur with exercise

OR

- If the patient has palpitations associated with chest pain, suggestive of angina

OR

- If the patient has a history of heart disease
  - R/O contraindications to ETT (e.g., unstable angina, severe aortic stenosis, hypertrophic cardiomyopathy, prolonged QT interval) before ordering.
→ Echocardiogram:
- If the exam suggests valvular or other cardiac structural abnormality

TREATMENT/MANAGEMENT

→ If an EKG is normal and symptoms are suggestive of stress or stimulant use, reassure the patient that the cardiac exam is normal and her symptoms are amenable to appropriate therapy (e.g., stress reduction, elimination of stimulants).
→ If the work-up suggests an underlying illness or disease (e.g., anemia [see the **Anemia** chapter in Section 10] or hyperthyroidism [see the **Thyroid Disorders** chapter in Section 10]), initiate appropriate evaluation.
→ If an EKG is normal and the patient is moderately symptomatic (e.g., persistent palpitations, tachycardia, tremors), may begin low-dose beta blocker therapy (e.g., atenolol 25–50 mg p.o. QD; see **Table 6E.1, Pharmacologic Therapy for Hypertension [Selected Agents]** in the **Hypertension** chapter) for symptom control.
→ If an EKG is normal and the patient's symptoms suggest situational stress, may begin (in consultation with a physician) low-dose anxiolytic therapy (e.g., alprazolam 0.25 mg p.o. BID) if appropriate (determined by patient reliability, clinic setting, follow-up). If symptoms suggest depression, may begin antidepressant therapy (e.g., paroxetine 20 mg p.o. QD) if appropriate.
NOTE: Selective serotonin reuptake inhibitor (SSRI) antidepressants may increase anxiety, nervousness, and palpitations. Use with caution.

CONSULTATION

→ Referral to or consultation with a cardiologist is indicated for:
- An abnormal EKG, including arrhythmias, frequent ectopy, or ischemic changes
- Evidence of structural cardiac disease
- Palpitations associated with syncope or near syncope; electrophysiologic studies may be indicated.

→ As needed for prescription(s).

PATIENT EDUCATION

→ Teach the patient how to take her radial or carotid pulse to assess for rate and regularity.

→ Advise the patient that healthy patients can have palpitations.

→ Educate the patient regarding stress reduction techniques to be used in reducing or eliminating palpitation:
- A regular exercise routine—e.g., 30 minutes of aerobic exercise 2–3 times/week (in a low-risk patient)
- Meditation and relaxation techniques useful for stress reduction

→ Advise the patient to decrease/eliminate stimulant use (e.g., cigarettes, alcohol, caffeine, recreational drugs).

→ Advise the patient regarding regular use of stimulant medications, including discontinuing medication or switching to another agent with fewer side effects. The patient may tolerate symptoms better after reassurance that palpitations are medication-related.

FOLLOW-UP

→ Re-evaluate the patient in 1–2 months if no discernible cause is found.

→ Re-evaluate the patient in 2–3 weeks if pharmacological therapy is begun.

→ Document in progress notes and on problem list.

BIBLIOGRAPHY

Barsky, A. 2001. Palpitations, arrhythmias, and awareness of cardiac activity. *Annals of Internal Medicine* 134(9 Part 2): 832–837.

Ehlers, A., Mayou, R., Sprigings, D. et al. 2000. Psychological and perceptual factors associated with arrhythmias and benign palpitations. *Psychosomatic Medicine* 62(5):693–702.

Goroll, A. 2000. Evaluation of palpitations. In *Primary care medicine: office evaluation and management of the adult patient*, 4th ed., eds. A. Goroll and A. Mulley. Philadelphia: Lippincott Williams & Wilkins.

Summerton, N., Mann, S., Ribgy, A. et al. 2001. New-onset palpitations in general practice: assessing the discriminant value of items within the clinical history. *Family Practice* 18(4):383–392.

Zimetbaum, P., and Josephson, M. 1998. Evaluation of the patient with palpitations. *New England Journal of Medicine* 338(19):1369–1373.

SECTION 7

Gastrointestinal Disorders

7-A Abdominal Pain 7-2
7-B Appendicitis. 7-11
7-C Cholecystitis 7-14
7-D Constipation 7-18
7-E Diarrhea 7-23
7-F Diverticular Disease 7-29
7-G Gastroesophageal Reflux and Heartburn. 7-33
7-H Gastrointestinal Bleeding. 7-39
7-I Hemorrhoids and Anal Fissures 7-43
7-J Hernia. 7-48
7-K Inflammatory Bowel Disease 7-51
7-L Irritable Bowel Syndrome 7-60
7-M Peptic Ulcer Disease 7-64

Lisa L. Lommel, R.N., C., F.N.P., M.S., M.P.H.
Jeanne R. Davis, R.N., F.N.P., M.P.H.

7-A

Abdominal Pain

Abdominal pain may be classified as either acute or chronic. The term *acute abdomen* implies "any serious acute intra-abdominal condition (such as appendicitis) attended by pain, tenderness, and muscular rigidity, and for which emergency surgery must be considered" (Dirckx 2001). An acute onset of abdominal symptoms may or may not indicate an acute abdomen. Further, it is possible that while the onset of symptoms is considered acute, the patient's abdominal symptoms have been present for anywhere from minutes to weeks. In addition, acute abdominal symptoms may be the manifestation of a chronic health problem, such as chronic pancreatitis or vascular insufficiency (Martin et al. 1997). Clearly, if the pain is acute in onset *and* severity, the management goal is early diagnosis and timely referral to the appropriate specialist. In cases of chronic or recurrent pain, the goal is to provide an effective work-up to establish a diagnosis and treatment plan.

The major pathogenic mechanisms underlying abdominal pain include obstruction and perforation of the hollow viscus, peritoneal irritation, vascular insufficiency, mucosal ulceration/inflammation, altered bowel motility, capsular distention or inflammation, metabolic imbalance, nerve injury, abdominal wall injury, and referral from an extra-abdominal site (Richter 2000). In women of reproductive age, especially those with lower abdominal pain, gynecologic and obstetric etiologies must be considered in the differential diagnosis, as well as the common gastrointestinal and urinary causes (Robertson 1998).

Because the location of pain often does not coincide with the site of involvement, the provider should elicit a thorough history, perform a thorough physical examination, and be familiar with areas where abdominal pain commonly is referred or perceived (see **Table 7A.1, Common Anatomical Pain Sites for Specific Disease States**).

DATABASE

SUBJECTIVE

→ A complete description of the abdominal pain is needed, including:
- Onset, chronology/pattern of pain, location, characteriza-

tion (quality [patient to rate pain from 1–10] and quantity), radiation, setting, duration, aggravating and alleviating factors, history of similar episodes, frequency and interruptions in function

→ Associated symptoms:
- Fever, nausea, vomiting, distention, flatus, anorexia, dysuria, hematuria, urinary frequency, jaundice, stool pattern and characteristics, gynecological symptoms, and menstrual pattern

→ A comprehensive medical and surgical history:
- History of diagnostic testing or prior abdominal or pelvic surgery, dietary patterns/association of pain with meals, effect of pain on activity and sleep, recent travel, drug/alcohol ingestion (including prior treatments used to relieve the pain), family history, social history, psychological history, occupational history, and review of systems

→ Older patients are more likely to have serious causes of abdominal pain:
- Both mortality and misdiagnosis rise exponentially with each decade beyond age 50.
- Elderly patients with abdominal pain are more likely to have catastrophic illnesses rarely seen in younger patients (American College of Emergency Physicians 2000).

→ Historical findings and symptoms experienced in common pathogenic mechanisms of abdominal pain are found in **Table 7A.2, Abdominal Palpation**.

Obstruction

→ Acute small bowel obstruction:
- History of abdominal surgery or hernia is common
- Rapid onset of cramping, intermittent, mid-abdominal pain
- Pain may be severe in proximal obstruction
- Patient may be comfortable between bouts of pain
- Pain steady with complete obstruction
- Pain greatest with jejunal obstruction
- Flatus and small amounts of stool common at onset of obstruction; diarrhea with partial obstruction; inability to pass gas and stool with complete obstruction

Table 7A.1.   COMMON ANATOMICAL PAIN SITES FOR SPECIFIC DISEASE STATES

Right Upper Quadrant and Flank

Hepatitis	Pyelonephritis	Intestinal obstruction
Pancreatitis	Nephrolithiasis	Inflammatory bowel disease
Gastritis	Choledocholithiasis	Retrocecal appendicitis
Duodenitis	Duodenal ulcer	Gastric ulcer
Cholecystitis	Penetrating or perforating ulcer	Colon carcinoma

Epigastrium

Pancreatitis	Early appendicitis	Intestinal obstruction
Gastritis	Gastric ulcer	Mesenteric thrombosis
Duodenitis	Colitis	Colon carcinoma
Gastroenteritis	Penetrating or perforating ulcer	Aneurysm
Duodenal ulcer	Inflammatory bowel disease	

Left Upper Quadrant and Flank

Hepatitis	Pyelonephritis	Inflammatory bowel disease
Gastritis	Nephrolithiasis	Colon carcinoma
Pancreatitis	Diverticulitis	
Splenic enlargement, rupture, infarction	Intestinal obstruction	

Right Lower Quadrant and Flank

Appendicitis	Mittelschmerz	Endometriosis
Intestinal obstruction	Salpingitis	Ectopic pregnancy
Hernia	Ovarian cyst/torsion	Abdominal wall hematoma
Nephrolithiasis	Diverticulitis	Psoas abscess
Pyelonephritis	Inflammatory bowel disease	Leaking aneurysm
Cholecystitis	Penetrating or perforating ulcer	Mesenteric adenitis

Umbilical

Early appendicitis	Mesenteric adenitis	Aneurysm
Gastroenteritis	Inflammatory bowel disease	Mesenteric thrombosis
Pancreatitis	Intestinal obstruction	
Hernia	Abdominal wall hernia	

Left Lower Quadrant and Flank

Diverticulitis	Mittelschmerz	Abdominal wall hematoma
Intestinal obstruction	Salpingitis	Ectopic pregnancy
Hernia	Ovarian cyst/torsion	Leaking aneurysm
Pyelonephritis	Endometriosis	Psoas abscess
Nephrolithiasis	Appendicitis	

Hypogastrium

Cystitis	Ovarian cyst/torsion	Ectopic pregnancy
Diverticulitis	Endometriosis	Abdominal wall hematoma
Appendicitis	Nephrolithiasis	Colon carcinoma
Salpingitis	Inflammatory bowel disease	
Hernia	Intestinal obstruction	

Source: Reprinted with permission from Hickey, M.S., Kiernan, G.J., and Weaver, K.E. 1989. Evaluation of abdominal pain. *Emergency Medicine Clinics of North America* 7(3):437–452.

Table 7A.2. ABDOMINAL PALPATION

Finding or Sign	Description	Clinical Occurrence
Bassler's sign	Sharp pain elicited by pinching the appendix between the thumb of the examiner and the iliacus muscle	Chronic appendicitis
Beevor's sign	Upward movement of the umbilicus	Paralysis of the lower portions of the rectus abdominis muscles
Blumberg's sign	Transient abdominal wall rebound tenderness	Peritoneal inflammation
Ballance's sign	Presence of a dull percussion note in both flanks consistent on the left side but shifting with change of position on the right	Ruptured spleen
Carnett's sign	Disappearance of abdominal tenderness to palpation when anterior abdominal muscles are contracted	Abdominal pain of intra-abdominal origin
Chandelier sign	Intense lower abdominal and pelvic pain upon manipulation of the cervix	Pelvic inflammatory disease
Charcot's sign	Intermittent, right upper quadrant abdominal pain, jaundice, and fever	Choledocholithiasis
Chaussier's sign	Severe epigastric pain in gravid female	Eclampsia
Claybrook's sign	Transmission of breath and heart sounds through the abdomen	Ruptured abdominal viscus
Courvoisier's sign	Palpable, nontender gallbladder in the presence of clinical jaundice	Pancreatic or common bile duct malignancy
Cutaneous hyperesthesia	Increased abdominal wall sensation to light touch	Parietal peritoneal inflammation secondary to an inflammatory intra-abdominal pathology
Direct abdominal wall tenderness		Localized inflammation of the abdominal wall, peritoneum, or an intra-abdominal viscus
Fothergill's sign	Abdominal wall mass that does not cross the midline and remains palpable when the rectus muscle is tense	Rectus muscle hematoma
Iliopsoas sign	Elevation and extension of the leg against pressure of the examiner's hand causes pain	Appendicitis (retrocecal) or an inflammatory mass in contact with the psoas
Kehr's sign	Left shoulder pain when the patient is supine or in the Trendelenburg position. (**NOTE:** The pain may occur spontaneously or following the application of pressure to left subcostal region.)	Free blood in the peritoneal space
Kustner's sign	Palpable mass anterior to the uterus	Dermoid cyst of the ovary
McClintock's sign	Postpartum heart rate >100/minute	Postpartum hemorrhage
Murphy's sign	Palpation of the right upper abdominal quadrant during deep inspiration results in right upper quadrant abdominal pain	Acute cholecystitis
Obturator sign	Flexion of right thigh at right angles to trunk and external rotation of the same leg in the supine position results in hypogastric pain	Appendicitis (pelvic appendix); pelvic abscess; an inflammatory mass in contact with muscle
Puddle sign	Alteration in intensity of transmitted sound in the intra-abdominal cavity secondary to percussion when the patient is positioned on all fours and the stethoscope is gradually moved toward the flank opposite the percussion	Free peritoneal fluid
Rovsing's sign	Pain is referred to McBurney's point on applying pressure to the descending colon	Acute appendicitis
Subcutaneous crepitus		Subcutaneous empyema or gas gangrene
Sumner's sign	Increased abdominal muscle tone upon exceedingly gentle palpation of the right or left iliac fossa	Early appendicitis; nephrolithiasis; ureterolithiasis; ovarian torsion
Toma's sign	Right-sided tympany and left-sided dullness in the supine position as a result of peritoneal inflammation and subsequent mesenteric contraction of the intestine to the right side of the abdominal cavity	Inflammatory ascites

Source: Reprinted with permission from Hickey, M.S., Kiernan, G.J., and Weaver, K.E. 1989. Evaluation of abdominal pain. *Emergency Medicine Clinics of North America* 7(3):437–452.

- Distention is increased with a more distal obstruction
- Nausea, vomiting, weakness, anxiety
→ Large bowel obstruction:
  - More common in patients over 50 years old; often preceded by constipation or change in bowel habits
  - Bloating, distention, cramping pain, constipation, mild nausea, and vomiting
  - Diarrhea with partial obstruction
  - Usually less vomiting and less pain than small bowel obstruction, but more distention
→ Cystic duct obstruction:
  - Commonly presents with a history of biliary tract disease
  - Acute pain typical—known as biliary "colic"—lasting an hour or more after sudden onset in epigastric region/right upper quadrant (RUQ)
  - Pain may radiate to scapular region
  - Associated with nausea, vomiting, fever
  - May have only mild epigastric pain
  - Jaundice
→ Acute cholecystitis:
  - See the **Cholecystitis** chapter.
→ Common duct obstruction:
  - More likely to have epigastric pain than with cystic duct obstruction, pain less severe
→ Acute ureteral obstruction:
  - Sudden onset of crampy pain, pain initially in the back/flank that radiates to lower abdomen and groin
  - May have nausea, vomiting, anorexia, hematuria
  - Abdominal pain, fever, chills with development of pyelonephritis, bacteremia, or abscess
  - See the **Urinary Tract Disorders** chapters in Section 12 for other renal causes of abdominal pain.

Peritoneal Irritation

→ Peritonitis:
  - Localized injury from infection or chemical irritation may cause mild to severe, sharp, aching, or burning pain
  - Degree of pain and systemic reaction depends on nature and severity of insult
  - Spread of the irritant may cause generalized abdominal pain
  - Pain increased with coughing, palpation, or movement
  - May complain of malaise, nausea, and vomiting
→ Acute pancreatitis:
  - Gallstone pancreatitis more common in women
  - Alcoholic pancreatitis more common in men
  - May report alcohol intake or heavy meal immediately before attack
  - May have history of similar episodes or biliary colic
  - Epigastric pain with abrupt onset; steady, severe, and boring pain
  - Worse when walking and lying supine, better when sitting and leaning forward
  - Pain radiates to the back or costal margins and varies in intensity from mild to severe
  - Nausea and vomiting usually present

- Severe pain more common in left upper quadrant (LUQ)
- Sweating, weakness, and anxiety common with severe attack (Friedman 2002)
→ Chronic pancreatitis:
  - Symptoms may be identical to those of acute pancreatitis
  - History of acute pancreatitis
  - History of alcohol abuse
  - Episodes of epigastric pain, with radiation to lower thoracic or upper lumbar vertebral region
  - Pain can be dull or sharp and severe
  - Commonly associated with nausea and vomiting
  - May also have diarrhea, anorexia, flatulence, and weight loss
  - May complain of change in appearance of stools
  - Attacks may be hours to weeks long and become continuous
→ See the **Appendicitis** chapter.

Vascular Disorders

→ Acute arterial insufficiency from atherosclerosis or embolus:
  - Acute, sudden, periumbilical, or generalized abdominal pain
  - Subtle, early presentation common (several days of mild, constant pain initially)
  - May also present with severe, central abdominal pain with embolus
  - May have history of myocardial infarction (MI)
→ Chronic mesenteric insufficiency:
  - May precede acute episode of infarction, with bowel infarction being described as "severe" pain (Stone 1996)
  - Epigastric or periumbilical cramping or dull postprandial pain, lasting 1–3 hours
  - Symptoms are more extreme after a large and fatty meal
  - May have weight loss secondary to avoidance of eating
  - May be associated with nausea, vomiting, and bloating
  - Constipation and occult blood loss possible
→ Ruptured abdominal aortic aneurysm/aortic dissection:
  - Severe, acute abdominal pain radiating to back or genitalia
  - Symptoms of shock
  - Dissecting or ruptured abdominal aortic aneurysm often described as a "tearing" sensation
→ Mesenteric venous thrombosis:
  - Less common, but may present similarly to arterial occlusion, although slower progressive course

Mucosal Ulceration/Inflammation

→ Upper gastrointestinal (GI) tract ulceration. See the **Gastroesophageal Reflux and Heartburn**, **Peptic Ulcer Disease**, and **Inflammatory Bowel Disease** chapters.

Alteration in Bowel Motility

→ Dyspepsia:
  - Pain or discomfort in upper abdomen

- May have bloating, nausea, early satiety, postprandial fullness, heartburn, and belching
→ See the **Irritable Bowel Syndrome**, **Diverticular Disease**, and **Diarrhea** chapters.
→ Intestinal pseudo-obstruction (associated with Parkinson's disease): mimics symptoms of intestinal obstruction

Capsular Distention (Distention of the Capsule Surrounding an Organ)

→ Hepatic capsular distention from hepatitis, congestive heart failure
→ Fatty infiltration or subcapsular hematoma may cause aching pain in RUQ
→ Splenic capsular distention from blunt trauma may cause pain in LUQ

Metabolic Disturbances

→ Lead poisoning may cause abdominal pain that is cramping, wandering, poorly localized, and colicky
→ Rigid abdomen may be present
→ Porphyria
  - May mimic bowel obstruction with cramping abdominal pain and hyperperistalsis
  - Acute intermittent porphyria may present with moderate to severe abdominal pain, localized or generalized
  - Nausea, vomiting, and diarrhea usually present
  - Proximal muscle pain may be present
  - Neuropsychiatric symptoms possible
→ Angioneurotic edema: may result in severe, episodic abdominal pain
  - Diabetic ketoacidosis: may be associated with weakness, diaphoresis, mental status changes, severe abdominal pain, and vomiting
  - Systemic lupus erythematosus (SLE): may have an insidious onset, although when presenting acutely, may appear somewhat like porphyria (splenomegaly, abdominal pain [especially postprandial], peripheral neuropathies, photosensitivity) or with fever, anorexia, malaise, weight loss, arthralgias, rash, and arthritis.
→ See the **Type 1 Diabetes Mellitus** and **Type 2 Diabetes Mellitus** chapters in Section 10.

Nerve Injury

→ Abdominal pain may be secondary to mechanical obstruction or injury due to an intra-abdominal nerve (e.g., intra-abdominal cancers can invade pain-causing nerves).
→ Surgical procedures, such as hernia repair, can cause peripheral nerve injuries resulting in chronic recurrent pain.
→ Surgical scars can cause localized tenderness months after surgery secondary to neuroma formation (Suleiman et al. 2001).
→ Pain can be perceived as intra-abdominal but may be associated with nerve root irritation secondary to herpes zoster, either before the rash appears or with postherpetic neuralgia (DeBanto et al. 1999).

→ See also the **Varicella Zoster Virus** chapter in Section 11.

Abdominal Wall Pathology

→ Abdominal wall pain may be sharp initially, then become dull, nagging, and nonprogressive over time.
→ Symptoms may worsen when the abdominal wall is tensed (as with sneezing, coughing, or heavy lifting) (Suleiman et al. 2001).
→ History of trauma or overexertion (includes mild strains, contusions, hematomas, and penetrating wounds) (Stone 1996)
→ Myofascial tears can cause abdominal wall pain and are found in athletes or following heavy exertion.
→ Following surgery, trauma, or pregnancy, hematomas of the abdominal wall or rectus sheath can occur (Suleiman et al. 2001).
→ Traumatic injury to the abdominal wall:
  - May present with pain that is constant, aching, and exacerbated by movement and pressure on abdomen.
  - What appears to be a mild abdominal wall injury may be associated with underlying organ tears, rupture, or contusions (Stone 1996).
→ Pain along costal margin or subxiphisternal region associated with Tietze's syndrome (costal chondritis) may mimic epigastric or upper quadrant gastrointestinal disease.
→ See the **Hernia** chapter.

Referred Pain From Extra-Abdominal Site

→ Pulmonary (pulmonary infarction, pleuritis, pneumonia, pneumothorax, pulmonary embolism) or cardiac disorders (MI) may be interpreted as upper abdominal pain.
→ Cardiac pain may be noted in the epigastrium, chest, arm, shoulder, neck, or jaw.
→ Nausea and vomiting may be present with MI.
→ See the **Dysmenorrhea**, **Ectopic Pregnancy**, **Endometriosis**, **Pelvic Inflammatory Disease**, **Pelvic Masses**, **Pelvic Pain—Acute**, **Pelvic Pain—Chronic**, and **Urinary Tract Disorders** chapters in Section 12.

OBJECTIVE

→ A complete physical examination should be done and include targeted assessments: general appearance (assess for pallor, perspiration, restlessness, hands held tightly over abdomen, reluctance to move), vital signs (temperature, heart rate, blood pressure, respiratory rate, postural changes in blood pressure and heart rate), and cardiac, pulmonary, abdominal and renal, pelvic, and rectal examinations.
→ Assessment should include:
  - Pelvic exam: evaluate cervix (assess for cervical motion tenderness), assess for adnexal tenderness or masses and organomegaly
  - Digital rectal exam: masses, fecal impaction, tenderness, hemorrhoids, obtain stool for occult blood
  - Skin: jaundice, signs of chronic liver disease (spider angiomata, clubbing or spooning of fingernails), dehydration, edema, and dermatomal rash

- Chest: splinting, pleural friction rub, consolidation in lower lobes
- Heart: murmurs, enlargement, signs of heart failure or pericardial friction rub
- Abdominal examination (patient lying supine with knees bent, back flat) should include:
  - Inspection (ask patient to point to area of greatest pain with a single finger, assess for presence of distention, visible peristalsis, jaundice, scarring, abdominal wall masses)
  - Auscultation (altered bowel sounds, hepatic rub, or vascular bruit)
  - Percussion (hepatosplenomegaly, delineation of masses and free air)
  - Palpation beginning at region away from the maximal area of pain (assess for hepatosplenomegaly, masses, costovertebral angle tenderness [CVAT], external hernias, ascites [assess for fluid wave])
  - Assess for involuntary guarding, cough, rebound tenderness, rigid abdomen, perform special signs and maneuvers as appropriate (see **Table 7A.2**).
- Signs and symptoms of shock should be assessed in patients with suspected acute abdomen
→ Abdominal examination may be difficult to complete in patients who have moderate to severe degrees of anxiety or pain.
→ Must have high index of suspicion when examining the elderly, as usual physical findings of acute peritoneal irritation may be absent in the elderly.

Obstruction

→ Small bowel obstruction:
- Inspect for scars, hernias
- Patient appears restless during bouts of pain; tachycardia, temperature normal or mildly elevated
- Obstruction with or without perforation can cause postural changes in blood pressure and heart rate
- Tender, distended abdomen, especially with distal obstruction
- High-pitched, hyperactive bowel sounds
- A tender hernia may be present
- Stool guaiac usually negative
- Plain radiograph of the abdomen (supine and upright) shows distention of loops of small bowel with air-fluid levels, absence of gas in the large bowel (distal to the obstruction), elevated white blood cell (WBC) count, elevated hematocrit with signs of dehydration
→ Large bowel obstruction:
- Progressive abdominal distention and tympany, hyperactive bowel sounds
- Positive stool guaiac common with rectal examination (Richter 2000)
- WBC count may be normal or elevated
→ Acute ureteral obstruction:
- Diaphoretic, anxious
- Right- or left-sided, diffuse, flank or groin tenderness

- See the **Urinary Tract Disorders** chapters in Section 12 for other renal causes of abdominal pain.
→ Cystic duct obstruction:
- Acute cystic duct obstruction often steady and lasting over an hour after initial onset
- RUQ tenderness with or without jaundice
- Chills and spiking, intermittent fever with infection
- May have positive Murphy's sign (see **Table 7A.2**).
- Elevated WBC count (20,000–30,000/mm^3)
- Cholelithiasis: elevated alkaline phosphatase, bilirubin, and amylase levels commonly present during symptomatic episodes (Zackowski 1998)
- Acute cholecystitis: See the **Cholecystitis** chapter.
→ Common duct obstruction:
- Jaundice, emesis
- Tender RUQ, is less focal and deeper than acute cholecystitis
- Marked elevation of alkaline phosphatase is common, as is hyperbilirubinemia

Peritoneal Irritation

→ Peritonitis:
- Abdominal findings may include rebound tenderness, tenderness to palpation or percussion; rigid distention of abdomen; reduced or absent bowel sounds
- Rectal and vaginal tenderness
- Patient usually lies very still due to increase in pain with movement
- Peritonitis can cause postural changes in blood pressure and heart rate as a result of blood or fluid loss
- Low-grade fever
- Assess for psoas sign (see **Table 7A.2**)
→ Acute pancreatitis:
- Upper abdominal mass due to inflamed pancreas or pseudocyst may be palpated occasionally
- Elevated temperature, tachycardia, hypotension, pallor, or mild jaundice
- Abdominal distention possible
- Diffuse epigastric tenderness most often without guarding, but varying degrees of guarding are possible
- Usually no rigidity or rebound
- Moderate elevation in WBCs
- Bilirubin, serum lipase, and amylase may be elevated
- In severe acute pancreatitis, may present with hypotension, signs of shock, significant elevation of WBCs and hematocrit
→ Chronic pancreatitis:
- Tenderness over pancreas, mild guarding, steatorrhea
- Elevated serum amylase, serum lipase, and bilirubin (normal amylase level does not exclude diagnosis)
→ See the **Appendicitis** and **Diverticular Disease** chapters and the **Hepatitis—Viral** chapter in Section 11.

Vascular Disorders

→ Acute arterial insufficiency from atherosclerosis or mesenteric thrombus:

- Abdominal tenderness may be present but poorly localized.
- Early in the disorder, pain may be out of proportion to clinical findings.
- Diagnosis is usually evident with signs of peritonitis/shock.
- Specific to mesenteric thrombus, atrial fibrillation may be present and a tender mass may be felt in upper or midabdomen.

→ Chronic mesenteric insufficiency:
  - Symptoms may precede an acute episode of infarction (Richter 2000).
  - May have occult blood loss.
  - Abdominal bruits are fairly common, carotid or femoral bruit is possible.
  - Diagnosis is usually confirmed with arteriography.

→ Abdominal aneurysm or aortic dissection:
  - Abdominal aortic aneurysm: pulsatile mid-upper abdominal mass, with anterior-posterior and lateral movement
  - Ruptured abdominal aneurysm: sudden onset of symptoms with clinical signs of shock from blood loss (initially hypertensive, then hypotensive), lower extremity ischemia (Stone 1996)

→ Mesenteric venous thrombosis:
  - Pain complaints seem in excess of those elicited by physical exam

Mucosal Ulceration

→ See the **Peptic Ulcer Disease** chapter.

Altered Bowel Motility

→ See the **Irritable Bowel Syndrome, Diverticular Disease,** and **Diarrhea** chapters.

Capsular Distention

→ Hepatic capsular distention: enlarged liver, jaundice, ascites, other signs of chronic liver disease
→ Splenic distention: enlarged spleen

Metabolic Disturbances

→ Lead poisoning: hyperperistalsis, abdominal rigidity, encephalopathy, peripheral neuropathy, and anemia
→ Acute intermittent porphyria: soft abdomen, spleen may be enlarged, fever, elevated WBCs, range of neuropsychiatric symptoms
→ SLE: fever, "butterfly" rash and other dermatologic lesions possible, joint manifestations, splenomegaly, peripheral neuropathy
→ Ketoacidosis: "fruity breath," signs of dehydration, tachycardia, elevated WBCs (see the **Type 1 Diabetes Mellitus** and **Type 2 Diabetes Mellitus** chapters in Section 10)

Nerve Injury

→ A variety of objective findings may be associated with nerve injury depending on the etiology: Assess for pain in a dermatomal distribution and for hyperesthesia (both occur with nerve injury due to herpes zoster).

Abdominal Wall Pathology

→ Abdominal wall trauma may be evident or a mass may be palpated.
→ Area of tenderness may be localized to an area of 1–2 cm in diameter (a "trigger point") (Suleiman et al. 2001).
→ Carnett's sign (see **Table 7A.2**) will distinguish intra-abdominal versus abdominal wall pain.
→ Cutaneous nerve involvement will show impaired sensory function in the area of nerve distribution.
→ With herpes zoster pain in the dermatomal distribution, minimal associated symptoms are present, then hallmark rash appears after several days.
→ See the **Hernia** chapter.

Referred Pain From Extra-Abdominal Site

→ Objective findings of cardiac or pulmonary disorders are evident, with pain radiating from these regions.
→ See the **Dysmenorrhea, Ectopic Pregnancy, Endometriosis, Pelvic Inflammatory Disease, Pelvic Masses, Pelvic Pain–Acute, Pelvic Pain–Chronic,** and **Urinary Tract Disorders** chapters in Section 12.

ASSESSMENT

→ Abdominal pain
→ R/O obstruction (gastric outlet, small and large bowel, biliary and urinary tract)
→ R/O peritoneal irritation (infection, chemical irritation, systemic or local inflammatory process)
→ R/O vascular insufficiency (emboli, atherosclerotic narrowing, hypotension, aortic aneurysm dissection)
→ R/O mucosal ulceration (peptic ulcer disease, inflammatory bowel disease [IBD], gastric cancer)
→ R/O altered motility (gastroenteritis, IBD, irritable bowel syndrome, diverticular disease)
→ R/O metabolic disturbance (diabetic ketoacidosis, porphyria, lead poisoning)
→ R/O nerve injury (herpes zoster, root compression, nerve invasion or damage)
→ R/O muscle wall disease (trauma, myositis, hematoma)
→ R/O referred pain (pulmonary or cardiac)
→ R/O psychopathology (depression, anxiety)

PLAN

DIAGNOSTIC TESTS

→ Ideally, the initial diagnostic studies that are chosen by each clinician will aid in diagnosing acute and chronic disorders, and most importantly serious disorders that warrant immediate referral—e.g., obstruction, peritonitis, acute vascular insufficiency, metabolic disorders, and cardiac or pulmonary disease.
→ Complete blood count (CBC) with differential:
  - This is helpful in determining the presence of an acute infection.
  - Changes in the CBC may not occur in the elderly or the chronically ill, even in an intra-abdominal emergency.

- A markedly elevated WBC count is indicative of inflammation and/or infection, although it does not necessarily correspond to severity of the infection.
- A low WBC count may occur with a viral illness such as gastroenteritis.
- Leukocytosis and a shift to immature WBC's suggest an infectious process (a left shift without an attendant elevation in the WBC count may indicate a problem in the elderly).
- A low hematocrit may indicate the possibility of anemia due to a gastrointestinal malignancy or bleeding, especially with a positive stool occult blood.
- Anemia can also be present with IBD, ischemic colitis, and lead poisoning (Zackowski 1998).
- An elevated hematocrit may indicate dehydration.
- Because the CBC is a nonspecific test, management must not rest on this result alone.

→ Serum electrolytes may be helpful with severe or persistent vomiting and diarrhea.

→ Amylase:
- Often elevated in cases of pancreatitis
- May be elevated in intestinal obstruction (strangulated), perforated ulcer, intra-abdominal abscess, and biliary tract disease (Richter 2000, Stone 1998)

→ Serum lipase may be increased with stomach, gallbladder, pancreatic, or renal disease.

→ Antinuclear antibody (ANA), anti-DNA to rule out SLE

→ Stool for occult blood should be done on all patients.

→ Stool examination for ova and parasites and bacterial cultures may be ordered in cases of diarrhea.

→ Sudan red stain for fecal fat may be ordered (see the **Diarrhea** chapter).

→ Urinalysis:
- Red cells in the urine, along with flank pain, suggest a ureteral stone.
- Bacteria and white cells suggest an inflammation of the urinary tract.
- Ketonuria is common when the patient has not eaten or is in diabetic ketoacidosis.

→ Urine hCG: Rule out pregnancy in every woman of reproductive age with lower abdominal pain.

→ Urine samples to be checked for coproporphyrin for suspected lead poisoning and porphyria.

→ Tests for renal function (24-hour urine and serum samples for calcium, uric acid, blood urea nitrogen [BUN], creatinine, urine oxalate, citrate, electrolytes) and hepatic function (hepatitis screen, liver function studies including alkaline phosphate and bilirubin) may be ordered if clinical findings are suspicious for renal or biliary liver disorders.

→ Order a chest x-ray and electrocardiogram (EKG) in cases of upper abdominal pain, if clinical findings are suspicious for pulmonary or cardiac disease, or in elderly patients and those with cardiac risk factors with upper abdominal pain of unclear etiology.

→ The usual collection of radiographic views of the abdomen often includes an upright abdominal film; a kidney, ureter, and bladder (KUB) view; and an upright chest film (Martin et al. 1997).

- A plain radiograph of the abdomen (supine and upright):
  - Order if bowel obstruction is suspected:
    - Small-bowel obstruction may show distention of loops of bowel with high air-fluid levels, combined with absence of gas in large bowel distal to obstruction (Richter 2000).
    - Large bowel obstruction with an incompetent ileocecal valve may show distention and gas in the large and small bowel.
    - X-ray will assist in diagnosing: free air (which under the diaphragm indicates a perforated viscus); peritoneal bleeding, abscess or mass; tumor; biliary or renal stone; abdominal aortic calcification suggesting an aneurysm; and pancreatic calcification due to pancreatitis.
    - While only bowel obstruction and perforation can be accurately ruled out with plain films, plain films should be utilized when patients have moderate to severe abdominal pain or when any of the above conditions are suspected.

- Intestinal contrast studies (barium swallow or barium enema) can help with diagnosis of esophageal, gastric, duodenal, and colon disease (Stone 1998), but use with caution if obstruction or perforation is suspected.

- Upper GI series or endoscopy may be ordered when the patient does not respond to ulcer therapy or has symptoms of epigastric or periumbilical pain, melena, hematemesis, and weight loss.

- Colonoscopy/sigmoidoscopy are utilized to rule out diverticular disease, colon cancer, IBD, ulceration, and bowel obstruction or to locate source of bleeding.

- Intravenous pyelogram (IVP) may assist in diagnosing disease in the kidneys or ureters or in identifying a mass impeding these structures.

- Ultrasound can be used to assess a variety of conditions:
  - Renal ultrasound may assess for renal stone, tumor, or ureteral dilatation
  - Pelvic ultrasound for uterine or ovarian mass
  - Abdominal ultrasound:
    - Test of choice for suspected acute cholecystitis and choledocholithiasis
    - Useful in detecting biliary obstructions
    - Can be used to detect aortic aneurysm
  - Ultrasonography (plus needle biopsy if accessible) is the test of choice for suspected pancreatic cancer

- Computerized tomography (CT):
  - CT of abdomen, to assess for vascular disorders, may be ordered with physician consultation
  - Test of choice when diverticulitis is suspected
  - Used to assess biliary tree disease, abscess, masses and cysts
  - CT with IV contrast utilized in evaluating suspected dissecting aortic aneurysm, appendicitis

- Can be used for evaluation of suspected gastrointestinal, genitourinary, or pancreatic cancer
→ Endoscopic retrograde cholangiopancreatography (ERCP) is also used for detecting biliary disease, obstruction, and/or pancreatic cancer
→ Exploratory laparoscopy if diagnosis remains in question
→ See the **Dysmenorrhea, Ectopic Pregnancy, Endometriosis, Pelvic Inflammatory Disease, Pelvic Masses, Pelvic Pain—Acute, Pelvic Pain—Chronic**, and **Urinary Tract Disorders** chapters in Section 12 for additional diagnostic tests.

TREATMENT/MANAGEMENT

→ Patients with evidence of obstruction, peritoneal irritation, acute vascular insufficiency, metabolic disorders, and cardiac or pulmonary disease should be referred to a physician immediately.
→ Repeated histories and examinations may offer new data and allow for appropriate diagnosis, referral, and treatment.
→ Analgesia should not be given until an adequate diagnosis is made so that symptoms and/or signs of disease progression are not obscured.
→ See the **Gastrointestinal Disorders, Genitourinary Disorders, Dermatological Disorders, Respiratory/Otorhinolaryngological Disorders, Cardiovascular Disorders, Hematological/Endocrine/Immunological Disorders, Infectious Diseases**, and **Behavioral Disorders** sections for management of specific conditions.

CONSULTATION

→ Referral to a physician is warranted in patients with evidence of obstruction, peritoneal irritation, acute vascular insufficiency, metabolic disorders, and cardiac or pulmonary disease.
→ Consultation with a physician and/or referral is warranted when:
  - Undiagnosed abdominal pain is present.
  - Signs and symptoms do not follow the usual course of disease.
  - Impressive signs and symptoms are present (e.g., high fever, severe pain, shock, elevated WBCs, other laboratory test abnormalities, or patient is unable to eat or drink).
→ Referral to a mental health provider is warranted in cases of severe psychogenic disorder, depression, or neurosis.
→ As needed for prescription(s)

PATIENT EDUCATION

→ Patient education will depend on the etiology of abdominal pain. Refer to the appropriate chapter(s) for patient education regarding specific etiologies.

FOLLOW-UP

→ When the diagnosis is unclear and the patient is not ill enough for immediate referral or admission, close follow-up is important.

→ Chronic abdominal pain may require a methodical work-up and therapeutic trials.
→ Teach the American Cancer Society's recommendation for early detection of cancer in asymptomatic people (Zoorob et al. 2001):
  - Fecal occult blood test: yearly beginning at age 50

  AND
  - Digital rectal exam and flexible sigmoidoscopy: every 5 years beginning at age 50

  OR
  - Digital rectal exam and colonoscopy: every 10 years beginning at age 50

  OR
  - Digital rectal exam and double contrast barium enema: every 5–10 years beginning at age 50.
→ Document in progress notes and on problem list.

BIBLIOGRAPHY

American College of Emergency Physicians. 2000. Clinical policy: critical issues for the initial evaluation and management of patients presenting with a chief complaint of nontraumatic acute abdominal pain. *American College of Emergency Physicians* 36(4):406–415.

DeBanto, J.R., Varilek, G.W., and Haas, L. 1999. What could be causing chronic abdominal pain? *Postgraduate Medicine* 106(3):141–146.

Dirckx, J.H., ed. 2001. *Stedman's concise medical dictionary for the health professions*, 4th ed., p. 15. Baltimore: Lippincott Williams & Wilkins.

Friedman, L.S. 2002. Acute pancreatitis. In *Current medical diagnosis and treatment*, 41st ed., eds. L. Tierney, Jr., S. McPhee, and M. Papadakis, pp. 641–643. New York: Lange Medical Books/McGraw-Hill.

Hickey, M.S., Kiernan, G.J., and Weaver, K.E. 1989. Evaluation of abdominal pain. *Emergency Medicine Clinics of North America* 7(3):437–452.

Martin, R.F., and Rossi, R.L. 1997. The acute abdomen. *Surgical Clinics of North America* 77(6):1227–1243.

Richter, J.M. 2000. Evaluation of abdominal pain. In *Primary care medicine*, 4th ed., eds. A.H. Goroll and J.A. Mulley, pp. 375–384. Philadelphia: Lippincott Williams & Wilkins.

Robertson, C. 1998. Differential diagnosis of lower abdominal pain in women of childbearing age. *Lippincott's Primary Care Practice* 2(3):210–229.

Stone, R. 1996. Primary care diagnosis of acute abdominal pain. *Nurse Practitioner* 21(12):19–39.

_____. 1998. Acute abdominal pain. *Lippincott's Primary Care Practice* 2(4):341–357.

Suleiman, S., and Johnstone, D.E. 2001. The abdominal wall: an overlooked source of pain. *American Family Physician* 64(3):431–438.

Zackowski, S.W. 1998. Chronic recurrent abdominal pain. *Emergency Medicine Clinics of North America* 16(4):877–894.

Zoorob, R., Anderson, R., Cefalu, C. et al. 2001. Cancer screening guidelines. *American Family Physician* 63(6):1101–1112.

Lisa L. Lommel, R.N., C., F.N.P., M.S., M.P.H.
Jeanne R. Davis, R.N., F.N.P., M.P.H.

7-B

Appendicitis

Appendicitis is one of the most common causes of the acute surgical abdomen. The lifetime occurrence of appendicitis is approximately 7% (Hardin 1999, Stone 1998). The peak incidence of appendicitis occurs between 10–30 years old and is more common in males. It is uncommon after age 50, but when appendicitis does occur in this age group, it is associated with higher levels of complications and morbidity because of atypical presentation and delayed diagnosis and treatment (Pisarra 1999).

Obstruction of the appendiceal lumen by a fecalith, inflammation, foreign body, or neoplasm is thought to initiate appendicitis. Mucosal ulceration has been identified as an antecedent to obstruction in many cases. Once the obstruction occurs, the mucosa of the obstructed appendix gets inflamed and continues to secrete fluids. This, in turn, distends the appendix and increases pressure, causing pain, necrosis, and possibly perforation. Perforation is a serious complication of appendicitis because it can cause peritonitis and intra-abdominal sepsis. Delays in treatment are associated with perforation; this is more common among the elderly (Stone 1998).

DATABASE

SUBJECTIVE

→ Patient has negative history of appendectomy.
→ Symptoms usually begin with gradual, mild, intermittent, and cramping pain localized to either the epigastric or periumbilical area.
→ Within 12 hours, the pain spreads to the right lower quadrant (RLQ) where it is constant, increasing in severity and aggravated by cough or motion.
→ Nausea with one or two episodes of vomiting after onset of pain is very common.
→ Anorexia is also commonly associated with acute appendicitis.
→ Malaise, a feeling of constipation (even after a bowel movement), or sometimes diarrhea may develop after the pain has started.
→ Patient can usually point to a specific area of maximal tenderness.

→ Depending on the location of the patient's appendix, other symptoms may occur:
   ▪ Appendix adjacent to the bladder—urinary frequency and dysuria
   ▪ Retrocecal or pelvic appendix—minimal or absent abdominal tenderness and positive tenderness in flank or on rectal examination (Hardin 1999)
→ Obese or elderly patients may have a delay in the appearance of abdominal signs, and they may not experience sharp localization of symptoms.
→ The elderly may have vague symptoms and mild abdominal tenderness (Kraemer et al. 2000).

OBJECTIVE

→ Temperature is normal or slightly elevated (37.2–38° C, 99–100.4° F).
→ Temperature above 38.3° C (101° F) may indicate perforation or another diagnosis.
→ Tachycardia is present with an elevation of temperature.
→ Microscopic hematuria and pyuria may be present.
→ Light palpation or percussion can identify a point of maximal tenderness in RLQ.
→ Rebound tenderness and muscle rigidity or involuntary guarding in RLQ
→ Hyperesthesia of the skin in RLQ
→ When asked to cough, the patient may be able to identify the painful area precisely (a sign of peritoneal irritation).
→ Diminished or absent bowel sounds
→ Rigidity and tenderness are increased as the disease progresses.
→ There is a positive iliopsoas sign (retrocecal), obturator sign (pelvic appendix), Rovsing's sign, and Sumner's sign (see **Table 7A.2, Abdominal Palpation** in the **Abdominal Pain** chapter).
→ While the digital rectal exam is not consistently helpful in cases of appendicitis, it may be helpful in ruling out rectal, gynecologic, pelvic, and urologic disease (Stone 1998).

→ Tenderness on right side of rectal wall
→ Signs of perforation include:
- Pain persisting over 36 hours
- Increasing pain, tenderness, and spasm of RLQ followed by diffuse abdominal tenderness and evidence of generalized peritonitis or a localized abscess (tender mass in RLQ)
- Fever, malaise, tachycardia, and a white blood cell (WBC) count elevation of up to 20,000–30,000/μL with a prominent left shift (Hardin 1999)
- Perforation rarely occurs in the first eight hours.

ASSESSMENT

→ Acute appendicitis
→ R/O gastroenteritis
→ R/O mesenteric adenitis
→ R/O pelvic inflammatory disease
→ R/O ruptured graafian follicle or corpus luteum cyst
→ R/O acute diverticulitis
→ R/O perforated peptic ulcer
→ R/O acute cholecystitis
→ R/O ruptured ectopic pregnancy
→ R/O twisted ovarian cyst or ovarian torsion
→ R/O mittelschmerz
→ R/O nephrolithiasis
→ R/O acute salpingitis or tubo-ovarian abscess
→ R/O ureteral colic or pyelonephritis
→ R/O perforated colonic cancer
→ R/O ulcerative colitis or Crohn's ileitis
→ R/O intestinal obstruction
→ R/O abdominal aneurysm

PLAN

DIAGNOSTIC TESTS

→ Obtain complete blood count and differential:
- Elevated WBC count to 10,000–20,000/μL with increase in neutrophils is common (leukocytosis with a left shift).
- While moderate elevation in WBCs is common during an appendicitis attack, WBC count has low specificity for diagnosis of appendicitis (normal WBC count should not rule out possibility of acute appendicitis).
- WBCs >20,000/μL may indicate perforation.
→ C-reactive protein is commonly elevated (>0.8 mg/dL) in appendicitis.
- An elevated C-reactive protein level in combination with an elevated WBC count and neutrophilia are highly sensitive (97–100%) for appendicitis (Hardin 1999).
→ Urinalysis is helpful in ruling out genitourinary symptoms that can mimic appendicitis and help diagnose renal/ureteral calculi.
→ Urine or serum pregnancy test is essential.
→ While imaging studies may not always be performed in patients with typical appendicitis, they are commonly used and are very useful in patients with an equivocal diagnosis.
- Ultrasound:
  - Abdominal or transvaginal ultrasound (US) accurately diagnoses appendicitis in over 85% of cases (McQuaid 2002).
  - Demonstration of an enlarged and thick-walled appendix on ultrasound is diagnostic for appendicitis (if appendix cannot be seen, appendicitis cannot be excluded).
  - US performed for nonperforated appendicitis is more sensitive and specific than when utilized for evaluation of perforated appendicitis.
  - US is very useful in the exclusion of adnexal disease and for verifying other organic causes of abdominal pain (McQuaid 2002, Pisarra 1999).
- Computed tomography (CT):
  - CT is more accurate than ultrasonography for appendicitis and has been shown to improve provider decision-making in patients with moderate probability of appendicitis (Graff et al. 2001, Hardin 1999).
  - CT is very helpful when a suspected appendicitis presents atypically.
  - Evaluation by CT scan and clinical assessment combined has a higher sensitivity (98.3%) and specificity (95.8%) than either alone (Gwynn 2001).
  - CT can reliably diagnose appendicitis by visual identification of an abnormal appendix as well as by identifying periappendiceal inflammatory changes (especially useful in cases of suspected appendiceal perforation) (Gwynn 2001, McQuaid 2002).
- Plain abdominal radiograph:
  - In patients with suspected appendicitis, may reveal abnormalities in acute appendicitis
  - Is not sensitive or specific, is often misleading
  - Plain films should not be routinely obtained for patients with suspected appendicitis, although they can help diagnose other causes of abdominal pain (Hardin 1999, Rao et al. 1999).
→ As a result of the myriad presentations of appendicitis, in some cases diagnostic laparotomy or laparoscopy is required.

TREATMENT/MANAGEMENT

→ During close observation, the patient should rest, be given nothing by mouth, and should not be prescribed laxatives or narcotics that will interfere with the assessment of disease progression.
→ Once there is a strong suspicion of appendicitis or it is diagnosed, immediate referral to a surgeon is warranted.
→ Appendicitis is treated by surgical appendectomy via laparoscopy or laparotomy, depending on the preference of the surgeon and the patient's status.
→ If perforation has occurred, the choice of treatments varies.

CONSULTATION

→ Physician consultation (usually surgical) may be sought in diagnosis.

PATIENT EDUCATION

→ Explain the disease process, progression, and treatment plan.

→ Advise the patient about the probability of surgery if a diagnosis of appendicitis is made.

___

FOLLOW-UP

→ As indicated by the surgical team
→ Teach the American Cancer Society's recommendation for early detection of cancer in asymptomatic people (Zoorob et al. 2001):
  ▪ Fecal occult blood test: yearly beginning at age 50
                    AND
  ▪ Digital rectal exam and flexible sigmoidoscopy: every 10 years beginning at age 50
                    OR
  ▪ Digital rectal exam and colonoscopy: every 5–10 years beginning at age 50
                    OR
  ▪ Digital rectal exam and double contrast barium enema: every 10 years beginning at age 50.
→ Document in progress notes and on problem list.

BIBLIOGRAPHY

Graff, L., and Robinson, D. 2001. Abdominal pain and emergency department evaluation. *Medicine Clinics of North America* 19(1):123–136.

Gwynn, L.K. 2001. The diagnosis of acute appendicitis: clinical assessment versus computed tomography evaluation. *Journal of Emergency Medicine* 21(2):119–123.

Hardin, D.M. 1999. Acute appendicitis: review and update. *American Family Physician* 60(7):2027–2034.

Kraemer, M., Franke, C., Ohmann, Q. et al. 2000. Acute appendicitis in late adulthood: incidence, presentation, and outcome. *Langenbeck's Archives of Surgery* 385(7):470–481.

McQuaid, K.R. 2002. Appendicitis. In *Current medical diagnosis and treatment*, 41st ed., eds. L. Tierney, Jr., S. McPhee, and M. Papadakis, pp. 641–643. New York: Lange Medical Books/McGraw-Hill.

Pisarra, V.H. 1999. Recognizing the various presentations of appendicitis. *Nurse Practitioner* 24(8):42–53.

Rao, P.M., Rhea, J.T., Rao, J.A. et al. 1999. Plain abdominal radiography in clinically suspected appendicitis: diagnostic yield, resource use, and comparison with CT. *American Journal of Emergency Medicine* 17(4):325–328.

Stone, R. 1998. Acute abdominal pain. *Lippincott's Primary Care Practice* 2(4):341–357.

Zoorob, R., Anderson, R., Cefalu, C. et al. 2001. Cancer screening guidelines. *American Family Physician* 63(6): 1101–1112.

Lisa L. Lommel, R.N., C., F.N.P., M.S., M.P.H.
Jeanne R. Davis, R.N., F.N.P., M.P.H.

7-C

Cholecystitis

Cholecystitis is an inflammation of the gallbladder wall that occurs most often when a stone becomes lodged in the cystic duct. As a result, pressure inside the gallbladder rises, causing rapid distention, decreased blood supply, ischemia of the gallbladder wall, bacterial invasion with acute inflammation, and possible perforation. Approximately 90–95% of all cases of acute cholecystitis are associated with cholelithiasis (Ahmed et al. 2000, Beers et al. 1999). Gallstones found in the gallbladder are classified as cholesterol, pigmented, or mixed stones, based on their chemical composition. Up to 90% of gallstones are considered to be "cholesterol gallstones" (defined as being composed of more than 50% cholesterol). These develop when bile becomes saturated with cholesterol. Pigmented stones have less than 20% cholesterol. Common bile duct stones (choledocholithiasis) may form de novo in bile ducts or migrate to the common bile duct from the gallbladder.

Gallbladder disease is two to three times more common in women than men (Kalloo et al. 2001). While hereditary factors play a strong role in the development of gallbladder disease, other factors are known to increase the risk of gallstone development as well. These include elevated endogenous (secondary to puberty, pregnancy) or exogenous estrogens (oral contraceptives or postmenopausal hormone replacement therapy), obesity, rapid weight loss, hyperlipidemia, intestinal hypomotility disorders, long-term parenteral nutrition, certain drugs (HMG-CoA reductase inhibitors, ceftriaxone, octreotide), patients with spinal cord injuries, and those with diseases of the terminal ileum (Kalloo et al. 2001). Gallstones are not found in 5–10% of patients with acute cholecystitis. The pathogenesis of acute acalculous cholecystitis is not fully understood, but probably involves ischemia, biliary stasis, and chemical inflammation.

Repeated episodes of acute inflammation or chronic irritation of the gallbladder wall by stones may lead to chronic cholecystitis, which is characterized by varying degrees of chronic inflammation of the gallbladder. The gallbladder wall may become thick and infiltrated with inflammatory cells. The subsequent development of fibrosis leads to a loss of contractility and concentrating function of the gallbladder. The mucosa may be ulcerated and scarred, and the lumen may contain sludge or stones that may obstruct the cystic duct (Beers et al. 1999). Calculi are usually present.

Untreated or inadequately treated acute cholecystitis can rapidly progress to empyema, gangrene of the gallbladder wall with perforation, intra-abdominal abscess, or diffuse peritonitis. Risk factors associated with complications of gallbladder disease include diabetes, being disabled, over 60 years of age, or having stones greater than 2.5 cm or less than 0.5 cm.

DATABASE

SUBJECTIVE

Acute Cholecystitis

→ The patient may be asymptomatic.
→ Most patients with acute cholecystitis have had previous attacks of biliary pain.
→ The pain is sudden-onset, severe, and steady below the right costal margin or in the epigastric region, radiating to the back, the right scapula, or the right clavicular area, and it gradually subsides in 12–18 hours.
→ The pain of acute cholecystitis typically lasts longer than 3 hours, and after 3 hours, it moves from the epigastrium to the right upper quadrant (RUQ).
→ Pain is usually precipitated by a heavy, fatty meal and aggravated by deep inspiration.
→ Anorexia, nausea, and vomiting are common.
→ When the above symptoms are present and there is a recent history (past 2–4 weeks) of major surgery, acalculous cholecystitis should be considered (Friedman 2002).
→ In the elderly, localized tenderness may be the only presenting sign (with no pain or fever).

Chronic Cholecystitis

→ Patient usually has a long history of recurrent exacerbations with RUQ pain, fever, nausea, and vomiting (Kalloo et al. 2001).

→ Although dyspeptic symptoms, including fatty food intolerance, belching, and bloating, were thought to be due to chronic gallbladder disease, this has not been proven (Goroll 2000). Regardless, these symptoms are commonly reported by patients with gallstones.

→ Dark urine and light, clay-colored stools may occur in acute and chronic cholecystitis.

OBJECTIVE

Acute Cholecystitis

→ RUQ abdominal tenderness with involuntary guarding of right-sided abdominal muscles, with or without rebound tenderness

→ Decreased bowel sounds

→ The gallbladder may be palpable, although this is unlikely (Beers et al. 1999, Friedman 2002).

→ Low-grade fever

→ Positive Murphy's sign (see **Table 7A.2, Abdominal Palpation** in the **Abdominal Pain** chapter)

→ Complications are indicated by high fever, rigors, tachycardia, hypotension, leukocytosis, and rebound tenderness, which suggest empyema, gangrene of the gallbladder with perforation, intra-abdominal abscess, or diffuse peritonitis.

Chronic Cholecystitis

→ Mild or absent RUQ tenderness

→ Jaundice may be present

→ May have fever

ASSESSMENT

→ Cholecystitis—acute or chronic

→ R/O dyspepsia

→ R/O peptic ulcer

→ R/O pancreatitis

→ R/O hepatitis

→ R/O liver abscess

→ R/O appendicitis

→ R/O diverticulitis

→ R/O irritable bowel syndrome

→ R/O inflammatory bowel disease (IBD)

→ R/O right lower-lobe pneumonia/diaphragmatic pleurisy

→ R/O neoplasm of the stomach, pancreas, liver, or gallbladder

→ R/O angina/myocardial infarction

→ R/O Fitz-Hugh-Curtis syndrome

→ R/O cholangitis

→ R/O pleurisy

PLAN

DIAGNOSTIC TESTS

→ White blood cell count is usually high (12,000–15,000/μL), with a left shift.

→ Total serum bilirubin, alkaline phosphatase, and serum aminotransferases are often elevated.

→ Lipase is usually normal unless a stone obstructs the pancreatic duct and pancreatitis is also present.

→ Amylase elevation suggests (but does not confirm) gallstone pancreatitis (Beers et al. 1999).

→ Ultrasound (US):

- US of the gallbladder and biliary tree is the test of choice for evaluation of symptomatic patients with suspected acute cholecystitis.
  - US is particularly accurate for diagnosing cholelithiasis (Goroll 2000).
  - US provides >95% sensitivity and specificity for the diagnosis of gallstones that are >2 mm in diameter (Ahmed et al. 2000).
  - US can also show thickening of the gallbladder wall, as well as the presence of inflammatory fluid in/around the gallbladder.

→ Hepatobiliary scintigraphy (HIDA scan):

- An alternative to ultrasound for detection of acute cholecystitis
- Evaluates biliary excretion of intravenously injected nuclear isotope to determine patency of cystic duct
- Sensitivity and specificity approach that of ultrasound, but the cost is greater and the test takes more time.

→ Endoscopic retrograde cholangiopancreatography (ERCP):

- ERCP is indicated for patients with acute cholecystitis and elevated liver function tests or abnormally high levels of serum amylase and lipase in order to rule out suspected choledocholithiasis or gallstone pancreatitis before cholecystectomy (Kalloo et al. 2001).
- ERCP provides diagnostic and therapeutic options, and has a sensitivity and specificity of 95% for detection of common bile duct stones (Ahmed et al. 2000).

→ Oral cholecystogram:

- Ultrasound has generally replaced the oral cholecystogram for diagnosing acute cholecystitis, although this test has come back into use in patients who are being considered for lithotripsy or gallstone dissolution (Goroll 2000).

→ Computed tomography (CT)/magnetic resonance imaging (MRI):

- While CT of the gallbladder is not a first-line test to detect gallstones, CT and MRI are far superior to ultrasound in detecting complications of acute cholecystitis (perforation of gallbladder or biliary ducts, abscess formation, or pancreatitis).
- MRI and CT scans are comparable to ERCP in terms of diagnostic accuracy, but offer no therapeutic options.

→ Electrocardiograph to rule out cardiac symptoms

→ Chest x-ray to rule out pulmonary symptoms

TREATMENT/MANAGEMENT

Acute Cholecystitis

→ Referral to a physician is warranted for decision regarding surgical or nonsurgical treatment.

→ Patients with acute cholecystitis require hospital admission for complete bowel rest, parenteral fluids and nutrition, intravenous antibiotics, analgesics, and possibly cholecystectomy (Bagshaw 1999, Kalloo et al. 2001).

→ Medical therapy:

- Patients unwilling or too frail to undergo general anesthesia and surgery are candidates for medical therapy, which aims to dissolve stones by using bile acids, extracorporeal shock-wave lithotripsy, ether instillation, or a combination of modalities (Goroll 2000).
- Medical management may be chosen for the elderly, diabetics, or poor surgical candidates, although acute cholecystitis will usually subside on a conservative regimen.

→ Surgical intervention:

- Frequently the treatment of choice
- Because there is a high risk of recurrent attacks, cholecystectomy should be performed by either laparoscopy or laparotomy within 1–3 days after hospitalization, as long as the patient is hemodynamically stable (Ahmed et al. 2000).
- While laparoscopic cholecystectomy is becoming the technique of choice in cases of uncomplicated acute cholecystitis, conventional open cholecystectomy is still common (Goroll 2000).

Chronic Cholecystitis

→ Referral to a physician is warranted for a decision regarding surgical or nonsurgical treatment.

→ Surgical treatment of chronic cholecystitis is the same as for acute cholecystitis. If indicated, cholangiography can be performed during laparoscopic cholecystitis.

→ Nonsurgical methods include:

- Gallstone dissolution (chemical and physical)
  - Ursodeoxycholic (ursodiol) acids:
    - Oral bile salts that cause dissolution of some cholesterol stones—safe for long-term use, effective only in patients with functioning gallbladders
    - Results are best in those with a few small stones; 40% are stone free after 2 years (Goroll 2000).
    - Contraindicated in patients with inflammatory bowel disease or peptic ulcer disease
- Extracorporeal shock-wave lithotripsy:
  - Effective in the small percentage of patients who have a small number of calcium-containing stones (if stones are ≥3 cm and if patient has a functional gallbladder)
  - Is effective 95% of the time
  - After stone is shattered, follow-up with ursodeoxycholic acid agents to achieve full dissolution or stone passage (Goroll 2000)
- Methyl-tert-butyl ether:
  - Dissolves cholesterol stones, is used to treat highly selected populations with multiple or large cholesterol stones
  - Can dissolve stones in <3 days of continuous application
  - Instilled directly into gallbladder by way of a percutaneous catheter (is both difficult and potentially dangerous)
- Analgesics (e.g., meperidine) to control pain

- Rehydration with IV fluids and electrolytes
- Parenteral antibiotics

CONSULTATION

→ Referral to a physician is warranted to decide whether to treat patient surgically or nonsurgically.

→ As needed for prescription(s).

PATIENT EDUCATION

→ See the "Treatment/Management" section.

→ Explain the disease process and management plan.

→ Advise the patient regarding the purpose of tests ordered, and how/when the patient will be notified of results, as appropriate.

→ Counsel patient regarding a weight-reduction diet.

→ Some gallstone patients with dyspeptic symptoms feel better if they avoid fatty foods.

→ Multiple studies report that it is the number of calories consumed (rather than the proportion of calories coming from the intake of saturated fat/cholesterol) that correlates best with risk of gallstones (Goroll 2000).

→ Daily consumption of small amounts of alcohol (about 1 ounce/day) correlates with a 20% reduction in risk of symptomatic gallstone disease (Goroll 2000).

→ Medical treatment and risk of gallstone formation:

- Rises markedly with use of estrogen and clofibrate
- A modest increase in relative risk of gallstones with thiazide intake
- Discuss the risk of recurrent episodes.

FOLLOW-UP

→ As indicated by case presentation

→ Teach the American Cancer Society's recommendation for early detection of cancer in asymptomatic people (Zoorob et al. 2001):

- Fecal occult blood test: yearly beginning at age 50

AND

- Digital rectal exam and flexible sigmoidoscopy: every 5 years beginning at age 50

OR

- Digital rectal exam and colonoscopy: every 10 years beginning at age 50

OR

- Digital rectal exam and double contrast barium enema: every 5–10 years beginning at age 50.

→ Document in progress notes and on problem list.

BIBLIOGRAPHY

Ahmed, A., and Cheung, R.C. 2000. Management of gallstones and their complications. *American Family Physician* 61(6): 1673–1688.

Bagshaw, E.J. 1999. Abdominal pain protocol: right upper quadrant pain. *Lippincott's Primary Care Practice* 3(5): 486–492.

Beers, M., and Berkow, R. 1999. *The Merck manual of diagnosis and therapy*, 17th ed. Whitehouse Station, N.J.: Merck & Co.

Friedman, L.S. 2002. Acute cholecystitis. In *Current medical diagnosis and treatment*, 41st ed., eds., L.M., Tierney, Jr., S.J. McPhee, and M.A. Papadakis, pp. 707–708. New York: Lange Medical Books/McGraw-Hill.

Goroll, A.H. 2000. Management of asymptomatic and symptomatic gallstones. In *Primary care medicine*, 4th ed., eds. A.H. Goroll and J.A. Mulley, pp. 447–453. Philadelphia: Lippincott Williams & Wilkins.

Kalloo, A.N., and Kantsevoy, S.V. 2001. Gallstones and biliary diseases. *Primary Care* 28(3):591–603.

Zoorob, R., Anderson, R., Cefalu, C. et al. 2001. Cancer screening guidelines *American Family Physician* 63(6):1101–1112.

Lisa L. Lommel, R.N., C., F.N.P., M.S., M.P.H.

7-D

Constipation

Constipation is one of the most common gastrointestinal complaints seen in primary care. Historically, constipation has been defined as a frequency of defecation of two times a week or less. However, individuals may describe constipation in a variety of ways. Many individuals who describe themselves as constipated complain about the characteristics of defecation, including excessive straining or discomfort, or the passage of hard, pellet-like stools. These individuals may or may not have a frequency of defecation that is within the normal range. Other individuals describe the characteristics of defecation as normal but with a less-than-normal frequency (Wald 2000). An international committee recently developed a definition of chronic functional constipation that includes defecatory characteristics as well as frequency (see **Table 7D.1, Rome II Criteria for Functional Constipation**).

The normal physiologic process of defecation depends on the coordinated activity of the proximal and mid colon to reduce the volume of material, the sigmoid colon and rectum to accommodate material until evacuation, and the muscles of the pelvic floor and sphincter to achieve evacuation. These activities are controlled by the enteric and autonomic nervous system. Constipation can develop if one or more of these mechanisms are disordered (Schiller 2001).

Constipation is highly prevalent in women and becomes more common with age, with a sharp rise in individuals over age 65. Risk factors associated with constipation are inactivity (although exercise is not shown to be an effective treatment), number of medications being taken, low income, low education level, depression, and history of physical or sexual abuse (Locke III et al. 2000, Stark 1999). There is no established relationship between constipation and decreased dietary fiber or fluid intake. However, colonic transport may be influenced by decreased caloric intake. Many diseases as well as several drugs slow transit time through the colon. (See **Table 7D.2, Diseases Associated with Chronic Constipation** and **Table 7D.3, Drugs Associated With Constipation**). In addition, constipation may develop as a physiologic process of aging due to deterioration in nerve function, relaxation of support musculature, decreased

sensation, and decreased mobility. Trauma to the pelvic nerve and/or support musculature during childbirth may also increase women's risk for constipation.

DATABASE

SUBJECTIVE

→ Patient may have a history of:
- Decreasing frequency of bowel movements
- Straining at defecation
- Hard, dry stools that are difficult to express
- A sense of incomplete evacuation
- Abdominal pain, bloating, or flatulence
- Emotional tension, inability to relax

Table 7D.1. ROME II CRITERIA FOR FUNCTIONAL CONSTIPATION

Two or more of the following for at least 12 weeks in the preceding 12 months:
- Straining with at least 25% of defecations
- Lumpy or hard stools in at least 25% of defecations
- Sensation of incomplete evacuation with at least 25% of defecations
- Sensation of anorectal blockage in at least 25% of defecations
- Manual maneuvers to facilitate at least 25% of defecations
- Less than 3 defecations per week

There are no loose stools present, and there are not sufficient criteria for irritable bowel syndrome (see the **Irritable Bowel Syndrome** chapter).

Source: Adapted with permission from Rome II Criteria Committee. 2000. *Rome II: the functional gastrointestinal disorders*, 2nd ed., eds. D. Drossman, E. Corazziari, N. Talley et al. McLean, Va.: Degnon Associates. Available at: http://www.romecriteria.org. Accessed on August 1, 2002.

→ Patient may recite history of contributing factors:
- Dietary: inadequate fiber, low fluid intake
- Physical inactivity
- Pregnancy
- Advancing age
- Mechanical, endocrine, metabolic, neurologic, psychogenic disorders causing constipation (see **Table 7D.2**)
- Prescription and/or recreational drug use (see **Table 7D.3**)

OBJECTIVE

→ Abdominal exam:
- A mass or fullness may be palpated over the large intestine.
- Bowels sounds may be hyperactive or absent.
→ Pelvic exam:
- Rectocele may be present.
- Rectal discharge may be present (suggesting a sexually transmitted infection).
→ Inspection of the anus during attempted defecation:
- Prolapse of the rectal mucosa may be present.

→ Digital exam should be done to evaluate resting anal tone, sensitivity, reflexes, and contracting muscle strength:
- Dry, hard stool may be felt on rectal exam.
- Hemorrhoids, fistulas, or fissures may be present and felt on rectal exam.
→ Neurological exam:
- Rule out focal deficits.
- Signs of mechanical, metabolic, endocrine, neurologic, or psychogenic disorders may be present (see **Table 7D.2**).

ASSESSMENT

→ Constipation, episodic or chronic
→ R/O irritable bowel disease
→ R/O slow transit constipation
→ R/O rectal outlet obstruction
→ R/O organic constipation (mechanical obstruction or drug side effect)
→ R/O constipation secondary to systemic disease

Table 7D.2. DISEASES ASSOCIATED WITH CHRONIC CONSTIPATION

Functional Constipation

Pelvic floor dysfunction
Colonic inertia (slow-transit constipation)
Hypertonic internal anal sphincter
Irritable bowel syndrome

Neurogenic Disorders

Autonomic neuropathy
Cauda equina syndrome
Hirschsprung's disease
Intestinal pseudo-obstruction
Multiple sclerosis
Parkinson's disease
Spinal cord injury
Cerebral vascular disease

Endocrine and Metabolic Disorders

Diabetes mellitus
Hypothyroidism
Hypercalcemia
Hyperkalemia
Hypomagnesemia
Porphyria
Systemic sclerosis
Heavy metal poisoning
Uremia

Mechanical Obstruction

Colon cancer
External compression from malignant lesion
Rectocele, if large
Postsurgical abnormalities, including adhesions
Megacolon
Anal fissure/strictures, painful hemorrhoids
Inflammatory bowel disease
Mucosal intussusception
Rectal prolapse
Infectious proctitis

Psychosocial Dysfunction

Eating disorders
Cognitive impairment
Depression
Situational stress
Anxiety
Somatization
Phobias

Other Conditions

Pregnancy
Degenerative joint disease
Immobility
Cardiac disease
Laxative abuse

Source: Compiled from Schiller, L.R. 2001. Gastrointestinal disorders in the elderly. *Gastroenterology Clinics* 30(2):497–515; Wald, A. 2000. Constipation. *Advances in Gastroenterology* 84(5):1232; Locke, G.R. III, Pemberton, J.H., and Phillips, S.F. 2000. American Gastroenterological Association medical position statement: guidelines on constipation. *Gastroenterology* 119(6):1770; Browning, S.M. 1999. Constipation, diarrhea, and irritable bowel syndrome. *Primary Care* 26(1):114–115; and Richter, J.M. 2000. Approach to the patient with constipation. In *Primary care medicine*, 4th ed., eds. A.H. Goroll and A.G. Mulley, Jr., p. 422. Philadelphia: Lippincott Williams & Wilkins.

PLAN

DIAGNOSTIC TESTS

→ History is a hallmark in diagnosing constipation.

→ A recent or unexplained change in bowel habits not associated with a definable cause (i.e., medication) requires an evaluation to rule out organic cause.

→ Obtain stool for occult blood.

→ TSH to rule out hypothyroidism

→ Serum calcium to rule out hypercalcemia

→ CBC

→ Serum glucose

→ Creatinine

→ Anoscopy may identify anal fissures, fistulas, or hemorrhoids.

→ Plain supine and upright films of the abdomen to rule out obstruction with acute onset of constipation.

→ Flexible sigmoidoscopy, colonoscopy, barium radiographs, radiopaque marker studies, and/or anorectal manometry may be indicated for unexplained or chronic constipation not responding to treatment. Physician consultation/referral is indicated for these tests.

TREATMENT/MANAGEMENT

→ See the "Patient Education" section.

Table 7D.3.   DRUGS ASSOCIATED WITH CONSTIPATION

Anticholinergics
Anticonvulsants
Antidiarrheal agents
Antiemetics: 5-HT$_3$ antagonists
 Granisetron
 Ondansetron
Antihistamines
Antihypertensives
Anti-Parkinson drugs
Calcium channel blockers
Cation-containing agents
 Aluminum (antacids, sucralfate)
 Bismuth
 Calcium (antacids, supplements)
 Iron supplements
Diuretics
Nonsteroidal anti-inflammatory agents
Opiates
Tricyclic antidepressants

Source: Compiled from Wald, A. 2000. Constipation. *Advances in Gastroenterology* 84(5):1233; and Locke, G.R. III, Pemberton, J.H., and Phillips, S.F. 2000. American Gastrointestinal Association technical review on constipation. *Gastroenterology* 119(6):1768. ©2000 American Gastroenterological Association.

→ First-line treatment for constipation is nonpharmacologic. Results are unlikely before several weeks of a treatment program. This program should be considered life-long to prevent and/or manage future constipation events. The treatment plan includes diet, physical activity, and treatment for other conditions.

→ Diet (see **General Nutrition Guidelines**, Section 16):
 ■ Fluid intake: increase water to 6–8 glasses/day.
 ■ Fiber: increase intake of bran, whole grain products, raw fruits and vegetables.
 ■ Avoid constipating foods: milk, cheese, rice, and bananas.

→ Physical activity: patients should be encouraged to be as physically active as possible, although increased activity may not improve constipation.

→ Treatment for conditions or change of medications that may be causing constipation. See **Tables 7D.2** and **7D.3**.

→ If nonpharmacologic treatments are not effective, bulk or osmotic laxatives are added next. See **Table 7D.4, Summary of Medications Commonly Used for Constipation**. NOTE: Psyllium, calcium polycarbophil, and methylcellulose should be well diluted and consumed before meals or at bedtime.

→ When patients fail to respond to bulk or osmotic laxatives, stimulant laxatives may be considered. NOTE: Stimulant laxatives have the potential for abuse. Continuous daily use may produce diarrhea causing hyponatremia, hypokalemia, and dehydration, especially in the elderly. When used only 2–3 times a week, they can be safe and effective for long periods (Wald 2000).
 ■ Laxatives should not be used in patients with undiagnosed abdominal pain or with possible intestinal obstruction or fecal impaction.

→ In patients not responding to oral laxatives, tap water or phosphate enemas are safe. NOTE: Water intoxication and dilutional hyponatremia with weakness, shock, convulsions, and coma may occur in children and elderly with megacolon who are given large tap water enemas (Wald 2000).
 ■ Caution should be employed in giving phosphate enemas to patients with renal dysfunction because hypocalcemia and hyperphosphatemia may occur (Wald 2000).

→ Biofeedback programs in adults with constipation related to pelvic floor dysfunction has been found to have a success rate >75%. Dieticians and behavioral psychologists make up the program team (Locke III et al. 2000).

→ Treatment for specific disease that contributes to constipation should be completed (see **Table 7D.2**).

→ Referral to a mental health provider may be indicated if depression, anxiety, or other disorders are present.

CONSULTATION

→ Physician consultation is warranted for obstruction, impaction, or failure to respond to conservative treatment, and for certain causative disorders.

→ As needed for prescription(s).

PATIENT EDUCATION

→ Advise patients to record bowel habits and food intake for a few weeks to assess for true constipation versus patient misconceptions.

→ Reassure patients and educate about normal range of bowel habits.

→ Advise patients against excessive use of laxatives and cathartics.

→ Advise patients to avoid prolonged straining at stool or sitting on toilet for prolonged periods.

→ Advise moderate exercise.

→ Advise regular toileting habits, especially in the morning and after meals when colonic activity is highest.

→ Advise that during periods of lifestyle alteration (e.g., bed rest, travel), constipation can be avoided by engaging in prevention activities (e.g., increase in fluids, fiber, and exercise).

→ Advise patients that bran should be taken with a meal and that a beverage must be taken after consuming bran. Bran can cause abdominal bloating and flatulence. Starting with small amounts of bran and increasing to tolerance level can minimize symptoms.

FOLLOW-UP

→ Assess bowel activity and related lifestyle habits on subsequent visits.

→ Teach the American Cancer Society's recommendation for early detection of cancer in asymptomatic people (Zoorob et al. 2001):

→ Fecal occult blood test: yearly beginning at age 50

AND

→ Digital rectal exam and flexible sigmoidoscopy: every 5 years beginning at age 50

OR

→ Digital rectal exam and colonoscopy: every 10 years beginning at age 50

OR

→ Digital rectal exam and double contrast barium enema: every 5–10 years beginning at age 50.

→ Document in progress notes and on problem list.

Table 7D.4. SUMMARY OF MEDICATIONS COMMONLY USED FOR CONSTIPATION

Type	Generic Name	Trade Name	Dosage	Time of Onset to Action
Bulk: fiber	Bran		1 cup/day	
	Psyllium	Metamucil®, Perdiem® with fiber	1 tsp up to TID	
	Methylcellulose	Citrucel®	1 tsp up to TID	
	Calcium polycarbophil	FiberCon®	2–4 tablets QD	
Osmotic: stool softener	Docusate sodium	Colace®	100 mg BID	12–72 hrs
Hyperosmolar agents	Sorbitol		15–30 mL QD or BID	24–48 hrs
	Lactulose	Chronulac®	15–30 mL QD or BID	24–48 hrs
	Polyethylene glycol	Golytely®, Colyte®, Miralax®	8–32 oz QD	0.5–1 hr
Suppository	Glycerin		Daily, as needed	0.25–1 hr
	Bisacodyl	Dulcolax®	Daily, as needed	0.25–1 hr
Stimulants	Bisacodyl	Dulcolax®	10 mg suppositories up to 3/day	0.25–1 hr
	Anthraquinones	Senokot®	2 tablets p.o. QD to 4 tablets BID	8–12 hrs
		Perdiem®	1–2 tsp QD	8–12 hrs
		Pericolace®	1–2 tablets QD	8–12 hrs
Saline laxative	Magnesium	Milk of Magnesia®	15–30 mL QD or BID	1–3 hrs
		Haley's MO® (with mineral oil)	15–30 mL QD or BID	1–3 hrs
Lubricant	Mineral oil		15–45 mL p.o. QD	6–8 hrs
Enemas	Mineral oil retention enema		100–250 mL/rectum QD	6–8 hrs
	Tap water enema		500 mL/rectum QD	5–15 min
	Phosphate enema	Fleet®	1 Unit/rectum QD	5–15 min
	Soapsuds enema		1,500 mL/rectum	2–15 min

Source: Reprinted with permission from Locke, G.R. III, Pemberton, J.H., and Phillips, S.F. 2000. American Gastrointestinal Association technical review on constipation. *Gastroenterology* 119(6):1773.

BIBLIOGRAPHY

Browning, S.M. 1999. Constipation, diarrhea, and irritable bowel syndrome. *Primary Care* 26(1):113–139.

Locke, G.R. III, Pemberton, J.H., and Phillips, S.F. 2000. American Gastrointestinal Association technical review on constipation. *Gastroenterology* 119(6):1761–1766.

_____. 2000. American Gastroenterological Association medical position statement: guidelines on constipation. *Gastroenterology* 119(6):1770.

Richter, J.M. 2000. Approach to the patient with constipation. In *Primary care medicine*, 4th ed., eds. A.H. Goroll and A.G. Mulley, Jr., pp. 420–424. Philadelphia: Lippincott Williams & Wilkins.

Rome II Criteria Committee. 2000. *Rome II: the functional gastrointestinal disorders*, 2nd ed., eds. D. Drossman, E. Corazziari, N. Talley et al. McLean, Va.: Degnon Associates. Available at: http://www.romecriteria.org. Accessed on August 1, 2002.

Schiller, L.R. 2001. Gastrointestinal disorders in the elderly. *Gastroenterology Clinics* 30(2):497–515.

Stark, M.E. 1999. Challenging problems presenting as constipation. *American Journal of Gastroenterology* 94(3):567–574.

Thompson, W.G., Longstreth, G.F., and Drossman, D.A. 1999. Functional bowel disorders and functional abdominal pain. *Gut* 45(Suppl. II):1143–1147.

Wald, A. 2000. Constipation. *Medical Clinics of North America* 84(5):1231–1245.

Zoorob, R., Anderson, R., Cefalu, C. et al. 2001. Cancer screening guidelines. *American Family Physician* 63(6):1101–1112.

Lisa L. Lommel, R.N., C., F.N.P., M.S., M.P.H.
Jeanne R. Davis, R.N., F.N.P., M.P.H.

7-E

Diarrhea

While there is no clear agreement on how *diarrhea* is defined, it is most often measured in terms of frequency, consistency, and weight. Excessive stool frequency is the most widely used criterion for diarrhea (Fine et al. 1999). Three or more bowel movements per day (Chassany et al. 2000, Mathan 1998, Schiller 2000) and/or a stool weight of greater than 200 g/day (DeBruyn 2000, Schiller 2000) or 300 g/day (Beers et al. 1999) are generally considered to be abnormal. Diarrhea is the result of excess fecal water, and it can be due to myriad causes, including medication, exposure to pathogens, surgery, or an inflammatory process (Beers et al. 1999). These causes produce:

→ *Osmotic diarrhea:* when unabsorbable water-soluble molecules remain in the bowel, causing increased nonabsorbable intraluminal water—as seen in sugar or lactose intolerance or with poorly absorbed salts such as laxatives. Sugar substitutes (sorbitol and mannitol) can cause osmotic diarrhea.

→ *Secretory diarrhea:* when the small and large bowel secrete more electrolytes and water than they can absorb. This can be due to bacterial toxins, enteropathogenic viruses, bile acids (e.g., after ileal resection), unabsorbed dietary fat, and some medications or hormones. Five percent of secretory diarrhea is caused by microscopic colitis. Microscopic colitis refers to a syndrome of chronic watery diarrhea associated with a normal gross appearance of the surface of the colon when viewed by endoscopy, but histological analysis of the colonic mucosa reveals an increased number of inflammatory cells (Fine 1998).

→ *Exudative diarrhea:* intestinal loss of serum proteins, blood, mucus, or pus (secondary to impaired colonic absorption and inflammation of the mucosa), which can be associated with ulcerative colitis, shigellosis, and cancer.

→ *Decreased absorption time:* Decreased absorption time is caused by a decreased absorptive surface (as with bowel/gastric resection) or by decreased contact time (secondary to certain medical conditions such as hyperthyroidism and irritable bowel syndrome or medications that speed transit time), leading to excess fecal water.

Diarrhea is also classified and treated by its duration (acute versus chronic). *Acute diarrhea* is defined as diarrhea lasting for less than four weeks (Dupont 1997, Schiller 2000). The most common causes include infection, drug reactions, and alterations in diet. The course of acute diarrhea is usually self-limited, unless the patient is immunocompromised. *Chronic diarrhea* is commonly defined as diarrhea lasting at least one month (Dupont 1997, Fine et al. 1999).

DATABASE

SUBJECTIVE

→ Stool characteristics:
- Loose, liquid stools
- Blood, mucus, pus, or grease in stools
- Urgency to defecate (with or without fecal incontinence)
- Increase in frequency of stools
- Volume usually perceived as large

→ Associated symptoms:
- Abdominal pain
- Cramping before, during, and/or after defecation
- Increase in flatulence
- Abdominal bloating
- Nausea, vomiting
- Weight loss
- Fever
- Increased heart rate
- Rash
- Symptoms of dehydration: thirst, decreased urine output, dry mouth, postural lightheadedness

→ Historical evidence/symptoms of common causes of diarrhea include:
- Recent foreign or domestic travel
- Exposure to a rural water supply (including swimming in or drinking from a lake or a stream)
- Exposure to others with diarrhea
- Occupation: exposure to children or nontoilet-trained infants (e.g., in day care center)

- Sexual preferences/activity
- Psychogenic factors:
  - Nervousness or anxiety
- Drugs:
  - Ingestion of magnesium-containing antacids, metoclopramide, chemotherapeutic agents, bile acid resins, laxative use/abuse
  - Recent use of antibiotics: Colitis can develop when normal bowel flora is suppressed by antibiotic use, allowing *Clostridium difficile* to proliferate and cause mild to severe, profuse, watery stools.
  - Illicit drug use/alcohol abuse
- Infection:
  - Usually abrupt onset
  - Associated symptoms: headache, anorexia, fever, nausea, vomiting, malaise, myalgia
  - Diarrhea of viral etiology has an incubation period of 48–72 hours and lasts 1–3 days.
- Dietary factors:
  - Digestion of poorly absorbable carbohydrates (e.g., sorbitol, mannitol) or fats (steatorrhea)
  - Excessive intake of fruits or caffeine-containing foods, herbal teas
  - Lactase deficiency with intolerance to milk, causing bloating and/or cramping
  - Consumption of raw meats, eggs, or shellfish; unpasteurized milk or juice
  - Food allergy, which can cause diarrhea after ingestion of certain foods
- Other intestinal factors:
  - Relationship of defecation to meals/time of day: Assess if there is passage of stools/fecal urgency during the night and whether symptoms wake patient from sleep.
  - Fecal impaction (more common in elderly), which may cause a period of absent stools
- Chronic diarrhea:
  - Consider inflammatory bowel disease (IBD) or malignancy with symptoms of bleeding, fever, or weight loss.
  - Consider acquired immunodeficiency syndrome (AIDS) if diarrhea >1 month, with unexplained weight loss and history of at-risk behaviors.
  - Irritable bowel syndrome, idiopathic IBD, malabsorption syndrome, laxative overuse, chronic infections, and idiopathic secretory diarrhea are the most frequent diagnoses made in patients with chronic diarrhea.
- Gastrointestinal surgery:
  - Dumping syndrome:
    - Refers to the early delivery of a large amount of liquid or food to the small intestine
    - Is usually due to resective gastric operations
    - Dumping syndrome may cause sweating, lightheadedness, tachycardia, and diarrhea following food ingestion.
- See the **Inflammatory Bowel Disease**, **Irritable Bowel Syndrome**, **Diverticular Disease**, and **Abdominal Pain** chapters; the **Type 1 Diabetes Mellitus**, **Type 2 Diabetes Mellitus**, and **Thyroid Disorders** chapters in Section 10; and the **Hepatitis—Viral** chapter in Section 11.

OBJECTIVE

→ Vital signs:
  - Depending on the extent of dehydration secondary to diarrhea, may find orthostatic pulse and blood pressure changes, elevation in temperature, and/or weight loss
  - Other signs of volume depletion: dry mucous membranes, decreased skin turgor, absent jugular venous pulsations, altered sensorium
→ Abdominal exam:
  - Abdominal tenderness, distention; occasionally will have guarding, rebound
  - Increased bowel sounds (though may be decreased as in cases of fecal impaction)
  - Hepatosplenomegaly
→ Pelvic exam
→ Rectal exam:
  - Assess sphincter/pelvic floor muscle function, fissures, hemorrhoidal tags, inflammation, ulcers
  - Fecal occult blood testing
→ Consider evaluation of thyroid, lymph nodes, cardiovascular system

ASSESSMENT

→ Diarrhea
→ See **Table 7E.1, Differential Diagnosis of Diarrhea**.

PLAN

DIAGNOSTIC TESTS

→ Usually no diagnostic testing is recommended if the history and physical examination suggest viral illness.
→ Complete blood count with differential:
  - Indicated if:
    - Diarrhea persists more than a few weeks
    - Positive fecal occult blood test
    - History of rectal bleeding
    - Patient is immunocompromised
    - Complications are present
  - May have leukocytosis with excess immature white blood cells with bacterial infection, neutropenia, salmonella
  - Lymphocytosis with viral pathogens
→ Serum electrolytes, blood urea nitrogen, creatinine for mineral/volume depletion
→ Check thyroid-stimulating hormone if other signs/symptoms of hyperthyroidism are present (e.g., tachycardia, tremor, increased appetite, weight loss, nervousness).
→ Evaluation of stool:
  - For history and clinical findings suggestive of bacterial or parasitic infection, obtain:
    - Stool culture
    - Stool for ova and parasites (especially *Giardia lamblia*)

- Obtain stool for occult blood
- Patients with recent history of antibiotic ingestion should have stools examined for *Clostridium difficile* toxin (enzyme-linked immunosorbent assay [ELISA] or indirect fluorescent antibody [IFA]).
- Quantitative stool collection and analysis:
  - To work up chronic diarrhea, a 48- or 72-hour quantitative stool collection may be utilized:
    - To characterize magnitude of diarrhea volume
    - To assess for evidence of fat in stool if fat malabsorption is present (better to obtain a 72-hour quantitative stool-fat determination)
    - To identify or rule out other possible etiologies of diarrhea

→ Endoscopy:
  - Sigmoidoscopy is recommended when blood or pus is present, if unable to attribute diarrhea to acute bacterial infection, or if inflammatory bowel disease (especially ulcerative colitis) is suspected.
  - Colonoscopy should be substituted for sigmoidoscopy if Crohn's disease or neoplasia is suspected.
  - Upper endoscopy is recommended to rule out a small intestinal malabsorptive disorder, as well as Crohn's disease and other possible etiologies of diarrhea.

→ Radiology:
  - Barium enema and upper GI series may be indicated to demonstrate anatomic abnormalities (blind loops, fistulas, tumors), Crohn's disease, or jejunal diverticulosis

Table 7E.1.   DIFFERENTIAL DIAGNOSIS OF DIARRHEA

Acute Diarrhea	Chronic or Recurrent Diarrhea	
Viruses	**Protozoa**	**Malabsorption**
	Giardia lamblia	Sprue
Bacterial Toxins	*Entamoeba histolytica*	Intestinal lymphoma
Staphylococcus	*Cryptosporidium*	Bile salt malabsorption
Clostridium		Whipple's disease
	Inflammation	Pancreatic insufficiency
Bacteria	Ulcerative colitis	Lactase deficiency
Salmonella	Crohn's disease	Other disaccharidase deficiencies
Shigella	Ischemic colitis	Alpha-beta lipoproteinemia
Escherichia coli (including O157:H7)	Pseudomembranous colitis	
Campylobacter	Collagenous colitis	**Postsurgical**
Yersinia	Lymphocytic colitis	Postgastrectomy dumping syndrome
Bacillus cereus		Enteroenteric fistulas
Vibrio parahaemolyticus	**Drugs**	Blind loops
Vibrio cholerae	Laxatives	Parasympathetic denervation
Listeria	Antibiotics	Short-bowel syndrome
	Quinidine	Bile and diarrhea
Protozoa	Guanethidine; other	
Giardia lamblia	antihypertensive agents	**Other**
Entamoeba histolytica	Caffeine	Cirrhosis
Cryptosporidium	Digitalis	Diabetes mellitus
Microsporidia		Heavy-metal intoxication
	Functional	Other neurogenic diarrheas
Drugs	Irritable bowel syndrome	Hyperthyroidism
Laxatives	Diverticulosis	Addison's disease
Antibiotics		Pellagra
Caffeine	**Tumors**	Scleroderma
Alcohol	Bowel carcinoma	Amyloidosis
Antacids	Villous adenoma	
	Islet cell tumors	
Functional	Carcinoid syndrome	
Anxiety	Medullary carcinoma of thyroid	
Acute presentations of chronic or recurrent diarrhea (see "Chronic or Recurrent Diarrhea" entries)		

Source: Reprinted with permission from Richter, J.M. 2000. Evaluation and management of diarrhea. In *Primary care medicine*, 4th ed., eds. A.H. Goroll and A.G. Mulley, pp. 408–420. Philadelphia: Lippincott Williams & Wilkins.

- Computed tomography (CT):
  - CT is performed in patients with chronic diarrhea to assess for pancreatic cancer or evidence of chronic pancreatitis in the presence of malabsorption, or in patients with abnormal pancreatic function tests.
→ Additional diagnostic studies may be needed for specific suspected etiologies (e.g., serologic testing for amebic disease, testing for food allergies, etc.).

TREATMENT/MANAGEMENT

Acute Diarrhea

→ Usually acute benign diarrhea is self-limited and will resolve spontaneously within a few days.
→ Hydration:
  - Hydrate with oral fluids rich in electrolytes and sugar to facilitate the absorption of water.
  - IV therapy is necessary if adequate hydration cannot be maintained orally.
→ Boiled starches/cereals (potatoes, noodles, rice, wheat) with a small amount of salt added, crackers, bananas, or soup during episodes of watery diarrhea may be helpful.
→ Many authorities recommend excluding milk products early in the illness because lactase on the bowel mucosal surface may be diminished by inflammation, although clinical lactose intolerance is not commonly found in cases of acute diarrhea.
→ When stools are formed, the patient's diet may return to normal as tolerated.
→ Can use antidiarrheal agents to reduce stool frequency and abdominal cramping, unless severe diarrhea is present (see "Antidiarrheal Agents," below).
→ If there is a high suspicion of an infectious organism (bacteria, protozoa) based on community prevalence or likely environmental exposures, treat empirically with antibiotics.

Chronic Diarrhea

→ If the patient is taking medications that may be causing diarrhea, re-evaluate the need for their use.
→ Eliminate foods causing diarrhea (e.g., caffeine, milk products).
→ Vitamin therapy is recommended for patients with malnutrition and steatorrhea.
→ Malabsorption as a result of pancreatic insufficiency responds to enzyme supplements.
→ Dumping syndrome may respond to small, frequent feedings.
→ Pseudomembranous colitis responds to antibiotic therapy.
→ Discontinue chronic laxative use.
→ Chronic diarrhea of unknown etiology after work-up may be treated with a trial of therapy for irritable bowel syndrome (see the **Irritable Bowel Syndrome** chapter).
→ Diarrhea of psychogenic origin may be managed with psychotherapy.
→ See the **Inflammatory Bowel Disease**, **Irritable Bowel Syndrome**, **Diverticular Disease**, and **Abdominal Pain** chapters; the **Type 1 Diabetes Mellitus**, **Type 2 Diabetes**

Mellitus, and **Thyroid Disorders** chapters in Section 10; and the **Hepatitis—Viral** chapter in Section 11.
→ If diagnostic testing has failed to confirm a diagnosis, or if a specific treatment of a diagnosis has failed to produce a cure, consult with a physician.

Antidiarrheal Agents

→ Treatment with antidiarrheals has *not* been shown to slow the clearance of pathogens (Schiller 2000).
→ Bismuth subsalicylate:
  - 30 mL p.o. or 2 tablets p.o. up to 8 tablets/day for symptomatic relief is appropriate for treatment of acute diarrhea (DuPont 1997).
  - Cannot be combined with antimicrobials.
  - Side effects: black stools and tongue. Remind the patient that this agent contains salicylates.
  NOTE: Bismuth can bind with some medications and reduce their absorption.
→ Kaolin and pectin (over-the-counter drug):
  - Prescribe as directed on the package.
  - Efficacy of this agent is questionable.
→ Narcotics:
  - Assess for addiction risk prior to treatment.
  - Loperamide hydrochloride:
    - A peripherally acting opiate
    - Treatment of choice in acute diarrhea episodes
    - Good safety profile in healthy adults
    - Dose: 4 mg p.o. initially, then 2 mg p.o. after each unformed stool (maximum 8 mg/day [over-the-counter dose] or 16 mg/day [prescription dose], use for ≤2 days) (DuPont 1997)
  - Diphenoxylate:
    - Indicated for acute diarrhea, when fever is absent or low-grade
    - Dose: 2 tablets (4 mg) p.o. QID, use for ≤2 days (DuPont 1997)
    - May cause objectionable cholinergic side effects
  - Tincture of opium:
    - Indicated for acute diarrhea, when fever is absent or low grade
    - Useful in HIV-associated diarrhea (DuPont 1997), use for ≤2 days (DuPont 1997)
    - Dose: 0.5–1.0 mL p.o. every 4–6 hours for ≤2 days
  NOTE: These agents should be avoided in patients with high fever, bloody stools, or both (dysentery), with chronic diarrhea, or when there is a possibility of acute surgical abdomen (especially diverticulitis, obstruction).
→ Anticholinergics:
  - Include belladonna tincture, atropine, and propantheline, which can decrease peristalsis and are useful with diarrhea due to irritable bowel syndrome
  - See the **Irritable Bowel Syndrome** chapter.

Antibiotic Therapy

→ Antibiotic therapy is appropriate for certain types of bacterial and parasitic infections, especially if there is a high prevalence of bacterial/protozoal infection in the community or if the patient recently traveled to a high-risk area. (The choice of antibiotic treatment for specific bacteria or parasites is beyond the scope of this chapter.)

Fluid Therapy and Diet Alteration

→ In nondehydrated, otherwise healthy people with acute diarrhea, sport drinks, diluted fruit drinks with saltine crackers, soups, and broths will meet the fluid and salt needs in most cases.

→ See the diet recommendations above.

Traveler's Diarrhea

→ In the majority of episodes of acute diarrhea, including traveler's diarrhea, the routine use of antimicrobials is not recommended, as this condition is usually self-limiting.

→ Drug prophylaxis for traveler's diarrhea (Ansdell 1999, Banerjee et al. 2001, Juckett 1999, Richter 2000, Sack 2002):

- Bismuth subsalicylate can be used to prevent traveler's diarrhea (may have antibacterial, antisecretory, and antitoxin properties). Dosage:
  - 60 mL or 2, 262 mg tablets p.o. QID
  - Review side effects (black stools), contraindications, and risks of long-term use (>3 weeks) with the patient. **NOTE**: Bismuth can bind with some medications and reduce their absorption.
- Antibiotics:
  - Appropriate as a prophylactic treatment for traveler's diarrhea for individuals who are at high risk of complications if they become dehydrated. (Drug prophylaxis against traveler's diarrhea may be taken for up to 3 weeks.)
    - Doxycycline 100 mg p.o. QD with food
      OR
    - Trimethoprim/sulfamethoxazole DS, 1 tablet p.o. QD
      OR
    - Norfloxacin 100–400 mg QD
      OR
    - Ciprofloxacin 250–500 mg p.o. QD

→ Medical treatment for traveler's diarrhea (Banerjee et al. 2001, Juckett 1999, Richter 2000):

- Mild traveler's diarrhea can be treated with:
  - Loperamide: 2, 2 mg tablets p.o. initially, then 1 tablet after each loose stool (maximum 8 mg dose in 24 hours)
    PLUS
  - Ciprofloxacin (750 mg p.o. for 1 dose) or other fluoroquinolone (will usually relieve mild cases of traveler's diarrhea in less than 24 hours)
- Moderate traveler's diarrhea can be treated with:
  - Loperamide (2 mg p.o. after each loose stool, up to 16 mg/day)
    PLUS
  - Ciprofloxacin 500 mg p.o. BID for 3 days
    OR
  - Norfloxacin 200 mg p.o. BID for 3 days

OR

- Trimethoprim/sulfamethoxazole DS 1 tablet p.o. BID for 3 days (higher risk of antibiotic resistance with trimethoprim/sulfamethoxazole DS)
- Severe traveler's diarrhea: Consult with a physician.

CONSULTATION

→ Consultation with and/or referral to a physician is warranted:

- For acute severe diarrhea or when the patient is unable to maintain oral hydration (hospital admission and parenteral fluid replacement may be necessary)
- For elderly patients or those with chronic or debilitating illnesses
- In cases of chronic diarrhea when unable to establish diagnosis
- As needed for prescription(s)

PATIENT EDUCATION

→ Educate the patient about the pathophysiology and management plan for diarrhea.

→ Advise the patient to continue with hydration throughout her recovery period.

→ Review signs/symptoms of dehydration.

→ Recommend foods that are easily digestible: high-carbohydrate substances such as bananas, rice, baked potatoes, and applesauce.

→ Advise patients with possible contagious diarrhea to maintain good hygiene (i.e., wash hands with soap and water after using the bathroom).

→ Review the side effects of medicines.

→ Review how to prevent traveler's diarrhea. Patient should avoid:

- Tap water/ice cubes
- Unpasteurized milk
- Uncooked vegetables
- Unpeeled fruit
- Raw or undercooked meat or seafood

→ To relieve perineal discomfort, advise the patient to:

- Take sitz baths for 10 minutes 2–3 times/day
- Use absorbent cotton (instead of wash cloths or paper products) to:
  - Gently dry perineal area after bath
  - Wash rectal area (with warm water) after bowel movements
- Avoid the use of soap
- Clean perineal area with witch hazel pads
- Advise the patient that a short course of 0.5–1.0% hydrocortisone cream for perianal inflammation may be helpful.

→ Advise the patient to minimize narcotic therapy in the treatment of diarrhea.

→ See the **Inflammatory Bowel Disease, Irritable Bowel Syndrome, Diverticular Disease, Diarrhea—Infectious, Abdominal Pain, Type 1 Diabetes Mellitus, Type 2 Diabetes Mellitus, Thyroid Disorders**, and **Hepatitis—Viral** chapters.

FOLLOW-UP

→ As indicated by case presentation
→ Recommend that the patient return to the clinic and/or contact clinician if:
  ▪ Fever persists, worsens, or is ≥101.3° F or 38.5° C
  ▪ Abdominal pain persists or worsens
  ▪ Bloody stools present
→ Teach the American Cancer Society's recommendation for early detection of cancer in asymptomatic people (Zoorob et al. 2001):
  ▪ Fecal occult blood test: yearly beginning at age 50
              AND
  ▪ Digital rectal exam and flexible sigmoidoscopy: every 5 years beginning at age 50
              OR
  ▪ Digital rectal exam and colonoscopy: every 10 years beginning at age 50
              OR
  ▪ Digital rectal exam and double contrast barium enema: every 5–10 years beginning at age 50.
→ Document in progress notes and on problem list.

BIBLIOGRAPHY

Ansdell, V. 1999. Prevention and empiric treatment of traveler's diarrhea. *Medical Clinics of North America* 83(4):945–973.

Banerjee, S., and Lamont, J.T. 2001. Traveler's diarrhea. In *Textbook of primary care medicine*, 3rd ed., ed. J. Noble, pp. 1016–1018. St. Louis, Mo.: Mosby.

Beers, M., and Berkow, R. 1999. *The Merck manual of diagnosis and therapy*, 17th ed. Whithouse Station, N.J.: Merck & Co.

Chassany, O., Michaux, A., and Bergmann, J. 2000. Drug-induced diarrhea. *Drug Safety* 2(1):53–72.

DeBruyn, G. 2000. Infectious disease: Diarrhea. *Western Journal of Medicine* 172:409–412.

DuPont, H. 1997. Practice guidelines: guidelines on acute infectious diarrhea in adults. *American Journal of Gastroenterology* 92(11):1962–1975.

Fine, K.D. 1998. Diarrhea. In *Feldman, Sleisenger and Fordtran's gastrointestinal and liver disease*, 6th ed., eds. M. Feldman, B.F. Scharschmidt, M.H. Sleisenger et al., pp. 128–149. Philadelphia: W.B. Saunders.

Fine, K., and Schiller, L. 1999. American Gastroenterological Association technical review on the evaluation and management of chronic diarrhea. *Gastroenterology* 116(6): 1464–1486.

Juckett, G. 1999. Prevention and treatment of traveler's diarrhea. *American Family Physician* 60(1):119–124.

Mathan, V. 1998. Diarrhoeal diseases. *British Medical Bulletin* 54(2):407–419.

Richter, J.M. 2000. Evaluation and management of diarrhea. In *Primary care medicine*, 4th ed., eds. A.H. Goroll and A.G. Mulley, pp. 408–420. Philadelphia: Lippincott Williams & Wilkins.

Sack, D.A. 2002. Acute infectious diarrhea. In *Rakel: Conn's current therapy*, 54th ed., eds. R.E. Rakel and E.T. Bope, pp. 12–18. Philadelphia: W.B. Saunders.

Schiller, L. 2000. Diarrhea. *Medical Clinics of North America* 84(5):1259–1274.

Zoorob, R., Anderson, R., Cefalu, C. et al. 2001. Cancer screening guidelines. *American Family Physician* 63(6):1101–1112.

Lisa L. Lommel, R.N., C., F.N.P., M.S., M.P.H.
Jeanne R. Davis, R.N., F.N.P., M.P.H.

7-F

Diverticular Disease

Diverticular disease is an umbrella term used to describe the condition in which diverticula (with or without complications) are present. Diverticula are herniations of the mucosa and submucosa that occur through a relatively weak area in the muscle lining. Diverticula can occur anywhere in the colon, but up to 90% of patients have involvement in the sigmoid colon, where it is narrowest and intraluminal pressures are greatest. Diverticula vary in number from one to several dozen or more (Stollman et al. 1999b). They are typically 5–10 mm in diameter but can exceed 2 cm. While individuals with diverticular disease are usually asymptomatic, approximately 20–25% will manifest clinical illness (Cheek et al.1999, Stollman et al. 1999a).

Diverticula can lead to one of several diagnoses: *asymptomatic diverticulosis*, *symptomatic uncomplicated diverticulosis*, *acute diverticulitis*, or *complicated diverticulitis*. The vast majority of patients with diverticulosis remain asymptomatic, with diverticula found incidentally on barium enema or other diagnostic tests done for other indications. Individuals with symptomatic uncomplicated diverticulosis may experience nonspecific symptoms.

Diverticulitis, which is defined as inflammation and/or infection associated with diverticula, develops in up to 25% of patients with diverticula. Acute diverticulitis is usually caused by the obstruction of a single sac (by undigested food residue or a fecalith), which causes the sac to distend and perforate. Mucous secretions accumulate and overgrowth of normal colonic bacteria can lead to microabscesses and microperforations, causing local inflammation.

Complicated diverticulitis occurs when there is macroperforation of the diverticula, which can cause formation of an abscess, fistula, stricture, gastrointestinal (GI) bleeding, obstruction, and, rarely, generalized peritonitis. The consequences and sequelae of diverticulitis are more severe in immunocompromised patients, although this population does not experience an increased frequency of diverticular disease.

The prevalence of diverticular disease increases with age. Only 2–5% of individuals under age 40 experience diverticulosis, while 30% of individuals do so by age 60 and 50–65% or more over age 85 (Ferzoco et al. 1998, Marinella et al. 2000, McQuaid 2002). There is no gender predilection.

Diverticular disease is very common in developed countries such as the United States, Europe, and Australia, and is thought to be related to the western diet. Diets low in fiber, causing increased intestinal transit time, smaller stool volume, and elevated colonic pressure, are thought to cause diverticula to form. In addition, it is thought that altered colonic motility may play a role in diverticular disease, also leading to higher resting pressures in patients with diverticulosis. It is not clear how hereditary factors contribute to diverticular disease.

DATABASE

SUBJECTIVE

→ Symptomatic uncomplicated diverticulosis: Nonspecific symptoms may include the following:
   ▪ Abdominal pain (usually left lower quadrant [LLQ], which reflects the propensity for this disorder to occur in the sigmoid colon)
   ▪ Flatulence, bloating
   ▪ Changes in bowel habits (constipation, diarrhea, and/or passage of mucus)
→ Acute diverticulitis:
   ▪ LLQ abdominal pain most common
   ▪ Occasionally will have right lower quadrant (RLQ) abdominal tenderness
      • This may be due to cecal diverticulitis (uncommon) or due to a redundant sigmoid colon.
      • Asian patients present with right-sided diverticula/ pain predominantly (Ferzoco et al. 1998, Goroll 2000, Kennedy et al. 1998).
   ▪ Fever, malaise
   ▪ Alterations in bowel habits (e.g., diarrhea, constipation)
   ▪ Dysuria and urinary frequency (induced by bladder irritation from nearby inflamed sigmoid colon)
   ▪ Immunosuppressed patients may present with much more subtle signs/symptoms and have a higher risk of complicated disease.

→ Complicated diverticulitis:
- Pneumoturia, recurrent cystitis, fecaluria—possibly due to a colovesical fistula (results from perforation of diverticula into bladder)
- Inability to have a bowel movement (obstipation), abdominal distention, and colicky pain (bowel obstruction)
- Rectal bleeding (possibly due to erosion into a blood vessel)
- Fever

→ Symptoms of diverticular disease may be recurrent or chronic.

OBJECTIVE

→ Diverticulosis: clinical findings are commonly absent with diverticulosis, although it is possible to find fullness or mild tenderness in the LLQ with a thickened, palpable sigmoid and descending colon.

→ Diverticulitis: signs of diverticulitis depend on disease severity.
- Fever
- Abdominal tenderness, usually LLQ tenderness (although right-sided signs do not preclude diverticulitis), may have guarding and/or rebound tenderness
- Sausage-shaped mass palpable on abdominal, rectal, or pelvic examination
- Positive psoas and obturator sign possible with intra-abdominal abscess
- Decreased bowel sounds
- Tachycardia
- Elevated white blood cell (WBC) count and erythrocyte sedimentation rate
- Trace blood in stool may be present, but profuse lower GI bleeding is very uncommon

ASSESSMENT

→ Diverticulosis
→ R/O diverticulitis
→ R/O appendicitis
→ R/O irritable bowel syndrome
→ R/O inflammatory bowel disease
→ R/O ischemic or pseudomembranous colitis
→ R/O complicated peptic ulcer disease
→ R/O gynecological disorders
→ R/O carcinoma
→ R/O colonic obstruction
→ R/O urologic disorders
→ R/O infectious enterocolitis

PLAN

DIAGNOSTIC TESTS

→ Complete blood count (CBC)
→ Urinalysis
→ Stool occult blood test (commonly positive with diverticulitis, but a positive result should never be attributed solely to diverticulosis without further work-up)

→ Diverticulosis:
- Diagnosis of asymptomatic or mildly symptomatic uncomplicated diverticulosis:
  - It is usually not necessary to perform imaging studies in a patient with nonspecific symptoms of colonic dysfunction.
  - The incidental identification of diverticulosis by barium enema (BE), colonoscopy, or computerized tomography (CT) scanning does not require any further diagnostic evaluation.

→ Diverticulitis:
- If a clear clinical picture of mild diverticulitis is suspected based on history and physical exam, no additional tests are needed to diagnose diverticulitis (American Society of Colon and Rectal Surgeons 1995).
- If the diagnosis is uncertain, the choice of diagnostic tests depends on availability, feasibility, and clinician preference.
  - CT:
    - CT is considered to be the diagnostic study of choice by most clinicians for immediate confirmation of acute diverticulitis, supplanting BE (Cheek et al. 1999, Kennedy et al. 1998, Stollman et al. 1999a).
    - Although CT is more expensive than BE, it has proven to be safer and more sensitive and cost effective than BE.
    - CT can rule out the presence of abscess/fistulas, although it has limitations (may miss small abscesses or fail to distinguish between inflammatory and neoplastic masses).
    - CT is suggested if the initial clinical evaluation does not yield a diagnosis in the patient with acute abdominal pain.
  - Contrast enema:
    - In the past, BE was the standard test in patients with symptoms suggesting colonic disease (able to provide the number/location of colonic diverticula).
    - Currently, the use of BE requires caution, as a significant diagnostic error rate is associated with its use, as well as the risk of dislodging an obstructive diverticular plug with use of insufflation (possibly leading to perforation).
    - BE should not be performed during an acute attack, if a mass is present, or with signs of peritoneal irritation.
    - BE still remains a useful complementary study to CT scans.
  - Endoscopy:
    - Colonoscopy or sigmoidoscopy is indicated to rule out other pathology included in the differential diagnosis (e.g., carcinoma, polyps, inflammatory bowel disease).
    - Endoscopy should not be performed during the acute phase.
    - While it can demonstrate the presence of diverticula, its usefulness is limited, as diverticula are almost always extraluminal.

- Plain radiographs:
  - Plain abdominal x-ray or chest x-ray is indicated in acute attacks to evaluate for evidence of free air (signifying perforation) and to exclude ileus, bowel obstruction, soft tissue mass, and pneumoperitoneum.
- Ultrasonography:
  - May be useful in diagnosis of acute diverticulitis, but is usually used as a second-line diagnostic tool behind CT
  - It is useful to rule out pelvic/gynecologic pathology in females.

TREATMENT/MANAGEMENT

→ Incidentally identified diverticulosis in an asymptomatic patient:
  - A high-fiber diet is commonly recommended (and may be beneficial).
→ Symptomatic uncomplicated diverticulosis:
  - High-fiber diet or fiber supplements (e.g., bran powder, 15 g/day) (Goroll 2000):
    - While data show that diverticula do not regress with increased fiber intake, there is some amelioration of symptoms in patients with uncomplicated disease.
    - Consider bulk additives such as psyllium or methylcellulose if the patient is unable to tolerate bran (1 tablespoon daily, increasing to 1 tablespoon TID, with 8–16 ounces of water per dose) (see the **Constipation** chapter).
    - Although whole pieces of fiber (e.g., nuts, seeds) have traditionally been avoided in the diet secondary to a perceived risk that they become entrapped in diverticula, no controlled studies support this belief (Stollman et al. 1999a).
  - Anticholinergic and antispasmodic agents:
    - May improve symptoms by diminishing muscular contraction
    - May have a possible unwanted side effect of constipation
→ Diverticulitis:
  - Mild acute diverticulitis, which is defined as temperature <38.3° C/101° F and WBCs <13,000–15,000 µL, may be managed on an outpatient basis after physician consultation.
    - Rest and clear liquids to rest bowel
    - Broad-spectrum antibiotic (should cover Gram-negative rods and anaerobes). Common regimens include:
      - Amoxicillin/clavulanate 500 mg p.o TID or 875 mg p.o BID for 7–14 days (Gilbert et al. 2002)
        OR
      - Metronidazole 500 mg p.o TID–QID
        PLUS
        ➤ Ciprofloxacin 500 mg p.o BID for 7–14 days
        OR
        ➤ Trimethoprim-sulfamethoxazole 160/800 mg p.o. for 7–14 days (Stollman et al. 1999a)
      NOTE: This treatment should be reserved for patients with a clear diagnosis of diverticulitis who are able to tolerate oral antibiotics.

- Mild, nonopiate analgesic for pain (e.g., acetaminophen 500 mg tablets, 2 p.o. every 4–6 hours as needed, maximum dose 4,000 mg/24 hours)
- Monitor temperature, pain, assess abdomen for signs of peritonitis, and monitor WBC count for elevation.
→ Moderate-severe acute diverticulitis or complicated diverticulitis warrants referral to a physician for hospitalization, intravenous antibiotic therapy, bowel rest, and evaluation for possible surgical intervention.
→ Recurrent attacks of diverticulitis or the presence of perforation, fistula, or abscess require surgical intervention and referral.

CONSULTATION

→ Consultation with physician for diagnosis of diverticular disease
→ Consultation with physician for management of diverticulosis and mild diverticulitis
→ Consultation with nutritionist as indicated for diet plan
→ Referral to appropriate specialist for diagnostic tests
→ Referral to physician for management of recurrent disease or complications
→ As needed for prescription(s)

PATIENT EDUCATION

→ Explain the pathophysiology, risk factors, and treatment plan.
→ Advise the patient to call if she has temperature elevation, abdominal pain, or bleeding.
→ Advise the patient to avoid laxatives, enemas, and opiates because of the risk of constipation (Goroll 2000).
→ Advise the patient to avoid foods that may increase risk of obstruction, including nuts, seeds, corn, popcorn, cucumbers, tomatoes, figs, and strawberries.
→ Inform the patient that flatulence and bloating caused by bran intake will subside with continued use.

FOLLOW-UP

→ Patients treated at home should be told to call their clinician or go to an emergency facility if increasing pain, fever, bleeding, or inability to tolerate oral fluids occurs.
→ Patients with mild diverticulitis should be followed closely and monitored for increasing temperature, elevated WBC count, pain, change in abdominal exam, or signs of peritonitis. Consultation with a physician should be considered if there is no improvement within 48 hours.
→ Teach the American Cancer Society's recommendation for early detection of cancer in asymptomatic people (Zoorob et al. 2001):
  - Fecal occult blood test: yearly beginning at age 50
    AND
  - Digital rectal exam and flexible sigmoidoscopy: every 5 years beginning at age 50
    OR
  - Digital rectal exam and colonoscopy: every 10 years beginning at age 50
    OR

- Digital rectal exam and double contrast barium enema: every 5–10 years beginning at age 50.
→ Document in progress notes and on problem list.

BIBLIOGRAPHY

American Society of Colon and Rectal Surgeons. 1995. Practice parameters for sigmoid diverticulitis. *Diseases of the Colon and Rectum* 38(2):125–132.

Cheek, C., and Radley, S. 1999. Diverticulosis: fiber is the key. *Practitioner* 243:321–324.

Ferzoco, L., Raptopoulos, V., and Silen, W. 1998. Acute diverticulitis. *New England Journal of Medicine* 338(21):1521–1526.

Gilbert, D.N., Moellering, R.C., and Sande, M.A. 2002. *The Sanford Guide to Antimicrobial Therapy 2002*, pocket edition. Hyde Park, Vt.: Antimicrobial Therapy Inc.

Goroll, A.H. 2000. Management of diverticular disease. In *Primary care medicine*, 4th ed., eds. A.H. Goroll and J.A. Mulley, pp. 493–495. Philadelphia: Lippincott Williams & Wilkins.

Kennedy, M., and Zarling, E. 1998. Answers to 10 key questions on diverticular disease of the colon. *Comparative Therapeutics* 24(8):364–369.

Marinella, M., and Mustafa, M. 2000. Acute diverticulitis in patients 40 years of age and younger. *American Journal of Emergency Medicine* 18(2):140–142.

McQuaid, K.R. 2002. Diverticular disease of the colon. In *Current medical diagnosis and treatment*, 41st ed., eds. L. Tierney, Jr., S. McPhee, and M. Papadakis, pp. 657–658. New York: Lange Medical Books/McGraw-Hill.

Stollman, N., and Raskin, J. 1999(a). Diagnosis and management of diverticular disease of the colon in adults. *American Journal of Gastroenterology* 94(11):3110–3121.

——. 1999(b). Diverticular disease of the colon. *Journal of Clinical Gastroenterology* 29(3):241–252.

Zoorob, R., Anderson, R., Cefalu, C. et al. 2001. Cancer screening guidelines. *American Family Physician* 63(6):1101–1112.

7-G
Gastroesophageal Reflux and Heartburn

Gastroesophageal reflux is a normal physiologic event that results from the regurgitation of gastric contents into the esophagus. *Gastroesophageal reflux disease* (GERD) describes a spectrum of signs and symptoms that can range from mild heartburn to severe dysphagia and odynophagia. It is not well understood why a normal physiologic event becomes symptomatic and, for some individuals, chronic and severe.

Heartburn is the most common symptom of GERD. It presents as a retrosternal burning sensation caused by irritation from the reflux of stomach acid into the esophagus. It is estimated that 36% of the population has heartburn at least once a month (Richter 2000). For many of these individuals, the symptoms are transient, but for some they persist.

The etiology of GERD is multifactorial. The underlying cause in most individuals is an inappropriate relaxation of the lower esophageal sphincter (Fendrick 2001). Several factors contribute to GERD-related symptoms. First, the material being refluxed is highly caustic. Acidic gastric material and bile acids from the duodenum are the primary offending agents in the development of GERD; the length of the exposure is an important factor. Except for rare cases of *Zollinger-Ellison syndrome* (a triad of peptic ulcer, hyperacidity, and pancreatic tumors), most patients with GERD do not have qualitatively and quantitatively abnormal secretion of gastric acid and digestive juices (Szarka et al. 1999). A second factor influencing the development of GERD symptoms is a breakdown in the normal local esophageal defense mechanisms, either by an innate susceptibility of esophageal lining cells to resist acid injury, by the destruction of local defenses by prolonged acid exposure, or both. Finally, many individuals with GERD have functional abnormalities of the lower esophageal sphincter. Hormonal, neural, anatomical, and dietary factors have been implicated, as have esophageal motility disorders and delayed gastric emptying. The role of hiatal hernia remains controversial, although the incidence of prolonged reflux appears to increase with hiatal hernia (Scott et al. 1999). Reflux is increased in pregnancy due to the reduced sphincter pressure caused by increased circulating levels of progesterone and estrogen and increased abdominal pressure.

Reflux esophagitis refers to inflammation of the esophagus secondary to injury of the mucosa by refluxed acid, bile, or pancreatic enzymes. Complications of esophagitis include strictures, ulcerations, and bleeding—which is sometimes significant enough to result in anemia. *Barrett's esophagitis* is the most significant complication of GERD. Barrett's esophagitis is a premalignant change that consists of metaplastic columnar epithelialization of the distal esophagus caused by long-standing, severe reflux. Patients with Barrett's esophagitis are at 30–125 times higher risk of developing adenocarcinoma of the esophagus (Richter 2000).

Other complications of GERD include a chronic cough, sinusitis, laryngitis, loss of dental enamel, intrinsic or nocturnal asthma, or recurrent aspiration pneumonia (Theodoropoulos et al. 1999).

Gastroesophageal reflux may accompany peptic ulcer disease (particularly in gastric hypersecretory conditions). With the recent discovery that *Helicobacter pylori* causes gastric and peptic ulcers, patients with symptoms of GERD and peptic ulcer disease should be evaluated for ulcer disease and *H. pylori* (Richter 2000, Schoenfeld 1998).

GERD is usually a chronic illness that persists over the patient's lifetime. Continuous medical therapy, including lifestyle changes, will become a part of the patient's daily life. Appropriate maintenance therapy is an important factor in managing a patient with GERD.

DATABASE

SUBJECTIVE

→ Most common symptoms include:
  - Heartburn: retrosternal ache or burning pain radiating upward; onset usually within 30–60 minutes of eating (especially large meals)
  - Symptoms are usually worse at night. Inciting or aggravating factors include lying down, bending over, obesity, and tight clothing. Symptoms may be relieved by drinking water or milk, or taking antacids.

- Recurring or persistent vomiting
- Chest pain: reflux may trigger chest pain that can mimic cardiac pain (chest heaviness or pressure that may radiate to the neck, shoulder, or jaw).
- Regurgitation: fluid or food particles regurgitated, especially at night with soiling on pillow (water brash)
- Coughing or strangulation feeling, especially at night
- Hoarseness and sore throat, particularly in the morning
- Nausea
- Hiccups
- Globus ("lump in throat")
- Belching

→ Patients should be screened for more severe symptoms if the above-mentioned symptoms occur more than twice a week (DeVault 1999).

→ Symptoms that may indicate a more serious problem are:
- Chest pain
- Odynophagia
- Shortness of breath
- Dysphagia
- Weight loss

→ History may include:
- Scleroderma, diabetes mellitus, or hiatal hernia, which may predispose to reflux
- Adult onset asthma—especially when associated with nocturnal coughing, wheezing, or dyspnea (may be caused by pulmonary aspiration of gastric contents)

OBJECTIVE

→ The examination is usually unremarkable.

→ Teeth may show signs of dental erosion due to acid reflux.

→ Respiratory exam may reveal wheezing due to aspiration of regurgitated stomach contents.

→ Conduct cardiovascular exam to rule out masked cardiac pain and disease.

→ The epigastrium should be examined to rule out a mass.

→ A stool exam for occult blood may be positive.

→ Decreased hematocrit and hemoglobin may be present with bleeding.

→ Sclerodactyly, calcinosis, and telangiectasis may suggest scleroderma.

ASSESSMENT

→ Gastroesophageal reflux disease

→ R/O esophagitis including Barrett's

→ R/O ischemic heart disease

→ R/O esophageal spasm

→ R/O peptic ulcer disease

→ R/O cholelithiasis

→ R/O esophageal infection in an immunocompromised host (*Candidia albicans*, cytomegalovirus, herpesvirus)

→ R/O scleroderma

→ R/O diabetes mellitus

→ R/O anemia

→ R/O Zollinger-Ellison syndrome

PLAN

DIAGNOSTIC TESTS

→ Diagnosis of reflux is made if the symptoms are typical and there is an absence of clinical finding for other diseases.

→ CBC

→ Stool for occult blood as indicated

→ Ambulatory pH monitoring has been considered the gold standard for diagnosis of GERD.
- The pH monitor is placed in the esophagus above the lower esophageal sphincter and the pH is monitored over a 24-hour period. During that time period, the patient writes down the time and situation in which the symptoms occur. Symptoms that are associated with a lowered pH assist in the diagnosis of GERD.
- Testing is considered useful in the following situations (Kaynard et al. 2001):
  • Evaluation of normal or equivocal endoscopic findings in patients whose symptoms are refractory to proton pump inhibitors.
  • Consideration of antireflux surgery in a patient whose endoscopic findings are negative for GERD
  • Evaluation of patients whose antireflux surgery failed to control symptoms
  • Detection of reflux in patients with chest pain after cardiac evaluation showed no symptoms
  • Evaluation of patients with ear, nose, throat, or pulmonary symptoms after proton pump treatment failure
  • Documentation of GERD after diagnosis of adult-onset, nonallergic asthma
- A recent study demonstrated a potential for the proton pump inhibitor omeprazole (Prilosec®) in the diagnosis of GERD. Symptom relief after 14 days of 40 mg p.o. per day was shown to be as specific as pH monitoring in the diagnosis of GERD (Fass 2000).
- Endoscopy with biopsy should be considered (Kaynard et al. 2001):
  • To assess extent of damage resulting from esophageal disease
    NOTE: Only 50% of patients with GERD have microscopic evidence on endoscopy.
  • If symptoms are not improved with a full-dose therapeutic trial of proton pump inhibitor, see the "Treatment/Management" section.
  • In patients with significant weight loss, occult blood loss, dysphagia, odynophagia, frequent vomiting
  • With esophageal symptoms in an immunocompromised patient
  • In older patients with onset of new symptoms with long-standing GERD
  • With evidence of gastrointestinal bleeding or iron deficiency anemia
  • To diagnose and/or treat complications of GERD such as esophagitis and strictures
  • In patients with at least 10 years of GERD symptoms to screen for Barrett's esophagitis

- Every 2–3 years after two negative endoscopic exams of patients with changes of Barrett's esophagitis without dysplastic transformation
- Every six months for one year, then every year with the finding of low-grade dysplasia
  NOTE: High-grade dysplasia indicates consideration of surgery (Gopal 2001).
■ Air contrast barium esophagram may be indicated to assess for stricture or tumor in a patient with severe or long-standing disease (Fendrick 2001).

TREATMENT/MANAGEMENT

→ The goal of treatment is to minimize the exposure of the esophagus to refluxate, which will alleviate symptoms and heal the esophagus, preventing complications and maintaining remission.
→ Healthy patients with uncomplicated reflux can be treated empirically with nonpharmacologic measures. Pharmacologic measures can be added as needed.
→ For patients failing to respond to pharmacologic measures, older patients, or if heartburn is accompanied by dysphagia, weight loss, anemia, or positive stool occult blood, a more extensive work-up is indicated (see the "Diagnostic Tests" section).
→ A step-wise management approach has been developed. When the lower step does not relieve symptoms, the next step is recommended. Step 1, lifestyle modifications, is advised as a general measure that should be continued throughout therapy and maintenance (Richter 2000).

Step 1

→ Lifestyle modification:
■ Head of the bed should be elevated with 6-inch blocks under the bedposts.
  NOTE: Pillows do not effectively elevate the head and chest.
■ Avoid foods high in fat or carbohydrates. Other foods that may cause symptoms are peppermint, chocolate, spicy foods, citrus fruits and juices, tomato-based products, onions, and garlic.
■ Avoid smoking, alcohol, and coffee.
■ Reduce weight if obese
■ Avoid recumbency for 3 hours after meals.
■ Avoid large meals near bedtime or before exercise.
■ Avoid tight belts, girdles, bending over, and lifting.
■ Avoid drugs, if possible, that decrease sphincter tone, including theophylline compounds, calcium channel blockers, meperidine anticholinergics, β-2-antagonists, prostaglandins, dopamine, nitrates, diazepam, and morphine.
■ Avoid drugs, if possible, that may injure the esophageal mucosa, including tetracycline, quinidine, potassium chloride tablets, nonsteroidal anti-inflammatory drugs, and biphosphonates.
■ Relaxation training to reduce stress

Step 2

→ Add pharmacologic therapy as needed—helpful for mild, intermittent, or infrequent symptoms or for symptom prevention
■ Antacids after meals and at bedtime (see **Table 7G.1, Composition of Selected Commonly Used Antacids and Antirefluxants**).
  • Antacids and alginic acid (an antirefluxant that can be purchased alone or in combination with an antacid) together are more effective than antacid alone.
  • Antacids may be taken alone or in combination with histamine H_2 blockers.
    NOTE: Antacids should not be taken at the same time as H_2 blockers due to decreased absorption of H_2.
■ Antacids provide immediate acid neutralization while the H_2 blockers provide sustained acid suppression.
■ Antacids may reduce the absorption of certain drugs, including fluoroquinolones, tetracycline, and ferrous sulfate.
→ Over-the-counter histamine H_2 -receptor blocker (see **Table 7G.2, Medications Used in the Treatment of Gastroesophageal Reflux Disease**).
■ H_2 blockers provide acid suppression.
■ Over-the-counter H_2 blockers are about one-half the dosage of prescription H_2 blockers. They can be especially helpful when taken before an activity that may cause reflux (e.g., heavy meal, exercise).
NOTE: Cimetidine (and to a lesser extent ranitidine) may cause inhibition of the cytochrome P450 system, which may alter levels of drugs metabolized by this pathway (theophylline, phenytoin, warfarin, propranolol, calcium channel blockers, chlordiazepoxide, diazepam, metronidazole, lidocaine, protease inhibitors, and certain tricyclic antidepressants) (DeVault 1999, Scott et al. 1999, Szarka et al. 1999).

Step 3

→ Switch to full prescription dosages of histamine H_2 blocker or proton pump inhibitor for symptom relief and to heal esophagitis when the disease is mild to moderate. (See **Table 7G.2, Medications Used in the Treatment of Gastroesophageal Reflux Disease**.)
→ Treatment should continue for 6–12 weeks for healing. If symptoms are relieved, patients can step down to Step 2 (while continuing with Step 1).
→ Proton pump inhibitor is the first line therapy for endoscopically documented erosive esophagitis.

Step 4

→ Prokinetic drugs have been developed in an attempt to increase lower esophageal sphincter pressure and stop reflux. These drugs have limited usefulness due to their side effects. When combined with H_2 blockers or proton pump inhibitors, the therapeutic benefit is small, the cost is higher, and the risk of side effects may increase (see **Table 7G.2**) (DeVault 1999).

- Metoclopramide:
  - Most useful in patients with reflux without severe heartburn and those with gastroparesis
  - One-third of patients cannot tolerate it because of central nervous system side effects (drowsiness, irritability, and extrapyramidal effects).

OR

- Bethanechol:
  - Not well tolerated because of cholinergic effects. Contraindicated in patients with asthma.

OR

- Cisapride:
  - Serious side effects, including cardiac arrhythmias and potentially dangerous drug interactions, have limited the use of this drug. Available only through Limited Access Program, (877) 795-4247.

Step 5

→ Surgery (fundoplication procedure) for incapacitating, refractory disease

Maintenance Therapy

→ Long-term management of GERD often requires pharmacologic therapy in addition to Step 1 lifestyle modifications.

→ In patients with mild symptoms, antacids or over-the-counter histamine H_2 receptor blockers may be used to control symptoms over the long term.

→ In patients with nonerosive, moderate to severe symptoms, H_2 blockers may control symptoms (Scott et al. 1999). While H_2 blockers may successfully control more severe symptoms initially, proton pump inhibitors are often required for long-term control.

- Patients with endoscopically documented esophagitis often require long-term proton pump inhibitor therapy after symptoms are relieved and the esophagitis has healed. The lowest effective proton pump inhibitor dose should be used to maintain remission (Scott et al. 1999).

- The effectiveness of long-term proton pump therapy for reducing the risk of developing Barrett's esophagitis has not been established.

Table 7G.1.   COMPOSITION OF SELECTED COMMONLY USED ANTACIDS AND ANTIREFLUXANTS

Medication	Active Ingredient	Dosage
AlternaGel®	Aluminum hydroxide (600 mg/5 mL)	5–10 mL (maximum 90 mL/day)
Amphojel®	Aluminum hydroxide (320 mg/5 mL)	10 mL (maximum 60 mL/day)
Gaviscon® tablets	Aluminum hydroxide (80 mg) Magnesium trisilicate (20 mg) Alginic acid	2–4 chewed tablets up to 4 times daily
Gaviscon® extra strength tablets	Aluminum hydroxide (160 mg) Magnesium carbonate (105 mg) Alginic acid	2–4 chewed tablets up to 4 times daily
Maalox®	Aluminum hydroxide (225 mg/5 mL) Magnesium hydroxide 200 mg/5 mL)	10–20 mL up to 4 times daily
Maalox® Plus Tablets	Aluminum hydroxide (350 mg) Magnesium hydroxide (250 mg) Simethicone (25 mg)	1–3 chewed tablets up to 4 times daily
Mylanta®	Aluminum hydroxide (200 mg/5 mL) Magnesium hydroxide (200 mg/5 mL) Simethicone (20 mg/5 mL)	10–20 mL up to 4 times daily
Mylanta® Gelcaps	Calcium carbonate (311 mg)	2–4 capsules up to 4 times daily
Mylanta® Gas	Simethicone (40, 80, or 125 mg capsules)	4–125 mg chewed up to 4 times daily
Tums®	Calcium carbonate (500 mg)	No more than 16/day
Tums® EX	Calcium carbonate (750 mg)	No more than 12/day
Tums® Anti-gas/Antacid	Calcium carbonate (500 mg) Simethicone (20 mg)	No more than 16/day

Source: Reprinted with permission from DeVault, K.R. 1999. Overview of medical therapy for gastroesophageal reflux disease. *Gastroenterology Clinics of North America* 28(4):831–845. © 1999 with permission from Elsevier Science (USA).

- The safety of long-term proton pump inhibitor therapy has not been definitively determined. The modest increase in circulating gastrin levels seen in some patients on long-term proton pump therapy does not seem to be clinically significant, but no long-term data are available yet (Kaynard et al. 2001).

- Patients with *Helicobacter pylori* infection who are on long-term proton pump therapy may be at risk for atrophic gastritis (a risk for carcinoma). These patients should be treated for *Helicobacter pylori* infection (Richter 2000) (see the **Peptic Ulcer Disease** chapter).

CONSULTATION

→ Consultation with a physician may be sought when the patient's symptoms are not relieved by conservative measures.

→ Consultation with a physician is warranted for atypical symptoms and if a therapeutic trial does not improve symptoms.

→ Consultation or referral to a physician should be considered for evaluation of relapse of symptoms.

→ Referral to a physician is warranted for diagnostic evaluation.

→ As needed for prescription(s).

PATIENT EDUCATION

→ See the "Treatment/Management" section.

→ Explain the pathophysiology of reflux, the chronic and recurrent nature of the disease, aggravating factors, and necessity of following conservative measures.

→ Advise the patient to continue with medication as prescribed until otherwise directed, even after symptoms have subsided.

Table 7G.2.   MEDICATIONS USED IN THE TREATMENT OF GASTROESOPHAGEAL REFLUX DISEASE

Drug	Dosage
Over-the-Counter: H2-Receptor Blockers	
Nizatidine (Axid® AR)	75 mg p.o. BID
Famotidine (Mylanta® AR, Pepcid® AC)	10 mg p.o. BID
Cimetidine (Tagamet® HB)	200 mg p.o. BID
Ranitidine (Zantac® 75)	75 mg p.o. BID
Prescription: H2-Receptor Blockers	
Cimetidine (Tagamet®)	400 mg p.o. BID 800 mg p.o. BID
Famotidine (Pepcid®)	20 mg p.o. BID 40 mg p.o. BID
Nizatidine (Axid®)	150 mg p.o. BID
Ranitidine (Zantac®)	150 mg p.o. BID to QID 300 mg p.o. BID
Prokinetic Agents	
Cisapride (Propulsid®) Available only through limited access program. Call (877) 795-4247	10 mg p.o. BID to QID 20 mg p.o. QID
Metoclopramide (Reglan®)	10 mg p.o. QID
Bethanechol	25 mg p.o. QID
Proton Pump Inhibitors	
Lansoprazole (Prevacid®)	15 mg p.o. QD 30 mg p.o. QD
Omeprazole (Prilosec®)	10 mg p.o. QD 20 mg p.o. QD
Pantoprazole (Protonix®)	40 mg p.o. QD
Rabeprazole (Aciphex®)	20 mg p.o. QD

Source: Compiled from Scott, M., and Gelhot, A.R. 1999. Gastroesophageal reflux disease: diagnosis and management. *American Family Physician* 59(5):1161–1169; and Fendrick, A.M. 2001. Management of patients with symptomatic gastroesophageal reflux disease: a primary care perspective. *American Journal of Gastroenterology* 96(Suppl. 8):S29–S33.

→ Help the patient quit alcohol and smoking by referring her to appropriate support services—i.e., Alcoholics Anonymous, Nicotine Anonymous, and the American Cancer Society. (See the **Alcoholism and Other Drug Problems** and **Smoking Cessation** chapters in Section 14.)

→ Instruct the patient about methods of stress reduction (See the **Stress Management** chapter in Section 14.)

FOLLOW-UP

→ Re-evaluate the patient 4–6 weeks after initiating treatment.

→ Initial pharmacological therapy should be maintained for 12 weeks.

→ At every visit, reinforce adherence to conservative measures.

→ Withdraw one pharmacological agent at a time to determine if maintenance treatment is required at a minimum level.

- Up to 45% of patients relapse after discontinuing medication.
- Some patients may require a maintenance dose of a particular drug.
- If maintenance is required, determine the minimal treatment necessary to avoid symptoms.

→ Teach the American Cancer Society's recommendation for early detection of cancer in asymptomatic people (Zoorob et al. 2001):

- Fecal occult blood test: yearly beginning at age 50
  AND
- Digital rectal exam and flexible sigmoidoscopy: every 5 years beginning at age 50
  OR
- Digital rectal exam and colonoscopy: every 10 years beginning at age 50
  OR
- Digital rectal exam and double contrast barium enema: every 5–10 years beginning at age 50.

→ Document in progress notes and problem list.

BIBLIOGRAPHY

DeVault, K.R. 1999. Overview of medical therapy for gastroesophageal reflux disease. *Gastroenterology Clinics of North America* 28(4):831–845.

Fass, R. 2000. Emperical trials in treatment of gastroesophageal reflux disease. *Digestive Diseases* 18(20):20–26.

Fendrick, A.M. 2001. Management of patients with symptomatic gastroesophageal reflux disease: a primary care perspective. *American Journal of Gastroenterology* 96(Suppl. 8):S29–S33.

Gopal, D.V. 2001. Another look at Barrett's esophagitis. *Postgraduate Medicine* 110(3):57–66.

Kaynard, A., and Flora, K. 2001. Gastroesophageal reflux disease. *Postgraduate Medicine* 110(3):42–53.

Richter, J.M. 2000. Approach to the patient with heartburn and reflux (gastroesophageal reflux disease). In *Primary care medicine*, 4th ed., eds. A.H. Goroll and A.G. Mulley, Jr., pp. 394–399. Philadelphia: Lippincott Williams & Wilkins.

Schoenfeld, P.S. 1998. Acid peptic diseases in the era of *Helicobacter pylori*. *Lippincott's Primary Care Practice* 2(4): 358–368.

Scott, M., and Gelhot, A.R. 1999. Gastroesophageal reflux disease: diagnosis and management. *American Family Physician* 59(5):1161–1169.

Szarka, L.A., and Locke, G.G. 1999. Practical pointers for grappling with GERD. *Postgraduate Medicine* 105(7):88–105.

Theodoropoulos, D.S., Lockey, R.F., Boyce, Jr., H.W. et al. 1999. Gastroesophageal reflux and asthma: a review of pathogenesis, diagnosis, and therapy. *Allergy* 54:651–661.

Zoorob, R., Anderson, R., Cefalu, C. et al. 2001. Cancer screening guidelines. *American Family Physician* 63(6):1101–1112.

Lisa L. Lommel, R.N., C., F.N.P., M.S., M.P.H.
Jeanne R. Davis, R.N., F.N.P., M.P.H.

7-H

Gastrointestinal Bleeding

Gastrointestinal (GI) bleeding is defined as bleeding originating anywhere in the upper or lower GI tract. Upper GI bleeding originates proximal to the ligament of Treitz (Peter et al. 1999). The ligament of Treitz is a fibromuscular band that widens the angle of the duodenojejunal flexure. It is often used as the anatomic dividing point when differentiating between upper and lower GI bleeding. The most common cause of upper GI bleeding is peptic ulcer disease (PUD) (Fallah et al. 2000, Pianka et al. 2001). Lower GI bleeding refers to blood loss distal to the ligament of Treitz, with 95% of cases occurring in the colon (McQuaid 2002, Pianka et al. 2001). Hemorrhoids are thought to be the most common cause of lower GI bleeding (Pianka et al. 2001).

In the majority of cases, resolution of both upper and lower GI bleeding occurs spontaneously (Zuckerman et al. 2000). Regardless, GI bleeding can be life-threatening. For this reason, it is critical to distinguish between those patients who need immediate hospitalization and those who can be managed on an outpatient basis. Risk factors for poor outcome in patients with GI bleeding include: age older than 60 years, ongoing bleeding, and hypotension (systolic blood pressure <100 mm Hg) (Zuckerman et al. 2000). In all cases of GI bleeding, cancer risk assessment and screening are critical components of the work-up.

DATABASE

SUBJECTIVE

→ Each presenting symptom is a manifestation of the source and rate of bleeding, as well as an indication of whether there is underlying or coexistent disease; therefore it is important to obtain a comprehensive medical history.

→ The patient may complain of tarry, dark-colored stools (melena), bright red or maroon blood per rectum (hematochezia), or vomiting fresh or changed blood, which may appear like coffee grounds (hematemesis).

→ Occasionally, GI bleeding is occult and only detectable by chemical testing of the stool.

→ The most common presentation of upper GI bleeding is hematemesis or melena (McQuaid 2002).

■ Hematemesis almost always originates proximal to the ligament of Treitz (Beers et al. 1999, Pianka et al. 2001, Richter 2000).

■ Melena is typically seen with upper GI bleeding but can occasionally occur in the small bowel or right colon.

→ Lower GI bleeding:

■ Hematochezia
  • Usually indicates lower GI bleeding
  • Often signifies mild bleeding, commonly from an anorectosigmoid source
  • Patient typically complains of fresh blood mixed with solid brown stool or bright red blood dripping into toilet after a bowel movement.
  • Rarely, these symptoms result from a brisk upper GI bleed (Beers et al. 1999, Zuckerman 2000).
  • If the patient complains of acute, painless, large-volume maroon or bright red bleeding (especially patients who are over 50 years old), consider diverticulosis or vascular ectasias.
  • Bloody diarrhea in combination with crampy abdominal pain, urgency, or tenesmus is characteristic of inflammatory bowel disease (IBD), infectious colitis, or ischemic colitis.

→ Bleeding symptoms:
  ■ Assess whether there is a history of bleeding, easy bruising, or ecchymosis.
  ■ Assess nature/duration of bleeding.

→ Associated symptoms:
  ■ Assess for presence of abdominal pain, vomiting, diarrhea, constipation, urgency, frequency, tenesmus, change in bowel habits, weight loss, fever, weakness, dysphagia, history of frequent nose bleeds, anorexia, shortness of breath.

→ Past medical history:
  ■ Assess for history of PUD, liver disease, IBD, hemorrhoids, polyps, radiation to abdomen or pelvis, cardiopulmonary disease, renal disease, cancer, bleeding disorders, prior abdominal or pelvic surgery.

→ Intake of medication/food:
- Use of aspirin, alcohol, nonsteroidal anti-inflammatory drugs (consider ulceration or gastritis)
- Use of other medications (anticoagulants, corticosteroids, alendronate, potassium chloride)
- A false-positive result on a stool guaiac test can be produced by the use of glycerol guaiacolate (an expectorant) or a by a recent meal of rare red meat (Richter 2000).
- Black stools can result from bismuth (Pepto-Bismol), iron, or charcoal intake.
- A recent intake of beets can cause red-colored stools.

→ See the **Peptic Ulcer Disease, Abdominal Pain, Diarrhea, Gastroesophageal Reflux and Heartburn, Hemorrhoids and Anal Fissures, Inflammatory Bowel Disease, Irritable Bowel Syndrome**, and **Diverticular Disease** chapters.

OBJECTIVE

A complete physical exam may be indicated, depending on patient's symptoms. The exam should focus on:

→ Examination of nasopharynx for sources of bleeding

→ Assessment for signs of delirium secondary to an acute bleed (especially in the elderly) (Pianka et al. 2001)

→ Enlargement or fixation of lymph nodes

→ Assessment of skin for pallor, ecchymoses, petechiae, telangiectases, and/or stigmata of chronic liver disease (e.g., jaundice, palmar erythema, spider angiomata)

→ Cardiac and pulmonary exam:
- Assess for evidence of valvular heart disease (can be associated with a GI bleed).
- Assess for evidence of hemodynamic stability: orthostatic changes and tachycardia:
  - Postural hypotension: an orthostatic fall in blood pressure ≥10 mmHg and/or
  - An increase in heart rate >10 beats/minute on moving from supine position to standing (suggests blood volume loss) (Richter 2000)
  - If the patient has a coexistent disease or is taking medications that can cause changes in peripheral vascular resistance, the clinician must interpret these signs cautiously.
  - Assess for signs of congestive heart failure ("high output" congestive heart failure associated with severe anemia).

→ Abdominal exam:
- Assess for ascites, hepatosplenomegaly, abdominal scars, evidence of a mass, bowel sounds, tenderness, peritoneal signs.
- Visual exam of the external anus and anoscopy may show evidence of bleeding, hemorrhoids, or fissure.
- Digital rectal exam: assess for mass, hemorrhoids, fissures, fistula.
- Assess for occult blood in stool.
- See the "Diagnosis" section for performance of nasogastric aspiration and lavage in patients suspected of upper GI bleeding.

→ See also the **Peptic Ulcer Disease, Abdominal Pain, Diarrhea, Gastroesophageal Reflux and Heartburn, Hemorrhoids and Anal Fissures, Inflammatory Bowel Disease, Irritable Bowel Syndrome**, and **Diverticular Disease** chapters.

ASSESSMENT

→ R/O epistaxis

→ R/O respiratory tract bleeding

→ R/O gastritis

→ R/O gastric ulcer

→ R/O hemorrhagic esophagitis

→ R/O gastroesophageal reflux disease

→ R/O Barrett's esophagus

→ R/O arteriovenous malformations

→ R/O celiac disease

→ R/O Dieulafoy's lesions

→ R/O Meckel's diverticulum

→ R/O aortoenteric fistula

Common Causes of Lower GI Bleeding

→ R/O hemorrhoids

→ R/O anal fissures

→ R/O gastrointestinal malignancy

→ R/O ischemic colitis

→ R/O angiodysplasia (vascular ectasia)

→ R/O IBD

→ R/O diverticular disease

→ R/O polyps

Common Causes of Upper GI Bleeding

→ R/O Mallory-Weiss tear (associated with vigorous vomiting)

→ R/O esophageal or gastric varices (associated with chronic liver disease)

→ R/O other vascular anomalies

→ R/O gastric or duodenal erosions

→ R/O PUD

→ R/O gastrointestinal malignancy

PLAN

DIAGNOSTIC TESTS

→ Fecal occult blood test:
- GI bleeding is often detected with a fecal occult blood test.

→ CBC:
- An initial low hematocrit in the face of stable vital signs may represent chronic anemia or subacute bleeding rather than acute hemorrhage.
- An equilibration period can take 24–72 hours before concentrations reflect blood loss.
- Hemoglobin and hematocrit may not accurately reflect amount of blood loss at time of presentation in a person with active GI bleeding.

→ Renal function studies to rule out factors that may exacerbate bleeding:

- BUN/creatinine ratio:
  - While a BUN/creatinine ratio >33–36 is suggestive of an upper GI hemorrhage, some consider this to be an unreliable test (Fallah et al. 2000, Peter et al. 1999).
- → Serum electrolytes
- → Liver function tests to rule out chronic liver disease, which may exacerbate bleeding:
  - Bilirubin, alkaline phosphatase, albumin, aspartate transaminase (AST), alanine transaminase (ALT)
- → Coagulation studies:
  - Prothrombin time (PT), partial thromboplastin time (PTT), and platelet count to rule out factors that may exacerbate bleeding
- → Blood type and cross match if transfusion is needed
- → Nasogastric aspiration and lavage:
  - Nasogastric aspiration may be helpful in patients without hematemesis who have suspected upper GI bleeding or if location of bleeding is in question (Fallah et al. 2000)
  - Aspiration of fresh blood and failure to clear blood with lavage are indicators of persistent bleeding (Fallah et al. 2000).
  - While a bloody aspirate confirms an upper GI source, nasogastric aspiration may be negative in the presence of a heavy upper GI bleed.
  - Is limited by lack of specificity and sensitivity
- → Endoscopy:
  - The initial work-up of most cases of occult bleeding should not require testing other than colonoscopy and/or upper endoscopy.
  - Upper endoscopy:
    - Useful for patients with symptoms referable to the upper GI tract (heartburn, dyspepsia, dysphagia, vomiting, weight loss), for suspected acute brisk upper GI bleed, for patients with hematochezia and hemodynamic instability, and for patients with suspected esophagitis, Mallory-Weiss tears, or gastritis (McQuaid 2002, Pianka et al. 2001, Richter 2000).
    - Some clinicians will perform a "screening" endoscopy for patients with cirrhosis due to high risk of hemorrhage secondary to esophageal varices.
    - Endoscopic technology has made upper endoscopy both diagnostic and therapeutic.
    - Small bowel biopsy can be performed during upper endoscopy (Zuckerman et al. 2000)
    - Endoscopy can achieve hemostasis in >90% of cases of acute upper GI bleeding (Fallah et al. 2000).
    - Visualization of the bleeding site can provide information to aid in efforts to predict a patient's prognosis for indicators of mortality, such as the need for surgery and the patient's risk of rebleeding (Peter et al. 1999, Zuckerman 2000).
  - Colonoscopy:
    - The diagnostic procedure of choice for patients with hematochezia who are at risk for colon cancer and whose bleeding is not explained by anorectal pathology

- Most patients over age 50 with bleeding are candidates for colonoscopy (Richter 2000).
- Can be both diagnostic and therapeutic
- Appropriate for evaluating a positive result found on fecal occult blood test, as colonic adenomas and carcinomas are the most common GI neoplasms
  - Detects >95% of colorectal polyps and cancer and permits polypectomy, tumor biopsy, or endoscopic cautery of vascular ectasias (McQuaid 2002)
- Not as useful with massive or ongoing lower GI hemorrhage; therefore, upper GI and perianal bleeding should be excluded first.
  - Flexible sigmoidoscopy:
    - Useful in work-up of hematochezia (for distal lesions)
    - Anoscopy and sigmoidoscopy:
      - Appropriate for an otherwise healthy person <45 years old with small volume bleeding to look for evidence of anorectal disease, IBD, or infectious colitis
      - If a lesion is found, no further evaluation is needed immediately unless bleeding persists or is recurrent (McQuaid 2002).
- → Barium study:
  - Air-contrast barium enema in combination with sigmoidoscopy is useful when colonoscopy is contraindicated.
  - Barium studies are also useful with an inconclusive endoscopy result, as a supplementary procedure for patients with inactive bleeding, with unexplained chronic blood loss, or with suspected small-bowel disease (Richter 2000).
- → Radiologic studies for acute lower GI bleeding (Pianka et al. 2001)
  - Nuclear medicine scan (technetium radionuclide scan):
    - May be indicated in the evaluation of active lower GI bleeding (Peter et al. 1999)
    - Is low risk and confirms ongoing bleeding so that angiography can follow, if needed
    - Detects intermittent or slower bleeds more accurately than does angiography
    - High false-negative rate, high rate of misidentification of lesions
  - Diagnostic angiography:
    - Helpful with massive bleed
    - Permits infusion of vasopressin or embolization into a bleeding artery
    - Can define lesions with abnormal vasculature
    - Limited usefulness if there is no evidence of bleeding on the bleeding scan

TREATMENT/MANAGEMENT

- → Primary management strategy is to treat underlying cause of GI bleeding
- → See the **Peptic Ulcer Disease**, **Abdominal Pain**, **Constipation**, **Diarrhea**, **Gastroesophageal Reflux and Heartburn**, **Hemorrhoids and Anal Fissures**, **Inflammatory Bowel Disease**, **Irritable Bowel Syndrome**, and **Diverticular Disease** chapters.

→ With a mild to moderate iron deficiency anemia and a negative endoscopic evaluation of the colon and upper GI tract, a trial of a diet high in iron-containing foods and ferrous sulfate supplementation is appropriate (see the **Anemia** chapter in Section 10) (McQuaid 2002).

→ Discontinue nonsteroidal anti-inflammatory drug or aspirin if ulcers or gastritis is suspected.

→ Surgical treatment may be indicated.

CONSULTATION

→ Consultation and/or referral to a physician are indicated if the patient has mild to moderate chronic or acute GI blood loss.

→ Consultation and/or referral to a physician are indicated if the patient has a comorbid condition that might be aggravated by anemia (e.g., ischemic heart disease).

→ Immediate referral to a physician is warranted in cases of acute hemorrhage, chronic unstable bleeding, profound anemia, suspected hemodynamic instability, or significant abdominal pain with GI bleed.

→ As needed for prescription(s).

PATIENT EDUCATION

→ Educate the patient about the pathophysiology of, and management plan for, GI bleeding.

→ Educate the patient about the signs and symptoms of worsening blood loss or volume depletion.

FOLLOW-UP

→ Monitor the patient who has acute mild or chronic stable bleeding with periodic CBC.

→ At every visit, reinforce adherence to conservative measures.

→ Teach the American Cancer Society's recommendation for early detection of cancer in asymptomatic people (Zoorob et al. 2001):

- Fecal occult blood test: yearly beginning at age 50

AND

- Digital rectal exam and flexible sigmoidoscopy: every 5 years beginning at age 50

OR

- Digital rectal exam and colonoscopy: every 10 years beginning at age 50

OR

- Digital rectal exam and double contrast barium enema: every 5–10 years beginning at age 50.

→ Document in progress notes and on problem list.

BIBLIOGRAPHY

Beers, M., and Berkow, R. 1999. *The Merck manual of diagnosis and therapy*, 17th ed. Whitehouse Station, N.J.: Merck & Co.

Fallah, M.A., Prakash, C., and Edmundowicz, S. 2000. Acute gastrointestinal bleeding. *Medical Clinics of North America* 84(5):1183–208.

McQuaid, K.R. 2002. Gastrointestinal bleeding. In *Current medical diagnosis and treatment*, 41st ed., eds. L.M. Tierney, Jr., S.J. McPhee, and M.A. Papadakis, pp. 586–592. New York: Lange Medical Books/McGraw-Hill.

Peter, D.J., and Dougherty, J.M. 1999. Evaluation of the patient with gastrointestinal bleeding: an evidence-based approach. *Emergency Medicine Clinics of North America* 17(1):239–261.

Pianka, J.D., and Affronti, J. 2001. Management principles of gastrointestinal bleeding. *Primary Care* 28(3):557–575, vi.

Richter, J.M. 2000. Evaluation of gastrointestinal bleeding. In *Primary care medicine*, 4th ed., eds. A.H. Goroll and J.A. Mulley, pp. 404–408. Philadelphia: Lippincott Williams & Wilkins.

Zoorob, R., Anderson, R., Cefalu, C. et al. 2001. Cancer screening guidelines. *American Family Physician* 63(6):1101–1112.

Zuckerman, G.R. 2000. Acute gastrointestinal bleeding: clinical essentials for the initial evaluation and risk assessment for the primary care physician. *Journal of the American Osteopathy Association* 100(12 Suppl. Part 2):S4–S7.

Zuckerman, G.R., Prakash, C., Askin, M.P. et al. 2000. AGA technical review on the evaluation and management of occult and obscure gastrointestinal bleeding. *Gastroenterology* 118(1):201–221.

Lisa L. Lommel, R.N., C., F.N.P., M.S., M.P.H.
Jeanne R. Davis, R.N., F.N.P., M.P.H.

7-1

Hemorrhoids and Anal Fissures

In primary care practice, the assessment and treatment of anorectal symptoms is very common. While hemorrhoids and fissures commonly cause anorectal complaints, other etiologies for these symptoms, including inflammatory bowel disease (IBD), cancer, and infection, must be ruled out.

Anal Fissures

An *anal fissure* is a linear tear or rocket-shaped ulcerated area that most commonly occurs in the posterior midline of the distal anal canal. Up to 10% of fissures occur in the anterior midline area (this is seen more in postpartum women). Multiple fissures or fissures occurring in the lateral position are unusual, and if present, IBD, an infectious process, or immunosuppression should be considered.

Anal fissures are believed to be caused by trauma to the anal canal during defecation, perhaps secondary to straining, constipation, or increased internal sphincter tone. As acute anal fissures often have minimal inflammation, the majority will heal spontaneously in 2–3 weeks. Chronic anal fissures are usually deeper. A sentinel tag, hypertrophied anal papilla, induration, and/or anal stenosis are potential secondary changes associated with chronic anal fissures.

Hemorrhoids

Hemorrhoids are a very common condition, affecting half of patients over 50 years old, with no predilection for either gender (Goroll 2000). Hemorrhoids represent dilations of the anorectal vascular network. Possible causes of hemorrhoids include increased venous pressure secondary to upright posture, straining with bowel movements, arteriovenous communications in rectal tissue, and compromised fibrous tissue in the rectal mucosa, which can lead to prolapsed cushions of tissue. Factors associated with hemorrhoids include pregnancy, obesity, portal hypertension, chronic constipation, and a high-fat and low-fiber diet.

There are two major types of hemorrhoids, which are named based on their anatomic position and vascular origin. An *internal hemorrhoid* occurs above the dentate line and represents dilation of the superior hemorrhoidal plexus. When these vessels dilate, they become thin-walled and bulge into the lumen. Internal hemorrhoids are covered by rectal mucosa, which is not very pain sensitive.

Internal hemorrhoids are further classified into four groups. A *Stage I hemorrhoid* causes symptoms, but does not prolapse out of the anal canal. A *Stage II hemorrhoid* prolapses with bowel movements but reduces spontaneously. A *Stage III hemorrhoid* prolapses readily with bowel movements and sometimes with exertion, and requires manual reduction. A *Stage IV hemorrhoid* is a permanently prolapsed hemorrhoid (which is subsequently prone to thrombosis and infarction) (Goroll 2000, Hulme-Moir et al. 2001, McQuaid 2002).

External hemorrhoids are located below the dentate line and are covered by pain-sensitive squamous epithelium. External hemorrhoids derive from the inferior hemorrhoidal plexus (which includes the vessels in the dermis of the lower anal canal and the perianal skin).

A major complication of hemorrhoids is thrombosis, which can occur with internal or external hemorrhoids.

DATABASE

SUBJECTIVE

→ General history questions:
- Pain:
  - Pain may be sharp or dull; mild or severe; stabbing, burning, or aching.
  - Location of pain may be predominantly anal, anorectal (local anal pain plus rectal discomfort and tenesmus) or rectocolonic (rectal discomfort, tenesmus, and/or rectal discharge plus diarrhea, abdominal pain, bloating, and/or nausea).
- Bowel habits/symptoms:
  - Incomplete defecation, change in bowel habits (constipation or diarrhea)
- Associated symptoms:
  - Masses, nodules, discharge, rectal itching
  - Bleeding

- Assess extent, character, and timing of bleeding (e.g., pink staining on toilet tissue, bright red blood dripping into the bowl, or squirting blood).
  - Assess if blood coats the stool or is mixed with it.
  - Assess whether bleeding occurs with bowel movements and stops promptly, lasts longer than the bowel movement, or occurs between bowel movements.
- History:
  - Laxative use
  - Topical medications
- Health and social practices:
  - Sexual
  - Hygienic
  - Recent trauma

→ Anal fissures:
- Perirectal pain (sharp, searing, or burning) that is associated with defecation
- Pain is often severe and may last for a few minutes during, or persist for several hours after, defecation.
- Rectal bleeding: usually small amount of bright red blood that is not mixed with stool and is noted on toilet tissue only (dried blood or blood mixed with stool indicates other pathology).
- Pruritus ani accompanies anal fissures in 50% of cases (Jonas et al. 2001).
- Discharge is possible, but not common.
- Assess duration: considered chronic if fissure has failed to heal within 6 weeks.

→ Hemorrhoids:
- Uncomplicated hemorrhoids may produce no symptoms.
- Pain, bleeding, and/or a prolapsed mass are common presenting complaints.
- Assess history of hemorrhoids.

→ Internal hemorrhoids:
- Painless bleeding (bright red blood that ranges from streaks of blood visible on toilet paper or stool to bright red blood that drips into the toilet bowl after a bowel movement)
- Patient may experience prolapse with defecation, with or without spontaneous reduction, or with permanent prolapse (second-, third-, or fourth-degree).
- Discomfort and pain are unusual with internal hemorrhoids, occurring only when there is extensive inflammation and thrombosis of irreducible tissue.
- With prolapse, mucus and particles of stool may be deposited on the perianal skin, causing secondary pruritus.
- Chronically prolapsed hemorrhoids may result in perianal discharge that can cause irritation.

→ External hemorrhoids:
- Patient may feel an external anal mass, which is generally asymptomatic unless acutely thrombosed.
- Thrombosed external hemorrhoid:
  - Patient will have a relatively acute onset of exquisite pain, especially during defecation.
  - Symptoms may be precipitated by coughing, heavy lifting, or straining at stool.

- Pain is most severe within the first few hours but gradually eases over 2–3 days as edema subsides.
- Skin tag may be present in later stages.

OBJECTIVE

A thorough and gentle inspection of the anus and perianal region should be performed.

→ General:
- Anal skin should be assessed for erythema, eczema, psoriatic patches, an abscess, ulcerations, vesicles, fistulas, fissures, condylomata, nodules, hemorrhoids, skin tags, dermatitis, and inflammation.
- Palpate for enlarged lymph nodes (assess inguinal lymph nodes).

→ Fissures:
- Anoscopic and digital rectal exams, although recommended in patients with anal fissures, may be very painful. Can use a topical anesthetic (such as 2% lidocaine jelly) applied to the fissure to lessen discomfort (Vincent 1999).
- If a digital rectal exam is possible, check for masses (both fluctuant and firm), discharge, and ulcers.
- Test stool for occult blood.

→ Acute fissures:
- As the perianal skin is stretched, fissures will be visible at the anal verge, usually in the posterior midline but occasionally in the anterior midline.
- The fissure may be apparent as a linear or pear-shaped split in the lining of the distal anal canal, but spasm and pain of the anal sphincter may preclude an adequate view or exam.
- An early fissure has sharply demarcated, fresh mucosal edges, and there may be granulation tissue at its base.

→ Chronic fissures:
- Secondary changes, such as a sentinel skin tag (or "pile") protruding from the anus, hypertrophied anal papilla, or some degree of anal stenosis may be present with chronic fissures.
- Horizontal fibers of the internal sphincter muscle may be visible in the base of the mucosal defect.
- The area around the fissure may become sclerotic and appear white.
- The proximal end of the fissure may contain granulation tissue that is often confused with an anal polyp.
- With increasing chronicity, the margins of the fissure become indurated and there is a distinct lack of granulation tissue.
- If the patient has atypical or multiple fissures, consider other causes.

→ Hemorrhoids:
- Rarely will have a low hematocrit due to hemorrhoidal bleeding alone.

→ Internal hemorrhoids:
- The patient should be asked to squeeze and bear down, both during inspection and with digital examination, as this may cause internal hemorrhoids to protrude through the anus.

- Anoscopy provides optimal visualization of internal hemorrhoids.
- If an internal hemorrhoid is visible, assess for reducibility.
- To distinguish between prolapsed internal hemorrhoids and dilated or thrombosed external hemorrhoids: Internal hemorrhoids are covered by mucosa and external hemorrhoids by skin.
- With fourth-degree hemorrhoids, mucosa may be keratinized.
- Internal hemorrhoids may be palpable on digital examination of anal canal.

→ External hemorrhoids:
- External hemorrhoids are visible on perianal inspection, and will present as masses of varying sizes at the anal opening.
- When an external hemorrhoid is thrombosed, it may appear as a bluish perianal nodule covered with skin and may be up to several centimeters in size.
- Most external hemorrhoids are actually simple skin tags and do not contain dilated blood vessels.
- Skin tags are very common and may be the end result of a resolved thrombosed external hemorrhoid, the sentinel tag found distal to a chronic fissure, or an isolated finding.

ASSESSMENT

→ Hemorrhoid—internal: first-, second-, third-, or fourth-degree
→ Hemorrhoid— external
→ Anal fissure—acute or chronic
→ R/O infection (bacterial, viral)
→ R/O abscess
→ R/O carcinoma
→ R/O proctitis
→ R/O diverticular disease
→ R/O inflammatory bowel disease

PLAN

DIAGNOSTIC TESTS

→ Rectal examination and anoscopy are warranted for diagnosis of both anal fissures and hemorrhoids.
→ Topical anesthetic may be necessary for examination (as described in the "Objective" section above).
→ For patients over 40 years old, sigmoidoscopy or colonoscopy should be performed if patient has:
- Iron deficiency anemia (to rule out disease proximal to the sigmoid colon)
- Hematochezia (to rule out disease in the rectum or sigmoid colon that could be misinterpreted in the presence of hemorrhoidal bleeding)
- Rectal inflammation, fistulas, nonhealing fissures, or chronic rectal symptoms (see the **Inflammatory Bowel Disease** chapter)
→ Patients with atypical fissures (especially those that fail to heal), masses, nodules, and ulcerations should be referred for biopsy.

→ Stool guaiac testing is recommended to confirm presence of blood.
→ Hemoglobin/hematocrit is recommended to rule out anemia.
→ Rectal cultures as indicated to rule out sexually transmitted infections.
→ Consider an HIV test and serological test for syphilis for women at risk.
→ Additional testing may be warranted, depending on the patient's condition.

TREATMENT/MANAGEMENT

The following diet recommendations and general measures may be appropriate for patients with anal fissures and/or hemorrhoids.

→ General diet recommendations:
- High-fiber diet to prevent hemorrhoids and fissures: fresh fruit, vegetables, grains
- One of the best sources of fiber is wheat bran, although other grains are good sources.
- Water 6–8 glasses/day
→ General measures:
- Fiber supplements or stool softeners (or both) are helpful in some patients when the situation is acute or if the high-fiber diet alone is not enough to soften stools (McQuaid 2002, Orkin et al. 1999, Pfenninger et al. 2001):
  - Fiber supplements: psyllium or hydrophilic colloid as directed or bran powder (1–2 tbsp BID added to food or in 8 oz of fluid)

    OR

  - Stool softener: docusate sodium, 50–200 mg QD. Stool softeners are used to minimize straining and only short-term use is appropriate.
- Frequent warm sitz baths (20–30 minutes, TID–QID)
- Laxatives and enemas are generally not necessary and should be avoided.
- See the "Patient Education" section for additional treatment.
→ Acute anal fissures:
- Most anal fissures (>90%) are acute and relatively short-lived, resolving spontaneously or with simple conservative therapy (See "General Diet Recommendations" and "General Measures" listed above) (Jonas et al. 2001).
- Topical preparations:
  - The use of available topical preparations is controversial.
  - While there is support for using a topical corticosteroid alone (hydrocortisone [HC] ointment 1%) (McQuaid 2002), as well as support for the use of suppositories containing a topical corticosteroid and a local anesthetic (Pfenninger et al. 2001), other experts assert that topical preparations of corticosteroids with local anesthetics may not confer any benefit and may actually be harmful (anesthetics may delay healing and lead to skin sensitization) (Jonas et al. 2001). Therefore, consider consulting with an experienced clinician regarding treatment.

- Treatment may include the following:
  - Hydrocortisone ointment or cream 1% as directed
  - Oral analgesics if pain is moderate to severe, being aware that narcotics may aggravate constipation and that aspirin and nonsteroidal anti-inflammatory drugs may impair blood clotting and prolong bleeding
  - Anal pain caused by fissures can be treated symptomatically (e.g., lubricants such as mineral oil)
→ Chronic anal fissures:
  - Refer to physician if the patient has been diagnosed with a chronic fissure (if fissure has not healed with simple measures)
  - Pharmacologic treatment (consult with physician before prescribing):
    - Topical nitroglycerin ointment (0.2–0.5%), applied by fingertip to the anus and anal canal BID for 6–8 weeks (can decrease mean resting sphincter pressure)
    - Injection with botulinum toxin into the internal anal sphincter
  - Surgical treatment:
    - If pharmacologic treatment fails, surgical treatment may be necessary.
    - Chronic or recurrent fissures may benefit from partial, lateral, internal sphincterotomy, with risk of minor incontinence.
→ Internal hemorrhoids:
  - Treatment of internal hemorrhoids is based on symptoms and degree of internal hemorrhoidal prolapse.
  - Initially place patient on conservative therapy (see general diet recommendations and general measures listed above).
  - For edematous, prolapsed hemorrhoids, perform gentle manual reduction and consider topical analgesic treatments (suppositories or ointments).
  - Mucoid discharge may be treated effectively by the local application of a cotton ball tucked next to the anal opening after bowel movements.
  - Surgery:
    - Consultation with a physician may lead to a decision to fix internal loose tissue and reduce blood flow in enlarged columns by rubber band ligation, infrared coagulation, or sclerotherapy.
    - Laser treatment is not considered beneficial.
    - Surgical excision reserved for patients with chronic severe bleeding due to Stage III or IV hemorrhoids or acute thrombosed Stage IV hemorrhoid.
→ External hemorrhoids:
  - Management and treatment are based on symptoms; if patient has no major symptoms and does not notice the hemorrhoid, no treatment is necessary.
  - Hemorrhoids that cause minimal symptoms may be managed with methods aimed at reducing constipation/ straining and reducing local irritation.
  - All patients, regardless of severity or treatment choice, should follow the general diet recommendations listed above.
  - If the patient is experiencing severe pain or discomfort, referral to a physician is warranted (treatment may include rubber-band ligation, sclerotherapy, cryotherapy, infrared photocoagulation, bipolar diathermy, or surgery).
  - In most cases, it is not necessary to remove hemorrhoids to treat them effectively (Goroll 2000).
→ Over-the-counter (OTC) preparations:
  - Inflammation and itch symptoms: Consider a suppository preparation containing a steroid (e.g., HC) for a limited period of time. For predominantly external symptoms, prescribe 1% or 2.5% HC cream.
  - Severe pain: topical anesthetics—choose one that is minimally sensitizing (e.g., pramoxine, not benzocaine).
  - Preparation H ingredients are not shown to have any beneficial effect on hemorrhoids.
  - OTC creams and suppositories can be used but may be harmful to anal mucosa with prolonged use.
    - Anusol® ointment (with or without 1% hydrocortisone): Rub into anal area up to TID–QID.
    - Astringent compresses (e.g., witch hazel pads) prn
→ Thrombosed external hemorrhoids:
  - Consult with physician for treatment and management.
  - Treatment is directed at immediate pain relief because most will resolve on their own.
  - For first few hours, can recommend that patient lie prone with a cold pack applied to a thrombosed hemorrhoid.
  - After inflammation decreases, recommend warm sitz baths TID–QID.
  - May need to prescribe oral analgesics (may need codeine) and stool softeners.
  - During the first 2–3 days of the process, the patient may report fairly severe pain, which gradually improves as tension reduces in the distended vessels.
  - If the patient is in significant pain, if the lesion has ulcerated, or if conservative therapy has not been successful within 3 days, refer for surgical removal of clot.

CONSULTATION

→ Referral to a physician is warranted:
  - If the symptoms are severe and not reduced with nonsurgical intervention
  - For hemorrhoids that bleed repeatedly and produce intractable pain or become thrombosed (Goroll 2000)
  - If the patient has inflammatory proctitis or a fistula
  - If there is a nonhealing or atypical fissure, a nodule, or ulcerations
  - As needed for prescription(s)

PATIENT EDUCATION

→ Advise the patient to avoid straining at stool or sitting on the toilet for a prolonged period of time.
→ Advise the patient to eat a high-fiber diet (see the general diet recommendations listed above).
→ Recommend a regular time to have bowel movements.
→ Avoid vigorous wiping or straining.
→ Warm sitz baths

→ Advise the patient to maintain a regular exercise program.

→ If appropriate, advise the patient to discontinue anal intercourse at least until the symptoms are under control, and when doing so in the future, to use a generous amount of lubrication with penetration.

FOLLOW-UP

→ In 1–2 weeks, re-evaluate patients with moderate to severe symptoms to assess management plan. If symptoms are not improved, consider referral for surgical treatment.

→ Re-evaluate patients with thrombosed hemorrhoid in one week.

→ For patients in whom a rectal examination or anoscopy could not be performed because of severely painful fissures, allow for healing of the acute stage and re-examine.

→ At every visit, reinforce adherence to conservative measures.

→ Teach the American Cancer Society's recommendation for early detection of cancer in asymptomatic people (Zoorob et al. 2001):

- Fecal occult blood test: yearly beginning at age 50

    AND

- Digital rectal exam and flexible sigmoidoscopy: every 5 years beginning at age 50

    OR

- Digital rectal exam and colonoscopy: every 10 years beginning at age 50

    OR

- Digital rectal exam and double contrast barium enema: every 5–10 years beginning at age 50

→ Document in progress notes and on problem list.

BIBLIOGRAPHY

Goroll, A.H. 2000. Approach to the patient with anorectal complaints. In *Primary Care Medicine*, 4th ed., eds. A.H. Goroll and J.A. Mulley, pp. 447–453. Philadelphia: Lippincott Williams & Wilkins.

Hulme-Moir, M., and Bartolo, D.C. 2001. Hemorrhoids. *Gastroenterology Clinics of North America* 30(1):183–197.

Jonas, M., and Scholefield, J.H. 2001. Anal fissure. *Gastroenterology Clinics of North America* 30(1):167–181.

McQuaid, K.R. 2002. Anorectal diseases. In *Current medical diagnosis and treatment*, 41st ed., eds. L.M. Tierney, Jr., S.J. McPhee, and M.A. Papadakis, pp. 668–673. New York: Lange Medical Books/McGraw-Hill.

Orkin, B.A., Schwartz, A.M., and Orkin, M.A. 1999. Hemorrhoids: what the dermatologist should know. *Journal of the American Academy of Dermatology* 41(3):449–456.

Pfenninger, J.L., and Zainea, G.G. 2001. Common anorectal conditions: Part II. Lesions. *American Family Physician* 64(1):77–88.

Vincent, C. 1999. Anorectal pain and irritation. *Primary Care* 26(1):53–68.

Zoorob, R., Anderson, R., Cefalu, C. et al. 2001. Cancer screening guidelines. *American Family Physician* 63(6):1101–1112.

7-J

Hernia

A *hernia* is an abnormality in the musculofascial integrity of the abdominal wall that allows abdominal structures to protrude. The groin hernia is the most common location, but hernias can also occur in the abdomen. The overall incidence of groin hernias in adults is about 12 times more common in males than females (McIntosh et al. 2000). Approximately 96% of groin hernias are inguinal and 4% are femoral (Bax et al. 1999). It is often not clear whether a hernia is the result of a congenital defect or secondary to trauma or injury. A hernia that presents after trauma may be due, in part, to a previously asymptomatic congenital defect. Factors that increase intra-abdominal pressure, such as coughing, heavy lifting, or straining, may contribute to the appearance of the hernia.

The most common types of groin hernias in adults are inguinal and femoral. *Inguinal hernias* are further described as direct and indirect hernias. The *direct inguinal hernia* enters through the wall of the canal. Direct inguinal hernias increase in incidence with age and are the least likely of the external hernias to become strangulated (Goroll et al. 2000). The *indirect inguinal hernia* passes through the internal abdominal inguinal ring into the inguinal canal and exits through the external inguinal ring. The indirect inguinal hernia is the most common hernia in both sexes.

Femoral hernias pass through the femoral canal inferior to the inguinal ligament and become cutaneous in the fossa ovalis. These hernias are at greater risk of becoming incarcerated and are more common in older patients and in patients with previous hernia repairs. Femoral hernias are more common in females than males, by a ratio of 4:1 (McIntosh et al. 2000). Women may be predisposed to them due to a weakness in the pelvic floor musculature following childbirth. Femoral hernias account for less than 5% of all groin hernias, but 40% of these present as emergencies with incarceration or strangulation (McIntosh et al. 2000). It is often difficult to distinguish between groin hernias on examination, especially when the hernia is strangulated and the sac is large.

The most common ventral hernia is the *umbilical hernia.* The umbilical hernia passes through the umbilical ring and is considered to be congenitally acquired. Because the large bowel is frequently involved, strangulation and incarceration are common. Umbilical hernias are more common in women. They are associated with obesity, multiparity with prolonged labor in women, and large intra-abdominal tumors and cirrhosis with ascites in both genders (Goroll 1999, Mensching et al. 1996).

A *strangulated hernia* is an irreducible hernia in which the blood supply to the entrapped bowel has been compromised, resulting in obstruction and infarction. Fixation and rigidity of the hernial ring is associated with increased risk of strangulation (often seen in femoral hernias). Risk of strangulation has also been found to be higher in hernias of recent onset—both femoral and inguinal.

DATABASE

SUBJECTIVE

→ Patients are often asymptomatic.
→ Irreducible or incarcerated hernia may present with mass while supine, associated with higher degrees of pain.
→ Strangulated hernia may present with colicky abdominal pain, nausea, vomiting, and symptoms of obstruction.
→ Reducible hernias:
  ▪ Usually present when standing or with increase intra-abdominal pressure with coughing or Valsalva maneuver.
  ▪ Mass disappears when supine.
  ▪ May have varying degrees of intermittent pain with radiation when mass is present.
→ Pain may be aggravated by physical exertion.
→ May notice a swelling or bulge over corresponding anatomical site:
  ▪ Indirect inguinal:
    • Mass, tenderness over the deep inguinal ring
  ▪ Direct inguinal:
    • Mass, tenderness over the external inguinal ring
  ▪ Femoral:
    • Mass, tenderness in the femoral region
  ▪ Umbilical:
    • Mass, tenderness at umbilicus

OBJECTIVE

→ Examine while patient is in supine and standing position, and while doing Valsalva maneuver.

→ Reducible hernias are evident when standing and reduce when supine.

→ Direct inguinal:
- Visible and/or palpable protrusion over external inguinal ring
- Examination of the external inguinal ring is difficult in women.

→ Indirect inguinal:
- Visible and/or palpable protrusion over inguinal ring
- Examination of external inguinal ring is difficult in women.

→ Femoral:
- Visible and/or palpable protrusion in femoral region
- Difficult to distinguish between femoral and indirect inguinal, especially if incarcerated or a large sac

→ Umbilical:
- Difficult to palpate when large amount of subcutaneous fat is present
- Visible and/or palpable protrusion at umbilicus
- Ask the patient to lift her lead from the exam table and bear down while supine.

→ An irreducible hernia may present with tenderness, discoloration, edema, fever, and signs of bowel obstruction (e.g., distention, tympany, and hyperperistalsis) (see the **Abdominal Pain** chapter).

→ Examine groin for lymphadenopathy or other masses that do not change with Valsalva maneuver.

ASSESSMENT

→ Hernia:
- Indirect inguinal
- Direct inguinal
- Femoral
- Umbilical

→ R/O inguinal lymphadenopathy

→ R/O intra-abdominal mass

→ R/O musculoskeletal disorder

→ R/O appendicitis

→ R/O ectopic pregnancy

→ R/O tubo-ovarian abscess or cysts

→ R/O skin abscess/lymphadenitis

PLAN

DIAGNOSTIC TESTS

→ Ultrasonography may be useful in differentiating a simple hernia from an incarcerated hernia, a pathologic lymph node, or other groin swelling; it may also be warranted in patients with symptoms but no palpable defect.

→ The sensitivity and specificity of sonography of the inguinal area with the patient supine and upright and during the Valsalva maneuver is approximately 90% (Bax et al. 1999).

TREATMENT/MANAGEMENT

→ Consultation with a physician and/or surgeon is warranted for evaluation if surgery is considered. Any hernia that is irreducible, incarcerated, or strangulated should undergo surgical repair.

→ Asymptomatic reducible inguinal hernias (depending on size) may be managed expectantly. See the "Patient Education" section.

→ Symptomatic, reducible inguinal hernias should undergo elective repair to relieve symptoms and prevent strangulation.

→ Femoral hernias should undergo elective repair due to a high incidence of strangulation.

→ Umbilical hernias without protrusion may be managed expectantly.

→ Umbilical hernias with protrusion should undergo elective repair due to the high incidence of strangulation.

→ An adult hernia presenting with a painful and irreducible mass that was previously reducible should undergo immediate reduction to prevent strangulation.
NOTE: Contraindications to reduction are fever, leukocytosis, or other signs of toxicity indicating a strangulated bowel (Mensching et al. 1996).

→ Exacerbating factors should be managed appropriately—e.g., cough caused by smoking should be managed by advising smoking cessation.

CONSULTATION

→ Consultation with a general practitioner and/or surgeon is warranted in all cases of hernia.

→ Referral to a surgeon is indicated for surgery.

PATIENT EDUCATION

→ Patients who are managed expectantly should be advised to seek care for signs and symptoms of incarceration or strangulation—e.g., tenderness, discoloration, edema, fever, or signs of bowel obstruction (see the **Abdominal Pain** chapter).

→ Education should be provided for factors that may be contributing to the occurrence of the hernia (e.g., coughing caused by smoking). A referral for smoking cessation should be made.

FOLLOW-UP

→ Patients who are being managed expectantly and who are knowledgeable about signs and symptoms of complications can be followed routinely.

→ Follow-up may be indicated for factors contributing to the occurrence of the hernia.

→ Teach the American Cancer Society's recommendation for early detection of cancer in asymptomatic people (Zoorob et al. 2001):
- Fecal occult blood test: yearly beginning at age 50
  AND
- Digital rectal exam and flexible sigmoidoscopy: every 5 years beginning at age 50

OR
- Digital rectal exam and colonoscopy: every 10 years beginning at age 50

OR
- Digital rectal exam and double contrast barium enema: every 5-10 years beginning at age 50

→ Document in progress notes and on problem list.

BIBLIOGRAPHY

Bax, T., Sheppard, B.C., and Crass, R.A. 1999. Surgical options in the management of groin hernias. *American Family Physician* 59(4):893–906.

Goroll, A.H., and Mulley, A.G. 2000. Approach to the patient with an external hernia. In *Primary care medicine*, pp. 431–434. Philadelphia: Lippincott Williams & Wilkins.

McIntosh, A., Hutchinson, A., Roberts, A. et al. 2000. Evidence-based management of groin hernia in primary care—a systematic review. *Family Practice—An International Journal* 17(5):442–447.

Mensching, J.J., and Musielewicz, A.J. 1996. Abdominal wall hernias. *Emergency Medical Clinics of North America* 14(4): 739–756.

Zoorob, R., Anderson, R., Cefalu, C. et al. 2001. Cancer screening guidelines. *American Family Physician* 63(6):1101–1112.

Lisa L. Lommel, R.N., C., F.N.P., M.S., M.P.H.
Jeanne R. Davis, R.N., F.N.P., M.P.H.

7-K

Inflammatory Bowel Disease

The term *inflammatory bowel disease* (IBD) refers to a number of chronic, relapsing inflammatory disorders involving the gastrointestinal (GI) tract. The two most common conditions are *ulcerative colitis* (UC) and *Crohn's disease* (CD). Inflammatory bowel disease is more common in developed, Western countries than elsewhere. Approximately 600,000 people in the United States have some form of IBD (Botoman et al. 1998). Onset of IBD occurs most commonly between the ages of 20–40 (Langmead et al. 2001). Both UC and CD are more common among the Ashkenazi Jewish population of the United States and Europe (Kelly et al. 2001).

The etiology of IBD is not clearly understood but is thought to be due to a combination of genetic factors and abnormalities in immune regulation. Among family members of IBD patients, the prevalence of IBD is 50 times higher than in the population overall (Kelly et al. 2001). In addition, environmental factors are thought to play a role in its development. Bacterial, viral, and perhaps dietary antigens may trigger an ongoing enteric inflammatory response. Tobacco use also plays a role in IBD (with cigarette smoking appearing to decrease the risk of UC and increase the risk of developing or exacerbating CD) (Langmead et al. 2001). Exacerbations and remissions are typical of both disease states (Brown 1999, Stotland et al. 1998).

UC and CD may represent a group of heterogeneous disorders rather than distinct disease entities. A diagnosis of "indeterminate colitis" can be made for the 5–15% of patients with IBD who cannot be reliably diagnosed with UC or CD (Chutkan 2001). Extraintestinal involvement may occur with both UC and CD. The most common symptomatic extraintestinal manifestation of IBD is an asymmetric migratory arthralgia affecting the knees, hips, ankles, or elbows (Kelly et al. 2001). Other extraintestinal manifestations of IBD involve the skin (erythema nodosum, pyoderma gangrenosum), the joints/bones (arthritis, enteropathic arthropathy, sacroileitis, ankylosing spondylitis), the eyes (episcleritis, uveitis), the kidneys (oxalate stones and uric acid stones), the hepatobiliary tract (gallstones, sclerosing cholangitis, cholangiocarcinoma, pericholangitis, fatty infiltration), and the blood (anemia, thromboembolic events).

UC is a chronic, recurrent, inflammatory condition characterized by diffuse inflammation of the mucosal surface of the colon. Rectal involvement has been estimated to occur 95–100% of the time (Chutkan 2001, Kelly et al. 2001, McQuaid 2002). Involvement may extend proximally in a confluent and contiguous manner to involve part or all of the colon. Approximately 40–50% of cases are confined to the rectum (proctitis) or rectosigmoid region (proctosigmoiditis), 30% extend up to the splenic flexure (left-sided colitis), and less than 20% extend more proximally (extensive colitis or pancolitis) (McQuaid 2002). In general, the extent of colonic involvement does not progress over time. Patients with UC typically have symptomatic flare-ups and remissions. Those with pancolitis tend to have more severe symptoms. Complications of UC include toxic colitis, toxic megacolon (or toxic dilation, which can lead to perforation, hemorrhage, generalized peritonitis, and septicemia), and colon cancer. There is no known cure for UC, except surgery.

Crohn's disease is a chronic, recurrent disease characterized by transmural inflammation (extending through all layers of the bowel wall) involving any segment of the GI tract from mouth to anus. Lesions start out as discrete superficial ulcerations with hyperemia and edema. As the disease advances, these lesions coalesce, become deeper, and are accompanied by swelling of the intervening mucosa. Distribution of bowel inflammation is discontinuous, and diseased segments of bowel are characteristically sharply demarcated from adjacent normal bowel (known as "skip areas"). Approximately half of all cases involve small bowel and colon (usually the terminal ileum and adjacent proximal ascending colon [ileocolitis]), one-third of cases involve only the small bowel (usually the terminal ileum [ileitis]), and 20% of cases affect only the colon (McQuaid 2002). Less than 5% have clinically significant involvement of the upper GI tract (Bitton 2002).

Major complications of CD include fibrostenotic obstruction, enteric and perianal fistulas, abdominal and perianal abscess, perforation, perineal suppuration, and GI cancer. Risk of GI cancer depends on the location and duration of disease of the affected area. Patients with multiple bowel resections or with involvement of certain areas of the GI tract may have malabsorption of fat, bile acids, vitamins, and minerals. This disease is chronic and lifelong.

DATABASE

SUBJECTIVE

→ General history:
- Onset of symptoms (abrupt versus insidious)
- Duration of symptoms (relapsing and remitting symptoms versus continuous)
- Fatigue and/or malaise commonly associated with exacerbations of IBD
- Intolerance to dairy products
- Known immunosuppression
- Use of tobacco
- Receptive anal intercourse
- Radiation exposure
- Recent travel
- Recent antibiotic use
- Contact with others who have similar symptoms
- Family history of GI symptoms or disease

→ History should include a complete review of systems, as extraintestinal manifestations of IBD can involve multiple body systems.

Ulcerative Colitis

→ The hallmark symptom of UC is bloody diarrhea, with rectal bleeding being the presenting complaint in 90% of patients (Kam 1998).

→ In mild cases, symptoms include:
- Gradual onset of relatively infrequent diarrhea (<4 bowel movements [BMs]/day)
- Minimal and intermittent blood in stools
- No significant abdominal tenderness
- No systemic symptoms

→ In moderate cases, symptoms include:
- Frequent liquid stools (4–6 BMs/day)
- Blood and/or pus in stools
- Abdominal pain, tenderness, and cramping
- Fecal urgency
- Mild fever during exacerbations

→ With ulcerative proctitis, symptoms include:
- Chief complaint is rectal bleeding
- Fecal urgency, tenesmus, rectal pain, pruritus ani
- Diarrhea or constipation

→ In severe cases, symptoms include:
- More than six diarrheal BMs/day
- Large amount of blood in stool, with concomitant symptoms of anemia
- Weight loss, anorexia
- Rapid heartbeat
- Fever
- Abdominal pain, tenderness
- Symptoms of dehydration to varying degrees
- Complications may cause a wide range of symptoms

(e.g., secondary to hemorrhage, pericolitis, toxic dilatation, perforation, and carcinoma) and/or due to extra-intestinal involvement.

Crohn's Disease

→ Symptoms vary, depending on the location and extent of the disease.

→ Symptom onset may be subtle.

→ May notice associated manifestations (e.g., weight loss) before GI symptoms

→ Diarrhea and abdominal pain (especially in the right lower quadrant of abdomen) are cardinal symptoms of Crohn's disease.
- Assess if pain precedes evacuation of liquid stools and/or follows food intake.
- Associated symptoms: nausea, abdominal distention

→ Assess for fever, chills, nocturnal sweats.

→ Oral CD:
- Lesions in mouth: Edema and linear ulcers are the most common manifestation.
- Ulcers can be severe/painful and can impair nutritional status.

→ Gastroduodenal CD:
- Manifestations are rare—<5% of patients are affected.
- Symptoms are most commonly associated with other disease locations, usually the small intestine.
- Symptoms may include cramping pain that follows food intake, early satiety, nausea, abdominal distention, and/or postprandial vomiting.

→ Small and large bowel CD:
- Small bowel and ileocolitis:
  - Assess for abdominal pain (possibly right lower quadrant [RLQ]), diarrhea, low-grade fever, fatigue, obstructive symptoms, nausea, vomiting, weight loss, postprandial pain (if fibrostenotic disease).
  - Significant/constant pain and fever may signify abscess.
- Colonic:
  - Symptoms of CD are difficult to distinguish from UC.
  - Bloody diarrhea, hematochezia, weight loss, fever, rectal symptoms (fecal urgency, tenesmus, passage of mucus, pus, and blood) are possible.
- Perianal disease:
  - Hemorrhoidal tags, draining fissures or fistulas (suggested by rectal discharge, perianal pain, or both)
- Intestinal obstruction:
  - Due to narrowing of small bowel suggested by postprandial bloating, loud bowel sounds, vomiting, intermittent colicky pain
- Fistulas with or without infection:
  - Sinus tract can penetrate through the bowel and form fistulas at a number of locations.
  - Suggested by fever, chills, dysuria, pneumaturia, frequent urinary tract infections, tender abdomen, weight loss
- Steatorrhea in cases of fat and bile salt malabsorption

→ Complications of CD can present with a variety of symptoms (related to obstruction, enteric or perianal fistulas, abdominal or perianal abscess, perforation, and perianal suppuration).

OBJECTIVE

Ulcerative Colitis

→ Clinical findings depend on the severity of illness.
→ In mild cases, patient may present with:
  - Slightly tender or normal abdominal examination
  - Fever (less common with mild UC)
  - Normal laboratory values
→ In moderate to severe cases, patient may present with:
  - Abdominal tenderness, especially along course of colon
  - Abdominal distention
  - Decreased bowel sounds
  - Rectal examination revealing irritation, hemorrhoids, fissures, and spasm
  - Signs of dehydration and undernutrition to varying degrees
  - Tachycardia
  - Pallor
  - Fever
→ Laboratory findings reflect severity of disease:
  - Positive blood in stool
  - Stool negative for bacteria and parasites
  - Decreased hemoglobin and hematocrit, which reflect amount of blood loss
  - White blood cell (WBC) count and C-reactive protein and/or erythrocyte sedimentation rate (ESR) elevated in moderate to severe cases and with complications
  - Electrolytes reflect severity of disease with decrease in potassium, magnesium, and sodium
  - Decreased albumin, calcium, and total protein in moderate to severe cases
  - Abnormal liver function studies in severe cases
→ Patient may present with enlarged lymph nodes.

Crohn's Disease

→ Clinical findings depend on the severity of the illness.
→ Patient may present with:
  - If small bowel is involved:
    - Mid-abdominal and RLQ tenderness
    - RLQ fullness or mass reflecting adherent loops of bowel
  - Anal fissures, fistulas, hemorrhoids, or abscesses
  - Aphthoid ulcers in mouth, soft palate, or perianal area
  - Rectovaginal fistulas
  - Enlarged lymph nodes
  - Fever
  - Physical manifestations of undernutrition
→ Laboratory findings reflect the severity of the disease:
  - Positive or negative blood in stool
  - Stool negative for bacteria or parasite
  - Macrocytic anemia (vitamin B_{12} malabsorption)
  - Decreased hemoglobin and hematocrit

  - Normal or elevated WBC
  - Elevated ESR and/or C-reactive protein
  - Decreased total protein and albumin in severe cases

ASSESSMENT

→ Inflammatory bowel disease
→ R/O infectious colitis (bacterial, viral, fungal, parasitic)
→ R/O drug-induced colitis
→ R/O radiation proctitis or colitis
→ R/O diverticular disease
→ R/O irritable bowel syndrome
→ R/O neoplastic disorder
→ R/O ischemic colitis
→ R/O appendicitis
→ R/O pelvic inflammatory disease
→ R/O ovarian cysts and tumors
→ R/O endometriosis
→ R/O other gynecologic etiologies
→ R/O AIDS

PLAN

DIAGNOSTIC TESTS

→ Diagnostic studies of stool
  - Culture
  - Examination for ova and parasites
  - Assessment for occult blood
→ Serology:
  - ESR and/or C-reactive protein
  - Complete blood count (CBC)
  - Depending on severity of disease:
    - Electrolytes
    - Total protein, albumin
    - Liver function studies
    - Serology tests to distinguish UC from CD:
      - Antineutrophil cytoplasmic antibodies with perinuclear staining (pANCA) are found in 60–70% of patients with UC and 5–10% of patients with CD.
      - Antibodies to the yeast *Saccharomyces cerevisiae* (ASCA) are found in 60–70% of patients with CD and 5–10% of patients with UC.
      - The combination of these two tests has 50% sensitivity and 97% specificity for diagnosing CD (if pANCA negative, ASCA positive), and 57% sensitivity and 97% specificity for diagnosing UC (if pANCA positive, ASCA negative) (Chutkan 2001, McQuaid 2002).
      - While this differentiation may be important when considering surgical intervention, the clinical utility of auto-antibody testing in IBD is still unproven.
→ Endoscopy:
  - Colonoscopy (Kelly et al. 2001, Richter 2000):
    - Colonoscopy: UC
      - Colonoscopy with biopsy is the examination of choice for UC, allowing for assessment of both the severity of colonic inflammation and ulceration as

well as the extent of disease involvement (assessed by appearance and histologic exam of mucosa).
- May reveal loss of normal vascular pattern and mild to moderate diffuse inflammation in mild UC.
- May reveal continuous, diffuse inflammation and granulomatous, superficial ulcerations in moderate-severe UC.
- Colonoscopy: CD
  - Colonoscopy with biopsy may be useful in differentiating CD from UC.
  - Colonoscopy may reveal ulcerated fissures and focal asymmetric abnormalities with "skip areas" between diseased segments.
  - Colonoscopy is the diagnostic study of choice to evaluate possible segmental colonic involvement.
  - Colonoscopy with biopsy is utilized for cancer screening.
- A small-bowel follow-through is needed for diagnosis and to delineate the extent of the disease in patients with CD.
- Upper intestinal endoscopy with biopsy is more sensitive than barium studies for diagnosis of gastroduodenal CD.
→ Radiographic studies:
- X-ray is useful in the diagnosis and management of Crohn's disease.
  - Barium enema complements colonoscopy; it is useful before surgery and to evaluate fistulas and narrow strictures.
- Computed tomography:
  - Useful in diagnosing CD, especially with a history of diarrhea and presence of a palpable mass
  - Useful for identification of transmural intestinal thickening in CD
  - Useful for identifying extramural complications (e.g., fistulas, abscesses)
→ Ultrasonography can help delineate gynecologic etiologies of symptoms.
→ Additional testing may be warranted to rule out extra-intestinal manifestations as well as complications of the disease.

TREATMENT/MANAGEMENT

→ The majority of patients with mild disease can be managed on an outpatient basis.
→ Hospitalization is warranted for patients with moderate to severe disease or major complications.

Nutritional Therapies

→ General measures include:
- Advise a low-residue diet, eliminating raw fruits and vegetables and fruit juices.
- Low-fiber diet may be helpful in patients with active symptoms (e.g., eliminating nuts, seeds, tough meat, and cole slaw in order to reduce risk of obstruction).
- Advise a low-fat diet for patients with steatorrhea (<80 g/day), although if steatorrhea is chronic, the patient may need increased fat intake.

- Trial elimination of lactose-containing foods (i.e., dairy products)
- Limitation of caffeine
- Balanced, high-calorie (2,500–3,000 kcal/day) and high-protein (120–150 g/day) diet for undernourished patients
- With severe exacerbations, elemental supplements (e.g., Ensure®, Sustacal®) or total parenteral alimentation may be warranted to rest the bowel.
- Home parenteral nutrition is widely available as an alternative to hospitalization.
- Enteral nutrition and further discussion of parenteral nutrition for patients with IBD are beyond the scope of this chapter.
- A multivitamin with iron, calcium, and magnesium aids in decreased absorption of fat-soluble vitamins.
- Folic acid supplementation (1 mg/day) is warranted when intake of green leafy vegetables and fresh fruits is poor or when the patient is being treated with sulfasalazine.
- Parenteral vitamin B_{12} therapy as indicated (may occur in CD or previous ileal resection) (Botoman et al. 1998)
- Parenteral iron therapy as indicated (oral therapy not well tolerated)
- Fiber supplements can decrease diarrhea in mild-moderate disease (e.g., 1–2 tsps of psyllium p.o. QD) (Richter 2000).

Supportive Therapy

→ Opiates:
- Useful for providing symptom relief of diarrhea during acute phase of IBD
- Must use with caution in acutely ill patients
- Loperamide:
  - Slows intestinal motility and affects water and electrolyte movement through the bowel
  - Is helpful as adjunctive therapy in patients with proctitis and diarrhea, in patients with chronic watery diarrhea without active disease, or in patients who have undergone certain types of surgery
  - Most effective and least addicting of opiates
  - Dosage 2–4 mg p.o., maximum dose 8 mg/24 hours, titrate as needed for stool frequency (Michetti et al. 1999)
- Codeine sulfate 15–30 mg p.o. with meals and at HS
- Deodorized opium tincture 0.5–0.75 mL (10–15 drops) p.o. titrated for effect
- Diphenoxylate 2.5–5 mg p.o. TID–QID
NOTE: Avoid use of antidiarrheal medications in acute IBD, avoid use with bloody diarrhea or suspected enteric infection and in severe disease (such as active pancolitis), and avoid prolonged use of these drugs in all patients.
→ Cholestyramine:
- Useful in patients who develop bile salt-induced diarrhea after ileal resection
- Exercise caution when using long-term
- Dose: 1 packet (4 g)/day, can titrate up to 4 packets/day until diarrhea is controlled (Bitton 2002)

- Do not give to patients with steatorrhea.
- Consult with physician.
→ Nicotine:
  - Transdermal nicotine patches may have some benefit in patients with mild to moderate active UC, although they do not help maintain remission of UC.
  - Side effects include nausea and headache (Bitton 2002).
  - Consult with physician.

Overview of Pharmacological Therapy

→ While UC and CD seem to be different entities, the same pharmacologic agents are used to treat both.

→ Despite extensive research, there are still no specific therapies for these diseases.

→ Before prescribing from the following list of pharmacologic agents, clinicians must refer to the *Physicians' Desk Reference (PDR)* for a thorough review of all side effects, interactions, warnings, precautions, contraindications, and required monitoring diagnostic studies.

→ Medication doses are listed in the following section under the specific disease.

NOTE: IBD treatment regimens may vary across sites and they are often individualized as needed to treat each patient's symptoms.

Aminosalicylates (5-ASAs)

→ Used for anti-inflammatory effects

→ These compounds tend to be more effective in UC.

→ Many of the 5-ASAs require monitoring tests to screen for adverse reactions.

→ Oral 5-ASAs:
  - Sulfasalazine:
    - Used for years to treat IBD
    - Particularly effective in treating mild or moderately severe UC, although used in treatment of CD as well (Bitton 2002)
    - Efficacy and side effects (e.g., headache, nausea, vomiting) are dose-dependent. Side effects are more common with sulfasalazine than newer aminosalicylates (Bitton 2002).
    - Dose is tapered up to achieve symptomatic relief while minimizing side effects (see the "Treatment/Management" sections of ulcerative colitis and Crohn's disease).
    - Hematologic monitoring and folic acid supplementation are needed with sulfasalazine secondary to impaired folate metabolism.
  - Mesalamine:
    - Two oral medications containing mesalamine are commonly used:
      - Pentasa®: available as 250 mg capsules, active in small bowel and colon
      - Asacol®: available as 400 mg tablets, effective for cecum and large bowel
    - Side effects are generally mild and reversible.
    NOTE: Mesalamine is more expensive but has fewer side effects than sulfasalazine.

- Olsalazine:
  - Used for colon disease only, not absorbed in small intestine
  - Rarely used since advent of mesalamine
- Balsalazide disodium:
  - Used for treatment of UC, delivers the active anti-inflammatory medication directly to the colon, where it works topically
  - Side effects include headache and/or abdominal pain
→ Topical 5-ASAs:
  - Topical mesalamine:
    - Available as rectal suppository and rectal suspension enema
    - Can deliver much higher concentrations of 5-ASA to the distal colon than oral compounds
    - Side effects are uncommon.
    - Enema is indicated for treatment of active, mild-moderate, distal UC; proctosigmoiditis; or proctitis.
    - Suppository indicated for treatment of active, mild-moderate, ulcerative proctitis.

Corticosteroids

→ Useful for short-term treatment of moderate to severe active disease

→ Oral formulations:
  - Prednisone:
    - Used for mild-moderate, active CD involving the ileum and/or ascending colon
    - Side effects may include adrenal suppression, bone thinning, mood alterations, weakened resistance to infection, impaired glucose tolerance, and cushingoid appearance.
  - Budesonide:
    - Improvements noted in terminal ileum and proximal small bowel (helpful in ileocolonic CD).
    - Can induce remission, is less likely to cause systemic side effects than other steroidal agents (Bitton 2002, McQuaid 2002)
    - Side effects include headache, respiratory infection, nausea, and symptoms of hypercorticism.
→ Topical formulations:
  - Hydrocortisone suppositories, foam, and enemas
    NOTE: Long-term use of steroid preparations is associated with significant side effects and toxicity.

Immunomodulators

→ Azathioprine and 6-mercaptopurine:
  - Both of these drugs are clinically equivalent and have similar side effect profiles.
  - Induce and maintain remission in patients with refractory IBD and are useful in complex, inoperable perianal disease (Bitton 2002)
  - Less evidence supporting efficacy in UC
  - Awareness of side effects is critical, but both are considered safer and better tolerated than long-term corticosteroid use.

- Monitor for neutropenia/myelosuppression.
- Slow onset of action (approximately 3–6 months)
- Consult with physician for use.
→ Methotrexate:
- Weekly intramuscular methotrexate has been shown to be helpful with chronic active CD, allowing for steroid reduction (Bitton 2002).
- Must be aware of side effects
- Diagnostic testing is necessary for monitoring for adverse reactions (see *PDR*).
- Patients taking methotrexate should receive folic acid: 1 mg/day (Bitton 2002).
- May be helpful in allowing tapering of corticosteroids in refractory UC.
- Consult with physician for use.
→ Cyclosporine:
- A potent immunosuppressive drug
- May be helpful in managing IBD
- Some evidence shows it can help patients who have fistulizing CD that is unresponsive to steroids or antibiotics, or patients with severe UC who do not respond to corticosteroids.
- Consult with physician for use.

Biologic Therapies
→ Infliximab:
- A genetically engineered antibody that neutralizes a protein that contributes to the inflammation in CD, halting further inflammation.
- Approved by the Food and Drug Administration for treating moderate-severe CD, and for CD patients with enterocutaneous fistulas
- May help with moderate-severe disease resistant to other forms of therapy
- Relapse common, safety/efficacy need to be established
- TB test needed prior to administration
- Consult with physician for use.

Antibiotics
→ Antibiotics are clearly beneficial in CD.
- Metronidazole is effective in managing Crohn's ileocolitis or colitis, as well as perianal fistulas and perineal disease (Bitton 2002).
- Ciprofloxacin is also helpful in CD.
→ There is no consistent evidence that antibiotics are beneficial with UC, except for treatment of superimposed infection.
NOTE: Avoid alcohol use while on metronidazole (can cause disulfiram-like reaction).

Ulcerative Colitis: Mild to Moderate Disease
→ Distal colitis (proctitis/proctosigmoiditis):
- 5-ASAs (topical or oral):
  • Topical 5-ASAs (Bitton 2002, Botoman et al. 1998, Kam 1998, Michetti et al. 1999):
    – Mesalamine enema or suppository very effective

– Dosage: mesalamine enema 4 g/60 mL per rectum at HS or mesalamine suppository 500 mg per rectum BID–TID
– Evaluate after 2–4 weeks for efficacy, taper to lowest dose to treat symptoms if efficacious (can taper to 1 enema every third night), consider a second topical preparation (steroid or a second mesalamine agent) if no response.
  • Oral 5-ASAs:
    – Oral agents to be used if topical treatment is ineffective (Bitton 2002)
    – Mesalamine: 800 mg p.o. TID (Asacol®) OR 1 g p.o. QID (Pentasa®)
                    OR
    – Olsalazine: 500 mg QD, maximum dose 3 g QD (Michetti et al. 1999)
                    OR
    – Sulfasalazine: start at 500 mg p.o. BID, increase over 1–2 weeks up to 4 g/day (2 g p.o. BID) for 2–4 weeks or until symptoms abate, then decrease to the smallest dose that maintains control of symptoms (usually 1 g p.o. BID).
- Topical corticosteroids (Bitton 2002, Kam 1998):
  • Corticosteroid enemas are beneficial in patients with ulcerative proctosigmoiditis.
  • Hydrocortisone suppository: 30 mg per rectum QD or BID
                    OR
  • Hydrocortisone acetate rectal foam: 90 mg per rectum at HS or BID for proctitis
                    OR
  • Hydrocortisone enema for proctosigmoiditis: 100 mg/ 60 mL at HS or BID
  NOTE: Taper down all use of steroids.
→ Extensive colitis: Consult with a physician.
- 5-ASAs:
  • Mesalamine:
    – Asacol® 2.4–4.8 g p.o. QD OR Pentasa® 2–4 g p.o. QD
                    OR
  • Olsalazine sodium 1–2 g p.o. QD
                    OR
  • Sulfasalazine 4 g p.o. QD
  • Within 4 weeks, should achieve a therapeutic response (this may only occur at maximal doses) (Bitton 2002).
- Consider oral corticosteroids in patients unresponsive to 5-ASAs in order to induce remission (consult with physician).

Ulcerative Colitis: Moderate-Severe Disease
→ Details of treatment/management of moderate-severe disease are beyond the scope of this chapter.
→ Refer to physician for management.
→ Refer to medical texts for further information.

Ulcerative Colitis:
Maintenance Therapy

→ Distal colitis:
  ■ 5-ASAs (topical or oral) (Bitton 2002, Kam 1998, Michetti et al. 1999):
    • Mesalamine suppositories 500 mg per rectum QD
      OR
    • Mesalamine enema per rectum 1 g at HS
      OR
    • Oral mesalamine: Asacol® 0.8–1.6 g p.o. QD OR Pentasa® 1.5 g p.o. QD
      OR
    • Sulfasalazine 1–3 g/day p.o. QD (taken as 1–1.5 g BID)
      OR
    • Olsalazine 1–2 g p.o. QD
  ■ Immunomodulators:
    • Azathioprine or 6-mercaptopurine (consult with physician)
→ Extensive colitis:
  ■ 5-ASAs:
    • Sulfasalazine 2–4 g p.o. QD
      OR
    • Mesalamine 1.2–2.4 g p.o. QD
      OR
    • Olsalazine 1–2 g p.o. QD
  NOTE: Some patients may need dual therapy with oral and rectal agents to maintain remission (Bitton 2002).
  ■ Oral corticosteroids as needed (consult with physician)
  ■ Azathioprine or 6-mercaptopurine (consult with physician)

Ulcerative Colitis:
Surgical Treatment

→ While UC can be cured with surgery, fewer than 10% of patients undergo surgical treatment for UC.
→ Surgery is required most often in patients with extensive colitis.
→ Indications for surgery:
  ■ Persistently active disease with an inadequate response to medical therapy or unacceptable medication-induced side effects
  ■ Colonic dysplasia or carcinoma
  ■ Fulminant colitis, toxic megacolon, colonic perforation, and persistent severe colonic hemorrhage are urgent indications for surgery.

Crohn's Disease:
Mild to Moderate Disease

→ 5-ASAs (Bitton 2002, Botoman et al. 1998, Langmead et al. 2001, McQuaid 2002, Michetti et al. 1999):
  ■ Mesalamine: 800 mg p.o. TID (Asacol®)
      OR
  ■ Mesalamine: 500 mg–1 g p.o. QID (Pentasa®)
      OR

  ■ Sulfasalazine 1.5–3 g p.o. BID
      OR
  ■ Olsalazine 500 mg p.o. BID for colon disease only
  ■ Patients who do not respond after 3–4 weeks of maximal treatment may benefit from the addition of ciprofloxacin (dose: 500 mg p.o BID for 3–4 months).
NOTE: Both mesalamine and sulfasalazine can induce remission in ileocolitis or colitis, although mesalamine is more effective in ileitis compared to sulfasalazine.
→ Antibiotics (Bitton 2002, McQuaid 2002):
  ■ Metronidazole (with or without ciprofloxacin):
    • Metronidazole has a potency similar to that of sulfasalazine.
    • Dose: 250 mg p.o. TID
    • Effective in treating patients with Crohn's ileocolitis or colitis, or perianal disease
    • Use if 5-ASAs are not effective
    • Advise patient to avoid alcohol while on metronidazole.
  ■ Ciprofloxacin:
    • Dose: 500 mg p.o. BID (Bitton 2002, McQuaid 2002)
  ■ Maintain patient on antibiotic for 3–4 months (Bitton 2002).
→ Corticosteroids:
  ■ Prednisone is especially efficacious with small bowel involvement.
  ■ Consider for patients with marked systemic symptoms and those who fail to respond to 5-ASA medications and antibiotics.
  ■ Use high doses initially (e.g., 40–60 mg p.o. QD) for an active flare-up, then taper after 2–3 weeks or once remission has been achieved (McQuaid 2002).
  ■ Chronic low doses of steroids are often required.
  ■ Steroids plus sulfasalazine are more effective than sulfasalazine alone in bringing an acute flare-up under control but are ineffective in preventing a relapse.
  ■ Budesonide (9 mg p.o. QD) can be used to induce remissions with somewhat fewer side effects than prednisone (for mild to moderate ileocolonic CD) (Bitton 2002, McQuaid 2002).
→ Immunomodulators:
  ■ Azathioprine or 6-mercaptopurine:
    • Azathioprine (doses of 2–2.5 mg/kg/day p.o.) or 6-MP (1–1.5 mg/kg/day p.o.) are effective for treating the active disease, as well as the long-term treatment of CD, especially if the disease is unresponsive or frequent recurrences need chronic steroids.
    • Consult with a physician for prescribing, especially if higher doses are needed.
  ■ Infliximab: consult with physician.

Crohn's Disease:
Oral

→ Topical therapy alone, with hydrocortisone in methylcellulose, pectin or gelatin, or sucralfate
→ Viscous lidocaine occasionally used, swish in mouth

Crohn's Disease:
Gastroduodenal

→ Omeprazole, sucralfate, or H2-receptor antagonists may induce partial or even complete remission in these patients. (See *PDR* for dosage schedule.)

Crohn's Disease:
Severe, Refractory, Steroid-Dependent, Perianal, or Fistulizing Disease

→ Refer to specialist for management.
→ Details of treatment/management of moderate-severe disease are beyond the scope of this chapter.
→ Refer to medical texts for further information.

Crohn's Disease:
Maintenance Therapy

(Botomon et al. 1998, McQuaid 2002)

→ Aminosalicylates:
  ■ Mesalamine:
    • Pentasa® shown to be useful in maintaining remission of CD at dose of 4 g p.o. QD
    • Asacol® shown to be useful in maintaining remission of CD at dose of 800 mg p.o. TID
→ Metronidazole: At 10–20 mg/k/day, it is the drug of choice for perianal disease.
  NOTE: High dosages of metronidazole may need to be maintained for a prolonged period. Patient should be aware of potential side effects, including paresthesias (Kelly et al. 2001).
→ Azathioprine or 6-mercaptopurine: consult with physician.
→ Infliximab: consult with physician.

Crohn's Disease:
Surgery

(Brown 1999, Chutkan 2001, Kelly et al. 2001)

→ Approximately 65–75% of patients with Crohn's colitis will have at least one resectional surgery.
→ Probability of surgery is 70–75% at 20 years and 90% at 30 years from time of onset of symptoms.
→ As surgery does not cure the patient with CD (unlike UC), CD is likely to recur.
→ Indications for surgery:
  ■ Intractable disease, colonic stricture, perforation, obstruction, fistulas, malignancy, perianal disease/fistulas, and severe bleeding

CONSULTATION

→ The majority of patients with IBD should be managed in consultation with a gastroenterologist for diagnosis and to evaluate the extent of the disease.
→ After the initial diagnosis, patients with mild, limited UC that is responding well to medical treatment may not require regular consultation and management by a specialist.

→ Referral to a physician who is experienced in treating IBD is warranted for surgical indications, conditions unresponsive to medical therapy, or moderate to severe UC and for most patients with CD.
→ Referral to a physician is warranted for colonoscopy and x-ray procedures.
→ Referral to a psychotherapist as indicated for anxiety or depression.
→ Consultation or referral to a nutritionist for education.
→ Referral to appropriate specialist for evaluation of extra-intestinal manifestations (most commonly gastroenterology, rheumatology, or dermatology).
→ As needed for prescription(s).

PATIENT EDUCATION

→ See the "Treatment/Management" section.
→ Explain the pathogenesis, treatment plan, chronicity, and course of disease. Include the patient's family in the education.
→ Women with IBD should be counseled to consult with their obstetrician to discuss fertility, timing of pregnancy, and risks related to active IBD.
→ For patients who have a colostomy or ileostomy (temporary or permanent), special teaching and support need to be provided about the physical and emotional aspects of living with a stoma.
→ Address psychosocial issues:
  ■ Discuss concerns regarding incontinence, cancer, and social isolation.
  ■ Provide a supportive relationship and observe for signs of depression from chronic illness.
  ■ Discuss the role of psychosocial stress as potentially impacting the course of IBD, as well as ways to manage life stressors.
  ■ Resources for education and support services for patients and their families:
    • Crohn's and Colitis Foundation of America (CCFA) (800) 932-2423
      www.ccfa.org
    • National Digestive Diseases Information Clearinghouse (301) 654-3810
      www.niddk.nih.gov
→ Advise the patient regarding a nutritious diet (see "Nutritional Therapies" in the "Treatment/Management" section).
  ■ Encourage small, regular, frequent meals.
  ■ Advise quitting smoking and alcohol intake: refer to appropriate support services if indicated (i.e., American Cancer Society, Nicotine Anonymous, Alcoholics Anonymous).
→ Advise a regular exercise program.
→ Patients can be taught to adjust their medications within a prearranged set of guidelines and limits, allowing them a more active role in their own care.
→ Discuss the increased risk of osteoporosis associated with IBD (secondary to corticosteroid use, and possible calcium and vitamin D malabsorption).

→ Discuss the increased risk of colon cancer among UC patients and the need for colon cancer surveillance (see the "Follow-up" section).

→ Discuss the increased risk for small bowel adenocarcinoma (and possibly for colon cancer) among CD patients and the need for colon cancer surveillance (see the "Follow-up" section).

FOLLOW-UP

→ The patient should be followed closely during exacerbations.

→ During remission, evaluations are warranted every 3–6 months to document:
  - Number of exacerbations (if any)
  - Weight
  - Proctoscopy or sigmoidoscopy
  - Appropriate lab tests

→ Follow up with monitoring tests as appropriate for specific medications (refer to *PDR*).

→ Colon cancer surveillance:
  - Ulcerative colitis (Bitton 2002, Kelly et al. 2001):
    - Increased incidence of colon cancer after 8–10 years is approximately 5%.
    - Colonoscopy with directed biopsy should be performed 8–10 years after diagnosis of extensive colitis and 12 years after diagnosis of left-sided colitis.
    - Surveillance colonoscopies should be performed every 1–2 years thereafter if biopsies are negative.
  - Crohn's disease:
    - In CD of the colon, cancer risk increases with an increasing area of involvement and longer duration.
    - In small bowel disease, cancer risk increases with longer duration.
    - Cancer surveillance (colonoscopy with directed biopsy) should start approximately 8–10 years after diagnosis of extensive colitis.
    - Upper GI and small-bowel x-ray with colonoscopy should be performed every two years.
    - Colonoscopic screening may be appropriate for patients with longstanding, extensive Crohn's colitis, but no established screening protocols exist for intestinal carcinoma in CD.

→ Testing for occult blood in stool as an indicator of malignancy is inappropriate because many patients with IBD experience blood loss.

→ Document in progress notes and on problem list.

BIBLIOGRAPHY

Bitton, A. 2002. Inflammatory bowel disease. In *Rakel: Conn's Current Therapy 2002*, 54th ed., eds. R.E. Rakel and E.T. Bope, pp. 478–485. Philadelphia: W.B. Saunders.

Botoman, V., Bonner, G., and Botoman, D. 1998. Management of inflammatory bowel disease. *American Family Physician* 57(1):57–72.

Brown, M. 1999. Inflammatory bowel disease. *Primary Care* 26(1):141–170.

Chutkan, R. 2001. Inflammatory bowel disease. *Gastroenterology* 28(3):539–556.

Kam, L. 1998. Ulcerative colitis in young adults. *Postgraduate Medicine* 103(1):45–59.

Kelly, C.P., and Michetti, P.F. 2001. Inflammatory bowel disease. In *Textbook of primary care medicine*, 3rd ed., ed. J. Noble, pp. 983–990. St. Louis, Mo.: Mosby.

Langmead, L., and Rampton, D. 2001. A GP guide to inflammatory bowel disease. *Practitioner* 245(1620):224–229.

McQuaid, K.R. 2002. Inflammatory bowel disease. In *Current medical diagnosis and treatment*. 41st ed., eds. L. Tierney, Jr., S. McPhee, and M. Papadakis, pp. 648–657. New York: Lange Medical Books/McGraw-Hill.

Michetti, P., and Peppercorn, M. 1999. Medical therapy of specific clinical presentations. *Gastroenterology Clinics of North America* 28(2):353–370.

Richter, J.M. 2000. Management of inflammatory bowel disease. In *Primary care medicine*, 4th ed., eds. A.H. Goroll and A. Mulley, pp. 474–484. Philadelphia: Lippincott Williams & Wilkins.

Stotland, B., Cirigliano, M., and Lichtenstein, G. 1998. Medical therapies for inflammatory bowel disease. *Hospital Practice* 33(5):141–156.

7-L

Irritable Bowel Syndrome

Irritable bowel syndrome (IBS) is a common disorder that is a part of a larger diagnostic group of functional disorders with symptoms localized to the mid or lower gastrointestinal tract. Related disorders include functional abdominal bloating, functional constipation, functional diarrhea, and unspecified bowel disorder. This group of disorders is characterized by abdominal discomfort or pain associated with defecation or a change in bowel habits (Thompson et al. 1999).

Irritable bowel syndrome has no specific pathophysiological marker. The bases for irritable bowel syndrome are currently believed to be intestinal motor and sensory dysregulation and central nervous system dysfunction. The symptoms of IBS are the result of both abnormal intestinal motility and enhanced visceral sensitivity. Recent studies have shown a strong association between affective disorders and IBS. This supports the observation that some IBS patients do not always have gut-centered symptoms but may have more generalized alterations in smooth muscle activity and increased visceral sensation (e.g., as in urinary bladder hyperactivity) (Farthing 1998). Individuals often manifest "noncolonic" symptoms of IBS, including urinary symptoms of frequency and nocturia, dyspareunia, gastroesophageal reflux, noncardiac chest pain, back pain, and fatigue. Additionally, 40–60% of individuals diagnosed with IBS have depression and/or anxiety, suggesting that psychosocial factors may be a strong component of this syndrome (Farthing 1998).

Studies of the general population suggest that 10–20% of adults experience IBS symptoms. Less than one-half of these individuals will seek medical care for their symptoms. Irritable bowel syndrome constitutes a significant portion of a primary care provider's practice, with one-fourth of all gastrointestinal referrals relating to IBS. In Western societies, studies suggest a female to male ratio of 2:1. IBS is most commonly diagnosed between the ages of 20–40, and over time, up to 30% of individuals become asymptomatic. Individuals with IBS often miss days from school or work and their estimated overall estimated health care costs are considerable (Borum 1998, Dalton et al. 1997).

The diagnostic criteria for IBS were developed in Rome, Italy, by an international team of experts; they were recently updated. These clinical diagnoses are used to define subjects for clinical research. The diagnostic criteria for IBS are shown in **Table 7L.1, Rome II Diagnostic Criteria for Irritable Bowel Syndrome**.

DATABASE

SUBJECTIVE

→ A detailed history is key in diagnosing IBS (see **Table 7L.1**).

→ A hallmark symptom is abdominal pain relieved with defecation and associated with a change in consistency or frequency.

→ The patient may notice mucus in her stool and excessive flatulence.

→ Stool symptoms may be constipation-predominant, diarrhea-predominant, bloating-predominant, or a combination of constipation and diarrhea.

→ Abdominal bloating and feeling of incomplete evacuation of stool are common.

→ Symptoms wax and wane; they do not typically intensify over time.

→ Abdominal pain (described as "cramps," "grips," "twinges," and "colic") is poorly localized, migratory, variable in nature, and relieved with defecation.

→ Symptoms may be worsened by:
  ■ Meals
  ■ Tobacco
  ■ Certain dietary components such as alcohol, low dietary fiber, coffee, tea, citrus fruits, sorbitol-containing foods, and gas-producing foods
  ■ Medications such as antibiotics, β-blockers, bronchodilators, cardiac medications, diuretics, and narcotics
  ■ Stressful life events
  ■ Menses
  ■ Physical overexertion

→ Extra-intestinal symptoms such as nausea, heartburn, early satiety, loss of appetite, dyspareunia, headaches, backaches, lethargy, and urinary symptoms are commonly reported (Schmulson et al. 1999, Talley 1998).

→ Symptoms that are less suggestive of IBS (and should be investigated further) include the following: abdominal pain not associated with bowel symptoms, significant weight loss, rectal bleeding, steatorrhea, fever, anemia, or symptoms that awaken the patient from sleep.

→ The patient may miss school or work related to pain and symptoms.

→ Inquire regarding history of laxative abuse.

→ Patient may have a history of depression, anxiety, physical or sexual abuse, or narcotic abuse.

→ Inquire regarding history of recent travel precipitating constipation (from inactivity, dehydration, or a change in diet) or diarrhea (from infection).

OBJECTIVE

→ Physical exam is usually within normal limits. Exceptions may include:
- Tenderness to abdominal palpation in the left lower quadrant in region of sigmoid colon
- Abdominal distention
- Tympanic percussion of abdomen due to air trapped in the colon
- Tenderness on rectal exam

Table 7L.1.   ROME II DIAGNOSTIC CRITERIA FOR IRRITABLE BOWEL SYNDROME

At least 12 weeks, which need not be consecutive, in the preceding 12 months of abdominal discomfort or pain that has two of three features:
- Relieved with defecation; and/or
- Onset associated with a change in frequency of stool; and/or
- Onset associated with a change in form (appearance) of stool
                    PLUS
- Diarrhea-predominant
  - 1 or more of items 2, 4, or 6 below and none of 1, 3, 5
- Constipation-predominant
  - 1 or more of 1, 3, or 5 and none of 2, 4, 6

1. Fewer than three bowel movements a week
2. More than three bowel movements a day
3. Hard or lumpy stool
4. Loose (mushy) or watery stools
5. Straining during a bowel movement
6. Urgency (having to rush to have a bowel movement)
7. Feeling of incomplete bowel movement
8. Passing mucus (white material) during a bowel movement
9. Abdominal fullness, bloating, or swelling

Source: Adapted with permission from Rome II Criteria Committee. 2000. *Rome II: the functional gastrointestinal disorders*, 2nd ed., eds. D. Drossman, E. Corazziari, N. Talley et al. McLean, Va.: Degnon Associates. Available at: http://www.romecriteria.org. Accessed on August 1, 2002.

ASSESSMENT

→ Irritable bowel syndrome

→ R/O inflammatory bowel disease, including Crohn's disease and ulcerative colitis

→ R/O constipating medications

→ R/O lactose intolerance

→ R/O infectious enteritis or gastroenteritis (e.g., *Giardia lamblia*, *Campylobacter jejuni*, salmonellosis, *Escherichia coli*)

→ R/O celiac spruce

→ R/O chronic pancreatitis

→ R/O peptic ulcer disease

→ R/O endometriosis

→ R/O endocrine disorders (hypo- or hyperthyroidism, diabetes)

→ R/O colon cancer

→ R/O laxative abuse

PLAN

DIAGNOSTIC TESTS

→ IBS is a diagnosis of exclusion.

→ CBC

→ Chemistry panel

→ Thyroid function studies

→ Stool for blood, ova and parasites, *Clostridium difficile*, bacterial culture, and fecal fat. Yield on all but occult blood studies is very low if stool is not loose.

→ Colonoscopy for patients with the following:
- Age greater than 40 years
- Family history of colon cancer or IBS
- Symptoms suspicious for neoplasm (Dalton et al. 1997)

→ Radiographic or endoscopic studies may be warranted if the patient has upper gastrointestinal tract symptoms.

→ Screening sigmoidoscopy to rule out tumors or mucosal disease

→ If suspicious for lactose intolerance (diarrhea and bloating two hours after ingesting a lactose-rich meal), consider a two-week trial of a lactose-free diet or a lactose breath hydrogen test.

→ A more detailed diagnostic evaluation should be considered for individuals with:
- Recent onset of symptoms (particularly in patients over age 50)
- Severe or disabling symptoms
- Recent change in symptoms
- Family history of colon cancer

TREATMENT/MANAGEMENT

→ Simethicone, charcoal, and/or Beano may decrease intestinal gas and abdominal bloating.

→ Low-dose tricyclic antidepressants may be helpful in patients with diarrhea- or pain-predominant IBS, including:
- Imipramine
- Desipramine
- Amitriptyline

→ Selective serotonin reuptake inhibitors (SSRIs) tend not to cause constipation and may be helpful when constipation is predominant (Camilleri 2001, Verne et al. 1997). These medications are usually used in patients with frequently occuring or continual symptoms. A 2–3 month trial is usually needed before the therapeutic effect can be assessed (Camilleri 2001). These include:
- Paroxetine
- Fluoxetine
- Sertraline

→ For treatment of depression or anxiety, consider:
- Biofeedback
- Psychoactive medications
- Psychotherapy
- Hypnotherapy
- Cognitive-behavioral therapy, either alone or in combination with any of the treatments listed immediately above.
- Avoid implying that the symptoms are psychogenic. Instead, explain that these treatments may help the patient cope with a chronic, uncomfortable illness.

→ For abdominal pain:
- Anticholinergic medications (Verne et al. 1997):
  • Dicyclomine 10–20 mg p.o. TID–QID
  • Use with caution when constipation is predominant.
- Hyoscyamine sulfate (Verne et al. 1997):
  • Short-acting agent is given in a dose of 0.125–0.25 mg orally or sublingually before meals.
  • Long-acting agent is given in a dose of 0.375–0.75 mg BID.
- These medications may be given 30–60 minutes before meals to prevent postprandial abdominal pain.

→ For constipation:
- Increase dietary fiber and bulking agents with psyllium (Metamucil®, Fiberall®) 15–25 g p.o. daily (taken with a large amount of fluid).

→ For diarrhea:
- Loperamide 4 mg p.o. initially, followed by 2 mg p.o. after passage of each unformed stool (Camilleri 2001) **NOTE:** May induce constipation, should be tritrated for each individual patient. Liquid formula is less constipating.
- Diphenoxylate with atropine 2.5 mg p.o. QID (McQuaid 2001)

CONSULTATION

→ Physician consultation may be needed for IBS treatment plan.
→ Physician referral is warranted for sigmoidoscopy or radiographic studies.
→ Physician referral may be indicated for disabling symptoms or refractory disease.
→ Referral to a psychotherapist is warranted for patients with serious pathology.

PATIENT EDUCATION

→ Reassure the patient that IBS is a benign syndrome and does not progress or increase the risk for any other disease.

→ Teach the patient to complete a daily diary for 2–3 weeks that monitors dietary intake, exacerbating factors, stressors, and emotional responses. This will help to identify management strategies and may give the patient a sense of control over the illness (Dalton et al. 1997).
→ Advise a high-fiber, low-fat diet.
→ Advise the patient to limit foods that exacerbate symptoms (i.e., sorbitol-containing foods, alcohol, caffeine, gas-producing foods, carbonated beverages, citrus fruits, and fatty foods).
→ Avoid milk and milk products only in patients with lactose intolerance.
→ Advise patients to avoid fad food and diets.
→ Advise patients to avoid medications that exacerbate symptoms, including:
- Antibiotics
- β-blockers
- Cardiac medications
- Bronchodilators
- Diuretics
- Narcotics
- Medications stimulating diarrhea (fermentable fibers, magnesium-containing antacids) and constipation-producing agents (calcium channel blockers, aluminum containing antacids, bismuth subsalicylate, sucralfate, anticholinergics, calcium supplements) should also be avoided.

→ Advise regular meal intake.
→ Advise routine toileting, especially with constipation.
→ Review interventions to reduce stress.
→ Encourage regular exercise.

FOLLOW-UP

→ Referral for management of depression, anxiety, history of physical or sexual abuse, or narcotic abuse.
→ Patients with severe symptoms or significant psychosocial impairment should be referred to a gastrointestinal specialist.
→ Organizations for referral include:
- International Foundation for Functional Gastrointestinal Disorders (IFFGD)
  P.O. Box 17884
  Milwaukee, Wis. 53217
  (414) 964-1799
  Toll free: (888) 964-2001
- National Digestive Diseases Information Clearinghouse (NDDIC)
  2 Information Way
  Bethesda, Md. 20892-3570
  (301) 654-3810

→ Teach the American Cancer Society's recommendation for early detection of cancer in asymptomatic people (Zoorob et al. 2001):
- Fecal occult blood test: yearly beginning at age 50
                    AND
- Digital rectal exam and flexible sigmoidoscopy: every 5 years beginning at age 50

OR
- Digital rectal exam and colonoscopy: every 10 years beginning at age 50

OR
- Digital rectal exam and double contrast barium enema: every 5–10 years beginning at age 50

→ Document in progress notes and on problem list.

BIBLIOGRAPHY

Borum, M.L. 1998. Gastrointestinal disease in women. *Medical Clinics of North America* 82(1):21–50.

Camilleri, M. 1999. Therapeutic approach to the patient with irritable bowel syndrome. *American Journal of Medicine* 107(5A):27S–32S.

_____. 2001. Management of the irritable bowel syndrome. *Gastroenterology* 120(3):652–668.

Dalton, C.B., and Drossman, D.A. 1997. Diagnosis and treatment of irritable bowel syndrome. *American Family Physician* 55(3):875–880.

Farthing, M.J.G. 1998. New drugs in the management of the irritable bowel syndrome. *Drugs* 56(1):11–21.

McQuaid, K. 2001. Alimentary tract. In *Current medical diagnosis and treatment*, 41st ed., eds. L.M. Tierney, Jr., S.J. McPhee, and M.A. Papadakis, pp. 559–661. New York: Lange Medical Books/McGraw-Hill.

Rome II Criteria Committee. 2000. *Rome II: the functional gastrointestinal disorders*, 2nd ed., eds. D. Drossman, E. Corazziari, N. Talley et al. McLean, Va.: Degnon Associates. Available at: http://www.romecriteria.org. Accessed on August 1, 2002.

Shaw, B. 1996. Management and treatment of gastrointestinal disorders. *Journal of Nurse-Midwifery* 41(2):155–172.

Schmulson, M.W., and Chang, L. 1999. Diagnostic approach to the patient with irritable bowel syndrome. *American Journal of Medicine* 107(5A):21S–26S.

Talley, N.J. 1998. Irritable bowel syndrome: disease definition and symptom description. *European Journal of Surgery* (Suppl.)583:24–28.

_____. 1999. Irritable bowel syndrome: definition, diagnosis and epidemiology. *Baillieres Clinical Gastroenterology* 13(3):371–384.

Thompson, W.G., Longstreth, G.F., Drossman, D.A. et al. 1999. Functional bowel disorders and functional abdominal pain. *Gut* 45 (Suppl. II):II43–II47.

Verne, G.N., and Cerda, J.J. 1997. Irritable bowel syndrome. *Postgraduate Medicine* 102(3):197–208.

Zoorob, R., Anderson, R., Cefalu, C. et al. 2001. Cancer screening guidelines. *American Family Physician* 63(6):1101–1112.

Lisa L. Lommel, R.N., C., F.N.P., M.S., M.P.H.
Jeanne R. Davis, R.N., F.N.P., M.P.H.

7-M
Peptic Ulcer Disease

Peptic ulcer disease (PUD) can be defined as a break or excoriation of the gastrointestinal (GI) mucosa. Peptic ulcers typically form in the gastric or duodenal mucosa when the mucosa is vulnerable to gastric acid and pepsin. Ulcers may range in size from several millimeters to several centimeters, but are usually over 5 mm in diameter (McQuaid 2002). By definition, ulcers extend through the muscularis mucosae.

Duodenal ulcers are five times more common than gastric ulcers, and over 95% of these ulcers are located in the bulb or pyloric channel (McQuaid 2002). In the stomach, benign ulcers usually occur in the antrum and at the junction of the antrum and body on the lesser curvature. While the incidence of duodenal ulcer disease has declined over the past 30 years, the incidence of gastric ulcers seems to be increasing (McQuaid 2002).

Among the American adult population, the lifetime prevalence of ulcers is approximately 10%, and they occur slightly more commonly in men than in women (1.3:1) (McQuaid 2002). Although ulcers can occur in any age group, duodenal ulcers most commonly occur between the ages of 30–55, while gastric ulcers are more likely between the ages of 55–70.

Atypical symptoms, complex treatment issues, and higher complication and mortality rates make managing elderly patients with PUD more difficult. Complications among the elderly are more common because the elderly are more likely to have delayed diagnosis and treatment, to have comorbid medical conditions, to use multiple medicines (including ulcerogenic medicines, such as nonsteroidal anti-inflammatory drugs), and be malnourished.

Factors Contributing to the Development of PUD

Helicobacter Pylori

H. pylori is a bacterial infection that is the most common cause of peptic ulcer. Its pathogenic role in PUD (duodenal and gastric) is widely recognized. While only one in six patients infected with *H. pylori* develops ulcer disease, between 90–99% of patients with duodenal ulcers and 80% of patients with gastric ulcers are infected with this Gram-negative bacterium (Anderson et al. 2000, Goroll 2000, McQuaid 2002, Meurer et al. 2001). *H. pylori* is mainly transmitted in childhood, secondary to direct person-to-person exposure (fecal-oral or oral-oral) (Freston 2000, Smoot et al. 2001).

H. pylori puts individuals at risk for ulcer disease, as infection leads to increased acid secretion and reduced mucosal protection. As the population ages, the frequency of *H. pylori* colonization of the gastric mucosa increases. The prevalence of infection is only 10% at age 20, but rises to 50% at age 60 (Anderson et al. 2000, Linder et al. 2001). Complications arising secondary to *H. pylori* infection include ulcer perforation and bleeding. In addition, *H. pylori* infection is strongly associated with antral gastritis and is a known risk factor for gastric carcinoma and mucosa-associated lymphoid tissue (MALT) lymphoma of the stomach. Because of this association, *H. pylori* has been classified by the World Health Organization's International Agency for Research on Cancer as a group I carcinogen and a definite cause of gastric cancer in humans (Anderson et al. 2000, Meurer et al. 2001).

Nonsteroidal Anti-Inflammatory Drugs (NSAIDs)

NSAIDs are the second most common cause of gastric and duodenal ulcers. While NSAIDs are especially likely to increase the risk of gastric ulcers in all age groups, the elderly are particularly vulnerable. While the mechanisms of NSAID-related GI tract toxicity are thought to be multifactorial, GI injury is due primarily to the inhibition of prostaglandin synthesis of the gastric mucosa. As prostaglandins play a role in protecting the gastric mucosa, inhibition of prostaglandin production leaves the gastric mucosa vulnerable to gastric acid, pepsin, and bile salts, leading to mucosal damage and ulceration. In addition, NSAIDs have a direct erosive effect on GI mucosa.

While the risk of PUD generally increases with the dose and duration of NSAID use, up to one-quarter of complications are observed within the first month of therapy (Goroll 2000).

Further, NSAIDs are associated with a five- to seven-fold increased risk of gastric ulceration in the first three months of use (Meurer 2001). With chronic NSAID use, the relative risk of gastric ulcers is increased 40-fold (McQuaid 2002). Patients at greatest risk for developing ulcers from NSAIDs include those with a history of ulcer disease or upper GI bleeding, age greater than 60 years old, concomitant use of corticosteroids or anticoagulants, chronic major-organ impairment, and high doses of or use of multiple NSAIDs. While the risk is small, it is possible to develop serious complications from NSAID-induced ulcers, including perforation, bleeding, or obstruction.

Interaction Between NSAIDs and H. Pylori

The interaction between *H. pylori* and NSAIDs is complex and controversial. It is not clear whether the relationship between *H. pylori* and NSAIDs as risk factors for PUD is independent, synergistic, or antagonistic. The influence of other factors (i.e., past exposure to NSAIDs, a history of ulcer complication[s], or concurrent use of acid-suppressant therapy) must be considered (Chan 2001, Leong et al. 2001). It is clear that ulceration and ulcer complications are reduced with the eradication of *H. pylori* in NSAID users.

→ Acid-induced ulcers:
  ■ Zollinger-Ellison syndrome: More than 90% of patients with this rare syndrome develop peptic ulcers secondary to hypergastrinemia and acid hypersecretion, which is caused by a gastrin producing tumor (gastrinoma). Zollinger-Ellison syndrome is commonly suspected in patients with multiple ulcers. While less than 1% of PUD is caused by gastrinomas, over two-thirds of gastrinomas are malignant.
→ Idiopathic ulcers:
  ■ Recent studies indicate that as *H. pylori*-associated ulcers are identified and treated, the percentage of idiopathic ulcers is increasing. Currently, 30–40% of peptic ulcers have no obvious cause and fall into the idiopathic category (Smoot et al. 2001).
→ Other risk factors for PUD:
  ■ Tobacco use:
    • Retards the rate of ulcer healing and increases the frequency of recurrences
  ■ Chronic alcohol abuse:
    • While alcohol can compromise the mucosal barrier and cause gastritis, there is no clear evidence it is associated with PUD. Regardless, patients with alcohol-related cirrhosis are at increased risk for ulcer formation and complications.
  ■ Glucocorticosteroids:
    • High-dose steroid therapy (>30 mg/day) may increase the risk of PUD, although without concomitant NSAID use, the overall risk is very small.
  ■ Heredity:
    • Seems to play some role in the development of PUD
  ■ Chronic disease states:
    • Chronic lung disease (chronic obstructive pulmonary disease, cystic fibrosis), systemic mastocytosis, myelo-

proliferative disorders, Crohn's disease, chronic renal failure, liver cirrhosis, basophilic leukemia, malignancy, viral infections (herpes simplex, cytomegalovirus), and cocaine use have been associated with PUD (Smoot et al. 2001).
  ■ Stress:
    • In specific circumstances, stress has also been implicated in ulcer disease.
    • Stress secondary to severe illnesses has been associated with gastric ulcers.
    • Life stressors in otherwise healthy people have not been shown to be a cause of ulcers (although they may be associated with stomach pain and increased acid secretion).
→ Complications of PUD:
  ■ The most common complication of PUD is hemorrhage, followed by perforation (Beers et al. 1999, Linder et al. 2001). Both occur more frequently among the elderly. Other complications include gastric outlet obstruction, ulcer penetration into contiguous structures, stomach cancer, and MALT lymphomas (Beers et al. 1999).

DATABASE

SUBJECTIVE

→ Obtain a complete medical and family history, with a focus on the following:
  ■ Assessment of abdominal symptoms:
    • The cardinal feature of peptic ulcer (gastric and duodenal) is epigastric abdominal pain described as dull, aching, burning, "hunger-like," nonradiating, and not severe.
    • The classic symptoms of PUD are commonly absent in the elderly. When older patients present with complications of PUD, the symptoms may be nonspecific and nonlocalizing.
    • With ulcer penetration, patients may complain of changes in the intensity and rhythmicity of their ulcer symptoms, with the pain becoming more severe and constant. The pain may radiate to the back and is unresponsive to antacids or food.
    • Sudden, severe, generalized abdominal pain may indicate ulcer perforation, although elderly or debilitated patients and those on chronic steroid therapy may experience minimal initial symptoms and present later with bacterial peritonitis, sepsis, and shock.
    • It is possible for an ulcer-related upper GI hemorrhage to cause no symptoms.
    • Approximately 10% of patients taking NSAIDs will develop abdominal discomfort, although most people who develop serious GI complications secondary to NSAID use have no history of abdominal discomfort (McQuaid 2002, Smoot et al. 2001).
    • Gastric ulcer pain is most likely to radiate from the epigastrium to the back or substernal area.
  ■ Timing of pain:

- PUD symptoms typically occur as clusters of daily symptoms lasting for a few weeks and separated by pain-free periods (periodicity).
- While clinical history cannot accurately distinguish duodenal from gastric ulcers, certain symptoms can be more typical of a certain type of ulcer.
  - Two-thirds of duodenal ulcers and one-third of gastric ulcers cause nocturnal pain that awakens the patient.
  - Duodenal ulcer pain is classically relieved by food, is absent before breakfast, and starts 2–3 hours after eating, while gastric ulcer pain is more likely to be precipitated by food (although a patient can have the opposite symptoms with both types of ulcers).
- A change from a patient's typical rhythmic discomfort to constant or radiating pain may reflect ulcer penetration or perforation.
- Associated symptoms:
  - *H. pylori* is most commonly asymptomatic, but the patient may have abdominal distention or bloating, belching, nausea, flatulence, and halitosis.
  - Nausea and anorexia may occur with gastric ulcers.
  - Melena and hematemesis commonly occur with a bleeding ulcer.
  - Gastroesophageal reflux symptoms, diarrhea, steatorrhea, and weight loss may occur in patients with Zollinger-Ellison syndrome.
  - Hematemesis; passage of bloody or black, tarry stools; weakness, syncope, and thirst can be caused by blood loss secondary to hemorrhage (Beers et al.1999).
  - Alarm signs for gastric cancer or complicated ulcer disease include rectal bleeding or melena, weight loss >10% of body weight, dysphagia, anorexia, and/or early satiety.
- Medication/drug use:
  - Assess for history of:
    - NSAID or aspirin ingestion
    - Anticoagulant use
    - Steroid use
    - Alcohol, drug, and tobacco use

OBJECTIVE

→ Physical examination is often normal in uncomplicated PUD.
→ Mild, localized epigastric tenderness to deep palpation may be present.
→ Fecal occult blood testing is positive in one-third of patients with PUD (McQuaid 2002).
→ Assess for signs of shock; hypotension; ill-appearing, rigid abdomen; hyperactive bowel sounds initially (which progress to hypoactive and possibly silent); and rebound tenderness (may indicate perforated ulcer).
→ Hemorrhage may produce postural hypotension, tachycardia, and pallor.
→ Physical findings associated with peritonitis, including fever and leukocytosis, may be diminished or completely absent in the elderly.

ASSESSMENT

→ Peptic ulcer disease
→ R/O nonulcer dyspepsia
→ R/O ulcer perforation
→ R/O hemorrhage
→ R/O atypical gastroesophageal reflux
→ R/O biliary tract disease
→ R/O Zollinger-Ellison syndrome
→ R/O acute pancreatitis
→ R/O acute cholecystitis/choledocholithiasis
→ R/O esophageal rupture
→ R/O gastric volvulus
→ R/O ruptured aortic aneurysm
→ R/O carcinoma
→ R/O cardiac disease
→ R/O irritable bowel syndrome
→ R/O liver disease
→ R/O Mallory-Weiss tear

PLAN

DIAGNOSTIC TESTS

→ Diagnosis is most often made on clinical findings.
→ Laboratory tests are normal in uncomplicated PUD but may be ordered to exclude ulcer complications or confounding disease entities.
  - CBC: Anemia may occur with acute blood loss from a bleeding ulcer or from chronic blood loss. Leukocytosis suggests ulcer penetration or perforation.
  - BUN: An elevation in BUN may be the result of absorption of blood nitrogen from the small intestine (McQuaid 2002).
  - Amylase: An elevated serum amylase in a patient with severe epigastric pain suggests ulcer penetration into the pancreas.
  - Fasting serum gastrin level: A fasting serum gastrin level is the most sensitive and specific method for identifying Zollinger-Ellison syndrome.
    - Levels >100–150 pg/mL indicate Zollinger-Ellison syndrome.
    - Histamine H_2 receptor antagonists should be withheld for 24 hours and proton pump inhibitors (PPIs) withheld for one week before a gastrin level is measured.
    - A fasting serum gastrin should be drawn:
      - If ulcers are refractory to standard therapy
      - With giant ulcers (>2 cm)
      - Multiple duodenal ulcers
      - If ulcers are associated with diarrhea or with complications
      - For patients with peptic ulcers who are *H. pylori*-negative and are not taking NSAIDs
→ Endoscopy:
  - Upper endoscopy is the procedure of choice for diagnosing duodenal and gastric ulcers, as well as for the evaluation of GI bleeding.

- Endoscopy is reserved for use in patients with alarm signs (e.g., rectal bleeding or melena, weight loss >10% of body weight, dysphagia, anorexia, and/or early satiety) or with persistent symptoms despite appropriate empiric therapy.
- Endoscopy provides better diagnostic accuracy than barium radiography and allows for biopsy in order to assess for the presence of malignancy and *H. pylori* infection.
- Endoscopic diagnostic methods for *H. pylori* include histology, culture, and biopsy urease tests.
  - Steiner's stain of gastric antral biopsy specimen (histologic identification of organisms) is considered the "gold standard."
  - Culture for detection of *H. pylori* is rarely necessary in clinical practice (it is time and labor-intensive) but useful for managing and treating failures.
  - Rapid urease test (urease activity of biopsy specimen) is highly specific and simple.
- 3–5% of benign-appearing gastric ulcers are malignant (duodenal ulcers are virtually never malignant and do not require biopsy) (McQuaid 2002).
- Endoscopy appears to be safe in the elderly, with complication rates similar to those in younger patients.
→ Imaging:
- Radiographic studies can be used to diagnose peptic ulcers, although with less sensitivity than endoscopy.
  - When these are performed, the double-contrast technique is the radiographic study of choice.
  - These studies have limited accuracy in distinguishing benign from malignant gastric ulcers.
  - All gastric ulcers diagnosed by x-ray should be re-evaluated with endoscopy after 8–12 weeks of therapy.
- Upright or decubitus films of the abdomen may reveal free intraperitoneal air when ulcer perforation has occurred.
→ Testing for *H. pylori*-induced ulcers:
- The decision to test for the presence of *H. pylori* is based on intention to treat.
- Numerous diagnostic tests are available to determine if patients are infected with *H. pylori* (Smoot et al. 2001):
  - Laboratory serology tests
  - Urea breath tests
  - Stool antigen tests
  - Rapid urease assays
  - Histology
  - Bacterial culture
- Overall, the sensitivity and specificity of most of these tests are excellent.
- The most frequently used tests are antibody assays that use serum or whole blood.
- The "gold standard" is direct identification of *H. pylori* by culture; the sensitivity of culture, though good, is not ideal.
→ Testing for *H. pylori* is recommended if the following criteria are met (Anderson et al. 2000):
- If there is evidence of active duodenal or gastric ulcer
- If the patient is asymptomatic but has a documented history of ulcer disease and is on antisecretory therapy

- If there is a family history of gastric cancer
- If low-grade gastric (MALT) lymphomas are present
- Although asymptomatic individuals should not be tested for *H. pylori,* if an asymptomatic person has a positive *H. pylori* test result, some clinicians recommend eradication therapy because *H. pylori* is classified as a group I carcinogen (Anderson et al. 2000).
→ Choosing a diagnostic test to rule out *H. pylori* infection:
- Specific antibody test:
  - If the patient has known, uncomplicated PUD
  - If the patient has dyspepsia, a prior history of PUD, and was not previously treated with eradication therapy
  - If the patient has undifferentiated dyspepsia (without endoscopy)
  - If the patient is asymptomatic with a history of documented PUD not previously treated with eradication therapy
- Stool antigen or urea breath test:
  - If the patient has dyspepsia and a history of PUD treated for *H. pylori*
→ Serology testing:
- In the office setting, initial serology testing is convenient and cost-effective.
- Laboratory-based or office-based ELISA tests detect IgG antibodies to *H. pylori,* although the sensitivity and specificity of clinic-based serologic tests are lower than lab-based tests.
- Antibody tests may remain positive for months after the successful eradication of the infection, so they are not recommended to prove that eradication therapy has been successful.
→ The urea breath test:
- Measures urease activity
- Can be used for initial diagnosis of infection and as a reliable test of cure
- Can detect presence/absence of active *H. pylori* infection with greater accuracy than the serologic test
- Is usually administered on an outpatient basis in the hospital
- Sensitivity is reduced by acid suppression with PPIs (withhold these for 2–4 weeks before administering the test)
→ Stool antigen:
- Measures *H. pylori* antigens
- Detects current *H. pylori* infection with approximately 95% accuracy
- Can be used for an initial diagnosis of infection and for evaluating treatment success when performed 4–6 weeks after completing antibiotic therapy
- Is relatively convenient

TREATMENT/MANAGEMENT

→ Pharmacologic agents used to treat PUD:
NOTE: See the *Physicians' Desk Reference (PDR)* for details regarding indications, warnings, drug interactions, contraindications, side effects, and varying dosages.

→ Acid-antisecretory agents:
  ■ PPIs:
    • Omeprazole 10 mg, 20 mg, 40 mg
    • Rabeprazole sodium 20 mg
    • Lansoprazole 15 mg, 30 mg
    • Pantoprazole sodium 40 mg
      – These should be administered 30 minutes before meals (usually breakfast).
      – These result in >90% healing of duodenal ulcers after 4 weeks and 90% of gastric ulcers after 8 weeks of treatment when given once daily.
  ■ PPIs provide faster pain relief and more rapid ulcer healing compared with H_2 receptor antagonists; however, nearly equivalent overall healing rates may be achieved with longer courses of H_2 receptor antagonists.
  ■ PPIs are safe in short-term therapy.
  ■ Long-term use may lead to a mild decrease in vitamin B_{12} and iron absorption of unclear significance.
  ■ Histamine H_2 receptor antagonists:
    • Cimetidine 100 mg (over-the-counter [OTC]), 200 mg, 300 mg, 400 mg, 800 mg
    • Ranitidine 75 mg (OTC), 150 mg, 300 mg
    • Famotidine 10 mg (OTC), 20 mg, 40 mg
    • Nizatidine 150 mg, 300 mg
      – Effective in the treatment of PUD, but PPIs are preferred because they are more efficacious.
      – All inhibit nocturnal acid output, but are less effective at inhibiting meal-stimulated acid secretion.
      – All are well-tolerated.
    • For uncomplicated PUD, administer once daily p.o. at bedtime as follows (McQuaid 2002):
      – Ranitidine OR nizatidine 300 mg
                OR
      – Famotidine 40 mg
                OR
      – Cimetidine 800 mg
    • Ulcer symptom relief usually occurs within 2 weeks.
    NOTE: There is the risk of interaction when cimetidine is co-administered with other agents metabolized by cytochrome P450 enzymes.
→ Agents enhancing mucosal defenses:
  ■ Sucralfate, bismuth, misoprostol, and low doses of aluminum-containing antacids promote ulcer healing through the enhancement of mucosal defensive mechanisms.
  ■ These agents are not used as a first-line therapy for active ulcers.
  ■ Because they provide rapid relief of ulcer symptoms, antacids are commonly used as needed to supplement antisecretory agents during the first few days of treatment.
  ■ Sucralfate, 1 g p.o. QID, is sometimes added to antisecretory therapy in patients with refractory ulcers.
  ■ Bismuth salts:
    • Inhibit pepsin, increase secretion of mucus, and form a barrier to the diffusion of acid in the ulcer crater

    • Lead to detachment of *H. pylori* from gastric epithelium and will disrupt bacterial cell walls, causing the bacterium to lyse
  ■ Misoprostol:
    • A prostaglandin analog that stimulates gastroduodenal mucus and bicarbonate secretion
    • Effective as a prophylactic agent in reducing the incidence of gastroduodenal ulcers in patients taking nonselective NSAIDs
    • Dose: 200 mcg p.o. QID with food for duration of NSAID therapy
    • Causes diarrhea in 10–20% of patients
    • With the advent of PPIs and cyclooxygenase-2 (COX-2) selective NSAIDs, is now less commonly used
→ Agents that promote healing through eradication of *H. pylori*
  ■ Treatment of *H. pylori*-induced ulcers:
    • Goals of treating *H. pylori* include relief of dyspeptic symptoms, promotion of ulcer healing, and eradication of *H. pylori* infection in order to reduce the risk of ulcer recurrence and complications.
    • With successful eradication of *H. pylori* with antibiotics, ulcer recurrence rates are reduced from approximately 85% to 5–20% at 1 year.
    • Despite this, eradication of *H. pylori* has proved difficult.
    • Combination regimens that employ 2–3 antibiotics with a PPI, H_2 receptor antagonist, and/or bismuth are required to achieve adequate rates of eradication and to reduce the number of failures due to antibiotic resistance.
    • Continued therapy for 14 days is the most reliable and effective regimen and is recommended in the United States.
    • Therapies employing only 1–2 antibiotics cannot be recommended (secondary to antibiotic resistance and high clinical failure and recurrence rates).
    • There is less resistance to amoxicillin or tetracycline, while resistance to metronidazole and clarithromycin has been increasing (McQuaid 2002, Smoot et al. 2001).
    • It is advisable to include amoxicillin as first-line therapy in most patients, reserving metronidazole for penicillin-allergic patients.
    • No resistance seems to develop to bismuth.
    • Because patient adherence to therapy is critical, simpler regimens with BID dosing may be more successful in eradicating the *H. pylori* organism.
    • Because of concern with resistance, people who need to be treated a second time should be treated using different antibiotics.
  ■ Treatment regimens to eradicate *H. pylori*:
    • Regimen one:
      – Lansoprazole 30 mg p.o. BID for 2 weeks
                OR
      – Omeprazole 20 mg p.o. BID for 2 weeks PLUS
      – Clarithromycin 500 mg p.o. BID for 2 weeks PLUS
      – Amoxicillin 1 g p.o. BID for 2 weeks OR metronidazole 500 mg p.o. for 2 weeks

- Regimen two:
  - Bismuth subsalicylate 525 mg (2 tablets) p.o. QID for 2 weeks PLUS
  - Metronidazole 250 mg p.o. QID for 2 weeks PLUS
  - Tetracycline 500 mg p.o. QID for 2 weeks PLUS
  - H_2 receptor antagonist for 4 weeks
- Regimen three:
  - Bismuth subsalicylate 525 mg (2 tablets) p.o. QID for 2 weeks PLUS
  - Metronidazole 500 mg p.o. BID OR metronidazole 250 mg p.o. QID for 2 weeks PLUS
  - Tetracycline 500 mg p.o BID–QID for 2 weeks PLUS
  - Lansoprazole 30 mg p.o. every morning for 2 weeks OR omeprazole 20 mg p.o. every morning for 2 weeks

  NOTE: Continue treatment with PPI QD OR H_2 receptor antagonist for 4–8 weeks to promote healing.
- Regimen four:
  - Ranitidine bismuth citrate 400 mg p.o. BID for 2 weeks PLUS
  - Clarithromycin 500 mg p.o BID for 2 weeks PLUS
  - Metronidazole 250 mg p.o. QID for 2 weeks
- After completing antibiotics, consider an antisecretory agent for 2–4 weeks (for duodenal ulcer) or 4–6 weeks (for gastric ulcer) to ensure ulcer healing (Anderson et al. 2000, McQuaid 2002, Meurer 2001, Meurer et al. 2001, Smoot et al. 2001).

NOTE: Avoid alcohol use while on metronidazole (potential for antabuse-like reaction).

NOTE: Eradication of *H. pylori* can fail secondary to:
- The use of ineffective regimens (when clinicians use dual therapies despite evidence that triple and quadruple regimens are superior in efficacy and cost-effectiveness)
- Patient noncompliance (less common than suboptimal prescribing)
- Increasing resistance to antibiotics

→ Treatment of NSAID-induced ulcers:
- Ulcer healing is delayed if the NSAID is continued.
- Both gastric and duodenal ulcers respond rapidly to therapy with H_2 receptor antagonists or PPIs once NSAIDs are eliminated.
- PPIs:
  - Uncomplicated duodenal ulcer:
    - Omeprazole 20 mg p.o. QD for 4–8 weeks OR
    - Lansoprazole 15 mg p.o. QD for 4–8 weeks OR
    - Rabeprazole sodium 20 mg p.o. QD for 4–8 weeks
  - Uncomplicated gastric ulcer:
    - Omeprazole 40 mg p.o. QD for up to 8 weeks OR
    - Lansoprazole 30 mg p.o. QD for up to 8 weeks
- H_2 receptor antagonists:
  - Uncomplicated duodenal ulcer:
    - Cimetidine 800 mg p.o. QD at HS for 6 weeks OR
    - Ranitidine or nizatidine 300 mg p.o. QD at HS for 6 weeks OR
    - Famotidine 40 mg p.o. QD at HS for 6 weeks

- Uncomplicated gastric ulcer:
  - Cimetidine 400 mg p.o. BID OR 800 mg p.o. QD at HS for 8 weeks OR
  - Ranitidine OR nizatidine 150 mg p.o. BID for 8 weeks OR
  - Famotidine 20 mg p.o. BID OR 40 mg p.o. QD at HS for 8 weeks
- Prophylactic treatment for asymptomatic, low-risk, chronic NSAID users remains controversial.

→ For high-risk patients who require long-term NSAIDs:
- If a nonselective NSAID cannot be stopped, a PPI can be used daily to heal the ulcer. The lowest dose possible of the NSAID should be used. Omeprazole heals and prevents ulcers more effectively than ranitidine among people taking NSAIDs for ulcers.
- "Double" doses of H_2 receptor antagonists (e.g., ranitidine 300 mg p.o. BID) and standard doses of PPIs (e.g., omeprazole 20 mg p.o. up to QID) are effective prophylactic agents for the duration of NSAID use.
- The COX-2 inhibitors, celecoxib and rofecoxib, have been shown to have less GI toxicity (and a significantly lower incidence of peptic ulceration) than older NSAIDs. Although there remains some risk of GI toxicity with the COX-2 inhibitors, the patient should switch to a COX-2 selective inhibitor if possible.
- Low-dose aspirin may compromise the benefits gained by using COX-2 inhibitors (Hawkey 2001).
- Attention should be paid to other risk factors for ulceration and bleeding, such as the concurrent use of corticosteroids or anticoagulants.
- Misoprostol is approved for the prevention of NSAID-induced ulcers in persons at high risk of developing ulcers, but it is associated with diarrhea, even at lower than optimal doses.

→ Acid induced ulcers:
- Idiopathic:
  - Idiopathic ulcers should be treated in the same way that ulcers were treated prior to the discovery of *H. pylori*. Either PPIs or H_2 receptor antagonists may be used (for 6–8 weeks). With the recurrence of ulcers, antisecretory treatment should be restarted, with PPIs being the preferred choice for maintenance therapy.
- Zollinger-Ellison syndrome:
  - Ulcer disease in these patients can be managed with PPIs. Surgical resection of gastrinomas is the treatment of choice for these patients.

→ Nonulcerative dyspepsia:
- People with abdominal pain in the absence of ulcer disease after work-up for ulcers are known as having non-ulcer dyspepsia.
  - It is not recommended that this population be tested and treated for *H. pylori* infection.
  - Once *H. pylori* testing has been done and found to be positive in a person (regardless of their diagnosis), it is recommended that treatment be offered, as *H. pylori* has been classified as a carcinogen.

- There is no evidence that *H. pylori* eradication in patients with nonulcer dyspepsia improves symptoms.
→ Surgery:
  - Rates of surgery for treatmentof PUD have declined over the past 2–3 decades as a result of medical treatment.
  - Surgical intervention for PUD complications is now rare, although it remains an option for the treatment of refractory disease and its complications.
  - Indications for surgery include perforation, obstruction that does not respond to medical therapy, uncontrolled or recurrent bleeding, suspected malignant gastric ulcer, and symptoms refractory to medical management (Beers et al. 1999).

CONSULTATION

→ Physician consultation may be sought for management of typical symptoms of peptic ulcer disease.
→ Refer/consult with physician regarding ulcers that are refractory to medical therapy.
→ Refer/consult with physician if symptoms are atypical.
→ Refer/consult with physician if there is evidence of a bleeding ulcer.
→ Immediate referral is warranted in cases of obstruction, acute hemorrhage, or perforation.
→ As needed for prescription(s).

PATIENT EDUCATION

→ Explain risk factors, physiology, treatment regimens, and consequences of inadequate treatment.
→ Advise the patient to continue with medication as prescribed, even after symptoms have subsided.
→ Advise the patient about the specific details of various treatment regimens.
→ Advise the patient regarding a nutritious diet and regular meal intake. A bland or milk diet is not necessary.
→ Encourage limiting only those foods that cause discomfort.
→ Assist the patient in discontinuing alcohol and smoking with referral to appropriate support services if necessary (i.e., Alcoholics Anonymous, American Cancer Society, etc.).
→ Remind the patient that NSAID and aspirin use are commonly implicated in refractory ulcers.
→ Teach the patient the signs/symptoms of ulcer disease complications, and encourage her to seek help if these symptoms occur.

FOLLOW-UP

→ Re-evaluate the patient in 4–6 weeks and after completing the medication regimen.
→ Stress the importance of returning to the clinic for follow-up if symptoms persist, as nonhealing gastric ulcers may indicate the presence of an undiagnosed gastric malignancy.
→ Follow up to ensure the drug regimen is being followed.
→ Follow up to ensure eradication of *H. pylori*.
→ Follow-up testing (i.e., urea breath or stool antigen test) is

recommended for patients who do not respond to therapy or for those with a history of ulcer complications or cancer.
→ A follow-up endoscopy may be needed 8–12 weeks after the start of therapy to document complete healing of ulcers.
→ Patients with a history of ulcer complications, gastric MALT lymphoma, or early gastric cancer should undergo a routine posttreatment urea breath test or endoscopy to ensure successful eradication. These patients will usually be followed in collaboration with a gastroenterologist.
→ Routine, noninvasive follow-up testing can be considered in patients who have persistent symptoms following eradication therapy. The stool antigen test, performed four weeks following therapy, should be considered.
→ If symptoms resolve with eradication therapy, there is no need for test of cure (for uncomplicated ulcer disease or undifferentiated dyspepsia).
→ At every visit, reinforce adherence to conservative measures.
→ Teach the American Cancer Society's recommendation for early detection of cancer in asymptomatic people (Zoorob et al. 2001):
  - Fecal occult blood test: yearly beginning at age 50
                     AND
  - Digital rectal exam and flexible sigmoidoscopy: every 5 years beginning at age 50
                     OR
  - Digital rectal exam and colonoscopy: every 10 years beginning at age 50
                     OR
  - Digital rectal exam and double contrast barium enema: every 5–10 years beginning at age 50
→ Document in progress notes and on problem list.

BIBLIOGRAPHY

Anderson, J., and Gonzalez, J. 2000. *H. pylori* infection. *Geriatrics* 55(6):44–49.

Beers, M., and Berkow, R. 1999. *The Merck manual of diagnosis and therapy,* 17th ed. Whitehouse Station, N.J.: Merck & Co.

Chan, F.K.L. 2001. *Helicobacter pylori* and nonsteroidal anti-inflammatory drugs. *Gastroenterology Clinics* 30(4):937–952.

Freston, J.W. 2000. Management of peptic ulcers: emerging issues. *World Journal of Surgery* 24(3):250–255.

Goroll, A.H. 2000. In *Primary care medicine,* 4th ed., eds. A.H. Goroll and J.A. Mulley, pp. 434–447. Philadelphia: Lippincott Williams & Wilkins.

Hawkey, C.J. 2001. NSAIDs and COX-2 inhibitors: What can be learned from large outcome trials? The gastroenterologist's perspective. *Clinical and Experimental Rheumatology* 19(6 Suppl. 25):S23–S30.

Leong, R.W.L., Chan, F.K.L., and Sung, J.J.Y. 2001. *Journal of Gastroenterology* 36:731–739.

Linder, J.D., and Wilcox, C.M. 2001. Acid peptic disease in the elderly. *Gastroenterology Clinics* 30(2):363–376.

McQuaid, K.R. 2002. Peptic ulcer disease and Zollinger-Ellison syndrome. In *Current medical diagnosis and treatment,*

41st ed., eds. L.M. Tierney, Jr., S.J. McPhee, and M.A. Papadakis, pp. 618–626. New York: Lange Medical Books/ McGraw-Hill.

Meurer, L.N., 2001. Treatment of peptic ulcer disease and non-ulcer dyspepsia. *Journal of Family Practice* 50(7):614–619.

Meurer, L.N. and Bower, D.J. 2001. Management of *Helico-bacter pylori* infection. *American Family Physician* 65(7): 1327–1339.

Smoot, D.T., Go, M.F., and Cryer, B. 2001. Peptic ulcer disease. *Gastroenterology* 28(3):487–503.

Zoorob, R., Anderson, R., Cefalu, C. et al. 2001. Cancer screening guidelines. *American Family Physician* 63(6):1101–1112.

SECTION 8

Musculoskeletal
Disorders

8-A Common Disorders of the Musculoskeletal System—Introduction . . **8-2**

8-B Fibromyalgia **8-3**

8-C Osteoarthritis **8-8**

8-D Rheumatoid Arthritis **8-12**

8-E Bursitis and Tendinitis **8-15**

8-F Shoulder Pain **8-18**

8-G Elbow Pain **8-23**

8-H Wrist, Hand, and Finger Pain **8-27**

  → Carpal Tunnel Syndrome **8-27**

  → De Quervain's Disease **8-30**

  → Osteoarthritis of the Basilar Joint of the Thumb **8-31**

  → Trigger Fingers **8-32**

  → Ganglion Cysts **8-33**

8-I Hip Pain **8-36**

8-J Knee Pain **8-39**

  → Acute Knee Pain **8-39**

  → Chronic Knee Pain **8-43**

8-K Ankle Pain **8-48**

8-L Foot Pain **8-52**

8-M Low Back Pain **8-58**

  → Acute Low Back Pain **8-59**

  → Chronic Low Back Pain **8-69**

8-N Table 8N.1. Anti-inflammatory and Analgesic Medication **8-74**

Diane C. Putney, M.N., R.N., C.F.N.P.

8-A

Common Disorders of the Musculoskeletal System— Introduction

Orthopedic problems account for an estimated 10% of all visits to primary care providers. Symptoms and injuries involving the musculoskeletal system are the second most common reason that patients visit primary health care facilities (Snider 1997). The majority of musculoskeletal problems do not require surgical intervention. Therefore, conservative treatment can generally be successfully initiated and managed by the primary care provider.

The musculoskeletal ailments that compel women to seek medical consultations in primary care facilities generally include: *osteoarthritis* or *degenerative joint disease*, *tendinitis*, *bursitis*, *intra-articular cartilage problems*, *nerve compression* and *overuse syndromes*, and *low back pain*.

In addition, there are a number of related conditions that defy anatomic specificity, such as *rheumatoid arthritis* and *fibromyalgia*, that appear predominately in women, often with devastating sequelae. These chapters focus on the more typical clinical presentations that face the primary care provider.

Therapeutic evaluation of joint pathology requires a basic but precise knowledge and understanding of musculoskeletal anatomy and function. Palpable bony prominences serve as landmarks for the underlying involved bursae, tendons, ligaments, and nerves—locations that are of crucial importance when administering parenteral treatments such as cortisone injections. Thus, the author has included relevant descriptions of anatomy and pathophysiology with respect to the diagnoses or problems under specific consideration within the context of their clinical presentation.

BIBLIOGRAPHY

Snider, R.K., 1997. *Essentials of musculoskeletal care.* Rosemont, Ill.: American Academy of Orthopedics.

Diane C. Putney, M.N., R.N., C.F.N.P.

8-B
Fibromyalgia

Fibromyalgia (FM) is a chronic, non-inflammatory rheumatological condition in which the predominant feature is severe, widespread muscle pain throughout the axial skeleton. Non-articular in its presentation, this controversial ailment accounts for approximately 23% of all consultations to rheumatology clinics in the United States, Canada, Mexico, Spain, and Australia (White et al. 2000). Fibromyalgia affects at least 2% of the U.S. population (Puttick 2001) and is seven times more prevalent in women than men (White et al. 2000).

In 1990 the American College of Rheumatology (ACR) adopted the following three criteria for diagnosing FM: the presence of widespread pain for at least three months; pain in the cervical, thoracic and lumbar spine, as well as the anterior chest; and pain in at least 11 of 18 tender points on digital palpation (Leventhal 1999) (see **Figure 8B.1, Tender Points in Fibromyalgia Syndrome**).

It is not unusual for persons with FM to remain symptomatic for as long as eight years before an accurate diagnosis is rendered (White et al. 2000), even though these patients may have made extensive use of the health care system during that time.

Despite the ongoing controversy surrounding the etiology, diagnosis, and treatment of FM, it has emerged as a significant world health problem. Individuals with FM generally rate their functional status, health, and quality of life lower than those with osteoarthritis, rheumatic arthritis, systemic lupus erythematosus, and scleroderma. Twenty-five percent of persons with FM receive disability benefits (White et al. 2000).

The etiology of FM is unknown. It has been observed that patients with FM have a decreased pain threshold and an increased sensitivity to both biological and psychological influences (Neeck et al. 2000). This reduced pain threshold, which occurs at the level of the central nervous system, makes the person vulnerable to a plethora of ensuing abnormalities; and anatomic dysfunction, psychological changes and painful, tense musculature along the axial skeleton all occur (Neeck et al. 2000).

The biochemical discrepancies in persons with FM probably involve certain hormonal deviations in the hypothalamic pituitary-adrenal axis that are precipitated by the chronicity of painful stimuli. These stimuli result in hyperactivity of the corticotropin-releasing hormone neurons (CRH). About one-third of persons with FM have demonstrated subnormal insulin growth factor levels (IGF), which in turn decrease growth hormone secretion (Millea et al. 2000). An increase in a neurotransmitter associated with enhanced pain perception, identified only as "P," present in cerebral spinal fluid, further suggests that disparities in the autonomic and endocrine stress response systems contribute to the underlying etiology (Millea et al. 2000). Additionally, the sleep disturbances regularly experienced by persons with FM are caused by an apparent electrophysiological derangement during stage IV sleep. This triggers an alteration in the circadian rhythms and its associated neurotransmitters, cortisol and megaton (Friedberg et al. 2001, White et al. 2000).

A recent Israeli study concluded that 21.6% of the research subjects with FM sustained a significant neck injury within a year of the onset of their symptoms (White et al. 2000). However, any evidence supporting this theory is both inconsistent and insufficient, as is scientific inquiry regarding possible immunological defects in persons with FM (Friedberg et al. 2001).

Research focused on the relationship between psychopathology and FM deserves consideration due to the high incidence of depression in these patients. Whether or not depression coexists with FM; is a psychological reaction to chronic, severe pain; or is an antecedent to the disease continues to be a matter of ongoing debate (Friedberg et al. 2001, White et al. 2000).

Certainly, the limited efficacy of current treatment, along with a paucity of specific identifiable pathology to satisfactorily explain the physical pain, emotional distress, and functional disability lends stature to the biopsychosocial model of pain. This includes the suggestion of a predisposing FM personality type. The person acquiring a diagnosis of FM has been described as a compulsive overworker and overachiever who lacks assertiveness. One study suggests these self-imposed high standards of accomplishment precipitate a conversion reaction-type illness in the patient, which in turn, accommodates her subconscious desire to rescue herself from life's overwhelming responsibilities (Friedberg et al. 2001).

Contemporary research appears to negate the presumption that FM is psychosomatic in origin. However, persons with FM who take antidepressant medication are three times more likely to experience symptomatic improvement (Leventhal 1999). The fatigue and pain experienced by persons with FM is notably more debilitating than those with a primary diagnosis of depression. Antidepressant medication provided adequate symptomatic relief in only one-third of persons with FM (Leventhal 1999). Regardless of the specific intervention employed, less than 50% of all persons with FM actually benefit from treatment, and only 3% ever experience complete remission of their symptoms (Leventhal 1999).

Figure 8B.1.   TENDER POINTS IN FIBROMYALGIA SYNDROME

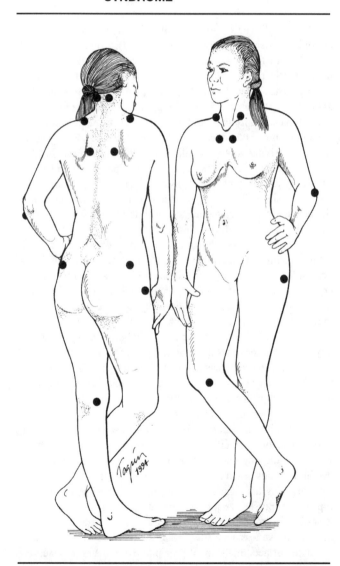

Source: Reprinted with permission from Goroll, A.H. 2000. *Primary care medicine*, 4th ed., eds. A.H. Goroll and J.A. Mulley. Philadelphia: Lippincott Williams & Wilkins.

It is likely that this general failure of conventional treatment has prompted the abundant use of alternative therapies among at least 91% of patients with FM (Leventhal 1999). These treatments may include dietary regimens, chiropractic and massage therapy, and specific food supplements, most notable SAMe (S-adenosyl-L-methionine). SAMe is a naturally occurring salt that is present in all body tissues. It has been found to provide significant symptomatic improvement when administered in either oral or parenteral form (Leventhal 1999).

The controversy surrounding the actual legitimacy of FM has led to a continuum of denunciation as a bona fide disease entity. The existing consensus among scholars of this phenomenon appears to be limited to the following facts: the cause of FM is unknown; there is no cure; FM is not progressive or life-threatening; and FM does not result in permanent alterations within the musculoskeletal system. With respect to treatment, symptoms can be controlled to a moderate degree at best.

Finally, there is general agreement that patients with FM are best served by a comprehensive treatment approach that gives consideration to symptomatic pain relief, psychological distress, sleep disturbances, and the social context in which the symptoms occur (Earnshaw et al. 2000).

DATABASE

SUBJECTIVE

→ Demographics:
- Women between the ages of 20–60 (Snider 1997).
- Incidence is equal among black and Caucasian persons (Friedberg et al. 2001).
- Latinos have twice the incidence of black or Caucasian people (Friedberg et al. 2001).

→ 55% of patients with FM report abrupt onset of symptoms.

→ Symptoms may include the following:
- Widespread pain for at least three months delineated as follows (Leventhal 1999, Merchant et al. 2001, Puttick 2001, Snider 1997):
  - Pain on both the right and left sides of body
  - Pain above and below the waist
  - Pain along the axial skeleton
- Pain is exacerbated by physical activity but not relieved by rest.
- Sleep disturbances occur, leading to generalized fatigue.
- Morning stiffness
- Anxiety
- Depression
- Irritable bowel symptoms
- Urinary frequency
- Paresthesias in the hands and feet that are non-dermatomal
- Diminished pain threshold
- Perception of swelling in hands and feet
- Headaches
- Memory and concentration difficulties
- Frequent drug reactions and hypersensitivities
- Dysmenorrhea
- Reynaud's-type symptoms (Leventhal 1999, Puttick, 2001, Snider 1997)

- Approximately 80% of patients with FM have symptoms of chronic fatigue syndrome (Wilke 2000).

OBJECTIVE

→ General:
- A diagnosis of FM is based primarily on symptoms as reported by the patient. Objective findings may elude description.
- Patients with FM may have made many visits to health care providers (Puttick 2001).

→ Tenderness at 11 or more of 18 points along the axial skeleton (as designated by the ACR) to palpation with enough force to cause blanching of the thumbnail beds (see **Figure 8B.1**). Tender points have no palpatory characteristics that distinguish them from the surrounding tissue (Leventhal 1999, Merchant et al. 2001, Puttick 2001, Snider 1997).

→ Palpation at the specific points characteristically elicits much more tenderness than when palpating inflamed rheumatoid arthritis (Smythe 2000).

→ Normal joint exam (Snider 1997)

→ Normal diagnostic tests, which may include laboratory work, as well as radiographs and various imaging studies (Fan et al. 1992, Snider 1997)

→ No evidence of inflammation throughout the musculoskeletal system (i.e., erythema, edema, warmth) (Millea et al. 2000)

ASSESSMENT

→ Fibromyalgia

→ R/O bursitis, tendinitis

→ R/O peripheral nerve entrapment syndromes (i.e., carpal tunnel syndrome)

→ R/O hypothyroidism

→ R/O primary clinical depression

→ R/O anxiety disorder

→ R/O somatization disorder

→ R/O chronic fatigue syndrome (Friedberg et al. 2001, Wilke 2001)

→ R/O polymyalgia rheumatica (Puttick 2001, Salvarani et al. 2000)

→ R/O myofascial pain syndrome

→ R/O HIV (Fan et al. 1992)

→ R/O rheumatoid arthritis

→ R/O systemic lupus erythematosus

PLAN

DIAGNOSTIC TESTS

→ Indicated lab tests may include the following (Fan et al. 1992):
- CBC
- ESR
- Creatine kinase
- TSH
- RF (rheumatoid factor)
- ANA (antinuclear antibody)

→ Nerve conduction studies (NCS) and electromyograms

(EMGs) may be ordered to rule out nerve entrapment syndromes or peripheral neuropathies.

TREATMENT/MANAGEMENT

→ The patient with mild symptoms of FM and without sleep disturbances may derive therapeutic benefit solely from having her illness identified, and therefore legitimized (Millea et al. 2000).

→ Pharmacological therapy remains the primary treatment modality (Hadhazy et al. 2000).
- Antidepressants:
  - Agents that affect neurotransmitter metabolism at the receptor site are the most successful in managing pain for patients with FM (Leventhal 1999).
  - Clinicians should consider treatment with antidepressants, even if a depressive disorder is not evident (O'Malley et al. 1999).
  - Tricyclic antidepressants inhibit the reuptake of serotonin, a neurotransmitter that modulates both pain and sleep.
    - Amitriptyline, one of the original antidepressants, is the most widely prescribed medication for the treatment of FM.
      ➤ Dose 10–50 mg p.o. every HS (Snider 1997)
      ➤ 25–30% of patients with FM experience significant relief of symptoms (Millea et al. 2000).
    - Fluoxetine 20 mg p.o. every HS (Millea et al. 2000)
    - Amitriptyline and fluoxetine are more effective when prescribed together for the treatment of FM than either drug alone (Leventhal 1999, Millea et al. 2000).
  - Dosing is highly individualized.
- Analgesics:
  - Cyclobenzaprine 10–40 mg p.o. every HS (Millea et al. 2000)
  - Chronic opioid analgesic therapy (COAT) is reserved for patients with severe pain, significant functional impairment, and when other therapies have failed (Millea et al. 2000).
- Nonsteroidal anti-inflammatory drugs (NSAIDs) are prescribed in at least 90% of patients diagnosed with FM, despite the consistent failure of NSAIDs to diminish their pain (Leventhal 1999). (See **Table 8N.1, Anti-inflammatory and Analgesic Medications**.)
- Corticosteroids: approximately 25% of FM patients are treated with various steroid preparations, although their effectiveness has yet to be demonstrated.

→ Alternative pharmacological treatment (O'Malley et al. 1999):
- S-adenosyl-L-methionine (SAMe):
  - A naturally occurring salt that is present in all body tissues
  - SAMe has been used in the treatment of FM for the past 25 years.
  - Its effectiveness has been demonstrated with oral and parenteral preparation.
  - Dosage: 800 mg p.o. QD (Sierpina 2002)

- Malic acid (Wolf, Janet. Personal communication. Fibromyalgia Self-help Group. Kaiser Permanente. San Diego, Calif. 2001):
  - An organic dicarboxylic acid
  - Involved in the generation of adenosine triphosphate
  - Dose: 2,400 mg/day
  - Should be administered with magnesium sulfate, vitamins B_1 and B_6
- S-hydroxytryptophan:
  - A serotonin substrate
  - Dose: 100 mg QD
- Growth hormone injections: studies have demonstrated significant improvement in symptoms, but the cost of such treatment would be prohibitive.
- Chlorella pyrenoidosa (Millea et al. 2000):
  - A unicellular green algae that grows in fresh water
  - Dose:
    - 10 g/day or
    - 100 mL of extract/day
→ Non-pharmacological and mind-body therapies (MBTs) (Buskila 2000, Hadhazy et al. 2000):
- There is no evidence that justifies utilizing MBTs in place of other conventional therapies.
- Its use is only recommended in conjunction with drug therapy.
- If FM patients are going to benefit from MBTs, improvement will generally be noted within 3–24 weeks. (Hadhazy et al. 2000, Leventhal 1999).
- Severely depressed patients are not expected to respond favorably to mind-body therapies (Hadhazy et al. 2000).
- Exercise:
  - Aerobic exercise three times a week has been shown to decrease pain, but does not improve sleep disturbances or fatigue.
  - Patients with fibromyalgia syndrome may have difficulty complying with an exercise regimen.
- Biofeedback:
  - Biofeedback has been shown to significantly reduce the number of tender points (see **Figure 8B.1**).
  - The effects of biofeedback are enhanced when used concurrently with relaxation training and exercise.
- Relaxation training, meditation, and cognitive restructuring are briefly mentioned in the literature on FM. According to one study, patients who underwent 3–24 weeks of these therapies reported general overall improvement.
- Acupuncture has demonstrated therapeutic efficacy in all seven published studies in the literature (Nasir 2002).
→ No known therapy for FM has ever resulted in more than modest improvement (White et al. 2000).

CONSULTATION

→ Rheumatological consultation should be considered when the patient's FM symptoms are severe, debilitating, and adversely compromising their basic functional capacity.

→ Psychiatric consultation should be sought if the clinician suspects the patient has a serious psychological disturbance.

PATIENT EDUCATION

→ General:
- FM is not life-threatening or progressive (Snider 1997).
- The pathophysiology of FM does not cause permanent changes in the musculoskeletal system.
- Treatment is an ongoing process rather than the management of a single episode (Millea et al. 2000).
- Symptoms of FM can be controlled to a moderate degree.
- Despite the perceived as well as actual level of disability, FM patients should be encouraged to maintain regular employment and involvement in their customary social activities (Puttick 2001).
→ At least 20% of patients treated with antidepressant medication develop side effects (Leventhal 1999).
- Weight gain: which often results from the increased appetite associated with mood elevation
- Constipation
- Orthostatic hypotension
- Urinary retention
- Somnolence
- Fluoxetine: can precipitate states of agitation and weight loss
- In the event that opioids are prescribed, advise the patient of the following potential complications (Leventhal 1999):
  - Dependency
  - Habituation
  - Toxicity

FOLLOW-UP

→ Exacerbations of FM symptoms can be precipitated by stress, which may necessitate prescribing a series of alternative treatments (Millea et al. 2000).
→ During routine follow-up evaluations, clinicians should consider prescribing antidepressant therapy, even when a depressive disorder is not apparent.
→ FM support groups and classes have contributed to re-establishing a sense of well-being among patients because they validate the legitimacy of their symptoms (Snider 1997).
→ A slight majority of patients do not have a discernable psychiatric illness (i.e., depression). Therefore clinicians must evaluate the degree of emotional distress resulting from chronic pain. Ongoing assessment of adequate pain control and the need for medication adjustments are a necessary part of follow-up.

BIBLIOGRAPHY

Buskila, D. 2000. Fibromyalgia, chronic fatigue syndrome, and myofascial pain syndrome. *Current Opinion in Rheumatology* 12:113–123.

Close, D. and Beckenham, K. 2001. Fibromyalgia syndrome. Letters to the editor. *Rheumatology* 40:348.

Earnshaw, S.M., MacGregor, G., and Dawson, J.K. 2001. Fibromyalgia–monotheories, monotherapies and reductionism. Letters to the editor. *Rheumatology* 40:348–349.

Fan, P.T., and Blanton, M.E. 1992. Clinical features and diagnosis of fibromyalgia. *Journal of Musculoskeletal Medicine* 9:24–42.

Friedberg, F., and Jason, L.A. 2001. Chronic fatigue and fibromyalgia: clinical assessment and treatment. *Journal of Clinical Psychology* 57:433–455.

Hadhazy, V.A., Ezzo, J., Creamer, P. et al. 2000. Mind–body therapies for the treatment of fibromyalgia. A systematic review. *Journal of Rheumatology* 27:2911–2918.

Leventhal, L. 1999. Management of fibromyalgia. *Annals of Internal Medicine* 13:850–858.

Merchant, R.E., and Andre, C.A. 2001. A review of recent clinical trials of the nutritional supplement Chlorella pyrenoidosa in the treatment of fibromyalgia, hypertension, and ulcerative colitis. *Alternative Therapies* 7:79–91.

Millea, P.J., and Holloway, R.L. 2000. Treating fibromyalgia. *American Family Physician* 62:1575–1587.

Nasir, L.S. 2002. Acupuncture. *Primary Care: Clinics in Office Practice* 29:1–11.

Neeck, G., and Crofford, L.J. 2000. Neuroendocrine perturbations in fibromyalgia and chronic fatigue syndrome. *Rheumatic Diseases Clinics of North America* 26:989–1002.

O'Malley, P.G., Jackson, J.L., Santoro, J. et al. 1999. Antidepressant therapy for unexplained symptoms and symptom syndromes. *Journal of Family Practice* 48:980–990.

Puttick, M.P.E. 2001. Rheumatology: 11. Evaluation of the patient with pain all over. *Canadian Medical Association Journal* 164:223–227.

Salvarani, C., Cantini, F., and Olivieri, I. 2000. Distal musculoskeletal manifestations in polymyalgia rheumatica. *Experimental Rheumatology* 18:551–552.

Schwalm, A. 2001. *Drug facts and comparisons*. St. Louis, Mo.: Wolters Kluwer Company.

Sierpina, V.S., and Carter, R. 2002. Alternative and integrative treatment of fibromyalgia and chronic fatigue syndrome. *Clinical Family Practice* December 4(4):853.

Smythe, H. 2000. Fibromyalgia: can one distinguish it from malingering? More work needed; more tools supplied. *Journal of Rheumatology* 27:2536–2540.

Snider, R.K. 1997. *Essentials of musculoskeletal care*. Rosemont, Ill.: American Academy of Orthopedics.

White, K.P., Carette, S., Harth, M. et al. 2000. Trauma and fibromyalgia: Is there an association and what does it mean? *Seminar on Arthritis and Rheumatism* 29:200–216.

Wilke, W.S. 2001. Can fibromyalgia and chronic fatigue syndrome be cured by surgery? *Cleveland Clinic Journal of Medicine* 68:277–279.

Wright, M.G. 2000. Letters to the editor. *Rheumatology* 40:348.

8-C

Osteoarthritis

Osteoarthritis (OA), or *degenerative joint disease* (DJD) is the most common musculoskeletal disorder in persons over age 50 (Paget 2000). There is some disparity in the literature as to whether the incidence of OA is equal in both genders. However, the consensus of opinion suggests that of the 70% of persons over age 65 who are afflicted with OA the vast majority are women (Brief et al. 2001, Buckwalter et al. 2001, Hungin et al. 2001). Race is not a differentiating factor. Osteoarthritis affects approximately 21 million Americans and has an impact that is far-reaching and devastating (Adler et al. 2001, Estes et al. 2000). It accounts for the greatest cause of medical disability in persons over age 65 and is the chief complaint precipitating more than 7 million doctor visits annually in the United States (Adler et al. 2001, Buckwalter et al. 2001).

Osteoarthritis can be classified into primary and secondary conditions, each one involving at least one of four distinct pathological processes: degeneration of intra-articular cartilage as evidenced by joint space narrowing; the formation of new bone at the base of the cartilage and in the joint margins, the latter commonly referred to as *osteophytes* or *bone spurs*; *sclerosis*, or thickening of the ends of the bones; and the formation of fluid-filled areas of bone called *cysts* (Adler et al. 2001, Buckwalter et al. 2001).

The precise pathophysiology of OA is not known. However, OA is no longer considered to be a normal consequence of aging. Rather, it is more than likely a complex process involving wear and tear of cartilage—the thick, cushioning between the ends of bones—certain genetic predispositions, as well as biomechanical risk factors such as occupation, high level athleticism, and body habitus, to name a few (Brief et al. 2001, Loughlin 2001). The cumulative effect of OA is pain, diminished function, and social incapacity. Since cartilage has no pain receptors, the pain is thought to emanate from the involved synovium, or lining of the joints and soft tissue structures, and it is mediated by prostaglandin action as well as various efferent nerve endings (Hungin et al. 2001).

It is common practice for clinicians practicing in primary care settings to refer persons with painful, arthritic joints to an orthopedic surgeon for consultation and treatment, despite the fact that comparatively few of these patients will require surgery. Since the vast majority of persons with OA need long-term, conservative care focusing on alleviating pain and improving function, they may be better served by primary care providers (Buckwalter et al. 2001).

DATABASE

SUBJECTIVE

→ OA commonly occurs in patients (Estes et al. 2000):
- Over 40 years of age
- With a history of previous trauma to the affected joint
- With a history of obesity (Manek 2001)

→ Symptoms include:
- Pain and swelling in the affected joint, aggravated by weight-bearing activity and going up and down stairs
- Pain at rest, which can interfere with sleep in the advanced stages
- Decreased range of motion (ROM) and buckling of the knee in the affected joint as the disease advances
- Stiffness, especially after prolonged periods of sedentary activity
- Symptoms are exacerbated by damp, cold weather (Estes et al. 2000)
- Inability to grasp objects, turn door handles, twist open jars due to pain and stiffness (Kozin 2000)
- OA can develop in any synovial joint. The most commonly affected joints include (Buckwalter et al. 2001):
  - Distal interphalangeal (DIP) and first carpal metacarpal (CMC) joints of the hand (Estes et al. 2000)
  - First metatarsophalangeal (MTP) joint of the foot
  - Wrist
  - Acromioclavicular joint
  - Hip
  - Lumbar and cervical spine
  - Knee

OBJECTIVE

→ Patient may present with:
- Swelling of the affected joint due to joint effusion (Adler et al. 2001)
- Painful ROM
- Joint line tenderness
- Crepitus
- Joint deformity
  - *Heberde's nodes* at the distal interphalangeal joints (DIPS)
  - *Bouchard's nodes* at the proximal interphalangeal joints (PIPS)
  - Decreased ROM (Estes et al. 2000)
  - Joint contracture
  - Periarticular muscle spasm
- Joint subluxation (Buckwalter et al. 2001)
- Muscle atrophy in the involved extremity

ASSESSMENT

→ Osteoarthritis
→ R/O rheumatoid arthritis
→ R/O systemic lupus erythematosus (SLE)
→ R/O intra-articular cartilage tear
→ R/O gout
→ R/O tendinitis
→ R/O bursitis
→ R/O nerve compression syndrome
→ R/O chondrocalcinosis—calcium pyrophosphate deposition disease, a condition that often co-exists with OA, and has a greater incidence in women (Stucki et al. 1999)
→ R/O osteonecrosis

PLAN

DIAGNOSTIC TESTS

→ X-rays of the affected joint. Radiographs are currently the standard of reference for detecting and quantifying the extent of joint destruction from OA (Backhaus et al. 1999). **NOTE:** See sections on individual joint problems for specific views.
- Characteristic x-ray findings may include (Buckwalter et al. 2001, Estes et al. 2000):
  - Joint space narrowing
  - Osteophyte formation
  - Subchondral sclerosis, which gives the ends of the bones a dense, white appearance
  - Subchondral cyst formation, or small, lucent areas of bone
  - Subluxation, or partial dislocation of the joint
  - Loose bodies, or calcified pieces of intra-articular cartilage
→ Bone scan
→ CT (computerized tomography)
→ MRI
→ Laboratory studies:

- ESR
- UA
- CBC
- RF (rheumatoid factor)
- ANA (anti-nuclear antibody)
→ Synovial fluid analysis for glucose, cell count and differential, culture and sensitivity, crystals, and cytology as indicated to rule out infection or crystal-induced arthropathies

TREATMENT/MANAGEMENT

→ Acetaminophen has been identified by the American College of Rheumatology (ACR) to be the most appropriate initial treatment for OA based on the overall cost, therapeutic efficacy, and toxicity profile (Manek 2001).
- 500–1000 mg p.o. BID
- May be increased up to 1000 mg p.o. BID
- Should not exceed 4 g in 24 hours
→ Nonsteroidal anti-inflammatory drugs (NSAIDs) for 2–6 weeks. (See **Table 8N.1, Anti-inflammatory and Analgesic Medication**.)
- The patient's response to NSAIDs is idiopathic. When the patient has unpleasant side effects from one NSAID, or fails to demonstrate a therapeutic benefit or a reduction in symptoms within two weeks, a different NSAID should be considered.
- NSAIDs should be prescribed with caution in patients with a history of peptic ulcer disease, gastrointestinal bleeding, persons with diabetes and congestive heart failure who may have renal insufficiency, as well as asthmatics in whom the use of NSAIDs have been known to induce bronchospasm (Buckwalter et al. 2001).
- In patients with a history of gastric ulcers, consider prescribing one of the following medications concomitantly (Gotzsche 2000):
  - Cimetidine 400 mg p.o. BID
  - Omeprazole 20–40 mg p.o. BID
  - Misoprostol 800 mg p.o. BID
- Aspirin or enteric-coated aspirin is an effective NSAID, but it requires frequent dosing (QID) to maintain a therapeutic blood level, and is no longer considered the treatment of choice.
→ COX-2 inhibitors are one of the newer classes of anti-inflammatory drugs used to treat arthritic conditions. The inhibition of the COX-2 enzyme is anti-inflammatory without affecting the cytoprotective gastric prostaglandin COX-1, thereby sparing the gastric mucosa (Manek 2001, Scheiman 2001). (See **Table 8N.1.**)
- Patient selection (Scheiman 2001):
  - Persons with a history of gastrointestinal ulcer complications
  - Persons receiving anti-coagulant therapy
  - Advanced age
- COX-2 inhibitors are comparable to COX-1 or traditional NSAIDs in therapeutic efficacy (Paget 2000).

- Celecoxib is contraindicated for persons with a history of allergy to sulfonamides (Manek 2001).
- With consideration applied to the above information, the two most widely prescribed COX-2 inhibitors may be prescribed as follows:
  - Rofecoxib 12.5–25 mg p.o. BID
  - Celecoxib 100–200 mg p.o. BID
→ Glucosamine and chondroitin: classified as a food supplement in the U.S. Both are molecules which exist in intra-articular cartilage, the latter playing a role in maintaining adequate fluid content, and therefore its elasticity and resistance (Brief et al. 2001).
  - Glucosamine and chondroitin are generally taken conjointly in doses of 500 mg and 400 mg, respectively, TID (Brief et al. 2001).
  - Glucosamine and chondroitin can be taken as an adjunctive therapy in treating OA. There is no need for patients to discontinue regular use of prescribed NSAIDs (Schardt 1998).
  - Despite a preponderance of evidence that supports the therapeutic efficacy of glucosamine and chondroitin, the Arthritis Foundation has declined to advocate its use (Brief et al. 2001, McAlindon 2000).
→ Oral analgesics may be prescribed with caution on a prn basis, or regular dosing to reduce the amount of NSAIDs required to relieve symptoms (Buckwalter et al. 2001). (See **Table 8N.1**.)
  - Propoxyphene, napsylate, and acetaminophen 1–2 tablets p.o. every 6–8 hours
  - Hydrocodone bitartrate, and acetaminophen 1–2 tablets p.o. every 6–8 hours
  - Acetaminophen with codeine #3, 1 tablet p.o. every 6 hours
→ Intra-articular steroid injections can be administered, as needed, approximately every 3–4 months by a qualified clinician.
→ Intra-articular injections of hyaluronic acid, one of the more contemporary forms of treatment in the U.S., should be considered for persons with OA of the knee only, specifically, persons who have failed to derive benefit from all other reasonable forms of conservative treatment, including steroid injections.
  - Theoretically, hyaluronan, a component of proteoglycan aggregates found in intra-articular cartilage, provides symptomatic relief by increasing joint lubrication and retarding cartilage degeneration (Buckwalter et al. 2001).
  - Hyaluronic acid is generally administered intra-articularly once a week for 3–5 weeks.
  - Hyaluronic acid administration ideally should not exceed two series of treatments annually (Manek 2001).
→ Capsaicin: a pepper plant derivative, is a topical over-the-counter preparation for persons with more localized areas of OA (Manek 2001).
→ Physical therapy should be prescribed to increase muscle strength and range of motion.
→ Application of ice packs for 25-minute periods TID–QID,

unless the person has peripheral neuropathy or peripheral vascular disease.
→ Bracing and splinting extremities to promote rest, help prevent deformity, and reduce spasm.
→ Lateral heel wedge shoe inserts for patients with medial compartment osteoarthritis in the knee(s) redistribute body weight across the lateral side of the tibia, which can decrease pain and increase joint stability.
→ Custom made "unloader braces" can be prescribed to persons with advanced OA of the knee whose medical condition or age preclude consideration for knee arthroplasty. The brace shifts body weight from the diseased to the healthy knee compartment, which reduces pain and increases joint stability (Buckwalter et al. 2001).
→ Cane, walker, or crutches as indicated to relieve loading forces on diseased joints.
→ Weight reduction of 5.1 kg (11.25 lbs) over a 10-year period has been noted to reduce symptomatic knee arthritis in women by more than 50% (Buckwalter et al. 2001, Manek 2001).
→ At least one million persons in the U.S. receive acupuncture treatments for OA, despite limited evidence of its therapeutic efficacy (Ezzo et al. 2001).

CONSULTATION

→ Orthopedic consultation, if conservative measures of treatment have failed, for consideration of the following:
  - Joint replacement
  - Osteotomy
  - Arthroscopic debridement and/or lavage of joints
  - Joint fusion
  - Arthroplasty
  - Removal of a loose body
  - Physician consultation if conservative management of arthritic condition may interfere or compromise treatment of the patient's other medical problems (e.g., diabetics with neuropathies)

PATIENT EDUCATION

→ Provide the patient with appropriate explanations regarding the diagnosis, pathophysiology, and natural history of OA that has resulted in her symptoms.
→ Weight loss and dietary counseling may be indicated. Refer the patient to the appropriate services and/or nutritionist. (See **General Nutrition Guidelines**, Section 16.)
→ Prescribe a regular exercise regimen to increase muscle strength in the extremities of involved joints.
  - Encourage non-weight-bearing forms of exercise (e.g., swimming, bicycling, stretching) and weight-resistance training.
  - Explain the effects of physical activity on joints:
    - Inadequate activity results in osteoporosis, decreased ROM, and muscle atrophy. This will precipitate increased joint loading and subsequent progression of the disease (Buckwalter et al. 2001).

→ Recommend shoes with adequate shock absorption and extra depth and width (Manek 2001).

→ Educate patients with respect to the potential side effects of NSAIDs, including COX-2 inhibitors and analgesics.

- Recommend taking medication directly after meals to avoid gastro-intestinal disturbances.
- Caution patients against combining different NSAIDs.
- Acetaminophen can cause rashes and hepatotoxicity in large doses.
- Mild narcotics can result in somnolence, habituation, and dependency.

→ Potential side effects of glucosamine and chondroitin include the following (Brief et al. 2001):

- Gastro-intestinal disturbances
- Headache
- Sensation of heaviness in the lower extremities
- Heart palpitations
- Fatigue
- Skin reactions

→ Patients receiving corticosteroid injections should be advised of the following:

- Diabetic patients may note an increase in their blood sugar for several days after the injection.
- Approximately 50% of patients experience moderate to severe pain in the affected joint that may last from several hours to a week. This complication is not indicative of the eventual success of the treatment and is self-limiting with ice applications and joint elevation.

→ Adverse side effects of hyaluronic acid injections occur in approximately 8% of patients receiving this treatment (Buckwalter et al. 2001). These patients will complain of severe pain, swelling, and warmth in the knee that may persist for several hours to a week.

→ Patients must be instructed on the proper use of canes crutches, walkers, orthotic devices, braces, and splints.

- Inappropriate, or overuse of wrist splints and knee braces can cause eventual weakness of the surrounding musculature, joint deformities, and increased pain.

→ Instruct the patient to put her affected joints through their full range of motion every 15–20 minutes to minimize stiffness (Estes et al. 2000).

→ Applications of heat improve joint mobility, but can increase edema in already inflamed joints (Estes et al. 2000); the general recommendation is to apply ice packs for 25 minutes immediately following a 10-minute application of moist heat.

FOLLOW-UP

→ The patient should return for a follow-up visit 4–6 weeks after conservative treatment is initiated.

→ Serum creatinine, and liver function studies should be monitored routinely—in consultation with the patient's internist—when the patient at risk is maintained indefinitely on NSAIDs.

→ The patient is encouraged to seek medical follow-up when she fails to experience adequately sustained relief of symptoms.

→ Document in progress notes and on problem list.

BIBLIOGRAPHY

Adler, J., Kalb, C., Peraino, K. et al. 2001. Arthritis: what it is, why you get it and how to stop the pain. *Newsweek* September 3(138):38–46.

Backhaus, M., Kamradt, T. Sandrock, D. et al. 1999. Arthritis of the finger joints: a comprehensive approach comparing conventional radiography, scintigraphy, ultrasound, and contrast-enhanced magnetic resonance imaging. *Arthritis and Rheumatism* 42:1232–1245.

Brief, A.A., Maurer, S.G., and Di Cesare, P.E. 2001. Use of glucosamine and chondroitin sulfate in the management of osteoarthritis. *Journal of the American Academy of Orthopaedic Surgeons* 9:71–78.

Buckwalter, J.A., Stanish, W.D., Rosier, R.N. et al. 2001. The increasing need for nonoperative treatment of patients with osteoarthritis. *Clinical Orthopaedics and Related Research* 385:36–45.

Estes, J.P., Bochenek, C., and Fassler, P. 2000. Osteoarthritis of the fingers. *Journal of Hand Therapy* 13:108–123.

Ezzo, J., Hadhazy, V., Birch, S. et al. 2001 Acupuncture for osteoarthritis of the knee. *Arthritis and Rheumatism* 44: 819–825.

Gotzsche, P.C. 2000. Non-steroidal anti-inflammatory drugs. *British Medical Journal* 320:1058–1061.

Hungin, A.P, and Kean, W.F. 2001. Nonsteroidal anti-inflammatory drugs: overused or underused in osteoarthritis? *American Journal of Medicine* 110:85–115.

Kozin, S.H., and Michlovitz, S.L. 2000. Traumatic arthritis and osteoarthritis of the wrist. *Journal of Hand Therapy* April–June:124–135.

Loughlin, J. 2001. Genetic epidemiology of primary osteoarthritis. *Current Opinion in Rheumatology* 13:111–116.

Manek, N.J. 2001. Medical management of osteoarthritis. *Mayo Clinic Proceedings* 76:533–539.

McAlindon, T.E., LaValley, M.P., Gulin, J.P. et al. 2000. Glucosamine and chondroitin for treatment of osteoarthritis: a systematic quality assessment and meta-analysis. *Journal of the American Medical Association* 283:1469–1475.

Paget, S.A. 2000. Arthritis therapies: where are they now? *Arthritis Trends* 7–15.

Schardt, D. 1998. Relieving arthritis pain. Can supplements help? *Nutrition Action Healthletter* 25:3–5.

Scheiman, J.M. 2001. The COX-2 inhibitors: as safe as first thought? *Journal of Musculoskeletal Medicine* 18:348–356.

Simon, L.S. 2000. Cyclooxygenase-2 inhibitors. What role in arthritis? *Arthritis Trends* 17–27.

Stucki, G., Hardegger, D., Böhni, U. et al. 1999. Degeneration of the scaphoid-trapezium joint: a useful finding to differentiate calcium pyrophosphate deposition disease from osteoarthritis. *Clinical Rheumatology* 18:232–237.

Wickersham, R. 2000. *Drug facts and comparisons*. St. Louis, Mo.: Wolters Kluwer.

8-D
Rheumatoid Arthritis

Rheumatoid arthritis (RA) is an inflammatory systemic musculoskeletal disease that affects three times as many women as men, and approximately 1% of the United States population as a whole (Ramsburg 2000). Rheumatoid arthritis can occur at any age, although most frequently in women in their 30s–60s.

The economic devastation that RA has in our society is underscored by the annual $8.7 billion dollar toll that it exacts on our health care system. The physical impact of the disease prohibits at least 50% of persons from maintaining gainful employment within 10 years after a diagnosis is made (Paget 2000, Ramsburg 2000). Fortunately, pharmacological research over the past decade, especially into the immunotherapy targeting proinflammatory cytokines, has led to a greater understanding of the pathophysiology of RA (Jorgensen et al. 2000).

The underlying pathophysiology of RA involves the interaction between various proteins, including cytokines, which are tissue-damaging enzymes, and adhesion molecules within the synovial membranes. The triggering event most likely involves an infectious agent such as a virus (Paget 2000). Specifically, tumor necrosis factor (TNF), the dominant cytokine in the pathogenesis of RA, precipitates a massive inflammatory reaction within the synovium, which results in diminished bone formation, increased bone reabsorption, and the secretion of protein-degrading enzymes. These enzymes proceed to destroy the intra-articular cartilage and underlying bone, eventually culminating in the chronic pain, deformity, and limited functional capacity so characteristic of the RA patient (Jorgensen et al. 2000, Ramsburg, 2000).

The goal of RA management is to prevent synovial inflammation, because it is the persistence of inflammatory properties such as erythema, warmth, and edema that induce bony destruction and disease progression (Paget 2000).

The development of disease-modifying-antirheumatic drugs (DMARDs) over the past two decades has resulted in our ability to actually change the course of the disease (Paget 2000). It stands to reason, therefore, that the significance of early disease detection and initiation of treatment cannot be understated.

The seven criteria formulated by the American College of Rheumatology in 1987 to distinguish RA from other rheumatological diseases are: 1) morning stiffness of at least one hour's duration, 2) the presence of arthritis in three or more joints, 3) arthritis in the hands, 4) symmetrical joint swelling, 5) the identification of rheumatoid nodules, 6) a positive serum rheumatoid factor (RF), and 7) x-ray findings which demonstrate bone lesions characteristic of RA (Ramsburg 2000). At least four of these criteria must be met before a legitimate diagnosis of RA can be made. In addition, patients with RA may present with extreme fatigue and depression, the significance of which is often minimized by characterizing their symptoms as psychosocial, and unfortunate delays in diagnoses can result. Once the diagnosis of RA has been established, medical management of the patient is usually overseen by the primary care clinician in consultation with a rheumatologist.

DATABASE

SUBJECTIVE
(Ramsburg 2000)

→ Women between the ages of 25–60

→ Morning stiffness for at least one hour

→ Joint pain and swelling which often migrates from one joint to another, typically affecting the hands and feet

→ Constitutional symptoms include: fever, general malaise, extreme fatigue, depression, and weight loss

→ Positive family history of RA

OBJECTIVE

→ Positive RF is present in 75–90% of people with RA (Snider 1997); considered significant if titer is ≥1:160

→ Clinical laboratory parameters that have a direct impact on the level of cytokines include (Paget 2000):
  ▪ Elevated sedimentation rate (ESR)
  ▪ C-reactive protein level
  ▪ Hemoglobin level
  ▪ Platelet count

→ The degree of joint inflammation present is determined by counting the number of swollen, tender joints (Paget 2000).

→ The presence of rheumatoid nodules—small, firm, often irregular lesions appearing on the dorsum of the distal upper extremities (Ramsburg 2000, Snider 1997)

→ Ulnar deviation of the fingers is often noted by having the patient extend her hands in a pronated neutral position.

→ The dorsum of the metacarpal phalangeal joints (MCPs) demonstrate a swollen appearance and a boggy texture.

→ Joint contractures, or the inability to fully extend a joint can result from painful motion as well as spontaneous rupture of the extensor tendons in the fingers.

→ Symmetrical involvement of the smaller joints is most typical (Snider 1997).

→ Comorbid conditions of RA often include (Snider 1997):
  ▪ Carpal tunnel syndrome
  ▪ Episcleritis
  ▪ Pulmonary interstitial disease

ASSESSMENT

→ Rheumatoid arthritis
→ R/O systemic lupus erythematosus (SLE)
→ R/O hepatitis
→ R/O lyme disease
→ R/O seronegative arthropathies, such as OA
→ R/O seronegative spondyloarthropathies
→ R/O gout
→ R/O polymyalgia rheumatica
→ R/O infection

PLAN

DIAGNOSTIC TESTS

→ Laboratory (Backhaus et al. 1999):
  ▪ RF (rheumatoid factor)
  ▪ ESR
  ▪ CBC
  ▪ Uric acid
  ▪ ANA (antinuclear antibody)
  ▪ HLA-327
  ▪ C-reactive protein

→ Radiographic findings (Backhaus et al. 1999, Williamson et al. 2001):
  ▪ Periarticular osteopenia
  ▪ Bony erosions at the joint margins
  ▪ Evidence of distal radial ulnar disease
  ▪ Joint space narrowing
  ▪ Dislocation of MCP joints in the hands

→ Synovial fluid analysis may be performed to rule out infection or crystal-induced arthropathies:
  ▪ Gram stain
  ▪ Culture and sensitivity
  ▪ Glucose count
  ▪ Cell count
  ▪ Crystal identification

→ Excisional biopsy of suspicious nodules can confirm their pathology as rheumatoid.

TREATMENT/MANAGEMENT

→ It is assumed for the purposes of this chapter that pharmacological treatment of the patient with RA, specifically when proposing the use of DMARDs, will be administered in consultation with a rheumatologist.

  ▪ Methotrexate is considered to be the most effective and widely prescribed DMARD to date (Paget 2000, Ramsburg 2000):
    • Decreases the number of bony erosions
    • Usual dosage 20–30 mg p.o. weekly (Paget 2000)
    • Contraindicated in pregnant women and those with renal insufficiency

  ▪ Leflunomide: a pyrimidine inhibitor that is clinically equivalent to methotrexate (Ramsburg 2000):
    • Inhibits the progression of joint damage by reducing the proliferation of T-cell lymphocytes
    • Dosage: loading dose of 100 mg p.o. QD for 3 days, followed by 20 mg p.o. QD
    • The majority of treatment involves combination drug therapy. In addition to methotrexate, the following drugs may be prescribed in consultation with a rheumatologist (Paget 2000):
      – Plaquenil
      – Sulfasalazine
      – Cyclosporine

→ Tumor necrosis factor antagonists (TNF-α's): these biological agents are the newest class of drugs, still in the process of being developed to treat RA, and involve the administration of synthesized versions of the soluble form of TNF receptor (sTNFR), a naturally occurring anti-inflammatory agent (Ramsburg 2000).

  ▪ Although the first known TNF-α has been FDA-approved since 1998, TNF-α's are not yet standard treatment for RA patients.

  ▪ TNF-α's must be administered either intravenously or subcutaneously due to their diminished potency with oral consumption.

  ▪ There are two TNF-α's referred to in the literature at present:
    • Infliximab
    • Etanercept

→ Oral corticosteroids (prednisone) are sometimes prescribed for the treatment of RA to control exacerbations or episodic flare-ups. An initial dose of 60 mg p.o. tapering by 10 mg/day over 10–14 days constitutes a typical regimen.

  ▪ DMARDs can be prescribed concurrently with prednisone, but NSAIDs must be stopped because the combination with prednisone can increase the risk of gastrointestinal bleeding.

→ With the exception of DMARDs, TNF-α's, and oral corticosteroid preparations, the remainder of pharmacological and non-pharmacological treatment for RA parallels that of OA (see the "Treatment/Management" section in the **Osteoarthritis** chapter). Caution should be taken to omit instructions for the application of ice packs in RA patients.

→ Celecoxib is the one COX-2 inhibitor presently approved for the management of RA (Simon 2000.) (See **Table 8N.1, Anti-inflammatory and Analgesic Medication**.)

CONSULTATION

→ Rheumatologist:
- For consideration of DMARDs and TNT-α's, which are capable of actually arresting and altering the course of the disease, prompt referral to a rheumatologist is necessary.

→ Orthopedist:
- Orthopedic referral is indicated when all reasonable means of conservative treatment fail, and the evaluation of specific joint pathology requires consideration for arthroscopic debridement, bony resection, fusion and grafting or, total joint arthroplasty, carpal tunnel release, or tendon transfers and repairs.

→ Internist:
- Regular consultation with the patient's internist or primary care provider as indicated.

PATIENT EDUCATION

→ Educate the patient on the potential complications of prednisone (Ramsburg 2000):
- Weight gain
- Cataracts
- Osteoporosis
- Mood alterations
- Skin frailty

→ Persons taking DMARDs should observe the following:
- Abstinence from alcohol consumption is necessary.
- Potential side effects include:
  - Ulcers of the oral mucosa
  - Nausea and vomiting
  - Anorexia
  - Fatigue
  - General malaise
  - Infertility
  - Irreversible alopecia
- The most typical side effect experienced from TNF-α's is that of soft tissue irritation at the injection site, but side effects may also include (Paget 2000, Ramsburg 2000):

- Triggering of autoimmune disorders
- URIs
- Headaches
- Diarrhea
- Tumor development
- Persons receiving TNF-α's must avoid live vaccines.

→ In addition to the above information, see the "Patient Education" management section of the **Osteoarthritis** chapter.

FOLLOW-UP

→ There is no clinical usefulness in follow-up RF titers once a positive result has been established.

→ When taking DMARDs, patients will require regular monitoring of their CBC, LFT's every 4–8 weeks, and creatinine levels approximately every 12 weeks (Ramsburg 2000).

→ See the "Follow-up" section of the **Osteoarthritis** chapter for additional recommendations regarding routine evaluation of the patient with RA.

BIBLIOGRAPHY

Backhaus, M., Kamradt, T., Sandrock, D. et al. 1999. Arthritis of the finger joints: a comprehensive approach comparing conventional radiography, scintigraphy, ultrasound, and contrast–enhanced magnetic resonance imaging. *Arthritis and Rheumatism* 42:1232–1245.

Jorgensen, C., Noel, D., Apparailly, F. et al. 2000. Stem cells for repair of cartilage and bone: the next challenge in osteo-arthritis and rheumatoid arthritis. *Annals of the Rheumatic Diseases* 60:305–309.

Paget, S.A. 2000. Arthritis therapies: where are we now? *Arthritis Trends* 7–15.

Ramsburg, K.L. 2000. Rheumatoid arthritis. *American Journal of Nursing* 100:40–43.

Simon, L.S. 2000. Cyclooxygenase-2 inhibitors. What role in arthritis? *Arthritis Trends* 17–27.

Snider, R.K. 1997. *Essentials of musculoskeletal care.* Rosemont, Ill.: American Academy of Orthopedics.

Williamson, L., Mowat, A., and Burge, P. 2001. Screening for extensor tendon rupture in rheumatoid arthritis. *British Society for Rheumatology* 40:420–423.

Diane C. Putney, M.N., R.N., C.F.N.P.

8-E
Bursitis and Tendinitis

Bursitis and *tendinitis* are generic terms that, until the present day, were applied to a number of vague painful musculoskeletal conditions that often defied more specific diagnoses. Bursitis can be generally described as the inflammation of a bursa—a disk-shaped, soft tissue structure, filled with synovial fluid that is situated between bony prominences, ligaments, and tendons (Adkins et al. 2000).

There are more than 160 bursae throughout the body. Their purpose is to decrease friction between bony prominences and tendoligamentous structures and facilitate gliding of these structures over one another (Snider 1997). Inflammation of the synovial tissue lining of the bursa can result in chronic friction, and occurs from direct trauma or in association with an underlying systemic disease such as rheumatoid arthritis (RA) (Foye et al. 2001, Slawski et al. 1997).

Diagnostic imaging techniques, research, and advances in medical practice have led to a more sophisticated understanding of musculoskeletal pathophysiology, leaving the diagnosis of bursitis for a few discrete clinical syndromes involving the musculoskeletal syndrome. Most patients with bursitis can be successfully managed by the primary care provider; very few patients need surgery.

Tendinitis is the inflammation of a tendon itself; *tenosynovitis* refers to inflammation of the tendon sheath. Repetitive motion of the tendon results in microtrauma and diminished vascularity of the entire soft tissue structure, or tendinitis. (Tytherleigh-Strong et al. 2001). The terms bursitis and tendinitis are used interchangeably due to the close structural proximity of tendons and bursae, as well as their functional interrelationship within the joint complex. The two conditions often present with similar signs and symptom and require the same medical management.

DATABASE

SUBJECTIVE

→ Demographics:
- Bursitis and tendinitis predominate in persons over the age of 30, although they may appear in persons of any age (Biundo et al. 2001, Foye et al. 2001). There does not appear to be any predilection by race.
- The patient often has a history of gout, RA, systemic lupus erythematosus (SLE), diabetes mellitus (DM), intra-articular disease, or biomechanical abnormalities such as leg length discrepancy (Adkins et al. 2000).
- Work related risk factors for bursitis and tendinitis include those that require the individual to perform repetitive, forceful activities that involve gripping; that maintain an awkward, static posture; that use implements that cause vibration; or to sustain prolonged exposure to cool temperatures (Piligian 2000).

→ Symptoms:
- Localized, aching pain in the affected extremity, aggravated by:
  - Vigorous use of the extremity
  - Rising after prolonged sedentary activity
  - Lying on the affected area at night
- Swelling, which may be:
  - Chronic: onset is gradual and often the result of microtrauma, or from athletic activity involving repetitive, forceful, gross motor movements of the upper and lower extremities.
  - Acute: onset is sudden and the result of trauma, infection, or an exacerbation of an underlying disease process such as RA (Snider 1997) or acute calcific tendinitis.

OBJECTIVE

→ Superficially inflamed bursae—such as the olecranon at the elbow, or the pre-patellar bursa over the anterior knee—are typically enlarged, regular, and fluctuant.

→ The presence of erythema and warmth may indicate gout, or less often, infection.

→ Chronically inflamed superficial bursae are usually nontender.

→ Severe tenderness of the bursa or the affected joints may be noted with a history of acute trauma or indicate an infectious process (Foye et al. 2001, Snider 1997).

→ Pain elicited by specific movements directed by the examiner, with and without applied resistance, is often the most specific indicator of which tendon or bursa is involved (Piligian 2000).

→ Limited active ROM at the extremes of flexion and extension of the affected extremity is not uncommon (Tytherleigh-Strong et al. 2001).

→ Muscle atrophy is typically noted in patients with a long-standing history of the condition who have not yet received or responded to treatment.

ASSESSMENT

→ Bursitis:
- Shoulder
  - Subacromial
  - Subdeltoid
  - Subscapularis
- Elbow
  - Olecranon
- Hip
  - Trochanteric
  - Iliopsoas
- Knee
  - Prepatellar
  - Pes Anserinus
- Foot
  - Retrocalcaneal

→ Tendinitis:
- Shoulder
  - Supraspinatus
  - Biceps
- Elbow
  - Lateral epicondylitis
  - Medial epicondylitis
- Wrist
  - de Quervain's tenosynovitis
- Hip
  - Gluteus medius tendinitis
- Knee
  - Quadriceps tendinitis
- Ankle
  - Anterior and posterior tibialis tendinitis
  - Peroneus longus and brevis tendinitis
- Foot
  - Achilles tendinitis

→ R/O tendon or intra-articular cartilage tear

→ R/O degenerative joint disease

→ R/O radiculopathy

→ R/O infection

→ R/O nerve compression syndrome

→ R/O gout

→ R/O fracture

→ R/O tumor

→ R/O chondrocalcinosis

PLAN

DIAGNOSTIC TESTS

→ Radiographs of the affected joint:
- Calcifications can sometimes be discerned in the involved bursa, tendon, or between joints.
- Soft tissue swelling or an effusion can indicate a fracture or an inflammatory process.
- Osteophyte formation and joint space narrowing indicate arthritic changes or a previous history of trauma.

→ Bone scans and MRIs are not routinely obtained in the course of evaluating bursitis and tendinitis, but they may be employed to rule out more serious pathology or to confirm a chronic disease process (Foye et al. 2001).

→ Fluid aspiration:
- Bloody fluid is often present if there is a history of trauma. It may also be noted in chronically inflamed bursa.
- Cloudy or purulent aspirate should alert the examiner to the possibility of gout or infection, and a culture and sensitivity as well as a gram stain should be obtained.

→ Laboratory: if symptoms are chronic, more than one joint is involved, or infection is suspected, the following are indicated:
- CBC
- ESR
- ANA (antinuclear antibody)
- RF (rheumatoid factor)
- Uric acid

TREATMENT AND MANAGEMENT

→ A 2–6 week course of NSAIDs would be appropriate for conditions that:
- Do not involve significant loss of joint motion
- Have endured for less than three weeks
- Have not appreciably interfered with the person's work or activities of daily living (see **Table 8N.1, Anti-inflammatory and Analgesic Medication**).

→ Injection of corticosteroids in conjunction with local anesthetic affords considerable and dramatic relief from symptoms approximately 90% of the time (Snider 1997).
- A person's response to corticosteroids is highly individualized however, and sometimes it can take up to two weeks for discomfort to resolve.

→ Physical therapy is generally indicated if there is loss of range of motion and muscle weakness (Foye et al. 2001, Piligian 2000).

→ Temporary immobilization of the affected joint with braces, splints, slings, casts, and crutches as indicated. Immobilization should be limited to seven days.

→ Phonophoresis, a technique that uses ultrasound to administer cortisone transdermally, is sometimes effective (Snider 1997).

→ Regular applications of ice—usually 25 minutes QID, especially before and after engaging in aggravating activity—are helpful in reducing inflammation and pain.

- This is contraindicated if the patient has a compromised peripheral vascular system or an underlying rheumatological disorder.
→ Compression bandages or Ace Wrap bandages can be applied following the aspiration of a superficial bursa (e.g., olecranon).
→ Consider prescribing the use of full-length arch supports for patients who have pain involving weight-bearing joints (i.e., hip, knee, ankle, and foot) (Adkins et al. 2000).

CONSULTATION

→ Referral to an orthopedist for further consultation is indicated when the patient has no significant or sustained relief from conservative treatment.
→ The patient should be referred to a rheumatologist when the condition is chronic, involves multiple joints, or an underlying rheumatological condition is suspected.
→ The younger, competitive athlete may benefit from consultation with a sports medicine clinician when training techniques appear to be the cause of chronic musculoskeletal problems.
→ Consultation from a neurologist or physiatrist is necessary when nerve entrapment or nerve compression syndromes are being considered.
→ The patient may desire an orthopedic surgical consultation to have an unsightly, chronically enlarged bursa excised.
→ A qualified clinician may need to be consulted for the proper administration of a cortisone injection when indicated or to aspirate a joint or bursa for diagnostic purposes.

PATIENT EDUCATION

→ Educate the patient regarding the pathogenesis of bursitis or tendinitis.
→ Education with respect to the proper use of NSAIDs is an important variable in maintaining the patient's compliance.
- The fact that NSAIDs are anti-inflammatory agents and not narcotic "pain pills" requires emphasis as patients often express concern about becoming dependent on medication.
  • This is especially important in light of the fact that 2–6 week courses of treatment with NSAIDs are the usual recommendation for musculoskeletal disorders, and non-compliance can be high if patients fear dependency.
→ Activity modification is essential and is determined by the joint involved, aggravating factors, and the patient's response to treatment.
→ Emphasize the importance of complying with prescribed physical therapy or rehabilitation programs.

→ Discuss proper use of orthopedic appliances such as arch supports and slings.
→ The patient for whom a cortisone injection is proposed must be instructed on its indications, actions, and potential side effects.
→ Explain the differences between cortisone and anabolic steroids.
- Cortisone, along with a local anesthetic such as lidocaine or marcaine, is sometimes the first treatment of choice and can often produce prompt and dramatic symptom resolution.
→ The patient should be advised to stretch the involved extremity at least three times a day.

FOLLOW-UP

→ Re-evaluation with the primary care provider is appropriate 3–6 weeks after a cortisone injection, and 6–8 weeks following a course of anti-inflammatory medication or physical or occupational therapy.
→ Orthopedic appliances may require modification, adjustment, or discontinuation.
→ The patient is encouraged to seek medical follow-up when conservative treatment fails to adequately relieve symptoms or the condition worsens.
→ Document in progress notes and on problem list.

BIBLIOGRAPHY

Adkins, S.B., and Figler, R.A. 2000. Hip pain in athletes. *American Family Physician* 61:2109–2118.

Biundo, J.J., Irwin, R.W., and Umpierre, E. 2001. Sports and other soft tissue injuries, tendinitis, bursitis, and occupation–related syndromes. *Current Opinion in Rheumatology* 13:146–149.

Foye, P.M., and Stitik, T.P. 2001. Trochanteric bursitis. *eMedicine Journal.* Accessed online at: http://emedicine.com/sports/topic137.htm on June 1, 2003.

Piligian, G., Herbert, R., Hearns, M. et al. 2000. Evaluation and management of chronic work-related musculoskeletal disorders of the distal upper extremity. *American Journal of Industrial Medicine* 37:75–93.

Slawski, D.P., and Howard, R.F. 1997. Surgical management of refractory trochanteric bursitis. *American Journal of Sports Medicine* 25:86–89.

Snider, R.K. 1997. *Essentials of musculoskeletal care.* Rosemont, Ill.: American Academy of Orthopedics.

Tytherleigh-Strong, G., Hirahara, A., and Miniaci, A. 2001. Rotator cuff disease. *Current Opinion in Rheumatology* 13:135–145.

Diane C. Putney, M.N., R.N., C.F.N.P.

8-F
Shoulder Pain

The shoulder, which serves as the point of attachment between the upper extremity and the axial skeleton, is comprised of three joints: the sternoclavicular (SC), acromioclavicular (AC), and the much larger glenohumeral joint (GHJ). The rather shallow placement of the humeral head into the glenoid fossa allows the GHJ the greatest range of motion of any joint in the human body (Tytherleigh-Strong et al. 2001). The GHJ derives its stability from static structures that include the glenoid labrum, glenohumeral ligaments, and a thick fibrous capsule. This stability is reinforced by the dynamic rotator cuff tendons and scapular muscles (Levine et al. 2000), The four rotator cuff tendons originate from the scapula, and insert around the humeral head, which permits the multidirectional movement of the shoulder. The subscapularis tendon allows for internal rotation of the humerus, while the infraspinatus and teres minor facilitate its external rotation. Finally, the supraspinatus tendon facilitates shoulder abduction along with the deltoid muscle (McLaughlin et al. 2001).

Rotator cuff pathology accounts for the greatest number of shoulder problems encountered by primary health care providers (Morrison et al. 2000). *Subacromial impingement* (the pathological process by which repetition of rotator cuff compression between the humeral head and the anterior-inferior aspect of the acromion) had long been considered to be the primary etiology of rotator cuff disease, but controversy has arisen because more contemporary studies suggest that the pathogenesis is multifactorial (McLaughlin et al. 2001, Tytherleigh-Strong et al. 2001).

The most significant factor in *primary impingement*, which is the anatomic encroachment on the rotator cuff tendon, is the shape of the acromion, specifically the presence of a bony prominence—a hook on its anterolateral undersurface (Tytherleigh-Strong et al. 2001).

Secondary impingement can result from alterations in normal biomechanics of the shoulder that accumulate with age or from forceful repetitive stresses that occur with extremes of motion in the younger athlete (McLaughlin et al. 2001, Tytherleigh-Strong et al. 2001).

When evaluating patients with shoulder pain, consideration should be given to their age, chronicity of symptoms, and the specific components of their chief complaint (Snider 1997). Patients age 30 and younger can have shoulder pain that is associated with an unstable joint. This instability, which is due, in part, to diminished tension of the glenohumeral ligaments, may be the underlying cause of chronic pain and apprehension associated with shoulder movement. The unstable shoulder can ultimately result in a frank dislocation (Levine et al. 2000). Injuries involving varying degrees of AC joint separation are more prevalent in younger patients (Snider 1997).

Rotator cuff impingement syndrome typically plagues middle-aged persons, as does the phenomenon of *frozen shoulder*, a condition of unknown etiology where both active and passive movement of the shoulder becomes constricted over a protracted period of time, usually ranging from 12–36 months. Of note is that approximately 70% of the 2% of the general population who develop frozen shoulder are women (Hannafin et al. 2000).

Degenerate rotator cuff tears, generally the result of chronic impingement syndrome, as well as degenerative joint disease of the GHJ and ACJ are conditions that predominate in persons over age 50 (Mantone et al. 2000, McLaughlin et al. 2001, Snider 1997). *Rotator cuff arthropathy*, while typically affecting the dominant arm, will demonstrate bilateral involvement 60% of the time (Jensen et al. 1999).

The prevalence of shoulder problems as well as the complexity of the shoulder joint itself make the evaluation of shoulder pain one of the more challenging examinations in primary care. This chapter addresses the more common shoulder pathologies encountered in a primary care setting.

DATABASE

SUBJECTIVE

→ History of trauma; common mechanisms of injury include:
  ■ A fall on an outstretched arm often precipitates a rotator cuff tear (Morrison et al. 2000).
  ■ A direct blow to the shoulder can result in:
    • Anterior shoulder dislocation
    • AC joint separation

- Proximal humerus fracture
- Clavical fracture
  - Forceful hyperextension or flexion of the arm can result in rotator cuff injuries and dislocations (McLaughlin et al. 2001).
→ The patient with an occupation that requires repetitive and heavy overhead lifting
→ The athlete who engages in recreational and competitive sports that involve repetitive and forceful abduction, flexion, and extension of the shoulder:
  - Volleyball
  - Tennis
  - Basketball
→ Pain:
  - Rotator cuff disease
    - Pain aggravated by (Tytherleigh-Strong et al. 2001):
      – Overhead movements
      – Abduction and forward flexion of the arm past 60°
      – Sleeping on affected shoulder
    - Pain typically radiates into the deltoid region
  - Frozen shoulder (Hannafin et al. 2000, Nofsinger et al. 1999):
    - Women age 40–60
    - Recent history of open heart surgery
    - History of diabetes mellitus
    - 20–30% of patients with a history of frozen shoulder on opposite side
    - History of cardiovascular accident
    - Sudden onset of pain
    - No history of trauma
    - Severe limitation of movement in all directions
  - Acute calcific tendinitis (Hannafin et al. 2000, Nofsinger et al. 1999):
    - Women age 30–60
    - Persons with sedentary occupations
    - Sudden onset of pain
    - No history of trauma
    - Severe limitation of movement in all directions
  - Osteoarthritis of the GHJ (Buckwalter et al. 2001):
    - Pain after prolonged sedentary activity
    - Pain aggravated by activity
    - Pain diminished by rest
  - Osteoarthritis or inflammation of the AC joint (McLaughlin et al. 2001):
    - Pain is aggravated by moving the arm across the chest.
  - Cervical radiculopathy (Sari-Kouzel et al. 1999):
    - Sudden onset of pain
    - Pain radiates into the scapula, down the arm, past the elbow.
→ Loss of motion (Hannafin et al. 2000):
  - Can occur, to varying degrees, in all shoulder pathology
  - In frozen shoulder:
    - The onset is insidious.
    - Motion is restricted in all directions.
  - In the arthritic shoulder, diminished ROM is progressive over many years.

→ Weakness (Levine et al. 2000, Mani et al. 2000, Morrison et al. 2000):
  - Onset is sudden in:
    - Rotator cuff tears
    - Fractures
    - Dislocations
  - Gradual onset of weakness occurs when motion is restricted over time. This will lead to the disuse atrophy seen in (Hannafin et al. 2000, Jensen et al. 1999):
    - Chronic rotator cuff disease
    - Frozen shoulder
    - Osteoarthritis
→ Instability: The patient will complain of:
  - Feeling as though the shoulder is catching
  - The sensation that the shoulder is "coming out of the joint"
→ Popping, snapping, grinding:
  - Remote history of trauma, especially dislocation
  - Occurs with chronic inflammatory conditions:
    - Rotator cuff disease
    - Osteoarthritis
→ Paresthesias:
  - Can occur in the forearm in chronic rotator cuff impingement due to traction on the brachial plexus
  - Cervical radiculopathy: numbness and tingling radiates down the arm and into one or more fingers
  - Acute anterior shoulder dislocation
  - Labral lesion

OBJECTIVE

→ A full neck examination should always precede the shoulder examination, to discern whether neck motion is causing the "shoulder pain" and is therefore more consistent with cervical disk disease.
  - Positive *Spurling's sign*: the patient complains of severe neck pain radiating down the arm with paresthesias in the hand when the examiner presses with a downward motion on the top of the person's head in cervical radiculopathy (Sari-Kouzel et al. 1999).
  - A positive *Impingement sign* can be elicited by the following methods:
    - Passive abduction of the affected arm to 90° with external rotation of the shoulder produces pain (McLaughlin et al. 2001).
    - Pain with active or passive forward flexion of the arm
    - Shoulder pain is resolved after the administration of 10 cc of 1% or 2% lidocaine into the subacromial bursa with a 25-gauge, 1 ½ inch needle (Tytherleigh-Strong et al. 2001). Unless the practitioner is trained in administrating these injections, the patient may require referral to a qualified clinician.
→ The patient's active ROM should be determined in forward flexion (FF), abduction, internal rotation (IR), and external rotation (ER).

- Achievement of full passive range of motion will exclude frozen shoulder, where movement is restricted in all directions, and to a lesser degree in osteoarthritis.
- Pain elicited with FF and abduction of the shoulder is typical of OA in the ACJ.
- Pain produced with resisted forward flexion with arms tested in both pronation (supraspinatus tendon) and supination (biceps tendon) is consistent with rotator cuff impingement (Mani et al. 2000).

→ Point tenderness over:
- The ACJ suggest OA
- The subacromial sulcus and greater tuberosity of the humeral head suggests rotator cuff disease
- The biceps tendon where it sits in the bicipital groove when an isolated biceps tendinitis exists
- Anterior and posterior shoulder suggests OA of the GHJ
- The inferior medial border of the scapula suggests scapulothoracic bursitis

→ Crepitus (Tytherleigh-Strong et al. 2001):
- Palpated over the subacromial bursa with internal and external rotation of the shoulder in the scapular plane suggests impingement syndrome
- Over the anterior and posterior shoulder suggests osteoarthritis

→ Weakness, easily discerned by having the patient resist external rotation, is often noted in chronic shoulder conditions where the pain has interfered with normal use and function (Hannafin et al. 2000, Morrison et al. 2000).
- Chronic rotator cuff impingement
- Frozen shoulder
- Degenerative rotator cuff tears
- Patient may have a positive *Drop sign*: the patient's arm is actively or passively elevated to 180°.
  - If, when lowering the arm to 90° of abduction, the patient experiences sudden weakness and pain with a simultaneous drop of the arm by 40°, the test is considered positive, and a rotator cuff tear should be suspected.

→ Instability: a review of the many exam techniques available to determine shoulder instability and its associated lesions is beyond the scope of this chapter. There are two simple tests that can be employed to assess general instability:
  - *Apprehension sign*: with the patient's arm in external rotation and abduction, pull the hand backwards into further extension. The test is positive when the patient drops her arm to the side to avoid dislocation or subluxation (Snider 1997).
  - *Sulcus sign*: when the patient is seated, pull down firmly on her arm by gripping the distant humerus. A deepening of the acromiohumeral sulcus will indicate glenohumeral instability (Snider 1997).

→ Muscle atrophy around the shoulder can be observed in chronic shoulder conditions with associated limited range of motion and weakness (Tytherleigh-Strong et al. 2001).

ASSESSMENT

→ Impingement syndrome of the rotator cuff
→ R/O rotator cuff tear
→ R/O osteoarthritis of the acromioclavicular joint
→ R/O frozen shoulder
→ R/O osteoarthritis of the glenohumeral joint
→ R/O calcific tendonitis (Speed 1999)
→ R/O shoulder instability
→ R/O bicipital tendonitis
→ R/O cervical radiculopathy
→ R/O Paget's disease
→ R/O fracture
- Proximal humerus
- Clavical
- Scapula
→ R/O gout
→ R/O avascular necrosis of the humeral head

PLAN

DIAGNOSTIC TESTS

→ Radiographs:
- The standard shoulder x-ray series should generally include three views: anterior/posterior, axillary, and transcapular-lateral projections.
- Additional "special" views may be indicated when considering the various etiologies of shoulder pain.

→ MRI of the affected shoulder is rapidly becoming the standard presurgical test for the confirmation of rotator cuff tears, labral lesions, and chronic impingement syndrome.
- MRI is also used to document the existence of a cervical disk disease.

→ Arthrograms confirm the diagnosis of complete tears of the rotator cuff.
- Many orthopedic surgeons consider this test to be the most reliable.

→ CT scans with double-contrast medium are used to evaluate certain types of shoulder lesions, particularly those involving the labrum.

→ EMGs can be helpful in differentiating a neurological problem from the paresthesias that are sometimes associated with shoulder instability.

TREATMENT/MANAGEMENT

→ NSAIDs: A 2–6 week course is the general rule. (See **Table 8N.1, Anti-inflammatory and Analgesic Medication**.)
→ Unless contraindicated by history of recent trauma, or if an infection is suspected, steroid injections can and should be considered for most painful shoulder conditions. Referral to a qualified clinician may be required (Morrison et al. 2000).
→ Physical therapy is almost always indicated during some phase of treatment and generally consists of rotator cuff strengthening exercises and stretching routines. In the case of adhesive capsulitis, long-term and aggressive physical therapy is the main treatment (Mani et al. 2000).

→ The importance of daily application of ice packs, 25 minutes TID, should be emphasized.

- This is especially true for individuals who cannot tolerate NSAIDs or are otherwise experiencing only modest relief from any other medication.

→ Occasionally, immobilizing the shoulder in a sling for up to one week is beneficial—usually only if there is a history of acute strain or trauma. In the event of dislocations, the standard is six weeks of strict immobilization.

CONSULTATION

→ Referral to an orthopedic surgeon is recommended in the following instances (Mantone et al. 2000):

- A young to middle-aged adult with a documented full-thickness rotator cuff tear.
- An elderly patient with a full-thickness rotator cuff tear who presents with significant pain and disability, and who is not responding satisfactorily to conservative treatment.
- The patient with chronic rotator cuff impingement who has been symptomatic for at least 6 months, and has had no adequately sustained relief from conservative treatment.
- The person with DJD of the GHJ or AVN of the humeral head with significant pain and disability who desires consultation for a total shoulder arthroplasty (TSA).
- Patients with OA of the ACJ who demonstrate a poor response to nonoperative treatment and desire surgical intervention, which involves a resection of the distal clavical.

→ The patient with a frozen shoulder should be referred to an orthopedic surgeon when:

- Her response to conservative treatment has been inadequate for at least 6 months.
- She cannot tolerate the associated pain and disability.
- A significant disparity exists between the patient's history and complaints, and her clinical presentation.
- The patient is 30 years old or younger and has had more than one dislocation in the same shoulder, or is over age 30 and has a history of chronic shoulder dislocations. These patients are candidates for a shoulder stabilization procedure.

NOTE: It must be emphasized to the patient that a frozen shoulder is almost always self-limiting, and that surgical manipulation of the shoulder under anesthesia is not considered to be a routine procedure (Hannafin et al. 2000).

→ Prompt orthopedic consultation should be obtained when plain radiographs reveal suspicious lesions.

- Patients with acute fractures of the humerus and glenoid rim

→ A referral to a neurologist, neurosurgeon, or spine surgeon is indicated if a central cervical lesion is suspected and response to conservative treatment is inadequate.

→ A rheumatology consultation is suggested when the patient's shoulder problems are one of multiple sites of chronic musculoskeletal pain, and a rheumatological condition is suspected.

PATIENT EDUCATION

→ Explain the biomechanics of the patient's injury and the pathophysiology of her disease process.

→ Instruct the patient on the proper dosage, administration, actions, and potential side effects of NSAIDs. See the *Physicians' Desk Reference* (PDR). (Also see **Table 8N.1**.)

→ When treatment with steroid injections is indicated, advise the patient that cortisone can weaken the surrounding soft-tissue structures in the shoulder for up to 4 weeks.

- Caution the patient, therefore, to avoid strenuous and vigorous use of the affected upper extremity for this time period following injection.
  - This can include routine household chores such as vacuuming.
- Other potential side effects of steroid injections include:
  - Subcutaneous atrophy
  - Depigmentation of the skin at the injection site
  - Post-injection soreness or a "flare reaction" may persist from 1–72 hours
  - Temporary elevation of blood sugar levels in diabetic patients

→ The patient is discouraged from engaging in activities that require overhead lifting and repetitive external rotation and abduction of the arm until her discomfort resolves.

→ Encourage the patient to ice the affected shoulder before and after engaging in activities that may exacerbate symptoms.

- This is contraindicated by a vascular or rheumatological condition.

FOLLOW-UP

→ The patient should generally return for re-evaluation 4–6 weeks after conservative therapy is initiated.

→ When treatment for suspected gout or infection has been prescribed, the patient should return for follow-up in 24–48 hours. The patient should be referred for immediate orthopedic consultation when there is no discernable improvement in the patient's signs and symptoms.

→ The patient should be instructed to seek clinical re-evaluation when symptoms persist beyond 6 months, or become progressively disabling.

→ Document in progress notes and on problem list.

BIBLIOGRAPHY

Buckwalter, J.A., Stanish, W.D., Rosier, R.N. et al. 2001. The increasing need for nonoperative treatment of patients with osteoarthritis. *Clinical Orthopaedics and Related Research* 385:36–45.

Hannafin, J.A., and Chiaia, T.A. 2000. Adhesive capsulitis: a treatment approach. *Clinical Orthopaedics and Related Research* 327:95–108.

Jensen, K.L., Williams, G.R., Russell, I.J. et al. 1999. Current concepts review: rotator cuff tear arthropathy. *Journal of Bone and Joint Surgery* 81–A:1312–1324.

Levine, W.N., and Flatow, E.L. 2000. The pathophysiology of shoulder instability. *American Journal of Sports Medicine* 28:910–917.

Mani, L., and Gerr, F. 2000. Occupational and environmental medicine: work–related upper extremity musculoskeletal disorders. *Primary Care: Clinics in Office Practice* 27:1–18.

Mantone, J.K., Burkhead, W.Z., and Noonan, J. 2000. Nonoperative treatment of rotator cuff tears. *Orthopedic Clinics of North America* 31:295–311.

McLaughlin, R.E., and Fenlin, J.M. 2001 Reversing the cycle of subacromial impingement. *Journal of Musculoskeletal Medicine* 18:365–371.

Morrison, D.S., Greenbaum, B.S., and Einhorn, A. 2000. Conservative management of shoulder injuries. *Orthopedic Clinics of North America* 31:1–11.

Nofsinger, C.C., Williams, G.R., and Ianotti, J.P. 1999. Calcific tendinitis of the trapezius insertion. *Journal of Shoulder and Elbow Surgery* 8:162–164.

Sari–Kouzel, H., and Cooper, R. 1999. Managing pain from cervical spondylosis. *Practitioner* 243:334–338.

Snider, R.K. 1997. *Essentials of musculoskeletal care.* Rosemont, Ill.: American Academy of Orthopedics.

Speed, C.A., and Hazleman, B.L. 1999. Calcific tendinitis of the shoulder. *New England Journal of Medicine* 340:1582–1584.

Tytherleigh-Strong, G., Hirahara, A., and Miniaci, A. 2001. Rotator cuff disease. *Current Opinion in Rheumatology* 13:135–145.

Diane C. Putney, M.N., R.N., C.F.N.P.

8-G
Elbow Pain

The elbow is a hinge joint that permits extension, flexion, pronation, and supination of the forearm (Chen 2001). Structures that have important clinical significance include the ulnar collateral ligament (UCL), which is the main stabilizer against ulnar stress; the ulnar nerve with its superficial location behind the medial epicondyle; the lateral epicondyle, a pyramid-shaped bony prominence; and the lateral collateral annular ligament, which is the primary stabilizer of the elbow (Boyer et al. 1999).

Lateral epicondylitis, or tennis elbow, is the most common elbow condition that the practitioner will address in primary care. While tennis elbow effects approximately 50% of athletes engaged in overhead throwing sports, less than 10% are tennis players (Boyer et al. 1999, Field et al. 1998). The causes are thought to be multifactorial, with repetitive overuse activities and a direct blow to the elbow among the most typical (Boyer et al. 1999, Snider 1997). It is estimated that the incidence of tennis elbow among industrial workers is approximately 59 in 10,000 (Sevier et al. 1999). The condition is most prevalent in people aged 30–60; women in their 40s are the most vulnerable (Snider 1997).

The etiology of tennis elbow is, for the most part, idiopathic. From a biomechanical standpoint, repetitive gripping motions, coupled with multiple forearm rotations and wrist extensions will precipitate inflammation at the insertion of the extensor carpi radialis brevis (ECRB) (Ljung et al. 1999, Mani et al. 2000). Unchecked, persistent inflammation leads to tendon degeneration, or *tendinosis* (Snider 1997). The end result is a patient with a chronically painful elbow, which can be incapacitating and sometimes resistant to conventional means of conservative treatment. Approximately 75% of patients with tennis elbow will experience a complete resolution of symptoms within a year when treated conservatively (Bowen et al. 2001). The initial phase of treatment can begin with the primary care provider.

Medial epicondylitis, or golfer's elbow, is another common cause of elbow pain that affects middle-aged women. Also characterized as an overuse syndrome, golfer's elbow develops from inflammation at the insertion of the flexor-pronator musculature onto the medial epicondyle (Mani et al. 2000). The incidence of medial epicondylitis is about a third as prevalent as lateral epicondylitis. Although not as disabling as lateral epicondylitis, the related pathogenesis and treatment recommendations are the same (Pienimaki et al. 2002). The goals of treatment are to decrease inflammation and adverse loading forces and to promote healing, upper extremity strength, endurance, and flexibility (Sevier et al. 1999).

DATABASE

SUBJECTIVE

→ Women 30–60 years old
→ History of occupational tasks involving repetitive gripping motions, wrist extension, and supination and pronation of the forearm, as well as frequent use of tools that cause vibration (Mani et al. 2000, Sevier et al. 1999)
→ The individual may engage in regular competitive throwing sports, especially overhead throwing and pitching (Chen et al. 2001).
→ Pain is exacerbated by clutching heavy objects or even shaking hands (Boyer et al. 1999).
→ Pain can be present at night or at rest.
→ Onset of pain is usually gradual and often radiates into the forearm.
→ The patient may have weakness in the affected extremity, which is generally attributed to the limitations imposed by severe pain (Mani et al. 2000).
→ She may report a history of precipitating trauma, such as bumping the elbow against a wall.
→ Paresthesias in the ring and small fingers may exist from irritation of the ulnar nerve, which is positioned directly behind the medial epicondyle (Chen et al. 2001).
→ Stiffness and difficulty completely extending the elbow are typical (Pascarelli et al. 2001).
→ Vague discomfort that occurs centrally and distally within the forearm can suggest radial tunnel syndrome (Nagy 1997).

OBJECTIVE

→ Exquisite point-tenderness over the *lateral epicondyle* (in tennis elbow) and *medial epicondyle tenderness* (in golfer's elbow) or *ulnar nerve irritation* (Mani et al. 2000).
→ Pain is increased with resisted wrist extension, forearm pronation, and middle finger extension with lateral epicondylitis (Piligian et al. 2000).
  - Occasional swelling over the lateral epicondyle is noted.
  - Loss of full extension of the elbow may be evident in cases of lateral epicondylitis that have been longstanding and resistant to treatment.
  - *Chair test*: The patient is asked to lift a chair with one hand in a position of forearm rotation and wrist palmer flexion. The person with tennis elbow will experience severe pain in the lateral side of the elbow (Boyer et al. 1999).
→ Resisted wrist flexion and forearm pronation usually produces pain in medial epicondylitis.
→ When tapping over the medial side of the elbow causes paresthesias in the small and ring fingers, an ulnar nerve entrapment syndrome should be suspected (Snider 1997).
  - Web space atrophy between the fingers can signify longstanding *ulnar nerve entrapment* (Snider 1997).
→ Complaints of aching discomfort in the medial side of the elbow and the proximal forearm, as well as shooting pains in the ring and small fingers, numbness, tingling, and a cold sensation, may indicate *cubital tunnel syndrome* (entrapment of the ulnar nerve at the elbow) (Chen et al. 2001, Snider 1997).
→ If the pain is more localized to the proximal volar aspect of the forearm, *pronator syndrome* (compression of the median nerve by the pronator teres as it crosses the elbow) should be considered (Chen et al. 2001).
→ Complaints of medial elbow pain coupled with neck and shoulder pain may indicate *cervical radiculopathy* (Snider 1997).
→ Valgus or varus stress applied to the elbow may indicate an *ulnar* or *radial collateral ligament injury* (Chen et al. 2001).

ASSESSMENT

→ Lateral epicondylitis (tennis elbow)
→ Medial epicondylitis (golfer's elbow)
→ R/O carpal tunnel syndrome
→ R/O radial tunnel syndrome
→ R/O cervical radiculopathy
→ R/O cubital tunnel syndrome
→ R/O pronator syndrome
→ R/O olecranon bursitis
→ R/O degenerative joint disease
→ R/O radial head fracture
→ R/O osteochondral loose body
→ R/O synovitis of the elbow
→ R/O triceps tendinitis
→ R/O gout

PLAN

DIAGNOSTIC TESTS

→ X-rays: anterior/posterior, lateral, and oblique are standard views.
  - Usually normal when there is soft tissue involvement only. Radiographic abnormalities, especially small calcifications over the lateral epicondyle can be noted approximately 16% of the time in patients with elbow pain (Pomerance 2002).
  - X-rays may also reveal the presence of degenerative changes, gouty erosions, or the existence of a loose body or a fracture (Snider 1997).
→ Electromyography and nerve conduction studies should be obtained to rule out *peripheral neuropathy* or a *nerve entrapment syndrome* (Boyer et al. 1999, Davidson et al. 1998).
→ Aspiration of the olecranon bursa or the radial capitellar joint, and fluid analysis should be undertaken when *infection* is suspected (Snider 1997).
  - CBC, ESR, uric acid levels, antinuclear antibody, and RA can rule out an underlying rheumatological or metabolic problem. These conditions should at least be considered when the elbow pain is bilateral, chronic, and co-exists with multiple sites of musculoskeletal pain and swelling.
→ MRIs are ordered when ruling out the more serious pathology (i.e., tumors, tendon rupture) (Mani et al. 2000).

TREATMENT/MANAGEMENT

→ Initial treatment:
  - NSAIDs for 2–6 weeks (see **Table 8N.1, Anti-inflammatory and Analgesic Medication**).
  - Tennis and/or golfer's elbow splint: the effect is to produce a counterforce at the origin of the extensor carpi radialis brevis. This prevents the muscles from fully extending, thereby decreasing the stress on the tendons (Sevier et al. 1999).
→ The patient should be instructed to apply ice packs to her elbow 25 minutes BID–QID.
→ Physical therapy should be prescribed for chronic elbow pain. The treatment modalities employed may include:
  - Ultrasound: a method of delivering heat up to a depth of 2 cm to the joint and soft tissue structure to increase regional blood flow, resulting in diminished pain and muscle spasm (Sevier et al. 1999).
  - Phonophoresis: 10% hydrocortisone ointment is applied through the skin using ultrasound equipment (Boyer et al. 1999).
  - Electrical stimulation is applied with a transcutaneous electrical stimulation (TENS) unit to alleviate chronic pain (Sevier et al. 1999).
  - Rehabilitation programs should be delayed until the acute phase of the condition has subsided.
    - Exercises consist of repetitions of the wrist flexion, extension, supination, and pronation performed with the wrist suspended off the edge of a flat surface (Sevier et al. 1999).

- Initially the patient's other hand can be used to supply a traction force on the fingers of the affected extremity.
- The patient is then instructed to progress to a 1- or 2-pound hand-held dumbbell.
- The goals of this regimen are to increase strength and flexibility of the wrist and extensor tendons (Sevier et al. 1999).

→ Acupuncture has demonstrated good short-term results for relief of elbow pain (Boyer et al. 1999, Fink et al. 2002, Nasir 2002).

→ Cortisone injections for the relief of medial and lateral epicondylitis have a 90% success rate. Resolution of pain is most successful when the patient has been symptomatic for less than six months (Sevier et al. 1999, Smidt et al. 2002). Cortisone injections by a qualified clinician can and should be considered during any phase of the condition once the diagnosis has been established.

→ Occasionally, the application of a long-arm fiberglass or plaster cast, which immobilizes the wrist extensors for 2–3 weeks, can alleviate discomfort (Jensen et al. 2001).

- The use of a removable sling is helpful during the acute phase of symptoms.

CONSULTATION

→ The patient who attributes her symptoms to work-related activity requires a prompt referral to the occupational medicine department.

→ A referral to an orthopedist for surgical consultation is indicated when the following conditions exist (Boyer et al. 1999):

- Exercised-induced elbow pain for at least one year
- Inadequate response to all reasonable means of conservative treatment
- Activity-induced pain persisting after three cortisone injections
- The patient reports an unacceptable quality of life

→ Refer the patient to a neurologist for further consultation when neuromotor and sensory deficits are noted during the history and exam.

→ Consultation with a rheumatologist may be necessary if:

- Chronic lateral epicondylitis coexists with an underlying rheumatological condition, and
- No adequately sustained relief is derived from conservative treatment

PATIENT EDUCATION

→ Educate the patient on the pathogenesis of her elbow pain.

→ Instruct the patient on activities to avoid: pushing, pulling, and heavy lifting (Sevier et al. 1999).

→ Instruct the patient on proper application of a force-counterforce brace (this may vary with the actual type of brace prescribed) (Mani et al. 2000).

→ Advise the patient to apply ice before and after engaging in potentially aggravating activities.

→ Instruct the patient to lift with the forearm supinated as opposed to pronated.

→ When the cause of the patient's condition can be attributed to involvement in racquet sports, consultation on modifying her technique and/or equipment is indicated.

- Using a racquet with a large head instead of a small head
- Using a racquet that inhibits vibrating forces such as graphite

FOLLOW-UP

→ A follow-up appointment should be made 4–6 weeks after initiating conservative treatment.

→ An occupational consultant may be required to suggest necessary alterations in the patient's physical work environment if the condition is chronic and caused by work-related demands.

→ The patient should be encouraged to seek medical re-evaluation if symptoms continue for one year or more.

- Refer the patient for surgical consultation.

→ Document in progress notes and on problem list.

BIBLIOGRAPHY

Bowen, R.E., Dorey, F.J., and Shapiro, M.S. 2001. Efficacy of nonoperative treatment for lateral epicondylitis. *American Journal of Orthopedics* 30:642–646.

Boyer, M.I., and Hastings, H. 1999. Lateral tennis elbow: "Is there any science out there?" *Journal of Elbow Surgery* 8:481–491.

Chen, F.S., Rokito, A.S., and Jobe, F.W. 2001. Medial elbow problems in the overhead–throwing athlete. *Journal of the American Academy of Orthopaedic Surgeons* 9:99–113.

Davidson, J.J., Bassett, F.H., and Munley, J.A. 1998. Musculocutaneous nerve entrapment revisited. *Journal of Shoulder and Elbow Surgery* 7:250–255.

Field, L.D., and Savoie, F.H. 1998. Common elbow injuries in sport. *Sports Medicine* 26:193–205.

Fink, M., Wolkenstein, E., Karst, M. et al. 2002. Acupuncture in chronic epicondylitis: a randomized controlled trial. *Rheumatology* 41:205–209.

Jensen, B., Bliddal, H., and Danneskiold–Samsoe, B. 2001. Comparison of two different treatments of lateral humeral epicondylitis—"tennis elbow." A randomized controlled trial. *Ugeskrift for Laeger* 163:1427–1431.

Ljung, B.O., Lieber, R.L., and Friden, J. 1999. Wrist extensor muscle pathology in lateral epicondylitis. *Journal of Hand Surgery* (British Volume) 24:177–183.

Mani, L., and Gerr, F. 2000. Occupational and environmental medicine: work–related upper extremity musculoskeletal disorders. *Primary Care: Clinics in Office Practice* 27:1–18.

Nagy, L. 1997. The treatment of therapy–resistant lateral epicondylitis. *Swiss Surgery* 3:76–79.

Nasir, L.S. 2002. Acupuncture. *Primary Care: Clinics in Office Practice* 29:1–11.

Pascarelli, E.F., and Hsu, Y.P. 2001. Understanding work-related upper extremity disorders: Clinical findings in 485 computer users, musicians, and others. *Journal of Occupational Rehabilitation* 11:1–21.

Pienimaki, T.T., Siira, P.T., and Vanharanta, H. 2002. Chronic medial and lateral epicondylitis: a comparison of pain, disability, and function. *Archives of Physical Medicine and Rehabilitation* 83:317–321.

Piligian, G., Herbert, R., Hearns, M. et al. 2000. Evaluation and management of chronic work–related musculoskeletal disorders of the distal upper extremity. *American Journal of Industrial Medicine* 37:75–93.

Pomerance, J. 2002. Radiographic analysis of lateral epicondylitis. *Journal of Shoulder and Elbow Surgery* 11:156–157.

Sevier, T.L., and Wilson, J.K. 1999. Treating lateral epicondylitis. *Sports Medicine* 28:375–380.

Smidt, N., Assendelft, W.J., van der Windt, D.A. et al. 2002. Corticosteroid injections for lateral epicondylitis: a systematic review. *Pain* 96:23–40.

Snider, R.K. 1997. *Essentials of musculoskeletal care.* Rosemont, Ill.: American Academy of Orthopedics.

Diane C. Putney, M.N., R.N., C.F.N.P.

8-H

Wrist, Hand, and Finger Pain

Evaluation and treatment of *wrist*, *hand*, and *finger pain* in the primary care setting will be presented together in this chapter. Most people use them together and are unable to distinguish the specific location of a problem. Careful history and examination by the primary care provider can help identify the etiology and location of the patient's condition.

Approximately 90% of hand and wrist problems evaluated in the primary care setting are comprised of *carpal tunnel syndrome* (CTS), *trigger fingers* (TF), *osteoarthritis of the basilar joint of the thumb, or the first carpal metacarpal joint* (CMC), *ganglion cysts*, or *radial carpal osteoarthritis of the wrist. De Quervain's stenosing tenosynovitis*, a painful wrist condition involving inflammation of the extensor tendon sheath that runs over the radial styloid, is also included because it predominantly affects women.

Carpal tunnel syndrome (CTS) accounts for at least 90% of all peripheral nerve entrapment syndromes (Arle et al. 2000, Snider 1997, Wong 2001). The incidence of CTS, which is at least three times more frequent in women (D'Arcy et al. 2000) may be well established. However its etiology remains a matter of ongoing debate within the medical community.

In spite of the high profile CTS maintains as a work-related musculoskeletal disorder (WRMD), exact causes of the condition are idiopathic (Lincoln et al. 2000). Advances in imaging techniques have augmented our understanding of the pathophysiology of CTS. It has been generally understood, for example, that the carpal tunnel, a rigid fibro-osseous structure comprised of eight bones bound ventrally by the transverse carpal ligament, is vulnerable to increases in hydrostatic pressure (Herbert et al. 2000). Swelling and inflammation of the median nerve branch, as well as the sheaths of nine flexor tendons that pass through the carpal tunnel, decreases tunnel volume causing nerve compression. Magnetic resonance imaging (MRI) of the wrist with CTS will depict flattening of the median nerve, bowing of the flexor retinaculum, and thickening of the involved flexor sheaths, as well as the deep palmer bursa (Jarvik et al. 2000). Median nerve compression precipitates the onset of intrinsic edema and ischemic changes that result in conduction slowing of the nerve (Arle et al. 2000).

Theoretically, any factor that structurally decreases the volume of the carpal tunnel can potentially result in median nerve compression (Herbert et al. 2000). These factors can involve anatomical variations such as a smaller carpal tunnel or larger adjacent muscles and blood vessels. Excessive adipose tissue, the synovial hypertrophy associated with rheumatoid arthritis (RA), as well as the degenerative changes characteristic of OA may also be present (Arle et al. 2000). The presence of any one of a number of underlying systemic disorders are also contributing factors in the onset and severity of CTS symptoms (e.g., pregnancy, RA, collagen vascular disease, congestive heart failure, diabetes, thyroid disease, obesity, sarcoidosis, menopause, gout, tuberculosis, scleroderma, renal disease, and alcoholism) (D'Arcy et al. 2000, Herbert et al. 2000, Laine 1999, Snider 1997).

Occupational activities that place the employees at risk for CTS include long periods of forceful wrist extension and flexion, using tools that cause vibration, and repetitive gripping (Mani et al. 2000, Piligian et al. 2000). Recent studies show that a wrist positioned in 90° of flexion results in the highest carpal tunnel pressure of all wrist positions (Arle et al. 2000).

The cumulative effect of any one of these occupational, metabolic, or biomechanical risk factors can result in the onset of carpal tunnel symptoms. The classic triad of pain, numbness, and tingling along the median nerve distribution of the hand remains the primary nexus in patient complaints leading to a diagnosis of CTS (Herbert et al. 2000, Mani et al. 2000). There is wide variation, however, in the frequency, intensity, and specific form of discomfort. Fortunately, the evaluation and treatment for CTS is not nearly as complex as its pathogenesis, and treatment continues to prove successful for managing CTS.

Carpal Tunnel Syndrome

DATABASE

SUBJECTIVE

→ Patient is likely between ages 30–60; incidence is rare under age 20 (Snider 1997).

→ The incidence of CTS is three times more prevalent in women (D'Arcy et al. 2000).

→ Patient may have a history of obesity, diabetes, thyroid disease, RA, systemic lupus erythematosus (SLE), alcoholism, pregnancy, menopause, renal disease, sarcoidosis, or gout (Mani et al. 2000).

→ Patients may have occupations requiring repetitive forceful grasping and pinching and use vibrating hand-held tools (Mondelli et al. 2002).

- Examples include seamstresses, butchers, grocery clerks, typists, word processors, musicians, meat packers, cooks, carpenters, and mechanics (Mani et al. 2000).

→ Gradual onset of symptoms is typical, although persons with volar wrist ganglion cysts can present with acute onset.

- Onset of symptoms is precipitated by activities that maintain the wrist in flexion such as driving, holding a phone receiver, and reading (Arle et al. 2000).
- Symptoms are usually worse at night or early morning.

→ The patient with CTS will complain of a variation of symptoms that can generally be characterized as:

- Pain in the wrist and hand that radiates into the thenar eminence of the palm, proximal forearm, elbow, and shoulder (Herbert et al. 2000, Snider 1997).
- Numbness and tingling or a burning sensation in at least two of the four digits, which include the thumb, index, long, and ring finger (Herbert et al. 2000).
- The patient most often will describe the numbness as intermittent. The complaint of ongoing numbness is an indication for immediate referral to an orthopedist for a surgical consultation (Arle et al. 2000).
- Morning stiffness in the fingers (Snider 1997)
- Perception of decreased grip strength and fine motor coordination (Snider 1997)
- Swelling in the hands and fingers (Snider 1997)

OBJECTIVE

→ Thenar atrophy: a concavity noted along the abductor pollicis brevis muscle (APB), which constitutes the thenar eminence (D'Arcy et al. 2000, Herbert et al. 2000).

→ Weakness of the motor branch of the median nerve can be discerned by having the patient resist thumb abduction with the thumbs positioned at right angles to the palm (D'Arcy et al. 2000, Mani et al. 2000).

→ Diminished sensation over the median nerve distribution. This can be detected with two-point discrimination (Herbert et al. 2000) or more simply, the *Stroke test*: light touch applied with a stroking motion over the tip of the index finger compared with that of the small finger.

→ Swelling over the volar aspects of the wrist.

→ Positive *Tinel's sign*: a painful electrical shock sensation is elicited in the hand and fingers upon gentle tapping on the volar aspects of the wrist (D'Arcy et al. 2000, Herbert et al. 2000, Snider 1997).

→ Positive *Phalen's test*: paresthesias develop in the median nerve distribution of the hand when the wrists are held in

90° of flexion for up to 60 seconds (D'Arcy et al. 2000, Herbert et al. 2000).

- There appears to be a growing consensus in the literature that the Tinel's sign and Phalen's test, both considered to be essential findings in diagnosing CTS for over 40 years, actually have poor specificity, and are of ultimately limited diagnostic value to the clinician, especially with respect to determining whether the patient is a candidate for surgery (Arle et al. 2000, Herbert et al. 2000).

→ Grip and pinch strength can be assessed using a dynamometer and pinch meter.

ASSESSMENT

→ Carpal tunnel syndrome
→ R/O median nerve entrapment at the elbow
→ R/O cubital tunnel syndrome, or ulnar nerve entrapment at the elbow
→ R/O peripheral ulnar neuropathy
→ R/O diabetic neuropathy
→ R/O osteoarthritis of the basilar joint of the thumb
→ R/O volar-radial wrist ganglion
→ R/O de Quervain's stenosing tenosynovitis
→ R/O C_6 cervical radiculopathy
→ Rheumatoid arthritis
→ R/O syringomyelia

PLAN

DIAGNOSTIC TESTS

→ Electrodiagnostic evaluations, which include nerve conduction studies (NCS) and electromyography (EMG), are the gold standard measure for confirming the diagnosis of CTS (Arle et al. 2000, Herbert et al. 2000, Snider 1997, Witt et al. 2000).

- These studies provide an objective measure of the capacity for a nerve to conduct an electrical impulse (Snider 1997).
- Prolongation of the distal motor latency, slowing of the median sensory or motor nerve conduction across the wrist, and denervation of the abductor pollicis brevis (PB) constitute a positive electrodiagnostic study (EDS) for CTS.
- Severe neurophysiologic impairment is not generally correlated with a poor prognosis (Padua et al. 2001).

→ Obtain x-rays when the patient demonstrates limited range of motion or a recent history of wrist trauma (Snider 1997).

→ Laboratory tests are not routinely ordered as part of the diagnostic work-up for CTS. Consideration should be given on a case by case basis to obtaining the following (Herbert et al. 2000, Snider 1997):

- Uric acid: to rule out gout
- RA, ANA: when considering rheumatoid arthritis, SLE
- CBC, ESR: to assess for infection or an inflammatory process
- FBS: when evaluating diabetic status
- Thyroid function studies
- Creatine level: to determine renal function

→ MRI of the wrist can be obtained to rule out the presence of an occult ganglion cyst, but is rarely employed during the course of routine evaluation of CTS.

TREATMENT/MANAGEMENT

→ The treatment recommendations should be determined on the basis of the severity of the patient's symptoms, the duration of the symptoms, previous response to treatment as reported by the patient or documented in the medical record, and the presence of any nerve damage (i.e., thenar atrophy).

→ For mild causes of CTS (i.e., when the symptoms are infrequent and do not interfere with function) the most common nonsurgical treatments include:
  ■ Wrist splints, worn at bedtime to maintain the wrist in a neutral position and inhibit the degree of nerve compression (Herbert et al. 2000, Snider 1997).
  ■ Cessation or reduction in performing aggravating occupational activities and cessation or reduction of nonoccupational exposures (Herbert et al. 2000).

→ There is minimal evidence of therapeutic efficacy for NSAIDs and analgesics for the conservative management of CTS (Herbert et al. 2000, Newport 2000). (See **Table 8N.1, Anti-inflammatory and Analgesic Medication**.)
  ■ A reasonable treatment trial is 3–6 weeks.

→ Steroid injections should be recommended for mild to moderate relief of CTS as they can result in dramatic and indefinite relief of symptoms about 81% of the time (D'Arcy et al. 2000). This injection almost always requires a referral to an orthopedist or other qualified clinician.
  ■ If injections are helpful, the patient can receive them approximately every four months as long as she continues to derive adequate therapeutic benefit from them. In addition, injections can have a diagnostic as well as a therapeutic value (Herbert et al. 2000).
  ■ A good therapeutic response to a cortisone injection is predictive of a favorable surgical result (Herbert et al. 2000). However a poor response to an injection does not necessarily mean that the patient will have unsatisfactory relief from surgery (Newport 2000).

→ The administration of diuretics, including vitamin B_6 (pyridoxine), especially to menopausal women with CTS symptoms, is of questionable benefit and has ceased to appear in the current literature review as a standard treatment option.

→ Occupational or hand therapy is often prescribed in the course of medical management for patients with CTS. Although the study of ultrasound and iontophoresis has demonstrated some scientific basis for treatment, the overall therapeutic efficacy is uncertain. When the patient insists on hand therapy, she should be advised that satisfactory relief of her symptoms could take many months.

CONSULTATION

→ Patients should be referred to an orthopedist for surgical consultation of confirmed CTS if the following conditions occur (Arle et al. 2000, Herbert et al. 2000, Lascar et al. 2000):

  ■ Failed conservative treatment or inadequately sustained relief
  ■ Intolerable pain
  ■ Ongoing numbness
  ■ APB or thenar atrophy, and decreased sensation over the median nerve distribution

→ The patient who describes her symptoms as job-related should be promptly referred to the occupational medicine department. It is important to adhere to workmen's compensation laws governing the reporting of industrial injuries. There are state-imposed statutes of limitations and certain diagnostic studies required by insurance carriers that must be observed. Inattention to this matter early in the course of evaluation can result in a host of medical-legal problems, delays in proper treatment, and possibly, compensation.

→ Consultation with a neurologist is appropriate if the patient is not responding to treatment and/or the exam results (including NCS) are equivocal, or at odds with the patient's chief complaint. There are a number of neurological conditions that can mimic CTS (Witt et al. 2000).

→ Patients with complaints of pain and swelling in multiple sites in the upper extremities and a positive ANA or RF should be referred to a rheumatologist for further consultation and management.

PATIENT EDUCATION

→ Explain the disease process and associated symptoms of CTS.

→ Educate patients on the proper use of wrist splints:
  ■ Splints should be worn at night to maintain the wrist in a neutral position.
  ■ Continuous use of splints, or wearing them during routine activities should be discouraged. Over-immobilization of the wrist can lead to weakening of the surrounding muscles and tendons.

→ Counsel regarding the importance of minimizing exposure to occupational risk factors and to aggravating activities of daily living.

→ When the patient's CTS is officially classified as industrial, she will receive specific education regarding appropriate work stations, use of hand tools, hand positioning, etc.

→ It is essential to emphasize the high degree of success of treating CTS and that lack of compliance with treatment and follow-up can potentially result in permanent median nerve damage.

→ Patients receiving corticosteroid injections need information regarding potential complications and side effects:
  ■ Post injection soreness of the wrist may occur the following day
  ■ A temporary elevation of blood sugar for diabetics

→ Advise the patient that injections of cortisone for the treatment of CTS can result in relief of symptoms about 81% of the time, although resolution of her symptoms is temporary (D'Arcy et al. 2000, Newport 2000).

→ Carpal tunnel release (CTR) surgery is indicated for moderate to severe CTS, and of all available treatment, has a superior outcome (Herbert et al. 2000).

FOLLOW-UP

→ It is essential that patients seek follow-up if:
  ■ No resolution of symptoms after an adequate trial of conservative treatment, generally considered to be six weeks
  ■ Numbness and tingling in the fingers has become persistent and unremitting
  ■ Decreased sensation in the fingertips or weakness in the thumb
→ Instruct diabetic patients to monitor their blood glucose levels judiciously because poorly controlled levels may exacerbate symptoms.
→ Document in progress notes and on problem list.

De Quervain's Disease

De Quervain's disease was originally thought to involve inflammation of the tendon sheaths of the extensor pollicis longus (EPL) and extensor pollicis brevis (EPB) and was known as *stenosing tenosynovitis*. In light of more recent studies, however, it has been demonstrated that the histopathology consists of peritendinous fibrosis and fibrocartilaginous metaplasia without inflammation (Piligian et al. 2000). The thickened sheaths cause constriction of the tendons as they glide through the retinaculum, causing pain and swelling on the radial aspect of the wrist (Snider 1997).

Potential causes of de Quervain's disease range from mild trauma to microtrauma that results from activities requiring repetitive ulnar deviation of the wrist. These biomechanics mean that athletes and individuals in certain occupations may be at risk (Biundo et al. 1997, Mani et al. 2000, Piligian et al. 2000).

De Quervain's disease more commonly presents in women age 30–60 (Piligian et al. 2000). Pregnant and postpartum women are also susceptible to the development of de Quervain's. The condition is often misdiagnosed as CTS, however, because CTS is the most common cause of wrist discomfort associated with pregnancy.

When the individual with de Quervain's disease fails to demonstrate relief from treatment, an underlying metabolic predisposition must be considered, including diabetes mellitus (DM), RA, hypothyroidism, gout, and systemic lupus erythematosus (SLE) (Herbert et al. 2000).

In approximately 30% of the cases of de Quervain's there is involvement of both wrists. The associated conditions of trigger fingers, stenosing flexor tenosynovitis, and CTS in individuals with de Quervain's disease have been well documented (Szabo et al. 1992).

De Quervain's disease is most often successfully managed with conservative measures. Early recognition and prompt initiation of treatment or appropriate referral to an orthopedist can save the patient weeks or months of wrist pain.

DATABASE

SUBJECTIVE

→ Women of any race age 30–60
→ Pregnant or within one year postpartum
→ Recent history of acute or recurrent wrist strain or trauma
→ History of RA, DM, thyroid disease, CTS, gout, or SLE
→ Pain may present as:
  ■ Pain on the dorsal-radial aspect of the wrist that is exacerbated by grasping movements
  ■ Thumb pain, not wrist pain, (since abduction of the thumb causes pain)
→ The patient may complain of a lump on the radial side of the wrist.
→ There may be swelling over the dorsal-radial aspect of the wrist.
→ The patient may have a painful clicking or catching sensation.

OBJECTIVE

→ Severe point tenderness over the radial styloid
→ Mild edema along the radial aspect of the wrist (Mani et al. 2000)
→ Occasionally crepitus can be appreciated over the first dorsal compartment that contains the EPB and EPL (Piligian et al. 2000).
→ Positive *Finklestein's test*: instruct the patient to make a fist enclosing her thumb in full flexion; with gentle force, pull the fist in an ulnar direction. The person with de Quervain's is likely to experience severe pain (Piligian et al. 2000, Snider 1997). It is important to note that this maneuver can also cause pain in the person who has osteoarthritis of the basilar joint of the thumb, or with *Wartenberg's syndrome*, a painful condition that involves entrapment of the superficial branch of the radial nerve (Mani et al. 2000).
→ A palpable thickening of the tendon sheath with nodularity may be discerned. This is a manifestation of the fibro-cartilaginous metaplasia of the tendon sheaths in the first dorsal compartment (Piligian et al. 2000).
→ Severe tenderness over the snuff box, or scaphoid, *not the* radial styloid, is pathognomonic for a scaphoid fracture if the patient reports recent history of wrist trauma. This point deserves special emphasis since there is a tendency in the literature to use the term snuff box and radial styloid interchangeably. An acute scaphoid fracture when not diagnosed in a timely manner can result in a disabling, protracted course of treatment for the patient.

ASSESSMENT

→ de Quervain's disease
→ R/O osteoarthritis of the basilar joint of the thumb
→ R/O carpal tunnel syndrome
→ R/O rheumatoid arthritis of the wrist
→ R/O radioscaphoid DJD
→ R/O scaphoid fracture (with a preceding history of trauma)
→ R/O gout
→ R/O dorsal-radial ganglion cyst

PLAN

DIAGNOSTIC TESTS

→ Radiographs:
  - Anterior/posterior (A/P), lateral, scaphoid, and oblique views are routinely obtained, but will be normal in the absence of a fracture, or a rheumatoid, gout, or osteoarthritic condition.
→ Laboratory: RF, ANA, uric acid level if underlying rheumatological or metabolic conditions are suspected.
→ Finklestein's test as previously described in the "Objective" section above.
→ Electromyography and nerve conduction studies may be required if a peripheral nerve entrapment syndrome is suspected.
→ Aspiration of discrete lesions noted on the tendon sheaths can distinguish a ganglion cyst from fibrosis.

TREATMENT/MANAGEMENT

→ A steroid injection into the first dorsal wrist compartment is generally considered to be the initial treatment of choice, and the appropriate referral to a clinician qualified to administer this injection should be made promptly if necessary (Mani et al. 2000).
  - An injection usually provides dramatic and immediate relief of symptoms.
  - The patient may require up to 3 injections before permanent relief is established.
→ Alternately, appropriate treatment can be initiated by prescribing a thumb-spica wrist splint to be worn for approximately 6 weeks, although the success rate of this intervention alone is poor.
→ A course of NSAIDs can be prescribed for 2–6 weeks when not medically contraindicated (Piligian et al. 2000) (See **Table 8N.1**.)
→ Prescribe applications of ice for 25 minutes BID–QID.
→ Phonophoresis treatments can be administered by a physical or occupational therapist.
→ Immobilizing the wrist in a thumb-spica short-arm cast for 6 weeks is a treatment option for patients who refuse injection and have failed other means of treatment.

CONSULTATION

→ Referral to an orthopedist or other qualified clinician is indicated for the administration of a steroid injection.
→ Referral to a hand surgeon is indicated for consideration of a surgical release of the first dorsal wrist compartment if the patient presents with a chronic history of de Quervain's and inadequately sustained relief from conservative treatment.
→ Referral to a rheumatologist may be indicated if the patient's symptoms are chronic, bilateral, and associated with multiple aches and pains in the upper extremities, or the overall presentation is one of an underlying rheumatological condition.
→ Refer to **Occupational Health**, Section 15, when the patient characterizes her condition as an industrial injury.

PATIENT EDUCATION

→ Educate the patient on the pathophysiology of de Quervain's disease.
→ Instruct the patient on the importance of minimizing exposure to activities that require repetitive, forceful ulnar deviation of the wrist and thumb abduction (Piligian 2000).
→ Inform the patient of potential side effects of steroid injections into the first dorsal compartment, which are generally limited to subcutaneous atrophy and skin depigmentation over the radial styloid (Snider 1997). These conditions are temporary and will resolve within about 8 months.

FOLLOW-UP

→ When the patient declines referral to an orthopedist for injection or surgical consultation, have her make a follow-up appointment with the primary provider 4–6 weeks following the initiation of more conservative treatment.
→ See the "Consultation" section above.
→ Document in progress notes and on problem list.

Osteoarthritis of the Basilar Joint of the Thumb

The pathogenesis of *osteoarthritis (OA) of the basilar joints* parallels that of most joint degeneration—i.e., destruction of intra-articular cartilage, osteophyte, and cyst formation, and sclerosis. However, these processes are thought to be exacerbated in the first CMC joint as a result of a combination of biomechanical factors such as ligamentous laxity as well as the anatomical construction of the joint itself (Barron et al. 2000, Snider 1997). Osteoarthritis of the basilar joint of the thumb has the highest incidence in women between the ages of 30–60. This condition affects about one in four women and predominates at a rate of 10–20 times that in men (Barron et al. 2000, Newport 2000).

A history of previous trauma, most typically a fracture or a dislocation of the thumb can predispose both men and women to developing basilar joint OA (Snider 1997). The cumulative effects of basilar joint instability, degenerative changes, and repetitive shearing and grasping forces on the CMC joint results in this chronically painful, sometimes disabling condition (Newport 2000).

DATABASE

SUBJECTIVE

→ Postmenopausal women, although women as young as 30 can become symptomatic.
→ The patient will complain of radial-sided pain in the thumb that is exacerbated by turning doorknobs, twisting jars, and any movements requiring a pincer grasp (Newport 2000).
→ Younger women, especially, note pain in the thenar eminence of the affected thumb that sometimes radiates proximally along the thumb side of the forearm (Barron et al. 2000).
→ The patient complains of diminished grip strength and fine motor coordination in the affected hand.

→ Occasionally patients will complain of what they perceive to be a painful "lump" at the base of the thumb. This is the bony protrusion of the first metacarpal as it subluxes out of the joint (Barron et al. 2000).

→ Concerns about "muscle cramping" in the thumbs are not uncommon.

OBJECTIVE

→ Positive *Shoulder sign*—prominence at base of the thumb resulting from dorsal subluxation of the joint (Barron et al. 2000)

→ Decreased web space between the thumb and index finger

→ Decreased pinch strength. This can be qualified with the use of a pinch meter.

→ Severe point tenderness over the first CMC joint

→ Positive *Grind test*: pain, crepitus, and instability is elicited in the base of the thumb by adducting and rotating the thumb (Barron et al. 2000).

→ Positive *Abduction stress test* (AST): instruct the patient to resist abducting her thumb against that of the examiner's (Johnson, James. Personal communication. Department of Orthopedic Surgery. Kaiser Permanente. South San Francisco, Calif. December, 2001).

→ Adduction contracture of the first CMC occurs in advanced stages.

→ Occasionally swelling over the first CMC is noted.

→ Disuse atrophy of the thenar muscles can be observed on occasion.

ASSESSMENT

→ Osteoarthritis of the basilar joint of the thumb

→ R/O carpal tunnel syndrome

→ R/O de Quervain's disease

→ R/O old scaphoid fracture

→ R/O volar or dorsal ganglion cyst

→ R/O radial carpal arthritis

→ R/O trigger thumb

PLAN

DIAGNOSTIC TESTS

→ The existence of osteoarthritis of the basilar joint of the thumb can be confirmed on radiographs that should include anterior/posterior, lateral, oblique, and basal-joint stress views.

→ Radiographic findings are the basis of the classification system which stages the disease (Barron et al. 2000):

- *Stage I*: normal with the exception of the trapezoid metacarpal joint (TMJ), which indicates the presence of synovitis
- *Stage II*: joint space narrowing and osteophyte formation
- *Stage III*: significant TMJ narrowing, subchondral sclerosis, and the presence of larger osteophytes
- *Stage IV*: advanced disease of the TMJ and scapho-trapezoid joint (STJ), which often includes joint subluxation

TREATMENT/MANAGEMENT

→ Initial treatment consists of immobilizing the first CMC with a removal thumb-spica splint and 2–6 week course of NSAIDs (see **Table 8N.1**).

→ The patient may benefit from thenar muscle strengthening exercises, generally initiated in consultation with an occupational or hand therapist.

→ The most effective nonoperative treatment for OA of the basilar joint of the thumb is the administration of a corticosteroid injection from a qualified clinician.

→ Activity modification should be encouraged (Newport 2000).

CONSULTATION

→ The patient should be referred to an orthopedic hand surgeon for consultation when conservative treatment has failed and she continues to have pain and disability.

PATIENT EDUCATION

→ Teach the general principles that apply to most osteo-arthritic conditions, emphasizing:

- Splint applications should be continuous for 3 weeks.
- Caution the patient to avoid using standard wrist splints that are readily obtainable in most drugstores. The complete exposure of the thumb permitted by these splints is likely to exacerbate the pain associated with OA of the basilar joint of the thumb (Barron et al. 2000).

→ Activity modification:

- Minimize pinch force.
- Employ writing implements with large diameters.
- Read using a bookstand as opposed to grasping the reading material.

→ Counsel regarding the potential side effects of NSAIDs.

→ Side effects of cortisone injection in the first CMC may include:

- Post-injection soreness
- Temporary depigmentation and subcutaneous atrophy at the injection site

Trigger Fingers

Flexor tendon entrapment of the thumb or fingers, or *trigger fingers* constitutes the most common complaint associated with hand pain that presents in the primary ambulatory care setting (Biundo et al. 1997). The condition is often misdiagnosed as an injury, tendinitis, or arthritis.

Triggering of digits results from the idiopathic thickening of the proximal part of the flexor tendon sheath. Mechanical irritation from compressive and sheer forces in the tendon causes inflammation, swelling, and pain at the level of the A-1 pulley on the palmar surface of the metacarpal-phalangeal (MCP) joint. Most often occurring in the thumb and middle or small fingers, the painful snapping of the digit is caused by the discrepancy between the thickened tendon sheath and the A-1 pulley (Moore 2000).

The nodular thickening becomes trapped under the MCP ligament in the flexed finger, making subsequent extension of the digit painful and difficult, often requiring manual, passive manipulation to extend and flex the digit (Snider 1997).

Trigger digits affect persons of all ages, including neonates, although the condition typically presents in women, usually after the fourth decade (Mani et al. 2000, Moore 2000).

Trigger fingers and thumbs can be associated with underlying endocrine disorders that have a significant inflammatory component such as hypothyroidism and diabetes, rheumatoid arthritis, carpal tunnel syndrome, and systemic lupus erythematosus (Mani et al. 2000, Moore 2000, Snider 1997). A traumatic event rarely causes this condition. Reports of work-related trigger digits are anecdotal in the literature, and the association with occupational risk factors has not been well established (Mani et al. 2000). Multiple trigger fingers may exist in the same person and simultaneously occur in both hands.

Spontaneous resolution of a triggering digit is reported to be approximately 20% (Moore 2000). Although the standard interventions for trigger finger treatment are sometimes beyond the scope of the practitioner in a typical primary care setting, it is essential that the clinician recognizes the existence of a trigger finger and arrange for its timely treatment.

DATABASE

SUBJECTIVE

→ The patient complains of pain and stiffness in the involved digit(s) that is often worse upon rising in the morning.
→ The patient will be unable to fully flex her finger (Mani et al. 2000).
→ The patient awakens with her finger locked in flexion.
→ The patient complains of a painful snapping in the involved finger.
→ The patient may note a "lump" at the base of the MCP on the affected digit.
→ There may be swelling in the digits.
→ The patient may have a history of diabetes, gout, rheumatoid arthritis, lupus, or carpal tunnel syndrome.

OBJECTIVE

→ The affected thumb or finger may be mildly edematous.
→ The examiner can palpate a tender nodule or thickening on the palmar surface of the metacarpal just proximal to the palmar digital crease (Mani et al. 2000).
→ The patient can usually reproduce the snapping or locking of the digit at will. Otherwise, the examiner may have the patient flex all fingers into a fist.
  ■ The patient is then instructed to extend the unaffected digits while the examiner holds the trigger finger in flexion and then releases the finger into extension.
→ The patient may be unable to actively flex the involved digit. This is particularly true when the thumb is involved.

ASSESSMENT

→ Trigger thumb or finger
→ R/O flexor tenosynovitis
→ R/O osteoarthritis of the basilar joint of the thumb

→ R/O de Quervain's stenosing tenosynovitis
→ R/O ganglion of the flexor tendon sheath of the finger

PLAN

DIAGNOSTIC TESTS

→ X-rays are indicated only in the event of a precipitating traumatic event.

TREATMENT/MANAGEMENT

→ The treatment for trigger thumb or finger is the prompt administration of an injection of cortisone into the affected flexor tendon sheath from a qualified clinician (Biundo et al. 1997, Mani et al. 2000). A steroid injection has a success rate of approximately 93% for up to 4 months, and a cure rate of 72% (Moore, 2000).
→ Although several authors have reported a 73–77% success rate when treating trigger fingers by splinting them in extension, these patients had mild symptoms for less than 6 months. An average of 3–9 weeks of splinting was required to resolve their symptoms (Moore 2000).
→ Physical and occupational therapy have demonstrated minimal therapeutic efficacy in treating trigger fingers.

CONSULTATION

→ The patient should be promptly referred to an orthopedist or other trained practitioner for the steroid injection when necessary.
→ The patient should be referred to an orthopedist for surgical consultation when there is inadequately sustained relief from conservative treatment or in cases where the affected digit is locked in flexion.

PATIENT EDUCATION

→ Educate the patient on the pathogenesis of trigger fingers. Emphasize that there is nothing she did to provoke this condition, and therefore, no preventive measures to avoid its reoccurrence.
→ Inform the patient that it sometimes requires up to 4 weeks after a steroid injection before the trigger digit resolves. Patients with diabetes mellitus may experience a temporary elevation in blood sugar following the injection.

FOLLOW-UP

→ If the patient does not experience at least 4 months of adequately sustained relief from injections, surgery, in the form of a trigger finger release (TFR) should be recommended. TFR is a simple, 30-minute office procedure, performed under local anesthesia, which almost always results in permanent resolution of the condition.

Ganglion Cysts

Ganglion cysts are the most common tumors that form in the human body (Cheng et al. 1999, Snider 1997). A ganglion cyst is a benign lesion arising either from a synovial sheath or a joint capsule, filled with a usually transparent viscous fluid containing a mixture of hyaluronic acid, glucosamine, albumin, and globulin. Most often ganglions will occur on the dorsum or volar aspects of the wrist and hands. The most common ganglion cysts that occur on the wrist and hand include the dorsal, volar, flexor tendon sheath, and mucous cysts.

Typically affecting women in the 20–40 age range, the ganglion cyst has no known etiology. In general, the presence of a ganglion does not present a functional disturbance for the patient. The patient will usually seek medical treatment or consultation for reassurance that she does not have cancer, or because she is concerned about the cosmetic appearance of the lesion.

The primary care practitioner can reassure the patient that ganglion cysts are not cancerous and explain the range of treatment options.

DATABASE

SUBJECTIVE

→ A female of any age, but typically age 20–40
→ A mass on the wrist, hands or fingers is present that may have initially caused pain and then has resolved over time
→ The mass fluctuates in size.
→ A history of trauma may be present.
→ The patient may feel as though there is a pebble in her hand when she grips (e.g., the steering wheel of her car).
→ A fingernail depression exists in the digit affected with a mucous cyst on the distal interphalangeal joint (DIP).

OBJECTIVE

→ Volar or dorsal ganglions can usually be readily observed on the wrist or hand.
→ The lesions are typically nontender, regular, firm, and movable.
→ Flexor tendon sheath ganglion cysts (FTSGC) must be palpated for identification due to their small size (i.e., approximately 2 mm). FTSGC can be located on the palmar aspect of the proximal flexion crease in the affected finger.
→ Volar and dorsal wrist ganglions can be transilluminated with a penlight. If the lesion does not transilluminate, other diagnoses should be considered.
→ Striations or concavities of the fingernails can be noted with the presence of a mucous cyst.

ASSESSMENT

→ Dorsal ganglion cyst
→ Volar ganglion cyst
→ Flexor tendon sheath ganglion cyst
→ Mucous cyst
→ R/O trigger fingers
→ R/O Dupuytren's disease
→ R/O giant cell tumor
→ R/O bone tumor
→ R/O foreign body
→ R/O rheumatoid nodule

PLAN

DIAGNOSTIC TESTS

→ The most accurate diagnostic method to confirm the diagnosis of a ganglion cyst is aspiration. If the lesion cannot be aspirated, the presence of a solid mass such as a benign giant cell tumor should be considered. Laboratory analysis is not generally indicated unless the aspirate is not readily identifiable.
→ X-rays should be obtained:
  ■ To confirm the presence of a mucous cyst. Mucous cysts are always associated with degenerative changes in the DIP. A small osteophyte is typically noted with the soft tissue mass of the cyst on an x-ray. Standard anterior/posterior and lateral views are sufficient.
  ■ To rule out the presence of a solid soft tissue mass that may be encroaching on the bone, or a foreign body
  ■ To rule out the existence of a bone tumor
→ MRIs can be obtained to determine the presence of an occult ganglion cyst.

TREATMENT/MANAGEMENT

→ When the diagnosis of a cyst is made that does not cause pain or functional disability in the patient, no treatment is needed.
→ Volar and dorsal ganglion cysts can be easily aspirated in the clinic by a qualified clinician. Aspiration of the lesion can provide a diagnostic as well as a therapeutic effect. Aspiration can result in indefinite resolution of the mass, and there is no limit to the number of aspirations that can be performed.
→ Flexor tendon sheath ganglion cysts (FTSGC) can be treated by rupturing the lesion with 0.5 cc of 1% lidocaine and a number 27-gauge needle. Refer the patient to a qualified clinician.
→ Mucous cysts can be aspirated, but this procedure does not typically resolve the chief complaint, which is pain and deformity of the fingernail. Mucous cysts are always associated with the underlying existence of a bone spur, which is the probable cause of the pain and deformity.

CONSULTATION

→ Refer the patient to an orthopedic surgeon if she desires surgical excision of the mass. With the exception of a volar-radial ganglion cyst on the wrist, the excision is generally an office procedure.
→ The patient should be referred to an orthopedist or another qualified clinician, when necessary, for aspiration or rupture of lesion. FTSGCs are generally the only candidates for rupture due to their small size.

PATIENT EDUCATION

→ Educate the patient on the pathogenesis of ganglion cysts and the associated implications, emphasizing that the lesions are totally benign. Reassure the patient that treatment for ganglions is not necessary except for a volar wrist ganglion that impinges on the median nerve, causing an acute carpal tunnel syndrome.

→ Provide information on the treatment options for cysts (i.e., aspiration or surgery).
→ Post-surgical complication may include:
  ■ Protracted pain and stiffness in the wrist
  ■ Swelling for several months following surgery
  ■ Recurrence of the lesion 10% of the time
  ■ The permanent presence of a scar
→ Reassure the patient that there is no evidence the ganglions will ever become malignant.

FOLLOW-UP

→ The patient is advised to obtain routine follow-up as desired for assessment or aspiration of the lesion.

BIBLIOGRAPHY

Arle, J.E., and Zagler, E.L. 2000. Surgical treatment of common entrapment neuropathies in the upper limbs. *Muscle and Nerve* 23:1160–1174.

Barron, O.A., Glickel, S.Z., and Eaton, R.G. 2000. Basal joint arthritis of the thumb. *Journal of the Academy of Orthopaedic Surgeons* 8:314–323.

Biundo, J.J., Mipro, R.C., and Fahey, P. 1997. Sports–related and other soft tissue injuries, tendinitis, bursitis, and occupation–related syndromes. *Current Opinion in Rheumatology* 9:151–154.

Cheng, C.A., and Rockwell, W.B. 1999. Ganglions of the proximal interphalangeal joint. *American Journal of Orthopedics* 28:458–460.

D'Arcy, C.A., and McGee, S. 2000. Does this patient have carpal tunnel syndrome? The rational clinical examination. *Journal of the American Medical Association* 283:3110–3117.

Herbert, R., Gerr, F., and Dropkin, J. 2000. Clinical evaluation and management of work–related carpal tunnel syndrome. *American Journal of Industrial Medicine* 37:62–74.

Jarvik, J.G., Kliot, M., and Maravilla, K.R. 2000. MR nerve imaging of the wrist and hand. Nerve repair and reconstruction. *Hand Clinics* 16:13–24.

Laine, D.E. 1999. Low back pain and carpal tunnel syndrome: two troublesome presentations in the workplace. *Advance for Nurse Practitioners* 7:49–50, 74.

Lascar, T., and Laulan, J. 2000. Cubital tunnel syndrome: a retrospective review of 53 anterior subcutaneous transpositions. *Journal of Hand Surgery* 5:453–456.

Lincoln, A.E., Vernick, J.S., Ogaitis, S. et al. 2000. Interventions for the primary prevention of work–related carpal tunnel syndrome. *American Journal of Preventive Medicine* 18:37–46.

Mani, L., and Gerr, F. 2000. Occupational and environmental medicine: work–related upper extremity musculoskeletal disorders. *Primary Care: Clinics in Office Practice* 27:1–18.

Mondelli, M., Giannini, F., and Giacchi, M. 2002. Carpal tunnel syndrome incidence in a general population. *American Academy of Neurology* 58:289–94.

Moore, J.S. 2000. Flexor tendon entrapment of the digits: trigger finger and trigger thumb. *Journal of Occupational and Environmental Medicine* 42:526–545.

Newport, M.L. 2000. Upper extremity disorders in women. *Clinical Orthopaedics and Related Research* 372:85–94.

Padua, L., Padua, R., Aprile, I. et al. 2001. Multiperspective follow–up of untreated carpal tunnel syndrome. *American Academy of Neurology* 56:1459–1466.

Piligian, G., Herbert, R., Hearns, M. et al. 2000. Evaluation and management of chronic work–related musculoskeletal disorders of the distal upper extremity. *American Journal of Industrial Medicine* 37:75–93.

Snider, R.K. 1997. *Essentials of musculoskeletal care.* Rosemont, Ill.: American Academy of Orthopedics.

Szabo, R.M., and Madison, M. 1992. Carpal tunnel syndrome. *Orthopedic Clinics of North America* 23:103–109.

Witt, J.C., and Stevens, J.C. 2000. Neurologic disorders masquerading as carpal tunnel syndrome. *Mayo Clinic Proceedings* 75:409–413.

Wong, S.M., Hui, A.C., Tang, A. et al. 2001. Local versus systematic corticosteroids in the treatment of carpal tunnel syndrome. *American Academy of Neurology* 56:1565–1567.

Diane C. Putney, M.N., R.N., C.F.N.P.

8-1

Hip Pain

Hip pain can be challenging to diagnose because patients tend to characterize any regional pelvic discomfort of a musculoskeletal nature as hip pain. Hip pain can originate from any of six sources, including the hip joint, the soft tissue structures surrounding the hip and pelvis, pelvic bones, sacroiliac joints, lumbar spine, or the visceral organs associated with the genitalia, gastrointestinal, and urinary tract (Rossi et al. 2001, Snider 1997). The hip joint itself, like the shoulder, is a ball-and-socket joint comprised of the acetabulum and the femoral head. Surrounding the hip joint is a network of large muscle groups that coordinate the movements of flexion, extension, abduction, adduction, and internal and external rotation. The sciatic and lateral femoral nerves, along with the trochanteric iliopsoas bursae, are the soft tissue structures surrounding the hip and pelvis (Adkins et al. 2000, Rossi et al. 2001, Snider 1997).

The hip-related problems that affect women have been referenced in the literature for several centuries. Presently there is a compendium of clinical entities that is gaining recognition as *regional pain syndromes of the hip.* While the etiologies of hip pain can be interrelated and are probably multifactorial, there are several important causes of lateral hip pain.

Trochanteric bursitis predominates as a diagnosis in middle-aged and elderly women, although reports in the literature suggest an increasing incidence among younger athletic persons (Slawski et al. 1997). The trochanteric bursa, which is positioned just lateral to the greater trochanter, is subjected to repetitive microtrauma secondary to friction between the greater trochanter and the iliotibial band during flexion and extension of the hip. The pathogenesis appears to involve a combination of degenerative microtears or tendinopathy of the gluteus medius and minimus muscles that may or may not coincide with inflammation of the bursa (Bradley et al. 1998, Kagan 1999, Kingzett-Taylor et al. 1999, Slawski et al. 1997). Conservative treatment resolves symptoms in the vast majority of women with trochanteric bursitis.

Lateral hip pain may be the chief complaint of the patient with early osteoarthritis (OA) of the hip (Kagan 1999). However, patients with hip OA, which involves diminution of intra-articular cartilage between the femoral head and acetabulum, typically have pain in the groin and the anterior lateral thigh. The causes of hip OA can involve trauma, infection, and heredity factors, as well as idiopathic conditions such as *rapidly destructive hip disease* (RDHD). RDHD is a rare phenomenon in which there is complete destruction of the hip joint that progresses over the course of several weeks (Flik et al. 2000, Snider 1997).

Avascular necrosis (AVN) of the hip is characterized by the death of a comparatively small area of the trabecular bone within the femoral head. A less common cause of hip pain, AVN usually afflicts women in the third through fifth decades of life (Snider 1997). The precise etiology of AVN is not certain. It has been documented that any one of a combination of risk factors, ranging from trauma to regular use of oral corticosteroids to alcoholism can contribute to the onset of this condition, which affects between 10,000–20,000 persons in the United States annually (Adkins et al. 2000, Snider 1997). The middle-aged woman who complains of a deep, dull, aching groin pain, with a history of current or previous risk factors, coupled with an exam absent of obvious abnormalities, should be evaluated for AVN of the femoral head.

DATABASE

SUBJECTIVE

→ Middle-aged or elderly women
→ Young adult women who are competitive athletes in sports involving running/cutting actions, gymnastics, or dancing (Foye et al. 2001).
→ The patient may have a history of rheumatoid arthritis (RA), spinal stenosis, lateral disc herniation, or degenerative joint disease (DJD) of the lumbar spine, hips, or knees (Bradley et al. 1998, Kagan 1998).
→ Complaints of hip pain are most often unilateral.
→ Pain in the lateral aspect of the thigh radiating into the buttock and groin suggests trochanteric bursitis, OA of the hip, AVN, or iliotibial band syndrome (Adkins et al. 2000, Kagan 1998).

- Pain is aggravated with weight-bearing and when lying on the side affected with trochanteric bursitis.
→ Pain after prolonged sitting is characteristic of trochanteric bursitis, piriformis syndrome, and OA of the hip (Rossi et al. 2001, Snider 1997).
→ Buttock and leg pain without low back pain is typical of piriformis syndrome, not sciatica. This can be associated with paresthesias (Rossi et al. 2001).
→ Groin pain radiating down the anterior thigh to the knee suggests OA of the hip.
→ Deep, aching groin pain in the patient with a history of alcoholism, drug abuse, previous trauma to the hip, regular oral steroid use for medical reasons (i.e., asthma or PMR) suggests AVN.
→ Persistent groin pain in a young athlete that increases with activity may indicate a stress fracture of the femoral neck (Adkins et al. 2000).
→ Complaints of a snapping sensation that occurs over the hip with walking or pivoting movements may indicate snapping hip syndrome (Snider 1997).

OBJECTIVE

→ The patient with hip pain should have a complete examination of the lumbar spine. When the "hip pain" is reproduced by spinal movements and not provocative hip maneuvers, especially when the pain radiates past the knee, the clinician should suspect lumbar radiculopathy.
→ Leg-length discrepancies can predispose a patient to develop regional hip pain syndromes. If the discrepancy exceeds 2 cm, corrective action may be required with a heel lift (Adkins et al. 2000).
→ Deep tendon reflexes and straight leg raises should be within normal limits when the condition only involves the hip.
→ The patient with trochanteric bursitis experiences severe point tenderness over the greater trochanter upon palpation (Kagan 1999, Kingzett-Taylor et al. 1999, Snider 1997).
→ The patient with piriformis syndrome will have pain with active external rotation and passive internal rotation of the hip and palpation over the sciatic notch (Adkins et al. 2000).
→ The patient with piriformis syndrome will have point tenderness over the piriformis muscle, a small muscle located deep within the buttock (Robb-Nicholson 2001).
→ The patient with hip OA will most likely demonstrate significant quadriceps atrophy on the affected side.
→ Pain with internal rotation of the hip, especially with decreased range of motion, suggests hip joint pathology, specifically OA, or AVN in the later stages (Foye et al. 2001).
→ The elderly patient who complains of knee pain despite a normal knee exam, including x-rays, may have severe hip OA.
→ An antalgic gait is characteristic of hip OA.
→ Flexion contractures of the hip are typical of OA and advanced AVN.
→ The reproduction of groin pain with hip abduction, internal and external rotation is typical of AVN (Adkins et al. 2000).

→ Tenderness over the gluteus medius muscle insertion is probably gluteus medius tendinitis (Kingzett-Taylor et al. 1999).
→ Pain to palpation over the ischial tuberosity may indicate ischial bursitis (Adkins et al. 2000).

ASSESSMENT

→ Trochanteric bursitis
→ Osteoarthritis of the hip
→ Avascular necrosis of the hip
→ R/O gluteal bursitis
→ R/O piriformis syndrome
→ R/O ischial bursitis
→ R/O iliopsoas bursitis
→ R/O DJD of the lumbar spine
→ R/O rheumatoid arthritis
→ R/O herniated lumbar spine
→ R/O femoral cutaneous nerve entrapment
→ R/O tumor
→ R/O stress fracture of the femoral neck
→ R/O groin strain
→ R/O rapidly destructive hip disease (RDHD)
→ R/O nonmusculoskeletal pathology (i.e., gynecological, gastrointestinal or urinary tract problems)

PLAN

DIAGNOSTIC TESTS

→ X-rays: anterior/posterior (A/P), pelvis, and lateral views of the affected hip are standard. Additional radiographs of the lumbar spine or sacroiliac joints may be indicated.
  - The classic findings of narrowing of the hip joint space, osteophyte formation, sclerosis, and the presence of cysts in the femoral head are identified in varying stages of hip OA.
  - The *Crescent sign*, or a lucent area in the subchondral bone of the femoral head is the earliest finding of AVN that can be noted on an x-ray.
→ An MRI should be obtained when AVN of the hip is suspected, or to rule out a fracture of the hip, spinal pathology, or a tumor, even if plain x-rays are normal.
→ A bone scan can be obtained in the case of chronic trochanteric bursitis to rule out the presence of more serious pathology.
→ Laboratory studies can be useful when considering the following medical conditions:
  - Infection, or osteomyelitis: CBC, ESR
  - Ankylosing spondylosis (rare in women): HLA-B$_{27}$
  - Rheumatoid arthritis: RA
  - Systemic lupus erythematosus: antinuclear antibody test (ANA)
  - Polymyalgia rheumatica: ESR

TREATMENT/MANAGEMENT

→ See the **Osteoarthritis** chapter for hip osteoarthritis.
→ Trochanteric and ischial bursitis and piriformis syndrome:

- NSAIDs for 2-6 weeks (see **Table 8N.1, Anti-inflammatory and Analgesic Medication**)
- Application of ice packs for 25 minutes TID
- Avoid aggravating activity
- Physical therapy for hip strengthening and stretching exercises
- An injection into the trochanteric or ischial bursa of a steroid preparation by a qualified clinician is the most effective treatment (Foye et al. 2001).

→ When AVN is identified, provide:
- Crutches, cane or walker to avoid weight bearing on affected extremity
- Pain control with NSAIDs or mild analgesics
- Referral to an orthopedic surgeon to evaluate for a total hip arthroplasty (THA)

CONSULTATION

→ The patient may require referral to a qualified clinician for administration of a steroid injection.
→ The patient should be referred to an orthopedic surgeon in the following instances:
- Failure of any chronic condition that is, or has become, refractory to all reasonable conservative treatment
- AVN is identified as the cause of hip pain
- The patient has a hip or femoral neck fracture

→ The patient with a bone tumor should receive prompt consultation from a musculoskeletal oncologist.
→ Depending on the severity of the patient's symptoms, the patient with symptomatic spinal pathology may require consultation from one or more of the following specialists:
- Neurologist
- Neurosurgeon
- Orthopedic spine surgeon
- Physiatrist

→ Referral to a rheumatologist should be considered following a positive antinuclear antibody test, or if rheumatoid arthritis, polymyalgia rheumatica, or, in rare instances, ankylosing spondylosis, are identified.

PATIENT EDUCATION

→ Educate the patient on the pathophysiology of her specific hip condition.

→ Refer to the chapters on **Osteoarthritis**, and **Bursitis and Tendinitis**.

FOLLOW-UP

→ The patient should have a follow-up visit with the primary provider 4–6 weeks after treatment is initiated, and as required for modifications in the treatment regimen.
→ The patient is instructed to seek medical consultation if she fails to experience adequately sustained relief from treatment or if symptoms progress.
→ Document in progress notes and on problem list.

BIBLIOGRAPHY

Adkins, S.B., and Figler, R.A. 2000. Hip pain in athletes. *American Family Physician* 61:2109–2118.

Bradley, D.M., and Dillingham, M.F. 1998. Bursoscopy of the trochanteric bursa. *Arthroscopy: The Journal of Arthroscopic and Related Surgery* 14:884–887.

Flik, K., and Vargas, J.H. 2000. Rapidly destructive hip disease: a case report and review of the literature. *The American Journal of Orthopedics* July 29:549–552.

Foye, P.M., and Stitik, T.P. 2001. Trochanteric bursitis. *eMedicine Journal*. Accessed online at: http://emedicine.com/sports/topic137.htm on June 1, 2003.

Kagan, A. 1999. Rotator cuff tears of the hip. *Clinical Orthopaedics and Related Research* 368:135–140.

Kingzett–Taylor, A., Tirman, P.F.J., Feller, J. et al. 1999. Tendinosis and tears of gluteus medius and minimus muscles as a cause of hip pain: MR imaging findings. *American Journal of Radiology.* 173:1123–1126.

Robb–Nicholson, C. 2001. By the way, doctor: what is piriformis syndrome? *Harvard Women's Health Watch.* March 8:8.

Rossi, P., Cardinali, P., Serrao, M. et al. 2001. Magnetic resonance imaging findings in piriformis syndrome: a case report. *Archives of Physical Medicine and Rehabilitation* 82:519–521.

Slawski, D.P., and Howard, R.F. 1997. Surgical management of refractory trochanteric bursitis. *American Journal of Sports Medicine* 25:86–89.

Snider, R.K. 1997. *Essentials of musculoskeletal care.* Rosemont, Ill.: American Academy of Orthopedics.

Diane C. Putney, M.N., R.N., C.F.N.P.

8-J

Knee Pain

The knee is the largest synovial joint in the human body. Primarily a weight-bearing, hinge-type structure, the knee is subject to countless repetitive biomechanical forces, including the routine, complex gross-motor movements of daily living; rigorous athletic endeavors; malalignment features; and impact absorbed from physical trauma (Adler et al. 2001, Williams et al. 2000). The structural vulnerability of the knee joint makes the complaint of *knee pain* one of the most common problems encountered in the primary care setting.

The knee is comprised of three compartments formed by the articulation of the medial and lateral femoral condyles with the medial and lateral tibial plateaus and patella respectively (Johnson 2000). Positioned between the articular surfaces of the distal femur and proximal tibia are the medial and lateral menisci—tough fibrous structures of protein, water, and molecules—which permit its main function of shock absorption (Adler et al. 2001). The menisci, along with the medial and lateral collateral ligaments (MCL and LCL) play lesser roles in stabilizing the knee (Williams et al. 2000). The anterior cruciate ligament (ACL) inserting on the front of the proximal tibia and the back of the distal femur, promotes the knee's rotational and anterior stability (Snider 1997). Posterior knee stability is the function of the posterior cruciate ligament (PCL)—a thick, short ligament that crosses the ACL from the anterior distal femur to the posterior proximal tibia. The patella ligament is a wide structure formed by the convergence of the ends of the four quadriceps muscles. Covering the patella, and inserting onto the tibial tubercle, this ligament is an important component in the extensor mechanism of the knee. Of the eight bursae positioned within and around the knee, the suprapatellar pouch, prepatellar, semimembranous, and pes anserinus bursae have primary clinical significance. No less important than its soft tissue and bony components are the surrounding quadriceps and hamstring muscle groups that support, stabilize, and permit flexion and extension of the knee.

Knee pain can be categorized as acute or chronic, as well as by the specific structures involved. The person with hip degenerative joint disease and an intervertebral disk prolapse at the third and fourth lumbar vertebrae can also experience pain that is referred to the knee (Snider 1997).

The age of the patient with knee pain can be a significant mediating variable when reviewing the patient's history, clinical findings, and formulating a reasonable diagnosis and treatment plan. For example, in patients over age 40, degenerative changes are more likely than overuse conditions.

The vast majority of acute and chronic knee pain, excluding fractures and infections, involve the patellofemoral complex, ligament and meniscal pathology, or degenerative joint disease. These more common painful knee conditions are the focus of this chapter.

Acute Knee Pain

Acute knee pain is most often the result of specific trauma to the bones such as the patella and proximal tibia; the surrounding soft tissue structures, which include the medial and lateral menisci, anterior cruciate and medial collateral ligaments; or the extensor mechanisms of the quadriceps tendon and patella ligament. Significant injuries to the lateral collateral and posterior cruciate ligaments are less common and less clinically significant. Atraumatic conditions that can cause sudden onset of knee pain include joint infection and gout.

More than 250,000 patients annually sustain a complete *anterior cruciate ligament (ACL) tear*. The fact that the ACL-deficient knee is more prevalent in women has been well documented. When women and men engage in competitive, noncontact sports with the same equipment while conforming to similar rules and regulations, the incidence of ACL injury among women exceeds men by an eight to two ratio (Griffin et al. 2000). The patient typically reports an incident during which the knee pivoted sharply, or was forcefully hyperextended. The trauma is experienced as an acutely painful pop or tearing sensation, followed by immediate swelling, and inability to continue the previous activity. The pain and swelling can be expected to diminish considerably over time, but the knee continues to buckle or give way. This should alert the clinician to the possibility of an ACL-deficient knee (Williams et al. 2000). Left untreated, the unstable knee can hasten the degeneration of intra-articular cartilage, increasing the risk of cartilage tears, and ultimately precipitate the premature onset of osteoarthritis (Griffin et al. 2000, Snider 1997, Williams et al. 2000).

A *medial collateral ligament (MCL) tear* can occur when a valgus force without rotation is applied to the knee, an event that is common during running/cutting sports such as soccer and football (Snider 1997). Unless an MCL tear, even when complete, is associated with an ACL rupture, significant meniscal injury, or fracture, the patient is expected to achieve full recovery in 6–12 weeks with conservative treatment (Griffin et al. 2000). The person with a medial or lateral meniscal injury will often provide a history of some trauma associated with the onset of her symptoms, which are typically pain and swelling of the knee. The event may well be recalled as minor in nature, such as squatting to retrieve an object. The activity preceding the onset of symptoms is often attributed to the present injury only in retrospect. As a result, the clinician may fail to even consider the possibility of a meniscal injury. The patient's complaints may be misdiagnosed as arthritis in a middle-aged or elderly person and patella femoral pain or tendinitis in the young adult. The classic history of popping and locking emphasized in the literature may or may not be apparent.

An anterior cruciate ligament tear or a medial collateral ligament or a meniscal injury can occur in isolation or simultaneously in varying combinations. None of these injuries are an orthopedic emergency or require urgent consultation. Conservative treatment can and should be instituted by the primary care provider. Even in the event of a complete ACL tear in a competitive athlete, surgical intervention is not routinely considered for at least six weeks after the injury. Measures such as pain control, icing, and expeditious use of physical therapy are appropriate conservative intervention. It is incumbent upon the primary care provider to reassure and educate the patent with a knee injury in this regard. Unless a fracture is identified or suspected, the benefits from the timely application of an ice pack will far outweigh the immediate acquisition of an MRI and orthopedic surgery referral—two demands frequently made by patients and acceded to by clinicians.

DATABASE

SUBJECTIVE

→ The patient with an ACL-deficient knee typically provides a history similar to the following:

- The average age of a patient with an ACL injury is 30–40 (Griffin et al. 2000).
- She has sustained a vigorous twisting or hyperextension force injury to the knee.
- Swelling begins rapidly following the injury (Williams et al. 2000).
- She is unable to immediately resume the activity that preceded the injury and complains of diminished range of motion.
- About one-third of the individuals with an ACL tear will

report the occurrence of a popping or tearing sensation at the time of the trauma (Snider 1997).

- The patient may complain that the knee gives out on her for weeks following the injury as she attempts to resume her regular activity level.
- The patient reports that her knee feels unsteady, weak, or untrustworthy even if it does not give way.
- The individual with an ACL-deficient knee who presents months, or even years, after the precipitating event often complains of mild knee pain and occasional swelling, particularly following vigorous activity (Williams et al. 2000).

→ The patient with an isolated medial collateral ligament tear describes a history of engaging in a running/cutting sport or skiing event, during which time she sustained a valgus force to the knee (Beaty 1999).

- The patient is often able to continue participation in her activity following the injury.
- She complains of pain with pivoting motions of the knee.
- Swelling and stiffness are minimal.
- Reports of instability, popping, or catching are uncommon with an MCL injury, unless other soft tissue structures have been damaged (Snider 1997).

→ The patient with a meniscal tear may recall a precipitating traumatic event involving the knee, such as a twisting injury, or severe pain that occurred when standing from a squatting position (Beaty 1999).

- Complaints of persistent knee pain with mild swelling, exacerbated by pivoting movements, walking up and down stairs, and vigorous activity are common.
- It is not unusual for the patient with a meniscal tear to report pain awakening her at night when turning in bed. Sometimes, a history to this effect may be the *only* complaint.
- The patient with a meniscal tear may describe an occasional to frequent painful popping or clicking sensation in the knee (Snider 1997).
- The sensation of the knee catching or buckling is common for patients with a meniscal injury.
- An authentic instance of the knee locking, a phenomenon most often associated with a meniscal tear in which a piece of torn cartilage forms a wedge in the knee that prevents its normal movement, is not especially common. Buckling and catching sensations may lead the patient to believe her knee is locking.
- The presence of a meniscal tear should not be discounted in patients who fail to recall any trauma or painful body mechanics prior to the onset of her symptoms.

→ The knee is the most frequently infected synovial joint (Snider 1997). The possibility of an infected knee should be considered when the patient describes the sudden onset of atraumatic knee pain that rapidly progresses, is unremitting, is exacerbated by any movement, and prevents her from bearing weight.

- The patient may have a low-grade fever.
- The patient may or may not complain of swelling.
- A history of diabetes is a significant risk factor.

→ The person who complains of the sudden onset of atraumatic knee pain, swelling, and redness may have gout, a form of crystalline deposition disease (Snider 1997).

- The patient may complain of fever.
- The patient may or may not have a history of prior gouty episodes in other joints.

OBJECTIVE

→ An antalgic gait: a gait in which the affected knee is flexed or in recurvatum (abnormal backward bending of the knee) with a medial or lateral thrust (Cole et al. 1999).

→ Quadriceps atrophy is typically noted in the knee with acute or chronic ACL-deficiency.

→ A moderate to large knee joint effusion is often present with an acute knee injury, in which case the patient's knee assumes a resting position of 15–20° of flexion (Johnson 2000).

→ Deep, confluent erythema over the knee is most typical of gout, but infection must also be ruled out.

→ Medial or lateral joint line tenderness can be appreciated in an acute meniscal injury.

→ Tenderness specifically along the MCL suggests an MCL strain.

- Medial and lateral knee stability is tested in both full extension and with the knee in 25–30° of flexion when the patient is lying supine on the exam table. The examiner alternately applies a valgus and varus force to the knee with firm palm pressure. If the joint line opens more than 10 mm while the knee is flexed, a grade III tear is suggested (Snider 1997).

→ An ACL-deficient knee should be suspected when the examiner elicits a positive Lachman's and anterior drawer test, and/or a pivot shift. Always test the unaffected knee first for comparison (Beaty 1999).

- *Anterior drawer test*: While the patient is lying supine with both knees flexed to 90° and the examiner sitting on the patient's feet for stabilization, the examiner pulls forward on the patient's tibia with both thumbs placed on either side of the inferior pole of the patella. Up to 2 mm of shift is normal. A 4 mm or more anterior shift indicates a disruption of the anterior or lateral ligaments.

- *Lachman's test*: the patient is lying supine on the examining table. The examiner may find it helpful to position his or her own internally rotated knee under the patient's thigh if the patient is large or has difficulty relaxing. Either way, grasp the proximal tibia and pull it forward while stabilizing the distal femur with the other hand. The examiner will note the absence of a firm end point in the ACL-deficient knee.

- *Pivot shift*: this can sometimes be a challenge to perform, unless the patient is completely relaxed. This maneuver is performed with the patient lying supine with the knee extended. The examiner applies a valgus stress while internally rotating the entire leg and gradually flexing the knee. In an ACL-deficient knee, the tibia will shift at least 10° anteriorly on the femur.

→ The patient with an acute ACL or meniscal injury typically has limited knee flexion secondary to pain.

→ When the patient's knee is genuinely locked, the knee cannot be actively or passively manipulated through full range of motion because a torn piece of cartilage is wedged in the joint.

→ A palpable, painful joint line clunk or pop can sometimes be palpated in the patient with a meniscal tear with the application of *McMurray's test*. The examiner internally and externally rotates the patient's flexed knee while she is lying supine (Snider 1997).

→ The patient with an infected knee joint may have a knee that is relatively normal in appearance; however, she typically experiences severe pain with manipulation of the joint to any degree. It is difficult to bear weight on the affected knee to any degree.

→ When the patient with a history of an acute injury is unable to fully extend her knee or perform a straight leg raise, the possibility of a ruptured extensor tendon mechanism must be considered (Snider 1997).

→ The patient with a posterior cruciate ligament tear may reveal the characteristic posterior sag on exam. With the patient lying supine and both knees flexed at 90° the examiner will note that the tibia "sags" back on the femur (Beaty 1999).

ASSESSMENT

→ Anterior cruciate ligament tear
→ Medial and/or lateral meniscal tear
→ Medial collateral ligament injury
→ R/O gout
→ R/O knee joint infection
→ R/O patellar dislocation
→ R/O patellar tendon rupture
→ R/O posterior cruciate ligament tear
→ R/O tibial plateau fracture
→ R/O patellar fracture
→ R/O osteochondral loose body

PLAN

DIAGNOSTIC TESTS

→ X-rays: anterior/posterior (A/P), and lateral x-rays are standard views when the patient presents with a history of acute trauma. In the event that a fracture has been ruled out, alternate x-ray views can be helpful.

- A/P standing to determine the extent joint space narrowing.
- Bilateral *Merchant's view* can reveal the presence of patellofemoral subluxation, dislocation, or patellar fracture.
  - Merchant's view is a tangential view of the patella taken with the knee flexed to 30° (Boden et al. 1997).
- With few exceptions, when soft tissue injuries of the knee are suspected, the patient's x-rays will not demonstrate acute bony abnormalities.
  - A small avulsion fracture of the tibial spine can sometimes be noted when there is an acute ACL tear where the ligament inserts onto the tibia.

- The presence of an intra-articular osteochondral fragment or loose body, when observed on a plain x-ray, may be the cause of painful locking or catching of the knee (Bianchi 1999).

→ MRI has become the gold standard diagnostic study to confirm or rule out soft tissue injuries. Unless an occult fracture or tumor is suspected, an MRI is rarely necessary. An MRI should be considered it the patient fails to adequately respond to a reasonable trial of conservative treatment over the course of at least six weeks, and referral to an orthopedist is imminent.

→ Bone scans may be obtained, in consultation with the orthopedist, to rule out an infection (Snider 1997).

→ Laboratory tests:
- To rule out infection: CBC, ESR
- Knee aspiration: gram stain, culture and sensitivity
- To rule out gout: uric acid level

TREATMENT/MANAGEMENT

→ The initial and ongoing management of acute knee injuries can vary significantly, given the patient's age, symptoms, athleticism, anxiety level, and tolerance of the condition. Unless the clinician suspects a fracture or an intra-articular knee infection, appropriate therapeutic intervention should be instituted by the primary care clinician (Beaty 1999).

→ Crutches can be provided for the patient who cannot bear weight on the affected knee.

→ Unless contraindicated, a 2-week course of NSAIDs should be prescribed (see **Table 8N.1, Anti-inflammatory and Analgesic Medication**).

→ Analgesics such as propoxyphene napsylate or hydrocodone bitartrate can be prescribed during the acute phase of the injury (see **Table 8N.1**).

→ Unless a fracture is suspected, the patient should not be discouraged from full weight-bearing as tolerated.

→ The application of a hinged knee brace can be prescribed for the patient with an acute ACL or grade III MCL tear for up to six weeks. Bracing is inappropriate for a meniscal tear.
- Immobilizing the knee following a ligament injury can actually inhibit the healing process in the bone-ligament-bone complex (Woo et al. 2000).

→ Physical therapy, beginning with controlled range of motion exercises, is vital to prevent arthrofibrosis and reestablish optimal function of the knee (Woo et al. 2000) and should be prescribed soon after a ligament injury.

CONSULTATION

→ Urgent orthopedic consultation should be obtained for the patient under the following conditions:
- The patient appears to have a *locked knee*. This must be distinguished from the patient's history of a locking knee. The patient with a locked knee will present to the examiner with a knee fixed in what is usually a position of mild flexion. The patient cannot move her knee because of a biomechanical obstruction—usually a torn or

displaced meniscus—not because it merely causes pain to do so. The patient with the locked knee will most often require an arthroscopic procedure to repair the meniscus.
- When it is determined that the patient has an infected knee, or when infection is highly suspected. The patient is taken to the operating room for immediate incision, drainage, and irrigation of the infected knee.
- When a fracture about the knee is noted on an x-ray.

→ Routine referral to an orthopedist should occur in the following instances:
- The patient has an ACL tear, complains of instability, and wants surgical reconstruction of the ligament. The ideal candidate for an ACL reconstruction is under the age of 55, not especially obese, and does not demonstrate more than mild degenerative changes on a plain x-ray.
- The patient has persistent knee pain and swelling in her knee, especially when this is accompanied by mechanical symptoms (i.e., catching, popping, or buckling).
- The patient has not responded adequately to conservative treatment after 6–10 weeks.

→ Obese individuals do not derive the same long-term benefit from surgical repair or reconstruction of soft tissue injuries as persons of normal body weight. Consider referral for dietary consultation.

PATIENT EDUCATION

→ Educate the patient about the pathophysiology of her specific injury.
- A complete rupture of the medial collateral ligament will heal in about 6–10 weeks with conservative treatment.
- Grade I and grade II MCL injuries heal within 11–20 days (Woo et al. 2000).
- Complete ACL tears will not heal with conservative treatment; however, unless the patient is younger than 40, active, athletic, or complaining of instability, surgery is not always the most appropriate treatment option.
  - Physical therapy can be used for quadricept and hamstring strengthening.
  - An ACL stabilizing brace can be used when engaging in recreational sports.
  - If the patient is over age 40 and asymptomatic, she may not require any treatment.
- Small meniscal tears usually will heal with conservative treatment (Snider 1997).
- The patient with a symptomatic, untreated meniscal tear is at risk of incurring further knee injury as well as osteoarthritis over the long term (Snider 1997, Williams et al. 2000).
- Whether instability from untreated ACL tears will eventually result in osteoarthritis remains a matter of controversy (Williams et al. 2000).

→ A patient with an acute knee injury should be instructed on the value of treating it with rest, ice, and elevation.

→ The American Academy of Orthopedic Surgeons has maintained the position for the past 20 years that there is no

evidence that prophylactic knee bracing will prevent injuries (Griffin et al. 2000).
→ The patient with acute knee injuries should be advised to cross train until her symptoms completely resolve:
  ▪ Swimming
  ▪ Biking
  ▪ Weight resistance training with the exception of leg extensions, deep squats and forward lunges
→ Certain medical conditions can hinder the healing process of ligament injuries (Woo et al. 2000):
  ▪ Poor circulation
  ▪ Infection
  ▪ Diabetes

FOLLOW-UP

→ Make a follow-up visit in 1–3 weeks, depending on the injury, severity of symptoms, and the patient's level of anxiety.
→ The patient should otherwise return for routine follow-up 4–6 weeks after the injury to have her need for orthopedic referral further assessed.
→ The patient who has sustained an acute knee injury should be advised to seek follow-up if her symptoms persist in spite of conservative treatment and she cannot resume her normal activity level after 10–12 weeks.

Chronic Knee Pain

With the possible exception of collateral ligament injuries, inadequately treated acute trauma to the knee can result in *chronic knee pain* and *instability*. Atraumatic knee problems in a young adult or adolescent female are most often due to one of a number of *patellofemoral pain (PFP) syndromes*. The patella, which is situated within the extensor mechanism comprised of the quadriceps muscles and tendon, is the largest sesamoid bone in the human body. While the quadriceps tendon functions as the primary dynamic stabilizer of the patella, the static or stationary stabilization is maintained by the medial patellofemoral ligament (MPFL) (Boden et al. 1997). The patella-femoral joint complex is subjected to a myriad of forces, which, given any number of structural and biomechanical factors, can precipitate the onset of PFP. These factors most often involve the cumulative trauma associated with repetitive squatting that occurs during sports requiring running/cutting maneuvers or patella compression from lateral tilt of the patella that is caused by a tight lateral retinaculum, obesity, or weight lifting. Chronic patellar subluxation is typically associated with malalignment of the lower extremities, such as a valgus gait and excessive foot pronation (Boden et al. 1997, Snider 1997). The abnormal tracking of the patient that occurs with flexion and extension of the knee can precipitate the onset of anterior peripatellar knee pain.

Even routine activities such as walking up and down stairs substantially increase the loading forces on the patella-femoral joint complex. This can be an underlying factor in a patella dislocation or over the course of time result in primary osteoarthritis (OA) of the patella-femoral joint (Juhn 1999).

A malalignment problem of the lower extremities is just one of a number of biomechanical and physiological precursors to the development of OA of the knee. Other risk factors include obesity, history of previous meniscectomy, and having sustained a knee injury before the age of 22 (Adler et al. 2001, Cole et al. 1999, Williams et al. 2000).

Osteoarthritis of the knee is characterized primarily by the degeneration of intra-articular cartilage with the simultaneous increase of water content. It is three times more prevalent in women than men, and is most likely to become symptomatic in the fifth decade of life (Adler et al. 2001, Snider 1997). The onset of symptoms can occur long after there is radiographic evidence of the disease. Osteoarthritis of the knee can affect any one or all three compartments (i.e., medial, lateral, and patellofemoral). (See the **Osteoarthritis** chapter.)

The pain associated with OA occurs with activity in the initial stages. There appears to be no relationship between activity and premature development of knee OA (Cole et al. 1999). As OA in the knee progresses, the patient will experience an increase in pain, including pain at rest and after prolonged sedentary activity, as well as the onset of mechanical symptoms such as catching and buckling of the knee. When patients decrease their activity level to avoid exacerbating the symptoms, atrophy of the quadriceps and hamstrings muscles result, leading to instability.

The primary care provider is in a unique position to evaluate the extent of the patient's knee arthritis within the context of her entire physical and emotional well-being. A meaningful discussion of factors that contribute to an appropriate treatment plan, as well as realistic expectations with respect to prognosis for both conservative and operative interventions should ensue between the patient and her primary care provider. Medical conditions such as obesity or unstable chronic pulmonary disease that can have a significant impact on the viability of treatment options should be addressed before the patient is referred to an orthopedist for surgical consultation.

Patellofemoral Pain Syndromes
DATABASE

SUBJECTIVE

→ The patient is likely to be under age 45.
→ The patient has a slender to medium build and engages in frequent athletic activity.
→ The patient is obese or has recently experienced sudden weight gain, including that associated with pregnancy.
→ The patient may report a history of minor trauma preceding the onset of her symptoms (Boden et al. 1997).
→ Occasionally the patient will reveal a remote history of a patellar dislocation.
→ A middle-aged patient has an occupation that requires repetitive squatting, kneeling, or climbing (i.e., custodian, gardener).
→ The patient complains of anterior or peripatellar knee pain, which is typically exacerbated by the following activities:
  ▪ Climbing up and down stairs or ladders

- Participation in running/cutting sports such as tennis or basketball
- Running or jogging several miles or more
- When getting up out of a chair after prolonged sitting, which is characterized as a positive *Theater sign* (Snider 1997).
→ The patient describes a "deep, aching pain" or "sharp, stabbing pain."
→ The pain subsides with rest.
→ The patient often complains of mechanical symptoms:
  - Sensation of giving way
  - Buckling
  - Catching
→ On occasion, the patient will report swelling.
→ The patient's history includes long-standing knee pain, which originated in her adolescence.

OBJECTIVE

→ The patient's gait will frequently demonstrate:
  - Femoral anteversion
  - Genu valgum: knock-knees
  - Internal tibial torsion: the patellae point toward each other
  - Exaggerated foot pronation: flat foot
→ The patient will typically have crepitus in both knees, which is appreciated by cupping the hand over the patella while passively flexing and extending the patient's knee (Boden et al. 1997).
→ A knee effusion is generally not evident, but the examiner may note a generalized puffy appearance over the anterior knee.
→ The patient often has pain when directed by the examiner to squat, duck walk, and hop.
→ The patient may have mild, diffuse medial and lateral joint line tenderness.
→ The patient with a lateral patellar tilt generally has increased Q-angles of the patella. The *Q-angle* is basically a measurement of the angle between the quadriceps and the patellar tendon (Beaty 1999).
  - The examiner draws a line from the tip of the anterior-superior-iliac spine to the center of the patella, and another line from the center of the patellae to the mid-tibial tubercle. The normal "Q-angle" is about 10° in men and 15° in women. The examiner sometimes notes atrophy of the vastus medialis obliquus (VMO) muscle.
→ The patellae are often hypermobile and easily subluxed when the examiner pushes the patella from side to side with the patient laying supine while the knees are in full extension. The patella should not displace more than half its width, medially or laterally.
→ When the patient's dislocation symptoms are reproduced upon the applications by the examiner of medial pressure on the patella, the patient is said to have a positive *Patellar apprehension test.*
→ Abnormal tracking of the patella can best be determined while the patient is sitting with her knees flexed over the

side of the exam table. The examiner grasps the patella and passively flexes and extends the patient's leg. The examiner will be able to palpate the lateral excursion of the patella as the patient brings her knee into full extension.
→ The presence of a tender thickened area of synovium located just medial to the patella with a palpable snap may reveal the presence of a plica syndrome. A plica can mimic a meniscal tear (Beaty 1999).
→ The patient with patellofemoral pain (PFP) will usually have normal range of motion.
→ Ligamentous stability and tibial rotation tests should be within normal limits in persons with PFP.

ASSESSMENT

→ Patellofemoral pain syndromes
→ R/O meniscal injury
→ R/O ACL or MCL injury
→ R/O plica syndrome
→ R/O patellofemoral osteoarthritis
→ R/O osteochondritis dissecans: a condition in which a small area of subchondral bone becomes necrotic. The lesion may remain within the bone, or disengage from the bone, settling into the joint space (Hixon et al. 2000).
→ R/O patellar tendinitis

PLAN

DIAGNOSTIC TESTS

→ X-rays: anterior-posterior weight-bearing, lateral, and Merchant's view, which is a tangential view of the patella taken with the knee flexed to 30° (Boden et al. 1997).
→ MRIs: may be obtained if the examiner suspects a meniscal or ACL injury.
→ Bone scan: can be helpful to determine the presence of inflammation or arthritic changes around and behind the patella, especially when routine radiographs are normal.
→ Laboratory tests:
  - RF
  - ANA
  - ESR
  - CBC
  - Aspiration of synovial fluid when indicated by the patient's history and exam.
→ CT scans are an excellent means of determining precise patellar malalignment (Boden et al. 1997), but the routine acquisition of such a study is not recommended.

TREATMENT/MANAGEMENT

→ Patellofemoral pain syndromes are most often successfully managed with conservative treatment.
→ The essential aspect of treatment is rigorous patient compliance to a quadriceps and hamstring strengthening program (Beaty 1999, Juhn 1999).
  - Weight resistance exercises:
    - Leg presses
    - 30° squats

- Hamstring curls
- Straight leg raises
- Stationary and regular bike riding are excellent methods of strengthening muscle groups without stress on the patellofemoral joint complex.

→ Avoid running/cutting activities for 4–6 weeks or until the pain subsides.

→ A course of NSAIDs for 2–6 weeks is recommended for persons who complain of experiencing pain most of the time regardless of their activity level (see **Table 8N.1**).

→ Applications of ice for 25 minutes QD–TID are recommended to facilitate the resolution of inflammation.

→ Semi-rigid medial arch supports are important for patients with a valgus gait or excessive foot pronation.

→ The patient may find it helpful to wear a patellar stabilization brace initially. These braces can vary considerably in their construction. The simplest and least cumbersome brace is referred to as Cho-Pat, which is essentially a Velcro strip applied snugly just below the patella. However, when the patient has severe lateral riding of the patella, a hinge brace with padded rings that force the patella into maintaining normal alignment may be prescribed.

CONSULTATION

→ Consultation with an orthopedic surgeon is recommended in the following instances:
- When the patient's symptoms have not adequately resolved with a minimum of six months of rigorous nonoperative treatment.
- Meniscal or ligament injury is suspected.
- A plica syndrome is present.
- A symptomatic osteochondritic lesion is demonstrated on the x-rays or MRI.
- A referral to a dietician or a bariatric surgeon may be required before the obese patient can significantly benefit from therapy.

PATIENT EDUCATION

→ Educate the patient on the pathophysiology and biomechanics of PFP syndromes.

→ The importance of maintaining a regular quadriceps and hamstring strengthening program, even when becoming asymptomatic, cannot be overemphasized.

→ Patients who are athletic require instruction in cross-training:
- Biking
- Swimming
- Weight resistance

→ Patients who weight train should avoid the following exercises at all times:
- Deep squats
- Leg extensions
- Forward lunges

→ Runners are less likely to become symptomatic if they adhere to the following:

- Run on level ground, not hills, and preferably on dirt, grass or sand, rather than concrete or asphalt.
- Wear good running shoes with semi-rigid cushioned medial arch supports.

→ The patient may require instruction on activity modification with respect to her occupational demands:
- The use of knee pads
- Sitting on a low stool with legs extended rather than squatting or kneeling

→ The patient requires proper instruction on the use of NSAIDs (see **Table 8N.1**).

→ When the patient is using a patellofemoral support, educate her on its proper application and use.

→ The patient should be discouraged from going up and down stairs when she has the option to do otherwise.

FOLLOW-UP

→ The patient with PFP should return for routine follow-up approximately 6–8 weeks following the initiation of treatment.

→ The patent should be advised to seek medical follow-up when her symptoms persist despite reasonable conservative treatment.

Osteoarthritis of the Knee
DATABASE
SUBJECTIVE

→ The average age of onset of knee OA in women is 40–45 (Adler et al. 2001).

→ The patient is often obese.

→ The patient sometimes provides a remote history of a significant knee injury, (e.g., fracture) (Adler et al. 2001).

→ The predominant complaint of the patient with knee OA is pain which typically occurs:
- In the affected compartment of the knee during the early stages (Cole et al. 1999, Snider 1997)
- In association with activity
- After prolonged sedentary activity
- When the weather becomes cold and damp
- When squatting or kneeling
- When going up and down stairs, or walking down hills
- After a prolonged period of weight-bearing
- At the extremes of flexion and extension
- At rest in the advanced stages (Cole et al. 1999)

→ Complaints of swelling are common.

→ Descriptions of mechanical symptoms are typical of moderate to severe OA, the presence of a loose body, or ligamentous injury (Snider 1997, Williams et al. 2000):
- Giving way
- Buckling
- Catching

→ Complaints of stiffness and limited range of motion are common in persons with OA.

→ The patient sometimes reveals a previous history of knee surgery (Williams et al. 2000). The relationship between a prior meniscectomy and the development of arthritis has been well documented (Cole et al. 1999, Williams et al. 2000).

→ Hip pain from OA and AVN typically radiates down the anterior thigh and into the knee. Knee pain can also be referred from the lumbar spine.

OBJECTIVE

→ Standard practice dictates that an examination of the hip is performed on a person with a chief complaint of knee pain.

- If the patient complains that the pain radiates past the calf and into the foot, especially when accompanied by paresthesias and a history of low back pain, the clinician should examine the spine to rule out a central lesion.

→ Gait (Cole et al. 1999)

- Genu varum or varus gait: "bowlegs," typical of long standing medial compartment disease of the knee, is the most common malalignment problem observed in the patient with knee DJD.
- Genu valgum or valgus gait: "knock knees," the patient likely has degenerative changes of the lateral knee compartment. This is more common in women and patients with associated RA (Snider 1997).
- The patient has trouble squatting due to pain that increases with duckwalking or hopping.

→ Quadriceps atrophy is noted, especially when the patient's symptoms have been long-standing.

→ Flexion contractures may be noted in patients with advanced knee OA. Contractures occur when there is at least minus 10° of extension, which is caused by the formation of fibrous bands within the hamstring tendons (Cole et al. 1999).

→ A knee effusion may be present to varying degrees and is a typical response to chronic inflammation.

→ The patient often has joint line tenderness located along the affected compartment.

→ The patient with severe knee OA can demonstrate laxity or pseudolaxity that is secondary to either previous ligament injury or unicompartmental OA. Pseudolaxity is a phenomenon that can be noted when the examiner is able to open up the joint line by applying a varus or valgus stress to the knee (Williams et al. 2000).

→ The patient's range of motion may be limited, and she will experience subsequent pain with flexion, a result of tight hamstring tendons and muscles.

→ Patellar tendon reflexes are generally normal.

→ The presence of a painful joint line click with tibial rotation can suggest a degenerative meniscal tear.

→ Morbid obesity is very common in patients with severe knee OA.

ASSESSMENT

→ Degenerative joint disease/osteoarthritis of the knee
→ R/O meniscal tear
→ R/O chondrocalcinosis

→ R/O RA
→ R/O PFP syndrome
→ R/O osteonecrosis
→ R/O loose body
→ Pes anserinus bursitis
→ R/O hip DJD
→ R/O L_3 or L_4 lumbar radiculopathy

PLAN

DIAGNOSTIC TESTS

→ X-rays:

- Anterior-posterior (A/P) weight-bearing view of both knees: demonstrates the extent of joint space narrowing, the presence of chondrocalcinosis, loose bodies, malalignment, and sometimes the existence of osteochondral lesions. This is considered an essential x-ray view when evaluating patients with knee OA.
- Lateral view: the clinician can observe degenerative changes along the posterior aspect of the patella, and further delineate the location of a loose body. This x-ray is a standard view to be obtained with any series of knee radiographs.
- Bilateral Merchant's view of the knees is the best radiograph to assess patellar malalignment as well as patellofemoral DJD.
- Notch views can be ordered to further evaluate the presence of osteochondral lesions.
- Hip x–rays are ordered as indicated, to rule out hip pathology.

→ MRIs can be obtained to determine the presence of meniscal pathology and osteochondral lesions. When plain radiographs demonstrate significant degenerative changes, an MRI, in general, cannot appreciably add to the diagnostic process.

→ Bone scans are helpful to rule out degenerative changes in the patient who demonstrates unicompartmental disease on an x-ray, when the patient is a potential candidate for a high tibial osteotomy. Bone scans can reveal the presence of inflammation, infection, or other lesions not apparent on plain x-rays.

→ Laboratory tests:

- RA, ANA, uric acid, ESR, CBC with differential, if indicated to rule out infection, autoimmune disease, or gout.
- Synovial fluid analysis, as indicated to rule out infection or gout:
  - Gram stain
  - Culture and sensitivity
  - Cell count
  - Crystals

TREATMENT/MANAGEMENT

→ See the **Osteoarthritis** chapter.

CONSULTATION

→ Referral to an orthopedic surgeon is indicated when:

- The patient presents with advanced degenerative joint

disease that has failed all reasonable means of conservative treatment and whose medical status does not preclude major surgery.

- The patient has an intra-articular loose body with a history of mechanical symptoms (i.e., locking, buckling, or giving way of the knee).
- The patient complains of pain and disability despite an adequate trial of reasonable nonoperative treatment.
- The patient likely has a degenerative meniscal tear or osteochondral lesion that remains symptomatic when an adequate trial of conservative treatment has failed to resolve symptoms.
- The patient would benefit from a cortisone injection or the administration of hyaluronic acid treatments that the clinician is not qualified to perform.

→ Prompt orthopedic consultation is mandated when:
- Aspiration of synovial fluid reveals purulent drainage.
- The patient has a locked knee that must (and can) generally be distinguished from a knee contracture.

→ A referral to a rheumatologist is indicated when:
- There is multiple joint involvement of OA.
- The patient has RA, systemic lupus erythematosus, or fibromyalgia.

PATIENT EDUCATION

→ See the **Osteoarthritis** chapter.

FOLLOW-UP

→ See the "Patellofemoral Pain Syndrome" section of this chapter.
→ See the **Osteoarthritis** chapter.

BIBLIOGRAPHY

Adler, J., Kalb, C., Peraino, K. et al. 2001. Arthritis: What it is, why you get it and how to stop the pain. *Newsweek* September 3(138):38–46.

Beaty, J.H. 1999. *Orthopaedic knowledge update.* Rosemont, Ill.: American Academy of Orthopaedic Surgeons.

Bianchi, S., and Martinoli, C. 1999. Detection of loose bodies in joints. *Radiologic Clinics of North America* 37:679–690.

Boden, B.P., Pearsall, A.W., Garrett, W.E. et al. 1997. Patellofemoral instability: evaluation and management. *Journal of the American Academy of Orthopaedic Surgeons* 5:47–57.

Cole, B.J., and Harner, C.D. 1999. Degenerative arthritis of the knee in active patients: evaluation and management. *Journal of the American Academy of Orthopaedic Surgeons* 7:389–402.

Ezzo, J., Hadhazy, V., Birch, S. et al. 2001 Acupuncture for osteoarthritis of the knee. *Arthritis and Rheumatism* 44: 819–825.

Griffin, L.Y., Agel, J., Albohm, M.J. et al. 2000. Noncontact anterior cruciate ligament injuries: risk factors and prevention strategies. *Journal of the American Academy of Orthopaedic Surgeons* 8:141–150.

Hixon, A.L., and Gibbs, L.M. 2000. Osteochondritis dissecans: a diagnosis not to miss. *American Family Physician* 61: 151–156.

Johnson, M.W. 2000 Acute knee effusions: a systematic approach to diagnosis. *American Family Physician* 61: 2391–2400.

Juhn, M.S. 1999. Patellofemoral pain syndrome: a review and guidelines for treatment. *American Family Physician* 60: 2012–2022.

Snider, R.K. 1997. *Essentials of musculoskeletal care.* Rosemont, Ill.: American Academy of Orthopedics.

Williams III, R.J., Wickiewicz, T.L., and Warren, R.F. 2000. Management of unicompartmental arthritis in the anterior cruciate ligament–deficient knee. *American Journal of Sports Medicine* 28:749–760.

Woo, S.L., Vogrin, T.M., and Abramowitch, S.D. 2000. Healing and repair of ligament injuries in the knee. *Journal of the American Academy of Orthopaedic Surgeons* 8:364–372.

8-K

Ankle Pain

The ankle, a hinge joint formed by the distal fibula, tibia, and talus, carries the entire weight of the body. The ankle joint incorporates very little muscle mass. It derives its mechanical support and stability almost entirely from its surrounding ligamentous and tendinous structures, including the posterior talofibular ligament (PTFL), distal tibiofibular ligament (DTFL), and two peroneal tendons on the lateral side.

Every day, at least 25,000 people sprain their ankle; at least 40% of sprains occur during athletic endeavors (Beaty 1999, Snider 1997). A *sprain*, in the most general sense, can be defined as a partial or complete tear of the affected ligament fibers. Sprains are caused when the supporting soft tissue structures fail to respond sufficiently to maintain joint integrity during physiological loading. Sprains involving the lateral anterior talofibular (ATFL) and calcaneofibular (CFL) ligaments comprise about 85% of these injuries, which typically occur on an inverted ankle with a simultaneously plantar flexed foot (Omey et al. 1999, Wolfe et al. 2001).

Medial ankle sprains, which are estimated to comprise between 1–5% of all ankle sprains, involve trauma to the deltoid ligament. Deltoid ligament injuries, which are often associated with a fibular fracture, rarely occur in isolation. Injures to the medial side of the ankle are likely to involve more trauma than lateral ankle sprains. These injuries involve eversion, external rotational or dorsiflexion forces that can precipitate acute fracture as well as chronic instability (Wolfe et al. 2001). Injury to the syndesmosis, the tough ligament that binds the distal fibular and tibia, are sometimes referred to as *high ankle sprains*, and are similarly considered to be more serious than the average sprain.

Lateral inversion sprains of the ankle are typically graded with respect to severity. *Grade I sprains* involve pain over the injured ligament with swelling and instability. *Grade II sprains* present with moderate to severe swelling and mild laxity in addition to pain. *Grade III sprains* are characterized by severe swelling, instability, and pain, and are likely the result of a complete ATFL tear as well as injury to the CFL.

Ankle sprains can more generally be classified as complicated or uncomplicated. Uncomplicated ankle sprains always include grades I and II, and occasionally grade III sprains. Complicated sprains are grade III sprains that require surgical repair of the tendon (Wolfe et al. 2001).

Ankle sprains can be associated with a host of nonligamentous injuries (both acute and chronic) that involve surrounding soft tissue and bony structures. These may include subluxation, tearing, or dislocation of the peroneal tendons that are located just behind the lateral malleolus. Sometimes misdiagnosed as a lateral ankle sprain, it is not unusual for the patient who sustains trauma to the peroneal tendon to delay seeking treatment for months following the injury (Beaty 1999, Omey et al. 1999). Achilles tendon ruptures must always be considered when evaluating any patient who presents with ankle pain preceded by trauma (Snider 1997).

Fractures of the ankle bone and adjacent bones in the foot can usually be confirmed radiographically. Avulsion fractures of the distal fibula and tibia, as well as to the base of the fifth metatarsal are among the more typical injuries that occur in this regard (Beaty 1999, Omey et al. 1999, Snider 1997, Wolfe et al. 2001). Osteochondral lesions of the talor dome sequelae, which are eventually manifested in as many as 22% of ankle sprains, cannot be discerned on x-rays for many weeks, and sometimes months, following the original injury (Wolfe et al. 2001).

DATABASE

SUBJECTIVE

→ The patient with the typical ankle sprain provides a history of the ankle twisting inward as she planted her foot (Omey et al. 1999, Snider 1997, Wolfe et al. 2001).

→ Reports of a tearing or popping sensation, along with immediate swelling indicate a more serious injury (Snider 1997, Wolfe et al. 2001).

→ When the patient with an ankle sprain has a history of prior multiple sprains involving the same joint, she should be evaluated for chronic ankle instability (Omey et al. 1999, Wolfe et al. 2001).

→ Catching, popping, and swelling with a remote history of ankle trauma are highly suggestive of an osteochondral lesion (Wolfe et al. 2001).

→ The patient who is unable to bear weight, especially when she describes an eversion-type injury to the ankle, may have a fracture or syndesmosis sprain (Omey et al. 1999).

→ When the patient presents with a chief complaint of weakness in the ankle with a history of a painful ankle injury followed by rapid resolution of the pain, an Achilles tendon rupture should be suspected (Snider 1997).

→ The patient who complains of pain and swelling which only occurs with weight-bearing, and resolves at rest may have a stress fracture of the distal fibula, tibia, or one of the bones in the foot (Wolfe et al. 2001).

→ When the patient presents with a history of chronic inversion ankle sprains, lateral ankle pain, and painful snapping across the ankle, the clinician should consider the possibility of injury to the peroneal tendons (Omey et al. 1999).

→ Pain in the region of the proximal fibula may indicate a maisonneuve fracture, which is often associated with a syndesmosis injury (Wolfe et al. 2001).

OBJECTIVE

→ The patient with a typical lateral inversion sprain (grades I & II) of the ankle may present with:
  ■ Tenderness over the anterolateral ankle (ATFL and CFL)
  ■ Minimal swelling
  ■ Ability to bear weight without pain
  ■ No evidence of instability
  ■ Mild ecchymosis around the ankle
  ■ Normal x-rays

→ Injury to the syndesmosis of the ankle, or a medial ankle sprain may include the following findings:
  ■ Positive *Squeeze test*: pain is elicited when the examiner compresses the distal tibia and fibula above the mid-calf (Beaty 1999).
  ■ Tenderness over the deltoid ligament
  ■ Tenderness over the syndesmosis
  ■ Positive *External rotation test*: the examiner externally rotates the foot while stabilizing the calf with the patient's leg flexed over the exam table (Wolfe et al. 2001).
  ■ Tenderness over the proximal fibula and an x-ray confirming a proximal fibula, or maisonneuve fracture (Wolfe et al. 2001)
  ■ Inability to bear weight (Beaty 1999)
  ■ Minimal swelling about the ankle
  ■ X-rays that demonstrate widening of the tibiofibular space in excess of 6 mm

→ When the patient has a more serious grade II or grade III sprain or chronic ankle instability, the examiner is likely to note the following:
  ■ Inability of the patient to weight-bear on the affected extremity
  ■ Positive *Anterior drawer test*: determines the integrity of the ATFL. With the patient sitting, the examiner grasps the heel, pulling it forward while placing posterior pressure on the tibia (Wolfe et al. 2001).
  ■ Positive *Talor tilt test*: this test is performed with the

patient's ankle in neutral dorsiplantar flexion and is considered pathopneumonic for a complete tear of the ATFL and CFL. When the examiner inverts the heel on the tibia and the amount of varus tilt exceeds that of the opposite ankle (Snider 1997).
  ■ X-rays: demonstrate a talor tilt of more than 6° when compared to that of the opposite ankle (Beaty 1999).
  ■ Decreased range of motion

→ The patient who is point-tender over the base of the fifth metatarsal may have:
  ■ A fracture of the base of the fifth metatarsal (Omey et al. 1999)
  ■ An avulsion of the peroneus brevis tendon (Wolfe et al. 2001)

→ The patient with injured peroneal tendons, including subluxation, will reveal the following clinical findings (Beaty 1999, Omey et al. 1999):
  ■ Swelling over the posterior lateral aspect of the ankle
  ■ The examiner can provoke peroneal tendon subluxation with forceful ankle dorsiflexion and eversion.
  ■ Point-tender behind the lateral malleolus
  ■ Negative anterior drawer test
  ■ An avulsion fracture of the posterior lateral malleolus can be noted on x-ray.

→ When the patient has a ruptured Achilles tendon, the objective clinical findings are likely to include:
  ■ The inability to toe-raise and/or toe-walk
  ■ Weak plantar flexion
  ■ Swelling from the calf to the heel (Snider 1997)
  ■ Positive *Thompson test*: with the patient in a prone position and the knees flexed to 90° the injured ankle will not plantar flex when the examiner squeezes the midposterior calf (Järvinen et al. 2001).

ASSESSMENT

→ Lateral ankle inversion sprain
→ R/O medial/syndesmosis sprain
→ R/O peroneal tendon injury
→ R/O midfoot sprain
→ R/O Achilles tendon rupture
→ R/O fracture of the distal fibula
→ R/O fracture of the proximal fibula
→ R/O fracture of the base of the fifth metatarsal
→ R/O avulsion fracture of the distal fibula, tibia, and base of the fifth metatarsal
→ R/O stress fracture of the distal fibula, tibia, or tarsal bones
→ R/O talor dome or osteochondral lesion
→ R/O bony structural abnormality such as an accessory navicular or tarsal coalition

PLAN

DIAGNOSTIC TESTS

→ X-rays: Ottawa Ankle Rules can be employed to determine whether radiographs of the injured ankle are indicated when the patient presents with the following (Wolfe et al. 2001):

- Point-tenderness in the posterior half of the distal 6 cm of the fibula or tibia, navicular bone, or the base of the fifth metatarsal
- Inability to bear weight

→ The standard x-rays views of the ankle include:
- Anterior/posterior (A/P)
- Lateral
- Mortise view

→ X-rays of the foot should be obtained to rule out tarsal and metatarsal fractures, if indicated:
- A/P
- Lateral
- Oblique

→ MRI can be obtained in the following instances:
- To rule out an occult fracture
- To confirm a ruptured tendon
- To confirm the presence of an osteochondral lesion

→ CT scans are useful to determine:
- The presence of a tarsal coalition
- Loose bodies

→ Bone scans can be helpful in elucidating the presence of:
- Stress fractures
- An inflammatory process
- Degenerative changes

→ EMGs can rule out peripheral neuropathies, nerve damage, or nerve entrapment conditions such as a tarsal tunnel syndrome.

TREATMENT/MANAGEMENT

→ Initial management of most ankle sprains includes RICE (Omey et al. 1999, Wolfe et al. 2001):
- *Rest*: crutches will decrease the loading force on the injured extremity.
- *Ice* on the affected area for approximately 25 minutes every 2–3 hours for at least the first 48 hours.
- *Compression*: to decrease ankle edema, apply a 3–4 inch Ace wrap which should begin at the toes and extend just above the level of the maximal calf circumference. Other means of compression include:
  - Strapping with nonelastic adhesive tape
  - Laced stabilizers such as a Swedo® ankle boot
  - Elastic ankle guard
- *Elevation*: the edematous extremity should be elevated approximately 25 cm above the heart until most of the swelling abates.

→ The patient can be advised to weight-bear as tolerated (Omey et al. 1999).

→ To avoid the usual complication of ankle stiffening in plantar flexion, the following devices are recommended (Wolfe et al. 2001):
- Air-stirrup ankle support. This can be purchased at most pharmacies that carry medical supplies (Omey et al. 1999).
- Plaster posterior splint molded to maintain the patient's ankle in a neutral position
  - Circumferential casting in a short leg walking cast, or

removable walking boot (a routine practice until the past decade) is rarely considered appropriate, even for grade III sprains (Beaty 1999, Omey et al. 1999, Wolfe et al. 2001).

→ NSAIDs or mild analgesics can be prescribed for inflammation and pain and should be prescribed for the week following the injury (see **Table 8N.1, Anti-inflammatory and Analgesic Medication**).

→ Rehabilitation of the injured ankle should begin as soon as the patient is able to tolerate it, and it must include four elements:
- Re-establishing full range of motion, up to 2 weeks after the injury.
  - Achilles tendon stretching
  - "Writing" the alphabet by actively moving the foot and avoiding ankle inversion
- Muscle and tendon strengthening exercises, 2–4 weeks after the injury (Snider 1997):
  - These exercises should incorporate full range of motion, and include ankle inversion sets and peroneal tendon sets (Omey et al. 1999).
  - Toe raises on both feet, followed by one foot at a time are the simplest exercises that the clinician can instruct the patient on before she starts physical therapy.
- Proprioceptive training: this phase of rehabilitation will assist the patient in regaining control and balance, and usually begins 4–6 weeks following the injury:
  - Instruct the patient to heel and toe walk for a total of 50 feet twice a day.
  - Walking on surfaces of varying texture and firmness facilitates proprioceptive skills (i.e., grass versus concrete).
- Re-establishing the prior level of activity in the athletic person (Snider 1997, Wolfe et al. 2001). This phase can generally begin six weeks after the injury.
  - Start with a routine of walking one-quarter mile, followed by jogging one-quarter mile 4 times a week, and increase jogging by one-eighth a mile a week.
  - When the patient can jog a full mile without pain, she can begin a jog/run routine, progressing in the same manner.

CONSULTATION

→ The primary care provider should obtain urgent orthopedic consultation given the following circumstances:
- Achilles tendon rupture
- Peroneal tendon tear or subluxation
- Ankle or foot fracture
- Syndesmosis sprain
- High index of suspicion for a grade III sprain
- Penetrating wound with suspicion of wound entering the joint space

→ Referral to an orthopedist should be made when:
- The patient has a history of recurrent ankle sprains or instability.

- The patient has a symptomatic osteochondral lesion evident on radiographs and confirmed on MRI.
- The patient's symptoms of pain, swelling, and weakness fail to diminish despite compliance with all reasonable means of conservative treatment for at least six weeks.

PATIENT EDUCATION

→ Educate the patient on the biomechanics of ankle sprains, as well as the implications of her specific injury.

→ Instruct the patient on the principles of RICE.

→ When an air stirrup is prescribed for the patient with an ankle sprain, she should be advised to wear it whenever weight-bearing, until she is pain free. This usually takes about 6 weeks.

→ The athletic patient should be instructed to wear her air stirrup whenever engaging in running/cutting sports for one year following the injury (Snider 1997).

→ The patient must be advised on the importance of wearing properly fitting shoes with an excellent arch support.

→ Educate the patient on the consequences of an inadequately rehabilitated ankle (Wolfe et al. 2001).
- Limited range of motion
- Recurrent pain and swelling
- Chronic ankle instability

→ The patient can be informed of the potential sequelae of ankle sprains:
- As many as 20% of patients with inversion ankle sprains will have recurrent ankle sprains, resulting in chronic ankle instability (Beaty 1999).

- Patients with grade III sprains are more likely to develop chronic instability as well as osteochondral lesions (Omey et al. 1999).

FOLLOW-UP

→ The patient with an ankle sprain should be scheduled for a follow-up visit 2–6 weeks after the injury, depending on her clinical presentation.

→ The patient is advised to seek medical follow-up if her symptoms persist six months after the initial injury.

→ When the patient has a grade III ankle sprain, usually at least six months of conservative treatment should be administered before surgical intervention is considered (Omey et al. 1999).

BIBLIOGRAPHY

Beaty, J.H. 1999. *Orthopaedic knowledge update*. Rosemont, Ill.: American Academy of Orthopaedic Surgeons.

Järvinen, T.A.H., Kannus, P., Paavola, M. et al. 2001. Achilles tendon injuries. *Current Opinion in Rheumatology* 13: 150–155.

Omey, M.L., and Micheli, L.J. 1999. Foot and ankle problems in the young athlete. *Medicine and Science in Sports and Exercise* 31:470–486.

Snider, R.K. 1997. *Essentials of musculoskeletal care*. Rosemont, Ill.: American Academy of Orthopedics.

Wolfe, M.W., Uhl, T.L., Mattacola, C.G. et al. 2001. Management of ankle sprains. *American Academy of Family Physicians* 63:93–104.

8-L

Foot Pain

Approximately 2 million persons a year in the United States seek medical treatment for heel pain (Dreeben 2001), and twice as many women as men. *Heel pain* has been given various names, including *heel spurs, calcaneal periostitis, calcaneodynia,* and most notably, *plantar fasciitis* (Dreeben 2001, Snider 1997). Plantar fasciitis is the most frequent heel pain condition for which women seek medical treatment (Pyasta et al. 2001).

The plantar fascia is a multilayered fibrous aponeurosis with medial, lateral, and central components. This structure originates from the medial calcaneal tuberosity, extends the tendon known as the flexor digitorum brevis, and splits into five bands, which underlie each toe, at the base of the proximal phalanges (Narvaez et al. 2000). The other soft tissue structures from which heel pain can emanate include the retrocalcaneal and retroachilleal bursae, tarsal tunnel, and plantar fat pads (Cornwall et al. 1999).

The plantar fascia serves as a biomechanical tie between the longitudinal arches calcaneus, and the first and second metatarsal heads. These three structures constitute the weight-bearing portions of the foot (Narvaez et al. 2000). In the case of plantar fasciitis, inflammation occurs between the calcaneus and the fascia (Snider 1997). What the layperson will typically characterize as a heel spur is actually an osteophyte on the inferior border of the calcaneus. This "traction spur" is the end result of the ossification occurring between this fascia and the adjoining muscles. This spur causes mechanical irritation that permeates throughout the plantar surface of the heel.

Plantar fasciitis is caused by minor trauma or repetitive strain. Subsequently, inflammation, microrupture and microhemorrhaging of collagen fibers, degeneration of these fibers, and then, ultimately, fibrosis occurs (Young et al. 2001).

Occasionally a patient will relate the onset of her symptoms to a particular event or set of circumstances. However, in most cases the examiner must take a thorough history to elucidate the recurring factors that contributed to this otherwise idiopathic condition. Long considered an overuse syndrome in athletes, the onset of symptoms can also be prompted by sudden changes in running surfaces, drastic advances in mileage, and ill-fitting or worn footwear.

Certain medical conditions pose an increased risk for heel pain, including diabetes, fibromyalgia, scleroderma, rheumatoid arthritis, gonorrhea, tuberculosis, and pregnancy (Barrett et al. 1999, Tisdel et al. 1999). Certain structural features such as the presence of extremely high or flattened medial arches or a congenitally shortened Achilles tendon also factor into the etiology of plantar fasciitis.

Although plantar fasciitis is the most common cause of heel pain, there are other sources of heel pain that should be considered in the examination. For example, if the patient experiences an abrupt onset of symptoms following a traumatic event, she may have experienced a partial or complete rupture of the plantar fascia. Psoriatic arthritis may also present with heel pain (Narvaez et al. 2000). Ankylosing spondylitis and Reiter's syndrome are two additional conditions that are rare in women, but must be considered in the male patient with heel pain.

Certain benign soft tissue lesions that can occur within the plantar fascia include plantar fibromatosis and xanthomas, both of which are associated with hyperlipidaemia. Bony lesions resulting in heel pain, with the exception of calcaneal fractures and bone bruises, are less common and include osteomyelitis, benign bone tumors, and primary lymphoma.

The patient with plantar fasciitis, which is unilateral in at least 85% of cases (Dreeben 2001), typically experiences transient symptoms with varying degrees of intensity over a protracted period of weeks or months. At the time of the patient's initial evaluation for heel pain, she is likely to describe her discomfort as agonizing and sometimes incapacitating. The clinician can reassure the patient that a diagnosis can be made promptly and treatment readily dispatched. The benign nature of the condition as well as the impressive success rate of conservative treatment can also be emphasized.

DATABASE

SUBJECTIVE

Proximal Plantar Fasciitis

(Barrett et al. 1999, Cornwall et al. 1999, Narvaez et al. 2000, Pyasta et al. 2001, Tisdel et al. 1999)

→ Women who are:
- Young and athletic
- Middle-aged
- Elderly

→ Obesity

→ Sudden weight gain

→ Pregnancy

→ Women with a history of:
- Diabetes
- Rheumatoid arthritis (RA)
- Systemic lupus erythematosus (SLE)
- Scleroderma
- Fibromyalgia (FM)
- Minor trauma

→ Pain is most severe after:
- Prolonged sedentary activity
- Weight-bearing for long periods of time

→ Pain is described as follows:
- Predominating in the plantar surface of the heel
- Gradual in onset
- Nonradiating

→ Pain is aggravated by:
- Ill-fitting shoe wear
- Sudden change in type of shoe wear (i.e. wearing shoes with lower heels after many years of high heels)
- Walking or running on hard surfaces

Distal Plantar Fasciitis

(Dreeben 2001)

→ Pain occurs distal to the origin of the plantar fascia and radiates throughout the longitudinal arch.

→ Pain is most pronounced in the mid-arch.

→ This condition is much less common than proximal plantar fasciitis.

Plantar Fascia Rupture

(Barrett et al. 1999, Dreeben 2001, Narvaez et al. 2000, Young et al. 2001)

→ Sudden onset of intense pain accompanied by popping or tearing sensation in the arch

→ Pain occurs distal to the plantar fascia-calcaneal attachment

→ Swelling

→ Athletes who engage in running/cutting sports

→ History of multiple cortisone injections into the heel

Heel Fat Pad Atrophy

(Dreeben 2001, Narvaez et al. 2000, Pyasta et al. 2001, Tisdel et al. 1999, Young et al. 2001)

→ Middle-aged and elderly women

→ Gradual onset

→ Pain on the plantar surface of the heel

→ Pain is nonradiating

→ Pain is aggravated by:
- Hard surfaces
- Uncushioned shoes

→ Obesity

→ History of multiple steroid injections into the heel

Tarsal Tunnel Syndrome

(Barrett et al. 1999, Lau et al. 1999, Pyasta et al. 2001)

→ Pain along the medial and lateral borders of the plantar surface of the calcaneus

→ A history of trauma resulting in a fracture of a foot or ankle bone is the most common cause.

→ Paresthesias that radiates from the heel through the arch and into the toes

→ Pain aggravated by weight-bearing

→ Insidious onset

Calcaneal Stress Fracture

(Narvaez et al. 2000, Pyasta et al. 2001)

→ Diffuse plantar heel pain

→ Most common presentation:
- Middle-aged adults
- Runners
- Military personnel
- History of:
  - Osteoporosis
  - Neurological disorders
  - Rheumatoid arthritis

→ Often precipitated by an abrupt increase in activity level

Infracalcaneal and Retrocalcaneal Bursitis

(Dreeben 2001, Narvaez et al. 2000, Young et al. 2001)

→ Posterior, nonradiating heel pain aggravated by dorsiflexion of the ankle

→ History of repetitive trauma

→ Higher incidence in women

Osteomyelitis

(Narvaez et al. 2000)

→ History of diabetes mellitus

→ History of arteriosclerosis

→ History of a precipitating penetrating wound

Plantar Fibromatosis

(Narvaez et al. 2000)

→ The patient complains of a lump on the sole of her foot, which may or may not cause pain.

OBJECTIVE

Proximal Plantar Fasciitis

(Barrett et al. 1999, Cornwall et al. 1999, Dreeben 2001, Narvaez et al. 2000, Pyasta et al. 2001, Tisdel et al. 1999, Young et al. 2001)

→ There is tenderness over the medial calcaneal tuberosity and approximately 1–2 cms distally along the plantar fascia.

→ Pain increases with passive dorsiflexion of the ankle and great toe.

→ The Achilles tendon is tight, as noted with passive dorsiflexion of the ankle.

→ There is occasional presence of edema in the adjacent fat pad.

→ X-ray findings:
  ▪ An inferior calcaneal spur can be noted in approximately 50% of symptomatic patients.
  ▪ About 15% of asymptomatic patients will have a calcaneal spur that can be noted on x-rays.

→ Obesity

→ Pes planus: flattened medial arches

→ Pes cavus: high medial arches

→ The patient's symptoms will be bilateral 15% of the time.

Distal Plantar Fasciitis
(Dreeben 2001)

→ Diffuse tenderness along the mid portion of the medial arch

→ Passive dorsiflexion of the metatarsal phalangeal joints (MTPs) increase the pain along the mid arch

→ The heel is nontender.

Plantar Fascia Rupture
(Barrett et al. 1999, Dreeben 2001, Narvaez et al. 2000, Young et al. 2001)

→ The plantar surface of the foot will be edematous within the first two weeks of the injury.

→ Presence of ecchymosis

→ Diffuse tenderness along the medial arch

→ Difficulty bearing weight

→ When the patient reports the occurrence of the injury as remote, the clinical presentation is similar to plantar fasciitis.

→ The nodule can usually be palpated on the plantar surface of the foot at the point of the rupture.

Heel Fat Pad Atrophy
(Dreeben 2001, Tisdel et al. 1999)

→ The maximal point tenderness is appreciated in the center of the plantar surface of the heel and tends to be more centrally located.

→ Typically, a prominent calcaneal tubercle can be palpated.

→ The presence of diminished soft tissue padding is noted over the plantar surface of the calcaneus.

Tarsal Tunnel Syndrome
(Barrett et al. 1999, Dreeben 2001, Kohno et al. 2000, Pyasta et al. 2001)

→ Tenderness along the plantar surface of the medial arch and the lateral border of the calcaneus

→ Positive *Tinel's sign*: the paresthesias are induced when the examiner taps the patient over the tarsal tunnel or just below the medial malleolus.

→ Positive nerve conduction studies (NCS) demonstrating the dysfunction of the posterior tibial nerve

→ Excessive foot pronation

→ Occasionally, motor weakness can be discerned.

Calcaneal Stress Fracture
(Barrett et al. 1999, Dreeben 2001, Narvaez et al. 2000, Pyasta et al. 2001)

→ Diffuse tenderness over the plantar surface of the heel

→ Tenderness over the bony prominence of the mid-calcaneus

→ Occasional presence of edema over calcaneus

→ X-rays:
  ▪ Typically normal during the first several weeks following the onset of symptoms
  ▪ Follow-up x-rays will reveal diagnostic features of a fracture less than 50% of the time.

Infracalcaneal and Retrocalcaneal Bursitis
(Dreeben 2001, Narvaez et al. 2000)

→ Distention of the bursae can provoke swelling behind the ankle with bulging on either side of the Achilles tendon insertion.

→ The bursa is tender to palpation at the level of the shoe counter.

→ Skin overlying the bursa is hypertrophic and erythematous.

→ X-rays: demonstrate obliteration of the normal retrocalcaneal fat.

→ There is maximal point tenderness in the central bursa.

Osteomyelitis
(Narvaez et al. 2000)

→ Low grade fever

→ Infection tends to originate over pressure points:
  ▪ Calcaneus
  ▪ Metatarsal heads

Plantar Fibromatosis
(Narvaez et al. 2000)

→ The presence of firm, fibrous, and most often bilateral nodules in the plantar arch

→ Occasional contractures in the plantar fascia

ASSESSMENT

→ Proximal plantar fasciitis

→ R/O distal plantar fasciitis

→ R/O ruptured plantar fascia

→ R/O tarsal tunnel syndrome

→ R/O calcaneal stress fracture

→ R/O infracalcaneal bursitis

→ R/O retrocalcaneal bursitis

→ R/O heel fat pad atrophy

→ R/O plantar fibromatosis

→ R/O osteomyelitis

→ R/O bone bruise

→ R/O calcaneal tumors

→ R/O Achilles tendinitis

PLAN

DIAGNOSTIC TESTS

→ Radiographs (Barrett et al. 1999, Cornwall et al. 1999, Dreeben 2001, Narvaez et al. 2000, Tisdel et al. 1999, Young et al. 2001):
  ▪ Lateral view of the calcaneus is generally adequate when:
    • There is no history of trauma.
    • The patient has been symptomatic for 6–8 weeks.
    • The signs and symptoms are confined to the area of the heel.
  ▪ Anterior/posterior, lateral and oblique views should be obtained when:
    • There is a history of trauma.
    • The pain and tenderness are diffuse.
    • To rule out other sources of foot pain
  ▪ X-rays will reveal the presence of an inferior calcaneal spur 50% of the time; otherwise x-rays will be normal.
  ▪ Less than 25% of patients with heel spurs documented by x-rays have heel pain.
→ Bone scan (Dreeben 2001, Pyasta et al. 2001, Tisdel et al. 1999):
  ▪ Will demonstrate increased uptake over the medial calcaneal tuberosity with plantar fasciitis
  ▪ A bone scan should be obtained:
    • To rule out the presence of a stress fracture
    • As a pre-surgical test when the patient's plantar fasciitis has been longstanding and surgery is being considered
    • To rule out osteomyelitis
→ EMG/NCS (Barrett et al. 1999, Tisdel et al. 1999)
  ▪ To rule out tarsal tunnel syndrome or other nerve involvement when paresthesias are present
→ MRI (Dreeben 2001, Narvaez et al. 2000):
  ▪ Indicated to rule out:
    • Calcaneal tumor
    • Rupture of the plantar fascia
    • Osteomyelitis
  ▪ Indicated to determine the presence of deeply infiltrating plantar fibromatosis
  ▪ Not indicated to confirm the diagnosis of plantar fasciitis, but when obtained, MRI may reveal:
    • Fascial thickening of the proximal portion that extends into the calcaneal surface
    • Normal tissue
→ Laboratory tests (Tisdel et al. 1999):
  ▪ May be indicated to rule out an underlying systemic condition:
    • CBC
    • ESR
    • ANA
    • RA
    • Uric acid

TREATMENT/MANAGEMENT

Plantar Fasciitis
(Barrett et al. 1999, Cornwall et al. 1999, Narvaez et al. 2000, Pyasta et al. 2001, Tisdel et al. 1999, Young et al. 2001)

→ In about 95% of the cases, plantar fasciitis will resolve with conservative treatment.
→ It is reasonable to continue conservative treatment for up to two years.
→ Medication:
  ▪ NSAIDs for 2–8 weeks (see **Table 8N.1, Anti-inflammatory and Analgesic Medication**).
  ▪ Narcotics and muscle relaxants are not appropriate.
  ▪ Topical NSAID creams are of questionable effectiveness.
→ Achilles tendon stretching for 3 minutes, TID–QID
→ Orthotics:
  ▪ Full-length semi-rigid arch supports:
    • Spenco®
    • Birkenstocks®
  ▪ Custom-made orthotics are indicated when the patient has:
    • Rigid pes planus
    • Pes cavus
    • Over-the-counter orthotics have not served to diminish symptoms.
  ▪ Heel cups:
    • Heel fat pad atrophy
→ Ice packs for 25 minutes TID
→ Contrast baths:
  ▪ Soak feet in warm water and Epsom salts for 10 minutes.
  ▪ Immediately immerse feet in ice water for 3 minutes.
→ Cortisone injection:
  ▪ Indicated when:
    • The patient's symptoms are severe.
    • Previous trials of conservative treatment have failed to relieve symptoms.
  ▪ Injections may be administered every 6–12 weeks for a maximum of 3 injections in the same location within one year.
  ▪ Injections should be administered at the point of maximal tenderness; avoid injecting into the fat pad.
  ▪ Injections are not appropriate for distal plantar fasciitis.
→ The use of a night splint which maintains the patient's foot in a neutral position:
  ▪ Apply at bedtime for 2–8 weeks.
  ▪ This can be custom-molded from plaster by an orthopedic technician when the provider has access to a cast room.
  ▪ A night splint can be purchased at most medical supply stores and occasionally at sports equipment stores.
→ The patient can be placed in a weight-bearing short leg walking cast for 4–6 weeks to immobilize the foot, permitting the plantar fascia to rest.
→ Physical therapy can be ordered in some instances for the administration of phonophoresis.

Plantar Fascia Rupture
(Dreeben 2001, Narvaez et al. 2000)
→ Rest
→ Total contact cast for six weeks to permit ambulation without pain
→ NSAIDs (see **Table 8N.1.**)

→ Arch supports
→ Physical therapy

Heel Fat Pad Atrophy

(Dreeben 2001, Young et al. 2001)

→ Hard heel cups to compress fat on the undersurface of the calcaneus
→ Injections are to be avoided
→ The patient should wear soft-soled shoes with good arch supports.

Tarsal Tunnel Syndrome

If symptoms are mild to moderate (Barrett et al. 1999, Narvaez et al. 2000, Tisdel et al. 1999)

→ Arch supports
→ NSAIDs (see **Table 8N.1.**)
→ Contrast baths
→ Sometimes a steroid injection into the tarsal tunnel will provide temporary relief.

Infracalcaneal and Retrocalcaneal Bursitis

(Dreeben 2001, Narvaez et al. 2000, Tisdel et al. 1999)

→ Heel pads
→ Arch support
→ NSAIDs for 2–6 weeks (see **Table 8N.1.**)
→ Applications of ice to the bursa for 25 minutes TID
→ Occasional cortisone injections into the bursae

Calcaneal Stress Fracture

→ If a calcaneal stress fracture is confirmed by an x-ray or other imaging study, instruct the patient to remain non weight-bearing and obtain orthopedic consultation.

Plantar Fibromatosis

(Narvaez et al. 2000)

→ Shoe inserts with cutout under the lesion to decrease pressure
→ Surgical excision of lesion is discouraged because:
  ▪ There is a high rate of reoccurrence of the lesion.
  ▪ Scar tissue can form at the healed incision and can cause as much aggravation as the original lesion.

CONSULTATION

→ It is reasonable for the clinician to recommend to the patient that she have a consultation with an orthopedic surgeon or a podiatrist for a plantar fascia release when:
  ▪ All reasonable means of conservative treatment over a 6-month period have failed.
  ▪ The patient's symptoms respond satisfactorily to treatment, but they recur for at least 2 years.
→ The patient should be referred to an orthopedic surgeon for a consideration of a tarsal tunnel release when she has symptomatic tarsal tunnel syndrome that:
  ▪ Has been confirmed on nerve conduction studies
  ▪ Has not responded satisfactorily to nonoperative treatment

→ Indications for an urgent referral to an orthopedic surgeon include:
  ▪ The presence of calcaneal fracture
  ▪ A high index of suspicion for osteomyelitis
  ▪ When MRI or x-ray reveal the presence of a lesion suggestive of a tumor
→ The patient may require a referral to a qualified clinician for the administration of a cortisone injection for plantar fasciitis or tarsal tunnel syndrome.

PATIENT EDUCATION

→ Educate the patient on the pathophysiology of her disease process, and advise that heel pain is often chronic, but it is usually self-limiting and resolves within 6–18 months (Young et al. 2001).
→ Lifestyle changes:
  ▪ Educate obese patients on the importance of weight reduction to reduce heel pain.
  ▪ The patient should be advised on the impact of activity modification:
    • Long recreational walks should be postponed until symptoms resolve.
    • Avoid running/cutting sports
    • Limit repetitive heavy lifting
    • Avoid weight-bearing for prolonged periods
→ Shoe wear and the use of orthotics:
  ▪ The patient is advised to wear footwear at all times, even around the house.
  ▪ Footwear for the patient with heel pain should include (Cornwall et al. 1999, Young et al. 2001):
    • Shoes with good arch supports
    • Shoes with soft, shock-absorbent soles
  ▪ Educate the patient on the appropriate use of orthotics.
→ The importance of daily heel cord stretching exercises cannot be overemphasized (Barrett et al. 1999, Young et al. 2001).
→ Educate patients taking NSAIDS on their indications, dosage, and potential side effects (see **Table 8N.1**).
→ When discussing a cortisone injection for plantar fasciitis, advise the patient of the potential complications, including (Dreeben 2001, Tisdel et al. 1999):
  ▪ Rupture of the plantar fascia (very rare)
  ▪ Heel fat pad atrophy, which is more likely to occur following multiple injections
  ▪ Post-injection soreness, which ensues approximately 50% of the time

FOLLOW-UP

→ Medical follow-up should be arranged for the patient approximately 6–8 weeks after treatment is initiated.
→ The patient should be advised to seek medical follow-up or consultation:
  ▪ For routine treatment as needed
  ▪ When her symptoms remain intractable and recurrent over time, despite consistent trials of adequate treatment regimens

BIBLIOGRAPHY

Barrett, S.L., and O'Malley, R. 1999. Plantar fasciitis and other causes of heel pain. *American Family Physician* 59:2200–2206.

Cornwall, M.W., and McPoil, T.G. 1999. Plantar fasciitis. Etiology and treatment. *Journal of Orthopaedic and Sports Physical Therapy* 29:756–760.

Dreeben, S. 2001. Heel pain in women: sorting through the possible causes. *Women's Health: Orthopedic Edition* 4:45–51.

Kohno, M., Takahashi, H., Segawa, H. et al. 2000. Neurovascular decompression for idiopathic tarsal tunnel syndrome: Technical note. *Journal of Neurology, Neurosurgery and Psychiatry* 69:87–90.

Lau, J.T.C., and Daniels, T.R. 1999. Tarsal tunnel syndrome: a review of the literature. *Foot and Ankle International* 20: 201–209.

Narvaez, J.A., Narvaez, J., Ortega, R. et al. 2000. Painful heel: MR imaging findings. *Radiographics* 20:333–352.

Pyasta, R.T., and Panush, R.S. 2001. Common painful foot syndromes. *Bulletin on the Rheumatic Diseases* 48:1–3.

Snider, R.K. 1997. *Essentials of musculoskeletal care.* Rosemont, Ill.: American Academy of Orthopedics.

Tisdel, C.L., Donley, B.G., and Sferra, J.J. 1999. Diagnosing and treating plantar fasciitis: a conservative approach to plantar heel pain. *Cleveland Clinic Journal of Medicine* 66:231–235.

Young, C.C., Rutherford, D.S., and Niedfeldt, M.W. 2001. Treatment of plantar fasciitis. *American Family Physician* 63:467–477.

8-M

Low Back Pain

Low back pain (LBP) refers to pain distal to the inferior border of the scapula and above the cleft of the buttocks (Van Tulder et al. 2000). Low back pain has a lifetime incidence of 60–90% and is second only to upper respiratory infections as a cause for work absenteeism in persons under age 55 (Atlas et al. 2001, Borenstein 2001, Della-Giustina et al. 2000, Jermyn 2001, Patel et al. 2000, Standaert et al. 2000). It is the most common cause of disability in persons age 35 and younger and accounts for one-third of all workers' compensation costs (Atlas et al. 2001, Jermyn 2001). Low back pain is ranked fifth among reasons for visits to primary care practitioners and is the chief reason patients see orthopedic surgeons or neurosurgeons (Atlas et al. 2001, Patel et al. 2000).

The cost of LBP in the United States (U.S.) is estimated at approximately $20 billion for direct health care costs and more than $60 billion when indirect costs including lost work-days, disability, and diminished job productivity are factored in (Atlas et al. 2001, Rosomoff et al. 1999, Patel et al. 2000, Della-Giustina et al. 2000). Surgery is medically justified less than 1% of the time (Rosomoff et al. 1999).

Red Flags

The initial focus of the primary care evaluation is to identify red flags indicating life-threatening conditions that will not resolve with routine management (Malanga et al. 1999). These conditions, which represent a small percentage of LBP, include *metastatic lesions of the spine, infection, spinal fractures, referred pain from visceral organ structures*, and *cauda equina syndrome*, which is a neurosurgical emergency (Della-Giustina et al. 2000).

Metastatic disease of the spine is the most prevalent neoplasm affecting the axial skeleton (Borenstein 2001). Patients with a history of cancer are at additional risk for developing a metastatic spinal lesion (Della-Giustina et al. 2000). Metastases and multiple myeloma should also be considered in young persons with a confirmed atraumatic spine fracture. Traumatic fractures of the spine are more typical of older persons with osteoporosis or a history of chronic and prolonged steroid use (Jermyn 2001).

When evaluating the possibility of spinal infection as a cause of acute LBP, persons at greatest risk are those who have an extraspinal infection. Approximately 56% of spinal infections occur in the lumbar segment, and *Staphylococcus aureus* is the most likely organism (Borenstein 2001).

Cauda equina syndrome results from compression of the spinal nerve roots that supply neurological function to the bladder and bowels (Borenstein 2001). Approximately 50% of cauda equina syndromes are secondary to tumors causing central canal stenosis (Jermyn 2001). In a younger adult, epidural compression is more typically related to a large, central, herniated disk. Other potential etiologies include spinal canal hematomas, abscesses, and trauma.

Low back pain that is referred from systemic or visceral organ disease is likely to be associated with pelvic pathology or retroperitoneal processes (Atlas et al. 2001). An uncommon cause of LBP requiring emergency consultation and treatment is a ruptured abdominal aoristic aneurysm (Della-Giustina et al. 2000). A review of the literature indicates that patients under age 20 and those over age 50 are at greater risk for a serious LBP condition (Bratton 1999, Della-Giustina et al. 2000).

Risk of Disability and Chronicity

Once any red flags are identified and the more serious causes of LBP are excluded by history, the clinician can then focus on identifying LBP syndromes that pose a risk of disability and chronicity (Atlas et al. 2001). This step generally involves designating the LBP as acute, having lasted less than six weeks in duration, subacute, up to 12 weeks, or chronic, of more than three months in duration (Della-Giustina et al. 2000).

Evaluating the LBP patient during the acute and subacute phase requires ruling out various myofascial pain syndromes and differentiating those that sometimes mimic nerve root compression syndromes such as sciatica (Rosomoff et al. 1999). In sciatic conditions, pain usually originates in the lumbar spine, radiates through the buttock and down the length of the entire lower extremity. This can be associated with sensory and motor deficits (Della-Giustina et al. 2000). Lumbar disk herniation, in which sciatica is present 95% of the time, accounts for only 2–3% of LBP (Patel et al. 2000, Postacchini 2001). Disk herniation most often involves the fourth and fifth lumbar, or the fifth lumbar and first sacral vertebrae (Atlas et al. 2001). Other causes of acute LBP may include *foraminal stenosis, lumbar stenosis, piriformis syndrome, intraspinal tumor,* or *infection* (Della-Giustina et al. 2000).

Mechanical Causes of Low Back Pain

The vast majority of acute LBP involves mechanical alterations in the spine (Atlas et al. 2001), and *lumbosacral sprain* or *strain* will be the likely diagnosis. These conditions result from abnormal loading forces on the lumbar spine that cause microtrauma to the muscle and ligamentous structures that are innervated with numerous pain receptors (Jermyn 2001).

Additional causes of acute and subacute mechanical LBP include *Type IV spondylolysis*—a condition featuring either a traumatic fracture in the neural arch of the pars interarticularis—or *isthmic spondylosis*, which is most prevalent in adolescent or young adult athletes. This is essentially a stress fracture caused by the cumulative effect of repetitive microtrauma to the spine from aggravating physical activity (Standaert et al. 2000).

Coccygodynia, or pain in the base of the spine (the coccyx), typically results from trauma (Jermyn 2001). It is not unusual for the discomfort from coccygodynia to become chronic. In rare occasions, the etiology of coccygodynia is a lesion such as an intraosseous lipoma or giant cell tumor (Jermyn 2001).

Nonmechanical causes of acute LBP may be metabolic in origin such as Parkinson's or Paget's disease, or they may be exacerbations of an underlying rheumatological condition. *Polymyalgia rheumatica* (PMR) and *ankylosing spondylosis* (AS) are two conditions that can precipitate an acute or chronic LBP condition (Atlas et al. 2001).

Chronic Low Back Pain

Approximately 1% of the U.S. population is disabled from chronic low back pain, 97.6% of which can be characterized as myofascial in origin (Rosomoff et al. 1999). Persons whose abdominal muscles are weak and who engage in repetitive heavy lifting also have an increased risk of developing chronic LBP, as well as those who perceive their general state of health as poor (Reilly 2001). There is also a strong association between cigarette smoking, disk disease, diminished bone mass, and prolonged healing time for fractures (Porter et al. 2000).

Diagnosing chronic LBP is complicated by a plethora of associated psychosocial factors. For example, it is estimated that 3–19% of patients with chronic LBP have a substance abuse problem. The relationship between depression and chronic LBP has also been well documented (Rosomoff et al. 1999). Other psychological phenomena include somatoform disorder, which occurs when the patient is preoccupied with her pain despite a complete lack of physical findings, and a temporal relationship with poor job satisfaction (Borenstein 1999, Patel et al. 2000, Rosomoff et al. 1999).

A review of the literature indicates that there may be a relationship between obesity and chronic low back pain. Obesity has also been found to make it more difficult for patients to comply with therapeutic programs to ameliorate LBP (Borenstein 1999). Additionally, it has been noted that 44–61% of women experience LBP during pregnancy (Borenstein 1999).

Repetitive trauma, infection, and/or heredity add to the psychosocial and environmental factors that lead to chronic LBP. The arthritic changes of lumbar degenerative disk disease, for example, result in diminished disk heights, ligamentous laxity, and tears in the annulus fibrosis, all of which contribute to chronic LBP (Snider 1997).

Degenerative lumbar spinal stenosis is a common cause of chronic LBP in older adults. Spinal stenosis generally occurs when there is progressive narrowing of the lumbar spinal canal and the neural foramen (Atlas et al. 2001). Spinal stenosis is, with rare exceptions, associated with degenerative joint disease (DJD). It affects men and women equally, most often beginning between ages 40–60 (Sheehan et al. 2001).

Degenerative spondylolisthesis occurs when biomechanical alterations in the facet joints, which include heavy bony overgrowth as well as thickening and calcification of the ligamentum flavum, cause slippage of a vertebral body anteriorly onto the one below it (Sheehan et al. 2001). This results in significant narrowing of the central spinal canal (Snider 1997).

Spondylolisthesis is a common cause of LBP in the adolescent and young adult athlete. The condition is most often caused by repetitive mechanical forces on the posterior aspects of the lumbar spine. Repetitive hyperextension motions of the lumbar spine, for example, can cause a stress fracture of the pars interarticularis (Omey et al. 2000).

Chronic low back pain can have a rheumatologic etiology, such as ankylosing spondylosis, which is common in women, or a metabolic origin as in Paget's disease. With increasing regularity, however, chronic LBP fits into a spectrum of pain syndromes with no clear etiology, such as fibromyalgia (Bratton 1999). Extreme, chronic LBP may persist even after multiple surgical interventions; this is referred to as failed back pain syndrome, which affects at least 40% of post-operative patients (Rosomoff et al. 1999).

The vast majority of low back pain is self-limiting and tends to resolve spontaneously over time. This chapter covers the most common forms of LBP that primary care providers encounter as well as the red flags that indicate potentially life-threatening situations.

Acute Low Back Pain

→ Obtain a comprehensive medical history.
→ Eliciting the OPQRST's of LBP may be helpful (Della-Giustina et al. 2000):
  ▪ **O**nset
  ▪ **P**alliative and provocative factors
  ▪ **Q**uality
  ▪ **R**adiation
  ▪ **S**everity
  ▪ **T**iming

→ Psychosocial factors, including past and present work history, nicotine dependency, and physical activity level must be addressed.

DATABASE
SUBJECTIVE

Identification of Red Flags

Metastatic Lesions

(Bratton 1999, Della-Giustina et al. 2000, Patel et al. 2000, Rosomoff et al. 1999)

→ Age 50 or older
→ Pain is often described as a dull, throbbing ache that progresses slowly.
→ Pain increases with recumbency or while coughing.
→ History of cancer. Most common primary sites include:
  - Breast
  - Prostate
  - Kidney
  - Lung
  - Thyroid
→ History of multiple myeloma
→ Neurological symptoms:
  - Radicular pain
  - Weakness
  - Paresthesias

Infection

(Della-Giustina et al. 2000, Patel et al. 2000, Standaert et al. 2000):

→ Immunosuppression
→ Presence of a urinary tract infection
→ Fever is not often present.
→ Can affect persons at any age
→ Pain in the lumbar spine and sacrum in 90% of patients
→ Aggravating and relieving factors vary considerably.
→ History of chronic skin infections
→ Presence or recent history of having an indwelling Foley catheter
→ Organ transplant patients
→ History of diabetes mellitus
→ Approximately 50% of patients with spinal infections are symptomatic for three months by the time a diagnosis is rendered.
→ History of intravenous drug use. A complaint of LBP in the intravenous drug-abusing patient should be considered to be intervertebral osteomyelitis or an epidural abscess until proven otherwise (Della-Giustina 2000).
→ Night sweats
→ Involuntary weight loss

Spinal Fractures

(Patel et al. 2000, Rosomoff et al. 1999)

→ History of significant trauma
→ History of prolonged use of a corticosteroid preparation
→ Age 50 or over
→ Presence of osteoporosis
→ Localized pain in the lumbar vertebrae when bending forward from the waist

Cauda Equina Syndrome

(Atlas et al. 2001, Della-Giustina et al. 2000, Jermyn 2001, Rosomoff et al. 1999)

→ Acute onset of bladder dysfunction (i.e., incontinence or retention)
→ Saddle anesthesia: diminished sensation in the anus, perineum, and genitals (Rosomoff 1999)
→ Loss of anal sphincter tone
→ Fecal incontinence
→ Global or progressive motor weakness in lower limbs
→ Sexual dysfunction
→ Back pain, which is not always present, tends to be mild

LBP from Systemic or Visceral Organ Disease

(Atlas et al. 2001)

→ History of cancer
→ Unexplained weight loss
→ Age 50 or older
→ Failed conservative treatment
→ Pain is unrelated to level or type of patient activity
→ Increased pain in recumbent position
→ Risk factors for coronary artery disease
→ Gastrointestinal or genitourinary symptoms

LBP Syndromes That Pose Risk of Disability and Chronicity

Lumbar Disk Herniation and Sciatica

(Atlas et al. 2001, Della-Giustina et al. 2000, Jermyn 2001, Patel et al. 2000, Snider 1997)

→ 95% of the time the fifth and the first sacral vertebrae are involved.
→ 30–50 years of age
→ Pain radiates from the lumbar spine into the lower posterior or lateral part of the legs into the ankle and foot.
→ Pain is often described as sharp, shooting, or burning in character.
→ Paresthesias may be present in the lower extremities.
→ Pain decreases when standing.
→ Pain is typically aggravated by:
  - Flexing forward
  - Sitting erect
  - Changing positions
  - Coughing and sneezing
→ Weakness in one or both lower extremities
→ Herniation of the second and third, or the third and fourth lumbar vertebrae:
  - More frequent in elderly patients
  - May be accompanied by abdominal pain
  - Typically associated with quadriceps weakness
  - Usually does not radiate below the knee
  - Involves less than 5% of lumbar disk herniations

Spondylolisthesis and Spondylolysis

(Jermyn 2001, Nelemans et al. 2001, Patel et al. 2000, Standaert et al. 2000)

→ Affects approximately 15% of adolescent athletes
→ Pain radiates from the lumbar spine into the coccyx and the posterior and lateral thigh.
→ Tends to be more frequent in:
  - Divers
  - Weight lifters
  - Wrestlers
  - Gymnasts
  - Jumpers
  - Throwing, track and field sports
  - Rowers
→ Pain can have an acute onset if preceded by trauma, or a gradual onset.
→ Pain can be aggravated by:
  - Forward flexion of the spine
  - Spinal extension
  - Spinal rotation
→ Can affect persons of any age, but is more prevalent in women over age 40.
→ Spondylosis is three times more prevalent in Caucasian than black persons.

Mechanical LBP

Low Back Strains and Sprains

(Jermyn 2001, Della-Giustina et al. 2000, Patel et al. 2000, Snider 1997)

→ Most prevalent in 20–40 year olds
→ Pain is aggravated by activity.
→ Pain is located in the lower back and can radiate into the buttocks and posterior thigh.
→ Pain is typically described as an ache or spasm.
→ Paresthesias are absent.
→ Onset of symptoms may be acute or gradual.
→ Onset of symptoms may be precipitated by an unusually rigorous spinal movement or some form of emotional distress.
→ The person has difficulty standing erect.
→ Pain is often ameliorated by frequent changes in position.
→ Risk factors for low back strain or sprain include:
  - Heavy lifting
  - Operating heavy equipment that causes vibrations
  - Sitting for prolonged periods of time
  - Poor general fitness level
  - Poor work satisfaction
  - Low-paying employment
  - Cigarette smoking
  - Personality disorders

Coccygodynia

(Jermyn 2001)

→ Pain localized in the base of the spine
→ Almost always precipitated by trauma, including childbirth

Iliopsoas Syndrome

(Biundo et al. 2001, Rosomoff et al. 1999)

→ Ipsilateral paraspinal pain
→ Pain radiating into the anterior thighs (Rosomoff 1999)

Piriformis Syndrome

(Robb-Nicholson 2001, Rosomoff et al. 1999, Rossi et al. 2001)

→ Pain in the lateral and anterior hip and buttock aggravated by:
  - Vigorous activity
  - Lying on the affected side
→ Pain is described as a "dull ache" in the buttock.
→ Pain radiates down the posterior thigh when going up and down stairs.

OBJECTIVE

→ Observe the patient's spontaneous and active gross motor movements and general demeanor.
→ Observe the patient's gait, posture, standing balance, ability to crouch, and any apparent leg length discrepancy.
→ Note any scars from previous surgeries, erythema, or other abnormal lesions.
→ Percussion and palpation of the back can facilitate localization of pain and troublesome masses.
→ An abdominal examination is recommended to determine the presence of bruits, pulsatile masses, or other irregular lesions (Standaert et al. 2000).
→ A rectal examination is advised when the patient presents with red flags or the coccyx is tender to palpation.
→ Range of motion (ROM) of the patient's lumbar-sacral spine and both hips and knees should be noted.
  - Painful, passive ROM of the lower extremities can help distinguish referred pain caused by a central lesion from pain caused by specific joint pathology (Malanga et al. 1999).
  - Painful, limited internal rotation of the hip, for example, is pathognomonic for osteoarthritis of the hip.
→ The most important component in the physical assessment of LBP is the neurological examination (Della-Giustina et al. 2000).
  - The purpose is to localize any nerve root lesions or neurological defects.
  - A limited exam is usually adequate, and should include:
    • Sensory testing: (light touch over various aspects of the foot)
    • Straight leg raises
    • Ankle reflexes and knee reflexes
    • Test the strength of dorsiflexion of the ankle and great toe: weakness is indicative of nerve root dysfunction at the level of the fourth and fifth lumbar vertebrae (Atlas et al. 2001).
    • A vascular examination should make note of peripheral pulses, skin color, and temperature (Jermyn 2001).
→ Obtain radiographic, laboratory, and neurological studies to rule out any number of underlying medical, orthopedic, or neurological conditions.

Identification of Red Flags

Metastatic lesions

(Patel et al. 2000, Rosomoff et al. 1999)

→ Severe guarding of lumbar motion in all planes

→ Fever

→ Localized tenderness

→ X-rays demonstrate bony erosions or blastic lesions

→ Laboratory studies are usually within normal limits, with the possible exception of:
  ▪ A low hemoglobin (Hgb) and hematocrit (Hct) level
  ▪ An elevated sedimentation rate (ESR)

Infection

(Della-Giustina et al. 2000, Patel et al. 2000, Rosomoff et al. 1999)

→ Vertebral point tenderness to palpation

→ Severe guarding of lumbar motion in all planes

→ Fever occurs in about 50% of patients with spine infection

→ Vertebral bodies tender to percussion

→ Decreased range of motion secondary to severe pain

→ Laboratory findings:
  ▪ Elevated sedimentation rate (ESR)
  ▪ Normal white blood cell count (WBC)
  ▪ Positive blood cultures:
    • *Staphylococcus aureus* 62.7% of the time
    • *Streptococcus* 19.6% of cases

Spinal Fractures

(Bratton 1999, Rosomoff et al. 1999)

→ Severe guarding of lumbar motion in all planes

→ Vertebral point tenderness to palpation

→ Radiographic findings:
  ▪ Evidence of fracture
  ▪ Osteoporosis

Cauda Equina Syndrome

(Atlas et al. 2001, Bratton 1999, Della-Giustina et al. 2000)

→ Severe unilateral or bilateral weakness in lower extremities

→ Bladder distention

→ Diminished deep tendon reflexes (DTRs)

→ Abnormal sensory exam particularly over the buttocks, perineum, and medial proximal thighs

→ Overflow incontinence secondary to urinary retention in ≥90% of cases

→ Decreased anal sphincter tone in 60–80% of patients

→ Inability to heel and toe walk

→ MRI findings:
  ▪ Presence of primary or metastatic tumors in central spinal canal about 50% of the time
  ▪ Hematomas in the central spinal canal
  ▪ Abscesses

NOTE: Acute transverse myelitis presents identically to cauda equina syndrome, and is impossible to distinguish without an MRI.

LBP From Systemic or Visceral Organ Disease

→ Parkinson's disease (Jermyn 2001)

  ▪ Brisk deep tendon reflexes (DTRs)
  ▪ Shuffling gait

→ Ankylosing spondylitis (Patel et al. 2000)
  ▪ Decreased range of motion in lower spine
  ▪ Tenderness over sacroiliac joints
  ▪ Laboratory findings:
    • Elevated sedimentation rate (ESR)
    • Positive HLA-B_{27} in 90% of patients
  ▪ Radiographic findings:
    • Narrowing of sacroiliac joints
    • Osteoporosis
    • Sacroiliitis

→ Abdominal aortic aneurysm (Bratton 1999, Della-Giustina et al. 2000, Malanga et al. 1999)
  ▪ The patient is writhing in pain.
  ▪ The patient is unable to find a position of comfort.
  ▪ Auscultation of a bruit
  ▪ Appreciation of a pulsatile mass in the abdomen (Bratton 1999)

  NOTE: This condition deserves special consideration in the elderly patient (Della-Giustina et al. 2000).

→ Hyperthyroidism, electrolyte imbalances, drug toxicity
  ▪ Brisk deep tendon reflexes all typically associated with metabolic abnormalities (Jermyn 2001).

→ Nephrolithiasis, spinal infection
  ▪ Observation of the patient writhing in pain (Malanga et al. 1999):

LBP Syndromes That Pose Risk of Disability

Lumbar Disk Herniation and Sciatica

→ Positive straight leg raises (SLRs): with the patient lying supine, the examiner raises one of her fully extended legs. If the patient experiences pain down her leg at ≤60° radiating past the knee (not a reproduction of her LBP) the test is positive (Della-Giustina et al. 2000).
  ▪ The pain is aggravated by dorsiflexion of the foot.
  ▪ The test is 80% sensitive for a herniated disk.

→ Positive SLR is not proof of a herniated disk. Non-neurological etiologies of positive straight leg raises (SLRs) include (Jermyn 2001):
  ▪ Tight hamstring muscles
  ▪ Muscle spasm
  ▪ Sprained posterior longitudinal ligament

→ Positive crossed SLR: reproduction of radicular pain in the opposite leg. This test is sensitive but nonspecific for a herniated disk.

→ Muscle weakness (Rosomoff et al. 1999):
  ▪ Inability to toe walk: S_1 nerve root
  ▪ Inability to heel walk: L_4-L_5 nerve roots
  ▪ Inability to perform a single squat and raise: L_4-L_5 nerve roots

→ Unilateral muscle atrophy noted in lower extremities
  ▪ A discrepancy of ≤2 cm in leg length is considered within normal limits (Rosomoff et al. 1999).

→ Asymmetrical DTRs (Patel et al. 2000)

→ Diminished sensation in lower extremities is nonspecific unless it follows a dermatome or is unilateral.
→ Positive electromyographies (EMGs)
→ Radiographic findings (Atlas et al. 2001):
  ▪ X-rays: narrowing of intervertebral disks
  ▪ MRI: disk herniation; nerve root entrapment
→ L_3-L_4 nerve root compression:
  ▪ Unilateral quadriceps weakness
  ▪ Decreased patellar tendon reflexes
  ▪ Decreased sensation in shin, anterior thigh
→ L_4-L_5 nerve root compression (Jermyn 2001):
  ▪ Weakness of great toe extension and ankles
  ▪ Inability to heel walk
  ▪ Numbness on the top of foot and first web space
→ S_1 nerve root compression (Jermyn 2001):
  ▪ Numbness in the lateral part of the foot
  ▪ Asymmetrical Achilles tendon reflexes
  ▪ Weakness of plantar flexion
→ Positive *Lasegue's sign*: with the patient lying supine, and her knees in full extension, the patient will experience increased LBP (Bratton 1999).
→ The presence of a *list*: the trunk shifts to one side when the patient is standing and flexing forward at the lumbar spine (Snider 1997).

Spondylolisthesis and Spondylosis
(Borenstein, 2001, Omey et al. 2000, Patel et al. 2000, Sheehan et al. 2001, Standaert et al. 2000)

→ Exaggerated curve of the lumbar spine
→ Palpable step-off between the spinous processes of the lumbar spine
→ Tight hamstring muscles
→ X-rays:
  ▪ Defects in the pars interarticularis—i.e., forward displacement of the posterior elements of the vertebrae
  ▪ Disk degeneration noted in the elderly patient
  ▪ Heavy bony overgrowth at the facet joints
  ▪ Marked thickening and calcification of the ligamentum flavum
→ Point tenderness in lumbar spine, especially L_4-L_5
→ Hyperlordosis
→ Flexibility of the spine is usually within normal limits.
→ Forward flexion of the spine should not increase pain.
→ Neurological exam is generally within normal limits.
→ The patient's symptoms can usually be reproduced by instructing the patient to stand on one leg and lean backwards.

Mechanical LBP

Low Back Strains and Sprains
(Della-Giustina et al. 2000, Jermyn 2001, Snider 1997)

→ There is decreased range of motion in the lumbar spine.
→ Trigger point tenderness exists over paravertebral muscle groups and upper border of the buttocks.

→ Palpation does not reproduce symptoms.
→ There is no midline vertebral tenderness.
→ There is decreased lumbar lordosis.
→ Pain increases with forward flexion.
→ There are no neurological findings.
→ Laboratory studies are within normal limits.
→ X-rays are usually normal but may show diminished lumbar lordosis.
→ The patient has difficulty standing erect.

Coccygodynia
(Jermyn 2001)

→ Point tenderness at the base of the spine
→ Normal imaging studies

Iliopsoas syndrome
(Adkins et al. 2000, Rosomoff et al. 1999)

→ Stooped posture
→ Flattened lordotic curve
→ Limited extension of the lumbar spine
→ Point tenderness over the femoral triangle and pelvis
→ Pain can be reproduced with active and passive flexion/extension of hip.

Piriformis Syndrome
(Adkins et al. 2000, Robb-Nicholson 2001, Rosomoff et al. 1999, Rossi et al. 2001)

→ Positive *Freiberg's maneuver*: forceful passive internal rotation of the patient's fully extended leg causes pain.
→ Tenderness over the sciatic notch
→ Weakness with abduction and external rotation of the hip on the affected side
→ Palpation of the piriformis muscle feels tight on rectal exam (Rosomoff 1999).

PLAN

DIAGNOSTIC TESTS

→ When ordering diagnostic studies, it is important to consider the extent to which the results will influence management of the patient's problem (Atlas et al. 2001).
→ X-rays are generally of negligible benefit in evaluating acute LBP.
  ▪ Degenerative changes typically begin in patients age 40 or older (Wang et al. 2000).
  ▪ Less than one in 2,500 patients age 50 or younger yielded unexpected findings on plain x-rays according to one study (Atlas et al. 2001).
→ Indications for ordering spine x-rays are as follows (Atlas et al. 2001, Bratton 1999, Della-Giustina et al. 2000, Patel et al. 2000):
  ▪ History of significant trauma
  ▪ Neurological deficits
  ▪ Constitutional symptoms
    • Temperature $\geq 38°$ C
    • Unexplained weight loss of more than 10 pounds in 6 months

- Medical history of:
  - Cancer
  - Regular or frequent corticosteroid use
  - Drug and/or alcohol abuse
- High index of suspicion for spondylarthropathy
→ When the patient is not improving after a reasonable course of conservative treatment (i.e., 6–8 weeks)
→ When the patient is seeking monetary compensation for her LBP
→ Standard x-rays views include:
  - Anterior/posterior (A/P) views of the lumbar-sacral spine, or coccyx if indicated
  - Lateral view of the lumbar-sacral spine or coccyx if indicated
  - Additional views should be obtained when instability of the spine may be the cause of pain (Atlas 2001).
    - Flexion/extension views of the lumbar spine
  - Oblique views, which may be obtained to more thoroughly evaluate the patency of the neural foramina are rarely indicated due to:
    - Additional cost
    - Increased and unnecessary exposure to radiation
    - Oblique projections provide additional information in less than 8% of cases (Della-Giustina 1999).
→ X-rays of adjacent musculoskeletal structures may be indicated for:
→ Sacroiliac joints
→ Hips
→ Coccyx
→ Potential x-ray findings may include:
  - Determination of disk herniations on lateral projections if the rim of the disk is calcified in a way that outlines a disk fragment (Milette 2000).
  - Anterior displacement of one vertebra over the other in spondylolisthesis can be noted on the lateral projections (Atlas et al. 2001).
  - Defects involving the pars interarticularis, described in the literature as a "collar on a Scotty dog" in appearance, on the lateral or oblique views in spondylosis (Standaert et al. 2000).
  - The patient with a spinal infection may have the following x-ray findings (Della-Giustina et al. 2000):
    - Normal for the first two weeks
    - Over the next 2–8 weeks there is progressive:
      - Bone demineralization
      - Bony destruction
      - Irregularity of vertebral end plates
      - Disk space narrowing
  - Vertebral fractures
    - Compression
    - Secondary trauma
  - Malignant tumors
    - Ewing's sarcoma
    - Osteosarcoma
    - Metastatic lesions

- Degenerative changes
  - Disk space narrowing
  - Osteophyte formation
  - Sclerosis
  - Cyst formation
→ Bone scan (Atlas et al. 2001, Della-Giustina 1999, Wang et al. 2000, Malanga et al. 1999, Omey et al. 2000, Rosomoff et al. 1999)
  - Indications for obtaining a bone scan include:
    - Determining the presence and location of:
      - Infection
      - Occult fracture
      - Bony neoplasms
      - Monitoring of certain spinal diseases
  - Bone scans are contraindicated during pregnancy.
  - Bone scans should generally be followed by a CT scan or MRI.
→ CT scans (Atlas et al. 2001, Della-Giustina 1999, Della-Giustina et al. 2000, Wang et al. 2000, Malanga et al. 1999)
  - Indications for obtaining a CT scan:
    - To better evaluate bony detail of the spine, especially the facet joints
    - To identify infections
    - To determine the presence of a tumor
    - To determine the presence of conjoined nerve roots and differentiate them from a herniated disk
    - When the presence of metallic objects preclude an MRI
    - When a fracture is suspected
  - Limitations of CT scanning include:
    - When cauda equina is suspected, CT is not adequate for evaluating the spinal cord and canal.
    - Inferior visualization of the subarachnoid space
  - A CT scan in conjunction with a myelogram is highly sensitive to spinal cord compression and is the preferred alternative study if MRI is not available.
→ Myelogram: An air contrast medium is injected into the spinal column under fluoroscopic examination.
  - Indications for obtaining a myelogram (Atlas et al. 2001, Milette 2000):
    - Visualization of the spinal cord and disk protrusions
    - Exploration of the subarachnoid space
    - Permits examination of the entire lumbar region and intrathecal structures
  - In general, with the current availability of MRI, there are few indications for myelogram, and it probably should not be ordered by the primary care provider.
→ MRI:
  - MRI combines the advantages of CT, CT-myelography, and CT-myelogram (Wang et al. 2000).
  - MRI is considered the most accurate study for evaluating soft tissue structures, including nerves (Atlas et al. 2001).
  - MRI is indicated when the following conditions are suspected (Bratton 1999, Malanga et al. 1999, Rosner 2001):
    - Lumbar disk herniation

- Infection
- Tumor
- Progressive neural dysfunction
- Nerve root impingement (Malanga et al. 1999)
- Cauda equina syndrome (Bratton 1999)
- Limitations of MRI (Della-Giustina 1999):
  - Lack of 24-hour access to MRI
  - When the patient is claustrophobic and an open MRI is unavailable
  - MRI is contraindicated in patients with:
    - Pacemakers
    - Intracardial wires
    - Mechanical heart valves
    - Aneurysm clips
    - Metallic fragments in the eyes
→ *Diskography*: an invasive procedure whereby a contrast medium is injected into a disk. If the contrast leaks, it is diagnostic of an annular tear (Milette 2000).
  - Indications for diskography are (Malanga et al. 1999):
    - To localize a symptomatic disk
    - To determine whether a disk is contained or uncontained
    - As a preoperative test before a surgical spinal fusion
  - Diskography should not be considered before the patient has been symptomatic for at least three months, and is therefore not recommended for the evaluation of acute LBP (Rosomoff et al. 1999).
  - Diskography is not considered a routine test and should only be ordered in consultation with a spine surgeon.
→ Electrodiagnosis:
  - Electromyography (EMG) and nerve conduction studies (NCS)
    - Indications (Wang et al. 2000, Malanga et al. 1999, Rosomoff et al. 1999):
      - To differentiate peripheral neuropathy from radiculopathy
      - To determine the extent of nerve injury
      - To predict the course of recovery
      - To determine whether structural abnormalities are of functional significance
      - To detect radicular lesions
  - Positive findings are usually not manifested for 2–4 weeks following the onset of symptoms (Patel et al. 2000).
  - EMG abnormalities are present to some extent in approximately 80% of patients (Atlas et al. 2001).
→ Laboratory tests are occasionally indicated in the course of evaluating low back pain (Atlas et al. 2001, Bratton 1999, Della-Giustina et al. 2000, Patel et al. 2000).
  - CBC may be obtained to consider:
    - Infection
    - The presence of a metastatic lesion
    - Visceral causes of LBP
  - ESR can be elevated in the following conditions:
    - Infection
    - Metastatic tumor

- Inflammatory musculoskeletal conditions:
  - Rheumatoid arthritis (RA)
  - Polymyalgia rheumatica (PMR)
  - Systemic lupus erythematosus (SLE)
- Blood cultures are positive in over 40% of patients with spinal infections.
- Serum protein electrophoresis: abnormal values are suggestive of multiple myeloma.
- Urinalysis should be obtained when infection is suspected.
- When evaluating pathological fractures which result from underlying bone disease, additional lab tests may include:
  - Serum calcium levels
  - Alkaline phosphatase
  - Urinary hydroxyproline excretion
- Blood tests to confirm certain rheumatological conditions that may contribute to LBP:
  - RA: positive result when the patient has rheumatoid arthritis
  - ANA: a positive result is highly suggestive of SLE

ASSESSMENT

→ R/O metastatic lesions
→ R/O spinal infection
→ R/O fractures of the lumbar spine
→ R/O cauda equina syndrome
→ R/O LBP referred from visceral organ disease
→ R/O lumbar disk herniation
→ R/O spondylolisthesis and spondylosis
→ R/O low back sprains and strains
→ R/O coccygodynia
→ R/O iliopsoas syndrome
→ R/O piriformis syndrome
→ R/O systemic disease
  - Peripheral vascular disease
  - Peripheral neuropathy
  - Paget's disease
  - Osteoporosis

TREATMENT/MANAGEMENT

→ If red flags are identified, refer the patient to an appropriate specialist.
  - Cauda equina syndrome is a surgical emergency.
→ In primary care the focus is conservative care, education, and reassurance (Atlas et al. 2001).
→ Surgery is necessary in less than one in 200 patients with a specific diagnosis (Rosomoff et al. 1999).
→ More than 60% of patients with LBP significantly improve within seven days (Bratton 1999).
→ Most patients with LBP who maintain their normal activity level or resume it as soon as possible have superior outcomes overall (Bratton 1999, Della-Giustina et al. 2000, Malanga et al. 1999, Patel et al. 2000).
→ Activity modification:
  - Maintain normal activities as tolerated, avoiding those that induce pain (Della-Giustina 1999).

- If the patient is experiencing severe acute radiculopathy, 2–3 days of bed rest in the supine position is recommended (Patel et al. 2000).
  - Studies have demonstrated the detrimental effects of prolonged bed rest on bone, connective tissue, muscle groups, and cardiovascular fitness (Malanga et al. 1999).
- Sitting upright should be avoided when possible because this position exacerbates symptoms by raising intradiscal pressures (Patel et al. 2000).
- Standing for prolonged periods should be avoided (Patel et al. 2000).
- Low-stress aerobic exercise such as walking, biking, or swimming can usually be resumed within two weeks after the onset of LBP (Van Tulder et al. 2000).

→ Analgesia (see **Table 8N.1, Anti-inflammatory and Analgesic Medication**):
- Acetaminophen for initial treatment of mild to moderate pain (Della-Giustina 1999, Malanga et al. 1999):
  - Cost-effective
  - Well tolerated
  - High therapeutic index
- NSAIDs:
  - All NSAIDs have demonstrated comparable effectiveness in treating LBP (Borenstein 2001, Griffin et al. 2002, Van Tulder et al. 2000).
  - A 2–4 week course of NSAIDs is generally recommended (Patel et al. 2000).
  - NSAIDs are the most common medication prescribed for LBP (Rosner 2001).
  - NSAIDs are more effective during the first week of symptoms (Malanga et al. 1999).
  - NSAIDs can be combined with acetaminophen for the treatment of acute LBP (Della-Giustina et al. 2000).
  - When selecting an NSAID for a particular patient, the clinician must consider (Della-Giustina 1999):
    - Cost
    - Dosing schedule
    - Potential side effects
    - Contraindications
- Muscle relaxants:
  - Although muscle relaxants have proven to be more effective than placebo for the treatment of acute LBP, they are just as effective as NSAIDs (Atlas et al. 2001, Della-Giustina 1999).
  - In general, muscle relaxants have been shown to:
    - Induce increased range of motion of the lumbar spine
    - Enhance the patient's capacity for exercise (Jermyn 2001)
  - Common muscle relaxants prescribed for the treatment of acute LBP include (Barton 2001):
    - Tizandine
    - Cyclobenzaprine
    - Dantrolene
    - Carisoprodol
    - Baclofen

  - Orphenadrine
  - Diazepam
- Potential side effects of muscle relaxants include:
  - Dizziness in up to 70% of patients
  - Risk of dependency after one week of continuous use (Barton 2001)
- Opioids:
  - Opioids, in general, have not been proven to be more effective than acetaminophen for the treatment of LBP (Atlas et al. 2001, Rosomoff et al. 1999).
  - Six studies on the treatment of acute LBP failed to identify any significant therapeutic benefit of opioids over NSAIDs (Van Tulder et al. 2000). (See **Table 8N.1**.)
  - Opioids are typically prescribed for the treatment of moderate to severe LBP, and may include (Jermyn 2001):
    - Vicodin®: Hydrocodone bitartrate and acetaminophen (5 mg/500 mg)
    - Darvocet-N 100®: Propoxyphene napsylate and acetaminophen (100 mg/650 mg)
    - Tylenol® with codeine: Acetaminophen and codeine phosphate (300 mg/30 mg)
    - Percocet®: Oxycodone HCL and acetaminophen (7.5 mg/325 mg)
    NOTE: Refer to the *Physicians' Desk Reference* (PDR) for dosage schedule.
  - Opioids should be (Malanga et al. 1999):
    - Limited to pain that is unresponsive to alternative pharmacological treatment.
    - Prescribed in maintenance doses as opposed to prn.
    - Prescribed for a maximum of 1–2 weeks (Della-Giustina et al. 2000).
    - Potential side effects occur in about 50% of patients (Barton 2001):
      ➤ Sedation
      ➤ Habituation
- Antidepressants are not indicated for the treatment of acute LBP (Malanga et al. 1999, Rosomoff et al. 1999).
- Anticonvulsants are occasionally prescribed for persons with acute LBP to potentiate the effects of analgesics (Jermyn 2001).
- Oral corticosteroids:
  - Prescribed most often for persons with sciatica and/or a herniated disk (Della-Giustina 1999)
  - Not recommended for acute LBP that is not associated with radicular systems (Rosomoff et al. 1999)
  - The typical treatment regimen for oral corticosteroids is a prednisone taper—i.e., the patient takes a 10–14 day course of prednisone in decreasing doses, for example, 80 mg for 2 days, 70 mg for 2 days, etcetera.
  - Potential side effects of short term oral prednisone use include the following:
    - Mood lability
    - Weight gain
    - Urinary frequency
    - Insomnia

- Gastrointestinal disturbances
- Elevated blood glucose levels
■ Epidural steroid injections:
  • Epidural steroid injections, usually administered by an anesthesiologist, are typically given in a series of three, several weeks apart for the duration of the therapeutic response.
  • The use of epidural steroid injections for acute radicular LBP has not been well studied. The literature reports anywhere from a 10–66% percent rate of effectiveness (Della-Giustina 1999, Jermyn 2001).
  • The indications for epidural steroid injections for acute LBP are to:
    - Decrease nerve root inflammation secondary to disk disease (Malanga et al. 1999).
    - Decrease pain in patients with acute radicular LBP who have not improved after 4 weeks of more conservative therapy (Jermyn 2001).
  • Potential complications of epidural steroid injections (Sheehan et al. 2001):
    - Epidural hematomas
    - Meningitis
    - Arachnoiditis
    - Systemic effects of steroids may occur when the patient receives the injections on a regular and frequent basis.
→ Conventional physical therapy (PT):
  ■ Because most LBP will resolve within 2–4 weeks, PT should reasonably be delayed until that time (Atlas et al. 2001).
  ■ The goals of PT (Jermyn 2001, Malanga et al. 1999):
    • Restore flexibility of the lumbar spine
    • Increase range of motion of the lumbar spine
    • Improve functioning
    • Correct body mechanics
    • Strengthen the trunk
  ■ In addition to the standard stretching and strengthening program, physical therapists often administer other treatments that are purported to have analgesic and anti-inflammatory effects.
    • Transcutaneous electrical nerve stimulating (TENS):
      - The therapeutic value of TENS has yet to be proven (Rosomoff et al. 1999).
      - TENS should not be prescribed for the treatment of acute LBP (Atlas et al. 2001).
    • Ultrasound: a mechanical radiant energy system used to apply deep heat to the affected tissues.
      - Proponents claim it increases the length of periarticular ligaments and tendons (Patel et al. 2000).
      - Contraindications:
        ➤ Acute inflammatory conditions
        ➤ History of a laminectomy
        ➤ Over peripheral nerves
    • Spinal traction: a procedure whereby one and a half times the patient's body weight is used to distract the vertebral bodies in the lumbar spine (Malanga et al. 1999).

- Not recommended for acute LBP (Rosomoff et al. 1999).
- There is no convincing evidence that spinal traction is effective (Patel et al. 2000).
• Application of superficial heat:
  - Soothing, but not generally effective in relieving LBP (Rosomoff et al. 1999)
  - Can promote muscle relaxation (Patel et al. 2000)
  - Most effective during the early phase of treatment (Malanga et al. 1999)
  - Contraindications (Patel et al. 2000):
    ➤ Decreased peripheral circulation
    ➤ Peripheral neuropathy
    ➤ Presence of edema
    ➤ History of bleeding diathesis
• Application of ice (Patel et al. 2000, Malanga et al. 1999):
  - Provides some analgesic effect
  - Decreases edema in injured soft tissue
  - Anti-inflammatory effect
  - Contraindications:
    ➤ Diminished sensation
    ➤ Poor peripheral circulation
• Spinal manipulation (Malanga et al. 1999):
  - Can diminish acute pain within 1–4 weeks of initiating treatment.
  - Should be performed in conjunction with an exercise program
  - Should be discontinued if symptoms do not begin to resolve after 3 treatments
  - There is no evidence that continued treatments will prevent pain once the acute phase of LBP has run its course.
  - Manipulation has not been demonstrated to be more effective than conventional physical therapy (Della-Giustina et al. 2000).
  NOTE: There is little evidence that manipulation is more effective than placebo for the treatment of acute LBP (Rosner 2001).
• Exercise programs (Van Tulder et al. 2000)
  - There is strong evidence that exercise therapy is not effective for acute LBP.
  - Back exercises do not improve clinical outcomes for patients with acute LBP.
  - Despite the controversy, exercise programs are often prescribed for persons with acute LBP, and the treatment goals include (Bratton 1999):
    ➤ Preventing debilitation secondary to inactivity
    ➤ Improving activity tolerance
    ➤ Returning the patient to her highest level of functioning
• Miscellaneous treatment modalities:
  - Chiropractic treatment:
    ➤ There is some evidence that persons with acute LBP derive occasional benefit from this (Patel et al. 2000).

– Acupuncture:
  ➤ Based on the premise that there are patterns of energy flow called Qi through the body that are required for general health maintenance. Disruption of this flow is thought to cause disease (Malanga et al. 1999).
  ➤ Patients with sciatica have been shown to benefit from acupuncture.
  ➤ The therapeutic efficacy has not been well-established for persons with nonspecific LBP (Atlas et al. 2001).
– Lumbar corsets:
  ➤ In general, corsets are no longer considered to be appropriate for the treatment of LBP (Rosomoff et al. 1999).
  ➤ Corsets may have limited utility for treating compression fractures and some other acute spinal fractures (Patel et al. 2000).
  ➤ Lumbar supports have not demonstrated the capacity to prevent further spinal injury (Malanga et al. 1999).
– Massage therapy, diathermy, and biofeedback have not demonstrated any therapeutic benefit in the treatment of acute LBP (Bratton 1999, Della-Giustina et al. 2000).
– Alternative medicine: although no one form of alternative treatment has proven to be effective in the treatment of acute LBP, persons with LBP frequently seek out these therapies. It has been suggested that one of the most appealing aspects of alternative medicine practitioners is that these practitioners are more inclined to assert a specific diagnosis for the patient's LBP symptoms (Atlas et al. 2001).

CONSULTATION

→ Immediate orthopedic or neurosurgical consultation is required when any of the following conditions exist (Atlas et al. 2001, Patel et al. 2000):
  ▪ High index of suspicion for cauda equina
  ▪ Worsening neurological symptoms
  ▪ Intractable pain that is refractory to treatment
→ Referral to an orthopedic surgeon or a musculoskeletal oncologist should be made promptly when there is radiographic or laboratory evidence of (Atlas et al. 2001):
  ▪ Tumor
  ▪ Fracture
  ▪ Space occupying lesion
  ▪ Infection
→ The patient with metastatic spinal lesions should be referred to a neurosurgeon or musculoskeletal oncologist when (Borenstein 2001):
  ▪ She is demonstrating progressive neurological deficits.
  ▪ She has been resistant to radiation.
  ▪ The patient's pain is intractable.
  ▪ There is a need for a histological diagnosis.

→ Referral to an orthopedic spine surgeon or neurosurgeon should be considered when:
  ▪ The diagnosis is uncertain.
  ▪ The patient has been unresponsive to treatment.
  ▪ The patient is demonstrating a progressive neurological deficit and the following four criteria are met (Atlas et al. 2001):
    • The intensity of leg pain exceeds LBP
    • Positive straight leg raises
    • No therapeutic response to conservative treatment after 6 weeks for a herniated disk, or 12 weeks with spinal stenosis.
    • Imaging studies reveal a significant lesion that corresponds to the patient's symptoms (Della-Giustina et al. 2000).
→ Referral to a physiatrist or a spine surgeon is appropriate when (Atlas et al. 2001):
  ▪ Red flags have been excluded, and at least 6–8 weeks of conservative treatment have failed.
  ▪ The diagnosis is uncertain.
→ When the origin of the patient's LBP is likely from visceral organs, the patient should be referred to the appropriate specialist (Patel et al. 2000):
  ▪ Internist
  ▪ General surgeon
  ▪ Vascular surgeon
→ Patients with acute LBP who may have an underlying rheumatological condition should be referred to a rheumatologist.
→ Patients with LBP who may benefit from an epidural steroid injection should be referred to an anesthesiologist who is qualified to administer this treatment.

PATIENT EDUCATION

→ General principles:
  ▪ The success of most treatments for LBP depends on the patient's understanding of her condition and her role in minimizing the symptoms (Patel et al. 2000).
  ▪ Education regarding the patient's condition should include (Malanga et al. 1999):
    • A review of the basic relevant anatomy
    • Instruction on the biomechanics of the spine and how that relates to the patient's complaints
    • A description of the diagnostic studies indicated for the patient's specific complaint
  ▪ Written instruction reinforces verbal instruction.
  ▪ LBP is self-limiting most of the time.
→ Educate the patient on the potential side effects of prescribed medications and treatments.
→ Advise regarding spine care and injury prevention (Patel et al. 2000).
→ Advise that excess body weight has an adverse effect on treatment regimes for LBP (Patel et al. 2000).
→ Patients with LBP should be instructed to (Atlas et al. 2001):
  ▪ Avoid prolonged periods of sitting and standing.
  ▪ Stand up and move around every 30 minutes.

- Rise slowly from a sitting position to avoid the onset of pain and spasm.
- Refrain from engaging in strenuous activity (e.g., lifting and jogging) until symptoms have subsided for more than several days.
- Engage in low stress aerobic activity. Walking is the most therapeutic form of exercise.
- Utilize lifting techniques that emphasize lifting with large muscle groups in the lower extremities (i.e., quadriceps and hamstrings) (Jermyn 2001).
→ The single most predictive risk factor for future episodes of LBP is the occurrence of a prior episode (Malanga et al. 1999).

FOLLOW-UP

→ In the absence of red flags, follow-up with the primary care provider should occur about six weeks after the initial visit.
→ The patient with LBP should be advised to seek prompt medical follow-up if any of the following develop (Della-Giustina et al. 2000):
- Neurological symptoms
- Fever
- Worsening or unrelenting pain
- Loss of bowel or bladder functions (Bratton 1999)
→ Only 7% of LBP patients remain symptomatic after three months. They are then classified as chronic, and should be referred to a chronic pain facility (Rosomoff et al. 1999).

Chronic Low Back Pain

DATABASE

SUBJECTIVE

Spinal Stenosis

(Atlas et al. 2001, Capelle 2001, Patel et al. 2000, Sheehan et al. 2001, Snider 1997)

→ Pain originates in the lumbar spine, then radiates through the buttocks, and eventually downward into the calves.
→ The onset of symptoms is usually gradual, progressing slowly over the years.
→ The patient is typically affected beginning in her 50s–70s.
→ Pain is likely to increase with:
- Walking (pseudoclaudication)
- Extending the lumbar spine
- Standing
- Lying supine
→ Pain typically diminishes with:
- Forward flexion of the lumbar spine
- Sitting down
- Squatting
→ The patient may describe the leg pain as:
- Burning
- Cramping
- Bilateral

→ The patient often complains of her legs feeling weak, and may characterize the sensation as an "inability to find legs."
→ Complaints of paresthesias in the legs are described as:
- Numbness
- Tingling
- "Pins and needles"
→ In central canal spinal stenosis, neurological symptoms in the lower extremities are bilateral.
→ In foraminal spinal stenosis, the neurological symptoms are unilateral.

Lumbar Degenerative Disk Disease

(Patel et al. 2000, Snider 1997)

→ LBP that can radiate into one or both buttocks
→ Pain can be aggravated by mechanical symptoms.
→ The patient complains of stiffness when rising from a seated position.
→ The patient may complain of the intermittent presence of paresthesias in her lower extremities.
→ Typically presents in patients in their 30s–60s
→ Pain is relieved by rest.
→ History of smoking

Spondylolisthesis

(Omey et al. 2000, Patel et al. 2000, Snider 1997)

→ More common in women
→ Can occur at any age, but most typically begins in the third decade.
→ History of high level athletic endeavors, especially those that involve repetitive hyperextension of the spine:
- Gymnastics
- Dancing
- Diving
- Figure skating
→ Pain is exacerbated by:
- Forward flexion of the lumbar spine
- Heavy lifting
- Twisting
→ Spondylolisthesis may often simulate a herniated lumbar disk or spinal stenosis.
→ Usually there is no history of one particular incident of trauma.
→ Pain occurs in the lumbar spine, posterior and lateral aspects of thighs, and coccyx.

Spondylosis

(Jermyn 2001, Standaert et al. 2000)

→ Occurs in 3–6% of adult Caucasian persons
→ Affects up to 15% of adolescent athletes:
- Divers
- Weight lifters
- Wrestlers
- Gymnasts
- High jumpers
- Track and field sports
- Rowing

→ Onset of pain may be gradual or acute.

→ Pain is located in the lumbar spine and is usually nonradicular.

→ Pain increases with:

- Physical activity
- Lumbar spinal extension
- Rotational movements of the lumbar spine

Lumbar Disk Herniation and Sciatica

→ See the "Subjective" section of "Acute Low Back Pain, Lumbar Disk Herniation and Sciatica" in this chapter.

Psychogenic Pain

(Atlas et al. 2001, Patel et al. 2000, Rosomoff et al. 1999)

→ History of previous LBP

→ History of depression

→ History of substance abuse

→ Pending or past litigation

→ The patient is receiving workmen's compensation or state disability benefits

→ Lower socio-economic status

→ History of job dissatisfaction

→ History of inadequate response to treatment

→ Preoccupied with her LBP

OBJECTIVE

Spinal Stenosis

(Jermyn 2001, Patel et al. 2000, Rosomoff et al. 1999, Snider 1997)

→ Diminished knee and ankle reflexes that are asymmetrical

→ Unilateral great toe weakness with resisted dorsiflexion

→ Occasionally decreased sensation to pinprick and hot/cold temperature that is dermatomal

→ Decreased spinal extension

→ Unilateral decreased thigh and calf circumference

- Differences of up to 2 cm in leg length are within normal limits.

→ Radiographic findings may include:

- Asymmetrical narrowing of the joint spaces.
- Degenerative changes along the lumbar spine

→ MRI or CT will confirm narrowing of the spinal canal.

Lumbar Degenerative Disk Disease

(Patel et al. 2000, Snider 1997)

→ Tenderness along the lumbar spine and over the sacroiliac joints

→ Decreased spinal extension

→ X-ray findings include:

- Asymmetric narrowing of the joint spaces
- Osteophyte formation along the vertebrae
- Sclerotic subchondral bone

Spondylolisthesis

→ See the "Objective" section of "Acute Low Back Pain, Spondylolisthesis and Spondylosis" in this chapter.

Spondylosis

→ See the "Objective" section of "Acute Low Back Pain, Lumbar Disk Herniation and Sciatica" in this chapter.

Lumbar Disk Herniation and Sciatica

→ See the "Objective" section of "Acute Low Back Pain, Lumbar Disk Herniation and Sciatica" in this chapter.

Psychogenic Pain

(Patel et al. 2000, Snider 1997)

→ Patients with psychosomatic LBP may demonstrate any one of a number of positive *Waddell signs*: nonorganic clinical signs that indicate the presence of a functional component to the LBP:

- Superficial, nonanatomic tenderness
- Pain with simulated testing
  - Axial loading
  - Pelvic rotation
- Inconsistent responses to distraction
- Nonorganic regional disturbances (i.e., nondermatomal sensory loss)
- General emotional and physical overreaction to various examination maneuvers

→ Additional findings may include:

- Hypersensitivity to light touch
- Facial grimacing
- Diffuse tenderness in the lower back and sacroiliac region
- Deep tendon reflexes within normal limits
- Normal muscle strength
- Negative *sitting straight leg raises*: have the patient sit with her legs hanging over the edge of the exam table. Casually extend one of the patient's legs to about 90°. Unless the patient's sciatica is genuine, she will not react to this maneuver.

ASSESSMENT

→ R/O spinal stenosis

→ R/O lumbar degenerative disk disease

→ R/O spondylolisthesis

→ R/O spondylosis

→ R/O herniated intervertebral disk, sciatica

→ R/O psychogenic LBP

→ R/O fibromyalgia

→ R/O polymyalgia rheumatica

→ R/O compression fractures of the lumbar spine

→ R/O metabolic bone disease

→ R/O hip degenerative joint disease

PLAN

DIAGNOSTIC TESTS

→ See the "Diagnostic Tests" section of "Acute Low Back Pain" in this chapter.

TREATMENT/MANAGEMENT

→ See the "Treatment Management" section of "Acute Low Back Pain" in this chapter.

→ Approximately 90% of patients with LBP will recover within three months.

- A subset of the remaining 10% qualifies for the diagnosis

of failed back syndrome. At least 40% of them will have persistent or recurrent LBP or sciatica with associated levels of impairment, which exist even after spine surgery or noninterventional treatment (Rosomoff et al. 1999).

→ Managing the patient with chronic LBP includes behavior therapy such as:
- Psychotherapy
- Inpatient treatment for substance abuse
- Long term residence in a multidisciplinary pain treatment facility

→ Patients with chronic LBP who have undergone therapy in some form experience decreased pain intensity and increased functional capacity.

→ A review of behavioral patient outcomes suggests little support for one method of therapy over another (Van Tulder et al. 2001).

→ Behavioral therapy is effective only when the patient is motivated to change.

→ Due to the protracted duration of the symptoms, patients and providers are inclined to employ numerous conventional as well as alternative treatments in an effort to resolve the patient's LBP.

→ Multidisciplinary chronic pain centers (Rosomoff et al. 1999):
- Goals of the centers include:
  - Decrease or eliminate pain
  - Minimize the need for pain medication
  - Correct biomechanical abnormalities:
    – Posture
    – Gait
    – Range of motion
  - Diminish psychiatric or psychological impairment
  - Educate the patient with respect to how emotions, behavior, and attitudes affect the course of LBP
  - Improve the level of functioning in social, family and household roles
  - Restore vocational role functions
  - Educate the patient on methods to maintain functional level of rehabilitation and avoid reinjury
- Evidence has demonstrated that chronic pain clinics:
  - Improve symptoms in about 84% of patients with LBP within one year
  - Relief from pain is sustained over a significant period of time
  - Successfully return disabled patients to work

→ Operant conditioning (Van Tulder 2001):
- Reward adaptive behavior with positive reinforcement and withhold attention when the patient demonstrates behavior that focuses on her pain.
- This is time-contingent instead of pain-contingent pain management.
- This therapy requires the involvement of a spouse or significant other.

→ Respondent therapy:
- Designed to modify the physiologic response system to pain directly
- The patient is provided with a model of association

between tension and pain, and taught to replace muscle tension with a tension-incompatible reaction.
- Relaxation techniques
- Electromyographic biofeedback

→ Cognitive therapy:
- Designed to identify and modify the patient's cognition with respect to her pain and disability
- Cognitive restructuring techniques include:
  - Visual imagery
  - Attention diversion

→ Osteopathic therapy (Borenstein 2001):
- Considered for patients with chronic mechanical LBP who possess a high risk factor associated with conventional treatment such as manipulation

→ Dynamic lumbar stabilization (Capelle 2001):
- A technique that helps stabilize the lumbar spine in such a way that it will result in increased intervertebral disc space to accommodate the nerve roots branching off the spine.
- The technique involves physical therapy and strengthening exercises.
- Flattening the curve of the lumbar spine can enhance the duration of standing and walking.
- Patients with spinal stenosis are known to benefit from this treatment.

→ Prolotherapy (Malanga et al. 1999):
- The injection of a solution such as normal saline or 15% dextrose into loose tendons, ligaments, and joint capsules.
- The goal is to ignite the activation of fibroblastic activity to produce connective tissue within the affected area.
- This unconventional therapy is not used in general practice.

→ Chiropractic treatment may benefit some patients with chronic LBP (Patel et al. 2000).

Medication

→ Certain forms of medication are more widely prescribed for patients with LBP. These medications should be prescribed in consultation with a physician. The *PDR* should also be reviewed.
- Antidepressants (Jermyn 2001):
  - Address the underlying depression that often accompanies chronic LBP
  - Antidepressants may potentiate the affects of analgesia.
- Anticonvulsants (Jermyn 2001):
  - Powerful mood stabilizers
  - Potentiate the affects of analgesia

CONSULTATION

→ See the "Consultation" section of "Acute Low Back Pain" in this chapter.

→ Criteria for referral to a multidisciplinary chronic pain center (Rosomoff et al. 1999):
- The patient continues to experience significant pain after all other reasonable treatment trials.
- Severely diminished functional status

- The patient's perception of her LBP constitutes a disability
- Unchecked chemical or alcohol dependency
- Somatoform pain disorder

→ Patients with spinal stenosis should be referred to a neurosurgeon or orthopedic spine surgeon when the patient (Capelle 2001, Sheehan et al. 2001, Snider 1997):
  - Has failed conservative treatment
  - Experiences pseudoclaudication
  - Has bowel or bladder symptoms:
    - Urinary retention or loss of control
    - Fecal incontinence
  - Has progressive weakness in the legs

→ The goal of surgery for patients with chronic spinal stenosis is to enlarge that area of the spinal canal where the nerves are being compressed.

→ Surgery for spinal stenosis is generally well tolerated, even among elderly patients in their late 70s–80s.

PATIENT EDUCATION

→ See the "Patient Education" section of "Acute Low Back Pain" in this chapter.

→ Educate patients with chronic LBP for whom behavioral interventions are indicated on the purpose of the treatment and the importance of their compliance.

→ Emphasize the relationship between lifestyle changes and shorter states of functional disability:
  - Quitting smoking
  - Losing weight
  - Instituting and maintaining a regular exercise program
  - Maintaining an active routine as the limitations of LBP permits

FOLLOW-UP

→ See the "Follow-up" section of "Acute Low Back Pain" in this chapter.

BIBLIOGRAPHY

Adkins, S.B., and Figler, R.A. 2000. Hip pain in athletes. *American Family Physician* 61:2109–2118.

Atlas, S.J., and Deyo, R.A. 2001. Evaluating and managing acute low back pain in the primary care setting. *Spine* 16:120–131.

Barton, S. 2001. *Clinical evidence*. London: BMJ Publishing Group.

Biundo, J.J., Irwin, R.W., and Umpierre, E. 2001. Sports and other soft tissue injuries, tendinitis, bursitis and occupation–related syndromes. *Current Opinion in Rheumatology* 13:146–149.

Borenstein, D.G. 1999. Epidemiology, etiology, diagnostic evaluation and treatment of low back pain. *Current Opinion in Rheumatology* 11:151–160.

_____. 2001. Epidemiology, etiology, diagnostic evaluation and treatment of low back pain. *Current Opinion in Rheumatology* 13:128–134.

Bratton, R.L. 1999. Assessment and management of acute low back pain. *American Family Physician* 60:2299–2308.

Capelle, A.K. 2001. Spinal stenosis: severity determines treatment plan. *Mayo Clinic Health Letter* June 19:1–3.

Della–Giustina, D.A. 1999. Orthopedic emergencies. Emergency Department evaluation and treatment of back pain. *Emergency Medicine Clinics of North America* 17:877–893.

Della–Giustina, D., and Kilcline, B.A. 2000. Acute low back pain: a comprehensive review. *Comprehensive Therapy* 26:153–159.

Griffin, G., Tudiver, F., and Grant, W.D. 2002. Cochrane for clinicians: putting evidence into practice. Do NSAIDs help in acute or chronic low back pain? *American Family Physician* 65:1319–1321.

Jermyn, R.T. 2001. A nonsurgical approach to low back pain. *The Journal of the American Osteopathic Association* 101:S6–11.

Malanga, G.A., and Nadler, S.F. 1999. Nonoperative treatment of low back pain. *Mayo Clinic Proceedings* 74:1135–1148.

Milette, P.C. 2000. Imaging of low back pain I: Classification, diagnostic imaging, and imaging characterization of a lumbar herniated disk. *Radiologic Clinics of North America* 38:1267–92.

Nelemans, P.J., deBie, R.A., deVet, H.C. et al. 2001. Injection therapy for subacute and chronic benign low back pain. *Spine* 26:501–515.

Omey, M.L., Micheli, L.J., and Gerbino, P.G. 2000. Idiopathic scoliosis and spondylolysis in the female athlete. Tips for treatment. *Clinical Orthopaedics and Related Research* 372:74–84.

Patel, A., and Ogle, A.A. 2000. Diagnosis and management of acute low back pain. *American Family Physician* 61:1779–1790.

Porter, S.E., and Hanley, E.N., 2001. The musculoskeletal effects of smoking. *Journal of the American Academy of Orthopaedic Surgeons* 9:9–17.

Postacchini, F. 2001. Lumbar disc herniation: a new equilibrium is needed between nonoperative and operative treatment. *Spine* 26:601–602.

Reilly, P.A. 2001. Occupational low back pain. *Journal of Rheumatology* 28:225–226.

Robb–Nicholson, C. 2001. By the way, doctor: what is piriformis syndrome? *Harvard Women's Health Watch* March 8:8.

Rosner, A. 2001. Evidence–based clinical guidelines for the management of acute low back pain: Response to the guidelines prepared for the Australian Medical Health and Research Council. *Journal of Manipulative and Physiological Therapeutics* 24:214–220.

Rosomoff, H.L., and Rosomoff, R.S. 1999. Low back pain evaluation and management in the primary care setting. *Medical Clinics of North America* 83:644–662.

Rossi, P., Cardinali, P., Serrao, M. et al. 2001. Magnetic resonance imaging findings in piriformis syndrome: a case report. *Archives of Physical Medicine and Rehabilitation* 82:519–521.

Sheehan, J.M., Shaffrey, C.I., and Jane, J.A. 2001. Degenerative lumbar stenosis: the neurosurgical perspective. *Clinical Orthopaedics and Related Research* 384:61–74.

Snider, R.K. 1997. *Essentials of musculoskeletal care.* Rosemont, Ill.: American Academy of Orthopedics.

Standaert, C.J., Herring, S.A., Halpern, B. et al. 2000. Spondylolysis. *Physical Medicine and Rehabilitation Clinic of North America* 11:785–803.

Van Tulder, M.W., Ostelo, R., Vlaeyen, J.W.S. et al. 2001. Behavioral treatment for chronic low back pain: a systematic review within the framework of the Cochrane Back Review Group. *Spine* 26:270–281.

Van Tulder, M., Malmivaara, A., Esmail, R. et al. 2000. Exercise therapy for low back pain: a systematic review within the framework of the Cochrane Collaboration Back Review Group. *Spine* 25:2784–2796.

Wang, H., Koti, M., Smith, F.W. et al. 2000. Diagnosis of lumbosacral nerve root anomalies by magnetic resonance imaging. *Journal of Spinal Disorders* 14:143–149.

8-N

Anti-inflammatory and Analgesic Medication

Table 8N.1. ANTI-INFLAMMATORY AND ANALGESIC MEDICATION

Cyclooxygenase-2 (COX-2) Inhibitors					
Generic Drug Name	Trade Name	Usual Adult Dose	Maximum Adult Daily Dose	Available Dosage Forms	Comments
Celecoxib	Celebrex®	Osteoarthritis: 100 mg BID or 200 mg daily Rheumatoid arthritis: 100–200 mg BID	400 mg	Capsules: 100, 200 mg	
Meloxicam	Mobic®	7.5–15 mg daily	15 mg		"Preferential" COX-2 activity. Less selective than others in the class.
Rofecoxib	Vioxx®	Osteoarthritis: 12.5 mg daily (initial); 25 mg daily (maintenance) Pain or dysmenorrhea: 25 mg daily	50 mg	Tablets: 12.5, 25, 50 mg Oral suspension: 12.5 mg/5 mL, 25 mg/5 mL	
Valdecoxib	Bextra®	Arthritis: 10 mg daily Dysmenorrhea: 20 mg BID	40 mg	Tablets: 10, 20 mg	

Analgesics						
Narcotic Agents						
Generic Drug Name	Trade Name	Route	Usual Adult Dose	Available Dosage Forms	Dose equal to 10 mg IM of Morphine Sulphate	Comments
Codeine	Codeine	IV, IM, SC PO	15–60 mg every 4–6 hours 10–20 mg every 4–6 hours (for antitussive effect)	Injection: 30, 60 mg Oral solution: 15 mg/5mL Tablet: 15, 30, 60 mg	IM: 120–130 mg SC: 120 mg PO: 200 mg	Maximum daily dose is 360 mg. Has antitussive effects in lower doses (given orally). Often used in combination with other analgesics.

(continued)

Table 8N.1.   ANTI-INFLAMMATORY AND ANALGESIC MEDICATION *(continued)*

Generic Drug Name	Trade Name	Route	Usual Adult Dose	Available Dosage Forms	Dose equal to 10 mg IM of Morphine Sulphate	Comments
Hydrocodone	Vicodin®	PO	5–10 mg every 4–6 hours	Tablet: 2.5 mg with APAP 500 mg Tablet and/or capsule: 5 mg with APAP 400 or 500 mg, or aspirin 500 mg, or homatropine 1.5 mg Tablet: 7.5 mg with APAP 400, 500, 650, or 750 mg, or ibuprofen 200 mg Tablet: 10 mg with APAP 325, 400, 500, 650, 660 mg Elixir: 2.5 mg + APAP 167mg/5 mL Syrup: 5 mg hydrocodone + homatropine 1.5 mg/5 mL	5–10 mg	Only available in combination with acetaminophen, aspirin, homatropine, or ibuprofen.
Oxycodone	Roxicodone®, OxyContin®	PO	Immediate-release 5–15 mg every 4–6 hours	Capsule: 5 mg Tablet: 15, 30 mg Oral liquid: 20 mg/mL	5–10 mg	Also available in combination with aspirin (e.g., Percodan®) or APAP (e.g., Percocet®).
Propoxyphene	Darvon®	PO	Hydrochloride salt: 65 mg every 4 hours Napsylate salt: 100 mg every 4 hours	Capsule: 65 mg (HCl salt) Tablet: 100 mg (napsylate salt)	65 mg (HCl salt) 100 mg (napsylate salt)	100 mg of propoxyphene napsylate is equal to 65 mg of propoxyphene hydrochloride. Maximum daily dose of hydrochloride form is 390 mg. Maximum daily dose of napsylate form is 600 mg. Also available in combination with APAP (e.g., Darvocet®).

Non-Narcotic Analgesics						
Non-Salicylates						
Generic Drug Name	Trade Name	Usual Adult Dose	Maximum Adult Daily Dose	Prescription Strength	Nonprescription Strength	Comments
Acetaminophen	Tylenol®	325–650 mg every 4–6 hours	4,000 mg	NA	Tablets: 160, 325, 500, 650 mg Chewable tablets: 80 mg Drops: 80 mg/0.8 mL, 80 mg/1.66 mL, 100 mg/mL Elixir: 40, 80, 125, 160 mg/5 mL Liquid: 160 mg/5 mL, 500 mg/15 mL	Hepatotoxicity if overdosed and in persons with cirrhosis (limit dose to 2,000 mg/day in cirrhotics).

(continued)

Table 8N.1.   ANTI-INFLAMMATORY AND ANALGESIC MEDICATION *(continued)*

Salicylates*						
Generic Drug Name	**Trade Name**	**Usual Adult Dose**	**Maximum Adult Daily Dose**	**Prescription Strength**	**Nonprescription Strength**	**Comments**
Acetylsalicylic acid	Aspirin	325–975 mg every 4 hours	8,000 mg	Enteric coated tablets: 975 mg Slow release tablets: 800, 975 mg	Tablets: 325, 500 mg Chewable tablets: 81 mg Gum tablets: 227.5 mg Enteric coated tablets: 81, 165, 325, 500, 650 mg Slow release tablets: 81, 650 mg	Antagonizes effect of probenecid. Increases effect of sulfonylureas. Reduces renal clearance of methotrexate.
Choline magnesium trisalicylate	Trilisate®	500–1,000 mg every 12 hours	3,000 mg	Tablets: 500, 750, 1,000 mg Liquid: 500 mg/15 mL	NA	Antagonizes effect of probenecid. Increases effect of sulfonylureas. Reduces renal clearance of methotrexate.
Salsalate	Disalcid®	500–1,000 mg every 8 hours 750–1,500 mg every 12 hours	3,000 mg	Tablets: 500, 750 mg Capsules: 500 mg	NA	Antagonizes effect of probenecid. Increases effect of sulfonylureas. Reduces renal clearance of methotrexate.

Nonsteroidal Anti-inflammatory Drugs*						
Generic Drug Name	**Trade Name**	**Usual Adult Dose**	**Maximum Adult Daily Dose**	**Prescription Strength**	**Nonprescription Strength**	**Comments**
Diclofenac (immediate release)	Cataflam®	50 mg TID	200 mg	Tablets: 50 mg	NA	
Diclofenac (sustained release)	Voltaren®, Voltaren® XR	50 mg BID–TID 75–100 mg BID 100 mg daily	225 mg	Tablets, delayed release: 25, 50, 75, 100 mg	NA	
Diflunisal (also a salicylate)	Dolobid®	250–500 mg every 8–12 hours	1,500 mg	Tablets: 250, 500 mg	NA	Not metabolized to salicylate. Increases acetaminophen level by 50% when coadministered.
Etodolac	Lodine®, Lodine® XL	200–600 mg every 6–8 hours (maximum 1,200 mg/day)	1,200 mg	Tablets: 400, 500 mg Capsules: 200, 300 mg Tablets, extended-release: 400, 500, 600 mg	NA	Antacids reduce peak concentration by 20%. Long-acting form available.
Fenoprofen	Nalfon®	200–600 mg every 6 hours	3,200 mg	Capsules: 200, 300 mg Tablets: 600 mg	NA	Highly protein-bound (to albumin). Greater renal toxicity.

(continued)

Table 8N.1.   ANTI-INFLAMMATORY AND ANALGESIC MEDICATION *(continued)*

Generic Drug Name	Trade Name	Usual Adult Dose	Maximum Adult Daily Dose	Prescription Strength	Nonprescription Strength	Comments
Flurbiprofen	Ansaid®	50–100 mg every 6–8 hours (maximum 300 mg/day)	300 mg	Tablets: 50, 100 mg	NA	May cause CNS stimulation.
Ibuprofen	Motrin®, Rufen®	400–800 mg every 6–8 hours	3,200 mg	Tablets: 400, 600, 800 mg	Tablets: 100, 200 mg Chewable tablets: 50, 100 mg Capsules: 200 mg Suspension: 100 mg/2.5 mL, 100 mg/5 mL Drops: 40 mg/mL	Also approved for primary dysmenorrhea. Available in combination with hydrocodone (Vicoprofen®).
Indomethacin	Indocin®, Indocin® SR	25–50 mg BID–TID or 75 mg QD–BID (sustained release)	200 mg	Capsules: 25, 50 mg Capsules, sustained release: 75 mg Suspension: 25 mg/5 mL	NA	Available in suppository.
Ketoprofen	Orudis®, Oruvail®	50–75 mg every 6–8 hours	300 mg	Tablets: 12.5 mg Capsules: 25, 50, 75 mg Capsules, sustained-release: 100, 150, 200 mg	12.5 mg (Orudis® KT)	High rate of dyspepsia (11%). Available in sustained-release form.
Ketorolac	Toradol®	PO: 10 mg every 4–6 hours IM/IV: 30 or 60 mg initially, then 15–30 mg every 6 hours	PO: 40 mg IM/IV: 150 mg first day, then 120 mg daily	Tablets: 10 mg Injection: 15, 30 mg/mL	NA	Total duration of treatment should not exceed 5 days. 30 mg equal to 6–12 mg morphine sulfate but 10 times as expensive. 100% bioavailable. Indicated only as continuation of parenteral ketorolac, short-term.
Meclofenamate	Meclomen®	50–100 mg every 6 hours	400 mg	Capsules: 50, 100 mg	NA	High rate of diarrhea (10–33%). Also indicated to treat excessive menstrual bleeding.
Mefenamic acid	Ponstel®	500 mg, then 250 mg every 6 hours	1,000 mg	Capsules: 250 mg	NA	Also approved for primary dysmenorrhea.

(continued)

Table 8N.1.   ANTI-INFLAMMATORY AND ANALGESIC MEDICATION *(continued)*

Generic Drug Name	Trade Name	Usual Adult Dose	Maximum Adult Daily Dose	Prescription Strength	Nonprescription Strength	Comments
Nabumetone	Relafen®	500–750 mg BID; 1,000–2,000 mg daily	2,000 mg	Tablets: 500, 750 mg	NA	High rate of diarrhea (14%). Metabolized to active agent.
Naproxen	Naprosyn®, Naprelan®, EC-Naprosyn®	250–500 mg every 8–12 hours, or 250 mg every 6–8 hours, or 1,000 mg daily (controlled-release tablets)	1,250 mg first 24 hours, then 1,000 mg thereafter	Tablets: 250, 375, 500 mg Tablets, delayed-release: 375, 500 mg Suspension: 125 mg/5 mL	NA	Approved for acute gout. May increase effect of protein-bound drugs such as phenytoin, sulfonylureas, and warfarin. Available in QD dosage form.
Naproxen sodium	Anaprox®, Anaprox® DS	275–550 mg every 8–12 hours	1,375 mg first 24 hours, then 1,100 mg thereafter	Tablets: 220, 550 mg	Tablets: 220 mg (Aleve®)	Approved for acute gout. May increase effect of protein-bound drugs such as phenytoin, sulfonylureas, and warfarin.
Oxaprozin	Daypro®	600–1,200 mg daily	1,800 mg	Tablets 600 mg	NA	
Piroxicam	Feldene®	10–20 mg daily	20 mg	Capsules: 10, 20 mg	NA	High rate of dyspepsia (20%). May increase effect of protein-bound drugs such as phenytoin, sulfonylureas, and warfarin.
Sulindac	Clinoril®	150–200 mg every 12 hours	400 mg	Tablets: 150, 200 mg	NA	Approved for gout. Less renal toxicity.
Tolmetin	Tolectin®	400 mg every 6–8 hours, 600 mg every 8 hours	1,800 mg	Tablets: 200, 600 mg Capsules: 400 mg	NA	High rate of nausea (11%)

*Gastrointestinal (GI) irritation is a common adverse effect that can occur with all NSAIDs, even the newer agents that have greater receptor selectivity. Taking these medications with food will reduce the likelihood of GI irritation, and is especially recommended for the older, non-cyclooxygenase-2 (COX-2) selective agents.

Source: Adapted with permission from *Mosby's drug consult 2003: the comprehensive reference for generic and brand name drugs*, 13th ed., St. Louis, Mo.: Mosby. Accessed online from MD Consult at http://www.mdconsult.com. © 2003 Mosby. Permission granted by Elsevier.

References: Ellsworth, A.J. et al. 2000, 2001. *Mosby's medical drug reference*. St. Louis, Mo.: Mosby; Killion, K.H. et al. 2001, 2002. *Drug facts and comparisons*. St. Louis, Mo.: Wolters Kluwer; Lacy, C.F. et al. 2000. *Drug information handbook*, 8th ed. Cleveland, Ohio: AphA-Lexi-Comp; Manufacturers' package inserts; McEvoy G.K. et al. 2001, 2002. *AHFS drug information*. Bethesda, Md.: American Society of Health-System Pharmacists; United States Food and Drug Administration Center for Drug Education and Research. 2001, available at: http://www.fda.gov/cder.

SECTION 9

Neurological
Disorders

9-A Bell's Palsy **9-2**
9-B Dizziness **9-8**
9-C Face Pain **9-16**
9-D Headache **9-23**
        → Migraine Headache **9-26**
        → Cluster Headache **9-28**
        → Tension-Type Headache **9-29**
        → Temporal or Giant Cell Arteritis **9-30**
9-E Seizures **9-37**
9-F Temporomandibular Disorder **9-43**

9-A
Bell's Palsy

Bell's palsy is defined as a benign, unilateral, peripheral facial palsy of acute onset. It is the most common cause of nontraumatic facial paralysis in the world. Bell's palsy has been synonymous with the term *idiopathic facial paralysis*, but recent research implicates the reactivation of latent herpes simplex virus as the etiological agent of Bell's palsy.

Epidemiology

Bell's palsy affects 20–30 of every 100,000 people per year, with an overall incidence that is equal in males and females (Peitersen 1982). Bell's palsy is more common in young to middle-aged adults. In patients age 10–19, the condition is twice as common in females, with pregnant women having the highest rate. Bell's palsy is more common during the third trimester of pregnancy or in the immediate postpartum period. After age 40, Bell's palsy occurs more commonly in males. Diabetics are four times more likely to be affected than nondiabetics. In 10% of patients, Bell's palsy will recur, either on the same or opposite side. Sixty percent of patients will report a viral prodrome. There is a slight familial predisposition to Bell's palsy (Adour et al. 1978).

Anatomy

The seventh cranial nerve, also called the facial nerve, is a mixed motor, sensory, and parasympathetic nerve. This nerve supplies motor function to all of the facial muscles, supplies parasympathetic function to lacrimal and salivary glands, and carries sensory fibers from the anterior two-thirds of the tongue and from a portion of the external auditory canal.

The seventh cranial nerve originates in the brainstem and enters the temporal bone through the internal auditory meatus into the middle ear. Within this bony canal lies the geniculate ganglion from which innervation for tear production, salivation, and taste originates. The facial nerve then exits the skull via the stylomastoid foramen and passes through the parotid gland, subdividing to supply the facial muscles (see **Figure 9A.1, Distribution of the Facial Nerve**).

Bell's palsy is thought to be due to an inflammatory neuritis of the seventh nerve, as it passes through the bony canal within the temporal bone. It is hypothesized that inflammatory changes within the myelin sheath lead to ischemia and eventual neural degeneration. Magnetic resonance imaging (MRI) has confirmed swelling and enhancement of the geniculate ganglion and the facial nerve in Bell's palsy patients (Saatci et al. 1996).

Herpes simplex virus (HSV) has long been suspected as a possible cause of Bell's palsy. It is believed that after a primary herpes simplex infection, the HSV becomes dormant within the neural ganglion and is later reactivated, causing facial nerve paresis or paralysis without the characteristic herpetic rash.

Recent studies of patients with Bell's palsy have shown HSV genomes in samples of endoneurial fluid and posterior auricular muscle, strongly implicating HSV as the primary causative agent (Murakami et al. 1996).

Clinical Presentation

The onset of Bell's palsy is abrupt, with the initial symptom of unilateral facial paresis developing over 24–48 hours. Drooping of the brow and the corner of the mouth, widening of the palpebral fissure, and impairment of eye and mouth closure on the affected side are noted. Associated symptoms may include excessive tearing, hyperacusis (increased sense of hearing), dysgeusia (abnormal sense of taste), facial pain or retroauricular pain (which may be presenting symptoms before paralysis is evident) and mild pharyngeal sensory loss or weakness. Herpetic lesions are typically not present. These symptoms may continue to progress for up to 10 days, and full paralysis of the facial muscles may occur.

Peitersen (1982) studied the spontaneous course of 1,011 patients with Bell's palsy. Left untreated, 85% of patients showed some signs of improvement within three weeks and the remaining patients showed some sign of improvement within 3–6 months. Full recovery occurred in 71% of untreated patients. However, 16% of patients had moderate to severe disability, and 13% had minor residual signs or symptoms. The longer the delay in remission, the poorer the prognosis for full recovery. Other factors associated with a poorer outcome are: age over 60, the presence of severe ear pain, hyperacusis, or the comorbid association of diabetes, hypertension, or a psychiatric disorder (Adour et al. 1974).

Differential Diagnosis

There are many known causes of seventh nerve palsy, all of which need to be considered when examining a patient with suspected Bell's palsy (see **Table 9A.1, Selected Causes of Facial Paralysis**). *Ramsay Hunt syndrome*, also known as *herpes zoster oticus*, is a facial nerve palsy accompanied by a vesicular rash. Ramsay Hunt syndrome is caused by reactivation of the varicella zoster virus and is second to Bell's palsy as the most common cause of nontraumatic facial nerve paralysis. Because one-third of patients will not develop a rash for 2–14 days after the onset of facial palsy, Ramsay Hunt syndrome may be indistinguishable from Bell's palsy early in the course of the disease. Besides the distinctive vesicular rash, Ramsay Hunt syndrome tends to cause significant ear or facial pain and ipsilateral auditory or vestibular loss (see **Table 9A.2, Bell's Palsy Versus Ramsay Hunt Syndrome**). *Zoster sine herpete* is a version of Ramsay Hunt syndrome without rash (Sweeney et al. 2001).

Among other causes of facial weakness, stroke is one that commonly worries both patient and provider alike. The most significant difference between stroke and Bell's palsy is that the patient affected by stroke will *not* have weakness of the forehead muscles due to contralateral cortical innervation.

Adour et al. (1996) have noted that many patients with Bell's palsy have mild dysfunction in other cranial or cervical nerves. However, careful physical examination is needed, and if there is more than the mild involvement of the cranial nerves (see **Table 9A.3, Polyneuritis Manifestations of Bell's Palsy**) or other neurological findings are present, the diagnosis should be reconsidered.

Treatment

Although the majority of patients with Bell's palsy recover fully without treatment, the possibility of significant sequelae still exists. Prednisone, an anti-inflammatory agent, and acyclovir, an antiviral agent, have been used to reverse nerve inflammation and prevent denervation. Evidence regarding the benefit of these treatments is conflicting (Adour et al. 1996, De Diego et al. 1998). Recent practice recommendations from the American Academy of Neurology give support for the use of both prednisone and acyclovir to treat Bell's palsy. Although surgical decompression of the facial nerve has been a treatment option for many years, there is insufficient evidence for its use in treating Bell's palsy (Grogan et al. 2001).

For patients with persistent paralysis, botulinum toxin injections, tarsorrhaphy, lateral canthoplasty, or gold weight implants to the upper eyelid may be an option to improve facial appearance or protect the eye.

Figure 9A.1.   DISTRIBUTION OF THE FACIAL NERVE

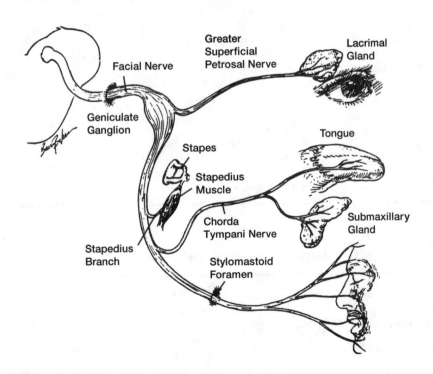

Source: Reprinted with permission from Alford, B.R., Jerger, J.E., Coats, A.C. et al. 1973. Neurophysiology of facial nerve testing. *Archives of Otolaryngology* 97:215. ©American Medical Association.

Complications

Complications from Bell's palsy include corneal ulceration, persistent facial weakness, facial spasm, abnormal facial movement (synkinesis), and abnormal lacrimation. "Crocodile tears," which is lacrimation triggered by gustatory stimuli, may occur and is attributed to aberrant regeneration of secretory fibers to the lacrimal gland.

DATABASE

SUBJECTIVE

→ Timing and onset
  ▪ Date of onset
  ▪ Rapidity of onset and progression of symptoms

→ Location of weakness
  ▪ Unilateral facial weakness, including the forehead
→ Associated symptoms may include the following:
  ▪ Facial or postauricular pain
  ▪ Facial numbness
  ▪ Eye irritation
  ▪ Increased sense of hearing
  ▪ Diminished or abnormal sense of taste
  ▪ Decreased tearing
  ▪ Drooling or inability to fully close lips
→ Associated symptoms indicating different etiology:
  ▪ Rash, fever, visual disturbance, speech or swallowing difficulty, numbness or weakness of extremities, ear

Table 9A.1. SELECTED CAUSES OF FACIAL PARALYSIS

Infectious	Traumatic	Neoplastic
Bell's palsy	Barotrauma	Acoustic neuroma
Cat scratch disease	Birth trauma	Carcinoma, locally invasive
Chickenpox	Facial injuries	Carcinoma, metastatic
Coxsackie virus	Surgical trauma	Cholesteatoma
Cytomegalovirus		Glomus jugulare tumor
Diphtheria	**Metabolic**	Leukemia
Encephalitis	Diabetes mellitus	Lymphoma
HIV infection	Hyperthyroidism	Meningioma
Influenza	Hypertension	Parotid tumors
Lyme disease	Pregnancy	Sarcoma
Malaria		
Meningitis	**Neurologic**	**Other**
Mononucleosis	Brainstem, cortical tumors	Alcoholism
Mumps	Guillain-Barré	Heavy metal toxicity
Otitis media, otitis externa, mastoiditis	Neurofibromatosis	Melkersson-Rosenthal syndrome
Poliomyelitis	Stroke	
Rabies		
Ramsay Hunt syndrome	**Autoimmune**	
Rubella	Multiple sclerosis	
Syphilis	Myasthenia gravis	
Tetanus	Sarcoidosis	
Tuberculosis	Sjögren's syndrome	
Varicella	Systemic lupus	

Table 9A.2. BELL'S PALSY VERSUS RAMSAY HUNT SYNDROME

Bell's Palsy	Ramsay Hunt Syndrome
Acute onset over 24–48 hours	Additional symptoms:
Unilateral facial paralysis/paresis, including muscles of the forehead	Severe facial or ear pain, which may be felt days before rash appears
Drooping of mouth, drooling	Dizziness and/or hearing loss
Post auricular pain	Vesicular rash on ear, tongue, hard palate, neck, face, or shoulder
Facial numbness	

discharge, tinnitus, hearing loss, vertigo, facial tics or altered mental status

→ Past medical history:
- Recent trauma, immunizations, viral illness or tick bite, pregnancy, malignancies, ear disease, hearing impairment, thyroid disease, diabetes, HIV infection, autoimmune disease

→ Family medical history:
- Facial paralysis, diabetes, hypertension, thyroid disease, cancer, autoimmune disease

→ Social history:
- Occupation, alcohol or drug history, HIV risk factors, activities that involve exposure to ticks

OBJECTIVE

→ Physical examination may include:
- Vital signs: temperature, pulse, respiration, blood pressure
- General appearance
- Skin: vesicular lesions or Lyme disease rash
- Eyes: tearing, redness, Bell's phenomenon (rolling upward of eyeball when trying to close affected eye), drooping of lower lid
- Ears: external ears and tympanic membranes may exhibit redness, discharge, or lesions
- Oral: mucosa is examined for lesions and salivary gland ducts for purulent discharge
- Salivary glands: check for redness, swelling or tenderness
- Neck: check for masses or adenopathy

- Neurological examination:
  - Determine if complete or partial facial paralysis is present.
  - Check for the exact area of facial muscle weakness, as weakness of both upper and lower face is consistent with Bell's palsy. Sparing of the forehead muscles suggests a central neurological problem.
  - Observe gait, check strength and symmetry of extremities and deep tendon reflexes.
  - Check cranial nerves II-XII: there may be very *mild* involvement of cranial nerves V, IX, X, or cervical nerves 2 or 3 (see **Table 9A.5, Cranial Nerve Testing**).

ASSESSMENT

→ Bell's palsy
→ See **Table 9A.1** for differential diagnoses.

PLAN

DIAGNOSTIC TESTS

→ Routine diagnostic tests may not be needed. However, the following diagnostic tests may be ordered to assist with differential diagnosis:
- Blood sugar, HgA1C, TSH, CBC, sedimentation rate, Lyme titer in endemic area, HIV test, VDRL, mono spot
- Audiogram may be considered if hearing loss is noted or if vertigo is reported by the patient.
- MRI or CT scan may be considered if a secondary cause of facial paralysis is suspected.

Table 9A.3.   POLYNEURITIS MANIFESTATIONS OF BELL'S PALSY

Cervical nerve 2 or 3	Retroauricular pain
Cranial nerve V (trigeminal)	Mild numbness or pain in trigeminal nerve distribution, mild masseter muscle weakness
Cranial nerve IX (glossopharyngeal nerve)	Mild numbness or dysesthesia of unilateral pharyngeal wall
Cranial nerve X (vagus nerve)	Mild unilateral motor weakness of palate or superior laryngeal nerve

Table 9A.4.   RED FLAGS IN BELL'S PALSY

Slow onset of paralysis

Paralysis that spares the forehead

Bilateral paralysis

Involvement of other cranial nerves, except as noted in Table 9A.3

Weakness or sensory loss of extremities

Significant hearing loss or vertigo

Associated tics and spasms

Paralysis that shows no improvement in 6 months

TREATMENT/MANAGEMENT

→ Prednisone 60 mg/day in 2 divided doses, for 5–7 days, at which time the patient is re-examined. If paralysis has stabilized and is partial, the dose may be stopped. If the paralysis has continued or is complete, the prednisone should be continued and tapered over the next 5 days.

→ Treat with acyclovir 200–400 mg 5 times a day for 10 days (Adour 1996).

→ If Ramsay Hunt syndrome is suspected, consider treatment with acyclovir 800 mg 5 times a day for 10 days (Sweeney et al. 2001).

→ If a diabetic is treated with prednisone, monitor blood sugars and adjust insulin dosage, if needed. For diabetics not on insulin, monitor blood sugars and consider adding short-term use of insulin during this time.

→ The usual precautions for corticoidsteroid use should be followed.

→ Moisturizing eye drops during the day and a moisturizing ointment at night should be used.

→ Careful taping of the lid at night may help to protect the cornea.

→ An eye patch and/or sunglasses will provide eye protection.

CONSULTATION

→ With neurologist or otolaryngologist, if the diagnosis is in question

→ With otolaryngologist if significant dizziness or hearing loss is reported

→ With ophthalmologist as needed for eye complications

PATIENT EDUCATION

→ Bell's palsy patients may be concerned regarding their appearance and prognosis. Offer reassurance that return of facial appearance and function within days to weeks is the norm.

→ Explain that abnormal tearing, salivation, drooling, altered taste or an increased sensitivity to sound may occur.

→ Instruct the patient about eye care to prevent corneal injury.

→ Instruct the patient about the usual precautions regarding medication side effects.

FOLLOW-UP

→ Patient is to follow up:
  ▪ In 5–7 days for recheck of the progression of the paralysis
  ▪ In 3–6 months if symptoms persist
  ▪ If eye pain, redness, or drainage occurs

Table 9A.5.   CRANIAL NERVE TESTING

Cranial Nerve (CN)		What to Test
CN II	Optic nerve	Visual acuity, visual fields
CN III	Oculomotor nerve	Pupillary reaction, extraocular movements (EOM)
CN IV	Trochlear nerve	EOM: downward, inward movement of eye
CN V	Trigeminal nerve*	V1: (sensory) facial sensation of forehead and nose. Corneal reflex (corneal sensation is carried on CN V, motor function carried by CN VI. Therefore, unaffected eye should blink in Bell's palsy.) V2: (sensory) upper teeth, gums and lip, cheek and side of nose V3: (sensory) lower teeth, gums and lip (motor) jaw clenching
CN VI	Abducens nerve	EOM: lateral deviation of eye Corneal reflex: unaffected eye should blink when affected cornea tested
CN VII	Facial nerve	Wrinkle forehead, raise eyebrows, close eyes tightly, show teeth
CN VIII	Vestibulocochlear nerve	Gross hearing, nystagmus and balance
CN IX*	Glossopharyngeal nerve	Sensory: posterior tongue and ear canal Motor: gag reflex, quality of voice
CN X*	Vagus nerve	Check movement of palate and pharynx: "say ah"
CN XI	Spinal accessory	Neck movement and shoulder shrugs
CN XII	Hypoglossal	Stick out tongue

*May be mildly affected in Bell's palsy

■ If the patient notes new or progressive symptoms
→ Document the extent of facial weakness and the neurological exam findings in the notes and on the problem list.

BIBLIOGRAPHY

Adour, K.K., Byl, F.M., Hilsinger, R.L. et al. 1978. The true nature of Bell's palsy: analysis of 1,000 consecutive patients. *Laryngoscope* 88:87–801.

Adour, K.K., Ruboyianes, J.M., Von Doersten, P.G. et al. 1996. Bell's palsy treatment with acyclovir and prednisone compared with prednisone alone: a double-blind, randomized, controlled trial. *Annals of Otology, Rhinology and Laryngology* 105:371–378.

Adour, K.K., Wingerd, J., Bell, D.N. et al. 1972. Prednisone treatment for idiopathic facial paralysis (Bell's palsy). *New England Journal of Medicine* 287:1268–1272.

Adour, K.K., and Wingerd, J. 1974. Idiopathic facial paralysis (Bell's palsy): factors affecting severity and outcome in 446 patients. *Neurology* 24:1112–1116.

Alford, B.R., Jerger, J.E., Coats, A.C. et al. 1973. Neurophysiology of facial nerve testing. *Archives of Otolaryngology* 97 Figure 1:214–219.

Billue, J. 1997. Bell's Palsy: an update on idiopathic facial paralysis. *Nurse Practitioner* 22(8):88–105.

De Diego, J.I., Prim, M.P., De Sarria, M.J. et al. 1998. Idiopathic facial paralysis: a randomized, prospective and controlled study using single-dose prednisone versus acyclovir three times daily. *Laryngoscope* 108:573–575.

Grogan, P.M., and Gronseth, G.S. 2001. Practice parameter: steroids, acyclovir and surgery for Bell's palsy (an evidence-based review). Report of the quality standards subcommittee of the American Academy of Neurology. *Neurology* 56(7):830–836.

Morrow, M. 2000. Bell's palsy and herpes zoster oticus. *Current Treatment Options in Neurology* 2:407–416.

Murakami, S., Mizobuchi, M., Nakashiro, Y. et al. 1996. Bell palsy and herpes simplex virus: identification of viral DNA in endoneurial fluid and muscle. *Annals of Internal Medicine* 124(1):27–30.

Peitersen, E. 1982. The natural history of Bell's palsy. *American Journal of Otology* 4(2):107–111.

Saatci, I., Sahinturk, F., Sennaroglu, L. et al. 1996. MRI of the facial nerve in idiopathic facial palsy (abstract). *European Radiology* 6(5):631–636.

Schirm, J., and Mulkens, P. 1997. Bell's palsy and herpes simplex virus. *Acta Pathologica Immunologica Scandinavica* 105:815–823.

Sweeney, C., and Gilden, D. 2001. Ramsay Hunt syndrome. *Journal of Neurological and Neurosurgical Psychiatry* 71:149–154.

Kathryn Zender, R.N., M.S.N., F.N.P.
Jacqueline Wish Gilbert, R.N., M.S., C.F.N.P.

9-B
Dizziness

Dizziness is a common problem encountered in the primary care setting. The term dizziness can describe a wide variety of sensory experiences related to disturbances of balance and equilibrium. It is helpful to divide dizziness into three categories of symptoms. *Vertigo* is a sense of rotational movement, *disequilibrium* is a feeling of unsteadiness or imbalance without the sensation of movement, and *lightheadedness* or *giddiness* is a sensation of swimming, floating, or swaying in the head or the surroundings. Patients may describe feeling faint (Wazen 2000).

All causes of dizziness may be associated with symptoms associated with the autonomic nervous system, including perspiration, nausea, pallor, and tachycardia. These symptoms also commonly occur in anxiety disorders, hysteria, and depression. Dizziness can be reproduced with hyperventilation and may be concurrent with panic, apprehensiveness, palpitations, breathlessness, and/or tremor. The challenge to the practitioner is to pinpoint the cause of the dizziness. Patients often have difficulty describing their symptoms in a manner that allows the practitioner to determine if the dizziness arises from the cardiopulmonary, peripheral vestibular, or central nervous systems. Therefore, a careful history revealing an accurate depiction of symptoms and a physical exam are necessary in order for the clinician to differentiate between the different types of dizziness. The most common cause for the failure of treatment for dizziness is misdiagnosis, leading to inappropriate treatment (Drachman et al. 1972).

Anatomical and Physiological Considerations

Vertigo

Any disease that interferes with the reception, transmission, and/or integration of sensory information can cause the perception of rotational movement or vertigo. For the human body to maintain balance and equilibrium, many fine adjustments are made below the level of awareness. These adjustments are responses to cues from the environment. Information is received and interpreted by sensory organs and is relayed via afferent impulses to the cerebellum and certain ganglionic centers in the brain stem. These centers integrate sensory data to allow for the subtle postural adjustments necessary to maintain balance (Wazen 2000).

There are structures in the eyes and ears that have the specific function of receiving sensory information. Dysfunction in these structures and organs, or in the transmission of sensory information to and from these organs, may result in the sensation of vertigo. Impulses from the retinas of both eyes and impulses from the ocular muscles provide visual cues regarding the position and movement of the body in relation to its surroundings. The peripheral vestibular system is located in the labyrinth of each ear. The labyrinth contains three semicircular canals, a utricle, and a saccule. This system detects angular acceleration, linear acceleration, and changes in the position of the head with respect to gravity. In each utricle and saccule there is a complex called the macula, which consists of a gelatinous layer within which calcium carbonate crystals (otoliths) are embedded. Hair cells project cilia into the macula, bending as the complex moves. The bending of these hair cells sends afferent impulses to the brain that give information about the position of the body (Adams et al. 1997, Baloh 1998, Hain 1997, Koelliker et al. 2001).

Disequilibrium

Disequilibrium describes the feeling of impaired balance and gait in the absence of any abnormal head sensation. Patients may describe it as dizziness in the feet. Disequilibrium is often due to impaired motor control. Five sensory modalities sample position and motion of the body: vision, vestibular sensation, proprioception, touch, and hearing, in descending order of importance. The disequilibrium type of dizziness is a common symptom in elderly patients. This can be attributed to the degeneration of one or more of the sensory organs. For example, an elderly person may have degenerative joint disease in the knee(s), cataracts, and decreased hearing. These deficits of the proprioceptive, visual, and hearing modalities can result in the person feeling unsteady or off balance. They may not notice the unsteadiness while sitting but have a more pronounced sensation when standing or walking (Drachman 1998, Hain 1997).

Lightheadedness or Presyncope

Lightheadedness describes a swaying, floating, or giddy sensation in the head. Patients may also describe a feeling of faintness. Lightheadedness often precedes a loss of consciousness or syncope. *Syncope* is defined as an abrupt but transient loss of consciousness accompanied by a loss of postural tone followed by a rapid recovery. As the attack develops, the patient begins to feel "badly," accompanied by striking pallor, perspiration, and sometimes nausea and vomiting. Vision may dim and a complete loss of consciousness may occur. This sequence of events is a consequence of a reduction in cerebral blood flow, cerebral oxygen utilization, or cerebral vascular resistance (Olshansky 1998). These reductions can be caused by the following:

→ Inadequate vasoconstrictor mechanisms, such as vasovagal syncope, postural hypotension, or micturation syncope
→ Hypovolemia (e.g. dehydration, blood loss)
→ Mechanical reduction in venous return to the heart such as valsalva, or cough
→ Reduced cardiac output
→ Cardiac arrhythmias
→ Altered state of brain oxygenation (e.g., anemia, hypoxia)
→ Emotional disturbances, (e.g., anxiety attacks, hysteria)
→ Metabolic disturbances, (e.g., hypoglycemia, hyponatremia) (Calkins 1997, Olshansky 1998, Pedley et al. 2000)

Common Disorders

Disorders resulting in dizziness can be broadly divided into three categories: peripheral vestibular, central neurological, and cardiovascular. Diagnostic evaluation typically includes obtaining historical evidence, physical findings, and lab results. Asking four complaint-specific questions usually narrows the diagnostic possibilities considerably. These questions should include the type (vertigo, disequilibrium, presyncope), the age of the patient, the relationship to position or motion, and the onset/frequency of the symptoms (Drachman 1998).

Peripheral Vestibular Disorders

Benign Paroxysmal Positional Vertigo (BPPV)
This condition is one of the most common causes of dizziness. It is benign and self-limiting. The attack consists of a brief sensation of rotational movement, usually lasting less than a minute and occurring with a change in position. Although the rotational sensation lasts only a short time, the patient may experience disequilibrium for hours in a severe attack. Benign paroxysmal positional vertigo can occur after head trauma or vestibular neuronitis, or it can be idiopathic. The symptoms may last several days to many months and can reoccur periodically. The pathophysiologic abnormality for BPPV occurs in the labyrinth. An otolith becomes dislodged from the macula and moves into the thick endolymph of the semicircular canals. As the head moves,

the otolith also moves as a result of gravitational forces when the head position changes. The movement of the otolith in the endolymph sends afferent impulses to the central nervous system (CNS). The CNS interprets these signals as angular acceleration of the head when none exists. These signals from the CNS cause the eyes to deviate in the opposite direction of the perceived acceleration resulting in the slow phase of nystagmus. This is followed by the fast phase of nystagmus, which is the subsequent corrective action of the eyes. It is the fast phase that determines the direction of the nystagmus. Benign paroxysmal positional vertigo can be diagnosed by obtaining a positive response to the Hallpike-Dix maneuver (see **Table 9B.1, Initial Evaluation Tests for Vertigo, Presyncope, Disequilibrium, and Lightheadedness**). Caloric testing is negative and hearing remains normal with BPPV (Adams et al. 1997, Baloh 1998, Drachman et al. 1972, Hain 1997, Koelliker et al. 2001, Ruff 1984, Wazen 2000).

Vestibular Neuronitis (Labyrinthitis)
Vestibular neuronitis is a benign disorder characterized clinically by a paroxysmal and usually single attack of vertigo without tinnitus or deafness. It most often occurs in young adults of either sex and is usually, although not always, associated with a nonspecific, viral upper respiratory infection. The onset of vertigo is abrupt and severe, accompanied by nausea and vomiting, nystagmus, and the need to remain immobile. The more severe symptoms of vertigo resolve after several days, but milder ones may persist for several weeks. Caloric testing reveals a reduced response on the affected side (Adams et al. 1997, Baloh 1998, Hain 1997, Ruff 1984, Wazen 2000).

Ménière's Syndrome
Ménière's syndrome is characterized by recurring episodes of vertigo, tinnitus, nausea, vomiting, and fluctuating hearing loss. The symptoms can occur separately or in combination, with variable periods of remission lasting several years. Vertiginous episodes last minutes to hours and are accompanied by nystagmus, nausea, and vomiting. Hearing loss begins as a unilateral, low-frequency, sensorineural type deficit and can improve between attacks. In severe cases it may progress to both ears with a complete loss of hearing. When the hearing loss is complete, the vertigo usually ceases, which can be explained by irreversible damage to the end organ (labyrinth). The significant pathological finding in patients with Ménière's syndrome is an increase in the volume of the endolymph causing distention of the entire endolymphatic system (endolymphatic hydrops). The association of hearing loss and vertigo occurs as a result of damage to the membranes in the endolymph and/or the eighth cranial nerve. It affects adults in early to mid life and men more often than women. Diagnosis can be confirmed with documentation of fluctuating hearing loss on audiograms (Adams et al., 1997, Baloh 1998, Hain 1997, Ruff 1984, Wazen 2000.)

Drug Toxicity
Drug toxicity can lead to any of the three types of dizziness: vertigo, disequilibrium, or lightheadedness. Aminoglycoside antibiotics can damage the fine hair cells of the vestibular system,

resulting in permanent vertigo and/or hearing loss. Salicylates, furosemide, quinine, and some anticonvulsants, antidepressants, and tranquilizers can cause dose-related dizziness. Use of illegal drugs, such as heroin, cocaine, methamphetamine, and marijuana, may also cause dizziness (Adams et al. 1997, Pedley et al. 2000, Wazen 2000).

Trauma

Vertigo can be the result of a head injury that damages either the peripheral or central vestibular system, or both. Headache, nausea, and dizziness are frequent symptoms after mild traumatic brain injury (MTBI) and may continue for weeks to months after the trauma. Whiplash or a significant blow to the head are two causes of MTBI. The mechanism of how MTBI affects vestibular function is poorly understood. It is currently believed that axonal damage in the frontal lobe is responsible for the symptoms. Brain CT scans obtained after this type of injury are usually normal (Baloh 1998, DeKruijk 2001, Ruff 1984, Wazen 2000).

Acoustic Neuroma

Acoustic neuroma, a Schwann-cell neoplasm, is the most common tumor that grows in the cerebellopontine angle. The earliest symptoms of this disorder are dizziness, tinnitus, and hearing loss. A CT scan with contrast or an MRI will distinguish this illness from Ménière's syndrome. The attacks of dizziness associated with acoustic neuroma are persistent rather than recurrent and are characterized by a sense of imbalance rather than true vertigo. Early diagnosis is important because current microsurgical techniques may allow for the removal of the tumor before it becomes too large in order to spare the facial nerve and preserve residual hearing (Wazen 2000).

Central Neurological Disorders

Migraine

Migraine is a common but seldom recognized cause of episodes of vertigo or lightheadedness. Baloh (1998) asserts most cases of benign paroxysmal vertigo and benign recurrent vertigo of

---

Table 9B.1.   INITIAL EVALUATION TESTS FOR VERTIGO, PRESYNCOPE, DISEQUILIBRIUM, AND LIGHTHEADEDNESS

VERTIGO:

Hallpike-Dix test: This provocative test will confirm the diagnosis of BPPV. Have the patient sit on the table or bed in a manner to allow the patient's head to hang off the edge when placed in the supine position. The examiner holds the sides of the patient's head and turns the head 45 degrees to the side being tested. The patient is then lowered to the supine position with the head turned and then also angled back off the bed or table 45 degrees. The patient should keep the eyes open and fixed on the examiner's face so the examiner may appreciate the character and severity of the nystagmus. Rotational nystagmus toward the affected ear, accompanied by vertigo, indicates a positive test. There is usually a latency period of 5–15 seconds before the nystagmus begins. The nystagmus lasts from 20 seconds to a minute and the severity will fatigue with repetition of the test. Once diagnosed, BPPV can be easily treated with Canalith repositioning maneuvers or the Epley or Semont maneuver (Brandt et al. 1994, Koelliker et al. 2001, Radtke et al. 1999).

Caloric testing: In caloric testing, the patient's head is tilted 30 degrees from the horizontal. The external ear canal is irrigated with water first at a temperature of 30° C and then at a temperature of 44° C. An intact tympanic membrane should be noted before irrigation. Irrigation with cold water will cause nystagmus toward the opposite ear being irrigated, and irrigation with warm water will cause nystagmus toward the ear being irrigated. A lack of the normal response indicates a problem with vestibular function. Hot water should never be used for irrigation (Calkins 1997).

Electronystagmogram (ENG): This test can help distinguish between peripheral and central causes of dizziness and can provide precise and quantitative information regarding vestibular function. Caloric testing and head movements are performed while eye movements are recorded with the eyes closed (Calkins 1997).

PRESYNCOPE:

Orthostatic blood pressure measurement: Obtain pulse and systolic and diastolic blood pressure measurements in the supine position and then recheck the measurements 1 minute and 5 minutes after moving to a standing position.

Electrocardiogram

DISEQUILIBRIUM:

Romberg and tandem gait tests

LIGHTHEADEDNESS:

Hyperventilation: Deliberate hyperventilation can reproduce symptoms of dizziness.

---

adulthood are caused by migraine. Episodes are cyclic, usually lasting 4–60 minutes. These episodes may or may not be associated with headache. Migraine is a diagnosis of exclusion. The diagnosis is confirmed by a positive response to treatment in a patient for whom all other etiologies have been ruled out. The mechanism for dizziness associated with migraine is not known. However, it is postulated that vasoconstriction involving the internal auditory artery or spreading depression resulting in neuronal dysfunction in key anatomic areas of the cortical brain may be the mechanism (Baloh 1998, Hain 1997).

Brainstem Disorders

Vertigo originating from brainstem abnormalities can be caused by vascular dysfunction, demylination, or neoplasm. This type of vertigo, as well as its accompanying nausea, vomiting, and nystagmus, are more protracted than they are when the vertigo originates from the peripheral vestibular system. Auditory function remains normal, but focal deficits in cranial nerves, and/or motor and sensory function, may be noted. Vertigo is a prominent symptom of transient ischemic attack and of brainstem infarction in the area of the vertebral-basilar arteries. These episodes of vertigo are abrupt and they are associated with other vertebral-basilar symptoms, most commonly visual disturbance, drop attacks, unsteadiness, and weakness (Adams et al. 1997, Drachman et al. 1972, Hain 1997, Ruff 1984). Demyelinating processes such as multiple sclerosis commonly cause injury to the brainstem that leads to dizziness. Multiple sclerosis is characterized by temporally separated episodes of neurologic impairment involving more than one region of the nervous system. Imaging of the brain and spinal cord, and evaluation of the cerebral spinal fluid are necessary to confirm a diagnosis (Drachman et al. 1972).

Degeneration

With aging, patients may experience degeneration of the organs responsible for maintaining balance. Past a certain age, which for each individual is different, degeneration of the fine hair cells and a decline in the number of nerve fibers occur in the vestibular system. Loss of function in sensory systems of vision, proprioception, and hearing, in combination with a decrease in the ability to integrate information from these systems, as well as a decrease in cerebral adaptive functions can contribute to disequilibrium in elderly people. Loss of proprioceptors occurring in degenerative joint disease can lead to balance problems, fear of falling, and decreased mobility. Older patients may describe more than one type of dizziness, making it difficult to attribute the symptoms to one diagnosis. Geriatricians are beginning to refer to dizziness in the elderly as a "geriatric syndrome" that results from impairment or disease in multiple systems (Drachman 1998, Lawson et al. 1999, Tinetti et al. 2000, Wazen 2000).

Cardiovascular

Presyncope or Syncope

Lightheadedness or dizziness usually precedes *syncope*, a brief loss of consciousness. If a patient has syncope in addition to dizziness, a cardiovascular diagnosis is likely an attributable cause.

Vasovagal Vasopressor Syncope

Vasovagal vasopressor syncope is a common, benign occurrence, caused by underfilling of the right side of the heart. Most often it occurs while standing as a result of pooling of the peripheral circulation. It can be triggered by emotional or situational events and is observed mostly in young, healthy adults. Weakness, nausea, pallor, diaphoresis, and blurred vision often accompany the premonitory symptom of dizziness. Young and otherwise healthy patients with a typical history of syncope do not need further workup. However, older patients presenting with comorbid illnesses, or in whom the dizziness is recurrent, should have other diagnoses ruled out (Calkins 1997, Drachman 1998, Drachman et al. 1972, Olshansky 1998, Pedley et al. 2000).

Orthostatic Syncope

Orthostatic syncope can occur in elderly patients suffering from progressive autonomic failure, multiple systems atrophy, and/or neuropathies. The attacks typically occur when the patient rises from the supine to standing position (Calkins 1997, Drachman 1998, Olshansky 1998).

Cardiac Syncope

Cardiac syncope occurs when there is either a vascular obstruction or disrhythmia in the heart. If the abnormality is severe enough to impede the heart's ability to adequately pump blood to the brain, the patient may have an abrupt drop attack, the hallmark of true cardiac syncope. Cardiac syncope usually is associated with underlying cardiac disease in less severe cases and may be accompanied by dyspnea, palpitations, angina, and dizziness (Calkins 1997, Drachman 1998, Drachman et al. 1972, Olshansky 1998, Pedley et al. 2000).

Psychophysiologic

Anxiety Disorders

Anxiety disorders may have symptoms of lightheadedness or vertigo. Hyperventilation occurring with panic attacks can explain the presyncopal lightheadedness. However, it does not explain the many complex sensory distortions of body movement, imbalance, and fear of falling that occur in people with anxiety disorders who do not experience hyperventilation. In patients with psychiatric illness, it can be difficult to determine if vertigo causes the acute anxiety or panic attack or if the panic attack causes hyperventilation and the associated lightheadedness. During an attack, patients may also experience paresthesias of the hands and face, blurred vision, dry mouth, tachycardia, palpitations, chest pains, and shortness of breath (Drachman et al. 1972, Panitch et al. 1998, Wazen 2000).

DATABASE

SUBJECTIVE

→ In determining the cause of dizziness, it is important to elicit the patient's understanding of the symptoms, frequency of symptoms, and precipitants as follows:

- Sensation of uncertainty or ill-defined lightheadedness (giddiness)

- Sensation of rotational movement (vertigo)
- Sensation of impending or actual fainting or loss of consciousness (syncope)
- Loss of balance or instability without any associated sensations of spinning (disequilibrium)
- A symptom pattern that:
  - Is paroxysmal or continuous
  - Affected by position or changes in posture
- Aural symptoms:
  - Tinnitus
  - Hearing loss
  - History of middle ear disease
- Visual symptoms:
  - Diplopia
  - Scotomata
  - Loss of vision
- Neurological symptoms:
  - History of central nervous system disease
  - Symptoms of numbness, weakness, ataxia
  - History of head injury
- Symptoms of psychoneurosis
- Associated nausea and vomiting
- History of recent upper respiratory infection
- History of drugs taken:
  - Alcohol
  - Marijuana
  - Antihypertensives
  - Psychotropics
  - Quinine
  - Furosemide
  - Cardiac medications

OBJECTIVE

→ Ear examination should include:
  - Auroscopic examination:
    - Checking for wax
    - Tympanic membrane assessment
  - Weber and Rinne tests
  - Eye examination should include:
  - Visual acuity
  - Fundoscopic exam
→ Neck examination should include:
  - Lymph nodes
  - Cervical spine
  - Thyroid
→ Cardiovascular examination should include:
  - Blood pressure: supine, standing, sitting
  - Cardiac dysrhythmia assessment
  - Auscultation of carotid arteries
→ Neurologic examination should include:
  - Cranial nerve testing
    - Second—visual fields
    - Third, fourth, and sixth—eye movements
    - Fifth—corneal reflex and facial sensation
    - Seventh—facial strength and symmetry

Table 9B.2. VESTIBULAR SUPPRESSANTS

Medication	Dosage
Diazepam	5–10 mg p.o. every 4–6 hours
Droperidol	2.5–5 mg IM every 12 hours
Promethazine	25–50 mg p.o. IM, supp every 4–6 hours
Prochlorperazine	5–10 mg p.o. or IM every 4–6 hours, or 25 mg supp every 12 hours
Meclizine	25 mg p.o. every 4–6 hours
Scopolamine	0.5 mg transderm every 3 days

NOTE: These medications may also increase dizziness.

Source: Adapted with permission from Hain, T. 1997. Vertigo and disequilibrium. In *Current therapy in neurologic disease*, 5th ed., eds. R.T. Johnson and J.W. Griffin, p. 10. St. Louis, Mo.: Mosby. © 1997, reprinted with permission from Elsevier.

  - Eighth—hearing
  - Ninth—palate movement
  - Eleventh—shoulder shrug
  - Twelfth—tongue protrusion
- Gait
- Coordination
- Reflex testing
- Romberg test
- Extra-ocular movement testing
- Finger-nose test
- Hallpike-Dix maneuver
- Caloric testing

ASSESSMENT

Types of Dizziness

→ Vertigo
  - Peripheral causes:
    - R/O benign paroxysmal positional vertigo (BPPV)
    - R/O vestibular neuronitis/labyrinthitis
    - R/O Ménière's syndrome
    - R/O drug toxicity
    - R/O trauma
    - R/O local ear dysfunction (e.g., otitis, cerumen impaction)
  - Central causes:
    - R/O migraine
    - R/O transient ischemic attacks
    - R/O acoustic neuroma
    - R/O multiple sclerosis
    - R/O posterior fossa tumor
→ Presyncope
  - R/O arrhythmia
  - R/O vasovagal reflex
  - R/O orthostatic hypotension

- R/O valvular heart disease
- R/O low cardiac output states (hypovolemia, congestive heart failure)
- R/O anemia
- R/O hypoglycemia
- R/O hypoxemia

→ Disequilibrium
- R/O cerebellar disease
- R/O Parkinsonism
- R/O drug toxicity (prescription and recreational)
- R/O altered visual acuity

→ Lightheadedness (giddiness)
- R/O anxiety
- R/O depression
- R/O panic disorders
- R/O hyperventilation
- R/O drug use

PLAN

DIAGNOSTIC TESTS

→ For benign dizziness, no specific lab tests are indicated. When indicated, the following tests may be considered, depending on the history and presentation:
- CBC, blood glucose, and TSH
- Electrocardiogram, Holter monitor
- Orthostatic blood pressure
- Audiometry
- Caloric tests
- Electronystagmography
- Rotational tests
- Extra-ocular movement testing
- Hallpike-Dix maneuver
- Romberg and tandem gait tests
- Hyperventilation
- Radiology:
  - Chest x-ray
  - CT scan or MRI/MRA of the head
- See **Table 9B.1**.
  NOTE: Abnormal CBC, blood glucose, and/or TSH may indicate metabolic problems and/or anemia. Electrocardiogram, Holter monitor, chest x-ray, and/or orthostatic blood pressure measurements may or may not be abnormal in dizziness arising from cardiovascular disorders. A diagnosis of multiple sclerosis must be confirmed by lesions noted on MRI studies and by abnormal CSF from lumbar puncture. Vertebrobasilar insufficiency and cerebellar hemorrhage can be confirmed with positive findings on MRI/MRA studies.

TREATMENT/MANAGEMENT

→ An optimal treatment plan depends on identifying the cause of dizziness.
→ For vertigo, several classes of drugs are effective in reducing symptoms.

- Drug therapy may be used to control autonomic symptoms (nausea and vomiting) or to suppress the vestibular system. Drug therapy should only be used in the first few days of an acute vertigo attack. (See **Table 9B.2, Vestibular Suppressants**.)
- BPPV can be treated using either the Epley or the Semont maneuver. (See **Table 9B.3, Canalith Repositioning Maneuvers**.)
- For presyncope, identify the precipitating factor (e.g., vasovagal attacks), avoid the inciting factor, and/or correct the cause by correcting the underlying disorder.
- For disequilibrium, treatment is determined by cause (e.g., someone with multiple sensory deficits may find eyeglasses, a cane, or a walker helpful).
- For dizziness related to psychological disorders, counseling as well as antidepressants may be advised.
- See "Patient Education" section.

CONSULTATION

→ Consultation with a physician is recommended when an underlying pathological condition is suspected or when severe symptoms are not responsive to palliative treatment.
→ Referral to a physician as appropriate when complex pathology is present.
→ As needed for prescription(s)

PATIENT EDUCATION

→ Explain the cause of dizziness based on examination findings.
→ Teach the patient how to perform the Epley or Semont maneuver for BPPV (see **Table 9B.3**).
→ Reassure the patient that dizziness may be a temporary manifestation of viral illness and is usually benign.
→ Advise the patient to reduce unnecessary sensory stimulation as indicated.
→ Advise the patient to avoid caffeine and nicotine, which can aggravate dizziness.
→ Advise the patient to avoid alcohol and recreational drugs.
→ Advise the patient to reduce movements that may exacerbate dizziness.
→ Discuss medication side effects as indicated.
→ If a psychological component is present, provide counseling and reassurance as indicated. Anxiolytic agents may be useful if symptoms persist.
→ Discuss safety measures to take during the course of dizziness and involve family members in the plan.
→ Recommend bed rest in a darkened room, with no reading or watching television.
→ Appropriate referral (cardiology, neurology, otolaryngology, psychiatry) may be necessary if the etiology is unclear or symptoms persist despite treatment.

FOLLOW-UP

→ Re-evaluate medication/management response within one to two weeks.

Table 9B.3.   CANALITH REPOSITIONING MANEUVERS

Patients with severe nausea and vomiting during the maneuvers may need to be medicated with an antiemetic before starting.

The Epley Maneuver:

With the patient seated, the patient's head is turned 45 degrees to the affected ear. The patient is then tilted backward to a supine position with the head in the same 45-degree rotation, hanging off the table. This should cause an attack of vertigo. The patient should be held in this position until the attack abates. Some authors suggest 4 minutes in this position. The head is then turned 90 degrees toward the unaffected ear. With the head remaining turned, the patient is rolled onto the side of the unaffected ear (the patient is now looking at the floor). This may provoke another attack of vertigo. The patient should remain in this position for 3 minutes. The patient is then moved to the seated position and the head is tilted down 30 degrees.

The Semont Maneuver:

With the patient seated, the head is turned 45 degrees horizontally toward the unaffected ear. The patient is then lowered into a position toward the affected ear, to lie on her side with the nose pointing upward. This position should induce a paroxysm of vertigo and nystagmus. The patient is left in this position for 3 minutes and then is quickly moved through the seated position to lie on the side of the unaffected ear with the nose pointed to the ground. Again, this position should produce vertigo and nystagmus. The patient is left in this position for 3 minutes before moving back to a seated position.

Putting the patient into these various positions allows for the movement of the displaced otolith to move out of semicircular canals and into the utricle where it will not induce the symptoms of vertigo and nystagmus.

These maneuvers have reported success rates of 66–100% for decreasing or alleviating symptoms. They can be repeated if symptoms don't resolve on the first attempt. Patients can also be taught to perform them if the symptoms return.

Source: Adapted with permission from Koelliker, P., Summers, R., and Hawkins, B. 2001. Benign paroxysmal positional vertigo: diagnosis and treatment in the emergency department—a review of the literature and discussion of Canalith-repositioning maneuvers. *Annals of Emergency Medicine* 37(4):392–398; and Radtke, A., Neuhauser, H., von Brevern, M.A. et al. 1999. A modified Epley's maneuver for self-treatment of benign paroxysmal positional vertigo. *Neurology* 53(6):1358–1360.

→ If not responsive to therapeutic plan, provide additional evaluation and consultation.

→ Document in progress notes and on problem list.

BIBLIOGRAPHY

Adams, R., Victor, M, and Ropper, A. 1997. *Principles of neurology*, 6th ed., eds. M. Wonsiewicz and M. Navrozov, pp. 295–310. New York: McGraw-Hill.

Baloh, R. 1998. Vertigo. *Lancet* 352:1841–1846.

Brandt T., Steddin S., and Daroff, R.B. 1994. Therapy for benign paroxysmal positioning vertigo, revisited. *Neurology* 44(5):796–800.

Calkins, H. 1997. *Current therapy in neurologic disease*, 5th ed., eds. R.T. Johnson and J.W. Griffin, pp. 5–7. St. Louis, Mo.: Mosby.

DeKruijk, J.R., Twinjnstra, A., and Leffers, P. 2001. Diagnostic criteria and differential diagnosis of mild traumatic brain injury. *Brain Injury* 15(2):99–106.

Drachman, D.A. 1998. Clinical crossroads: a 69-year old man with chronic dizziness. *Journal of the American Medical Association* 280:2111–2118.

Drachman, D.A., and Hart, C.W. 1972. An approach to the dizzy patient. *Neurology* 22:323–324.

Hain, T. 1997. Vertigo and disequilibrium. In *Current therapy in neurologic disease*, 5th ed., eds. R.T. Johnson and J.W. Griffin, pp. 8–14. St. Louis, Mo.: Mosby.

Koelliker, P., Summers, R., and Hawkins, B. 2001. Benign paroxysmal positional vertigo: diagnosis and treatment in the emergency department—a review of the literature and discussion of Canalith-repositioning maneuvers. *Annals of Emergency Medicine* 37(4):392–398.

Lawson J., Fitzgerald J., Birchall J. et al. 1999. Diagnosis of geriatric patients with severe dizziness. *Journal of the American Geriatrics Society* 47:12–17.

Olshansky, B. 1998. *Syncope: mechanisms and management*, eds. B. Grubb and B. Olshansky, pp. 15–71. Armonk, N.Y.: Futura Publishing.

Panitch, K., and Thompson, T. 1998. *Psychiatry for primary care physicians*, eds. L. Goldman, T. Wise, and D. Brody, pp. 97–117. Chicago: American Medical Association.

Pedley, T.A., and Ziegler, D.K. 2000. *Merritt's textbook of neurology*, 10th ed., ed. L.P. Roland, pp. 12–17. Philadelphia: Lippincott Williams & Wilkins.

Radtke A., Neuhauser H., von Brevern M.A. et al. 1999. A modified Epley's maneuver for self-treatment of benign paroxysmal positional vertigo. *Neurology* 53(6):1358–1360.

Ruff, R.L. 1984. *Signs and symptoms in neurology,* ed. P.D. Swanson, pp. 119–131. Philadelphia: J.B. Lippincott.

Tinetti, M., Williams, C., and Gill, T. 2000. Dizziness among older adults: a possible geriatric syndrome. *Annals of Internal Medicine* 132:337–344.

Wazen, J.J. 2000. *Merritt's textbook of neurology*, 10th ed., ed. L.P. Rowland, pp. 32–38. Philadelphia: Lippincott Williams & Wilkins.

9-C

Face Pain

Face pain is a common condition often seen in the primary care setting. Face pain can present as an acute or chronic problem and has many possible causes that overlap between areas of medical and dental specialization (see **Table 9C.1, Selected Causes of Face Pain**). In order to effectively diagnose and treat a patient with face pain, a multidisciplinary approach is often needed.

Face pain most often originates from diseased teeth or sinuses (Raskin 1988). However, there are many other causes of face pain that may be difficult to diagnose, especially when the pain is chronic.

Anatomy and Processing of Pain

The trigeminal nerve (CN V) provides sensation to most of the face. It has three major sensory nerve branches: the ophthalmic branch (VI), the maxillary branch (VII), and the mandibular branch (VIII) (see **Figure 9C.1, Borders of Territory of Sensory Nerves to the Head**). A motor portion of the trigeminal nerve supplies the muscles of mastication. Sympathetic and parasympathetic fibers are also carried by the trigeminal nerve.

Head and facial pain is processed through the trigeminal system, the upper cervical spinal cord, and by the seventh, ninth, and tenth cranial nerves. Pain originating in these structures can be referred anywhere in the head or face. Sensory nerve fibers relay impulses from these structures to the thalamus and the cerebral cortex, where perception of pain is determined by interaction between the cortex, thalamus, and limbic systems.

Recent research suggests that chronic pain, including chronic face pain, is a result of central nervous system sensitization, including within the trigeminal system, which causes neuronal hyperexcitability. It is believed that this process contributes to the amplification and prolongation of pain in the chronic pain state (Ren et al. 1999). Further research has also demonstrated the importance of numerous neurochemical substances in the modulation and processing of pain (Saper et al. 1999) and has important implications for the effective treatment of face pain conditions.

Neurological Causes of Face Pain

Headaches

Headache disorders often cause face pain. For details regarding these conditions, see the **Headache** chapter.

Neuralgias

Neuralgia is pain that originates in a nerve. There are a variety of neuralgia conditions that can cause face pain, including trigeminal, glossopharyngeal, and occipital neuralgia. The pain is typically described as sharp, brief, lancinating, or electric-like pain. The duration of the pain is usually 30 seconds and is characterized by refractory periods that follow the paroxysms of pain. According to Raskin (1988), there may a low-level constant ache with neuralgia as well.

Trigeminal neuralgia, also known as *tic douloureux*, is characterized by sudden, brief, severe, lancinating pain in the distribution of the trigeminal nerve, most often the maxillary (VII) or mandibular branches (VIII). Touch or movement of the face often provokes the pain (see **Figure 9C.2, Characteristic Trigger Zones of Trigeminal Neuralgia**). Cold wind may also be a trigger. It is most commonly seen in patients over age 40, with an average age of over 60. The disorder can be persistent or remitting, and is thought to be caused by focal demyelination of the trigeminal nerve anywhere along its course. This demyelination is often due to vascular compression at the trigeminal nerve root (Saper et al. 1999).

Trigeminal neuralgia in a younger patient, or bilateral symptoms in patients of any age, should raise the suspicion of multiple sclerosis. Trigeminal neuralgia that is progressive or associated with other neurological symptoms, including hypesthesia or anesthesia, should alert the clinician to the possibility of a tumor in the cerebello-pontine angle or an aneurysm of the posterior cerebral artery. It is also important to rule out sphenoid sinusitis, dental pathology, and locally infiltrative tumors as a source of trigeminal pain.

Figure 9C.1.   BORDERS OF TERRITORY OF SENSORY NERVES TO THE HEAD

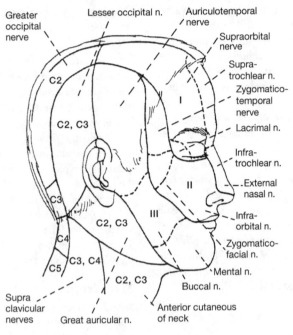

Cutaneous sensory supply to the head.
Border of the territory of each nerve.

Reprinted with permission from Loeser, J.D., Butler, S., Chapman, C.R. et al., eds. 2001. General considerations of pain in the head. *Bonica's management of pain*, 3rd ed., p. 836. Lippincott Williams & Wilkins.

Table 9C.1.   SELECTED CAUSES OF FACE PAIN

Dental	Otolaryngological	Rheumatological
Abscess	Ear disease	Fibromyalgia
Cracked tooth syndrome	Nasopharyngeal disease	Sjögren's syndrome
Impacted wisdom teeth	Salivary gland disease	Temporal arteritis
Periodontal disease	Sinus disease	
Postextraction syndromes		**Other**
Pulpitis	**Musculoskeletal**	Angina
	Myofascial pain	Atypical facial pain
Ophthalmological	Neck conditions	Carotidynia
Corneal injury	Temporomandibular disorder	Thoracic tumors, with referred pain to
Glaucoma		the face
Iritis	**Neurological**	
Optic neuritis	Diabetic neuropathy	
	Neuralgias	
	Headache conditions	
	Intracranial tumor	

Glossopharyngeal neuralgia causes a shock-like pain felt in the tongue or pharynx and is provoked by swallowing or talking. The pain may radiate to the ear, jaw, or upper neck. Syncope may occur in up to 2% of cases, due to stimulation of the vagus nerve during a pain paroxysm (Diamond et al. 1999).

Occipital neuralgia is another cause of face pain. The greater occipital nerve comes off of the second cervical nerve and can cause radiating pain over the posterior scalp, the vertex, and frontal and retro-orbital regions. The pain is described as a paroxysmal jabbing sensation in the distribution of the occipital nerve accompanied by paresthesias or dysthesia. It is thought to be caused by an infectious (viral), traumatic, or compressive disease of the occipital nerve.

Herpes zoster (*varicella zoster*) may also cause neuralgia. In this disorder, a reactivation of a latent varicella zoster infection causes a sustained aching pain. Hypesthesia and/or paresthesia may also occur in the affected area. The characteristic vesicular rash occurs some days later. The more common locations for zoster are the ear, involving the nervus intermedius, or the ophthalmic division of the trigeminal nerve. Postherpetic neuralgia may occur in elderly patients following the zoster infection. *Herpete zoster sine* is herpes zoster without rash.

Figure 9C.2.   CHARACTERISTIC TRIGGER ZONES OF TRIGEMINAL NEURALGIA

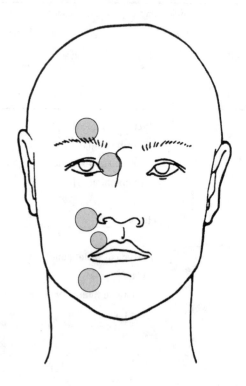

Adapted with permission from Raskin, N.H. 1988. Facial pain. *Headache*, 2nd ed., p.337. New York: Churchill Livingstone.

Diabetic neuropathy occasionally may cause pain in a facial distribution.

Otolaryngological Causes of Face Pain

Sinusitis

Sinusitis involves infection of one or more sinus cavities and is a common cause of face pain. Acute sinusitis often presents with purulent nasal discharge, cough, fever, and localized tenderness of the involved sinus cavity, either during or after an upper respiratory tract infection.

Typically, *frontal sinusitis* presents with localized pain in the supra-orbital or retro-orbital regions. In *maxillary sinusitis*, there may be pain in the malar region or pain may be referred to the teeth, ears, or forehead. Pain in sphenoid sinusitis is located in the vertex, occipital, and frontal and/or retro-orbital regions. *Ethmoid sinusitis* causes pain between and behind the eyes, which may radiate to the temple (Sjaastad 1988). Often, chronic sinusitis will not have these classic symptoms but may only present with vague face pain, a dull headache, or a toothache.

Sialadenitis

Sialadenitis causes pain in the submandibular or parotid areas. The pain typically worsens with eating. There may be localized tenderness or redness. The cause may be due to stasis of salivary flow, calculi, or infection. The submandibular glands are more susceptible to stone formation, while the parotid glands are more often affected by viruses such as mumps, cytomegalovirus, Coxsackie virus, or Epstein-Barr virus.

Autoimmune disorders such as Sjögren's syndrome and rheumatoid arthritis may be associated with salivary gland inflammation. Painless, firm swelling of the salivary gland may be indicative of benign or malignant tumors.

Otalgia

Otalgia may occur in association with face pain. The trigeminal nerve, the second and third cervical nerves, and the seventh, ninth, tenth cranial nerves are all involved in innervation of the ear. Referred pain to the ear and/or face can occur in numerous disorders. For example, tenth cranial nerve fibers may refer pain from pathology in the esophagus, lung, or thoracic cavity to the ear. When examination of the ear shows no obvious ear disease, consider pain from a referred source.

Table 9C.2.   FEATURES OF TRIGEMINAL NEURALGIA

- Electric shock-like paroxysms of pain
- Pain is triggered by touch, chewing, wind
- Refractory period after pain paroxysm
- Unilateral pain: usually VII or VIII branches
- No neurologic deficits

Other Otolaryngological Causes of Face Pain

Other otolaryngological causes of face pain include oral, nasopharyngeal, or sinus malignancies. These patients may complain of hoarseness, throat pain, dysphagia, and ear or facial pain. Risk factors include heavy alcohol use and smoking.

Dental Conditions Causing Face Pain

The most common cause of orofacial pain is the teeth and their surrounding structures (Graff-Radford 1996). Dental problems are often obvious by their location and triggering factors. Pulpitis, caused by dental caries, is a common cause of dental pain. Peridontitis and abscess may also cause orofacial pain. Typical symptoms of a dental problem include the provocation of facial pain by chewing or exposure of the teeth to hot, cold, or sweet foods. Pain may be specific to one tooth or may be poorly localized to the teeth or face. Pain may be transient or lingering.

Occasionally a dental problem such as cracked tooth syndrome may not show up on a dental exam or x-rays and may be difficult for the dentist to diagnose. This may require more than one dental evaluation before a correct diagnosis is reached. Other dental problems causing facial pain are impacted wisdom teeth and postextraction syndrome.

Musculoskeletal Conditions Causing Face Pain

Temporomandibular Dysfunction (TMD)

TMD encompasses a number of muscular or intra-articular temporomandibular joint (TMJ) disorders of the masticatory system. This is a disorder seen most often in young women. The most common symptoms of TMD are muscular face pain, preauricular pain, joint noises, and alteration in joint movement. The typical pain is described as a dull ache, which may be aggravated by use of the jaw (see the **Temporomandibular Disorder** chapter).

Myofascial Pain

Myofascial face pain is often seen in patients with fibromyalgia or bruxism and is characterized by hypersensitive trigger points within the muscles of the face (see the **Temporomandibular Disorder** chapter).

Many headache conditions have accompanying neck pain, but there are primary cervical disorders that also cause pain in the neck, head, and/or face. Cervical pain can radiate to the temporal or supraorbital area and may be referred to the contralateral side of the head. This pain is typically unilateral and often triggered or aggravated by neck movement or palpation of the cervical spine or surrounding structures. Its cause is postulated to be referred pain from myofascial trigger points in the neck muscles or inflammation of cervical spine facet joints or other neck structures (Saper et al. 1999).

Ophthalmological

Ophthalmological conditions such as *acute glaucoma*, *iritis*, *optic neuritis*, and corneal injury can cause face pain. It is usually obvious that the primary problem is with the eye. Ocular causes of face pain will be associated with a red eye, cloudy cornea, diplopia, enlarged pupil, or visual loss (Daroff 2000).

Atypical Facial Pain

Atypical facial pain is a chronic orofacial pain syndrome of unknown etiology. Surgical or dental procedures are often associated with the onset of the disorder. Some authors believe that most causes of this syndrome are of dental or myofascial origin (Friction 2000, Woda et al. 1999). The pain is felt as a continuous, deep, often burning pain. The pain may be reported as severe, but the patient may not appear uncomfortable. It is poorly localized, typically involving the eye, nose, cheek, temples, or jaw. This disorder affects women more frequently than men, and it may be associated with anxiety or depression. Most authorities agree that an exhaustive search for the cause of the pain should be undertaken before the diagnosis of atypical facial pain is made.

Other Causes of Face Pain

Angina due to coronary artery disease may mimic migraine type pain in the face or jaw. Anginal pain typically will occur during exertional activities and may be associated with symptoms of nausea, palpitations, diaphoresis, and dizziness (Kreiner et al.1999).

Carotidynia is a disorder in which the carotid artery periodically swells in the neck, may pulsate, and is painful and tender to the touch. Pain may radiate to the face and behind the ear and eye with symptoms lasting several days at a time. Icepick-like jabs may occur. It is more common in women age 40–50. Carotidynia occurs in two forms. The acute form is a self-limiting condition lasting days to weeks. In the chronic presentation, there is a pattern of periodic attacks. Some authorities believe carotidynia is a form of migraine (Diamond et al. 1999). Carotid dissection or aneurysm may acutely cause similar symptoms.

In rare occurrences, lung cancer may cause face pain. This has been described as severe, aching pain located in the aural-temporal area ipsilateral to the cancer. Associated findings include weight loss, elevated sedimentation rate, or digital clubbing (Capobianco 1995).

Temporal arteritis, also known as *giant cell arteritis*, is an important cause of face pain in patients over 50 years old. It is an autoimmune disorder that causes temporal artery inflammation and may be associated with polymyalgia rheumatica, a related inflammatory condition. Temporal arteritis may lead to visual loss or stroke, so it is crucial not to miss this diagnosis. Patients may complain of a headache or scalp or jaw pain. There may be pain and swelling at the temporal artery, visual disturbances, fever, or anemia. With rare exceptions, the erythrocyte sedimentation rate is elevated.

DATABASE

SUBJECTIVE

→ Age and sex of patient
→ Characteristics of pain:

- Onset: sudden or gradual
- Pattern: constant or intermittent
- Quality (sharp, dull, pulsating, etc.)
- Location and distribution of pain
- Severity and intensity (use of 1–10 pain scale is helpful)
- Timing: pattern with time of day, length of time of painful episode
- History of pain, course of pain, and current pain
- Effect on activities of daily functioning
- Aggravating and alleviating factors

→ Review of systems for presence of associated symptoms:
- Constitutional symptoms: weight loss, fever, weakness, syncope
- Skin: rash
- Head: headache
- Ears: ear pain or plugging
- Eyes: red eyes, visual disturbance, dry eyes
- Nose: nasal discharge or congestion
- Oral/TMJ: bruxism, dry mouth, oral lesions, pain with chewing (think TMJ, dental, temporal arteritis), TMJ joint sounds, tooth or gum pain, throat pain
- Neck: pain
- Chest: cough, breathing difficulty, pain
- Cardiac: chest pain (if appropriate, inquire into associated cardiac symptoms)
- GI: dysphagia, nausea or vomiting
- Musculoskeletal: joint pains, joint stiffness, myalgias
- Psychiatric: screen for anxiety, depression, and sleep disturbance

→ Past medical history:
- Allergies, cardiac disease, dental disease, depression, anxiety or stress, diabetes, headache disorder, malignancies, neurological disease, recent dental exam or x-rays, recent trauma (whiplash, surgery, dental procedures, or domestic violence), recent upper respiratory infection, rheumatological disease, sinus disease, or TMD.

→ Family medical history:
- Cardiac disease, depression or anxiety disorders, diabetes, headache disorders, malignancies, neurological disease or rheumatological disease

→ Social history/habits:
- Occupation, marital and family status, presence of stressors, history of smoking, use of alcohol, drugs, or caffeine

OBJECTIVE

→ Physical examination may include the following (palpating and percussing the face may trigger a painful neuralgia paroxysm, so use caution):
- Vital signs: temperature, pulse, respiration, and blood pressure
- General appearance
- Skin: Check for rash, swelling, or erythema.
- Head: Check for temporal artery tenderness, vesicular rash on face or scalp, percussion of the frontal and maxillary sinuses for tenderness.

- Ears: Check external ears and tympanic membranes for signs of redness, discharge, or lesions. Check if hearing is intact.
- Eyes: Check for redness, cloudiness of cornea, pupillary response, papilledema, and visual acuity if eye problem is suspected.
- Nose: Check nasal mucosa, septum and turbinates for redness, swelling or lesions.
- Oral: Check for lesions, salivary gland duct discharge and force bite test on tongue blade (if pain is felt on a particular tooth, suspect a dental problem).
- TMJ: Check for tenderness at preauricular area, restriction of mouth opening, joint noises, and pain with mouth opening.
- Salivary glands: Check for redness, swelling or tenderness. Check salivary gland ducts for purulent discharge as indicated.
- Neck: Check posture cervical muscle tenderness, range of motion of neck, for masses, cervical adenopathy, or carotid artery tenderness.
- Chest: Observe respiratory effort and auscultate breath sounds.
- Cardiac: Auscultate heart sounds and determine heart rate and rhythm.
- Musculoskeletal: Palpate for tenderness or muscle tension of the facial and neck muscles.
- Extremities: Check upper extremities, if indicated for strength and sensation, and clubbing of fingers.
- Neurological exam: Assess mental status. Observe gait, check balance, check strength and symmetry of extremities and deep tendon reflexes. Observe symmetry of facial muscles. Check cranial nerves II-XI, with emphasis on testing all sensory branches of the trigeminal nerve (see the **Bell's Palsy** chapter, **Table 9A.5, Cranial Nerve Testing**).

ASSESSMENT

→ Rule out the following disorders:
- Dental, musculoskeletal, neurological, ophthalmological, otolaryngological, rheumatological, and other causes of face pain (see **Table 9C.1**).

PLAN

DIAGNOSTIC TESTS

→ Diagnostic tests may include the following, based on history and exam:
- Cervical x-rays
- Chest x-ray to screen for thoracic tumor
- CT scan: is more accurate for diagnosis of sinus infection or tumor than are plain films
- MRI: to look for multiple sclerosis, cervical spine disease, or tumor
- Sinus x-rays to screen for sinus infection or nasopharyngeal abnormalities
- If cardiac disease is suspected, consider an electrocardiogram and exercise tolerance test.

→ Laboratory tests may include:
- Erythrocyte sedimentation rate is essential in patients over age 50 with complaint of headache or face or jaw pain. If the sedimentation rate is elevated, a temporal artery biopsy may be indicated.
- CBC with differential, blood sugar, HgbA1c. Other chemistry or serologies as appropriate.

TREATMENT/MANAGEMENT

→ For common otolaryngological disorders, acute herpes zoster, or TMD, see the appropriate chapter or textbook for management.

→ For dental, ophthalmological, cardiac disorders, tumor or suspected temporal arteritis, see "Consultation," below.

→ A general principle is to avoid narcotic analgesics in the treatment of chronic pain syndromes.

→ For treatment of trigeminal neuralgia or glossopharyngeal neuralgia:
- Carbamazepine has a 60–80% efficacy rate for trigeminal neuralgia. Pain may often improve within 24-48 hours. Start with 100 mg p.o. BID and increase by 100 mg p.o. every 3 days. Maximum dose is 1,200 mg/day.
- Side effects of carbamazepine include sedation, dizziness, ataxia, hepatic injury, and blood dyscrasias. Obtain baseline SGOT and CBC, repeat every 2 weeks for 6 weeks, then every 3 months. Serum carbamazepine levels may be monitored.
- Carbamazepine may interact with other medications; consult a pharmacist or pharmacology textbook as needed.
- Drug combinations may be needed for relief of symptoms. Other anticonvulsant medications commonly used are gabapentin and phenytoin. Baclofen, a centrally acting muscle relaxant, and tricyclic antidepressants may also be used. Consult a pharmacology textbook for dosing information.
- A variety of surgical techniques have been used to treat trigeminal neuralgia. These methods are reserved for refractory cases or when pain becomes unresponsive to medical therapy. Procedures include microvascular decompression, which involves a craniotomy approach, and the less invasive techniques of radiofrequency rhizotomy, glycerol injection, and gamma knife.

→ For diabetic facial neuropathy, postherpetic neuralgia, atypical facial pain, and chronic myofascial pain:
- A tricyclic antidepressant (TCA) is the first-line agent. Of commonly used TCAs, amitriptyline is the best-studied and is the first-line agent.
  - Amitriptyline may be started in small doses of 10–25 mg p.o. per night, with an increase of 1 pill every week until a dose of up to 75–80 mg p.o. per night is reached, until symptoms are relieved, or until medication side effects occur.
  - Side effects are sedation, dry mouth, and orthostatic hypotension.
- Capsaicin cream 0.025–0.075% applied locally to affected areas QID may provide some relief of neuropathic pain. It may cause burning or erythema at the application site. Expect capsaicin cream to take up to 2–6 weeks for full benefit.
- Lidocaine 5% gel or 4% cream applied topically to area QD may provide some relief of symptoms. Lidocaine may cause edema, erythema, or itching locally. Rare systemic reactions include dizziness, confusion, or sedation.
- In diabetic neuropathy, good blood sugar control is very important in both preventing neuropathy and managing pain (see the **Diabetes** chapters in Section 10).

→ For carotidynia: It is usually responsive to corticosteroids and analgesics, among other medications (Saper 1999). The chronic form is responsive to typical antimigraine measures (see the **Headache** chapter).

→ For occipital neuralgia: Nerve blocks have been shown to be helpful. Carbamazepine may also be effective. Surgical procedures are controversial but have been useful for some patients (Saper et al. 1999).

→ For patients with comorbid depression or anxiety: Consider treatment for these conditions (see the **Depression** and **Anxiety Disorders** chapters in Section 14).

CONSULTATION

→ For disorders that may require CT or MRI imaging, consultation with a neurologist may be useful.

→ If a dental or eye problem is suspected, referral to a dentist or ophthalmologist is the most appropriate action.

→ For atypical face pain, consultation with a dentist, otolaryngologist, neurologist, and/or face pain specialist may be indicated.

→ For glossopharyngeal neuralgia or carotidynia, consultation with a neurologist or otolaryngologist is recommended to rule out serious pathology.

→ For temporal arteritis, consultation with primary care physician or rheumatologist may be indicated. The treatment, with corticosteroids, is urgent to prevent irreversible complications of stroke or blindness. Referral to a surgeon for a temporal artery biopsy is also indicated.

→ For myofascial pain, referral to a physical therapist may be appropriate, except in cases of fibromyalgia (see the **Fibromyalgia** chapter in Section 8).

→ For suspected cardiac disease or malignancy, see the appropriate chapter or seek consultation with a physician.

→ Chronic pain programs may be indicated for patients with difficult-to-control chronic pain conditions.

→ For patients who have difficulty coping with stress, comorbid depression, or anxiety disorders, a referral to a mental health care provider may be helpful.

→ Obtain physician consultation if the diagnosis is uncertain or in cases of potential significant sequelae.

PATIENT EDUCATION

→ Review pertinent natural history of the disorder.

→ Explain that the use of anticonvulsants or antidepressants for chronic pain syndromes work on neuroreceptors to prevent pain. The dosage is gradually increased to achieve relief of symptoms with minimum side effects. It may take a month for these medications to work.

→ Review drug precautions and potential side effects with the patient.

→ Patients should wash hands after using capsaicin or lidocaine topicals and avoid getting product in their eyes.

→ For diabetes, good blood sugar control is essential for preventing neuropathic complications and pain control.

→ For trigeminal neuralgia, patients are advised to wear a scarf when outdoors to prevent wind from triggering an attack.

→ For musculoskeletal disorders, advise the patient about posture and muscle stretching and strengthening, and recommend the use of hot and cold packs to ease symptoms.

FOLLOW-UP

→ Determine follow-up based on the particular disorder and recommendations at the individual practice setting.

→ The patient should return if new or progressive symptoms occur or if the pain is not controlled.

→ Document in progress note and on problem list.

BIBLIOGRAPHY

Brown, R.S., and Bottomley, W.K. 1990. The utilization and mechanism of action of tricyclic antidepressants in the treatment of chronic facial pain: a review of the literature. *Anesthesia Progress* 37:223–229.

Capobianco, D.J. 1995. Facial pain as a symptom of non-metastatic lung cancer. *Headache* 35(10):581–585.

Daroff, R.B. 2000. The eye and headache. Presented at the Scottsdale Headache Symposium, American Headache Society January 30–February 1, 1986. Syllabus: pp. 583–595.

Diamond, M.L., and Soloman, G.D. 1999. *Diamond and Dalessio's the practicing physician's approach to headache*, 6th ed. Philadelphia: W.B. Saunders.

Friction, J. 2000. Atypical orofacial pain disorders: a study of diagnostic subtypes. *Current Review of Pain* 4:142–147.

Graff-Radford, S.B. 1996. Orofacial pain—an overview. *Journal of Back and Musculoskeletal Rehabilitation* 6:113–133.

Kreiner, M., and Okeson, J.P. 1999. Toothache of cardiac origin. *Journal of Orofacial Pain* 13(3):201–207.

Loeser, J.D., Butler, S., Chapman, C.R. et al., eds. 2001. *Bonica's management of pain*, 3rd ed. Philadelphia: Lippincott Williams & Wilkins.

Okeson, J.P. 1995. *Bell's orofacial pains*, 5th ed. Carol Stream, Ill.: Quintessence Publishing Co.

Raskin, N.H. 1988. *Headache*, 2nd ed. New York: Churchill Livingstone.

Ren, K., and Dubner, R. 1999. Central nervous system plasticity and persistent pain. *Journal of Orofacial Pain* 13(3):155–163.

Saper, J.R., Silberstein, S., Gordon, C.D. et al. 1999. *Handbook of headache management*, 2nd ed. Baltimore: Lippincott Williams & Wilkins.

Sjaastad, O. 1988. Classification and diagnostic criteria for headache disorders, cranial neuralgias and facial pain. *Cephalgia* 8(7):63–64.

Woda, A., and Pionchon, P. 1999. A unified concept of idiopathic orofacial pain: clinical features. *Journal of Orofacial Pain* 14(3):172–184.

9-D

Headache

Headache is one of the most common complaints in the general population, affecting up to 90% of the population yearly and 99% at some time during their lives (Silberstein et al. 1996). An estimated $17 billion per year in direct and indirect costs has been attributed to migraine. In addition, medical benefits and missed workdays from headache have cost American industry $50 million annually (Solomon et al. 1997).

Headache is a diffuse pain that can occur in different areas of the head and is not confined to the area of a nerve distribution (Clinch 2001). The major mechanisms of headache are vascular and meningeal inflammation, vascular dilatation, excessive muscle contraction, and traction on pain-sensitive structures (Pruitt 1995). Both vascular and muscular changes may occur in the same individual, and as a result more than one type of headache may be present. In such situations, the features of the predominant symptom pattern define the type of headache (e.g. tension-type versus migraine headache) (Weiss 1999).

The International Headache Society has classified headaches into three major groups (Headache Classification Committee of the International Headache Society [IHS] 1988). They are 1) psychological or functional headaches—the most prevalent types—which include tension-type headaches; 2) vascular headaches, which include migraine headaches; and 3) organic headaches, which include headaches caused by brain tumors and vascular inflammation.

In addition to this extensive classification system, a simpler system is often used in clinical settings. The simpler system classifies headaches as primary and secondary. Primary headaches are benign, usually recurrent, and not caused by organic disease. They include migraine with and without aura, tension-type headache, and cluster headache. Secondary headaches are caused by underlying organic disease, ranging from sinusitis to acute transient ischemic attack to cerebrovascular accident (Clinch 2001). (See **Table 9D.1, Headache Classifications**.)

In primary headaches, pain occurs when the cerebral vasculature, musculature, and/or some of the cranial nerves are irritated. A less understood feature seems to be abnormally low activity of the endogenous pain control system in parts of the brain. This hypoactivity disrupts brain neurotransmitter systems, leading to decreased serotonin levels and a sustained discharge of trigeminal pathways. A headache results. In migraine and cluster headaches, vascular dilatation contributes to the pain and may also be caused by the hypoactivity of the endogenous pain control system. Muscular overcontraction of the frontal and temporal muscles contributes to tension-type headaches. Teeth grinding, stress, and jaw clenching may also cause muscle tension. In the past, migraine, cluster, and tension-type headaches were considered to be separate types of headaches. It is now thought that these primary headaches are most likely all part of a broad spectrum of the same disease (Weiss 1999).

This section will include discussion of the diagnosis, treatment, and management of the most common types of headaches. These are the primary benign headaches of migraine, cluster, and tension-type, and the secondary headache of the inflammatory type related to temporal arteritis. Benign headaches usually do not require an extensive workup, but pathological ones do. However, each category of pathological traction and inflammation headache should be ruled out before a headache is classified as benign.

→ Headaches likely to be benign and not in need of further work-up may have the following characteristics:
- History of previous identical headaches
- Alertness and cognition are intact
- Neurological examination is normal
- Neck is supple
- Vital signs are normal
- Observation reveals continual improvement (Newman et al. 1998)

→ Headaches that may be pathologic and may require further work-up have the following characteristics:
- Most severe headache ever experienced
- First severe headache
- Vomiting precedes headache
- Fever or unexplained systemic signs
- Worsened by bending, lifting, coughing
- Onset after age 50

- Headaches increase in frequency and severity
- Headache following head trauma
- New-onset headache in a patient who has HIV or cancer, or risk factors for same
- Any abnormality on examination, including focal neurological symptoms or signs of disease
- Abnormal mental status, diminished level of consciousness
- Neck not completely supple
- Observation reveals no improvement or worsening (Newman et al. 1998)

The following general database is for reference when the presentation is headache and no diagnosis has yet been reached.

DATABASE

SUBJECTIVE

→ Age and circumstance of onset:
- Certain headache disorders are common to particular phases of life (e.g., migraine frequently begins in childhood).
- Circumstances surrounding onset (e.g., headaches prior to or during menstruation or ovulation, or headaches during pregnancy are often migrainous and more commonly without aura) (Moloney et al. 2000).

→ Location and laterality:
- Important clues to the type of headache are revealed by the location (e.g., cluster, migraine, and temporal arteritis

---

Table 9D.1. HEADACHE CLASSIFICATIONS

Primary Headaches	Secondary Headaches
<ul><li>Tension-type (most common)</li><li>Migraine (with and without aura)</li><li>Cluster</li></ul>	**Cerebrovascular** <ul><li>Hemorrhage (subarachnoid, cerebral, and cerebellar)</li><li>Infarction</li><li>Arteriovenous malformation (aneurysm)</li><li>Arteritis, vasculitis</li></ul>**Meningeal Irritation** <ul><li>Meningitis</li><li>Encephalitis</li></ul>**Intracranial Pressure Changes** <ul><li>Increased pressure</li><li>Neoplasm</li><li>Pseudotumor (benign intracranial hypertension)</li><li>Decreased pressure (postlumbar puncture)</li></ul>**Facial/Cervical Involvement** <ul><li>Sinusitis</li><li>Temporal arteritis</li><li>Narrow-angle glaucoma</li><li>Uveitis (dry-eye disorders)</li><li>Retrobulbar neuritis</li><li>Otitis</li><li>Trigeminal neuralgia</li><li>Dental pain</li><li>Parotitis</li><li>Cervical spine disorder</li></ul>**Systemic** <ul><li>Infection (noncephalic)</li><li>Allergy (foods, pollen)</li><li>Hormonal (premenstrual syndrome)</li><li>Toxin-induced (carbon monoxide)</li><li>Drug-induced (cocaine, alcohol)</li><li>Caffeine withdrawal</li><li>Exertional (coitus, cough)</li></ul>**Traumatic** <ul><li>Concussion and postconcussion</li><li>Hematoma (subdural, epidural)</li></ul>

Source: Reprinted with permission from Weiss, J. 1999. Assessing and managing the patient with headaches. *Nurse Practitioner* 24(7):19.

headaches characteristically are unilateral; muscle contraction pain is typically generalized and bilateral) (Silberstein et al. 2001a).

→ Prodromal events:
  - Warning symptoms prior to onset provide clues to the type of headache (e.g., aura, fluid retention, malaise, personality change, neck stiffness, irritable bowel symptoms, or sleep disturbance).
  - Migraine headaches characteristically present with prodromal events.

→ Precipitating factors:
  - Menstruation, alcohol consumption, cocaine use or withdrawal, oral contraceptives, or missed meals can be triggers for migraines.
  - New medication, bright lights, fatigue, loss of sleep, stress, food additives, and certain drugs often can provoke migraine headaches (Silberstein et al. 2001b).

→ Time of onset and duration:
  - Nocturnal awakening often is associated with vascular headache (e.g., hypertension-related headache).
  - Morning headaches may be migraine or muscular (due to jaw clenching, for example). They also may be due to withdrawal from caffeine, analgesics, or ergot preparations (Silberstein et al. 2001a).

→ Quality of the pain:
  - Pulsating, unilateral, throbbing pain usually is related to vascular headaches.
  - Band-like, bilateral pain usually is a symptom of muscle contraction headaches.
  - Intense, unilateral burning, boring, searing pain is associated with cluster headaches (Clinch 2001).

→ Frequency:
  - Muscular headaches often last the majority of a day and may happen daily.
  - Cluster headaches usually occur in brief attacks, lasting 30–90 minutes.
  - Migraine headaches in women usually occur once or twice a month at ovulation and/or menstruation (Silberstein et al. 2001b).

→ Accompanying symptoms:
  - Specific headache syndromes have specific symptoms (see discussions of specific types of headaches).

→ Relieving factors:
  - Vascular headaches can be relieved with rest and the application of cold.
  - Muscular headaches respond to heat, rest, and relaxation.
  - Determining what relieves the pain (e.g., caffeine) can be a diagnostic indicator (Silberstein et al. 2001b).

OBJECTIVE

→ Physical examination is usually normal because benign headaches are not associated with structural abnormalities.
  - Vital signs, including temperature, should be taken.
  - Head and neck examination should include:

  - Assess for craniocervical bruits over the eyes, carotid, and vertebral arteries.
  - Palpate for painful areas, rigidity, masses, or signs of trauma in the scalp, sinuses, and temporal arteries.
  - Eye examination should include:
    - Assess for glaucoma, optic atrophy, papilledema, impaired vision, retinal hemorrhage.
  - Nose, mouth, and dentition examination should include:
    - Assess for tenderness and jaw range of motion.
    - Check the temporomandibular joint for tenderness, crepitus, and range of motion.
  - Neurological examination should include:
    - Cranial nerves
    - Gait, deep tendon reflexes, meningeal signs, cerebellar testing, Romberg test
    - Mental status examination as indicated by history
    - Any neurological abnormalities will necessitate consultation/referral.

ASSESSMENT

→ Headache—primary
→ Headaches—secondary
→ See **Table 9D.1** for differential diagnosis.

PLAN

DIAGNOSTIC TESTS

→ Diagnostic testing in the majority of individuals with benign headaches is of limited value. However, when indicated by the history and physical, order the following:
  - Baseline laboratory tests should be within normal limits (WNL) if a benign headache:
    - Complete blood count (CBC)
    - Erythrocyte sedimentation rate (ESR)
    - Urinalysis (U/A)
    - Blood chemistry profile
  - Tests below will be WNL for benign headaches:
    - Sinus x-rays (CT scan is optimal versus x-ray)
    - Cervical spine x-rays
    - Tonometry
    - Lumbar puncture (LP)
    - Skull series
    - Brain scan, tomography, CT scan
    - Electroencephalogram (EEG)

→ For more details on pertinent diagnostics, see discussions of specific types of headaches.

TREATMENT/MANAGEMENT

→ First-line approaches are:
  - Establish good rapport with the patient.
  - Pay attention to precipitating, exacerbating, and relieving factors.
  - Provide psychological support.
  - Discuss relaxation therapy and stress management.

→ If the pain is quite severe and simple treatment measures have failed, medication can be given for:

- Symptomatic relief of an acute episode
- Abortive therapy to prevent a headache after warning signs have appeared
- Prophylaxis to reduce frequency, particularly if symptomatic therapy has failed
  Refer to **Table 9D.2, Pharmacological Therapies for Migraine Headache**; **Table 9D.3, Hormonal Therapies for Migraine Headache**; **Table 9D.4, Pharmacological Therapies for Cluster Headache**; and **Table 9D.5, Pharmacological Therapies for Tension-Type Headache** for treatment options.
→ Prophylaxis guidelines:
- Two or more incapacitating episodes per month
- Unresponsive to abortive therapy
- Complicated migraine with significant neurologic defects (Marks et al. 1997a)

CONSULTATION

→ Consultation with a physician is indicated for any presentation of headache that does not fall within the parameters of a clinician's experience or if there is a question about the diagnosis/treatment.
→ As needed for prescription(s)

PATIENT EDUCATION

→ Provide reassurance that most headaches do not represent a serious disease.
→ Include patient participation in the treatment plan. This is essential to ensure success.
→ Advise the patient that patience is necessary because several trials may be required to identify the best treatment.
→ Instruct the patient to keep a headache journal (if headaches are frequent) to detect a pattern.
→ Advise the patient that triggering factors and stresses may contribute to the headache.
→ Discuss the possibility of relaxation training, biofeedback, hypnosis, yoga, acupuncture, massage, and meditation as components of the treatment plan or as the main mode of treatment.
→ Explore lifestyle choices in work and domestic life to evaluate possible opportunities for stress reduction.
→ Consider psychotherapy.
→ Discuss medications and side effects.

FOLLOW-UP

→ While developing a treatment approach—such as medication, lifestyle changes, and adjunct therapy—follow-up should be frequent to evaluate management as determined by practitioner and client.
→ Document in progress notes and on problem list.

Migraine Headache

Migraine headaches afflict about 10% of all adults. There is a family history of migraine in two-thirds of patients (Pruitt 1995). They occur four times as often in women, with up to 25%

of women affected during their reproductive years. Up to 70% of headache cases in women are related to the menstrual cycle and often begin or terminate with menopause (Fettes 1997). About 16% of women will first develop migraines at the time of menopause. Migraine often improves during pregnancy but occasionally may worsen (Pruitt 1995).

Considerable evidence links estrogen to migraine headache. Consequently, these headaches are called menstrual migraines (MM) (Silberstein et al. 2001b). The predominant variant of MM is migraine without aura (IHS 1988). A migraine headache without aura is more likely to occur two days before the onset of menses and on the first two days of menses (Stewart et al. 2000). With advancing age, all types of migraines tend to decrease in number. However, hormone replacement therapy can exacerbate the condition or prevent natural improvement (Silberstein et al. 2001b).

Previously, migraines were classified as either *classic* or *common*. The 1988 IHS nomenclature distinguishes between migraine *with* or *without* aura. Neurological warning signs define a migraine with an aura. These signs often are visual and may occur 1–2 hours before the onset of a migraine attack. The prodrome may consist of photopsia (flashing lights and colors), teichopsia (shimmering, wavy lines), fortification spectrum (zigzag patterns), scotoma (blind spot), hemianopia (partial visual-field loss), and metamorphopsia (illusions of distorted size or shape) (Silberstein et al. 2001b).

More severe, less common forms of migraine are *hemiplegic* and *ophthalmoplegic*. A hemiplegic migraine has both motor and sensory symptoms in a unilateral distribution that continue after the headache is gone. Hemiplegic migraine may begin suddenly with hemiplegia or hemiparesis accompanied by confusion and aphasia. Recovery from paresis may take days to weeks, with multiple attacks resulting in permanent weakness. Oral contraceptive agents have been implicated in the exacerbation of hemiplegic migraine in women (Kumar et al. 1995).

An ophthalmoplegic migraine, a rare form of headache usually seen in children or young adults, is characterized by paralysis of the third, fourth, or sixth cranial nerves. Often there is third nerve paresis. One pupil is dilated, and there is difficulty moving the affected eye in any direction but outwards. This may last days or weeks after the headache is gone (Marks et al. 1997a).

DATABASE

SUBJECTIVE

→ Patient may have:
- Positive family history
- History of cyclic vomiting
- History of motion sickness
- Onset in early morning; headache lasts 2–12 hours, often ending in sleep
- Onset around first day of menstruation
- Onset in late childhood, early adolescence
- Onset at menopause
- Onset occurring after alcohol consumption
→ Symptoms may include:
- Photophobia

- Phonophobia
- Nausea, often with vomiting
- Throbbing pain, usually unilateral, along with the above symptoms

→ Sleep or resting in a dark room may terminate the attack.

→ Stress or the relaxation period after stress can increase the number of attacks.

→ Provoking factors may include:
  - Bright light, noise, alcohol, tension, strong scents, smoke, fasting, oral contraceptives, hormone replacement therapy, menstruation, certain foods

→ May be preceded by an aura:
  - Transient visual disturbance
  - Hyperacute sensoria

OBJECTIVE

→ Physical examination is usually normal because migraines are benign headaches and are not associated with structural abnormalities.
  - Vital signs, including temperature, should be taken.
  - Head and neck examination should include:
    - Check for meningeal signs.
    - Check for craniocervical bruits over the eyes, carotid, and vertebral arteries.
    - Palpate for painful areas, rigidity, masses, or signs of trauma in the scalp, sinuses, and temporal arteries.
  - Eye examination should include:
    - Check for glaucoma, optic atrophy, papilledema, impaired vision, retinal hemorrhage.
  - Nose, mouth, and dentition examination should include:
    - Check for tenderness, jaw range of motion, and the temporomandibular joint.
  - Neurological examination should include:
    - Cranial nerves
    - Gait, deep tendon reflexes, meningeal signs, cerebellar testing, Romberg test
    - Mental status examination as indicated by history
  - Neurological examination is typically normal. Any neurological abnormalities will necessitate consultation/referral.

ASSESSMENT

→ Migraine headache (with or without aura)
→ R/O tension-type headache
→ R/O cluster headache
→ R/O organic lesion

PLAN

DIAGNOSTIC TESTS

→ Laboratory studies are not routinely recommended.
→ Radiological studies are unnecessary in typical cases.

TREATMENT/MANAGEMENT

→ Nonpharmacological measures (see "Treatment/Management" in the initial section of this chapter):

- Investigate family and social circumstances for stress or psychological conflict in anticipation of stress reduction recommendations.
- Recommend activities that reduce stress:
  - Exercise
  - Relaxation techniques
  - Biofeedback
  - Acupuncture
  - Yoga
  - Meditation
  - Supportive counseling
  - A dark room, cold packs, and sleep to alleviate pain

→ For pharmacological measures for an acute attack, see **Table 9D.2**.

- Selective 5-HT$_1$ serotonin agonists (see **Table 9D.2**). These are contraindicated in cardiovascular, cerebrovascular, or peripheral vascular disease. Avoid use within 24 hours of other 5-HT$_1$ or ergots (Weiss 1999).
  - Mode of action includes vasoconstriction and reduction of plasma protein extravasation into perivascular space.
  - The patient must have an accurate diagnosis of migraine. Not for use in management of hemiplegic or basilar migraine.
  - Used for acute treatment, *not* prophylaxis.
    NOTE: Due to its short half-life, patients may get rebound headaches from use of this class of drug.
  - Refer to *Physicians' Desk Reference (PDR)* or drug package insert for further information. Consult physician prior to use.
- Ergot alkaloids, opioids, nonsteroidal anti-inflammatory drugs (NSAIDs) (see **Table 9D. 2**).
- For menses-associated migraine, any medication listed in **Table 9D.2** may be used. In particular, 5-hydroxytryptamine$_1$ (5-HT$_1$) agonists are helpful. A complete headache history will suggest the type and duration of preventive treatment, if indicated. Headaches that are exclusively or primarily limited to menses can be treated preventively with medication a few days before and during menses. NSAIDs are commonly used. Other oral medications may be used for prophylaxis, such as ergotamine tartrate (1 tablet BID or half a suppository at HS) or sumatriptan (25 mg TID) a few days before and at the start of menses (Bartleson 1999).
  - Another approach to menstrual migraine is to stabilize hormone levels. For women on oral contraceptive pills, eliminating the pill-free week when estrogen levels drop abruptly may be helpful. A transdermal estrogen patch a few days before menses or adding a low-dose oral estrogen during the pill-free week may prevent menstrual migraine (Moloney et al. 2000).
  - Migraines may be prevented in perimenopausal or menopausal women by providing a consistent hormone level with a continuous low-dose, combined estrogen-progestin regime (Moloney et al. 2000). (See **Table 9D.3** for hormonal approaches.)

→ For nonpharmacological measures for migraine prophylaxis, see "Treatment/Management."

→ For pharmacological measures for migraine prophylaxis, see **Table 9D.2**.

CONSULTATION

→ Consultation with a physician is indicated:
- For migraine headache unresponsive to treatment
- If there is uncertainty about diagnosis
- For headaches with a new pattern or features
- For complicated presentation of migraine
- For complex pharmacological regimens and narcotic use

→ As needed for prescription(s).

PATIENT EDUCATION

→ See "Patient Education" in the initial section of this chapter.

→ Explain causes of migraines. Reassure as to benign nature.

→ Advise the patient to avoid factors that trigger headaches:
- Foods—chocolate, certain cheeses, tomatoes, citrus fruits
- Alcohol—especially red wine
- Drugs—vasodilators, estrogens, monosodium glutamate, nitrites
- Glare or bright lights
- Emotional stress and acute changes in stress levels
- Minor head trauma
- Allergens
- Organic odors
- Climate change
- Irregular sleep patterns (lack of sleep or excessive sleep)
- Physical exhaustion
- Stress, relaxation after stress
- Exercise
- Hormonal changes:
  - Puberty
  - Menstruation
  - Climacteric
  - Pregnancy
- Hunger (Raskin et al. 2001)

→ Educate the patient about signs of impending attack so that treatment, if necessary, can be started as soon as possible.

→ Instruct the patient about medication usage.

→ Instruct about side effects of drugs, potential drug interactions, and potential for addiction.
- Overuse of ergotamine and most acute migraine medications may lead to a rebound or analgesic overuse headache. Their use should be limited (Silberstein et al. 2001b, Young et al. 1997).

FOLLOW-UP

→ Until a successful regimen is established to control headaches, frequent follow-up is recommended.

→ Document in progress notes and on problem list. Note known trigger factors and both successful and unsuccessful treatment plans. Develop contract for narcotic use, if necessary.

Cluster Headache (Histamine Headache, Horton's Headache, Migrainous Neuralgia)

A *cluster headache* is a vascular-type headache with such specific features that often history can be enough to make a diagnosis. The pain occurs around the eye, temples, neck, and face, and may extend into the shoulder on the same side. The pain is of a burning, boring, high-intensity nature, typically lasting 30 minutes to two hours. It tends to end suddenly. Profuse conjunctival watering and congestion, rhinorrhea, nasal obstruction, and increased perspiration are often associated with the pain.

Cluster headache sufferers are very sensitive to alcohol, aged cheeses, vasodilating agents, and drugs such as histamine or nitroglycerin. Cluster headache occurs more often in men than in women (6:1) with the onset typically later in life (20–50 years old) (Dodick et al. 2001).

The headaches occur in temporal clusters lasting 6–12 weeks. They may recur several months to a year later, often at the same time of year. Unlike other headaches, cluster headaches do not appear to be affected by hormonal changes, allergies, food sensitivities (except for aged cheeses, as mentioned), or stress (Dodick et al. 2001).

DATABASE

SUBJECTIVE

→ Symptoms include intense, nonthrobbing, sharp, boring, stabbing, or lancinating pain.
- Begin abruptly and last 30 minutes to two hours
- May occur daily, often at the same time of day
- Occur commonly in the evening, within two hours of falling asleep

→ Symptoms may also include:
- Associated ipsilateral conjunctival injection, eye tearing, and nasal stuffiness
- Sweating or reddening of affected side of face

→ There is no aura.

OBJECTIVE

→ Physical examination is usually normal because cluster headaches are benign and are not associated with structural abnormalities.

→ Refer to the physical examination procedures under "Objective" in the "Migraine" section of this chapter.

ASSESSMENT

→ Cluster headache

→ R/O migraine

→ R/O trigeminal neuralgia (see the **Face Pain** chapter)

→ R/O organic lesion

PLAN

DIAGNOSTIC TESTS

→ Diagnostic testing in the majority of individuals with benign headaches is of limited value.

→ Laboratory studies are not routinely recommended.

→ Radiological studies are unnecessary in typical cases.

→ For more details on pertinent diagnostics, see "Assessment" in the initial section of this chapter.

TREATMENT/MANAGEMENT

→ For abortive measures, see **Table 9D.4**.

→ For prophylactic measures, see **Table 9D.4**.

- For patients with episodic cluster, start early in the cluster period and continue until headache-free for at least 2 weeks (Mathew 1997).

→ See "Patient Education," below.

CONSULTATION

→ As necessary if the patient is unresponsive to treatment regimen

→ For change in pattern or features

→ As needed for prescription(s).

PATIENT EDUCATION

→ See "Patient Education" in the initial section of this chapter.

→ Advise the patient to avoid trigger factors.

→ Advise the patient to seek treatment at the first sign of a headache.

→ Advise the patient to be aware of possible side effects of medications.

FOLLOW-UP

→ At intervals, if the patient is being treated for chronic cluster headache

→ As necessary, if no relief with treatment regimen

→ Document in progress notes and on problem list.

Tension-Type Headache

Tension-type headaches are among the most prevalent causes of chronic and recurrent headache. Precipitants often include situational stress, anxiety, and depression. Over 90% are bilateral and described as a band-like or pressure sensation around the head (Pruitt 1995). Seventy-five percent of individuals with tension-type headaches are women. Family history of this disorder is often reported, although no genetic abnormality has been identified (Edmeads 1998). This type of headache may be episodic or chronic. When episodic, the pain may persist for several days (Raskin et al. 2001).

DATABASE

SUBJECTIVE

→ Symptoms may include:

- Ache, sensation of tightness, pressure, or constriction in the head, usually in the suboccipital, temporal, or bifrontal area
  - May experience hatband-like sensation
- Associated tightness in neck and/or shoulders

- Tenderness of upper border of the trapezius and other posterior shoulder, neck, and scalp muscles
- Neck muscles taut and contracted
- Associated nausea, photophobia, and photopsia

→ Headache is usually bilateral; rarely unilateral as in migraine.

→ Pain may be mild to incapacitating.

→ Pressure on tender muscles may increase headache intensity.

→ Headache may last hours to days; in chronic form, may persist months to years.

→ Headache often related to stress, depression, or anxiety.

→ There is positive family history in 40% of patients.

→ Symptoms can overlap with those of migraine without aura.

OBJECTIVE

→ Physical examination is usually normal because tension headaches are benign and not associated with structural abnormalities.

→ Refer to the physical examination procedures under "Objective" in the "Migraine" section of this chapter.

ASSESSMENT

→ Tension-type headache

→ R/O migraine without aura

→ R/O mass lesion

PLAN

DIAGNOSTIC TESTS

→ No diagnostic testing is indicated for this type of headache.

→ See "Diagnostic Tests" in the initial section of this chapter.

TREATMENT/MANAGEMENT

→ A supportive client/clinician relationship may enhance the outcome.

→ Nonpharmacological:

- Massage
- Heat
- Acupuncture/acupressure
- Biofeedback
- Relaxation training
- Physical therapy with transcutaneous electrical nerve stimulator (TENS) and ultrasound treatments
- Social support
- Exercise
- Yoga
- Stress reduction exercises (visualization/guided imagery)
- Counseling

→ Pharmacological measures:

- For abortive measures, see **Table 9D.5**.
- For prophylactic measures, see **Table 9D.5**.
- Other migraine drugs may be tried (see **Table 9D.2**).

CONSULTATION

→ Consultation with a physician is indicated for headaches if:

- They are unrelieved with nonpharmacological or common pharmacological treatment.
- They require the addition of analgesic combinations, antidepressants, or muscle relaxants.
- New pattern or features

→ As needed for prescription(s).

PATIENT EDUCATION

→ See "Patient Education" in the initial section of this chapter.

FOLLOW-UP

→ See "Follow-Up" in the initial section of this chapter.
→ Document in progress notes and on problem list.

Temporal or Giant Cell Arteritis

Temporal or *giant cell arteritis* is a systemic autoimmune disorder characterized by inflammation of the temporal artery, with headache, visual dysfunction, malaise, fever, and diffuse weakness (Marks et al. 1997b). It is a common disorder of the elderly. Women account for 65% of the cases (Raskin et al. 2001). Females over age 55 represent the typical patient, with a presentation of new onset unilateral headache, commonly over the temporal artery (Marks et al. 1997b). Irreversible blindness may occur unless treated early and very aggressively (Goroll et al. 1995).

DATABASE

SUBJECTIVE

→ Symptoms may include:
- Severe, unilateral, throbbing pain localized to the scalp, often noticed when brushing hair
- Pain with chewing (i.e., jaw claudication), sometimes resulting in weight loss
- Low-grade fever
- Joint pain and swelling (polymyalgia rheumatica)
- Night sweats
- Acute hearing loss
- Vertigo
- Visual changes

→ Symptoms may be:
- Of sudden onset
- Exacerbated by exposure to cold
- Worse at night

→ Patient may be asymptomatic.

OBJECTIVE

→ Refer to physical exam for migraine.
→ Specific objective components of temporal arteritis may include:
- Tender temporal arteries
- Reddened tender nodules or red streaking of the skin overlying the temple area

- Low-grade fever
- Myalgias
- Elevated ESR. Note that a normal ESR does not exclude temporal arteritis.

ASSESSMENT

→ Temporal arteritis
→ R/O other causes of headache

PLAN

DIAGNOSTIC TESTS

→ ESR: If greater than 40 mm/hour, a temporal artery biopsy should be seriously considered (Marks et al. 1997b).

TREATMENT/MANAGEMENT

→ Immediate, urgent treatment is required to prevent blindness.
→ Prednisone: 60–80 mg p.o./day (1 mg/kg/day):
- Should be started before biopsy results are received. Tapering begins when the sedimentation rate has been significantly reduced and symptoms are controlled.

→ Corticosteroid treatment may be required for as long 6–12 months (Marks et al. 1997b).
→ Monitor ESR periodically.
→ Observe for improvement in headache and scalp pain symptoms.

CONSULTATION

→ Comanagement with a physician is recommended.
→ Consultation with a rheumatologist is recommended if the temporal artery biopsy is negative but the presentation suggests temporal arteritis.
→ Referral to a physician is recommended for cases that do not respond to steroid therapy.
→ As needed for prescription(s).

PATIENT EDUCATION

→ Inform the patient of symptoms of arteritis.
→ Instruct the patient to report symptom occurrence immediately.
→ Educate the patient about the need to take prednisone to promote compliance.
→ Discuss side effects of steroids.
→ Involve the family in care as appropriate.

FOLLOW-UP

→ Close follow-up is recommended for assessing symptoms, monitoring for steroid toxicities, and supervising steroid taper.
→ Document in progress notes and on problem list.

Table 9D.2.   PHARMACOLOGICAL THERAPIES FOR MIGRAINE HEADACHE

Drug	Dosage	Comments
ABORTIVE MEASURES		
Ergotamine tartrate (Ergostat®, Ergomar®)	2 mg sublingually	• At the first sign of attack, 1 tablet under tongue; take subsequent doses at 30-minute intervals, no more than 3 tablets in 24 hours, and no more than 5 tablets/week.
Ergotamine tartrate with caffeine (Wigraine®, Cafergot®, Cafatine®)	2 mg suppository	• At the first sign of attack, 1 suppository at onset, repeat in 1 hour; maximum 2/day, 12/month. Use subnauseating dose initially (one-third of a 2 mg suppository) and repeat dose in 30–60 minutes. Limit use to no more than 2 days/week to avoid rebound headache. • For menstrual migraine, more frequent use is acceptable if use is restricted the rest of the month (Moore et al. 1997).
Ergotamine tartrate with caffeine (Cafergot®)	2 mg tablets p.o.	• Take 1–2 tablets, then 1 every 30 minutes up to 4 times. Maximum 6 tablets in 24 hours. No more than 10/week. A caffeine-containing preparation may have a more rapid onset. • Ergotamine therapy is contraindicated in coronary artery disease (CAD), severe hypertension (HTN), acute infection, renal or hepatic dysfunction, significant peripheral vascular disease (PVD), Raynaud's phenomenon, and pregnancy (Moore et al. 1997). • Side effects include nausea, vomiting, cramping, paresthesias, and rebound headache.
Dihydroergotamine (Migranal®)	0.5 mg nasal spray	• 1 spray/nostril, repeat in 15 minutes. Maximum dose: 6 sprays/24 hours or 15/week.
Dihydroergotamine (DHE 45®)	1 mg/mL for injection	• Use 0.5 mg IM, SC, or IV every hour for 3 hours. Maximum dose: 3 mg/24 hours. DHE is contraindicated in individuals with CAD, PVD, transient ischemic attacks, pregnancy, or sepsis. Should be avoided in women attempting pregnancy.
Codeine phosphate[1] (Tylenol #2–4®)	1 tablet p.o. 4 times a day	• Take 1 tablet every 6 hours as needed.
Oxycodone[1] (Tylox®, Percocet®)	1 tablet p.o. 4 times a day	• Take 1 tablet every 6 hours as needed.
Meperidine[1] (Demerol®)	50–150 mg p.o. SQ or IM	• Give 50–150 mg p.o., SQ, or IM, every 3-4 hours as needed.
Morphine sulfate[1] **Hydromorphone** (Dilaudid®)	10 mg IM 4 mg p.o. or IM	[1] Narcotic analgesics to be used with caution secondary to risk of habituation. May be an option for severe persistent headache when ergotamine therapy not possible.
Isometheptene mucate with dichloralphenazone and acetaminophen (Midrin®)	2 capsules p.o. initially	• Take 2 capsules p.o. initially and 1 capsule repeated hourly up to 5 capsules/12 hours. Helpful for those unable to take ergotamine. • Contraindicated during pregnancy or in CAD, liver or kidney dysfunction, PVD, glaucoma, severe HTN, or with a monoamine oxidase (MAO) inhibitor (Silberstein et al. 2001b). • Side effects: dizziness, liver toxicity
Ibuprofen (Motrin®)	200–800 mg p.o. every 4–6 hours	• 400–2,400 mg p.o./day in divided doses of no greater than 800 mg/dose. Treatment of choice for menstrual migraine. • Side effects: GI upset, bleed
Naproxen sodium (Naprosyn®, Anaprox®, Aleve®)	220–550 mg p.o. every 6–8 hours	• Maximum dose: 1,100 mg • Side effect: GI upset
Aspirin	500–1,000 mg p.o. every 4–6 hours	• Maximum dose: 4,000 mg in 24 hours • Side effect: GI upset
Acetaminophen (Tylenol®)	500–1,000 mg p.o. every 4–6 hours	• Maximum dose: 4,000 mg/24 hours • Side effect: liver toxicity
Butalbital (Fiorinal®, Esgic®)	1–2 tablets every 4–6 hours p.o. as needed	• Maximum dose: 6 tablets/24 hours • May be addictive.

(continued)

Drug	Dosage	Comments
Propoxyphene (Darvon®, Darvocet®)	1 tablet p.o. every 4–6 hours	• Maximum dose: 6 tablets/24 hours. • Is a controlled substance. May be addictive.

FOR NAUSEA

Drug	Dosage	Comments
Chlorpromazine (Thorazine®)	10–25 mg p.o. every 4–6 hours	• Treatment for nausea associated with migraine can also relieve pain.
Prochlorperazine (Compazine®)	5–10 mg p.o. or IM, 25 mg per rectum	
Metoclopramide (Reglan®)	5–20 mg p.o., IM, or IV	
Promethazine (Phenergan®)	12.5–25 mg p.o., IM, or per rectum	

SELECTIVE 5-HT$_1$ SEROTONIN AGONISTS FOR ACUTE ATTACK

Drug	Dosage	Comments
Sumatriptan[2] (Imitrex®)	6 mg SQ with autoinjector, may repeat in 1 hour	• Maximum dose: 12 mg/24 hours
	5–20 mg nasal spray, every 2 hours with 4 sprays of 5 mg each per nostril	• Maximum dose: 40 mg/24 hours
	25–100 mg tablets p.o., may repeat every 2 hours	• Maximum dose: 300 mg/24 hours
Naratriptan[2] (Amerge®)	1–2.5 mg p.o., may repeat in 4 hours	• Maximum dose: 5 mg/24 hours
Rizatriptan[2] (Maxalt®)	5–10 mg p.o., may repeat every 2 hours	• Maximum dose: 30 mg/24 hours. Comes in regular or oral-dissolving tablets.
Zolmitriptan[2] (Zomig®)	2.5 mg p.o., may repeat in 2 hours	• Maximum dose: 10 mg/24 hours [2] Side effects include taste disturbance, tingling, warm-hot sensations, dizziness, chest or neck discomfort. Contraindicated in cardiovascular, cerebrovascular, and peripheral vascular disease. Avoid use within 24 hours of other 5-HT$_1$s or ergots (Weiss 1999). Also, do not administer if taking MAO inhibitors (e.g., Marplan®, Nardil®, Parnate®), selective serotonin re-uptake inhibitors (e.g., Prozac®, Paxil®, Zoloft®), or lithium. Refer to *Physician's Desk Reference* or drug package insert.

PROPHYLACTIC MEASURES

BETA-BLOCKERS

Drug	Dosage	Comments
Propranolol[3] (Inderal®)	Initially 80 mg/day up to 160–240 mg in divided doses.	• Give BID–QID. • Maximum dose is 320 mg in 24 hours.
Timolol[3] (Blocadren®)	10–30 mg/day	
Nadolol[3] (Corgard®)	40–240 mg QD Maximum 240 mg/day	• Maximum dose 30 mg/day in divided doses. [3] Side effects include fatigue, drowsiness, nightmares, insomnia, depression, and bradycardia. Relative contraindications with asthma, depression, CHF, Raynaud's disease, and diabetes.
Atenolol[3] (Tenormin®)	50–100 mg QD Maximum 100 mg/day	

(continued)

Drug	Dosage	Comments
OTHERS		
Methysergide maleate (Sansert®)	2–8 mg p.o./day	• A second-line agent because of serious toxicity risk with prolonged use. • Side effects include nausea, muscle cramps, abdominal pain, weight gain, retroperitoneal and pleuropulmonary fibrosis.
Cyproheptadine (Periactin®)	4–20 mg p.o./day Give in divided doses.	• Has an atropine-like action. Use with caution with history of bronchial asthma, increased intraocular pressure, hyperthyroid, or cardiovascular disease.
CALCIUM CHANNEL BLOCKERS		
Verapamil[4] (Calan®)	40–240 mg TID	[4] Prophylactic effect takes 10–14 days. Full response in 2–4 weeks. • Side effects include hypotension, edema, headache, constipation, and nausea.
Nifedipine[4] (Procardia®)	30–180 mg p.o./day	
Diltiazem HCl[4] (Cardizem®, Dilacor®, Tiazac®)	120–480 mg/day Give in divided doses or in slow-release form.	
TRICYCLIC ANTIDEPRESSANTS (TCA)		
Amitriptyline[5] (Elavil®)	10–150 mg HS or divided doses	• Helpful if insomnia also occurs.
Nortriptyline[5] **HCL** (Pamelor®)	25–100 mg p.o./day in divided doses	[5] Side effects include nausea, flu-like symptoms, jitteriness, dry mouth, urinary retention, constipation, and orthostatic hypotension.
Doxepin[5] (Sinequan®)	25–100 mg p.o./day QD or in divided doses	
Protriptyline[5] (Vivactil®)	Start at 5 mg/day Dose: 5–60 mg	• In divided doses
OTHER ANTIDEPRESSANTS SSRIs		
Fluoxetine HCL[6] (Prozac®)	20–80 mg p.o./day	• SSRIs are not recommended for prevention of migraine. However, some headache experts use them. They are less effective than tricyclics (Noble et al. 1997).
Sertraline[6] (Zoloft®)	50–200 mg p.o./day	• Combining a SSRI and TCA in treating refractory cases of migraine can be beneficial (Silberstein et al. 2001b).
Paroxetine[6] (Paxil®)	10–50 mg/day No >50 mg/day	[6] Side effects include anxiety, insomnia, nervousness, fatigue, tremor, anorexia, nausea, vomiting, and light-headedness.
ANTIANXIETY		
Buspirone (BuSpar®)	7.5 mg BID Maximum 60 mg/day in divided doses	• Useful if patient is also anxious. Side effects include dizziness, nausea, headache, nervousness, lightheadedness, and excitement. • Not to be used concomitantly with MAO inhibitors.

Table 9D.3.   HORMONAL THERAPIES FOR MIGRAINE HEADACHE

Drug	Dosage	Comments
HORMONE THERAPY		
Estradiol transdermal system	.05 mg, .075 mg, 0.1 mg patches Lowest dose used to initiate therapy. Increase as needed.	• Estradiol or ethinyl estradiol is less likely to cause side effects than conjugated estrogens.
Conjugated estrogen (Premarin®)	0.3 mg/day 3 times a week	• Initiate 3 days before menses for menstrual migraine. Continue on the first day of menses and again on day 2. • Use continuously for perimenopausal and menopausal migraine. Combine with cyclic progesterones/progestins.
Micronized 17-beta estradiol	0.5–2.0 mg/day	
Esterified estrogen estropipate	0.3–2.5 mg/day 0.625–1.25 mg/day 0.75–3.0 mg/day 0.625–2.5 mg/day 0.625–1.25 mg estrogen with 1.25–2.5 mg methyl testosterone	• Begin at a low dose and increase as tolerated. • May exacerbate migraine more than other estrogens.
Danazol (Danocrine®)	200–600 mg/day	• Begin before menses starts. • Has many adverse effects and may precipitate menopausal symptoms.
Tamoxifen[1] (Nolvadex®) **Raloxifene**[1] (Evista®)	Currently under study	• May be helpful for resistant migraines. [1] Numerous adverse effects, including menopausal symptoms.

Source: Adapted with permission from Moloney, M.F., Matthews, K.B., Scharbo-Dehaan, M. et al. 2000. Caring for the woman with migraine headaches. *Nurse Practitioner* 25(2):17–39.

Table 9D.4.   PHARMACOLOGICAL THERAPIES FOR CLUSTER HEADACHE

Drug	Dosage	Comments
ABORTIVE MEASURES		
Inhaled oxygen	100% oxygen at 9 liters/minute for 10 minutes	• Preferred treatment at onset.
Sumatriptan (Imitrex®)	6 mg SQ (maximum 12 mg/24 hours) 20 mg nasal spray (maximum 40 mg/24 hours) 25–50 mg tablet every 2 hours (maximum 300 mg/24 hours)	• Most effective self-administered medication for symptomatic relief. • Nasal spray and p.o. are less effective. • Contraindicated in ischemic heart disease and uncontrolled hypertension. (See **Table 9D.2** for additional comments.)
Zolmitriptan (Zomig®)	5–10 mg p.o.	• An option for those who cannot tolerate oxygen or SQ sumatriptan or who prefer oral medication (Dodick et al. 2001).
Dihydroergotamine (DHE 45®)	0.5–1 mg IM, SC, or IV every hour for 3 hours 0.5 mg spray in each nostril. Repeat in 15 minutes (maximum of 6 sprays/24 hours).	• See **Table 9D.2** for contraindications. Provides prompt relief in 15 minutes.
Ergotamine tartrate (Ergostat®)	2 mg p.o. or rectally	• See **Table 9D.2** for contraindications.
Lidocaine HCL	1 cc of 4% nasal drops, may repeat once	• Useful as adjunctive therapy.
Cocaine HCL	In saline solution	• Less preferred because of potentially addictive properties (Mathew 1997).
PROPHYLACTIC MEASURES		
Prednisone	60 mg p.o./day for 3 days, tapered by 10 mg every third day over 18 days	• Give in a.m. to reduce sleep interference. • Side effects include weight gain, fluid retention, gastric irritation, hyperglycemia, and osteoporosis with chronic use.

(continued)

Table 9D.4.   PHARMACOLOGICAL THERAPIES FOR CLUSTER HEADACHE (continued)

Drug	Dosage	Comments
Ergotamine tartrate (Ergostat®)	1 mg p.o./day BID to prevent nocturnal attacks	• See **Table 9D.2** for contraindications.
Verapamil (Calan® SR)	240–720 mg p.o./day. Initial dose is 80 mg TID or 240 mg sustained-release.	• May combine with ergotamine. • See **Table 9D.2** for side effects.
Lithium carbonate	600–900 mg p.o./day	• Will require a full week before response. Blood lithium levels and renal and thyroid function must be monitored prior to and during treatment.
Valproic acid (Depakene®)	250 mg p.o. BID	• Side effects limit usefulness: lethargy, tremor, hair loss, weight gain (Mathew 1997). Baseline and follow-up CBC and liver function tests necessary to monitor for pancreatitis and platelet or liver dysfunction.
Methysergide maleate (Sansert®)	2–8 mg p.o./day	• See **Table 9D.2** for side effects. Potential for fibrotic complications. Not commonly used for more than 3 months.
Indomethacin (Indocin®)	25 mg p.o. TID	• Benefit usually within 48 hours.

Table 9D.5.   PHARMACOLOGICAL THERAPIES FOR TENSION-TYPE HEADACHE

Drug	Dosage	Comments
ABORTIVE MEASURES		
Ibuprofen[1] (Motrin®)	400–2,400 mg p.o./day Maximum 800 mg/dose	[1] May cause GI upset.
Naproxen[1] (Naprosyn®)	500 mg p.o. BID–QID	
Naproxen sodium[1] (Anaprox®)	275 mg p.o. BID–QID	
Aspirin	650 mg p.o. QID. Maximum 650 mg/dose	• May cause GI upset.
ANALGESIC COMBINATIONS		
ASA 325 mg/caffeine 40 mg/ butalbital 50 mg (Fiorinal®)	1–2 tablets p.o. immediately	• Maximum dose is 6/attack.
Acetaminophen 325 mg with caffeine and butalbital (Fioricet®)	1–2 tablets p.o. immediately	• Maximum dose is 6/attack.
PROPHYLACTIC MEASURES		
NONSTEROIDAL ANTI-INFLAMMATORY DRUGS (see ABORTIVE, above) **MUSCLE RELAXANTS**		
Cyclobenzaprine[5] (Flexeril®)	10–40 mg p.o./day in divided doses	[5] Short-term use only. May be habit-forming.
Diazepam[5] (Valium®)	2–10 mg p.o./day	
TRICYCLIC ANTIDEPRESSANTS		
Amitriptyline (Elavil®)	25–100 mg p.o./day	• See **Table 9D.2** for side effects.
Trazodone (Desyrel®)	50–150 mg p.o./day	
OTHER ANTIDEPRESSANTS **SSRIs**		
Fluoxetine (Prozac®)	20–80 mg p.o./day	• See **Table 9D.2** for side effects and other SSRIs.

BIBLIOGRAPHY

Bartleson, J.D. 1999. Treatment of migraine headaches. *Mayo Clinic Proceedings* 74(7):702–708.

Clinch, C.R. 2001. Evaluation of acute headaches in adults. *American Family Physician* 63(4):685–692.

Dodick, D.W., and Campbell, J.K. 2001 Cluster headache: diagnosis, management and treatment. In *Wolff's headache and other head pain,* eds. S.D. Silberstein, R.B. Lipton, and D.J. Dalessio, 7th ed., pp. 283–309. New York: Oxford University Press.

Edmeads, J. 1998. Headache and face pain. In *Internal medicine,* ed. J.H. Stein, 5th ed. pp. 1025–1033. St. Louis, Mo.: Mosby.

Fettes, I. 1997. Menstrual migraine. *Postgraduate Medicine* 101(5):67–77.

Goroll, A.H., May, L.A., and Mulley, A.G. 1995. Approach to the patient with polymyalgia rheumatic or temporal arteritis. In *Primary care medicine,* eds. A.H. Goroll, L.A. May, and A.G. Mulley, Jr., 3rd ed., pp. 807–810. Philadelphia: J.B. Lippincott.

Headache Classification Committee of the International Headache Society. 1988. Proposed classification and diagnostic criteria for headache disorders, cranial neuralgias, and facial pain. *Cephalgia* 8(Suppl 7):9–96.

Kumar, K.L,. and Cooney, T.G. 1995. Headaches. *Medical Clinics of North America* 79(2):261–286.

Marks, D.R., and Rapoport, A.M. 1997a. Diagnosis of migraine. *Seminars in Neurology* 17(4):303–306.

_____. 1997b. Practical evaluation and diagnosis of headache. *Seminars in Neurology* 17(4):307–312.

Mathew, N.T. 1997. Cluster headache. *Seminars in Neurology* 17(4):313–323.

Moloney, M.F., Matthews, K.B., Scharbo-Dehaan, M. et al. 2000. Caring for the woman with migraine headaches. *Nurse Practitioner* 25(2):17–39.

Moore, K.M., and Noble, S.L. 1997. Drug treatment of migraine: Part I. Acute therapy and drug-rebound headache. *American Family Physician* 56(8):2039–2048.

Newman L.C., and Lipton, R.B. 1998. Emergency department evaluation of headache. *Neurologic Emergencies* 16(2): 285–303.

Noble, S.L., and Moore, K.L. 1997. Drug treatment of migraine: Part II. Preventive therapy. *American Family Physician* 56(9):2279–2286.

Pruitt, A.A. 1995. Approach to the patient with headache. In *Primary care medicine,* eds. A.H. Goroll, L.A. May, and A.G. Mulley, Jr., 3rd ed., pp. 821–829. Philadelphia: J.B. Lippincott.

Raskin, N.H., and Peroutka, S.J. 2001. Headache including migraine and cluster headache. In *Harrison's principles of internal medicine,* eds. E. Braunwald, A.S. Fauci, D.L. Kasper et al., 15th ed., pp. 68–72. New York: McGraw-Hill.

Silberstein, S.D., and Lipton, R.B. 1996. Headache epidemiology: emphasis on migraine. *Neurologic Clinics* 14(2): 421–434.

Silberstein, S.D., Lipton, R.B., and Dalessio, D.J. 2001a. Overview, diagnosis and classification of headache. In *Wolff's headache and other head pain*, eds. S.D. Silberstein, R.B. Lipton, and D.J. Dalessio, 7th ed., pp. 6–26. New York: Oxford University Press.

Silbertstein, S.D., Saper, J.R., and Freitag, F.C. 2001b. Migraine: diagnosis and treatment. In *Wolff's headache and other head pain,* eds. S.D. Silberstein, R.B. Lipton, and D.J. Dalessio, 7th ed., pp. 121–237. New York: Oxford University Press.

Solomon, G.D., Cady, R.K., Klapper, J.A. et al. 1997. Standards of care for treating headache in primary care practice. National Headache Foundation. *Cleveland Clinic Journal of Medicine* 64:337–383.

Solomon, S.R., and Newman, L.C. 2001. Episodic tension-type headaches. In *Wolff's headache and other head pain,* eds. S.D. Silberstein, R.B. Lipton, and D.J. Dalessio, 7th ed., pp. 238–246. New York: Oxford University Press.

Stewart, W.F., Lipton, R.B., Chee, E. et al. 2000. Menstrual cycle and headache in a population sample of migraineurs. *Neurology* 55:1517–1523.

Weiss, J. 1999. Assessing and managing the patient with headaches. *Nurse Practitioner* 24(7):18–35.

Young, W.B., Silberstein, S.D., and Dayno, J.M. 1997. Migraine treatment. *Seminars in Neurology* 17(4):325–333.

Robin Taylor, R.N., M.S.N., F.N.P.
Jacqueline Wish Gilbert, R.N., M.S., C.F.N.P.

9-E
Seizures

Seizures are episodic, paroxysmal, involuntary alterations of behavior, movement, or sensation occurring when an abnormally active group of central nervous system (CNS) neurons discharge in an excessive and hypersynchronous pattern. Seizures can cause generalized convulsive activity; motor, sensory, autonomic, or psychic manifestations; or indiscernible experiential phenomena. It is important to distinguish seizures from *epilepsy*, a chronic condition of recurrent, unprovoked seizures caused by an underlying CNS disorder (Fauci et al. 2000, Valente 2000).

Approximately one in 11 people will have at least one seizure during their lifetime, most often in early childhood or late adulthood, but only one in 100 people will have epilepsy (Valente 2000). Any normal brain can be susceptible to seizure activity given the appropriate circumstances, and there are individual differences in susceptibility to seizures.

Seizures (also termed *ictal events*) are classified according to the focus of onset, clinical manifestations, and electroencephalographic (EEG) changes. There are two major categories: *partial (focal) seizures* and *generalized seizures*. Accurate seizure classification is essential for correct diagnostic and treatment decision-making. Seizure classification cannot always be made based on history or clinical observation. Scalp or intracranial EEG during seizure activity is sometimes necessary for accurate diagnosis (Fauci et al. 2000).

Partial seizures are restricted to discrete areas of the cerebral cortex and cause motor, sensory, autonomic, or psychic manifestations. Partial seizures can be *simple* (without impairment of consciousness) or *complex* (with impairment of consciousness). Partial seizures can spread throughout the cerebral cortex and become secondary generalized seizures. Complex partial and secondarily generalized seizures are often immediately preceded by a stereotypical simple partial seizure, also called a warning or an aura (Fauci et al. 2000). Complex partial seizures are typically followed by several seconds to hours of confusion, somnolence, or other impairment of consciousness. Complex partial seizures are the most common seizure type in adults (Schachter 1997).

Generalized seizures arise from both cerebral hemispheres simultaneously in a symmetric fashion. Primary generalized seizures are bilateral, clinical, and electrographic events without any detectable focal onset. *Absence seizures (petit mal)* cause brief lapses of consciousness and subtle, bilateral motor signs (such as rapid blinking) without loss of postural control. Absence seizures typically begin in childhood (Fauci et al. 2000). *Generalized tonic-clonic seizures (grand mal)* often begin without warning, though patients sometimes experience a prodrome, or symptom such as headache, for 1–2 days before the seizure (Schachter 1997). Generalized tonic-clonic seizures begin with a sudden generalized onset of rigid tonic muscle tone, impaired respirations, cyanosis, increased heart rate, blood pressure, and pupillary size. Generalized tonic-clonic seizures have a tonic phase and then a clonic phase of generalized jerking movements of the extremities. Each phase usually lasts less than one minute. Tonic-clonic seizures are typically followed by muscle flaccidity, increased salivation, stridor, incontinence, confusion, somnolence, or other impairment of consciousness lasting up to several hours. *Atonic seizures* are characterized by sudden, brief loss of postural tone, usually without post-ictal confusion. *Myoclonic seizures* are sudden, brief muscle contractions involving part or all of the body (Fauci et al. 2000).

Identifiable causes of seizures include congenital malformations, head trauma, brain tumors, CNS infection, alcohol or drug use, cerebrovascular disease (including ischemia), birth trauma, hypoxia, metabolic disorders, fever in infants or young children, or other damage to the brain. Partial seizures are often associated with structural brain abnormalities. Generalized seizures can result from cellular, biochemical, or more widespread structural abnormalities. However, in approximately 50% of individuals who develop seizures, there are no specific structural or biochemical abnormalities and, therefore, the cause is considered idiopathic. A genetic predisposition is found in individuals with idiopathic epilepsy. Up to half of all cases of epilepsy are refractory to treatment with anticonvulsant medications (Fauci et al. 2000, Valente 2000, Yoon 2000).

DATABASE

SUBJECTIVE

→ Patient may have history of:
- Symptoms of any kind of seizure activity, including:
  - Sudden loss of consciousness accompanied by staring and blinking; immediate regaining of consciousness
  - Period of confusion or amnesia
  - Brief jerks in arms or legs
  - Sudden loss of muscle tone causing an unbroken fall
  - Initial cry, respiratory arrest, cyanosis, tonic-clonic convulsions, relaxation followed by deep sleep
  - Incontinence
  - Presence of aura before seizure
- Alcohol use
- Drug use
- Electrolyte or metabolic disorders
- Acute infection
- Sleep deprivation
- Closed head trauma (seizures my develop within a two-year period)
- Open head trauma (seizures may develop at any time after injury)
- Cardiac arrhythmias
- Mitral or aortic valve disease
- Vascular malformation
- Tumor or stroke

→ Patient may have a family history of seizures or a personal history of febrile seizures.

OBJECTIVE

→ Assess vital signs, including postural changes in blood pressure and pulse.
→ Perform a complete neurological examination:
- Focal findings that localize CNS disease
- Mental status
- Motor function
- Cranial nerves
- Coordination

→ Assess for:
- Head trauma
- Papilledema
- Carotid disease
- Acute infection or systemic illness
- Cardiac dysrhythmias or valvular problems
- Manifestations of alcohol or drug use
- Manifestations of diabetes
- Chronic liver or renal disease
- Organomegaly (metabolic storage diseases)
- Limb asymmetry (early brain injury)
- Hyper- or hypothyroidism
- Neurocutaneous syndromes

ASSESSMENT

→ R/O disorders that mimic seizures:
- Syncopal attacks:
  - Vasovagal syndrome
  - Cardiac arrhythmias
  - Valvular heart disease
  - Heart failure
  - Hypotension
- Transient ischemic attacks
- Migraine
- Nerve compression
- Hyperventilation
- Metabolic disturbances:
  - Alcohol toxicity
  - Delirium tremens
  - Hypoglycemia
- Psychological disorders:
  - Acute psychosis
  - Panic attacks
  - Psychogenic seizures
  - Sleep disorders
- Movement disorders

→ R/O infection
→ R/O tumor
→ R/O trauma
→ R/O cerebral vascular accident
→ R/O drug overdose
→ R/O diabetic ketoacidosis
→ R/O nonketotic hyperosmolar hyperglycemia

PLAN

DIAGNOSTIC TESTS

→ Routine blood tests including CBC, electrolytes, glucose, calcium, magnesium, kidney and liver functions, oxygen saturation, VDRL or RPR, and urinalysis are indicated.
→ EEG is indicated. Only positive recordings are useful. A negative EEG does not exclude seizure or epilepsy (Valente 2000).
→ Toxicology screen of blood and urine is recommended if drug/alcohol use is suspected.
→ Neuroimaging studies, preferably head MRI, are indicated to assess for cortical dysplasias, infarcts and tumors if acute brain injury, new seizures, or a significant change in the pattern of seizures (Schachter 1997).
→ Lumbar puncture is indicated if there is any suspicion of encephalitis, meningitis, cerebrospinal fluid infiltration of tumor, or CNS syphilis, and in patients with HIV.

TREATMENT/MANAGEMENT

→ Therapy for seizure disorders focuses on complete seizure control with a minimum of adverse effects (Schachter 1997).
- This approach is initiated after any underlying cause of seizures has been ruled out or treated (e.g., brain tumor or encephalitis).
- Treatment is usually not recommended after a single seizure, unless a known cause is identified that cannot be reversed (Fauci et al. 2000).

- More than 18 anticonvulsant drugs (AEDs) are available in the United States for treatment of epilepsy.
- Accurate diagnosis of the type of seizure, once established, will determine the choice of AEDs.
- Most AEDs have similar cognitive side effects, including sedation, ataxia, and diplopia. Serious, idiosyncratic adverse effects such as liver toxicity, rash, and bone marrow suppression can occur. Baseline CBC and liver function tests should be done prior to AED initiation (Fauci et al. 2000).
- See **Table 9E.1, Commonly Used Antiepileptic Drugs.**
- In choosing AEDs, consider that:
  - AEDs should be titrated gradually until seizures are controlled or unacceptable side effects develop.
  - "Maximum tolerated dose" of one AED (monotherapy) is the goal of AED therapy. Monotherapy at maximum tolerated dose should be maintained until seizures recur or toxicity develops.
  - Rarely is there a "best" drug for a seizure type.
  - A given patient may not tolerate a particular drug.
  - A combination of two AEDs may be necessary if one AED at maximum tolerated dose does not provide optimal control. Up to 30% of patients with seizures may require more than one AED (Schachter 1997).
- → Factors involved in choosing AEDs:
  - Age:
    - Chronic effects in young adults make some choices less desirable.
  - Gender:
    - Some AEDs may lessen the effectiveness (by increasing the clearance) of low-dose oral contraceptives. Some AEDs present potential teratogenic risks during pregnancy and lactation (Schachter 1997).
  - Compliance:
    - Tailor to the patient's needs and schedule.
  - Cost:
    - Some AEDs are not covered by third-party payers. AEDs approved within the last 10 years are significantly more expensive than earlier AEDs.
- → Seizures are best controlled when the serum level of the AED is constant. AEDs with a long half-life can be taken once a day, whereas AEDs with a short half-life should be taken more frequently.
- → Routine serum AED levels are not indicated. AED levels should be checked if toxicity or noncompliance is suspected, or if seizures recur for unknown reasons.
- → Serum levels can be helpful to establish a baseline for therapeutic level and to detect noncompliance or other causes of lowered serum drug levels, should seizures recur. The therapeutic range of serum drug levels is only a guide during titration and ongoing treatment. Some patients require levels above the normal range for seizure control without adverse drug reaction, whereas others achieve seizure control or develop toxicity at doses below the therapeutic range (Valente 2000).

- The serum drug level should be checked during the steady state.
- → Discontinuation of drug therapy may be considered for individuals who are seizure-free for two years.
  - This must be done gradually over several months, with close monitoring.

CONSULTATION

- → Medical and neurological consultation is recommended, particularly during the initial evaluation and development of a treatment plan. If seizures continue to occur after three months, care should be assumed by an epileptologist. When the client is stable, primary management can be resumed.
- → As needed for prescription(s)

PATIENT EDUCATION

- → Explain possible restrictions that may be placed on the patient's lifestyle (e.g., driving).
  - Laws vary from state to state, but generally a person must be seizure-free for one year before she may reapply for a driver's license.
- → Educate regarding seizure disorders and possible societal stigmas. Allay fears and maintain dialogue regarding patient concerns.
- → Recommend that the patient carry a medical information card and/or wear a medical alert bracelet or necklace.
- → Explain signals that may indicate when a seizure may occur (e.g., headache, malaise, or some other vague symptom).
- → Stress the importance of taking medications.
- → Recommend that the patient keep a calendar of seizures, including date and time of seizure, triggers, symptoms, change in other medications, lifestyle or diet, and missed AED doses (Schachter 1997).
- → Educate family members and patient about the signs and symptoms of AED toxicity:
  - Anorexia
  - Visual symptoms (double vision)
  - Numbness of extremities
  - Dizziness
  - Behavioral problems
  - Fever
  - Drowsiness
  - Rash
  - Ataxia
  - Irritability
  - Gastric distress
- → Monitor and advise regarding AED levels as needed.
- → Educate family members about emergency measures to take during a seizure:
  - Protect head
  - Place person on bed or floor
  - Avoid objects in the mouth
  - Do not forcibly restrain
  - Remove eyeglasses and loosen clothing around head and neck

Table 9E.1.   COMMONLY USED ANTIEPILEPTIC DRUGS

Generic Name	Trade Name	Principal Uses	Typical Dosage and Dosing Intervals	Half-Life	Therapeutic Range	Adverse Effects		Drug Interactions
						Neurologic	Systemic	
Phenytoin (diphenylhydantoin)	Dilantin®	Tonic-clonic (grand mal) Focal onset	300–400 mg/day (3–6 mg/kg, adult; 4–8 mg/kg, child) QD–BID	24 hours (wide variation, dose dependent)	10–20 µg/mL	Dizziness Diplopia Ataxia Incoordination Confusion	Gum hyperplasia Lymphadenopathy Hirsutism Osteomalacia Facial coarsening Skin rash	Level increased by isoniazid, sulfonamides. Level decreased by enzyme-inducing drugs. Altered folate metabolism
Carbamazepine	Tegretol® Carbatrol®	Tonic-clonic Focal onset	600–1,800 mg/day (15–35 mg/kg, child) BID–QID	10–17 hours	6–12 µg/mL	Ataxia Dizziness Diplopia Vertigo	Aplastic anemia Leukopenia Gastrointestinal irritation Hepatotoxicity Hyponatremia	Level decreased by enzyme-inducing drugs. Level increased by erythro-mycin, propoxyphene, isoniazid, cimetidine
Valproic acid	Depakene® Depakote®	Tonic-clonic Absence Atypical absence Myoclonic Focal onset	750–2,000 mg/day (20–60 mg/kg) BID–QD	15 hours	50–150 µg/mL	Ataxia Sedation Tremor	Hepatotoxicity Thrombocytopenia Gastrointestinal irritation Weight gain Transient alopecia Hyperammonemia	Level decreased by enzyme-inducing drugs*
Lamotrigine	Lamictal®	Focal onset Tonic-clonic Atypical absence Myoclonic Lennox-Gastaut syndrome	150–500 mg/day BID	25 hours 14 hours (with enzyme-inducers) 59 hours (with valproic acid)	Not established	Dizziness Diplopia Sedation Ataxia Headache	Skin rash Stevens-Johnson syndrome	Level decreased by enzyme-inducing drugs* Level increased by valproic acid
Ethosuximide	Zarontin®	Absence (petit mal)	750–1,250 mg/day (20–40 mg/kg) QD–BID	60 hours, adult 30 hours, child	40–100 µg/mL	Ataxia Lethargy Headache	Gastrointestinal irritation Skin rash Bone marrow suppression	
Gabapentin	Neurontin®	Focal onset	900–2,400 mg/day TID–QID	5–9 hours	Not established	Sedation Dizziness Ataxia Fatigue	Gastrointestinal irritation	No known significant interaction
Topiramate	Topamax®	Focal onset Tonic-clonic	400 mg/day BID	20–30 hours	Not established	Psychomotor slowing Sedation Speech or language problems Fatigue Paresthesias	Renal stones (avoid use with other carbonic anhydrase inhibitors)	Level decreased by enzyme-inducing drugs

(continued next page)

Drug	Brand	Seizure Type	Dose	Half-Life	Therapeutic Level	CNS Side Effects	Other Side Effects	Drug Interactions
Tiagabine	Gabitril®	Focal onset Tonic-clonic Lennox-Gastaut syndrome	32–56 mg/day BID–QID	7–9 hours	Not established	Confusion Sedation Depression Dizziness Speech or language problems Paresthesias Psychosis	Gastrointestinal irritation	Level decreased by enzyme-inducing drugs*
Phenobarbital	Luminol®	Tonic-clonic Focal onset	60–180 mg/day (1–4 mg/kg, adult; (3–6 mg/kg, child) QD	90 hours (70 hours in children)	10–40 µg/mL	Sedation Ataxia Confusion Dizziness Decreased libido Depression	Skin rash	Level increased by valproic acid, phenytoin Enhances metabolism of other drugs via liver enzyme induction
Primidone	Mysoline®	Tonic-clonic Focal onset	750–1,000 mg/day (10–25 mg/kg) BID–TID	Primidone, 8–15 hours Phenobarbital, 90 hours	Primidone, 4–12 µg/mL Phenobarbital, 10–40 µg/mL	Same as phenobarbital		
Clonazepam	Klonopin®	Absence Atypical absence Myoclonic	1–12 mg/day (0.1–0.2 mg/kg) QD–TID	24–48 hours	10–70 ng/mL	Ataxia Sedation Lethargy	Anorexia	Level decreased by enzyme-inducing drugs*
Felbamate	Felbatol®	Focal onset Lennox-Gastaut syndrome	2,400–3,600 mg/day, (45 mg/kg, child) TID–QID	16–22 hours	Not established	Insomnia Dizziness Sedation Headache	Aplastic anemia Hepatic failure Weight loss Gastrointestinal irritation	Increases phenytoin, valproic acid, active carbamazepine metabolite
Levetiracetam	Keppra®	Focal onset	1,000–3,000 mg/day BID	6–8 hours	Not established	Sedation Fatigue Incoordination Psychosis	Anemia Leukocytopenia	None known
Zonisamide	Zonegran®	Focal onset	200–800 mg/day	50–68 hours	Not established	Sedation Dizziness Confusion Headache	Anorexia Renal stones	Level decreased by enzyme-inducing drugs*
Oxcarbazepine	Trileptal®	Focal onset	900–2,400 mg/day BID	10–17 hours (for active metabolite)	6–12 µg/mL	Fatigue Ataxia Dizziness Diplopia Vertigo Headache	See carbamazepine	Level decreased by enzyme-inducing drugs* May increase phenytoin

*Phenytoin, carbamazepine, phenobarbital

Source: Adapted with permission from Fauci. A., Braunwald, E., Isselbacher, K. et al. 2000. Seizures and epilepsy. In *Harrison's principles and practices of internal medicine,* 14th ed., pp. 360–369, 2354–2369. New York: McGraw-Hill.

- Make the immediate environment as safe as possible.
→ Educate family members about measures to take after the seizure:
  - Turn the person on her side to allow saliva or vomitus to drain.
  - Allow person to rest undisturbed.
  - Call for help if an injury occurs, apnea does not spontaneously resolve, or if loss of consciousness persists.
→ Recommend that the patient abstain from drugs and alcohol and avoid certain stimulants, such as coffee and tobacco.
→ Stress the importance of adequate and regular meals.
→ Stress the importance of adequate rest with regular sleep schedule.
→ Encourage regular exercise.
→ Advise that the patient avoid dangerous sports (e.g., swimming alone, scuba diving, mountain climbing, hang gliding, or snow sports) where a momentary loss of consciousness could be fatal.
→ Advise that the patient avoid jobs involving potentially dangerous work, such as operating heavy machinery or working underground or underwater.
→ Advise genetic counseling when one or both partners have epilepsy and desire children.
→ Advise women of childbearing age of the slightly higher risk of maternal complications during pregnancy and delivery. Also advise that some AEDs can increase the risk of fetal abnormalities.
→ Inform the patient about the availability of additional information from the following organizations:

  - Epilepsy Foundation of America
    4351 Garden City Drive
    Landover, Md. 20781

(800) EFA-1000
www.efa.org

- American Epilepsy Society
  342 North Main St.
  West Hartford, Conn. 06117
  (860) 586-7505
  www.aesnet.org

FOLLOW-UP

→ Evaluate the stability of the patient's status based on the number and frequency of seizures.
→ Monitor serum drug levels as needed.
→ Follow up more frequently if drug levels and symptoms are poorly controlled.
→ Refer as indicated under "Consultation," above.
→ Note seizure disorder on problem list and treatment regimen in progress notes.

BIBLIOGRAPHY

Fauci, A., Braunwald, E., Isselbacher, K. et al., eds. 2000. Seizures and epilepsy. In *Harrison's principles and practices of internal medicine,* 14th ed., pp. 2354–2369. New York: McGraw-Hill.

Schachter, S.C. 1997. Management of epilepsy: pharmacologic therapy and quality-of-life issues. *Postgraduate Medicine* 101(2):133–153.

Valente, L. 2000. Seizures and epilepsy: optimizing patient management. *Clinician Reviews* 10:(3):79–104.

Yoon, Y. 2000. New antiepileptic drugs and preparations. *Emergency Medicine Clinics of North America* 18(4):755–765.

Laura Hutkins, R.N., M.S., F.N.P., C.S.
Wendy L. Berk, C.A.N.P.

9-F
Temporomandibular Disorder

Temporomandibular disorder (TMD), formerly known as temporomandibular joint (TMJ) syndrome, is a common problem encountered in primary care. It involves one or both temporal-mandibular joints and their poorly understood structures of nerves, muscles, cartilage, fluid, and bone. The disorder is characterized by mild to severe pain with jaw movement, and/or limited range of motion of the jaw. Most cases are mild and self-limited and resolve with minimal medical intervention. The nurse practitioner can do a lot to reassure affected patients and teach them self-care to facilitate healing and prevent reoccurrence. A small minority of patients needs further treatment. An even smaller subset develops chronic TMD. For reasons that are unclear, the majority of patients who seek treatment for TMD are women age 15–40.

The TMJ is a complex synovial joint located between the temporal and mandibular bones. It is surrounded by a highly innervated fibrous capsule. Separating the joint into upper and lower compartments is the disc, which is a fibrous structure. The purpose of the disc is to cushion and stabilize the joint as it moves. The posterior attachment of the disc to the fossa (the retrodiscal tissue) is well vascularized and innervated, and it can be the location of pain when there is TMJ dysfunction.

Two movements are characteristic of the TMJ. When the jaw opens, a rotational movement is followed by a gliding translation. The disc and the condyle normally move together with the disc facilitating the movement, acting similar to a cushion. Dysfunction and pain can occur when the condyle and disc do not coordinate and the disc becomes an impediment to the motion. This may result in a clicking sensation or noise within the joint. Sometimes patients may experience jaw locking in the closed position (closed lock) due to a displaced disc and/or muscle trismus. The jaw can also become locked in an open position (open lock) when the condyle gets stuck in front of the disc or beyond the articular eminence.

Subluxation, degenerative joint changes, and connective tissue disease such as rheumatoid arthritis, osteoarthritis, psoriatic arthritis, or gout can also affect the TMJ. The jaw joint is very adaptable, however, and many people function well with significant structural abnormalities, even when the disc is displaced.

Muscular pain is the major symptom of TMD. The major muscles that cause movement of the TMJ are the temporalis, masseters, and medial pterygoids for closing the jaw and the lateral pterygoids and digastrics for opening the jaw.

The cause and effect relationship between muscle pain and disc derangement or injury remains unclear. A displaced disc may cause muscle spasm and/or muscle spasm resulting in a pulled-forward displaced disc. Thus, pathology in either the TMJ or the muscles of mastication may lead to secondary changes in the other structure, which then results in further pain (National Institutes of Health [NIH] 1996).

There is no clear consensus about predisposing or risk factors for TMD, and there are no scientifically established anatomic risk factors for developing the condition (Goldstein 1999). However, nonfunctional movements of the mandible (parafunctions) are universally accepted as contributing to dysfunction in certain individuals. These parafunctions include bruxism (clenching and grinding), lip biting, nail chewing, and tongue thrusting.

Bruxism during sleep is common but may be unrecognized by patients unless they are asked to monitor themselves or a bed partner mentions it. It should be considered if the TMJ pain seems worse in the morning. Psychological stress or problems with occlusion may be etiological factors for bruxism. Severe bruxism can lead to TMJ muscle spasm as well as tooth loosening and enamel damage.

Dysfunction of the cervical area (e.g., poor posture, degenerative changes, muscle tightness, and active trigger points) can cause referred pain to the jaw and changes in occlusion. Ligament laxity has been postulated as a predisposing factor, but studies to date have been inconclusive.

Malocclusion was once thought to be a causative factor for TMD, but there is no evidence that orthodontic treatment decreases or increases the risk of developing TMD. Malocclusion may, however, aggravate an ongoing condition. Malocclusion may need to be addressed if conservative measures fail. Lack of posterior teeth can cause abnormal loading of the TMJ and contribute to pain and dysfunction.

Trauma is acknowledged as a contributor to TMD. Occasionally, TMD symptoms can begin after a dental appointment or other situation where the mouth is held open for a long time. Also, a history of family violence is not uncommon. It may be unclear if the physical violence initiated the symptoms or if the resulting stress is the major contributing factor.

Anxiety and depression have been associated with TMD. However, as with most chronic pain, it is difficult to differentiate between physical and psychological symptoms. The clinician needs to be alert for abuse of prescription pain medications and muscle relaxants in chronic pain patients. In addition, caffeine and stimulant abuse can increase muscle tension and worsen TMD symptoms.

Because TMD affects mainly young women, new onset of jaw pain in a patient over 50 years old should alert the clinician to other possible diagnoses. Reasonable diagnostic considerations in older patients include temporal arteritis, tumor, connective tissue disease, facial neuralgia, and angina.

The key to treating TMD is to support the patient through the current episode of pain and allow healing to occur by itself. Treatment should focus on relieving pain, reducing inflammation, and restoring function. For severely affected individuals, referral to a multidisciplinary team composed of specialists in dentistry, behavioral medicine, and physical therapy is recommended. In most settings, this option is not available and referrals are made to the specialty with the most experience managing TMD. There is no evidence that any particular treatment or specialty is associated with superior outcomes (Christensen 2001).

DATABASE

SUBJECTIVE

→ Temporomandibular disorder, in all instances, includes the following symptoms:
  - Pain with jaw movement
  - Pain with palpation
  - Limitation of jaw range of motion (ROM) if pain is minimal
→ Temporomandibular disorder also may present with these symptoms:
  - Joint noises
  - Jaw movement, limitation, or deflection
  - History of locking
  - Headache
  - Ear discomfort/eustachian tube dysfunction/tinnitus
→ Symptom history should include:
  - Side of pain
  - Quality of the pain (e.g., achy, burning, throbbing, sharp)
  - Pattern of pain (e.g., worse in the morning)
  - Duration of symptoms
  - Precipitating factors:
    • Trauma
    • Dental examination/nerve block

  - Recent surgery that may have included prolonged wide mouth opening during intubation for general anesthesia
  • Stress
- Specific pain triggers and exacerbators, including pain with:
  • Chewing
  • Opening mouth
  • Hot or cold foods
  • Talking
  • Exercise
  • Neck movement
- Other aggravating factors (e.g., stress, position, job, school, weather)
- Associated symptoms, including:
  • Neck pain
  • Ear symptoms, such as pain, plugging, tinnitus
  • Headache
  • Tooth pain
  • Sinus discomfort/drainage
  • Numbness
  • Weakness
  • Herpetic rash
- Jaw function, including:
  • Locking—open or closed
  • Joint noise
→ Medical history should include:
- Trauma, such as:
  • Motor vehicle accident
  • Surgery or dental work
  • Physical assault or injury
- Dental history, including:
  • Braces
  • Bridge work or dentures (a loose fit may contribute to bruxism)
  • Tooth extraction, root canal
  • Splint
  • Clenching/grinding
- Other medical problems, particularly:
  • Diabetes
  • Hypertension
  • Thyroid disorder
  • Sleep disorder
  • Psychiatric disorder such as depression/anxiety
  • Connective tissue disorder/joint laxity
  • Heart disease
  • Headaches
  • Arthritis
  • Vasculitis
→ Family history, including:
- Connective tissue disease
- Headache
→ Substance use, including:
- Alcohol
- Smoking
- Street drugs, particularly stimulants
- Caffeine

→ Medication use, including:
- Analgesics
- Decongestants
  - These act as stimulants and can cause poor sleep and bruxing
- Prescription medications

→ Social factors, including:
- Occupation, especially shift work (irregular circadian rhythms can exacerbate stress)
- Home life, especially stressors and faulty coping mechanisms
- Hobbies, especially sports that cause clenching or activities that cause poor posture

OBJECTIVE

→ Include portions of the physical examination appropriate to the symptoms:
- Blood pressure
- Skin:
  - Look for vesicular rash (herpes zoster)
- Facial symmetry
- Ears:
  - Gross hearing
  - Ear canal for swelling, redness, pain, or discharge
  - Tympanic membrane
- Throat:
  - Include tongue, palate, buccal mucosa
    - Linea alba on the buccal mucosa can indicate bruxism, as can a scalloped tongue.
  - Observe for mucosal lesions
- Salivary glands:
  - Note size, consistency, pain.
  - A ductal stone may be palpated or purulent drainage may be seen.
- Teeth:
  - Look for missing teeth, wear marks, state of repair, tooth pain with percussion or biting gauze (the latter may indicate fracture).
- Mandible abnormalities:
  - Malocclusion, mandible asymmetry, retrognathia, prognathia, mandible pain.
- TMJ:
  - Palpate for pain in both open and closed positions.
  - Note deviation of the jaw when opening and closing the mouth. Hypomobility of one TMJ will cause the mandible to deviate to that side in a "C" movement when opening.
  - Measure ROM. This can be done fairly accurately without specialized instruments using a tongue blade. Mark the points measured on the blade, then line up the points on a millimeter ruler to determine the measurement.
    - First, measure maximal interincisal opening by having the patient open as wide as possible. Rest the tongue blade between the central incisors of the maxilla and mandible.

- Next, ask the patient to protrude the mandible. Using the tongue blade, mark the distance from the maxillary incisors to the mandibular incisors.
- Lastly, measure the lateral excursion of the mandible by asking the patient to move the mandible as far as possible to one side and then the other, with the teeth just barely apart.
- Mark the tongue blade at the midline point, which is the point between the maxillary incisors, and at the most deviated mandibular point, which is between the mandibular incisors. Compare your measurements to normal, which are:
  - Maximal interincisal opening: 35–50 mm (minimal functional opening is about 20 mm)
  - Protrusion: 8–10 mm
  - Laterotrusion: 8–10 mm

- Assess for joint noises (with and without stethoscope):
  - Click/pop or crepitus. It is difficult to ascertain the exact cause of the click or pop on physical examination.
  - These noises can be caused by fossa/disc/condyle incoordination or structural bony and soft tissue irregularities.
  - Note the timing, coordination, and consistency in opening and closing. Early opening clicks and pops have a better prognosis than late opening noises.
  - Crepitus is often associated with degenerative conditions such as osteoarthritis. Joint noises in and of themselves are not indicative of pathology, as they are common in the general population.
- Test joint loading:
  - Have the patient bite down on a cotton roll or two tongue blades placed between the posterior teeth. Repeat on each side.
  - Pain on the opposite side is a positive test and can indicate joint pathology. Pain on the same side of forced biting indicates tension forces on the capsule and ligament (Palmer et al. 1998).
- Neck:
  - Posture
  - Pain with palpation and ROM
  - ROM
  - Radicular symptoms with movement
  - Thyroid
  - Carotid arteries (e.g., pain, swelling, bruits)
- Neurological:
  - Symmetry of facial muscles
  - Facial sensation
  - Symmetry of tongue
  - Symmetry of palate
  - Gag reflex
  - Other cranial nerves, as appropriate
- Muscle screening examination:
  - Masseters
  - Temporalis

- Suboccipitals
- Trapezius
- Sternocleidomastoid

ASSESSMENT

→ TMD
→ R/O temporal arteritis
→ R/O atypical facial pain
→ R/O trigeminal neuralgia
→ R/O inflammatory joint disease

PLAN

DIAGNOSTIC TESTS

→ Laboratory:
- Erythrocyte sedimentation rate (ESR) or C-reactive protein for patients over 50 years old (to rule out temporal arteritis, which has symptoms that can mimic TMD)
- Rheumatoid factor, antinuclear antibody (ANA), uric acid if appropriate for TMJ crepitation (which may suggest inflammatory joint disease)

→ Radiology:
- X-rays should be done if there is significant trauma or if significant joint pathology is suspected.
- Other imaging studies that may yield information but are rarely useful in treatment decisions include:
  - Panorex
    - If accessible, this is inexpensive and is very helpful in visualizing mandibular tumors, fractures, dental abnormalities, the maxillary sinuses, and, grossly, the TMJ. Plain TMJ films and mandible films are less informative.
  - TMJ tomograms
    - This is best for arthritic findings.
    - It also can visualize the position of the condyle in the fossa.
  - MRI
    - This is a very expensive test that provides the clearest picture of soft tissue such as the disc.
    - An MRI should only be used if surgery is contemplated, on the recommendation of the oral surgeon.

TREATMENT/MANAGEMENT

→ Non-TMD disorders—treat or refer appropriately
→ TMD and jaw-related disorders:
- Joint noises as isolated findings do not need further treatment or follow-up. Approximately 35% of people have a TMJ click without pain or dysfunction, suggesting that this may be a normal variation (Goldstein 1999).
- Treatment options for TMD pain are varied and should be based on physical findings and history. Most TMD is self-limited and will eventually resolve with or without treatment. Current treatment is not evidence-based nor is there any evidence that one treatment is preferable to another (NIH 1996). The goal of most treatment is to relieve pain and to facilitate healing. Treatment options include education in self-care, prescription medication, physical therapy, behavioral therapy, and dental splints.

- Education and self-care (See **Appendix 9F.1, Self-Help for Jaw Pain**):
  - Local applications of heat or cold
  - Massage
  - Acupressure
- Drug therapy:
  NOTE: Medication for TMD should be prescribed at regular intervals for a designated period of time rather than prn. As-needed dosing may provide brief periods of relief with more frequent pain cycles and predispose the patient to overuse or abuse the drug (Dimitroulis 1998).
  - Non-narcotic analgesics
  - Tricyclics can be useful both for pain and for bruxism if given at HS.
  - Muscle relaxants as appropriate, such as cyclobenzaprine, 10 mg p.o. at HS, or carisoprodol, 350 mg p.o. QID.
    NOTE: Advise patients that muscle relaxants can cause drowsiness and to avoid taking them with other central nervous system depressants. Also advise patients of their potential for addiction (Elder 1991). Cyclobenzaprine is similar to tricyclics and may cause similar side effects.
  - Nasal steroids if allergic rhinitis is present, as mouth breathing can cause the mandible to protrude slightly.
- Behavioral therapy can be useful to modify habitual nonfunctional jaw movements that may exacerbate TMJ muscle spasm:
  - Relaxation training
  - Biofeedback
  - Hypnosis
- Physical therapy can provide:
  - TMJ mobility improvement
  - Upper-cervical, soft-tissue techniques
  - Demonstration of proper posture
  - Exercise program to establish a physiologic rest position for the jaw
  - Modalities to reduce inflammation and spasm, such as ultrasound.
- Dental splints:
  - Clear acrylic or rubber devices that are fitted on the maxillary teeth or occasionally the mandibular teeth
  - May help prevent bruxing, decompress the TMJ joint, decrease muscle tension, and stabilize the joint.
  - Can be used for bruxers, myofacial pain, open locking, mild to moderate closed locking, and protection of inflamed joints.
  - Worn continuously except for eating. Night bruxers and patients with milder symptoms may wear them only while sleeping.
  - The cost to the patient, which may be considerable, must be considered before a referral is made to the dentist.
  - Over-the-counter splints such as athletic bite guards are not recommended for long-term use because they can

change occlusion over time. However, they sometimes can relieve pain in mild cases for limited periods of time.

→ Surgery is rarely indicated.
 ▪ Arthroscopy, including lysis and lavage techniques, has the potential to smooth or remove destroyed or damaged joint structures. Disk perforation and severely damaged disks cannot be repaired. At best, surgery creates a starting point for the body's own healing or adaptation (Lambert et al. 1997).
→ In very severe cases when all appropriate treatments have been attempted, chronic pain programs can teach patients how to live satisfactory lives with their pain.

CONSULTATION

→ Consult a physician when the patient does not exhibit typical symptoms and signs, and/or when the diagnosis is unclear.
→ Refer to an otolaryngologist patients over 60 years old with new onset of symptoms.
→ Refer to a neurologist patients with complaints of numbness, paresthesia, and motor dysfunction.
→ Refer to a mental health professional patients with a severe emotional component.
→ Refer to a rheumatologist patients with significant connective tissue disease.
→ Refer patients to the emergency room or to a dental consultant for prolonged open lock needing jaw manipulation.
→ Refer to a dentist for splint.
→ Refer to physical therapy for severe muscle spasm and/or limited ROM.
→ Refer to a maxillofacial surgeon for:
 ▪ Progressive closed lock without pain
 ▪ Major mandible deformities
 ▪ Patients who have already had TMJ surgery
 ▪ Continued pain and decreased functioning unrelieved by six months of splint therapy
 ▪ Jaw pain and progressively decreasing function with connective tissue disease

 ▪ Acute new closed lock that is not primarily myofascial. These patients are candidates for arthrocentesis.
→ As needed for prescription(s)

PATIENT EDUCATION

→ See **Appendix 9F.1.**

FOLLOW-UP

→ Mild cases can be followed easily in a primary care setting. For moderate to severe cases, a team approach is preferred.
→ Document in progress notes and on problem list.

BIBLIOGRAPHY

Christensen, D. 2001. Moving temporal mandibular joint research into the 21st century. *TMJ Science* 1(1):9–18.

Dimitroulis, G. 1998. Temporal mandibular disorders: a clinical update. *BMJ* 317:190–194.

Elder, N.C. 1991. Abuse of skeletal muscle relaxants. *American Family Physician* 44:1223–1226.

Goldstein, B.H. 1999. Temporomandibular disorders, a review of current understanding. *Oral Surgery, Oral Medicine, Oral Pathology* 88(4):379–385.

Lambert, G.M., Dykgraff, L.C., and Stegenga, B. 1997. Etiology and natural progression of articular temporomandibular disorders. *Oral Surgery, Oral Medicine, Oral Pathology* 83(1):72–76.

National Institutes of Health (NIH). 1996. Management of temporomandibular disorders. *NIH technological statement online 1996,* April 29–May 1. Available at: http://www.consensus.nih.gov/ta/018/018_statement.htm. Accessed on August 1, 2002.

Palmer, M.L., and Epler, M.E. 1998. Face and temporomandibular joint. *Fundamentals of musculoskeletal assessment techniques,* 2nd ed. Philadelphia: Lippincott Williams & Wilkins.

Stohler, C.S. 1997. Phenomenology, epidemiology, and natural progression of the muscular temporomandibular disorders. *Oral Surgery, Oral Medicine, Oral Pathology* 83(1):77–81.

APPENDIX 9F.1

Self-Help for Jaw Pain

1. Stick to a soft diet. Cut your food into small pieces. Do not eat chewy foods such as French bread, bagels, licorice, or tough meat. Avoid crunchy food such as nuts, raw vegetables, popcorn, and corn nuts. Limit thin foods such as tortillas or lettuce, which require grinding to chew. If you are experiencing a lot of pain, process foods in a blender.

2. Never chew gum or ice.

3. Avoid creating a suction force inside your mouth as when drinking with a straw, smoking, or sucking hard candy.

4. Stop habits such as biting your lower lip or nails or chewing on pens or pencils.

5. Avoid sticking out your tongue (e.g., licking ice cream cones).

6. Do not grind or clench your teeth. Try to keep your teeth apart with your tongue gently resting against the roof of your mouth as it does when you say the word "mine."

7. Resist the temptation to open your mouth wide when you yawn or eat thick sandwiches.

8. Maintain good posture. Protrusion of the jaw and neck will change the position of your bite. Avoid resting your jaw in your hand.

9. Sleep on your back or on your side if this doesn't cause pain. Stomach sleeping will put additional strain on the jaw and neck.

10. Shun all sources of caffeine, which increases muscle tension.

11. Do not cradle the phone between your jaw and shoulder or carry uneven loads, such as heavy purses.

12. Wear sunglasses to prevent squinting of the facial muscles.

13. Exercise regularly, especially by walking and swimming, to help reduce pain. Avoid exercise that causes clenching, such as weight lifting and scuba diving. Avoid jarring activities such as horseback riding.

14. Learn and practice relaxation techniques, which can lessen pain. Enroll in a stress management class.

15. Notice which activities worsen your symptoms.

16. Educate yourself about TMJ and other ways to manage your symptoms. Resources:
    → Web sites:
      - www.tmj.org
      - www.tmjoints.org

    → The following books contain helpful suggestions on self-care for TMJ:
      - Goddard, Greg. 1991. *TMJ, the jaw connection*. Aurora Press.
      - Taddey, John. 1990. *TMJ, the self-help program*. Surrey Park Press.
      - Uppgaard, Robert. 1998. *Taking control of TMJ*. New Harbinger Publications.

Source: Wendy L. Berk. Permission is granted to reproduce this appendix for patients as needed.

SECTION 10

Hematological/ Endocrine/ Immunological Disorders

10-A Anemia **10-2**
10-B Chronic Fatigue Syndrome **10-14**
10-C Osteoporosis **10-18**
10-D Systemic Lupus Erythematosus **10-25**
10-E Thyroid Disorders **10-33**
10–F Type 1 Diabetes Mellitus **10-40**
10–G Type 2 Diabetes Mellitus **10-51**

Ellen M. Scarr, R.N., C., M.S., F.N.P., W.H.N.P.
Michelle M. Marin, R.N., M.S., A.N.P.

10-A

Anemia

Anemia is defined as an inappropriately low hemoglobin (Hgb) or hematocrit (Hct) relative to an individual's oxygen supply and demand. The World Health Organization (WHO) laboratory definition of anemia, based upon a population mean in both developed and developing countries, includes adult male Hgb less than 13 g/dL, menstruating female Hgb less than 12 g/dL, and pregnant female Hgb less than 11 g/dL (Goroll 2000a). Hgb values vary with age, sex, altitude at time of sampling, and hydration status. Hgb and Hct are slightly lower in blacks, while Asians, Caucasians, and Native Americans have similar values (Groer 2001).

By WHO definition, one-third of the world's population is anemic, including 35% of all women and 51% of pregnant women, as well as 18% of males and 40% of children under the age of 12 (Dugdale 2001). Anemia is also common in the United States, affecting 9% of women between the ages of 15–44 and 5.5% of elderly women (Black 2000). The most common types of anemia in this country are iron-deficiency anemia, anemia of chronic disease, and thalassemia (Dugdale 2001).

Anemia is a sign of disease, not a separate disease entity itself. In most individuals, anemia occurs in the context of a variety of symptoms and signs reflecting the primary illness.

Correct identification of the underlying etiology is essential and treatment must be specific to the cause.

Anemia may be classified by cell morphology or pathogenesis. *Cell morphology* refers to cell size, as determined by the mean corpuscular volume (MCV). Anemias classified by morphology are designated microcytic, normocytic, and macrocytic (see **Table 10A.1, Classification of Common Anemias by Morphology**). Classification based on *pathogenesis* refers to the etiology of the anemia: 1) excessive red blood cell (RBC) loss or destruction, and 2) decreased RBC production (see **Table 10A.2, Classification of Common Anemias by Pathogenesis**). For common anemias, morphological classification is useful and will be used in this chapter.

Common Microcytic Anemias

Iron-deficiency anemia, the most common anemia worldwide, develops when the iron supply to the bone marrow falls short of that required for RBC production. As a result, Hgb synthesis is defective. Factors contributing to iron-deficiency anemia include increased requirements during infant and adolescent growth spurts, pregnancy, and lactation; inadequate dietary

---

Table 10A.1. CLASSIFICATION OF COMMON ANEMIAS BY MORPHOLOGY

Microcytic	Normocytic	Macrocytic
Anemia of chronic disease (may be normocytic)	Anemia of chronic disease	Megaloblastic anemia
Iron-deficiency anemia	Aplastic anemia	Folate deficiency
Sideroblastic anemia	Hemolytic anemia	Vitamin B_{12} deficiency
Thalassemias	Sickle cell disease	Pernicious anemia
Alpha (α) thalassemia		Nonmegaloblastic anemia
Beta (β) thalassemia		Chronic liver disease
		Drug induced

Sources: Compiled from Bonner, H., Bagg, A., and Cossman, J. 2001. The blood and lymphoid organs. In *Essential pathology*, 3rd ed., ed. E. Rubin. Philadelphia: Lippincott Williams & Wilkins; and Linker, C. 2002. Blood. In *Current medical diagnosis and treatment*, 41st ed., eds. L. Tierney, Jr., S. McPhee, and M. Papadakis. New York: Lange Medical Books/McGraw-Hill.

intake, notably among impoverished and elderly people, vegetarians, and alcoholics; decreased absorption due to chronic intestinal malabsorption, atrophic gastritis, or gastrectomy; or blood loss through menstruation, gastrointestinal bleeding, regular blood donation, or chronic hemoglobinuria (Linker 2002).

Iron-deficiency most often develops insidiously as requirements exceed the amount of stored or absorbed iron. Initially, iron stores are depleted without compromising erythropoiesis, as indicated by a decrease in serum ferritin, the body's main iron storage protein. As iron depletion continues, serum total iron binding capacity gradually rises, and serum iron levels and saturation fall (see **Table 10A.3, Laboratory Findings in Microcytic Anemia**).

Eventually, iron reserves become so depleted that the iron supply is inadequate for RBC production and iron-deficiency anemia develops. As anemia develops, the MCV gradually falls; the lower the MCV, the more severe the anemia. The RBCs become small (*microcytic*), pale (*hypochromic*), and progressively more distorted in shape (*poikilocytic*), correlating with the restricted hemoglobin production. Symptoms of iron-deficiency anemia usually do not occur until the Hgb is <10 mg/dL (Groer 2001). If inadequate iron intake and/or blood loss are gradual, the onset of iron-deficiency anemia typically is insidious. If precipitous blood loss accounts for the anemia, its onset is typically sudden. Iron-deficiency anemia responds to iron replacement, a factor that differentiates it from other microcytic anemias.

A second common cause of microcytic anemia is *thalassemia*. The thalassemias are a heterogeneous group of inherited anemias that occur most commonly in patients with Mediterranean, African, Middle Eastern, and Southeast Asian heritage (Mandell 1999). These autosomal dominant disorders result in defective synthesis of either the alpha (α) chains of normal hemoglobin (the α-*thalassemias*) or beta (β) chains of normal hemoglobin (the β-*thalassemias*). The severity of the anemia depends on the type of inherited thalassemia and the amount of abnormal hemoglobin production. All thalassemias result in varying degrees of microcytosis and hypochromia (Bonner et al. 2001) (see **Table 10A.3**).

In normal inheritance, each parent contributes a genetic code for the production of the various globin chains that comprise hemoglobin; the combination of these chains produces the different types of hemoglobin. Hemoglobin A, which makes up 98% of adult hemoglobin, is made of two α and two β chains. Hemoglobin A_2 is made of two α and two delta (δ) chains, and comprises 1–2% of adult hemoglobin. Hgb F, the major fetal hemoglobin that makes up less than 1% of normal adult hemoglobin, is made of two α chains and two gamma (γ) chains.

In the α-*thalassemias*, α chain synthesis is impaired, resulting in an excess production of β chains, which accumulate to form tetramers (known as hemoglobin Barts in infants and hemoglobin H in adults) (Buetler 1998). Normally, four genes code for the production of α globin chains. In the α-*thalassemias*, one or more of these genes are missing or defective. The severity of the anemia is determined by the number of missing or defective genes.

In the most severe form of α-thalassemia, α-*thalassemia major*, no genes for α globin chain synthesis are inherited. This causes a condition known as *hydrops fetalis*, which is incompatible with life. Infants die in utero (usually between 28–40 weeks gestation) or at birth (Dugdale 2001). The red blood cells contain only hemoglobin Barts (four gamma chains) and are incapable of delivering adequate amounts of oxygen to the tissues.

A second form of α-thalassemia is *hemoglobin H disease*, in which only one gene for α globin chain synthesis is inherited and three of the genes have been deleted or mutated. There is chronic hemolysis of varying severity, resulting in a microcytic,

---

Table 10A.2.   CLASSIFICATION OF COMMON ANEMIAS BY PATHOGENESIS

Decreased RBC Production	Increased RBC Destruction

Stem cell disorders:
    Aplastic anemia
    Myelodysplasia syndromes
    Paroxysmal nocturnal hemoglobinuria
Precursor cell disorders:
    Iron-deficiency anemia
    Megaloblastic anemias (e.g., pernicious anemia, vitamin
      B_{12} deficiency, folate deficiency)
    Thalassemias (alpha and beta)
Progenitor cell disorders:
    Anemia of chronic disease
    Chronic renal failure
    Pure RBC aplasia
	Intrinsic hemolysis:
	    Enzyme disorders (e.g., G_6PD deficiency, pyruvate kinase
	      deficiency)
	    Hemoglobinopathies (e.g., sickle cell disease)
	    Membrane defects (e.g., acanthocytosis, hereditary
	      spherocytosis, hereditary elliptocytosis)
	Extrinsic hemolysis:
	    Acute blood loss
	    Antibody-mediated destruction (e.g., drug-induced, erythroblastosis fetalis, warm and cold reacting antibodies)
	    Mechanical destruction (e.g., macroangiopathic
	      [artificial heart valve], microangiopathic [disseminated
	      intravascular coagulation, thrombotic thrombocytopenic
	      purpura], hypersplenism)

Sources: Compiled from Bonner, H., Bagg, A., and Cossman, J. 2001. The blood and lymphoid organs. In *Essential pathology*, 3rd ed., ed. E. Rubin. Philadelphia: Lippincott Williams & Wilkins; and Linker, C. 2002. Blood. In *Current medical diagnosis and treatment*, 41st ed., eds. L. Tierney, Jr., S. McPhee, and M. Papadakis. New York: Lange Medical Books/McGraw-Hill.

hypochromic anemia, and splenomegaly. Onset is usually noted during childhood or, if the disease is mild, it may not be noted until adulthood. Usually individuals with this disorder are hematologically stable except when hemolysis is increased by infection or exposure to oxidative drugs.

In α-thalassemia trait, two α globin chain genes are present, which usually allows for near normal erythropoiesis (Buetler 1998). These individuals are typically clinically stable,

may have a mild hemolytic anemia with mild microcytosis and hypochromia, and are asymptomatic or minimally symptomatic.

The silent carrier state results from the deletion of only one α globin gene. Probably the most common single gene defect in the world, the silent carrier state affects 30% of blacks (Dugdale 2001). There is essentially normal erythropoiesis, with an asymptomatic microcytosis and normal (or low-normal) Hgb.

Table 10A.3.   LABORATORY FINDINGS IN MICROCYTIC ANEMIA

	Iron Deficiency	Alpha Thalassemias			Beta Thalassemias	
		Hgb H Disease	Minor / Trait	Silent Carrier	Major	Minor
Hemoglobin	↓	↓ (6–10 g/dL)	N/↓ (12–15 g/dL)	N	↓	↓
Hematocrit	↓	↓ (22–32%)	↓ (28–40%)	N	↓ (<10%)	↓ (28–40%)
MCV	↓	↓ (60–70%)	↓ (60–80%)	N	↓	↓ (55–75%)
Ferritin	↓ (< 30 µg/L)	N	N		N	N
Iron	↓ (< 30 µg/dL)	N	N		N	N
Total Iron Binding Capacity	↑	N	N		N	N
Transferrin Saturation	↓ (< 15%)	N	N		N	N
Reticulocyte Count	↓	↑				N / slight ↑
Peripheral Smear	Microcytosis Hypochromia Anisocytosis* Poikilocytosis* Target cells*	Markedly abnormal: Microcytosis Hypochromia Poikilocytosis Target cells	Mildly abnormal: Microcytosis Hypochromia Poikilocytosis Target cells (rare) Acanthocytes		Bizarre: Microcytosis Hypochromia Poikilocytosis (severe) Target cells Basophilic stippling Nucleated RBCs	Mildly abnormal: Microcytosis Hypochromia Target cells
Hgb A		70–95%	85–95%	98–100%	↓↓↓ / —	
Hgb A₂		—	N	N	—	↑ (4–8%)
Hgb F		—	N	N	↑↑↑	↑ (1–5%)
Hgb H		5–30%	—	—		

↑ increased   ↓ decreased   — absent   N within normal range   * late finding

Sources: Compiled from Fischbach, F. 2000. *A manual of laboratory and diagnostic tests*, 6th ed. Philadelphia: Lippincott Williams & Wilkins; and Linker, C. 2002. Blood. In *Current medical diagnosis and treatment*, 41st ed., eds. L. Tierney, Jr., S. McPhee, and M. Papadakis. New York: Lange Medical Books/ McGraw-Hill.

The α-thalassemias are seen most commonly in persons from China and Southeast Asia, and less commonly in blacks. If at risk, women of childbearing age should be screened for the α-thalassemias to prevent the more serious forms of the disorder in the fetus.

In the β-thalassemias, gene mutations reduce the synthesis of β-globin chains. The excess α chains do not form tetramers as the β chains do in the α-thalassemias. Instead, these excess α chains attach to and damage the red cell membrane. Here, too, the severity of the β thalassemia varies with the type of mutation, of which there are many variants.

Patients who are homozygous for β thalassemia have *β-thalassemia major*, also known as *Cooley's anemia*. There is a marked reduction in or complete absence of β globin chain synthesis. Affected individuals, usually of Mediterranean descent (mostly Greek and Italian), and less commonly Asians and blacks, appear healthy until approximately six months of age, when Hgb F changes to Hgb A (Linker 2002). Severe microcytic, hypochromic anemia develops, as well as bony deformities, growth retardation, jaundice, and hepatosplenomegaly. Dependent on transfusion therapy, these patients previously died in their 20s from secondary iron overload, but the use of iron chelating agents to reduce this complication from transfusion has improved the prognosis for this disorder. In a milder form of homozygous β thalassemia, *β-thalassemia intermedia*, individuals can survive without regular transfusions except in times of bodily stress.

Patients who are heterozygous for β thalassemia develop *β-thalassemia minor*. With one abnormal β chain, these individuals have a lifelong, asymptomatic, mild anemia with marked microcytosis. Only during pregnancy may these individuals require supportive transfusions due to the iron deficiency associated with pregnancy compounding the inherited anemia.

Common Normocytic Anemias

Anemia of chronic disease (ACD) is the most common normocytic anemia and is second only to iron-deficiency anemia in worldwide prevalence of anemia due to any cause (Brill et al. 2000). ACD is the most common anemia in the elderly and should be suspected in any woman with a known chronic illness. ACD is associated with chronic infectious disorders (e.g., tuberculosis, human immunodeficiency virus [HIV]), chronic inflammatory disorders (e.g., rheumatoid arthritis, systemic lupus erythematosus), and malignancies. The anemia is multifactorial, the result of an inadequate amount of iron available to the developing erythroblast, a reduced RBC life span, an impaired bone marrow response to erythropoietin, and suppression of erythropoietin production by inflammatory cytokines such as tumor necrosis factor, interleukins and prostaglandins (Bonner et al. 2001). ACD is a moderate anemia that is usually normocytic, although it can be microcytic and hypochromic, making it difficult to differentiate from iron-deficiency anemia. However, in ACD, the iron stores are normal or increased, and the ferritin level is normal. (See **Table 10A.4, Laboratory Findings in Normocytic Anemia.**)

The *hemolytic anemias* are a group of disorders associated with defects in the RBC membrane, which lead to membrane

Table 10A.4.   LABORATORY FINDINGS IN NORMOCYTIC ANEMIA

	Anemia of Chronic Disease	Hemolytic Anemia
Hemoglobin	Slightly ↓ (9–11 mg/dL)	↓
Hematocrit	Slightly ↓ (30–40%)	↓
MCV	N/slightly ↓	N
Ferritin	N/↑	
Iron	↓	
Total Iron Binding Capacity	↓	
Transferrin Saturation	↓	
Reticulocyte Count	N	↑
Peripheral Smear	Nondiagnostic	
Other		↑ Indirect/total bilirubin ↑ LDH ↓ Haptoglobin + Urine hemosiderin

↑ increased   ↓ decreased   N within normal range

Sources: Compiled from Fischbach, F. 2000. *A manual of laboratory and diagnostic tests*, 6th ed. Philadelphia: Lippincott Williams & Wilkins; and Linker, C. 2002. Blood. In *Current medical diagnosis and treatment*, 41st ed., eds. L. Tierney, Jr., S. McPhee, and M. Papadakis. New York: Lange Medical Books/McGraw-Hill.

instability and a shorted RBC lifespan. With the reduction in RBCs, the bone marrow attempts to compensate by increasing RBC production and releasing immature RBCs (reticulocytes). Anemia develops when the bone marrow can no longer compensate for the hemolysis, due either to the bone marrow's impaired function or the red cells' extremely short survival. Once active bleeding is excluded, an increase in the number of reticulocytes (*reticulocytosis*) with a falling or stable hematocrit is suggestive of hemolysis (See **Table 10A.4.**)

There are many causes of hemolytic anemia, including intrinsic causes, which are usually inherited, and the more common extrinsic causes. Inherited intrinsic causes include G_6PD deficiency (common in southern Mediterraneans and people of African descent), hereditary spherocytosis, and hemoglobinopathies such as sickle cell disease (Brill et al. 2000). Extrinsic causes include autoimmune diseases, malignancy, mechanical causes (e.g., prosthetic heart valves), infections, liver disease, disseminated intravascular coagulation (DIC), and numerous drugs known to precipitate hemolysis (e.g., methyldopa, penicillins, erythromycin, cephalosporins, acetaminophen) (Bonner et al. 2001, Linker 2002).

Common Macrocytic Anemias

The macrocytic anemias are classified as *megaloblastic* or *nonmegaloblastic*. Megaloblastic anemias are disorders caused by impaired DNA synthesis and are characterized by the presence of macrocytes (MCV >100 fL), hypersegmented neutrophils (five or more lobes), and abnormal bone marrow (Snow 1999). (See **Table 10A.5, Laboratory Findings in Macrocytic Anemia.**)

Megaloblastic anemia is most commonly a result of either vitamin B_{12} or folate (folic acid) deficiency. Vitamin B_{12} is found in all food products of animal origin (e.g., meat and dairy) and is stored in the liver. Given body stores of vitamin B_{12} and the small amount of daily loss, even a diet devoid of all animal products would not result in vitamin B_{12} deficiency for 3–6 years (Babior et al. 1998). Thus, dietary vitamin B_{12} deficiency is extremely rare except in strict vegans.

The most common cause of vitamin B_{12} deficiency is *pernicious anemia*. In pernicious anemia, a defect in the gastric mucosa results in the deficient formation of intrinsic factor, a substance that binds ingested vitamin B_{12} and allows its absorption in the terminal ileum (Mandell 1999). This disease rarely manifests itself before age 35; onset is usually in patients over 60 years old. Pernicious anemia may be acquired (autoimmune) or congenital; it is most common in those of Scandinavian or northern European ancestry and occurs to a lesser degree in blacks, Asians, and Hispanics (Babior et al. 1998).

Other causes of vitamin B_{12} deficiency include malabsorption secondary to subtotal gastrectomy or terminal ileal resection, various ileal inflammatory and neoplastic disorders, blind loop syndrome (where there is an overgrowth of vitamin B_{12}-consuming microorganisms in a surgically devised blind loop of intestine), or the fish tapeworm *Diphyllobothrium latum*, which ingests vitamin B_{12} (Bonner et al. 2001).

Individuals with an inadequate intake of folate-rich foods are likely to develop *folate-deficiency anemia*. Folate deficiency as a result of poor diet is not common in the developed world; folate is present in most fruits and vegetables, as well as many foods that are fortified with folate. Usually, daily requirements

Table 10A.5. LABORATORY FINDINGS IN MACROCYTIC ANEMIA

	Vitamin B_{12} Deficiency/Pernicious Anemia	Folate Deficiency Anemia
Hemoglobin	↓	↓
Hematocrit	↓	↓
MCV	↑ (110–140fL)	↑ (110–140fL)
Folate	N	↓ (<150 ng/mL)
Vitamin B_{12}	↓ (usually <100 pg/mL)	N
Peripheral Smear	Markedly abnormal: Anisocytosis Poikilocytosis Macro-ovalocytes Hypersegmented neutrophils	
Other	May see pancytopenia with ↓ WBC count	

↑ increased   ↓ decreased   N within normal range

Sources: Compiled from Fischbach, F. 2000. *A manual of laboratory and diagnostic tests*, 6th ed. Philadelphia: Lippincott Williams & Wilkins; and Linker, C. 2002. Blood. In *Current medical diagnosis and treatment*, 41st ed., eds. L. Tierney, Jr., S. McPhee, and M. Papadakis. New York: Lange Medical Books/McGraw-Hill.

are easily met by diet, and body folate stores are adequate for about three months (Goroll 2000a). Individuals at risk for folate-deficiency include alcoholics, anorectics, and those who eat no fruits or vegetables.

Folate deficiency because of poor absorption is rare, as folate is absorbed throughout the intestinal tract. However, patients with intestinal mucosal abnormalities may not absorb folate adequately, or iron, which can exacerbate the anemia (Mandell 1999). In addition, individuals who have increased need for folate due to exfoliative skin diseases (e.g., psoriasis), pregnancy, chronic hemolysis, or drug therapy (either inhibitors of DNA synthesis or folate antagonists) may also require folate replacement.

Nonmegaloblastic anemias are also marked by macrocytosis but lack the other morphological characteristics of megaloblastic anemias and are found with disorders such as liver disease, alcoholism, and hypothyroidism, as well as with the use of antiretroviral medications (Linker 2002, Snow 1999).

DATABASE

SUBJECTIVE

→ Symptoms may include:
- General: fatigue, decreased exercise tolerance, insomnia
- Central nervous system: dizziness, postural faintness, headache, irritability
- Respiratory: shortness of breath, dyspnea on exertion
- Cardiovascular: palpitations, chest pain, claudication
- Gastrointestinal: anorexia, nausea
- Skin: pallor

→ Most anemias are of insidious onset, and symptoms may not develop until Hgb and Hct are ≤50% of normal (e.g., <7–8 mg/dL). Rapid onset of anemia may produce symptoms at lesser levels of anemia (Dugdale 2001).

→ Marked fatigue and decreased exercise tolerance may be the earliest symptoms.

→ Certain anemias may present with additional characteristic symptoms.
- Iron-deficiency: craving of non-nutritive substances (e.g., clay, starch, ice, dirt) (*pica*), glossitis, cheilosis, dysphagia (from esophageal webbing), brittle nails, bleeding (epistaxis, hemoptysis, hematemesis, menorrhagia, metrorrhagia, hematochezia, melena, hematuria)
- Anemia of chronic disease: symptoms associated with malignancy, liver disease, chronic infection, or inflammation (e.g., fever, weight loss, lymph node swelling, night sweats, jaundice)
- Hemolysis: jaundice, icterus, dark urine
- Vitamin B_{12} deficiency: glossitis, anorexia, diarrhea, peripheral nerve paresthesias, ataxia, vertigo, diminished vibratory and position sense, mental status changes
- Folate deficiency: similar to vitamin B_{12} deficiency except no neurologic abnormalities

→ History may reveal:
- Recurrent or lifelong anemia
- Past use of hematinics such as iron, folate, vitamin B_{12}
- Surgeries such as splenectomy, ileal resection, cardiac valve replacement, or gastrectomy

- Chronic disorders (e.g., heart disease, renal disease, gastritis)
- Chronic infections (e.g., tuberculosis, parasitic infestations)
- Inflammatory diseases (e.g., collagen vascular diseases)
- Malabsorptive disorders (e.g., ileitis, colitis)
- Autoimmune disorders (e.g., rheumatoid arthritis, systemic lupus erythematosus)
- Closely spaced pregnancies

→ Family history may reveal:
- Sickle cell disease
- Thalassemia
- G_6PD deficiency
- Pernicious anemia
- Splenectomy

→ Current medications may include:
- Nonsteroidal anti-inflammatory drugs (NSAIDs)
- Oral contraceptives
- Steroids
- Sulfa compounds
- Antimalarials
- Anticonvulsants
- Cancer chemotherapy
- Antiretroviral therapy
- Current use of hematinics such as iron, folate, vitamin B_{12}
- Vitamin supplements

→ Social history may include:
- Diet inadequate in iron or folate-rich foods
- Alcohol and recreational drug use
- Toxic exposures through occupation, home environment, or hobbies
- Travel
- Regular blood donation
- HIV risks

OBJECTIVE

→ Vital signs:
- Exam may reveal:
  - Recent weight loss
  - Orthostatic blood pressure changes
  - Increased pulse rate
  - Increased respiratory rate
  - Fever

→ Skin/nails:
- Exam may reveal:
  - Pallor
  - Petechiae
  - Telangiectasia or spider angiomas
  - Jaundice
  - Koilonychia
  - Brittle nails
  - Brittle hair

→ Mucous membranes:
- Exam may reveal:
  - Cheilosis
  - Stomatitis
  - Smooth tongue or glossitis

→ Lymph nodes:
- Exam may reveal:
  • Lymphadenopathy
→ Eyes:
- Fundoscopic exam may reveal:
  • Increased vessel tortuosity
  • Hemorrhage
  • Exudate
→ Cardiovascular:
- Exam may reveal:
  • Murmur
  • Increased point of maximal impulse (PMI)
  • Gallop
  • Bounding peripheral pulses
  • Widened pulse pressure
→ Respiratory:
- Exam may reveal:
  • Rales
  • Basilar dullness (effusions)
→ Abdomen:
- Exam may reveal:
  • Splenomegaly
  • Hepatomegaly
  • Liver tenderness
→ Central nervous system (CNS):
- Exam may reveal:
  • Decreased vibratory sense
  • Decreased position sense
  • Diminished fine motor skills
  • Abnormal reflexes (hypo- or hyperreflexia)
  • Impaired memory
  • Confusion
→ Extremities/skeletal:
- Exam may reveal:
  • Bone tenderness
  • Structural deformity (facial, cranial)
  • Pedal edema
→ Pelvic:
- Exam may reveal:
  • Abnormal bleeding (vaginal, cervical)
→ Rectal:
- Exam may reveal:
  • Dark or tarry stool
  • Bright red blood per rectum or on stool
  • Guaiac positive stool

ASSESSMENT

→ Anemia
- R/O microcytic anemia
- R/O normocytic anemia
- R/O macrocytic anemia

PLAN

DIAGNOSTIC TESTS

→ Based on the history and physical exam, consider screening target populations for anemia:

- CBC or Hct/Hgb for women with heavy menses
- CBC, Hgb electrophoresis with quantitative Hgb A_2 and F for those at risk for thalassemias or hemoglobinopathies
- G_6PD prior to beginning oxidant medications, such as antimalarials (primaquine or dapsone), in blacks or individuals of Mediterranean descent
- Stool guaiac: take three stool samples for individuals over the age of 40.

Initial Evaluation of Anemia

→ Decreased Hgb and Hct are indicative of anemia.
→ Assess the MCV to determine morphologic classification of the anemia, which will guide further diagnostic studies.
- Microcytic: MCV <80 fL
- Normocytic: MCV 80–100 fL
  • If both macrocytic and microcytic RBCs are present, an electronically calculated MCV may "average" them together, incorrectly identifying the cells as normocytic. An elevated red cell size distribution width (RDW) is a clue to this. If concomitant macro- and microcytosis is suspected, ask for manual peripheral smear evaluation.
- Macrocytic: MCV >100 fL
  • Nonmegaloblastic: MCV >100 fL, <115 fL
  • Megaloblastic: MCV >115 fL; macro-ovalocytes and hypersegmented neutrophils present
→ Depending on clinical picture, may repeat CBC to verify anemia.
→ Stool guaiac x 3 should be performed if not previously obtained.
- If stool guaiac is positive, identify source of bleeding with appropriate diagnostic testing and refer as indicated.

Evaluation of Microcytic Anemia

→ Based on patient history and physical examination, consider iron-deficiency anemia, the thalassemias, or anemia of chronic disease.
→ Obtain serum ferritin level.
- Best indication of decreased iron stores; helps differentiate between iron-deficiency anemia and anemia of chronic disease
- Serum iron, total iron-binding capacity (TIBC), transferrin saturation are often ordered with ferritin but add little additional information, as they lack its sensitivity and specificity. These tests should not be routinely ordered in the evaluation of microcytosis (Goroll 2000a).
- Ferritin level <30 is indicative of absent iron stores.
→ If ferritin level is normal or elevated, consider hemoglobin electrophoresis (depending on individual patient risk profile). Consider peripheral smear for RBC morphologic abnormalities.
- Diagnosis is determined by abnormal amounts of Hgb A, Hgb A_2, and/or Hgb F. Alpha thalassemia trait is a diagnosis of exclusion, as Hgb electrophoresis is normal.
- Microcytosis is more pronounced in thalassemia than in iron-deficiency anemia.

→ If hemoglobin electrophoresis is normal (or not appropriate to obtain), order iron, transferrin saturation, and TIBC.
- In anemia of chronic disease, serum iron and transferrin saturation are low.

→ Calculate Mentzer index (MCV/RBC) to help differentiate between thalassemia and iron deficiency.
- Mentzer >13 suggests iron deficiency anemia.
- Mentzer <13 suggests thalassemia.

Evaluation of Normocytic Anemia

→ Obtain reticulocyte count.
- The reticulocyte count differentiates bone marrow failure (and RBC underproduction) from RBC loss.
  - Normally expressed as a percent of the individual's RBC count, the reticulocyte count alone does not adequately mirror the degree of marrow compensation and must be adjusted to the level of anemia.
  - Correct for anemia by multiplying the reticulocyte count by the Hct and divide by 0.45.
- An elevated reticulocyte count is found with hemolysis or blood loss; work-up as appropriate.
  - For hemolysis, obtain bilirubin, haptoglobin, and lactate dehydrogenase (LDH); consider direct Coombs' test (for drug-related hemolysis), G_6PD in patients at risk (e.g., taking sulfonamides or antimalarials), hemoglobin electrophoresis for sickle cell disease.
  - For blood loss, diagnostic testing as indicated to determine bleeding source.
- A low normal or decreased reticulocyte count is found with metabolic diseases such as myxedema (obtain thyroid stimulating hormone [TSH]) and alcoholic liver disease (obtain liver function tests [LFTs]).
- A severely depressed reticulocyte count warrants bone marrow investigation for aplastic anemia, parvovirus infection, or sideroblastic disease.

Evaluation of Megaloblastic Anemia

→ Megaloblastic anemia:
- Obtain peripheral smear. The presence of hypersegmented polymorphonuclear lymphocytes (PMNs), with five or more lobes, is an early sign of megaloblastic anemia.
- Obtain vitamin B_{12} and folate levels.
  - Always obtain both values; vitamin B_{12} can be inaccurately low in folate deficiency.
- Vitamin B_{12} levels <100 pg/mL indicate vitamin B_{12} deficiency.
  - Order or refer for oral Schilling test to confirm diagnosis. Schilling test differentiates vitamin B_{12} deficiency due to malabsorption from pernicious anemia. Other diagnostic testing may include anti-intrinsic factor antibodies, serum gastrin levels, and endoscopy (in pernicious anemia).
→ Nonmegaloblastic anemia:
- Obtain reticulocyte count to assess bone marrow activity.

TREATMENT/MANAGEMENT

→ In the treatment of anemia, the empiric use of iron in the absence of iron deficiency is not useful and may actually be harmful to some patients (Little 1999).

Iron-Deficiency Anemia

→ Evaluate contributing factors.
- While menstrual blood loss is a common cause of iron-deficiency anemia in a woman of reproductive age, gastrointestinal blood loss should be investigated in any woman, old or young, with iron-deficiency anemia.
→ Document Hgb/Hct and ferritin level prior to therapy.
→ Begin ferrous iron replacement with a daily total of 150–200 mg of elemental iron (Little 1999).
- Simple ferrous salts are absorbed most efficiently. Absorption of ferrous sulfate, gluconate, and citrate is equivalent; agents differ in the amount of elemental iron that is available.
  - Ferrous sulfate 325 mg (65 mg elemental iron) 1 p.o. TID
    - Treatment of choice. Least expensive, most available elemental iron.
  - Ferrous gluconate 325 mg (36 mg elemental iron) 1 p.o. TID
  - For patients who have achlorhydria or have had a gastrectomy, liquid iron therapy may prevent iron malabsorption (ferrous sulfate elixir 220 mg/5 mL supplies 44 mg of elemental iron).

NOTE: Iron is absorbed best if taken on an empty stomach 1 hour before or 1–2 hours after meals or at bedtime. Foods, antacids, and sucralfate inhibit iron absorption (Goroll 2000b). Vitamin C improves absorption. Gastrointestinal side effects (nausea, vomiting) are common within 1 hour after ingestion; constipation, diarrhea, and abdominal cramping may also occur when iron is first started. To avoid these side effects, begin with a suboptimal dose and increase gradually or advise the patient to take iron just after meals. Taking with food can decrease side effects but will also decrease absorption by 40–66% (Little 1999). It may be necessary to switch to another preparation with less elemental iron to decrease gastrointestinal discomfort.

→ If moderate to severe anemia, a precipitous drop in Hgb, or in patients with evidence of organ dysfunction such as angina or heart failure (e.g., high-output heart failure), consider transfusion. Watch for volume overload, especially in patients with history of hypertension and/or cardiovascular disease.

→ In moderate to severe anemia, check reticulocyte count in 1 week.
- It increases within 5–10 days and will be directly proportional to the severity of the anemia.

→ When the anemia is not severe, assess the Hgb in 1 month. Hgb level increases halfway to normal within 3 weeks and should return to baseline by 2 months (Linker 2002). Ferritin level is a more accurate measure of the body's iron stores; when >50 µg/L, adequate iron replacement has occurred (Little 1999).

→ Continue therapy for 4–6 months after Hgb is normal to replace bone marrow iron stores (continue iron until serum ferritin level is >50 µg/L) (Little 1999).

■ Women with ongoing iron requirements (e.g., heavy menses) may benefit from maintenance therapy (ferrous sulfate 325 mg QD).

→ If the patient does not respond, consider: poor compliance, poor absorption (caffeinated beverages [especially tea], antacids, H_2 blockers, proton pump inhibitors, tetracyclines), concurrent infection, malignancy or inflammatory process, concurrent lead poisoning, thalassemia, vitamin B_{12} or folate deficiencies, wrong diagnosis (e.g., anemia of chronic disease), or continued bleeding that exceeds the rate of erythropoiesis.

→ If oral ferrous sulfate is ineffective, consider referral for intravenous iron dextran treatment. Avoid intramuscular use of iron because of inconsistent absorption and injection site problems (including the development of sarcomas) (Goroll 2000b, Little 1999).

Thalassemia Anemia

→ Document Hgb A, Hgb A_2, and Hgb F levels by Hgb electrophoresis. If concurrent iron-deficiency anemia is suspected or documented, iron stores may need to be replete before the Hgb A_2 levels will be elevated on electrophoresis.

→ Hgb A, Hgb A_2, and Hgb F levels will be normal in alpha thalassemia. Thus, this is a diagnosis of exclusion.

→ No treatment is required if patient is hematologically stable. Avoid inappropriate iron use.

■ For Hgb H disease, provide folate supplementation. Avoid iron and oxidative medications (e.g., sulfonamides).

■ For severe thalassemia, refer to hematologist for transfusion, iron chelation therapy, and possible splenectomy.

→ Patients with α and β thalassemia require genetic counseling.

Anemia of Chronic Disease

→ Diagnosis of exclusion—exclude associated deficiencies such as iron, folate, vitamin B_{12}.

→ Treat the underlying condition.

→ If the diagnosis is unclear despite an evaluation, consider a trial of iron therapy. If no hematological response occurs within 2 months, stop the iron therapy.

→ Erythropoietin therapy may be effective in some cases (e.g., chronic renal failure, malignancy, chronic inflammatory disorders). Therapy should be considered if patient is transfusion-dependent or symptoms improve with erythropoietin (e.g., quality of life is improved) (Linker 2002).

Hemolytic Anemia

→ Identify the etiology—inherited or extrinsic. Treatment depends on symptoms, rapidity of illness, and underlying etiology.

Vitamin B_{12} Deficiency Anemia

→ Vitamin B_{12} therapy is initiated with intramuscular cyanocobalamin (B_{12}) 100 µg every day for 1–2 weeks, then twice weekly for 1 month, then 100 µg monthly. Therapy is lifelong. Some providers decrease injections to every 3–4 months once replacement has been achieved (Goroll 2000b).

→ Parenteral vitamin B_{12} therapy has traditionally been preferred, although large doses of oral vitamin B_{12} (e.g., 1,000–2,000 µg daily) may provide adequate replacement. Even in the absence of intrinsic factor, 1–2% of oral vitamin B_{12} is absorbed (Little 1999, Smith 2000).

→ Intranasal cyanocobalamin gel is available and is an appropriate, albeit expensive, alternative for maintenance therapy (500 µg per week).

→ Response to treatment is often prompt. Reticulocyte count increases within 5–7 days. Hgb, Hct, and MCV normalize within 2 months.

→ Hypokalemia may occur as new RBCs take up potassium. Monitor potassium level in first week or two, particularly if anemia has been severe (Linker 2002). Potassium supplementation may be needed.

→ CNS symptoms and signs are reversible if they have been present for less than 6 months. Impairment of longer duration may take 12 months to clear. In some cases, neurologic deficits are permanent (Goroll 2000b, Little 1999).

→ Watch for increased incidence of atrophic gastritis, gastric cancer, autoimmune diseases (e.g., IgA deficiency, rheumatoid arthritis, Graves' disease), and iron deficiency in individuals with pernicious anemia.

→ There are no data to support the use of vitamin B_{12} injections (e.g., for complaints of fatigue) in the absence of documented deficiency; empiric B_{12} supplementation should be avoided.

Folate-Deficiency Anemia

→ Prior to beginning treatment, assess for vitamin B_{12} deficiency. Treatment with folate may temporarily alleviate clinical symptoms of vitamin B_{12} deficiency, allowing underlying asymptomatic neurologic injury to progress (Little 1999).

→ 1–2 mg folate p.o. QD for 4–5 weeks is usually adequate to replenish body stores. Patients with severe malabsorption may require parenteral therapy initially.

■ Assess the reticulocyte count 5–7 days after beginning folate therapy or reassess the Hgb/Hct levels several months after beginning treatment (they should normalize within 2 months).

■ If the underlying cause of the deficiency has not been reversed—as in patients with chronic liver disease, renal dialysis, or malabsorption—continue 1 mg folic acid a day indefinitely. Address alcohol abuse as needed. In patients with drug-induced folate deficiency, withdraw the offending drug if possible. If the drug needs to be continued (such as with oral contraceptives or dilantin), folate will usually reverse the anemia.

CONSULTATION

→ Consultation with a physician is indicated for:
- A transfusion
- Hospitalization
  - Severe anemia of unknown etiology (Hct <20–25%, Hgb >7 g/dL). Be particularly concerned about elderly patients or those with heart failure or angina pectoris.
  - Pancytopenia suggesting potential aplastic anemia
  - Rapidly developing anemia and active bleeding
  - Thrombotic microangiopathies (microangiopathic hemolysis with thrombocytopenia and extremely high LDH) may be life-threatening
- When the assessment, diagnosis, or treatment plan is in question
- As needed for prescription(s)

PATIENT EDUCATION

→ See the "Treatment/Management" section.
→ Discuss the underlying etiology of anemia and importance of participation in the treatment plan. Include family members in the management plan as necessary.
→ Discuss the importance of consistent follow-up.
→ Discuss medications: indications, regimens, and side effects.

Iron-Deficiency Anemia/ Folate-Deficiency Anemia

→ Discuss the importance of a nutritionally sound diet high in iron or folate. See **Appendix 10A.1, Patient Education Handout: Dietary Iron** and **Appendix 10A.2, Patient Education Handout: Dietary Folate**.
→ Refer to nutritionist as indicated. See also **General Nutrition Guidelines**, Section 16.
→ Iron replacement—advise patient that:
- Iron tablets may cause nausea, abdominal cramping, diarrhea. If unable to tolerate on an empty stomach, advise ingestion with a small amount of food (preferably foods high in vitamin C).
- Iron will cause black stools.
- Iron elixir may stain teeth.
  - Advise taking the drug through a straw and then rinsing mouth immediately afterwards.
- Iron may be hazardous to small children. Ensure proper storage.

Vitamin B₁₂ Deficiency

→ Advise the patient that lifelong treatment and regular follow-up visits every six months are necessary to ensure maintenance of hematopoiesis and early diagnosis of other diseases commonly associated with pernicious anemia.

FOLLOW-UP

→ See the "Treatment/Management" section for specific anemias.

→ Consider work-up for gastrointestinal blood loss with iron-deficiency anemia, particularly in postmenopausal women.
→ Referral for genetic counseling as indicated.
→ Referral to nutritionist as indicated.
→ Document in progress notes and on problem list.

BIBLIOGRAPHY

Babior, B., and Bunn, H. 1998. Megaloblastic anemias. In *Harrison's principles of internal medicine*, 14th ed., eds. A. Fauci, E. Braunwald, K. Isselbacher et al., pp. 653–659. New York: McGraw-Hill.

Black, S. 2000. Anemia. In *Primary care across the lifespan*, eds. D. Robinson, P. Kidd, and K. Rogers, pp. 61–68. St. Louis, Mo.: Mosby.

Bonner, H., Bagg, A., and Cossman, J. 2001. The blood and lymphoid organs. In *Essential pathology*, 3rd ed., ed. E. Rubin, pp. 551–594. Philadelphia: Lippincott Williams & Wilkins.

Brill, J., and Baumgardner, D. 2000. Normocytic anemia. *American Family Physician* 62(10):2255–2264.

Buetler, E. 1998. Disorders of hemoglobin. In *Harrison's principles of internal medicine*, 14th ed., eds. A. Fauci, E. Braunwald, K. Isselbacher et al., pp. 645–652. New York: McGraw-Hill.

Dugdale, M. 2001. Anemia. *Obstetrics and Gynecology Clinics of North America* 28(6):363–381.

Fischbach, F. 2000. *A manual of laboratory and diagnostic tests*, 6th ed. Philadelphia: Lippincott Williams & Wilkins.

Goroll, A. 2000a. Evaluation of anemia. In *Primary care medicine: office evaluation and management of the adult patient*, 4th ed., eds. A. Goroll and A. Mulley, pp. 509–518. Philadelphia: Lippincott Williams & Wilkins.

Goroll, A. 2000b. Management of common anemias. In *Primary care medicine: office evaluation and management of the adult patient*, 4th ed., eds. A. Goroll and A. Mulley, pp. 531–536. Philadelphia: Lippincott Williams & Wilkins.

Groer, M. 2001. Common hematologic disorders. In *Advanced pathophysiology: application to clinical practice*, ed. M. Groer, pp. 402–409. Philadelphia: Lippincott Williams & Wilkins.

Linker, C. 2002. Blood. In *Current medical diagnosis and treatment*, 41st ed., eds. L. Tierney, S. McPhee, and M. Papadakis, pp. 517–569. New York: McGraw-Hill/Appleton & Lange.

Little, D. 1999. Ambulatory management of common forms of anemia. *American Family Physician* 59(6):1598–1604.

Mandell, E. 1999. Anemias. In *Primary care: a collaborative practice*, eds. T. Buttaro, J. Trybulski, P. Bailey et al., pp. 922–940. St. Louis, Mo.: Mosby.

Smith, D. 2000. Anemia in the elderly. *American Family Physician* 62(7):1565–1572.

Snow, C. 1999. Laboratory diagnosis of vitamin B₁₂ and folate deficiency. *Archives of Internal Medicine* 159: 1289–1298.

APPENDIX 10A.1.

Patient Education Handout: Dietary Iron*

Iron is essential to the formation of hemoglobin (Hgb), which carries oxygen in the blood. When body iron stores are low, there are no physical symptoms. But as there is less iron to produce healthy red blood cells, iron-deficiency anemia develops. Symptoms of this anemia are weakness, pale skin, shortness of breath, and sometimes craving things that are not food, such as ice, clay, or soil.

→ Most balanced diets contain an adequate supply of iron except for patients in one of these groups:
- Menstruating women, especially if bleeding heavily. Blood loss increases the need for iron.
- Pregnant women, who have increased iron needs to support a growing fetus
- Dieters, who may not eat enough iron-containing foods
- Strict vegetarians, if adequate amounts of legumes, dried fruits, leafy greens, or enriched cereals are not eaten
- Endurance athletes, especially marathoners
- Infants and children growing rapidly

→ The type of iron found in meat and other animal products, called *heme* iron, is better absorbed by the body than the *nonheme* iron found in plant foods. Nonheme iron found in grains and vegetables is better absorbed when eaten at meals with foods high in vitamin C or with a small amount of heme-containing foods.

→ Individuals with iron-deficiency anemia should cook in iron pots and pans when possible. In such pots, the iron content of food can be increased from 2.4 times the amount for three-minute cooking time to 29 times the amount for a three-hour cooking time.

→ Minimum daily requirement for iron: 10–15 mg.

→ Minimum daily requirement for vitamin C: 60 mg.

Selected food items and their iron or vitamin C amounts are listed below to assist in meal planning.

mg	Iron Source	Quantity		mg	Vitamin C Source	Quantity
28.0	clams, cooked	3-½ oz.		85	Brussels sprouts	1 cup
12.4	bran flakes	1 cup		80	strawberries	1 cup
10.5	prune juice	1 cup		60	orange juice	½ cup
10.0	soybeans	1 cup		50	spinach, cooked	1 cup
7.5	rice bran	¼ cup		48	broccoli	1 cup
7.5	beef liver	3 oz.		45	cantaloupe	¼ cup
6.7	oysters	7–10 medium		43	cabbage	1 ½ cup
6.0	pinto beans	1 cup		40	cranberry juice	1 cup
5.4	scotch barley	1 cup		21	watercress	1 cup
4.0	spinach, cooked	1 cup		20	tomato juice	½ cup
4.0	black beans	1 cup		18	carrots, raw	3 large
4.0	croissant	1 whole		16	green beans, cooked	1 cup
4.0	almonds, whole	¾ cup		12	peaches, dried	5 halves
3.8	peaches, dried	5 halves				
3.7	pumpkin seeds	¾ cup				
3.2	blackstrap molasses	1 tbsp.				
3.1	roast beef	3 oz.				
3.0	chickpeas	1 cup				
2.3	tomato juice	1 cup				
2.0	raisins	½ cup				
2.1	butternut squash, baked	1 cup				
1.0	Brussels sprouts, steamed	8				

*This handout may be reproduced for patient use.

APPENDIX 10A.2.

Patient Education Handout: Dietary Folate*

Folate, or folic acid, is an important vitamin for tissue growth and red blood cell production. Most people get an adequate amount of folate because it is plentiful in foods, but some people need to adjust their eating to consume enough of this vitamin in their diet.

→ Populations at risk for folate-deficiency anemia include:
- Pregnant and lactating women
- Women taking birth control pills
- Persons with certain medical conditions such as hyperthyroidism, tropical sprue, chronic hemolytic anemia, and psoriasis
- People with poor diets or heavy alcohol consumption

→ Folate-rich foods include:
- Dark green, leafy vegetables
- Citrus fruits and juices
- Beans and other legumes
- Wheat bran and other whole grains
- Pork, chicken, and shellfish

*This handout may be reproduced for patient use.

10-B
Chronic Fatigue Syndrome

Chronic fatigue syndrome (CFS) is a poorly understood disease of unknown etiology, possibly triggered by a variety of stressors. It is characterized by a constellation of signs and symptoms dominated by disabling fatigue. The illness usually affects adults in their third and fourth decades of life, with a higher incidence noted in women compared to men (Reid et al. 2000). Chronic fatigue syndrome has been reported in children and adolescents, however (Tomoda et al. 2000). Syndromes similar to CFS have been described in the literature for over two centuries.

Initially, CFS was thought to occur as a result of some type of chronic viral infection such as Epstein-Barr virus (EBV), human-T-lymphotrophic viruses I and II (HTLV-I, HTLV-II), and human herpes viruses types 6 (HHV-6) and 7 (HHV-7) (Greenlee et al. 2000, Reeves et al. 2000). Other proposed theoretical causes include immune dysfunction, psychiatric disorders (e.g., somatization disorder, depression), muscle dysfunction, and possibly endocrine dysfunction, about all of which there are conflicting data in the literature. However, preliminary evidence may link CFS to neurobiologic and functional abnormalities (De Becker et al. 2000, Komaroff 2000, Manu 2000, Neeck et al. 2000, Tomoda et al. 2000). Thus far, there is no evidence that CFS is transmitted through close household or intimate contact.

Diagnosing CFS is difficult because generalized, persistent fatigue is one of the most frequently reported problems in primary care settings, with an estimated prevalence as high as 24%. Additionally, it is a subjective symptom that is difficult to quantify and qualify. In the majority of individuals presenting with fatigue lasting for several weeks, there is no medical cause identified (Fukuda et al. 1994).

Although general fatigue is a hallmark symptom of CFS, other symptoms and signs must also be present to make the diagnosis. To clarify the criteria essential for a diagnosis of CFS, the Centers for Disease Control and Prevention (CDC) developed a working case definition as a guideline for practitioners and researchers (see **Table 10B.1, CDC Working Case Definition of Chronic Fatigue Syndrome or Idiopathic Chronic Fatigue**). This definition requires the patient be evaluated and demonstrate four or more of the criteria in order to meet the CDC definition of CFS (CDC 2000, Fukuda et al. 1994). Patients with unexplained chronic fatigue who are clinically evaluated and who fail to meet the CFS criteria may be diagnosed with idiopathic chronic fatigue. The reason(s) for failing to meet CFS criteria must be documented (CDC 2000, Fukuda et al. 1994).

DATABASE

SUBJECTIVE

→ Symptoms may include (CDC 2000, Fukuda et al. 1994, Neeck et al. 2000, Reeves et al. 2000, Reid et al. 2000):
- Fatigue:
  - Of new onset
  - Not a result of ongoing exertion
  - Not substantially improved by rest
  - Prolonged (≥24 hours) generalized fatigue after exercise that the patient had been able to tolerate prior to the onset of symptoms
- Mild fever, which may be recurrent
- Sore throat
- Enlarged, tender cervical lymph nodes
- Myalgia
- Chills
- Muscle weakness
- Migratory joint pain without edema or erythema of joints
- Headaches—generalized and different from headaches experienced by patient prior to onset of fatigue
- Impaired memory, forgetfulness, irritability, problems with concentration or thinking clearly, depression
- Insomnia or hypersomnia (excessive sleeping)

→ Symptoms reportedly develop within a few hours to a few days.

→ Patient denies a history of other conditions that may produce similar symptoms (e.g., malignancy, infection, autoimmune disorders, chronic diseases, neuromuscular disease, fungal or parasitic diseases, psychiatric disease, allergies, substance abuse, or drug side effects).

Table 10B.1.   CDC WORKING CASE DEFINITION OF CHRONIC FATIGUE SYNDROME OR IDIOPATHIC CHRONIC FATIGUE

Clinically evaluated, unexplained chronic fatigue cases can be separated into either the chronic fatigue syndrome (CFS) or idiopathic chronic fatigue on the basis of the criteria listed below.

Chronic Fatigue Syndrome Criteria

The presence of unexplained persistent or relapsing chronic fatigue that is:
- Of new or definite onset (i.e., has not been lifelong)
- Not the result of ongoing exertion
- Not substantially alleviated by rest
- Associated with a substantial reduction in previous levels of occupational, educational, social, or personal activities

AND

The presence of 4 or more of the following symptoms, all of which must have persisted or recurred during 6 or more consecutive months of illness and must not have predated the fatigue:
- Self-reported impairment in short-term memory or concentration severe enough to cause substantial reduction in previous levels of occupational, educational, social, or personal activities
- Sore throat
- Tender cervical or axillary lymph nodes
- Muscle pain
- Multijoint pain without joint swelling or redness
- Headaches of a new type, pattern, or severity
- Unrefreshing sleep
- Postexertional malaise lasting more than 24 hours

The method used to establish the presence of these and any other symptoms should be specified.

Idiopathic Chronic Fatigue Criteria

A case of idiopathic chronic fatigue is defined as clinically evaluated, unexplained chronic fatigue that fails to meet the CFS criteria. The reason(s) for failing to meet the criteria should be specified.

Source: Centers for Disease Control and Prevention. 2000. Chronic fatigue syndrome (CFS) definition. Available at: http://www.cdc.gov/ncidod/diseases/cfs/defined. Accessed on January 20, 2002.

OBJECTIVE
→ Patient may appear depressed, anxious, or with normal affect.
→ Patient may present with (CDC 2000, Fukuda et al. 1994, Neeck et al. 2000, Reeves et al. 2000, Reid et al. 2000):
  ■ Low-grade temperature elevation:
    • Oral temperature of 37.6°C to 38.6°C/99.6°F to 101.4°F
  ■ Enlarged and/or tender anterior or posterior cervical and/or axillary nodes. Lymph nodes >2 cm in diameter require further evaluation to rule out other pathology.

ASSESSMENT
→ Chronic fatigue syndrome
→ R/O idiopathic chronic fatigue
→ R/O anemia
→ R/O chronic infections (e.g., mononucleosis, hepatitis, tuberculosis)

→ R/O fibromyalgia
→ R/O endocrine disease (e.g., thyroid dysfunction, diabetes mellitus)
→ R/O autoimmune disease
→ R/O renal disease
→ R/O malignancy
→ R/O human immunodeficiency virus (HIV) infection
→ R/O psychiatric disease
→ R/O neuromuscular disease

PLAN
DIAGNOSTIC TESTS
→ The following tests should be considered routinely in the evaluation of a patient with CFS to rule out other causes for the symptomatology (CDC 2000, Fukuda et al. 1994, Neeck et al. 2000, Reeves et al. 2000, Reid et al. 2000):
  ■ Complete blood count (CBC) with differential, indices, and platelet count: within normal limits (WNL) in patients with CFS

- Urinalysis: WNL
- Purified protein derivative (PPD): negative
- Chemistry panel (electrolytes, liver function, BUN, creatinine, calcium, and fasting glucose): WNL
- Sedimentation rate: frequently <5 mm/hour
- Thyroid function tests: WNL
- Antinuclear antibodies: may demonstrate a low-level positive result
- Syphilis tests (VDRL or RPR): nonreactive

→ The following additional tests should be considered to rule out other causes of symptomatology based on the patient's history and physical examination:

- Antithyroid antibodies: may demonstrate a low-level positive result
- Lyme disease serology: negative
- Hepatitis serologies: negative
- HIV antibody: negative

  NOTE: HIV antibody testing may need to be repeated at 3–6 months after the initial test is done if the patient reports a recent history of possible exposure (see the **Human Immunodeficiency Virus-1 Infection** chapter in Section 11).

- Chest x-ray: WNL
- Skin testing for anergy (e.g., Candida, mumps, and/or tetanus): may not demonstrate a reaction to antigens
- Lymph node biopsy as indicated: WNL
- Serologies and cultures as indicated: WNL/negative
- Cosyntropin (Cortrosyn®) stimulation test (to rule out adrenal insufficiency): WNL
- Magnetic resonance imaging (MRI) (to rule out demyelinating disease): WNL
- Stool for ova and parasites: WNL
- Fecal occult blood: negative
- Quantitative immunoglobulins: WNL
- Lumbar puncture: WNL
- Evaluation for myasthenia gravis (e.g., acetylcholine receptor antibody test, electrophysiological tests): WNL

TREATMENT/MANAGEMENT

→ Multiple therapeutic interventions have been attempted in the treatment of CFS, but few have been studied adequately to demonstrate proven efficacy.

- Nevertheless, clinicians managing the care of patients with CFS do attempt to treat some CFS symptoms with treatments that have proven effective in other diseases to help diminish some of the debilitating effects of CFS.

→ Initiation and gradual increase in physical exercise up to 30 minutes a day has demonstrated substantial improvement in physical functioning and fatigue in patients with CFS (Reid et al. 2000).

→ Cognitive behavioral therapy by skilled therapists has demonstrated a beneficial effect on level of functioning in CFS patients (Reid et al. 2000).

→ Because sleep disturbances can contribute to an increase in other symptoms associated with CFS, attempts to relieve these sleep disorders are important and should include non-pharmacological recommendations such as establishing a consistent bedtime, avoiding caffeine and other stimulants in the late afternoon or evening, a comfortable room temperature (usually a cool environment is beneficial), and avoiding late snacks and daytime naps.

→ Pain associated with myalgias, arthralgias, and neuralgias can be quite severe and require pharmacological interventions with nonsteroidal anti-inflammatory drugs (NSAIDs) including:

- Naproxen 250–500 mg p.o. BID
- Naproxen sodium 275–550 mg BID
- Ibuprofen 400 mg p.o. TID–QID

  NOTE: Warn patients about potential side effects (e.g., gastritis, gastrointestinal bleeding, hepatotoxicity) and drug interactions. Consult the *Physicians' Desk Reference* for additional information.

→ Depression may require therapeutic interventions—including individual or group counseling—which are often common with other types of chronic diseases. If antidepressants are to be used, their initiation should be under the supervision of a physician managing the patient's psychiatric care.

→ Other therapies have been tried in CFS patients without evidence of efficacy, including: vitamin and mineral therapy, antiviral therapy (e.g. acyclovir), immunoglobulin therapy, and kutapressin (a porcine liver extract) (Reid et al. 2000).

→ Other documented pathology (e.g., thyroid dysfunction, anemia) should be treated as indicated.

NOTE: Although a patient may have CFS, other illnesses also can occur and warrant appropriate evaluation and treatment.

CONSULTATION

→ Consultation with a physician as indicated, but it is warranted if an underlying pathology is evident during work-up (e.g., malignancy, psychiatric disorder, thyroid disease).

→ As needed for prescription(s)

PATIENT EDUCATION

→ Educate the patient about CFS, including theoretical causes, diagnostic work-up required to document CFS, chronicity of illness, therapeutic options, prognosis, and community resources available, including:

- The Chronic Fatigue and Immune Dysfunction Syndrome (CFIDS) Association of America
  P.O. Box 220398
  Charlotte, N.C. 28222-0398
  (704) 362-2343
  www.cfids.org

- The National CFS and Fibromyalgia Association
  P.O. Box 18426
  Kansas City, Mo. 64133
  (816) 313-2000

- Centers for Disease Control and Prevention
  Department of Health and Human Services
  Public Health Service, CDC
  Atlanta, Ga. 30333
  (404) 332-4555 (Hotline)
  www.cdc.gov/ncidod/diseases/cfs

- National Institute of Allergy and Infectious Disease–CFS
  www.niaid.nih.gov/factsheets/cfs.htm

→ If other pathology is evident (e.g., anemia, thyroid disease), educate the patient about these specific problems, their causes, treatment options, prognosis, and follow-up as indicated.

→ Educate the patient's family about CFS, especially emphasizing the noncontagious nature of the disease.

FOLLOW-UP

→ Follow-up visits with the patient will vary and depend upon the patient's symptoms, success of chosen therapies, and/or need for additional consultation for evaluation of possible problems (e.g., psychiatric evaluations and/or therapy).

→ Document in progress notes and on problem list.

BIBLIOGRAPHY

Centers for Disease Control and Prevention (CDC). 2000. CFS definition. Available at: http://www.cdc.gov/ncidod/diseases/cfs/defined/defined3.htm. Accessed on January 20, 2002.

De Becker, P., Roeykens, J., Reynders, M. et al. 2000. Exercise capacity in chronic fatigue syndrome. *Archives of Internal Medicine* 160:3270–3277.

Fukuda, K., Strauss, S.E., Hickie, I. et al. 1994. The chronic fatigue syndrome: a comprehensive approach to its definition and study. *Annals of Internal Medicine* 121:953–959.

Greenlee, J.E., and Rose, J.W. 2000. Controversies in neurological infectious diseases. *Seminars in Neurology* 20(3):375–386.

Komaroff, A.L. 2000. The biology of chronic fatigue syndrome. *American Journal of Medicine* 108:169–171.

Manu, P. 2000. Chronic fatigue syndrome: The fundamentals still apply. *American Journal of Medicine* 108:172–173.

Neeck, G., and Crafford, L.J. 2000. Neuroendocrine perturbations in fibromyalgia and chronic fatigue syndrome. *Rheumatic Disease Clinics of North America* 26(4):989–1002.

Reeves, W.C., Stamey, F.R., Black, J.B. et al. 2000. Human herpesviruses 6 and 7 in chronic fatigue syndrome: a case-control study. *Clinical Infectious Diseases* 31:48–52.

Reid, S., Chalder, T., Cleare, A. et al. 2000. Extracts from "clinical evidence." Chronic fatigue syndrome. *British Medical Journal* 320:292–296.

Tomoda, A., Miike, T., Yamada, E. et al. 2000. Case report. Chronic fatigue syndrome in childhood. *Brain & Development* 22:60–64.

Kim K. O'Hair, R.N.P., M.S.N.

10-C
Osteoporosis

Osteoporosis is a "silent," systemic disease that results from the loss of total bone mass and the loss of microarchitectural integrity. These losses cause an increase in bone fragility and an increased risk of traumatic and nontraumatic bone fracture that may not be evident until a fracture occurs (McClung 1999). The National Osteoporosis Foundation (NOF) estimates that more than 1.3 million fractures per year occur in the United States as a result of osteoporosis, at an annual cost of more than $13.8 billion. The incidence of and cost associated with osteoporosis will rise as the population continues to live longer (NOF 1998). Because hip fracture incidence increases exponentially with increasing age, and the age of the population over 65 is expected to rise considerably in the next 40 years, the annual incidence of hip fracture is expected to rise to 840,000 per year by the year 2040 (McClung 1999).

About 70% of fractures experienced by the population age 45 or older are related to osteoporosis, with the greatest number of these experienced by postmenopausal women (NOF 1998). An estimated one-quarter of all women over age 60 will develop osteoporotic vertebral fractures, and about 15% of these osteoporotic women will experience hip fractures during their lifetime (Marcus et al. 1996). Women achieve maximum bone mass by age 20–30 and lose bone rapidly in the first five years after menopause (23% per year). This rate slows to less than 0.05% per year until the age of 70, when the rate accelerates again. By the age of 80, the average woman has lost approximately 35–40% of the bone mass she had in young adulthood (Marcus et al. 1996).

Osteoporosis can be defined qualitatively as microarchitectural changes that increase bone fragility with a resultant increase in the risk of fracture. Quantitatively, the World Health Organization (WHO) has defined osteoporosis as bone density 2.5 standard deviations below the mean for Caucasian women age 27–40 (National Institutes of Health [NIH] Consensus Statement Online 2000). However, osteoporosis can arise in any person who did not develop optimal bone mass in young adulthood (NIH Consensus Statement Online 2000).

Osteoporosis is further classified as primary or secondary. *Primary osteoporosis* occurs in both genders at all ages but commonly occurs postmenopausally in women, with a much later onset in men. *Secondary osteoporosis* is a result of medications, other diseases, or other conditions—examples include steroid-induced osteoporosis, and osteoporosis as a result of hypogonadism, untreated thyroid disease, or gastrointestinal absorptive diseases (Marcus et al. 1996, NIH Consensus Statement Online 2000). Any osteoporotic fracture can lead to a reduction in quality of life due to chronic and episodic pain, disability, and reduced functional independence (Kessenich 2000).

Pathophysiology

Throughout the life cycle, bone is continually being remodeled: Osteoblasts form new bone and osteoclasts resorb old bone. In postmenopausal women and elderly men, the resorption of bone outpaces the formation of new bone, resulting in a net loss of bone mass (Marcus et al. 1996). More rapid remodeling also causes more resorption of the trabeculae that form the supportive bone matrix of some bones, in particular the vertebrae. Once the trabeculae are resorbed, they cannot be reformed, reducing the strength of the vertebrae and increasing the risk of fracture (Marcus et al. 1996).

Morbidity and Mortality

The most common sites of osteoporotic bone loss are at the proximal femur, vertebrae, and distal forearm. Patients with hip fracture experience 10–20% excess mortality in the year following fracture (NIH Consensus Statement Online 2000). Up to 25% of hip fracture patients require long-term nursing home placement and only a third return to prefracture functional status (NIH Consensus Statement Online 2000).

The sequellae of vertebral fractures can include chronic back pain, loss of height, postural deformity, and kyphosis. Thoracic fractures can result in restrictive lung diseases and exacerbation of ongoing lung disease. Lumbar fractures may deform abdominal anatomy leading to abdominal pain and dysfunction. The cosmetic effect of these changes can result in depression and loss of self-esteem (NOF 1998). Depression, social isolation, anger, and frustration can also occur due to the reduction of daily activities, travel, and visiting friends and family.

Bone Density Evaluation

Measurement of bone mineral density (BMD) is the most common method used to establish a diagnosis of osteoporosis. Bone density is highly correlated to bone strength and risk of fracture. Bone mineral density of the hip, spine, radius, or calcaneus have been found to be equal predictors of fracture risk in general, although BMD of the hip is considered a better predictor of hip fracture than measurement at any other site (Cummings et al. 1998).

The WHO has set BMD measurements to develop the diagnostic criteria for osteoporosis. The T-score refers to the number of standard deviations (SDs) above or below the average BMD for healthy, Caucasian women age 27–40. The Z-score is the number of SDs above or below the average BMD for age- and gender-matched controls. A T-score of 0 represents the peak bone mass for a 27–40-year-old woman. The WHO has established that T-scores below –2.5 SDs constitute osteoporosis, that T-scores between –1.0 and –2.5 SDs indicate *osteopenia* (reduced bone mass with increased risk for osteoporosis), and that T-scores above –1.0 are within the range of normal values (NIH Consensus Statement Online 2000). The decision to obtain BMD evaluation should be based on individual risk assessment.

The NOF has developed evidence-based guidelines for BMD testing using the results of several prospective studies and meta-analyses of randomized trials (Cummings et al. 1998, NOF 1998). Candidates for BMD evaluation include:

→ All postmenopausal women under the age of 65 with one or more risk factors (other than menopause)

→ All women 65 years old or older

→ Postmenopausal women with current fractures (to establish the diagnosis and determine extent of disease)

→ Women who are considering medical therapy, where testing would facilitate decision-making

→ Women on antiresorptive therapy or other modalities for long periods of time, to assess effectiveness of the regimen

DATABASE

SUBJECTIVE

→ Risk factor identification, especially when the factor is independent of bone mineral density, can be used with BMD evaluation to improve prediction of fracture risk. Though NOF guidelines are delineated primarily for Caucasian women (due to the paucity of studies with significant numbers of subjects of other races or ethnicities), assessment of risk of osteoporosis should not be limited only to Caucasian women, but should include all races. The presence of multiple risk factors increases the probability of osteoporosis. The following risk factors have been adapted from several sources (Cummings et al. 1995, McClung 1999, NIH Consensus Statement Online 2000, NOF 1998):

- Low BMD: The lower the BMD, the greater the risk for osteoporotic bone fractures.
- Age: The number of fractures increases with age. The risk of hip fracture rises exponentially from 0.1% at age 65 to 1% by age 80.
- Race: Caucasian women have two to three times greater risk of hip fracture than African American or Hispanic women. Asian women have about 25–50% lower risk of hip fractures than Caucasian women, although their risk of vertebral fracture is almost equal to that of Caucasian women.
- Previous fracture: Women who have sustained a fracture of any type (since the age of 50) have twice the risk of sustaining another fracture of the same or any type. A finding of vertebral fracture on x-ray correlates to a three- to fourfold increase in future vertebral fractures as well as twice the risk of other types of fracture. This is an independent risk factor.
- Family history: The daughters of women who have sustained vertebral fractures will usually have a bone density 5% lower than the average. A maternal history of hip fracture also increases the risk of hip fractures by twofold, independent of BMD.
- Weight: Body weight is an important indicator. Obese women have higher estrogen levels and higher lifetime estrogen exposure. In addition, the extra weight results in greater stress on the bones and increased bone density. Women in the lowest 25% of body weight experience a two- to threefold greater risk of hip fracture than women in the heaviest 25% of body weight.
- Smoking: Smokers have a 50% greater risk of hip fractures, especially older smokers.
- Hypoestrogenism, as a result of menopause, surgery, or prolonged premenopausal amenorrhea, often results in low BMD. Late menarche, early menopause, and low estrogen levels have also been correlated with low BMD in several studies.
- Low lifetime calcium intake
- Medications: glucocorticoids, anticonvulsants, long-acting sedatives, overuse of thyroid supplements, lithium, chemotherapy, overuse of phosphate-binding antacids
- Inadequate exercise
- Impaired eyesight
- Alcoholism
- Recurrent falls
- Height: Taller-than-average women have an increased risk of fracture.

→ Because osteoporosis is most often a "silent" disease, patients with significant bone loss may present with minimal symptoms.

→ Symptoms may include (McClung 1999, NOF 1998):

- Spinal or other bone pain
- Loss of height
- Change in the fit of clothing, especially with increasing kyphosis

- Increased loss of adult teeth (Grodstein et al. 1999)
- Increased dental disease (Genco et al. 1999)

→ Gynecologic history:
- Menarche, regularity of cycles, age of menopause, status of uterus, ovaries, prolonged periods of amenorrhea, hypogonadism, chronic hypothalamic amenorrhea, polycystic ovarian disease

→ Family history:
- Maternal history of osteoporosis, loss of height, hip or spinal fracture

→ Major medical illnesses (Cummings et al. 1998, Marcus et al. 1996, NOF 1998):
- Cancer, multiple myeloma, systemic mastocytosis
- Gastrointestinal diseases including liver disease, anorexia or bulimia, gastric/bowel resection, malabsorptive disorders
- Endocrine diseases including hyperparathyroidism, thyroid disease (untreated or overtreated), Cushing's syndrome, rheumatic diseases, or arthritis
- Pulmonary diseases including asthma and obstructive lung disease
- Neurological conditions including Parkinson's disease, cerebrovascular accident (CVA), and seizure disorders
- Osteoarthritis
- Rheumatological diseases
- Visual impairment including cataracts, untreated refractive errors
- Presence of medical conditions requiring prolonged immobilization

→ Medications, current and previous therapies, complementary and alternative therapies, especially chronic corticosteroid use. (See "Risk Factors" above for additional medications.)

→ Lifestyle:
- Habits: smoking, recreational drug use, alcohol intake, level of physical activity, nutrition
- Nutrition: childhood and lifetime calcium intake and supplement use
- Exercise: type, frequency
- Sleep patterns, frequency of nocturnal rising, use of over-the-counter sleep medications

→ Mental health:
- Presence of depression, dementia, use of psychoactive drugs, use of long-acting sedative hypnotics, or selective serotonin re-uptake inhibitors

→ Psychosocial history:
- Living situation, including assessment of risk for falls
- Social support system
- Coping/stress management skills
- Assessment for physical or psychological abuse, current or potential

OBJECTIVE

→ Physical examination:
NOTE: Examination should be expanded to fit individual needs when appropriate.

- Mental/sensory status, affect, loss of cognitive or sensory function
- Height, weight, vital signs. Note stature, carriage, and gait. **NOTE:** The importance of yearly height measurement is emphasized.
- Visual acuity and fundoscopic examination as needed
- Neck: assess for nodules, lymphadenopathy, scars
- Spine: kyphosis, deformity
- Lungs: assess for presence of obstructive pulmonary diseases, asthma
- Abdomen: multiple skin folds may be indicative of vertebral compression fractures
- Extremities: assess muscle strength and muscle mass, sensory function
- Breast and pelvic examination if hormone replacement therapy is being considered or as needed

ASSESSMENT

→ R/O osteopenia
→ R/O osteoporosis
→ R/O fracture: traumatic or nontraumatic
→ R/O hyperparathyroidism
→ R/O subclinical hyperthyroid disease
→ R/O hypercalciuria
→ R/O gastrointestinal malabsorption conditions
→ R/O hypogonadism
→ R/O hematological disorders
→ R/O connective tissue or rheumatological diseases
→ R/O nutritional deficiencies
→ R/O alcoholism
→ R/O inappropriate use of glucorticoids
→ R/O anticonvulsant therapy

PLAN

DIAGNOSTIC TESTS

→ Radiologic studies:
- Dual-energy x-ray absorptiometry (DXA or DEXA): Used for hip, wrist and spine. Minimal radiation exposure (much less than chest x-ray). Highly reproducible. Note that BMD of the spine in women over age 65 is frequently increased due to osteoarthritic changes in the vertebrae.
- Single-energy x-ray absorptiometry (SXA) and peripheral dual-energy x-ray absorptiometry (pDXA or pDEXA): Used to measure BMD at forearm, finger, and heel. Relatively inexpensive, results not as reproducible.
- Quantitative computed tomography (QCT): Measures trabecular and cortical bone density at several body sites. Used as alternate to DXA to measure spinal BMD. More expensive. Relatively high radiation exposure.
- Ultrasound densitometry: Assesses BMD in patella, heel, tibia, or other peripheral bone. Not as precise as DXA. No radiation exposure, limited to peripheral skeleton.
- Radiographic absorptiometry: An older technology used to measure BMD of the hand. Not as reproducible, nor as precise, as DXA.

→ Laboratory tests for osteoporosis have been conducted for many years without great success in predicting fracture risk.
  - CBC with differential
  - Serum chemistry tests: calcium, alkaline phosphatase (biochemical markers of bone metabolism)
  - Thyroid function testing
  - 25-hydroxyvitamin D level (vitamin D deficiency)
  - Testing for other suspected causes of bone loss as appropriate

---

TREATMENT/MANAGEMENT/PREVENTION

→ The goals of treatment, management, and prevention are fourfold: to prevent further loss of bone, to prevent future fracture, to minimize symptoms, and to improve function and quality of life (McClung 1999, Woodhead et al. 1998).
  - Prevention is the most important of all treatment and management strategies for reducing the probability of osteoporotic fractures.
  - Women of all ages should be counseled and assessed for current and future risk of developing osteoporotic bone fracture.
  - Initial counseling and evaluation should begin in childhood and include emphasis on healthy nutrition, especially adequate intake of calcium and vitamin D, regular weight-bearing exercises, and avoiding tobacco use and alcohol abuse (NOF 1998).
  - It is important to note that all treatment and management strategies require life-long adherence for most patients (calcium and vitamin D requirements, reduction of risk of falls, etc.)
  - Fracture risk and osteoporosis have been found to recur, often rapidly, when any therapy or lifestyle modification is discontinued (NIH Consensus Statement Online 2000, NOF 1998).

→ Pharmacological therapy:
  - Calcium and vitamin D:
    • Adequate calcium and vitamin D intake are essential to the development of peak bone mass and overall maintenance of bone structure and integrity.
    • Optimal treatment of osteoporosis, with or without other drug therapy, requires calcium and vitamin D intake at the recommended levels (NIH Consensus Statement Online 2000).
    • All patients should be encouraged to maintain adequate intake of dietary calcium (1,200 mg/day, including supplements) and vitamin D (400 IU/day, may be increased to 800 IU in cases of vitamin D deficiency) (NIH Consensus Statement Online 2000, NOF 1998).
    • The importance of adequate calcium and vitamin D intake has been emphasized in the literature and clinical trials. This intervention is cost-effective, well-tolerated, and should accompany all other treatments (NIH Consensus Statement Online 2000, NOF 2001).
      – The typical American diet contains approximately 600 mg/day of calcium (NOF 1998).

➤ Supplementation or dietary modification may be needed to meet these recommendations.
➤ Many common foods have been supplemented with additional calcium and should be considered as sources of dietary calcium.
  - Vitamin D is readily available in fortified milk products.
    ➤ Sun exposure, with adequate sunscreen, also provides vitamin D precursors.
- Hormone therapy:
  • Estrogen replacement therapy (ERT) or hormone replacement therapy (HRT) have been the primary therapeutic approaches to prevention and treatment. Numerous cost-effective formulations are available.
    – Long-term HRT use has been associated with greater bone mass protection while short-term use of HRT for fracture prevention is controversial (Hully et al. 1998).
    – Smaller doses of HRT (0.3 mg conjugated equine estrogen [CEE] or its equivalent) have been found to have efficacy in bone mass protection and may provide a better-tolerated side effect profile (Ettinger et al. 1987).
    – Unfortunately, when a woman stops using HRT or ERT she begins to lose bone mass at the rapid rate noted in early menopause, and she may lose most of the protection against bone loss and fractures over the next 5–10 years (Cummings et al. 1998). (See the **Perimenopausal and Menopausal Symptoms and Hormone Therapy** chapter in Section 12.)
    – Women taking HRT with an intact uterus reduce their risk of developing endometrial cancer by the use of progestational agents such as medroxyprogesterone acetate or micronized oral progesterone, either cyclically or continuously.
    NOTE: Careful and complete counseling regarding risks and benefits is important. Side effect profile consideration should be evaluated prior to the initiation of therapy and periodically as needed (Writing Group for the PEPI 1996).
    – Recent large, randomized, and well-controlled studies have caused a re-evaluation of HRT.
      ➤ Results from the Heart and Estrogen/Progestin Replacement Study (HERS) have caused reconsideration of the effectiveness of HRT in the management of health concerns of postmenopausal women (Hulley et al. 1998).
        * For women with established coronary disease, it was shown that ERT provides no benefit and may cause harm.
        * An increased risk of thromboembolic events and gallbladder disease was also demonstrated with estrogen use.
    – The Women's Health Initiative (WHI), an ongoing, randomized, prospective, controlled hormone study

of postmenopausal women, has produced similar findings. The clinical arm evaluating the outcome of continuous conjugated equine estrogen (0.625 mg daily) and medroxyprogesterone acetate (2.5 mg daily) in women with intact uteri was discontinued when it was shown that the risks of this treatment exceeded the benefits.

➤ Risks of invasive breast cancer, coronary heart disease, stroke, and venous thromboembolic events were significantly increased.

➤ On the other hand, the WHI trial found significant decreases in the risk of spine and hip fractures (Writing Group for the Women's Health Initiative Investigators 2002).

– The North American Menopause Society (NAMS) Advisory Panel on Postmenopausal Hormone Therapy made a recommendation that, while many hormone regimes have been approved by the U.S. Food and Drug Administration (FDA) for the prevention of postmenopausal osteoporosis, there are risks associated with these regimes, and alternatives should be considered (NAMS 2002).

■ Bisphosphonates:

• The development of bisphosphonates has been of great significance in the prevention and treatment of osteoporosis. Bisphosphonates are very bone specific and are termed antiresorptive medications. Bisphosphonates slow osteoclast activity and the reduction of bone mass, thereby increasing BMD in a dose-dependent manner (Lin 1996). Reduction of vertebral fracture risk by 30–50% has been a consistent finding in many randomized clinical controlled trials and meta-analyses (NIH Consensus Statement Online 2000). Two bisphosphonates, alendronate and risedronate, have been approved by the FDA for prevention and treatment of osteoporosis (NOF 1998).

• A common feature of this class of drugs is the potential for causing gastric upset.

• All bisphosphonates are poorly absorbed from the stomach, and strategies to improve absorption are critical (Kessenich 2000).

– Alendronate:

➤ Particularly valuable for postmenopausal women with contraindications to HRT

➤ Must be taken on an empty stomach first thing in the morning with 8 oz. of plain tap water at least 30 minutes before any additional food or drink.

➤ Patients must remain upright following ingestion for the same period of time. Standard dosages are 10 mg p.o./day for osteoporosis treatment and 5 mg p.o./day for osteoporosis prevention.

➤ Alternately, a weekly dose of 70 mg p.o./week for treatment or 35 mg p.o./week for prevention may improve patient tolerance and compliance (NIH Consensus Statement Online 2000, NOF 1998).

– Risedronate:

➤ Women with pre-existing vertebral fracture taking this medication demonstrated a 60% reduction in risk of hip fracture (Harris et al. 1999).

➤ Prevention and treatment dosage is 5 mg p.o./day.

➤ Patients are advised to take risedronate between meals or prior to bedtime on an empty stomach with an 8 oz. glass of water and avoid food or further drink intake for at least 30 minutes.

➤ Patient must maintain an upright position for 30 minutes after ingestion.

➤ Dosage regimen is 400 mg p.o./day for 1 week, then 3 weeks without medication, repeated every 4 weeks.

■ Calcitonin:

• Osteoclast inhibitor that decreases bone resorption; it has FDA approval for the treatment of osteoporosis but not prevention.

• Delivered as a single daily intranasal spray of 200 units of salmon calcitonin; alternate nares each day to reduce nasal irritation (Overgaard et al. 1992).

• Found to increase spinal bone density by about 10–15%, but its efficacy may be much weaker than HRT or the bisphosphonates (Overgaard et al. 1992).

• Has demonstrated an analgesic effect for women with vertebral fractures and chronic back pain that make it more useful in this population (Overgaard et al. 1992).

• Considered as an alternate to HRT or bisphosphonates for women who have been unsuccessful with either therapy.

■ Selective estrogen receptor modulators (SERMs):

• SERMs have been shown to be effective in several clinical trials to reduce osteoporotic fractures.

– Raloxifene has been approved by the FDA for the prevention and treatment of osteoporosis at a dose of 60 mg p.o. QD (NOF 2001).
NOTE: Women taking raloxifene have shown a 60% decrease in relative risk for all breast cancers, and it may be an excellent choice for women with increased breast cancer risk (Cummings et al. 1999). The disadvantages of raloxifene include the increased risk of venous thrombolic events to the same degree that is seen with estrogen. In addition, SERMs have hypoestrogenic effects (hot flashes, vaginal dryness, sleeplessness, etc.) such as experienced in early menopause, and this can have an impact on drug compliance (NOF 1998).

– Tamoxifen (used for breast cancer treatment) is another SERM that has been identified as helpful in reduction of osteoporotic fracture.

➤ Dosage for women with high risk for breast cancer is 20 mg p.o./day.

➤ Not approved for treatment or prevention of osteoporosis but offers patients with breast cancer improvement in their fracture risk.

> Concerns regarding endometrial hyperplasia, thromboembolic events, and other estrogen-agonist side effects have limited its use (Cummings et al. 1999)

- Parathyroid hormone:
  - Parathyroid hormone (I-34) (PTH) may be the next advance in treating osteoporosis. Unlike other FDA-approved medication, PTH stimulates new bone formation and may have greater impact on bone density when used together with antiresorptive therapy. PTH was found to reduce the rate of new fractures and increase bone density in postmenopausal women (Neer et al. 2001). Though this drug shows promise, it has not yet received FDA approval.

→ Natural or complementary compounds:
- Interest in complementary and alternative medicines has greatly increased in the past several decades.
- Phytoestrogens (plant estrogens) are considered to act as naturally occurring SERMs and will bind to estrogen receptors but are less than 1% as potent as endogenous estrogens (Fugh-Berman 1999).
  - Studies regarding phytoestrogens have shown bone density increases or vertebral fracture reduction, but many trials have methodological problems (Fugh-Berman 2000).
  - While some phytoestrogens may have some weak estrogen effects and some anti-estrogen effects, randomized, well-controlled studies are limited.
  - In addition, the dosage and purity of commercial phytoestrogens and their possible adverse effects are not well identified. (An ongoing multicenter fracture study in Europe, which uses the incidence of fracture as a primary end-point, may be able to provide greater information regarding this product [Fugh-Berman 2000].)
  - Diets high in isoflavones (a class of dietary phytoestrogens) have been noted in some studies to increase lumbar bone density, without change noted in the hip or total body BMD (Fugh-Berman 1999).

→ Pain management:
- Due to their side-effect potential and potential for habituation, pain medications should be chosen carefully; they may increase the risk of falls, constipation, gastric distress, and likelihood of chronic use.
- Additional pain management measures should be carefully assessed for each individual. Such measures include applying heat or ice, massage, and stretching exercises.

→ Lifestyle modification:
- Prevention of fractures requires careful evaluation of risk of falls at home and outdoors.
- Patients should be advised to "fall-proof" their home. Modification of activities of daily living to reduce fall risk may also be required.
- Patients should avoid poor lighting, slippery floors, loose scatter rugs, and telephone or electrical cords in walkways.

- Furniture should be placed to minimize fall risk, grab-bars should be placed in bathrooms, and nonskid mats and adhesive strips should be placed as needed.
- Patients should wear low, broad-heeled shoes with flexible and soft soles rather than higher heeled shoes.
- Place night lights as needed in hallways.
- Commode chairs should be considered when appropriate.
- Walking aids such as canes and walkers are also useful when appropriate.
- Tobacco use should be avoided. Increased osteoporosis risk is yet another of the many reasons to stop smoking.
- Alcohol abuse (more than two to three alcoholic beverages/day) should be avoided. It may increase the incidence of falls and also reduce good nutritional intake (Cummings et al. 1995).
- Exercise, especially weight resistance training, is important throughout a woman's life to prevent osteoporosis.
  - Exercise improves mood, increases flexibility, increases muscle mass for better joint cushioning, and improves balance.
  - Exercise regimens should be adapted to the needs and abilities of the patient (NIH Consensus Statement Online 2000, NOF 1998).

CONSULTATION

→ Consultation with an osteoporosis specialist, endocrinologist, and/or pain management specialist should be considered as indicated.
→ Physical, occupational, psychological, or psychiatric therapies should be considered when appropriate.
→ Adolescent patients with hypogonadism or eating disorders may need consultation, as may patients with secondary osteoporosis, multiple medications, or complex medical conditions.

PATIENT EDUCATION

→ A detailed discussion of the etiology of osteoporosis, rationales for dietary change, and the need for weight-bearing exercise should be provided for better patient understanding and the promotion of patient compliance. Lifestyle modifications and assessment of household fall risk may require the participation of family members.
→ Numerous patient education materials are available in the literature and elsewhere. NOF offers many free educational papers and pamphlets. NOF may be contacted by telephone at (202) 223-2226 or at www.nof.org.

FOLLOW-UP

→ Patient compliance may be improved with telephone contact or a brief clinic visit several weeks after initiating any therapy or lifestyle modification. Yearly examinations may be adequate thereafter.
→ Follow-up abnormal test results. Monitor consultation compliance.

→ Psychiatric evaluation as needed to establish and treat depression or dementia.

→ In cases where elder abuse is suspected, follow site-appropriate protocols.

→ Document in progress notes and on problem list.

BIBLIOGRAPHY

Cummings, S.R., Black, D.M., Thompson, D.E. et al. 1998. Effect of alendronate on risk of fracture in women with low bone density but without vertebral fractures: results from the fracture intervention trial. *Journal of the American Medical Association* 280:2077–2082.

Cummings, S.R., Eckert, S., Krueger, K. et al. 1999. The effect of raloxifene on risk of breast cancer in postmenopausal women with established osteoporosis: results from the Multiple Outcomes of Raloxifene Evaluation (MORE) randomized trial. *Journal of the American Medical Association* 28:2189–2197.

Cummings, S.R., Nevitt, M.C., Browner, W.S. et al. 1995. Risk factors for hip fracture in white women: the study of osteoporotic fractures. *New England Journal of Medicine* 332:767–773.

Ettinger, B., Genant, H.K., and Cann, C.E. 1987. Postmenopausal bone loss is prevented by treatment with low-dose estrogen with calcium. *Annals of Internal Medicine* 106:40–45.

Fugh-Berman, A. 1999. Progesterone cream for osteoporosis. *Alternative Therapies in Women's Health* 1(5):63–65.

_____. 2000. Ipriflavone: mechanism and safety. *Alternative Therapies in Women's Health* 2(9):65–67.

Genco, R.J. and Grossi, S.G. 1999. Is estrogen deficiency a risk factor for periodontal disease? *Compendium of Continuing Education in Oral Hygiene* 6(6):10–12.

Grodstein, F., Colditz, G.A., and Stampfer, M.J. 1999. Tooth loss and hormone use in postmenopausal women. *Compendium of Continuing Education in Oral Hygiene* 6(6):5–7.

Harris, S.T., Watts, N.B., Genant, H.K. et al. 1999. Effects of risedronate treatment on vertebral and nonvertebral fractures in women with postmenopausal osteoporosis: a randomized controlled trial. Vertebral Efficacy With Risedronate Therapy (VERT) Study Group. *Journal of the American Medical Association* 282:1344–1352.

Hulley, S., Grady, D., Bush, T. et al. 1998. Randomized trial of estrogen plus progestin for secondary prevention of coronary heart disease in postmenopausal women. Heart and Estrogen/Progestin Replacement Study (HERS) Research Group. *Journal of the American Medical Association* 280:605–613.

Kessenich, C.R. 2000. Risedronate: a new bisphosphonate for the treatment of osteoporosis. *Nurse Practitioner* 25(3):106–108.

Lin, J.H. 1996. Bisphosphonates: a review of their pharmacokinetic properties. *Bone* 18(2):75.

Marcus, R., Feldman, D., Kelsey, J., eds. 1996. *Osteoporosis.* San Diego, Calif.: Academic Press.

McClung, B.L. 1999. Using osteoporosis management to reduce fractures in elderly women. *Nurse Practitioner* 24(3):26–42.

Medical Letter. 2000. Calcium supplements. *Medical Letter on Drugs and Therapeutics* 42(1075):29.

National Institutes of Health (NIH) Consensus Statement Online 2000. *Osteoporosis prevention, diagnosis, and therapy.* March 27–29, 2001.

National Osteoporosis Foundation (NOF). 1998. *Physician's guide to prevention and treatment of osteoporosis.* Washington, D.C.: National Osteoporosis Foundation.

_____. 2001. *National osteoporosis news pressroom.* Washington, D.C.: National Osteoporosis Foundation. Available at: http://www.nof.org/news/pressroom.htm. Accessed on October 14, 2002.

Neer, R.M., Arnaud, C.D., Zanchetta, J.R. et al. 2001. Effect of parathyroid hormone (I-34) on fractures and bone mineral density in postmenopausal women with osteoporosis. *New England Journal of Medicine* 334:1434–1441.

North American Menopause Society. 2002. *Amended report from the NAMS advisory panel on postmenopausal hormone therapy.* Available at: http://www.menopause.org/news.html. Accessed on October 14, 2002.

Overgaard, K., Hansen, M.A., Signe, B.J. et al. 1992. Effect of calcitonin given intranasally on bone mass and fracture rates in established osteoporosis: a dose-response study. *British Medical Journal* 305:556–561.

Physicians' desk reference. 2002. 56th ed. Montvale, N.J.: Medical Economics.

Woodhead, G.A. and Moss, M.M. 1998. Osteoporosis: diagnosis and prevention. *Nurse Practitioner* 23(11):18–35.

Writing Group for the PEPI. 1996. Effects of hormone therapy on bone mineral density: results from the Postmenopausal Estrogen/Progestin Intervention (PEPI) trial. *Journal of the American Medical Association* 276:1389–1396.

Writing Group for the Women's Health Initiative Investigators. 2002. Risks and benefits of estrogen plus progestin in healthy postmenopausal women: principal results from the Women's Health Initiative randomized controlled trial. *Journal of the American Medical Association* 288(3):321–333.

10-D

Systemic Lupus Erythematosus

Systemic lupus erythematosus (SLE) is an autoimmune multi-system disorder characterized by the presence of multiple autoantibodies directed at one or more components of cell nuclei (DNA, RNA, nuclear proteins, and protein-nucleic acid complexes). It is one of the disease entities within the lupus family of disorders. Patients with lupus erythematosus (LE) may have a disease limited to cutaneous forms (i.e., discoid lupus) or they may develop the systemic symptoms that characterize systemic disease. This chapter refers principally to SLE. The overall incidence of SLE in the United States is 124 per 100,000 population (Ruiz-Irastorza et al. 2001). There is a higher incidence of SLE in African Americans, Asian Americans, and Hispanic Americans compared to Caucasians (Schur 1996). Approximately 80% of cases occur in women between the ages of 15–40 with an incidence in this group estimated at 1 per 1,000 population. The overall sex distribution ratio (female:male) for SLE is 9:1 but increases to 15:1 during the reproductive years (Greenstein 2001). In addition, some individuals have a genetic predisposition that increases the risk for developing SLE.

Pathogenesis of SLE

SLE is a chronic systemic inflammatory connective tissue disease of autoimmune origin that presents in varied ways throughout the body in a pattern of relapse and remission (Gordon et al. 2001). The pathogenesis of SLE is secondary to an immune dysregulation of B cells that results in abnormally increased production of antibodies to nuclear antigens and other self-antigens that are not normally identified by the immune system as "abnormal." The target antigens for these autoantibodies are membranes, intracellular material, or nuclear material.

The autoantibodies produced in persons with SLE cause organ injury via one of two mechanisms: 1) direct target cell injury (e.g. hemolytic anemia) or 2) deposition of immune antibody/antigen complexes in tissue, thereby disrupting the tissue (e.g., nephritis). The deposition of immune complexes in vascular tissue contributes to an increased risk for thromboembolic events and osteonecrosis (Somers et al. 2002). The deposition of immune complexes in other organs initiates an inflammatory response that causes arthritis, skin lesions, pleurisy, pericarditis, cerebritis, or peritonitis. Although SLE can affect any body system, the majority of patients exhibit symptoms in only a few organs over several years.

Symptoms of SLE

Because SLE can affect multiple organ systems, the symptoms are diverse and differ in intensity and duration from one person to the next. The diagnostic criteria for SLE were developed by the American Rheumatoid Association in 1982 and revised by the American College of Rheumatology (ACR) in 1997 (Hochberg 1997, Tan et al. 1982). Diagnosis is based on the presence of four of the 11 criteria serially or simultaneously during any interval of observation (see **Table 10D.1, Diagnostic Criteria for Systemic Lupus Erythematosus**).

Ninety percent of individuals with SLE have constitutional symptoms with episodes of malaise, fatigue, anorexia, and low-grade fevers (see **Table 10D.2, Manifestations of Systemic Lupus Erythematosus**). Overall, however, the skin (dermatitis) and the musculoskeletal (polyarthritis) system are the most common organs affected. Dermatologic manifestations in hair, mucus membranes, or skin occur in 85–90% of patients with SLE at some point during the course of illness. Cutaneous findings are listed in four of the 11 diagnostic criteria (photosensitivity, oral ulcers, malar rash, and discoid rash). Interestingly, the hallmark "Malar rash" or "Butterfly rash" that appears on the upper cheeks and across the bridge of the nose occurs in only 30% of patients with SLE (Mills 1994). Other common dermatologic symptoms include patchy alopecia and Raynaud's phenomenon.

There are three LE-specific dermatologic presentations: acute cutaneous LE (ACLE), subacute cutaneous LE (SCLE), and chronic cutaneous LE (CCLE). ACLE lesions present acutely as erythema and edema. They can be widespread and frequently appear in a photodistribution pattern. All patients with ACLE have SLE. Lesions seen with SCLE are superficial and symmetrical and can affect sun-protected areas as well as those exposed to the sun. These lesions develop plaques and scaly papules that result in hypopigmentation when resolved. Approximately half the patients with SCLE have SLE. CCLE lesions or discoid lupus are discrete areas of erythematosus induration that develop into plaques with overlying scale, occurring most often in the head and neck areas. Less than 10% of patients with CCLE will develop systemic symptoms.

Ninety-five percent of patients with SLE have joint involvement, which ranges from mild arthralgia to inflammatory arthritis. Muscular atrophy or weakness can be secondary either to the disease itself or to prolonged therapy with corticosteroids. Osteonecrosis secondary to interruption of the blood supply to bone is a rare but debilitating complication of SLE.

The pulmonary, cardiovascular, and gastrointestinal symptoms associated with SLE are secondary to serositis or inflammation of serous membranes, including the linings of lung, heart, or, less frequently, abdominal cavity. Pleuritis occurs in 50% of patients and may be painless or noted in association with pleurisy. Lupus pneumonitis (acute or chronic) is more serious and usually occurs within the first three years following diagnosis (Medsger 1996). A similar proportion of patients will, at

Table 10D.1.   DIAGNOSTIC CRITERIA FOR SYSTEMIC LUPUS ERYTHEMATOSUS

The diagnosis of SLE requires four or more of the following 11 criteria serially or simultaneously during any interval of observation.

1. Malar (butterfly) rash
2. Discoid rash
3. Photosensitivity by patient history or medical observation
4. Oral or nasopharyngeal ulcers observed by a clinician
5. Arthritis: nonerosive, involving two or more joints
6. Serositis:
   - Pleuritis: pleuritic pain, rub heard by clinician or evidence of pleural effusion
     OR
   - Pericarditis documented by EKG or rub, or evidence of pericardial effusion
7. Renal disorder:
   - Persistent proteinuria >5 g/day or >3+ if not quantified
     OR
   - Cellular casts: red cell, hemoglobin, granular, tubular, or mixed
8. Neurologic disorder:
   - Seizures in the absence of drugs or metabolic derangements known to cause seizures
     OR
   - Psychosis in the absence of drugs or metabolic derangements known to cause psychosis
9. Hematologic disorder:
   - Hemolytic anemia with reticulocytosis
   - Leukopenia (<4,000 mm/μL on two or more occasions)
   - Lymphopenia (<1,500 mm/μL on two or more occasions)
     OR
   - Thrombocytopenia (<100,000 mm/μL) in the absence of drugs known to cause thrombocytopenia
10. Immunologic disorder:
    - Positive anti-DNA antibody to native DNA in abnormal titer
      OR
    - Positive anti-Sm (presence of antibody to Sm nuclear antigen)
      OR
    - Positive antiphospholipid antibodies based on:
      - An abnormal serum level of IgG or IgM cardiolipin antibodies
      - A positive test result for lupus anticoagulant using a standard method
        OR
      - A false-positive serologic test for syphilis known to be positive for at least 6 months and confirmed by *Treponema pallidum* immobilization or fluorescent treponemal antibody absorption test
11. Abnormal titer of antinuclear antibody by immunofluorescence or an equivalent assay at any point in time and in the absence of drugs known to be associated with "drug-induced lupus" syndrome

Source: Compiled from Tan, E.M., Cohen, S.S., Fries, J.F. et. al. 1982. The 1982 revised criteria for the classification of systemic lupus erythematosus. *Arthritis and Rheumatism* 25(11):1271–1277; and Hochberg, M.C. 1997. Updating the American College of Rheumatology revised criteria for the classification of systemic lupus erythematosus. *Arthritis and Rheumatism* 40(9):1725.

some point, develop nausea, vomiting, or abdominal pain from peritonitis, perforation, or pancreatitis, all of which are possible effects of the disease or adverse effects of nonsteroidal anti-inflammatory drugs (NSAIDs) used to treat the disease.

Serious organ system abnormalities occur in less than one-third of patients with SLE, but the presence or absence of significant major organ involvement determines the course and severity of disease (Mills 1994). The organ systems most often affected are the renal, hematologic, and central nervous system. Kidney involvement ranges from mild nephritis (asymptomatic proteinuria or hematuria) to glomerulonephritis and/or nephrotic syndrome. Approximately 5% of patients with significant renal disease will ultimately develop renal failure.

Hematologic manifestations of SLE include hemolytic anemia, thrombocytopenia, leukopenia or lymphocytopenia, and a variety of clotting abnormalities. A subset of patients with antiphospholipid syndrome will have autoantibodies (lupus anti-coagulant and/or anticardiolipin antibodies) directed toward cell membrane phospholipids on platelets that result in an increased risk for thromboembolic events.

Major central nervous system (CNS) complications usually occur only in patients with active systemic disease. Although the classic CNS symptoms associated with SLE are seizures, psychosis, and headaches, only migraine-type headaches are clearly linked to the disease process. The etiology of central (or peripheral) nervous system involvement can be multifactorial. Depression and cognitive dysfunction are common, and both can be exacerbated by corticosteroids, which are frequently prescribed for treatment of other symptoms of SLE. NSAIDs can cause aseptic meningitis. Patients with SLE and concomitant antiphospholipid syndrome are predisposed to thromboembolic complications such as transient ischemic attacks, cerebral vascular accidents, or focal neurologic events.

Table 10D.2. MANIFESTATIONS OF SYSTEMIC LUPUS ERYTHEMATOSUS

System	Symptoms	Frequency (%) at Onset	Anytime (%)
Constitutional	Fatigue	-	90
	Fever	36	80
	Weight loss	-	40–60
Integumentary	Malar (butterfly) rash	40	30
	Photosensitivity	29	25–58
	Alopecia	-	71
	Mucosal ulcerations	11	21–30
	Raynaud's phenomenon	18–33	60
	Purpura	-	15
	Urticaria	-	9
Musculoskeletal	Arthritis	44–69	95
	Arthralgia	77	85
	Myositis	3	3
Renal	Any	16–38	50–74
	Nephrosis	5	11–18
Gastrointestinal		-	18
Pulmonary	Pleurisy	16	30–45
	Effusion	-	24
	Pneumonia	-	29
Cardiac	Pericarditis	13	23–48
	Murmurs	-	23
	ECG changes	-	34
Central nervous system	Headache	12	36
	Organic brain syndrome	7	15–20
	Seizures	4	10–20

Source: Compiled from Schur, P.H. 1996. *The clinical management of systemic lupus erythematosus.* Philadelphia: Lippincott-Raven; and Weyand C.M., Wortmann, R., and Klippel, J.H. 1998. *Primer on the rheumatic diseases,* 11th ed. Atlanta, Ga.: Longstreet Press.

Clinical Course of SLE

The clinical course of SLE is variable and unpredictable, although the 10-year survival rate is greater than 90% (Mills 1994, Ruiz-Irastorza et al. 2001). Most patients will have periods of remission and relapse; thus, the course of lupus is expressed in terms of both activity and severity. *Activity* refers to the degree of inflammation whereas *severity* refers to the degree of impairment of a specific organ. An individual can have proteinuria from an acute inflammatory process in the kidney or from scarring secondary to prior acute episodes that results in impairment of function. The prognosis for men and children is less favorable than the prognosis for women. Persons with renal or CNS involvement have a poorer prognosis than those without manifestations in these organ systems (Gladman 1996). Infection is the most common cause of death and may be secondary to either the disease or prolonged treatment with immunosuppressive agents (Gladman 1996). The risk of life-threatening complications is greatest during the first five years following diagnosis.

Table 10D.3.   LABORATORY TESTS FOR SYSTEMIC LUPUS ERYTHEMATOSUS

Test	Definition	Clinical Implications
Antinuclear antibody (ANA)	• Detects a diverse number of antibodies to various cellular nuclear materials. • Reported as both a titer and pattern (speckled, homogenous, nucleolar, centromere, rim). • The patterns reflect the variability in immunofluorescence staining that different antibodies have.	• Useful screening test for diagnosis. • A negative ANA virtually excludes SLE. • A positive ANA indicates a need for more specific tests, as 32% of healthy individuals will have a positive ANA. • Titers are not sensitive indicators of disease, but high titers are more likely seen in patients with SLE. Low titers are more common in nonaffected individuals. • Patients with SLE can have a positive ANA with any pattern. Therefore, the pattern cannot make for a conclusive diagnosis.
Anti-dsDNA (anti-dsDNA)	• Detects presence of antibodies to double-stranded DNA. • Reported as titer.	• dsDNA antibodies are present in 30–50% of patients with SLE and are associated with systemic lupus and nephritis but not subacute cutaneous lupus or discoid lupus. • Anti-dsDNA is specific for SLE and therefore useful for diagnosis, although a negative anti-dsDNA does not rule out SLE. • Rising titers may be associated with disease progression.
Anti-Sm	• Antibodies to RNA protein that are found in plasma. • Reported as titer.	• Anti-Sm antibodies are specific for SLE and are one of the diagnostic criteria, but do not predict disease severity or clinical presentation. • Anti-Sm may appear with disease evolution.
Anti-Ro/SS-A and Anti-LA/SS-B	• Antibodies to RNA protein that are found in plasma. • Antigens originally termed SS-A and SS-B in patients with Sjögren's syndrome were found to be the same antigens as anti-Ro and anti-LA. • Reported as titer.	• Present in 30% (Ro/SS-A) and 15% (LA/SS-B) of patients with SLE. These antibodies are also seen in patients with Sjögren's syndrome. • Anti-Ro/SS-A alone is more common in SLE, whereas both antibodies are seen in Sjögren's syndrome. • Patients with anti-Ro/SS-A but not anti-LA/SS-B are more likely to have photosensitivity, nephritis, and thrombocytopenia. • Pregnant patients with either of these antibodies are at risk for neonatal SLE and congenital heart block. • Anti-LA/SS-B alone is associated with a decreased risk for nephritis.
Antiphospholipid antibodies: lupus anticoagulant (LAC) and anticardiolipin antibodies	• Antibodies directed toward the phospholipids on cell membrane. Cause platelet aggregation and thrombus formation. • Several tests for LAC: the Russell viper venom test (RVVT), activated PTT, and kaolin clotting time. • Reported as titer.	• Found in 5–10% of patients with SLE. Also present in drug-induced lupus and other autoimmune diseases. • Patients with LAC are at increased risk for thromboembolic complications, thrombocytopenia, and recurrent miscarriage. • Lupus anticoagulant was termed "anticoagulant" because this antibody causes prolongation of coagulation tests in vitro via interference in phospholipid cell membrane interactions in the coagulation cascade.

Source: Compiled from Shojania, K. 2000. Rheumatology: 2. What laboratory tests are needed? *Canadian Medical Association Journal* 162:1157–1163; Egner W. 2000. The use of laboratory tests in the diagnosis of SLE. *Journal of Clinical Pathology* 53:424–432; Hadi, H.A., and Treadwell, E.L. 1990. Lupus anticoagulant and anticardiolipin antibodies in pregnancy: a review 1. Immunochemistry and clinical implications. *Obstetrical and Gynecological Survey* 45(11):780–785.

Table 10D.4. DRUGS THAT CAN CAUSE LUPUS-LIKE SYNDROME

Definite Association	Possible Association
Chlorpromazine	Beta-blockers
Isoniazid	Captopril
Methyldopa	Hydralazine
Quinidine	Lithium
Procainamide	Penicillamine
	Phenytoin and other anticonvulsants

Laboratory Findings

The presence of autoantibodies to DNA, RNA, or occasionally other intracellular components is characteristic of several autoimmune disorders; therefore, there is no serologic test that confirms the diagnosis of SLE alone. Serologic data are only of value when interpreted in light of clinical findings.

The most common serologic test used to screen for SLE is the antinuclear antibody test (ANA). The ANA detects the presence of any antibody to nuclear material. More than 95% of patients with SLE will have a positive ANA. The absence of ANAs makes SLE highly unlikely. However, because ANA antibodies are common in persons with other connective tissue disorders and even in persons without disease, a positive test is not specific for SLE (Egner 2000, Shojania 2000).

Interpretation of tests for specific autoantibodies is difficult. Test values differ by type of assay and institutional reference ranges. The levels obtained do not correlate well with the severity of disease and their presence may vary in an individual over time. **Table 10D.3, Laboratory Tests for Systemic Lupus Erythematosus**, reviews the utility of various autoantibodies used in making the diagnosis of SLE.

Complications of SLE

Complications of SLE can be either secondary to the disease process or to the treatment and include osteonecrosis, atherosclerotic vascular disease, gastrointestinal (GI) disease, and myopathy. Osteonecrosis or avascular necrosis of the hip is a major source of morbidity in patients with SLE. This complication occurs if there is interruption of the blood supply to the bone. The poorly vascularized femoral and humeral heads are particularly vulnerable. Coronary atherosclerosis is more likely to occur in persons with SLE, independent of the classic risk factors such as smoking or hypertension (Karrar 2001).

Drugs used to treat SLE can have adverse effects as well. Corticosteroid treatment can result in osteoporosis and myopathy that manifest as muscle weakness. Treatment with NSAIDs has well known complications as well, which most often affect the GI system (i.e., peptic ulcer, GI bleeding). In addition, treatment with corticosteroids may increase the risk of NSAID-induced ulcers.

Differential Diagnosis of SLE

SLE has been called "the great imitator" because the clinical symptoms are nonspecific and overlap a great deal with other diseases. Therefore, the differential diagnosis is an important step in evaluating a patient with symptoms that are suggestive of SLE. The differential diagnosis includes other connective tissue disorders such as rheumatoid arthritis, mixed connective tissue disorder, scleroderma, and polymyositis. The issue is complicated by the fact that these diseases have overlapping features, and one can evolve into another (Wallace 1995). In addition, several medications can cause a lupus-like syndrome (see **Table 10D.4, Drugs that Can Cause Lupus-Like Syndrome**). Each year, approximately 15,000–20,000 cases of prescription drug-induced lupus are reported in the United States (Wallace 1995).

Management of SLE

The cornerstone of managing SLE is patient monitoring over time in order to detect flares and initiate treatment promptly. Treatment of SLE is tailored to specific symptoms and organ systems. Patient education and anticipatory guidance for managing activities of daily living are critical components of caring for patients with SLE.

Pharmacologic treatment of SLE should be managed by a physician specialist. A detailed discussion is beyond the scope of this chapter. The four classes of drugs most commonly used include anti-inflammatory agents, antimalarials, immunosuppressive agents, and cytotoxic agents. Drug therapy starts with the use of NSAIDs for treatment of arthritis, mild serositis, and musculoskeletal symptoms. Immunosuppressive drugs and cytotoxic drugs are used for patients with severe disease or major organ involvement. Cytotoxic drugs are used to suppress immune function and are generally reserved for persons with severe disease and/or those who have failed treatment with corticosteroids. Antimalarial drugs effectively treat skin rashes, mouth ulcers, and arthritis and are the drug of choice for SCLE (Gladman 1996). Corticosteroids are recommended for both their anti-inflammatory and immunosuppressive properties and thus are prescribed frequently.

Contraception, Pregnancy, and Hormone Replacement Therapy (HRT)

Historically, women with SLE have been counseled to avoid oral contraceptives or HRT because higher estrogen levels promote thrombogenesis and increase antiphospholipid antibody levels in mice (Boumpas 1995). The use of exogenous estrogens increases the risk of developing SLE in otherwise healthy women, but estrogens do not appear to exacerbate SLE per se. Although estrogens increase the risk of thromboembolism, women with SLE who do not have active nephritis or antiphospholipid syndrome may consider oral contraceptives (Lakasing et al. 2001, Mok et al. 2001a).

Pregnancy does not adversely affect the natural history of SLE. There are conflicting data on the incidence of flares during pregnancy, with some authors reporting an increase and some authors reporting no significant change (Silver et al. 1997). The exceptions are those women who conceive during a flare and those with active nephritis at the time of conception. In these two cases, the risk of flare during pregnancy can be as high as 55%, and pregnancy can accelerate the deterioration of renal status. Accordingly, women with SLE are counseled to delay pregnancy until a time of remission and should be referred to a perinatologist for preconceptional counseling (Mok et al. 2001b).

SLE can adversely affect the course of pregnancy. Women with SLE have an increased risk of miscarriage, pre-eclampsia, intrauterine growth retardation, and preterm birth (Hadi et al. 1990, Ostensen 2001). The fetus can develop neonatal lupus erythematosus or heart block. Both conditions are treatable and, if mild, usually resolve after birth (Rahman et al. 1998)

DATABASE

SUBJECTIVE

→ See **Table 10D.5, Screening Questionnaire for Systemic Lupus Erythematosus**.

→ The patient is most likely female and between puberty and menopause.

→ Symptoms may include:
- Constitutional symptoms:
  - Fatigue
  - Malaise
  - Anorexia and/or weight loss
  - Fevers (sudden onset of high fever, chills and musculoskeletal pain may represent a lupus flare)
- Pain:
  - Upon breathing (pleuritic)
  - Dyspnea, cough, fever (lupus pneumonitis)
  - Substernal pain aggravated by motion (pericarditis)
  - Persistent nontraumatic joint pain of variable duration (arthralgia)
  - Nausea and vomiting or abdominal pain (peritonitis)
  - Myalgias and "morning stiffness"
  - Monoarticular hip or shoulder pain (osteonecrosis)

- Dermatologic symptoms:
  - Malar (butterfly) rash or discoid rash (discoid rashes leave areas of hypo- or hyperpigmentation on resolution)
  - Alopecia

→ Past medical health history may include:
- Recurrent pregnancy loss
- Rashes following exposure to sun
- Pain and/or pallor in fingers or toes when exposed to cold
- Nocturia, change in urine color, or creation of foam with urination

→ Family history may include:
- History of SLE (10–20% of patients will have a first degree relative with SLE)

OBJECTIVE

→ Vital signs may be normal or the patient may have fevers. (Sudden onset of high fever, chills, and musculoskeletal pain may represent a lupus flare.)

→ Dermatologic findings may include:
- Malar rash (ACLE or SCLE)
- Rashes in photodistribution pattern (ACLE or SCLE)
- Scaly papules or plaques (SCLE)
- Diffuse areas of hypo- or hyperpigmentation (SCLE)
- Discoid lesions (CCLE)
- Hives
- Urticarial vasculitis
- Bullous skin lesions
- Telangiectasia
- Painless oral ulcers
- Alopecia (patchy, diffuse, scarring, or nonscarring)

→ Musculoskeletal findings may include:
- Nondeforming symmetrical joint pain, most often in digits and small joints
- Periarticular subcutaneous nodules along the extensor surfaces of the upper extremities

→ Cardiac findings may include:
- Pericardial friction rub (pericarditis)

Table 10D.5.   SCREENING QUESTIONNAIRE FOR SYSTEMIC LUPUS ERYTHEMATOSUS

1. Have you ever had arthritis or rheumatism for more than three months?
2. Do your fingers become pale, numb, or uncomfortable in the cold?
3. Have you had any sores in your mouth for more than two weeks?
4. Have you been told that you have low blood counts (anemia, low WBC count, or low platelet count)?
5. Have you ever had a prominent rash on your cheeks for more than a month?
6. Does your skin break out after you have been in the sun (not sunburn)?
7. Has it ever been painful to take a deep breath for more than a few days (pleurisy)?
8. Have you ever been told that you have protein in your urine?
9. Have you ever had a rapid loss of hair?
10. Have you ever had a seizure, convulsion, or fit?

Source: Adapted with permission from Schur, P.H. 1996. *The clinical management of systemic lupus erythematosus.* Philadelphia: Lippincott-Raven.

→ Pulmonary findings may include:
- Pleural friction rub (pleurisy)
- Rales (pneumonitis)
- Basilar dullness (pleural effusion)

→ Gastrointestinal findings may include:
- Diffuse tenderness
- Splenomegaly
- Hepatomegaly
- Pancreatitis

→ Renal findings may include:
- Mild disease—none
- Lupus nephritis—edema, hematuria, hypertension, or thrombocytopenia purpura

→ Hematologic findings may include:
- Fatigue (anemia)
- Easy bruising or spontaneous bleeding (thrombocytopenia)

→ Neurologic findings may include:
- Cognitive dysfunction
- Psychosis
- Seizures
- Organic brain syndrome
- Depression

→ Ob/gyn findings may include:
- Menorrhagia
- Recurrent spontaneous abortion
- Infertility

ASSESSMENT

→ Systemic lupus erythematosus
→ R/O drug induced lupus
→ R/O connective tissue disorders
- Rheumatoid arthritis
- Sjögren's syndrome
- Polymyositis
- Mixed connective tissue disorder
- Scleroderma
→ R/O viral hepatitis (B and C)
→ R/O syphilis
→ R/O parvovirus infection
→ R/O Stills disease
→ R/O CREST syndrome
→ R/O psoriatic arthritis

PLAN

DIAGNOSTIC TESTS

→ Lab tests should include: ANA, RF, VDRL, and urinalysis with evaluation of sediment.
→ Additional lab tests for differential diagnosis may include: anti-dsDNA, anti-RO/SS-A and anti-LA/SS-B, Russell Viper Venom test (or aPTT), anticardiolipin antibody.
→ Additional tests for specific symptoms may include:
- Muscle enzymes (R/O myositis)
- Liver function tests (elevated in active disease)
- 24-hour urinalysis for protein (nephritis or nephrotic syndrome)
- X-ray of digits does not reveal erosive changes (R/O rheumatoid arthritis)
- EKG findings typical of pericarditis may be present in patients with or without symptoms of pericarditis.
- Non-specific EKG abnormalities are indicative of conduction defects.
- Echocardiography may or may not reveal pericardial effusion.
- Chest x-ray may reveal pleural effusions (pleurisy), alveolar infiltrates (acute pneumonitis), or diaphragm elevation and fibrosis (chronic pneumonitis).
- Abdominal sonogram may reveal organomegaly and/or ascites.

TREATMENT/MANAGEMENT

→ Nonpharmacologic treatments include:
- Patient education
→ Pharmacologic treatments include:
- NSAIDs
- Corticosteroids
- Antimalarial drugs

CONSULTATION

→ Pharmacologic treatment should be initiated and monitored by an internist or rheumatologist. Treatment regimens are individualized and guided by clinical manifestations, which will vary from patient to patient and change over time within individuals.

PATIENT EDUCATION

→ Symptoms of lupus flare include malaise, poor appetite, weight loss or gain, fatigue, irregular or heavy menses, fever, mood changes, hair loss, oliguria, mouth sores, chest pain, edema, painful joints, shortness of breath, persistent headaches, nausea, and vomiting.
→ Patients with photosensitivity should be advised to use a high-factor protective sunscreen when unable to avoid sun exposure. The greatest support will come from using broad-spectrum sunscreens and wearing clothing made from tightly woven fabric.
→ Emotional support is necessary for patients and family members. NPs can help patients with SLE master the activities of daily living with appropriate assessment and guidance.
→ Patients on medications should be counseled about adverse side effects.
→ Diet:
- Encourage low-lipid diet (elevated risk for atherosclerosis)
- Calcium supplements (elevated risk for osteoporosis)
→ Sex, contraception, and pregnancy:
- IUDs contraindicated (elevated risk of infection)

- High-dose oral contraceptives contraindicated (elevated risk of migraines, phlebitis)
- Barrier methods safest
- Pregnancy associated with elevated risk of miscarriage, but pregnancy does not adversely affect the progress of SLE

→ Skin products:

- Sunscreen recommended with maximum SPF ratings (photosensitivity)
- Avoid medications that are photosensitizing sulfonamides, penicillin

→ Resource materials for SLE patients:

- Lupus Foundation of America
  1300 Piccard Drive, Suite 200
  Rockville, Md. 20850-4303
  (301) 670-9292
  (800) 558-0121
  www.lupus.org

- American Lupus Society
  260 Maple Court, Suite 123
  Ventura, Calif. 93003
  (805) 339-0443

- Bay Area Lupus Foundation
  2635 N. First St., #206
  San Jose, Calif. 95134
  (408) 954-8600
  www.balf.org

FOLLOW-UP

→ Document in progress notes and on problem list.
→ Return to clinic on a prn basis.

BIBLIOGRAPHY

Boumpas, D.T. 1995. Systematic lupus erythematosus: emerging concepts part 2: *Annals of Internal Medicine* 123:42–53.

Egner, W. 2000. The use of laboratory tests in the diagnosis of SLE. *Journal of Clinical Pathology* 53:424–432.

Gladman D.D. 1996. Prognosis and treatment of systemic lupus erythematosus. *Current Opinion in Rheumatology* 8:430–437.

Gordon, C., and Salmon, M. 2001. Update on systemic lupus erythematosus: autoantibodies and apoptosis. *Clinical Medicine* 1:10–14.

Greenstein, B.D. 2001. Lupus: Why women? *Journal of Women's Health and Gender Based Medicine* 10:233–239.

Hadi, H.A., and Treadwell, E.L. 1990. Lupus anticoagulant and anticardiolipin antibodies in pregnancy: a review 1. Immunochemistry and clinical implications. *Obstetrical and Gynecological Survey* 45(11):780–785.

Hochberg, M.D. 1997. Updating the American College of Rheumatology revised criteria for the classification of systemic lupus erythematosus. *Arthritis and Rheumatism* 40:1725.

Karrar, A., Sequeira, W., and Block, J.A. 2001. Coronary artery disease in systemic lupus erythematosus: a review of the literature. *Seminars in Arthritis and Rheumatism* 30:436–443.

Lakasing, L., and Khamashta, M. 2001. Contraceptive practices in women with systemic lupus erythematosus and/or antiphospholipid syndrome: What advice should we be giving? *Journal of Family Planning and Reproductive Health Care* 27(1):7–12

Medsger, T.A. 1996. In *The clinical management of systemic lupus erythematosus*, ed. P.H. Schur, pp. 87–93. Philadelphia: Lippincott-Raven.

Mills, J.A. 1994. Systemic lupus erythematosus. *New England Journal of Medicine* 333:1873–1896.

Mok, C.C., Lau, C.S., and Wong, R.W. 2001a. Use of exogenous estrogens in systemic lupus erythematosus. *Seminars in Arthritis and Rheumatism* 30:426–435.

Mok, C.C., and Wong, R.W. 2001b. Pregnancy in SLE. *Postgraduate Medical Journal* 77:157–165.

Ostensen, M. 2001. Rheumatological disorders. *Best Practice & Research Clinical Obstetrics and Gynecology* 15(6):953–969.

Rahman, P., Gladman, D.G., and Urowitz, M.B. 1998. Clinical predictors of fetal outcome in systemic lupus erythematosus. *Journal of Rheumatology* 25:1526–1530.

Ruiz-Irastorza G.A., Munther A.K., Castellino G. et al. 2001. Systemic lupus erythematosus. *Lancet* 357:1027–1032.

Schur, P.H. 1996. Historical perspective and changing history. In *The clinical management of systemic lupus erythematosus*, ed. P.H. Schur, pp. 5–6. Philadelphia: Lippincott-Raven.

Shojania, K. 2000. Rheumatology: 2. What laboratory tests are needed? *Canadian Medical Association Journal* 162:1157–1163.

Silver, R.K., and Branch, D.W. 1997. Autoimmune disease in pregnancy. *Clinics in Perinatology* 24:291–320.

Somers, E., Magder, L.S., and Petri, M. 2002. Antiphospholipid antibodies and incidence of venous thrombosis in a cohort of patients with systemic lupus erythematosus. *Journal of Rheumatology* 29(12):2531.

Tan, E.M., Cohen, S.S., Fries, J.F. et. al. 1982. The 1982 revised criteria for the classification of systemic lupus erythematosus. *Arthritis and Rheumatism* 25:1271–1277.

Wallace, D.J. 1995. *The lupus book: a guide for patients and their families.* New York: Oxford University Press.

_____. 1997. Differential diagnosis and disease associations. In *Dubois' lupus erythematosus*, 5th ed., eds. D.J. Wallace, and B.H. Hahn, p. 947. Baltimore, Md.: Lippincott Williams & Wilkins.

JoAnne M. Saxe, R.N., M.S., A.N.P., B.C.

10-E
Thyroid Disorders

The primary functions of the adult thyroid gland are to synthesize and secrete *L-thyroxine* (T_4) and 3,5,3'-triiodothyronine (T_3), active hormones that contribute to the regulation of an array of metabolic processes. These functions are orchestrated by a number of intrathyroidal and extrathyroidal influences (e.g., contributions from the hypothalamus and pituitary). Thus, when an individual presents with signs and symptoms suggestive of an altered circulation of thyroid hormones or enlargement of the gland (goiter), extrathyroidal factors/pathology should be suspected in addition to intrinsic thyroid gland pathology.

The three thyroid conditions that the primary care provider is most likely to encounter in ambulatory care settings are:

Primary Hypothyroidism

→ A condition caused by insufficient hormone secretion from the thyroid gland.
→ The most common causes of hypothyroidism are (Goroll 2000b, Tunbridge et al. 2000):
  ▪ Thyroid inflammatory diseases (e.g., chronic [Hashimoto's] thyroiditis, postpartum [subacute lymphocytic] thyroiditis, and subacute thyroiditis)
    • The initial presentation of thyroiditis, however, is often consistent with a diagnosis of thyrotoxicosis.
  ▪ Radioiodine-induced or surgically induced hypothyroidism
  ▪ Idiopathic thyroid atrophy

Thyrotoxicosis

→ A condition resulting from excessive serum concentrations of thyroid hormones (Dabon-Almirante et al. 1998).
→ The most common causes of thyrotoxicosis are:
  ▪ Primary hyperthyroidism
    • Diffuse toxic (hyperfunctioning) goiter (Graves' disease)
    • Toxic multinodular goiter
    • Toxic uninodular goiter
  ▪ Thyrotoxicosis without primary hyperthyroidism
    • Thyroid inflammatory diseases (e.g., Hashimoto's thyroiditis, postpartum thyroiditis, and subacute thyroiditis)

Thyroid Nodules

→ May be benign or malignant.

Primary hypothyroidism, a condition in which there is a loss of thyroid function secondary to pathology within the gland itself, accounts for 95% of all cases of hypothyroidism (Ross 1999). The prevalence of primary hypothyroidism for the general population ranges from 1–2%. Additionally, primary hypothyroidism is 10 times more common in women than men and is predominantly seen in women over age 50 (Tunbridge et al. 2000).

The most common cause of primary thyroid deficiency in iodine-replete regions is *Hashimoto's thyroiditis*, a chronic immune-mediated condition. In addition, a number of other thyroid inflammatory disorders, as part of the illness trajectory, may cause a longstanding hypothyroidism (e.g., some women with postpartum thyroiditis) or a self-limiting hypothyroidism (e.g., most women with postpartum thyroiditis and the vast majority of individuals with subacute thyroiditis). Approximately one-third of all cases of primary hypothyroidism are radioiodine-induced or surgically induced (Tunbridge et al. 2000.) Finally, a significant number of cases may be due to idiopathic thyroid atrophy.

Thyrotoxicosis can result from a variety of diseases. The most common diseases that cause ongoing overproduction of thyroid hormone(s) are Graves' disease, toxic multinodular goiter, and toxic uninodular goiter. Thyroid inflammatory diseases such as Hashimoto's thyroiditis, postpartum thyroiditis, or subacute thyroiditis may also produce a transient form of thyrotoxicosis. The prevalence of thyrotoxicosis, collectively, in women is approximately 2%, with the greatest prevalence in women over age 50 (Wang et al. 1997). Thyrotoxicosis, like hypothyroidism, is 10 times more prevalent in women than in men (Tunbridge et al. 2000).

In *diffuse toxic goiter (Graves' disease)*, extrathyroidal autoimmune processes stimulate excessive hormonal synthesis in the thyroid gland. This disorder usually occurs in women 20–50 years old (Jameson et al. 2001). Toxic multinodular goiter is a disease of the older adult, which often evolves from a longstanding simple goiter (thyroid enlargement without any clinical or laboratory manifestations of altered thyroid functions) (Siegel et al. 1998). In addition, an autonomously functioning single thyroid nodule (toxic uninodular goiter) is another relatively common disorder that may occur at any age but is more often noted in the older population.

A variety of thyroid inflammatory diseases may cause a transient and often mild form of thyrotoxicosis. Due to rapid destruction of thyroid tissue, a sudden release of thyroid hormones ensues, causing signs and symptoms consistent with thyrotoxicosis. Except for Hashimoto's thyroiditis, many thyroid inflammatory conditions reflect self-limiting conditions. After an individual proceeds through the cycles of hyperfunctioning and hypothyroidism, respectively, she recovers and returns to a euthyroid state (normal thyroid status). However, many individuals with Hashimoto's thyroiditis and a few women with postpartum thyroiditis eventually develop a permanent form of hypothyroidism.

Thyroid nodules are extremely common entities that often go undetected by the clinician because the nodules may be very small or located in a posterior region of the gland or because the clinician's physical examination was limited (Ross 1991, Wang et al. 1997).

Thyroid nodules may be functional (e.g., toxic uninodular goiter) or nonfunctional (e.g., benign follicular adenomas). The incidence of thyroid nodules, single and multiple, increases as one ages. Although these neoplasms are usually benign, a malignancy should be suspected, particularly if only one nodule is noted in an individual without any manifestations of an altered hormone status, and/or with a history of head, neck, or upper chest irradiation.

DATABASE
SUBJECTIVE

Primary Hypothyroidism

→ Signs and symptoms:
- Early manifestations include fatigue, a modest weight gain, dry skin, constipation, arthralgias/myalgias, heavy menses, or amenorrhea (menorrhagia is a more common presentation than amenorrhea, however), and/or cold intolerance.
- As the condition progresses, an individual will present with ongoing weight gain, notable dry skin, coarse hair, and/or hoarseness.
- Characteristic myxedematous presentations associated with severe hypothyroidism include the presence of lethargy, flat affect, daytime somnolence, continued weight gain, puffy and doughy skin, hair loss, dysphagia, dysarthria secondary to tongue enlargement, exaggerated hoarseness, decreased hearing, dyspnea, chest pain, severe constipation, joint complaints, hand pain and paresthesias (carpal tunnel syndrome), depressed mood, and/or an ataxic gait (rare).

→ Past health history may include (Jameson et al. 2001):
- Thyroiditis
- Autoimmune disorders that may coexist with primary hypothyroidism (e.g., Type I diabetes mellitus, pernicious anemia, systemic lupus erythematosus [SLE], and rheumatoid arthritis [RA])
- Thyroid surgery
- Radioiodine therapy
- Head, neck, and/or upper chest irradiation
- Neuroendocrine conditions (e.g., pituitary or hypothalamic tumors or disorders) that may cause secondary/extrathyroidal hypothyroidism
- Ingestion of medications that affect hormone synthesis (e.g., amiodarone, para-aminosalicylic acid, or lithium)
- Iodide administration

→ Patient may have a family history of thyroid disease and/or other endocrine disorders.
→ Personal/social and occupational/environmental health history may include:
- Iodine-deficient diet (now uncommon due to iodination programs in most communities where there is iodine-deficient soil)
- Childhood and/or work-related exposure to radiation or radioactive iodine

Thyrotoxicosis

→ Signs and symptoms:
- The most common manifestations are increased appetite, weight loss, generalized weakness, excessive perspiration, frequent bowel movements, irregular menses or amenorrhea, heat intolerance, insomnia, nervousness, and/or tremors.
- In the elderly population, the most common symptoms and signs are generalized weakness, weight loss, palpitations, tachycardia or atrial fibrillation, velvety smooth skin, and/or tremor (Dabon-Almirante et al. 1998).

→ Past health history may include:
- Thyroid disorders
- Neuroendocrine conditions (e.g., pituitary tumors)
- Thyroid surgery
- Antithyroid drug use (e.g., propylthiouracil or methimazole)
- Radioiodine therapy
- Ingestion of medications that affect thyroid function (e.g., thyroid hormone supplements, amiodarone or, rarely, lithium)
- Ingestion of iodine

→ Patient may have a family history of thyroid diseases.
→ Personal/social and occupational/environmental health history may include:
- A diet that is relatively high in iodine content (particularly for individuals who previously consumed an iodine-deficient diet due to geographic location [e.g., some regions of South America])

Thyroid Nodules

→ Signs and symptoms:
- If the nodular gland is hypofunctional, the individual may have signs and symptoms consistent with primary hypo-

thyroidism (see the previous discussion of "Primary Hypothyroidism").
- If the nodule(s) is/are autonomously functioning, the individual will often demonstrate signs and symptoms of thyroid hyperfunctioning (see the previous discussion of "Thyrotoxicosis").
- If the nodule(s) is/are nonfunctional, the individual will be without signs and symptoms of an altered thyroid status (euthyroid).
- If surrounding structures have been invaded by the nodule(s), either malignant or benign, the individual may present with complaints of hoarseness and/or dysphagia.

→ Past health history may include:
- Head, neck, and/or upper chest irradiation
- Goitrous thyroid conditions (e.g., Graves' disease)
- Thyroid surgery
- Intake of certain goiter-producing medications (e.g., lithium)
- Health historical data specific for hypothyroidism or thyrotoxicosis. (If the patient demonstrates signs and symptoms for these respective thyroid conditions, then elicit pertinent past health data consistent with hypothyroidism or thyrotoxicosis.)

→ Patient may have family history of goitrous thyroid conditions and/or thyroid cancer.

→ Personal/social and occupational/environmental history may include:
- Regular intake of dietary goitrogens (e.g., turnips or beets)
- Iodine-deficient or iodine-replete diet
- Work-related exposure to radiation or radioactive iodine

OBJECTIVE

Primary Hypothyroidism

→ The following findings may be noted on physical examination:
- Hypothermia if the individual is myxedematous
- Slight to moderate weight gain (usually no more than about 2–4 kg)
- Flat or blunted facial expressions
- Dry skin in early stages of hormonal depletion to pale, rough, and doughy skin with advanced depletion
- Coarse hair that tends to fall out or be brittle
- Periorbital swelling and loss of outer one-third of the eyebrows in myxedema
- Decreased auditory acuity with advanced disease
- Enlarged tongue with advanced disease
- Symmetrically enlarged and smooth thyroid gland, enlarged multinodular gland, or nonpalpable thyroid gland
- Bradycardia
- Signs of congestive heart failure (e.g., S_3, S_4, and jugular venous distention) with advanced disease
- Decreased bowel sounds
- Diminished tendon reflexes or a prolonged relaxation phase

- Depressed affect and poor attention span and/or somnolence

→ Results from commonly ordered diagnostic studies include:
- Altered blood tests:
  - Altered thyroid function tests (see **Table 10E.1, Common Thyroid Tests**)
  - Hyponatremia in severe disease
  - Increased serum cholesterol
  - Mild normocytic, normochromic anemia
- Usually a decreased uptake of radioisotopes, in comparison to normal tissue, via radioactive iodine uptake and/or thyroid scintiscan (see **Table 10E.1**)
- Electrocardiogram (EKG) changes secondary to a hypometabolic state (e.g., bradycardia) and/or pericardial effusion
- Chest x-ray and echocardiographic changes consistent with congestive heart failure in the elderly population, in persons with underlying heart disease, or in advanced thyroid disease

Thyrotoxicosis

→ Common findings on physical examination include (Dabon-Almirante et al. 1998):
- Restlessness
- Warm and moist skin
- Pretibial myxedema with Graves' disease
- Fine and silky hair
- Ocular signs from sympathetic hyperstimulation:
  - Diminished blinking
  - Lid lag
  - Inability to furrow the eyebrows on upward gaze
- Exophthalmus with Graves' disease
- Thyroid bruit
- Abnormal thyroid gland on palpation:
  - Diffusely enlarged with Graves' disease
  - Irregularly enlarged and multinodular gland with toxic multinodular goiter
  - Symmetrically enlarged, tender, or painless thyroid with thyroid inflammatory diseases
  - Single nodule with toxic uninodular goiter
- Tachycardia
- Systolic murmur
- Signs of congestive heart failure (e.g., S_3, S_4, and jugular venous distention)
- Increased bowel sounds
- Fine tremor of the tongue and hands and/or increased tendon reflexes

→ Results from commonly ordered diagnostic studies include:
- Altered thyroid function tests (see **Table 10E.1**)
- Elevated erythrocyte sedimentation rate (ESR) with some of the thyroid inflammatory disorders (e.g., subacute thyroiditis)
- Elevated white blood cell (WBC) count in some thyroid inflammatory diseases (e.g., subacute thyroiditis)
- Usually increased focal or diffuse uptake of radioisotopes in primary hyperthyroidism and low uptake in thyroiditis

Table 10E.1.   COMMON THYROID TESTS

Test	Definition	Clinical Implications	Comments
Serum free T$_4$ (FT$_4$)	Measurement of the metabolically active T$_4$ (unbound to thyroid-binding globulin)	• Decreased in primary hypothyroidism • Increased in thyrotoxicosis	May be increased by various drugs or conditions in individuals who are clinically euthyroid.
Free T$_4$ index (FT$_4$I)	Indirect measurement of FT$_4$	• Decreased in primary hypothyroidism • Increased in thyrotoxicosis • Aids the diagnosis of conditions related to altered thyroid-binding globulins but with unaltered thyroid hormone secretion	May be increased by various drugs or conditions in individuals who are clinically euthyroid.
Serum T$_3$	Measurement of bound and free serum levels of T$_3$	• Increased in T$_3$ thyrotoxicosis	May be increased by various drugs or conditions in individuals who are clinically euthyroid.
Highly sensitive thyroid stimulating hormone (TSH)	Measurement of TSH: an anterior pituitary hormone that stimulates growth and function of thyroid cells	• Sensitive and specific test for the initial assessment of thyroid dysfunction • Increased in primary hypothyroidism • Decreased in most forms of thyrotoxicosis	Values may be altered by certain drugs (e.g., aspirin and lithium).
Serum antithyroid antibodies (e.g., antithyroid peroxidase antibodies [also known as antithyroid microsomal antibody], antithyroglobulin antibodies, and anti-TSH receptor antibodies)	Measurement of immunologic markers for autoimmune thyroid diseases	• High titers of antithyroid peroxidase antibodies and/or antithyroglobulin antibodies are seen in Hashimoto's thyroiditis and Graves' disease. • Anti-TSH receptor antibodies are commonly seen in individuals with Graves' disease.	May be increased in clinically euthyroid individuals.
Radioactive iodine uptake (RAIU)	Measurement of thyroid function via uptake of radioactive iodine (^{123}I or ^{125}I)	• A study used to evaluate defects in thyroid hormone production. • Low uptake of radioactive iodine is noted in persons with hypothyroidism who are not iodine deficient, with thyroiditis, and with factitious thyrotoxicosis. • Increased uptake is often seen in individuals with Graves' disease, toxic multinodular and uninodular goiter.	• A variety of medications may interfere with uptake of the radioisotope. • This test is usually not necessary for the basic evaluation of most thyroid disorders. • Contraindications are iodine allergy, pregnancy, and/or lactation.
Thyroid scintiscan	Visualization of the thyroid gland via a scintillation camera after the administration of a radioactive isotope (e.g., ^{123}I or technetium-99m)	• This test provides information about the structure and function of the thyroid gland. • Increased uptake of the radioactive isotope is noted in a (hot) hyperfunctioning gland or nodule(s) (e.g., Graves' disease and toxic uninodular goiter, respectively). • Decreased uptake is seen in hypothyroidism and/or nonfunctioning (cold) nodule (e.g., thyroid cancer).	• A variety of medications may interfere with uptake of the radioisotope. • This test is usually not indicated for the evaluation of primary hypothyroidism. • Contraindications are iodine allergy, pregnancy, and/or lactation.
Thyroid ultrasonography	Ultrasonic visualization of the thyroid gland	Assists with the assessment of neck masses of questionable thyroid origin	Not an accurate tool for determining the status of nodules (benign versus malignant)

Sources: Compiled from Jameson, J.L., and Weetman, A.P. 2001. Disorders of the thyroid gland. In *Harrison's principles of internal medicine*, 15th ed., eds. E. Braunwald, A.S. Fauci, D.L. Kasper et al., pp. 2060–2084, New York: McGraw-Hill; and Pagana, K.D., and Pagana, T.J. 1998. *Manual of diagnostic and laboratory tests*. St. Louis, Mo.: Mosby.

Table 10E.2.   SUGGESTED APPROACH FOR THE ASSESSMENT OF THYROID DYSFUNCTION

Order the highly sensitive thyroid-stimulating hormone (TSH) test		
↓	↓	↓
Normal TSH → Are secondary causes of hypothyroidism suspected?	**Increased TSH →** Order a serum FT_4 or FT_4I	**Decreased TSH →** Order a serum FT_4 or FT_4I
No → No further testing is indicated. The patient is clinically euthyroid.	Decreased FT_4 or FT_4I — primary hypothyroidism	**Increased FT_4 or FT_4I—primary hyperthyroidism→** Order anti-TSH receptor antibodies • If the antibodies are elevated, the person has an autoimmune thyroid disease (e.g., Graves' disease). • If the antibodies are normal, the patient probably has a non-immune mediated form of thyrotoxicosis (e.g., toxic uninodular goiter). • Consult with a physician to determine the need for a thyroid scintiscan.
Yes → Order a serum FT_4	Increased FT_4 or FT_4I — pituitary (TSH-induced) thyrotoxicosis	**Normal FT_4 or FT_4I—subclinical hyperthyroidism or a rare form of primary hyperthyroidism called T_3 toxicosis →** Does the patient have signs and symptoms consistent with thyrotoxicosis?
Decreased FT_4 — Consult with a physician to determine the necessity for a thyrotropin-releasing hormone (TRH) stimulation test (for assessing the hypothalamic-pituitary function).	**Normal FT_4—subclinical hypothyroidism →** Order thyroid peroxidase antibodies • If the antibodies are elevated, the person has compensated chronic Hashimoto's thyroiditis (subclinical hypothyroidism). • If the antibodies are normal, consult with a physician to determine the necessity for a TRH stimulation test.	**Yes →** Order FT_3 • Increased FT_3-T_3 toxicosis • Consult with a physician to determine the need for a thyroid scintiscan. • **Normal →** Consult with a physician for other diagnostic considerations.
Normal FT_4 — No further testing is indicated. The patient is clinically euthyroid. Consult with a physician for other diagnostic considerations.		**No →** Order anti-TSH receptor antibodies • If the antibodies are elevated, the person has compensated Graves' disease (subclinical hyperthyroidism). • If the antibodies are normal, consult with a physician to determine the necessity for a TRH stimulation test.

Sources: Compiled from Jameson, J.L., and Weetman, A.P. 2001. Disorders of the thyroid gland. In *Harrison's principles of internal medicine*, 15th ed., eds. E. Braunwald, A.S. Fauci, D.L. Kasper et al., pp. 2060–2084, New York: McGraw-Hill; and Wartofsky, L. 1998. Diseases of the thyroid. In *Harrison's principles of internal medicine*, 14th ed., eds. A.S. Fauci, E. Braunwald, K.J. Isselbacher et al., pp. 2012–2035. New York: McGraw-Hill.

via radioactive iodine uptake and/or thyroid scintiscan (see **Table 10E.1**)
- EKG changes consistent with a hypermetabolic state (e.g., sinus tachycardia or atrial fibrillation)
- Chest x-ray and echocardiographic changes consistent with congestive heart failure in the elderly population or in persons with underlying heart disease

Thyroid Nodules

→ Findings on the physical examination are determined by the functional status of the thyroid gland.
- If the patient has a multinodular hypofunctioning gland (e.g., chronic [Hashimoto's] thyroiditis), she will have

objective findings of hypothyroidism (see "Hypothyroidism" in the "Objective" section).
- If the patient has a toxic uninodular goiter, then she will have physical findings consistent with a hyperfunctioning thyroid gland (see "Thyrotoxicosis" in the "Objective" section).
- If the patient has one or more thyroid nodules that are afunctional, she will be euthyroid.

→ Results from commonly ordered diagnostic procedures include:
- Altered thyroid function tests if the thyroid gland is hypo- or hyperfunctioning and/or inflamed (see **Table 10E.1**)
- Positive radioisotope uptake (a "hot" nodule) via thyroid

scintiscan in autonomously functioning nodules, which are almost always benign (see **Table 10E.1**)

- Negative to slight radioisotope uptake, which represents "cold" or "warm" nodularity, respectively, in nonfunctioning or hypofunctioning nodular glands
  - These nodules are also usually benign. However, more definitive diagnostic procedures (e.g., fine-needle aspiration [FNA] biopsy should be used for ruling out a malignancy, particularly if there is only one dominant nodule, because malignant nodules are more likely to be cold than hot [see **Table 10E.1**]).
- Malignant, benign, inadequate, or indeterminate/suspicious biopsy results via FNA
- Alterations in other blood tests, the chest x-ray, EKG, and/or echocardiogram if the individual demonstrates signs and symptoms consistent with hypothyroidism or thyrotoxicosis (see the respective "Objective" sections)

ASSESSMENT

→ Hypothyroidism (primary)
→ Thyrotoxicosis
- Primary hyperthyroidism or
- Thyrotoxicosis without hyperthyroidism
→ Thyroid neoplasms
- Benign
- Malignant
→ Rule out other possible causes for the patient's presentation:
- R/O pituitary disease
- R/O hypothalamic disease
- R/O cardiac disease
- R/O psychiatric conditions
- R/O nonthyroidal malignant neoplasm

PLAN

DIAGNOSTIC TESTS

→ See **Table 10E.1** and **Table 10E.2, Suggested Approach for the Assessment of Thyroid Dysfunction**.
→ Diagnostic thyroid studies include, but are not limited to: serum free T4, free T4 index, serum T3, highly sensitive thyroid-stimulating hormone (TSH), serum antithyroid antibodies, radioactive iodine uptake, thyroid scintiscan, and/or thyroid ultrasonography.
→ FNA biopsy is warranted if the patient has a solitary thyroid nodule or a multinodular gland suspected of having a cancerous nodule due to a history of head, neck, and/or upper chest irradiation or a rapid growth of part of the gland.

TREATMENT/MANAGEMENT

Primary Hypothyroidism

→ Consider discontinuing medications/exposures with an antithyroid effect (e.g., lithium).
→ Initiate oral hormone replacement with L-thyroxine in consultation with a physician (Goroll 2000b):
- Initial dosing:

- Young patients without underlying cardiac conditions: 50–100 μg per day
- Elderly patients and/or patients with heart disease: 25 μg per day
- Increase dosing gradually after checking the highly sensitive TSH:
  - 25–50 μg every 4–8 weeks until the highly sensitive TSH is within normal limits
→ Maintain full replacement of L-thyroxine, which is usually between 100–150 μg per day.
→ Hospital management is indicated when there is associated severe respiratory compromise, unstable angina, and/or congestive heart failure.
→ Monitor highly sensitive TSH every 6–12 months or as needed to assess adequacy of treatment (Goroll 2000b).

Thyrotoxicosis

→ Decrease iodine intake if it is thought to be contributing to hyperthyroidism.
→ Initiate use of beta-blocking agents (e.g., propranolol 20 mg QID) to control signs and symptoms related to hyperthyroidism (e.g., nervousness, palpitations, tremor, and heat intolerance) in consultation with a physician (Goroll 2000a).
- Use beta-blockers with caution for patients with congestive heart failure and/or obstructive airway disease unrelated to the thyrotoxicosis.
→ Refer to a physician for use of antithyroid agents (e.g., methimazole, propylthiouracil, or iodide) and/or ablative therapy (e.g., radioactive iodine [^{131}I] or subtotal thyroidectomy).
→ Hospital management is indicated when there is associated respiratory compromise, any hemodynamic instability (e.g., unstable angina, and/or congestive heart failure), and/or psychiatric decompensation.
→ Monitor the highly sensitive TSH after the individual is in remission and every 6–12 months to assess adequacy of treatment and to promptly detect treatment-induced hypothyroidism (Goroll 2000a).
→ Monitor anti-TSH receptor antibodies, if the patient has Graves' disease, every 6–12 months for early detection of any recurrence of this condition (Goroll 2000a).

Thyroid Nodules

→ Consider discontinuing goiter-producing medications.
→ If the patient has a solitary nodule or a distinct nodule within a multinodular gland, refer her to a physician for consideration of biopsy via fine-needle aspiration, thyroid scintiscan, and/or surgical and/or medical (L-thyroxine-suppressive or replacement therapy) treatment.
→ If the patient has a hypofunctioning multinodular goiter (e.g., chronic Hashimoto's thyroiditis), use the hypothyroidism treatment guidelines (see "Hypothyroidism" in the "Treatment/Management" section).
→ If the patient has a toxic multinodular goiter, use the thyrotoxicosis treatment guidelines (see "Thyrotoxicosis" in the "Treatment/Management" section).

CONSULTATION

Hypothyroidism

→ Physician consultation is indicated when:
- Considering invasive/uncommon diagnostic studies (e.g., thyrotropin-releasing hormone stimulation test)
- Initiating oral thyroid replacement therapy
- Considering treatment for subclinical hypothyroidism

→ Consultation with an occupational health provider (nurse practitioner or physician) is indicated if the hypothyroidism is suspected to be associated with a work-related exposure.

→ Physician referral is indicated for individuals who:
- Require hospitalization
- Are myxedematous
- Have secondary hypothyroidism
- Are not responding to conventional medical management

Thyrotoxicosis

→ Physician consultation is indicated when:
- Considering invasive/uncommon diagnostic studies (e.g., thyrotropin-releasing hormone stimulation test)
- Initiating beta-blocking agents
- Considering treatment for subclinical hyperthyroidism

→ Physician referral is indicated for the administration of anti-thyroid agents and/or ablative therapy.

Thyroid Nodules

→ Physician referral is indicated for the diagnostic evaluation and treatment of all patients who have a solitary nodule or a distinct nodule within a multinodular gland.

→ See "Hypothyroidism" and "Thyrotoxicosis," in the "Consultation" section, for recommendations for individuals with hypofunctioning multinodular goiters or toxic multinodular goiters, respectively.

PATIENT EDUCATION

→ Explain to the patient:
- The disease process (signs and symptoms and underlying etiologies)
- Diagnostic studies (preparation, procedure(s), after-care, and cost)
- Management/treatment (mechanism of action, use, precautions, adverse effects, and cost)
- The need for adhering to long-term management recommendations

→ Address the patient's and significant others' concerns and feelings regarding the disease process and/or management of the respective thyroid condition.

→ If indicated, refer the patient to a resource such as:
- Thyroid Foundation of America, Inc.
  410 Stuart St.
  Boston, Mass. 02116
  (800) 832-8321
  www.tsh.org

FOLLOW-UP

→ Emphasize the need for ongoing care for the respective thyroid condition.

→ Document thyroid condition in progress notes and on problem list.

BIBLIOGRAPHY

Dabon-Almirante, C.L.M., and Surks, M.I. 1998. Clinical and laboratory diagnosis of thyrotoxicosis. *Endocrinology and Metabolism Clinics of North America* 27(1):25–35.

Goroll, A.H. 2000a. Approach to patient with hyperthyroidism. In *Primary care medicine: office evaluation and management of the adult patient*, 4th ed., eds. A.H. Goroll and A.G. Mulley, pp. 630–654. Philadelphia: Lippincott Williams & Wilkins.

_____. 2000b. Approach to patient with hypothyroidism. In *Primary care medicine: office evaluation and management of the adult patient*, 4th ed., eds. A.H. Goroll and A.G. Mulley, pp. 653–660. Philadelphia: Lippincott Williams & Wilkins.

Jameson, J.L., and Weetman, A.P. 2001. Disorders of the thyroid gland. In *Harrison's principles of internal medicine*, 15th ed., eds. E. Braunwald, A.S. Fauci, D.L. Kasper et al., pp. 2060–2084. New York: McGraw-Hill.

Pagana, K.D., and Pagana, T.J. 1998. *Manual of diagnostic and laboratory tests.* St. Louis, Mo.: Mosby.

Ross, D.S. 1991. Evaluation of the thyroid nodule. *Journal of Nuclear Medicine* 32(11):2181–2192.

_____. 1999. Hypothyroidism: clinical presentation and interpretation of thyroid function tests. *Primary Care Case Reviews* 2(4):180–186.

Siegel, R.D., and Lee, S.L. 1998. Toxic nodular goiter. *Endocrinology and Metabolism Clinics of North America* 27(1):151–168.

Tunbridge, W.M.G., and Vanderpump, M.P.J. 2000. Population screening for autoimmune thyroid disease. *Endocrinology and Metabolism Clinics of North America* 29(2):239–253.

Wang, C., and Crapo, L.M. 1997. The epidemiology of thyroid disease and implications for screening. *Endocrinology and Metabolism Clinics of North America* 26(1):189–218.

Wartofsky, L. 1998. Diseases of the thyroid. In *Harrison's principles of internal medicine*, 14th ed., eds. A.S. Fauci, E. Braunwald, K.J. Isselbacher et al., pp. 2012–2035. New York: McGraw-Hill.

Margaret A. Scott, R.N., M.S.N., F.N.P.
Elisabeth O'Mara, R.N., M.S., A.N.P., C.D.E.

10-F

Type 1 Diabetes Mellitus

Diabetes mellitus (DM) is a group of disorders characterized by hyperglycemia. This hyperglycemia may be due to defects in insulin secretion, action, usage, and/or production. The American Diabetes Association (ADA), recognizing recent advances in the understanding of the etiology and pathogenesis of diabetes, now defines four classes of diabetes: *Type 1 diabetes mellitus, Type 2 diabetes mellitus, other specific types,* and *gestational diabetes mellitus.* Impaired glucose tolerance (IGT) and impaired fasting glucose (IFG) are not considered clinical entities but refer to metabolic stages between normal glucose regulation and hyperglycemia. These may signify risk factors for the development of diabetes mellitus, especially Type 2 DM (ADA 2001).

Type 1 diabetes mellitus, previously known as *insulin dependent diabetes mellitus* (IDDM) or *juvenile onset diabetes,* usually occurs before age 30 but can occur at any age. Onset of symptoms is frequently abrupt, and ketosis is common. The etiology of Type 1 DM is unknown, but genetics, environmental, and autoimmune factors contribute to its development. Treatment consists of insulin, dietary management and an exercise program (Schuman 1988).

Type 2 diabetes mellitus, previously known as *non-insulin dependent diabetes mellitus* (NIDDM), or *maturity onset* or *adult onset diabetes,* usually occurs after age 40 but may occur at any age. Approximately 75–80% of people with Type 2 DM are obese. Frequently, the patient does not develop symptoms and may have the disease for years before overt symptoms occur or a diagnosis is established. The etiology of Type 2 DM is considered multifactorial. Heredity plays a large role, predisposing the patient to beta cell dysfunction and insulin resistance. Treatment consists of diet alone, diet and oral medication, or diet and insulin.

Gestational diabetes mellitus (GDM) is hyperglycemia that develops during pregnancy. It places the fetus at greater risk of abnormalities at birth, including macrosomia, hypoglycemia, hypocalcemia, and hyperbilirubinemia. In addition, it places the fetus at greater risk for intrauterine death and neonatal mortality (Metzger 1991). Diagnosis is established with an oral glucose tolerance test during weeks 24–28 of gestation. The majority of women with GDM can maintain normal glucose levels through diet alone (Star et al. 1999). (See **Table 10F.1, Criteria for Diagnosis of Diabetes Mellitus.**)

Diabetes is estimated to affect over 16 million individuals in the United States, and it accounts for huge health care expenditures nationwide. Of these 16 million people, approximately 10% have Type 1 DM (U.S. Department of Health and Human Services [USDHHS] 1999). The etiology and pathogenesis of diabetes are complex and evolve as a consequence of pancreatic islet beta cell destruction in the context of genetic and environmental

Table 10F.1. CRITERIA FOR DIAGNOSIS OF DIABETES MELLITUS

1. Symptoms of diabetes plus casual plasma glucose concentration ≥200 mg/dL (11.1 mmol/L). Casual is defined as any time of day without regard to time since the last meal. The classic symptoms of diabetes include polyuria, polydipsia, and unexplained weight loss.

OR

2. FPG* ≥126 mg/dL (7.0 mmol/L). Fasting is defined as no caloric intake for at least 8 hours.

OR

3. 2-h PG[†] ≥200 mg/dL (11.1 mmol/L) during an OGTT.** The test should be performed as described by the World Health Organization (WHO 1985), using a glucose load containing the equivalent of 75 g anhydrous glucose dissolved in water.

In the absence of unequivocal hyperglycemia with acute metabolic decompensation, these criteria should be confirmed by repeat testing on a different day. The third measure (OGTT) is not recommended for routine clinical use.
* Fasting plasma glucose
** Oral glucose tolerance test
† Plasma glucose

Source: Reprinted with permission from American Diabetes Association. 2001. Clinical practice recommendations. *Diabetes Care* 24(1):S12. © 2001 American Diabetes Association.

susceptibility. Unlike Type 2 DM in which hyperglycemia results from insulin resistance and secretory defects, insulin deficiency in Type 1 DM becomes absolute and all individuals eventually require exogenous insulin administration to achieve glucose regulation (Powers 2001).

Based on results of recent clinical trials, most notably the Diabetes Control and Complications Trial (DCCT), the goals of therapy and approach to the management of Type 1 DM have changed dramatically in the last decade. The DCCT demonstrated that intensive treatment regimens and tight glucose control reduced the risks of development or progression of retinopathy, nephropathy, and neuropathy (the major chronic complications of DM) by 50–75%. Results further indicated that *any* improvement in glycemic control is beneficial in slowing the progression of complications, and provided the rationale for tight control, or the achievement of preprandial, bedtime, and glycated hemoglobin (HbA1c) levels as close to normal as possible as the goal of therapy (DCCT Research Group 1993, Powers 2001). (See **Table 10F.2, Glycemic Control for People with Diabetes.**) To this end, current ADA recommendations include frequent self-monitoring of blood glucose (SMBG), medical nutrition therapy (MNT), education in self-management and problem solving, and possible hospitalization for initiation of therapy. It is further emphasized that treatment goals and targets must be individualized to include such factors as age, lifestyle, cultural issues, occupation, cognitive abilities, presence and severity of complications of diabetes, ability to recognize hypoglycemic symptoms, and presence of comorbid conditions (ADA 2001).

In addition to receiving intensive counseling on dietary changes and exercise, all newly diagnosed Type 1 DM patients will require insulin. Dramatic changes in the approach to insulin therapy in Type 1 diabetics have occurred over the past decade. The recent addition of the rapid-acting insulin analogue lispro has allowed patients greater flexibility in insulin administration. The goal of flexible insulin therapy is to most closely mimic the normal physiologic insulin response. There are two components: a basal insulin (intermediate or long-acting insulins such as NPH, lente, or ultralente), which provides longer acting "basal" coverage of fasting hyperglycemia, combined with mealtime injections of short or rapid-acting insulins (regular or insulin lispro) to reduce postprandial hyperglycemia (Hirsch 1998, 1999). (See **Table 10F.3, Time Course of Action of Human Insulin Preparations.**) The number of injections can vary depending on the blood sugar goals and results and the patient's lifestyle and compliance (see **Figure 10F.1, Idealized Insulin Effects of Several Insulin Regimens**). Soon after the diagnosis of Type 1 DM is established and insulin and dietary therapy are prescribed, it is not uncommon for the individual to go through a "honeymoon period" during which little or no insulin is required. After this period, most adult patients require 0.5–1.0 units of insulin per kilogram of body weight per day. Some patients may be candidates for intensive insulin therapy (multiple daily injections) or continuous subcutaneous insulin injections (CSII) using insulin pumps, and should be referred to a diabetes specialty clinic or endocrinology as appropriate (Quinn 2001).

Table 10F.2.   GLYCEMIC CONTROL FOR PEOPLE WITH DIABETES*

	Normal	Goal	Additional Action Suggested
Whole blood values			
Average preprandial glucose (mg/dL)[†]	<100	80–120	<80/>140
Average bedtime glucose (mg/dL)[†]	<110	100–140	<100/>160
Plasma values			
Average preprandial glucose (mg/dL)[‡]	<110	90–130	<90/>150
Average bedtime glucose (mg/dL)[‡]	<120	110–150	<110/>180
HbA1c (%)	<6	<7	>8

* The values shown in this table are by necessity generalized to the entire population of individuals with diabetes. Patients with comorbid diseases, the very young and older adults, and others with unusual conditions or circumstances may warrant different treatment goals. These values are for nonpregnant adults.

"Additional action suggested" depends on individual patient circumstances. Such actions may include enhanced diabetes self-management education, comanagement with a diabetes team, referral to an endocrinologist, change in pharmacological therapy, initiation of or increase in self-monitoring of blood glucose, or more frequent contact with patient.

HbA1c is referenced to a nondiabetic range of 4.0–6.0% (mean 5.0%, SD 0.5%).

[†] Measurement of capillary blood glucose

[‡] Values calibrated to plasma glucose

Source: Reprinted with permission from American Diabetes Association. 2001. Clinical practice recommendations. *Diabetes Care* 24(1):S34. © 2001 American Diabetes Association.

Figure 10F.1. IDEALIZED INSULIN EFFECTS OF SEVERAL INSULIN REGIMENS

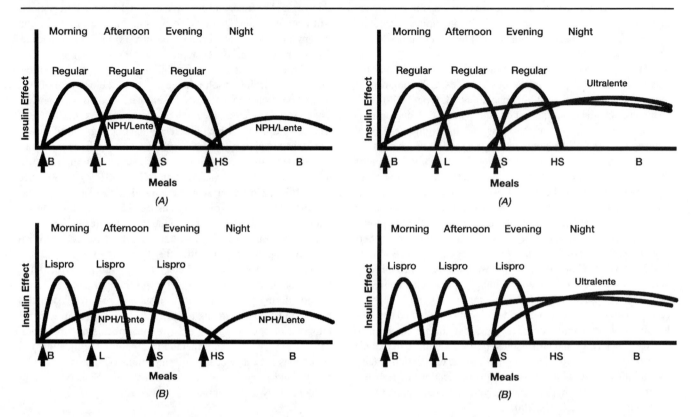

Idealized insulin effect provided by multiple dose regimens providing basal intermediate-acting insulin (NPH or lente) at bedtime and before breakfast, and preprandial injections of short-acting insulin (regular; A) or rapid-acting insulin (lispro; B). B, breakfast; L, lunch; S, supper; HS, bedtime snack. Arrow, time of insulin injection, 30 minutes before meals.

Idealized insulin effect provided by multiple-dose regimen providing basal, long-acting (ultralente) insulin and preprandial injections of short-acting insulin (regular; A) or rapid-acting insulin (lispro; B). B, breakfast; L, lunch; S, supper; HS, bedtime snack. Arrow, time of insulin injection, 30 minutes before meals.

Source: Reprinted with permission from Skyler, J.S. 1998. Insulin treatment. In *Therapy for diabetes mellitus and related disorders,* 3rd ed., ed. H.E. Lebovitz, pp. 186–203. Alexandria, Va.: American Diabetes Association.

Source: Reprinted with permission from Farkas-Hirsch, R. 1998. *Intensive diabetes management,* 2nd ed., p. 85. Alexandria, Va.: American Diabetes Association. *(continued)*

Table 10F.3. TIME COURSE OF ACTION OF HUMAN INSULIN PREPARATIONS

Insulin Preparation		Onset of Action (hours)	Peak Action (hours)	Effective Duration of Action (hours)	Maximum Duration of Action (hours)
Rapid-acting lispro (analog)		¼–½	½–1 ½	3–4	4–6
Short-acting regular (soluble)		½–1	2–3	3–6	6–8
Intermediate-acting NPH (isophane)		2–4	6–10	1–16	14–18
Intermediate-acting lente (insulin-zinc suspension)		3–4	6–12	12–18	16–20
Long-acting ultralente (extended insulin-zinc suspension)		6–10	10–16	18–20	20–24
Combinations	70/30–70% NPH, 30% regular	½–1	Dual	10–16	14–18
Combinations	50/50–50% NPH, 50% regular	½–1	Dual	10–16	14–18

Based on doses of 0.1–0.2 U/kg in the abdomen, for human insulin.

Source: Reprinted with permission from Farkas-Hirsch, R. 1998. *Intensive diabetes management,* 2nd ed. Alexandria, Va.: American Diabetes Association.

Figure 10F.1.   IDEALIZED INSULIN EFFECTS OF SEVERAL INSULIN REGIMENS (continued)

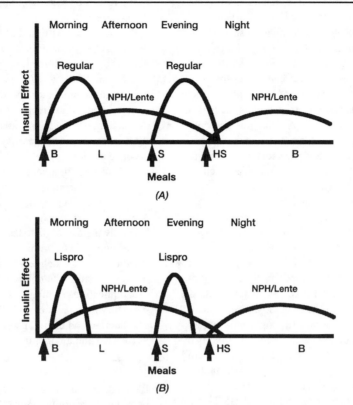

Idealized insulin effect provided by insulin regimen consisting of a morning injection of short-acting insulin and intermediate-acting insulin (NPH or lente), a presupper injection of short-acting insulin, and a bedtime injection of intermediate-acting insulin. A: regular insulin; B: lispro. B, breakfast; L, lunch; S, supper; HS, bedtime snack. Arrow, time of insulin injection, 30 minutes before meals.

Source: Reprinted with permission from Skyler, J.S. 1998. Insulin treatment. In *Therapy for diabetes mellitus and related disorders,* 3rd ed., ed. H.E. Lebovitz, pp. 186–203. Alexandria, Va.: American Diabetes Association.

Complications of Type 1 Diabetes Mellitus

Acute complications of Type 1 DM include *diabetic ketoacidosis* (DKA) and *hypoglycemia* (blood sugar <60 mg/dL). Diabetic ketoacidosis occurs in the environment of insulin deficiency and subsequent glucagon excess. Metabolically, it is characterized by hyperglycemia, ketosis, and acidosis. Symptoms and signs include nausea and vomiting, abdominal pain, thirst, polyuria, altered mental status, shortness of breath, tachycardia, dehydration, hypotension, abdominal tenderness, tachypnea, and lethargy. Diabetic ketoacidosis may result from undiagnosed diabetes, concomitant illness, undetected infections, stress, taking medication incorrectly, or, rarely, too much food. It may be life threatening and requires referral to a physician for hospitalization. The mortality rate with DKA is less than 5% (Centers for Disease Control and Prevention [CDC] 1991b).

Hypoglycemia is a complication resulting from therapy for diabetes, most commonly insulin in Type 1 diabetics. It occurs in an environment of insulin excess, caused by insulin administration, inadequate food intake, or too much exercise. Symptoms are usually gradual in onset and include weakness, irritability, shakiness, perspiration, and hunger. More advanced symptoms include confusion, restlessness, and visual changes, eventually leading to loss of consciousness and convulsions. It is treated with immediate ingestion of carbohydrates or administration of glucagon if severe. Frequent severe episodes of hypoglycemia place the patient at risk for permanent neurological changes and always warrant further investigation of possible preventable causes.

The chronic complications of diabetes mellitus are responsible for the considerable incidence of morbidity and mortality associated with the disease. Microvascular complications include nephropathy, retinopathy, and neuropathy, and the risks for development for all correlate with the duration of disease and degree of hyperglycemia. Diabetic nephropathy is the leading cause of end stage renal disease in the United States, accounting for approximately 40% of new cases (USDHHS 1999). In addition to tight glycemic control, several other interventions have been shown to be effective in decreasing the rate of progression. These include blood pressure targets of <130/80 mmHg, angiotensin converting enzyme (ACE) inhibitor therapy for all Type 1 patients with evidence of microalbuminemia, and dietary protein restriction for those with overt nephropathy (ADA 2001).

Similarly, diabetic retinopathy is the leading cause of blindness in the adult population (USDHHS 1999). Prevention through reduction of hyperglycemia remains the most effective intervention, in conjunction with annual comprehensive eye exams by an ophthalmologist or optometrist (ADA 2001).

Neuropathic complications range from peripheral neuropathy causing pain and decreased sensation to autonomic neuropathy potentially affecting gastrointestinal, cardiovascular, and genitourinary function. All forms are often refractory to treatment, which is mainly symptomatic. Prevention of sequelae such as ulceration and infection of the extremities is paramount. It mandates a thorough inspection of the feet and legs at all medical visits, as well as monofilament testing for sensory loss and rigorous patient education regarding foot care. Referral to a podiatrist specializing in diabetic foot care is also recommended.

Macrovascular complications (coronary artery disease, peripheral vascular disease, and cerebrovascular disease) in diabetics most often occur in association with risk factors such as smoking, dyslipidemia, hypertension, and obesity. The association between macrovascular disease and hyperglycemia is less well established than it is for microvascular disease, but the two are clearly related (Goroll et al. 2000). Since the risks for both heart disease deaths and stroke are up to 2–4 times greater in diabetics than nondiabetics, managing these risk factors is an integral component of care of the diabetic patient (USDHHS 1999). Current ADA recommendations include aggressive counseling regarding lifestyle modifications (weight loss, exercise, smoking cessation, reduction of dietary sodium), blood pressure goals of <130/80 mmHg, lowering LDL cholesterol to <100 mg/dL, lowering triglycerides to <400 mg/dL, and raising HDL cholesterol to >45 mg/dL in men and >55 mg/dL in women (ADA 2001). Prophylactic aspirin therapy (81–325 mg QD) is warranted in diabetics with coronary artery disease and should be considered in those with other coronary risk factors (Powers 2001).

DATABASE

SUBJECTIVE

→ People at risk for Type 1 DM include those with a family history of Type 1 DM.

→ Classic symptoms include increased thirst (polydipsia), frequent urination (polyuria), hunger (polyphasia), frequent infections (including vulvovaginal candidiasis in women), difficulty healing or resolving infections, fatigue, blurred vision, abrupt weight loss.

→ More advanced symptoms may include fruity odor to the breath, abdominal pain, vomiting, dehydration, labored breathing.

→ Elements of a comprehensive medical history of particular concern in patients with diabetes include (ADA 2001):
  ▪ Dietary habits, nutritional status, and weight history
  ▪ Details of previous treatment programs, including diabetes education

  ▪ Current treatment of diabetes, including medications, diet, and results of glucose monitoring, including HbA1c levels
  ▪ Exercise history
  ▪ Frequency, severity, and cause of acute complications such as ketoacidosis and hypoglycemia
  ▪ Prior or current infections, particularly skin, foot, dental, and genitourinary
  ▪ Symptoms and treatment of chronic complications associated with diabetes: eye, heart, kidney, nerve, sexual function, peripheral vascular, and cerebral vascular
  ▪ Other medications that may affect blood glucose concentration
  ▪ Risk factors for atherosclerosis: smoking, hypertension, obesity, hyperlipidemia, and family history
  ▪ Psychosocial, cultural, and economic factors that might influence the management of diabetes
  ▪ Family history of diabetes and other endocrine disorders
  ▪ Gestational history: history of spontaneous abortions, hyperglycemia, delivery of an infant weighing >4,000 g, toxemia, stillbirth, polyhydramnios, or other complications of pregnancy
  ▪ History and treatment of other conditions, including endocrine and eating disorders
  ▪ Tobacco and alcohol use

OBJECTIVE

→ Elements of a comprehensive physical examination of particular concern in patients with diabetes include (ADA 2001):
  ▪ Height and weight
  ▪ Blood pressure (with orthostatic measurements)
  ▪ Annual dilated retinal exam by an experienced ophthalmologist
  ▪ Thyroid palpation
  ▪ Cardiac examination
  ▪ Evaluation of pulses (with auscultation of carotids)
  ▪ Hand/finger examination
  ▪ Foot examination
  ▪ Skin examination (including insulin-injection sites)
  ▪ Neurological examination
  ▪ Dental and periodontal examination

→ If DKA is not present:
  ▪ May have a few of the classic findings as listed previously, or may be asymptomatic

→ If DKA is present, findings may include:
  ▪ Weight loss
  ▪ Fruity odor to the breath
  ▪ Warm, dry skin
  ▪ Dry mucous membranes
  ▪ Poor skin turgor
  ▪ Tachycardia
  ▪ Hypotension
  ▪ Tender abdomen
  ▪ Diminished or absent bowel sounds
  ▪ Hypothermia

- Hyperreflexia
- Somnolence
- Impaired consciousness

ASSESSMENT

- Type 1 diabetes mellitus
- R/O Type 2 diabetes mellitus
- R/O impaired glucose tolerance
- R/O chronic pancreatitis
- R/O Cushing's syndrome
- R/O acromegaly
- R/O pheochromocytoma
- R/O glucagonoma
- R/O drug-induced diabetes

PLAN

DIAGNOSTIC TESTS

→ Laboratory tests to include:
- Random blood glucose for diagnostic purposes; fasting plasma glucose for known diabetes
- White blood cell (WBC) count
- Sodium
- Potassium
- BUN and creatinine
- Bicarbonate
- pH
- Fasting lipid profile: total cholesterol, high-density lipoprotein (HDL), triglycerides, and low-density lipoprotein (LDL)
- HbA1c
- Thyroid stimulating hormone

→ Obtain urine to assess for:
- Ketones
- Glucose
- Protein
- Sediment
- Culture if sediment is abnormal or symptoms are present
- Microalbumin (timed specimen or albumin-to-creatinine ratio) in pubertal and postpubertal Type 1 patients who have had diabetes for at least 5 years

→ ECG

TREATMENT/MANAGEMENT

→ If there is no evidence of DKA, the individual may be managed on an outpatient basis.
- The ADA recommends formulating a management plan in conjunction with the patient, family, physician, and other members of the health care team, including a statement of short- and long-term goals and emphasizing patient self-management as much as possible.

→ Initiate insulin therapy.
- In newly diagnosed Type 1 patients, the total daily dose of insulin is calculated as 0.2–0.6 units/kg/day. Requirements usually increase to 0.5–1.0 units/kg/day.

- Once or twice daily insulin injections are no longer recommended. Multiple flexible insulin therapy programs exist (see **Figure 10F.1**). Approximately 40–50 % of the total daily dose comprises the basal insulin component, and the remainder is divided among the mealtime doses. Examples of 3- and 4-injection-per-day regimens are as follows:
  - Three injections per day with NPH or lente as basal insulin: short-acting regular insulin or lispro and intermediate-acting insulin (NPH or lente) before breakfast, short-acting regular insulin or lispro before the evening meal, and intermediate-acting insulin at bedtime. The administration of NPH or lente at bedtime reduces nocturnal hypoglycemia, and serum insulin levels before breakfast are higher (Hirsch 1999).
  - Three injections per day with ultralente as basal insulin: long-acting ultralente insulin divided equally in the morning and at dinner, with preprandial injections of short-acting regular insulin or lispro at each meal (Farkas-Hirsch 1998).
  - Four injections per day with NPH or lente as basal insulin: small doses of NPH or lente in the morning, a larger dose at bedtime, and short-acting regular insulin or lispro at each mealtime.
- Institute "action plans" to adjust insulin dose, depending on self-monitoring of blood glucose (SMBG) results (see **Table 10F.4, Sample Plan for Premeal Short-Acting [Regular] Insulin Dosing**).
- Prescribe glucagon kit (per physician's consultation).

→ Initiate antihypertensive therapy if blood pressure is >130/80 mmHg.
- Current recommendations include ACE inhibitors as first-line therapy, in combination with selective beta-blockers, calcium channel antagonists, and low-dose diuretics if necessary (Prisant 2001).

→ Initiate ACE inhibitor therapy for all normotensive Type 1 diabetics with microalbuminemia (ADA 2001).

→ Initiate lipid-lowering therapy with HMG-CoA reductase inhibitor (statins) in patients with LDL cholesterol ≥100mg/dL. Add resin if necessary to reach LDL goals (ADA 2001).

→ Initiate aspirin therapy (enteric-coated aspirin 81–325 mg/day) in patients with coexisting coronary heart disease and peripheral vascular disease. If not contraindicated, consider as primary prevention in patients with coronary risk factors (ADA 2001).

→ Refer to a registered dietitian to initiate/instruct about medical nutrition therapy (MNT). The goal of MNT is to assist diabetics in making changes in food intake and exercise to promote improved metabolic control and reduce complications. There is no single "ADA diet"; rather, approaches are individualized based on patient characteristics and goals (ADA 2001). Principles of MNT for Type 1 diabetes include:
- Synchronize food intake with insulin administration.
- Eat at consistent times.

- Learn types of foods and portion sizes.
- Use SMBG to adjust meal plan and insulin doses (Daly et al. 1998).
- Vary carbohydrate intake based on eating habits and glucose goals.
- Moderate daily protein intake to 10–20% of total calories.
- Moderate fat intake to <30% of total caloric intake, with <10% from saturated fat.
- Moderate total cholesterol to <300 mg/day.
- Adjust total caloric intake to achieve and maintain ideal body weight (ADA 2001).

- Drink alcohol in moderation only.
  - Alcohol may inhibit the liver's production of glucose during the fasting state and increase the hypoglycemia effect of insulin (Heins et al. 1992).
  - Limit alcohol intake to 1–2 drinks, 1–2 times per week (ADA 2001).
→ Prescribe an exercise program.
- Screening should include an exercise stress ECG in patients older than 35, a careful ophthalmologic exam to identify proliferative retinopathy, renal function tests, and a neurologic exam to determine peripheral neuropathy (Horton 1998).

Table 10F.4.   SAMPLE PLAN FOR PREMEAL SHORT-ACTING (REGULAR) INSULIN DOSING

Once insulin dosage is stable, use the following scheme for premeal alteration of dosage of regular insulin:

BG <50 mg/dL (<2.8 mmol/L)
- Reduce premeal short-acting insulin by 2–3 U.
- Delay injection until immediately before eating.
- Include at least 10 g of rapidly available carbohydrate in the meal.

BG 50-70 mg/dL (2.8–3.9 mmol/L)
- Reduce premeal short-acting insulin by 1–2 U.
- Delay injection until immediately before eating.

BG 70–130 mg/dL (3.9–7.2 mmol/L)
- Take prescribed premeal dose of short-acting insulin.

BG 130–150 mg/dL (7.2–8.3 mmol/L)
- Increase premeal short-acting insulin by 1 U.

BG 150–200 mg/dL (8.3–11.1 mmol/L)
- Increase premeal short-acting insulin by 2 U.

BG 200–250 mg/dL (11.1–13.9 mmol/L)
- Increase premeal short-acting insulin by 3 U.
- Consider delaying meal 15 minutes (to 45 minutes after injection).

BG 250–300 mg/dL (13.9–16.7 mmol/L)
- Increase premeal short-acting insulin by 4 U.
- Consider delaying meal 20–30 minutes (to 40–60 minutes after injection).

BG 300–350 mg/dL (16.7–19.4 mmol/L)
- Increase premeal short-acting insulin by 5 U. Delay meal 20–30 minutes (to 40–60 minutes after injection).
- Check urine ketones. If moderate to large, increase fluid intake and consider extra insulin (1–2 U). Recheck blood glucose and urine ketones in 2–3 hours.

BG 350–400 mg/dL (19.4–22.2 mmol/L)
- Increase premeal short-acting insulin by 6 U.
- Delay meal 20–30 minutes (to 40–60 minutes after injection).
- Check urine ketones. If moderate to high, increase fluid intake and consider extra insulin (1–2 U). Recheck blood glucose and urine ketones in 2–3 hours.

BG >400 mg/dL (>22.2 mmol/L)
- Increase premeal short-acting insulin by 7 U.
- Delay meal 30 minutes (to 50–60 minutes after injection).
- Check urine ketones. If moderate to high, increase fluid intake and consider extra insulin (1–2 U). Recheck blood glucose and urine ketones in 2–3 hours.

Planned meal is larger than usual
- Increase short-acting insulin by 1–2 U.

Planned meal is smaller than usual
- Decrease short-acting insulin by 1–2 U.

Unusual increased activity planned after eating
- Eat extra carbohydrate and/or decrease short-acting insulin by 1–2 U.

Unusually decreased activity planned after eating
- Consider increasing short-acting insulin by 1–2 U.

Plan assumes the following target goals in young, healthy Type 1 diabetics, and should be individualized for each patient:

Preprandial	70–130 mg/dL
1-h postprandial	100–180 mg/dL
2-h postprandial	80–150 mg/dL
0200–0400	100–140 mg/dL

BG = blood glucose

Source: Reprinted with permission from Skyler, J.S. 1998. Insulin treatment. In *Therapy for diabetes mellitus and related disorders*, 3rd ed., ed. H.E. Lebovitz, pp. 186–203. Alexandria, Va.: American Diabetes Association. © 1998 American Diabetes Association.

- ADA guidelines include blood glucose monitoring before and after exercise with accordant changes in insulin and carbohydrate as needed (ADA 2001).
- Recommend warm-up exercises for 5–10 minutes followed by aerobic exercise (50–70% of patient's maximum oxygen uptake) 3 times per week for 20–45 minutes and a cool-down period of 5–10 minutes (Horton 1998).
- SMBG (see the "Patient Education" section).

CONSULTATION

→ Physician referral required for DKA.

→ Physician consultation required for initiation of insulin therapy and adjustments of insulin dose.

→ Physician consultation required during or after loss of consciousness due to hypoglycemia.

→ Referral to nutritionist for instruction on medical nutrition therapy

→ Referral to appropriate specialist(s) when indicated (i.e., cardiologist, neurologist, nephrologist, ophthalmologist, podiatrist, perinatologist)

→ Referral to diabetes specialty clinic or endocrinologist if the patient is a candidate for intensive insulin therapy or continuous subcutaneous insulin infusion (CSII) therapy

→ Referral to social services when appropriate

PATIENT EDUCATION

→ SMBG
- Instruct the patient how to use the glucometer, including check strip, cleaning, and memory.
  - Advise the patient to bring the meter to all appointments. Recheck her technique at each visit.
- Instruct the patient how to use finger-sticking device and lancets.
  - Choose any finger.
    - Use sides of fingers and tips (avoid finger pads) and rotate sites.
  - Wash hands with soap and warm water.
    - Avoid using alcohol (unless in dirty environment) as it toughens skin.
  - Hang hand at side for 30–60 seconds to obtain blood sample more easily.
- Teach the patient how to record blood glucose results in her record book.
  - Advise the patient to bring her record book to all appointments.
  - Advise the patient what her target blood sugar range should be.

→ Instruct the patient about urine testing for ketones.
- Advise testing for ketones when blood glucose is >240 mg/dL or when the patient is ill.
- Advise the patient to call if ketones are moderate or large.
- Advise the patient to drink extra water if ketones are small.

→ Instruct about administering insulin.
- Instruction to include:
  - Types
  - Source
  - Dose
  - Onset
  - Peak
  - Duration
- Instruct about technique for drawing, measuring, and injecting insulin.
  - Do not aspirate prior to injecting.
- Instruct patient about site rotation.
  - Abdomen has best absorption, followed by arms, thighs, buttocks.
  - Stay in same region, same time of day.
  - Change site by 1 inch each time.
  - Do not use same site more than once every 3–4 weeks.
- Advise the patient to re-use needles if patient has good personal hygiene, has no acute illness or ongoing problems with infection, and is physically capable of safely recapping a syringe. Needles may be re-used until they become dull or bent (ADA 2001).
- Use a needle clipper device to dispose of needle. Discard syringe and lancets in a hard plastic or needle container.
  - Check local county policy for syringe take-back program.
- Advise about insulin storage.
- Keep bottles currently in use at room temperature, out of sunlight for up to 1 month, then discard. If stored, store in door of refrigerator and discard bottle after 3 months.
- Review symptoms, causes, treatment, and prevention of hypoglycemia with the patient and her family. Instruct the patient to carry at least 15 g of carbohydrate to be eaten or taken in liquid form in the event of a hypoglycemic reaction.
- Advise the patient to obtain a medical alert bracelet and explain the bracelet's purpose.
- Instruct the patient and her family members about using the glucagon kit.
- Advise the patient to call if her blood sugar is <60 mg/dL on a daily or weekly basis.

→ Review symptoms, causes, treatment, and prevention of hyperglycemia, including DKA.

→ Describe the importance of following the prescribed meal plan to improve blood sugar control.
- Encourage the patient to check blood sugars 1–2 hours after meals occasionally to see the effects of different foods on blood glucose.

→ Teach the patient about proper sick day management (e.g., colds, flu, infection):
- Explain that illness, stress, or infection may raise her blood sugar.
- Advise patient never to stop taking insulin, unless advised by her provider or if she is experiencing severe hypoglycemia.
- Advise patient to check blood sugar and urine ketones every 4 hours.
- Advise patient to call if blood sugar remains >300 mg/dL or <60 mg/dL or if she has trouble breathing or is vomiting (may be sign of DKA).

- Advise patient to drink extra liquids, ½–¾ cup every ½–1 hour.
- Advise patient to weigh herself daily and if there is more than 5-pound loss to call her provider.
- Advise patient to check her temperature and call her provider if temperature is >101°F (38.3°C).
- Advise patient to call if she is having trouble breathing (may be a sign of DKA).

→ Advise patient to have an ophthalmologic dilated retinal examination yearly.

→ Teach patient about proper foot care.

→ Recommend dental examination every 6 months.

→ Review local community resources and national organizations (refer to **Appendix 10F.1, Resources for Patients with Diabetes**).

→ Instruct patient regarding effects of smoking, alcohol, and drugs on diabetes. Counsel about lifestyle modification techniques when indicated.

→ Provide education for the patient's family about all aspects of diabetes care.

FOLLOW-UP

→ Number of visits will depend on blood glucose control, change in treatment program, and presence of complications.

→ May need to contact patient weekly to check on SMBG results.

→ See patient within several weeks or one month if major changes in insulin dose are made.

→ See patient every 3–6 months if she is maintaining treatment goals (see **Table 10F.2**).

→ Per recommendations of the ADA (2001), the interim history should include:
- Frequency, causes, and severity of hypoglycemia or hyperglycemia
- Results of regular glucose monitoring
- Adjustments by the patient of the therapeutic regimen
- Problems with adherence
- Symptoms suggesting development of the complications of diabetes
- Psychosocial status and lifestyle changes
- Other medical illnesses
- Current medications
- Tobacco and alcohol use

→ Physical examination should include:
- Yearly physical examination
- Check weight, blood pressure, and feet every visit, in addition to fundoscopic exam
- Ophthalmologic examination yearly if patient has had the diagnosis of Type 1 DM for more than five years
- Women planning pregnancy should have an eye examination before pregnancy and during their first trimester. Referral to a perinatologist for prepregnancy counseling is strongly advised.

→ Diagnostic tests should include:
- HbA1c at least twice yearly if the patient is meeting treatment goals, quarterly if she is not meeting glycemic goals or if there is a change in therapy
- Fasting cholesterol, HDL, triglycerides and calculated LDL yearly
- Creatinine, urinalysis yearly; after 5 years of Type 1 DM, obtain microalbuminuria by one of three methods (ADA 2001):
  - Albumin-to-creatinine ratio in random spot collection
  - 24-hour collection with creatinine
  - Timed (4-hour or overnight) collection

→ Patient education should include a review of:
- Diet—reasons for success or failure
- Exercise program—reasons for success or failure
- SMBG—technique and results (interpret results with patient)
- Hypoglycemic/hyperglycemic problems, symptoms, treatment, causes, and prevention
- Medications
- Birth control and family planning issues
  - Advise three months of normal HbA1c prior to conception
- Foot care, dental care (CDC 1991a)
- Habits: smoking, alcohol, drugs
- Psychological adjustment (CDC 1991a)
- Complications

→ See the "Treatment/Management" section.

→ Document in progress notes and on problem list.

BIBLIOGRAPHY

American Diabetes Association. 2001. Clinical practice recommendations. *Diabetes Care* 24(1):S1–S133.

Centers for Disease Control and Prevention (CDC). 1991a. *Take charge of your diabetes: A guide for patients.* Atlanta, Ga.: National Center for Chronic Disease Prevention and Health Promotion.

_____. 1991b. *The prevention and treatment of complications of diabetes mellitus, a guide for primary care practitioners.* Atlanta, Ga.: National Center for Chronic Disease Prevention and Health Promotion.

Conlon, P.C. 2001. A practical approach to Type 2 diabetes. *Nursing Clinics of North America* 36(2):193–202.

Daly, A., and Powers, M. 1998. Medical nutrition therapy. In *Therapy for diabetes mellitus and related disorders*, 3rd ed., ed. H.E. Lebovitz, pp. 121–133. Alexandria, Va.: American Diabetes Association.

Diabetes Control and Complications Trial (DCCT) Research Group. 1993. The effect of intensive treatment of diabetes on the development and progression of long-term complications in insulin-dependent diabetes mellitus. *New England Journal of Medicine* 329:977–986.

Eisenbarth, G.S., and Kahn, C.R. 1990. Etiology and pathogenesis of diabetes mellitus. In *Principles and practice of endocrinology and metabolism*, ed. K.L. Becker, pp. 1074–1084. Philadelphia: J.B. Lippincott.

Farkas-Hirsch, R. 1998. *Intensive diabetes management*, 2nd ed. Alexandria, Va.: American Diabetes Association.

Goroll, A.H., and Mulley, A.G. 2000. *Primary care medicine: office evaluation and management of the adult patient*, 4th ed. Philadelphia: Lippincott Williams & Wilkins.

Groop, L.C., Groop. P.H., and Stenman, S. 1990. Combined insulin-sulfonylurea therapy in treatment of NIDDM. *Diabetes Care* 13 (Suppl. 3):47–52.

Haire-Joshu, D., ed. 1992. *Management of diabetes mellitus*. St. Louis, Mo.: Mosby.

Heins, J.M., and Beeke, C.A. 1992. Nutritional management of diabetes mellitus. In *Management of diabetes mellitus*, ed. D. Haire-Joshu, pp. 21-73. St. Louis, Mo.: Mosby.

_____. 1998. Intensive treatment of Type 1 diabetes. *Medical Clinics of North America* 82(4): 689–719.

Hirsch, I.B. 1999. Type 1 diabetes and the use of flexible insulin regimens. *American Family Physician* 60(8):2343–2356.

Horton, E.S. 1998. Exercise. In *Therapy for diabetes mellitus and related disorders*, 3rd ed., ed. H.E. Lebovitz, pp. 150–159. Alexandria, Va.: American Diabetes Association.

Karam, J.H. 1993. Diabetes mellitus and hypoglycemia. In *Current medical diagnoses and treatment*, ed. L.M. Tierney, pp. 912–948. Norwalk, Conn.: Appleton & Lange.

Lebovitz, H.E. 1998. Diagnosis and classification of diabetes mellitus. In *Therapy for diabetes mellitus and related disorders*, 3rd ed., ed. H.E. Lebovitz, pp. 5–7. Alexandria, Va.: American Diabetes Association.

Metzger, B.E., ed. 1991. Proceedings of the Third International Workshop Conference on Gestational Diabetes Mellitus. *Diabetes* 40 (Suppl. 2):1–201.

Peters, A.L., and Davidson, M.B. 1991. Insulin plus sulfonylurea agent for treating Type 2 diabetes. *Annals of Internal Medicine* 115:45–53.

Powers, A.C. 2001. Diabetes mellitus. In *Harrison's principles of internal medicine*, 15th ed., ed. E. Braunwald, pp. 2109–2137. New York: McGraw-Hill.

Prisant, L.M. 2001. Cardiovascular disease: how to reduce the risk in patients with diabetes. *Consultant* 41(3):461–470.

Quinn, L. 2001. Pharmacologic management of the patient with Type 2 diabetes. *Nursing Clinics of North America* 36(2):217–242.

Schuman, C.R. 1988. Diabetes mellitus: definition, classification, and diagnosis. In *Diabetes mellitus*, 9th ed., eds. J.A. Galloway, J. Potvin, and C.R. Schuman, pp. 2–13. Indianapolis: Eli Lilly and Co.

Skyler, J.S. 1998. Insulin treatment. In *Therapy for diabetes mellitus and related disorders*, 3rd ed., ed. H.E. Lebovitz, pp. 186–203. Alexandria, Va.: American Diabetes Association.

Sobel, D.S., and Ferguson, T. 1985. *The people's book of medical tests*. New York: Summit Books.

Star, W.L., and Murphy, J. 1999. Gestational diabetes mellitus. In *Ambulatory obstetrics*, 3rd ed., eds. W.L. Star, M.T. Shannon, L.L. Lommel et al. San Francisco: University of California-San Francisco Nursing Press.

U.S. Department of Health and Human Services (USDHHS). 1999. *Diabetes statistics*. Washington, D.C.: the Author. Available at: http://www.niddk.nih.gov/health/diabetes/pubs/dmstats/dmstats.htm. Accessed on June, 6, 2001.

White, N.H., and Henry, D.N. 1992. Special issues in diabetes management. In *Management of diabetes mellitus*, ed. D. Haire-Joshu, pp. 249–309. St. Louis, Mo.: Mosby.

World Health Organization. 1985. *Diabetes mellitus report of a WHO study group*. Technical Report Serial No. 727. Geneva: World Health Organization.

APPENDIX 10F.1.

Resources for Patients with Diabetes

- American Diabetes Association
  (800) DIABETES
  (800) 342-2383
  www.diabetes.org

- American Association of Diabetes Educators
  (800) 338-DMED
  www.aadenet.org

- American Dietetic Association
  (800) 877-1600
  (800) 366-1655
  www.eatright.org

- Centers for Disease Control and Prevention
  Division of Diabetes Translation
  (877) 232-3422
  www.cdc.gov/diabetes

- National Institute of Diabetes and Digestive and Kidney Diseases of the National Institutes of Health
  National Diabetes Information Clearinghouse
  (301) 654-3327
  www.niddk.nih.gov

Margaret A. Scott, R.N., M.S.N., F.N.P
Elisabeth O'Mara, R.N., M.S., A.N.P., C.D.E.

10-G
Type 2 Diabetes Mellitus

Diabetes mellitus (DM) is a group of disorders characterized by hyperglycemia. This hyperglycemia may be due to defects in insulin secretion, action, usage, and/or production. The American Diabetes Association (ADA), recognizing recent advances in the understanding of the etiology and pathogenesis of diabetes, now defines four classes of diabetes: *Type 1 diabetes mellitus, Type 2 diabetes mellitus, other specific types,* and *gestational diabetes mellitus*. Impaired glucose tolerance (IGT) and impaired fasting glucose (IFG) are not considered clinical entities but refer to metabolic stages between normal glucose regulation and hyperglycemia. These may signify risk factors for the development of diabetes mellitus, especially Type 2 (see **Table 10F.1, Criteria for Diagnosis of Diabetes Mellitus** in the **Type 1 Diabetes Mellitus** chapter and **Table 10G.1, Categories of Glucose Tolerance**)(ADA 2001).

Type 1 diabetes mellitus, previously known as *insulin dependent diabetes mellitus* (IDDM) or *juvenile onset diabetes,* usually occurs before the age of 30 but can occur at any age. The onset of symptoms is frequently abrupt and ketosis is common. The etiology of Type 1 DM is unknown, but genetics and environmental and autoimmune factors contribute to its development.

Gestational diabetes mellitus (GDM) is hyperglycemia that develops during pregnancy. It places the fetus at greater risk of abnormalities at birth, including macrosomia, hypoglycemia, hypocalcemia, and hyperbilirubinemia. In addition, it places the fetus at greater risk for intrauterine death and neonatal mortality (Metzger 1991). Diagnosis is established with an oral glucose tolerance test during weeks 24–28 of gestation. The majority of women with GDM can maintain normal glucose levels through diet alone (Star et al. 1990).

Type 2 diabetes mellitus, previously known as *noninsulin dependent diabetes mellitus* (NIDDM), *maturity onset,* or *adult onset diabetes,* usually occurs after age 40 but may occur at any age. Approximately 75–80% of people with Type 2 DM are obese. Frequently, the patient does not develop symptoms and may have the disease for years before overt symptoms occur or a diagnosis is established. Ninety percent of the estimated 16 million individuals with diabetes in the United States have Type 2 diabetes, and the prevalence is increasing both nationally and globally. Prevalence data for certain ethnic and racial groups show an increased risk for Type 2 DM among African American, Hispanic American, Asian American, and Pacific Islander groups as compared with non-Hispanic whites. Native American populations have the highest rates (Quinn 2001a).

In addition to environmental factors (i.e., nutrition and physical activity), genetics play a larger role in Type 2 DM than in Type 1. Individuals who have a parent with Type 2 DM are at increased risk for developing the disease; this risk approaches 40% if both parents are affected. Similarly, identical twins share a 70–90% concordance rate for developing the disease (Powers 2001). Other significant risk factors include obesity, age greater than 45 years, history of IFG or IGT, history of GDM, or delivery of an infant who weighs more than nine pounds or 4,000 g, hypertension, and elevated lipids.

The pathogenesis of Type 2 DM is characterized by complex interactions between three primary abnormalities: impaired

Table 10G.1.   CATEGORIES OF GLUCOSE TOLERANCE

Fasting Plasma Glucose

Normal:	<110 mg/dL (<6.1 mmol/L)
Impaired fasting glucose:	≥100 mg/dL (≥6.1 mmol/L) and <126 mg/dL (<7.0 mmol/L)
Diabetes:	≥126 mg/dL (7.0 mmol/L)

2-h Postload Plasma Glucose (OGTT)

Normal:	<140 mg/dL (7.8 mmol/L)
Impaired glucose tolerance:	≥140 mg/dL (7.8 mmol/L) and <200 mg/dL (11.1 mmol/L)
Diabetes	≥200 mg/dL (11.1 mmol/L)

Source: Reprinted with permission from Lebovitz, H.E. 1998. Diagnosis and classification of diabetes mellitus. In *Therapy for diabetes mellitus and related disorders,* 3rd ed., ed. H.E. Lebovitz, p. 6. Alexandria, Va.: American Diabetes Association. © 1998 American Diabetes Association.

insulin secretion secondary to pancreatic beta cell dysfunction, insulin resistance in muscle and liver tissue, and increased hepatic glucose production (Feinglos et al. 1998). Individuals with Type 2 diabetes may be asymptomatic at the time of diagnosis. The diagnosis is often made by a routine urinalysis or random blood glucose. Recent epidemiological data suggest that Type 2 DM may be present up to 10 years prior to diagnosis and that as many as 50% of individuals with Type 2 diabetes have one or more diabetes-specific complications at diagnosis. When the typical symptoms of polyuria, polydipsia, and polyphagia do occur, they are usually much less acute than those seen in patients with Type 1 diabetes, and ketosis is rare (Schuman 1988). These data have prompted the ADA to revise screening guidelines for the disease (see **Table 10G.2, Criteria for Testing for Diabetes in Asymptomatic, Undiagnosed Individuals**).

Several studies have demonstrated the value of tight glycemic control in reducing the morbidity and mortality associated with Type 2 diabetes. Most notably, the United Kingdom Prospective Diabetes Study (UKPDS) concluded that intensive pharmacologic therapy to lower blood glucose levels to as near normal as possible significantly reduced the risks of progression of microvascular complications in Type 2 disease. While no statistically significant effect on cardiovascular complications was

Table 10G.2. CRITERIA FOR TESTING FOR DIABETES IN ASYMPTOMATIC, UNDIAGNOSED INDIVIDUALS

1. Testing for diabetes should be considered in all individuals at age 45 or older and, if normal, it should be repeated at 3-year intervals.

2. Testing should be considered at a younger age or be carried out more frequently in individuals who:
   - Are obese ($\geq 120\%$ desirable body weight or a BMI ≥ 27 kg/m^2)
   - Have a first-degree relative with diabetes
   - Are members of a high-risk ethnic population (e.g., African American, Hispanic American, Native American, Asian American, Pacific Islander)
   - Have delivered a baby weighing >9 lb. or have been diagnosed with GDM
   - Are hypertensive ($\geq 140/90$)
   - Have an HDL cholesterol level ≤ 35 mg/dL (0.90 mmol/L) and/or a triglyceride level ≥ 250 mg/dL (2.82 mmol/L)
   - On previous testing, had IGT or IFG

The OGTT or FPG test may be used to diagnose diabetes; however, in clinical settings the FPG test is greatly preferred because of ease of administration, convenience, acceptability to patients, and lower cost.

Source: Reprinted with permission from American Diabetes Association. 2001. Clinical practice recommendations. *Diabetes Care* 24(1):S15. © 2001 American Diabetes Association.

observed with tight glycemic control, the study did establish the importance of aggressive treatment of blood pressure in reducing both macro- and microvascular complications (ADA 2001, UKPDS 1998). Treatment strategies for Type 2 DM now focus on: 1) achieving glycated hemoglobin (HbA1c) levels of less than 7% through diet, exercise, and medications (see **Table 10F.2, Glycemic Control for People with Diabetes** in the **Type 1 Diabetes Mellitus** chapter); 2) aggressive treatment of coexisting hypertension, dyslipidemia, coronary heart disease, and obesity; and 3) screening for and management of chronic complications (nephropathy, neuropathy, and retinopathy).

Experts agree that treatment of Type 2 diabetes should begin with a targeted and systematic approach to diet and exercise (the ADA recognized term is *medical nutrition therapy* [MNT]). Weight loss and body fat reduction are associated with acute reductions in blood sugar and are thus considered the cornerstone of therapy for Type 2 diabetics. Caloric restriction has direct effects on the metabolic mechanisms responsible for alterations in glycemic control and has repeatedly been shown to reduce hepatic glucose production, enhance insulin secretion, and improve insulin action in the periphery (Feinglos et al. 1998). All newly diagnosed individuals should be referred to a registered dietician familiar with current ADA recommendations.

Strict adherence to dietary and lifestyle changes may sustain normoglycemia in some individuals; however, most require pharmacologic therapy within several months of diagnosis. The UKPDS demonstrated that only 15% of patients achieved glycemic targets with diet and exercise therapy alone (Riddle 1999). Given the marked heterogeneity in phenotypic expression of Type 2 diabetes, selection of pharmacologic agents based on specific patient characteristics is paramount in helping patients to achieve normoglycemia. In addition to insulin, there are now five classes of oral agents available in the United States to treat Type 2 diabetes. Differing mechanisms of action among the classes affords the provider more flexibility in targeting specific defects, and choice of agents should be based on patient characteristics and lifestyle issues. Type 2 diabetes is a chronic and progressive disorder, and most patients who are initially well-controlled with oral agents eventually require administration of exogenous insulin. As insulin becomes the mainstay of therapy, it may be beneficial to add metformin or a thiazolidinedione to decrease insulin resistance, thereby reducing the necessity for larger insulin doses (Goroll et al. 2000). Ongoing studies are evaluating the effectiveness of intensive insulin therapy regimens and continuous subcutaneous insulin infusion using insulin pumps in Type 2 diabetes (see the "Treatment/Management" section for "stepped care" approach, and **Table 10G.3, Comparison of Oral Agents for Type 2 Diabetes**).

Complications of Type 2 Diabetes Mellitus

Acute complications of Type 2 diabetes include hyperosmolar hyperglycemic nonketotic syndrome (HHNS) and hypoglycemia. The underlying causes of HHNS are insulin deficiency and inadequate fluid intake. The condition may be precipitated by silent myocardial infarction, sepsis, serious infections

Table 10G.3. COMPARISON OF ORAL AGENTS FOR TYPE 2 DIABETES

	Mechanism of Action	Starting Daily Dosage (mg/day)	Usual Maintenance Dose	Patient Considerations	Contraindications
Sulfonylureas					
Chlorpropamide	Increase insulin secretion	250	500 mg QD	Recommended for recently diagnosed patients who are not totally insulin deficient, those with FPG <300, not obese	Type 1 DM
Tolbutamide		1,000–2,000	1,000 mg TID		Pregnancy or lactation
Glimepiride		1–2	4 mg QD		Hypersensitivity to sulfonylureas
Glipizide		5	10 mg BID		Severe liver or kidney disease
Glyburide		1.5–5	5 mg BID		Caution in elderly or conditions causing hypoglycemia
Meglitinide					
Repaglinide	Increase insulin secretion	1.5–6	4 mg TID	Recommended for recently diagnosed patients with postprandial hyperglycemia, patients with sulfa allergy who cannot take sulfonylureas	Type 1 DM Pregnancy or lactation Renal or hepatic dysfunction
Biguanides					
Metformin	↓ hepatic glucose production; ↑ glucose utilization	500 mg BID	1,000 mg BID	Recommended for recently diagnosed patients who are obese	Serum creatinine >1.4 in women or 1.5 in men or abnormal creatinine clearance Acute or chronic metabolic acidosis CHF requiring pharmacologic therapy Severe hepatic dysfunction Heavy ETOH use
α-Glucosidase Inhibitors					
Acarbose	↓ glucose absorption	25 mg TID*	50 mg TID	Recommended for patients with postprandial hypergly-cemia, patients with renal impairment who cannot use metformin	Patients with gastrointestinal disorders Liver disease
Miglitol		25 mg TID*	50 mg TID		
Thiazolidinediones					
Rosiglitazone	↓ insulin resistance; ↑ glucose utilization	4	4 mg BID	Recommended for patients with marked insulin resistance (extreme obesity)	Liver disease or elevated LFTs (LFTs must be monitored before treatment, q 2 months for 1 year, and q 4 months thereafter) Type 1 DM Pregnancy or lactation Severe CHF
Pioglitazone		15–30	45 mg QD		

*With first bite of each meal

Sources: Compiled from Powers, A.C. 2001. Diabetes mellitus. In *Harrison's principles of internal medicine*, 15th ed., ed. E. Braunwald, pp. 2109–2137. New York: McGraw Hill; Quinn, L. 2001. Pharmacologic management of the patient with Type 2 diabetes. *Nursing Clinics of North America* 36(2):217–242; and Riddle, M.C. 1999. Oral pharmacologic management of Type 2 diabetes. *American Family Physician* 60(9):2613–2620.

such as pneumonia or pancreatitis, stroke, or certain pharmacologic agents (glucocorticoids, diuretics, phenytoin, beta-blockers, and calcium channel blockers) (Genuth 1998). HHNS is typically characterized by severe hyperglycemia (>1,000 mg/dL), hyperosmolarity, severe dehydration, and altered mental status (Powers 2001). Ketosis is rarely seen. HHNS may occur in individuals age 60 years or older who have Type 2 DM that is untreated or undiagnosed. Immediate referral to a physician for hospitalization is required because the mortality rate has been reported to be as high as 50% for these patients (CDC 1991b).

Hypoglycemia (blood glucose levels <60 mg/dL) is a complication resulting from therapy for diabetes (either insulin or oral agents). Symptom onset is usually gradual and includes weakness, irritability, shakiness, perspiration, and hunger. More advanced symptoms include confusion, restlessness, and visual changes, eventually leading to loss of consciousness and convulsions. It is treated with immediate ingestion of carbohydrates, or administration of glucagon if severe. It is less prominent in Type 2 diabetes than in Type 1, but should not be overlooked. All patients on oral or insulin therapy should be counseled regarding recognition of symptoms and treatment.

The chronic complications of diabetes mellitus are responsible for the considerable morbidity and mortality associated with the disease. Microvascular complications include nephropathy, retinopathy, and neuropathy. The risks of developing these correlate with the duration of disease and degree of hyperglycemia. Diabetic nephropathy is the leading cause of end stage renal disease in the United States and accounts for approximately 40% of new cases (USDHHS 1999). In addition to tight glycemic control, several other interventions have been shown to be effective in decreasing the rate of progression. These include blood pressure targets of <130/80 mmHg, ACE inhibitor therapy for all hypertensive Type 2 patients with evidence of microalbuminemia, and dietary protein restriction for those with overt nephropathy (ADA 2001).

Similarly, diabetic retinopathy is the leading cause of blindness in the adult population (USDHHS 1999). Preventing this complication by reducing hyperglycemia remains the most effective intervention, in conjunction with annual comprehensive eye exams by an ophthalmologist or optometrist (ADA 2001).

Neuropathic complications range from peripheral neuropathy causing pain and decreased sensation to autonomic neuropathy potentially affecting gastrointestinal, cardiovascular, and genitourinary function. All forms are often refractory to treatment, which is mainly symptomatic. Prevention of sequelae such as ulceration and infection of the extremities is paramount. It mandates a thorough inspection of the feet and legs at all medical visits, monofilament testing for sensory loss, and rigorous patient education regarding foot care. Referral to a podiatrist specializing in diabetic foot care is also recommended.

Macrovascular complications (coronary artery disease, peripheral vascular disease, and cerebrovascular disease) in diabetics most often occur in association with risk factors such as smoking, dyslipidemia, hypertension, and obesity. The association between macrovascular disease and hyperglycemia is less well-established than it is for microvascular disease, but the two are clearly related (Goroll et al. 2000). Since the risks for both heart disease deaths and stroke are up to 2–4 times greater in diabetics than nondiabetics, managing these risk factors is an integral component of care of the diabetic patient (USDHHS 1999). Current ADA recommendations include aggressive counseling regarding lifestyle modifications (weight loss, exercise, smoking cessation, reduction of dietary sodium), blood pressure goals of <130/80 mmHg, lowering LDL cholesterol to <100 mg/dL, lowering triglycerides to <400 mg/dL, and raising HDL cholesterol to >45 mg/dL in men and >55 mg/dL in women (ADA 2001). Prophylactic aspirin therapy (81–325 mg QD) is warranted in diabetics with coronary artery disease and should be considered in those with other coronary risk factors (Powers 2001).

DATABASE

SUBJECTIVE

→ Risk factors for Type 2 diabetes include (Powers 2001):
  ■ African American, Hispanic American, Asian American, Pacific Islander, or Native American origin
  ■ Family history of Type 2 diabetes
  ■ Obesity (≥20% over ideal body weight or body mass index [BMI] ≥27)
  ■ Age ≥45 years
  ■ Gestational diabetes mellitus or delivery of baby >4,000 g
  ■ Previously identified individuals with impaired glucose tolerance or impaired fasting glucose
  ■ Hypertension (blood pressure ≥140/90 mm Hg)
  ■ HDL cholesterol ≤35 mg/dL and/or triglycerides ≥250 mg/dL
  ■ Polycystic ovarian syndrome
→ Patient may be asymptomatic.
→ Symptoms may include frequent urination (polyuria), thirst (polydipsia), weight loss, blurred vision, or frequent infections (including vulvovaginal candidiasis in women).
→ Presenting symptoms of numbness, paresthesias, or visual problems may be chronic complications secondary to undiagnosed hyperglycemia.
→ Elements of a comprehensive medical history of particular concern in patients with diabetes include (ADA 2001):
  ■ Dietary habits, nutritional status, and weight history
  ■ Details of previous treatment programs, including diabetes education
  ■ Current treatment of diabetes, including medications, diet, and results of glucose monitoring, including HbA1c levels
  ■ Exercise history
  ■ Frequency, severity, and cause of acute complications such as HHNS and hypoglycemia
  ■ Prior or current infections, particularly skin, foot, dental, and genitourinary
  ■ Symptoms and treatment of chronic complications associated with diabetes: eye, heart, kidney, nerve, sexual function, peripheral vascular, and cerebral vascular
  ■ Other medications that may affect blood glucose concentration

- Risk factors for atherosclerosis: smoking, hypertension, obesity, hyperlipidemia, and family history
- Psychosocial and economic factors that might influence the management of diabetes
- Family history of diabetes and other endocrine disorders
- Gestational history: hyperglycemia, delivery of an infant weighing >4,000 g, toxemia, stillbirth, polyhydramnios, or other complications of pregnancy
- History and treatment of other conditions, including endocrine and eating disorders
- Tobacco and alcohol use

OBJECTIVE

→ Elements of a comprehensive physical examination of particular concern in patients with diabetes include (ADA 2001):
- Height and weight measurement, BMI
- Blood pressure determination (with orthostatic measurements)
- Annual dilated retinal exam by an experienced ophthalmologist
- Thyroid palpation
- Cardiac examination
- Evaluation of pulses (with auscultation of carotids)
- Foot examination
- Skin examination
- Neurological examination
- Dental and periodontal examination

ASSESSMENT

→ Type 2 versus Type 1 diabetes mellitus (depends on age, risk factors, presence of ketosis)
→ R/O impaired glucose tolerance
→ R/O hyperglycemia secondary to prescription medications (diuretics, glucocorticosteroids)
→ Following diagnosis, consider the following (although doubtful) as contributing factors:
- Cushing's syndrome
- Acromegaly
- Pheochromocytoma
- Glucagonoma

PLAN

DIAGNOSTIC TESTS

→ Screen individuals with one or more risk factors or symptomatic patients with fasting glucose (see **Table 10G.2**).
→ Laboratory tests to include:
- Random blood glucose for diagnostic purposes; fasting plasma glucose for known diabetes
- White blood cell (WBC) count
- Sodium
- Potassium
- Creatinine
- Bicarbonate
- Fasting lipid profile: total cholesterol, high-density lipoprotein (HDL), triglycerides, and low-density lipoprotein (LDL)

- Microalbumin (timed specimen or albumin-to-creatinine ratio) in all Type 2 patients
- HbA1c
- Liver function tests prior to initiating pharmacologic agents
- Thyroid stimulating hormone

→ Obtain urine to assess for:
- Ketones
- Glucose
- Protein, including microalbumin
- Sediment
- Culture if sediment is abnormal or symptoms are present

→ ECG

TREATMENT/MANAGEMENT

→ If there is no acute illness present and blood glucose is <240 mg/dL:
- Refer to a registered dietitian to initiate/instruct in medical nutrition therapy (MNT). The goal of MNT in Type 2 diabetes is to help diabetics make changes in food intake and exercise to promote weight loss, improve glucose and lipid levels, and reduce complications. There is no single "ADA diet"; rather, approaches are individualized based on patient characteristics and goals (ADA 2001). Principles of MNT for Type 2 diabetes include:
  - Modifying fat intake
  - Improving food choices
  - Restricting calories if obese
  - Varying carbohydrate intake based on eating habits and glucose goals
  - Daily protein intake should be 10–20% of total calories.
  - Fat intake should be <30% of total caloric intake, with <10% from saturated fat.
  - Total cholesterol should be <300 mg/day.
  - Total caloric intake is calculated to achieve and maintain ideal body weight (ADA 2001).
  - Alcohol is advised in moderation only.
    - Limit intake to 1–2 drinks, 1–2 times per week (ADA 2001).

→ Prescribe exercise program.
- Screening should include an exercise stress ECG in patients age 35 or older, a careful ophthalmologic exam to identify proliferative retinopathy, renal function tests, and a neurologic exam to determine peripheral neuropathy (Horton 1998).
- Recommend warm-up exercises for 5–10 minutes followed by aerobic exercise (50–70% of patient's maximum oxygen uptake) 3 times per week for 20–45 minutes and a cool-down period of 5–10 minutes (Horton 1998).

→ If blood glucose targets are not achieved after a 4–8 week trial of diet and exercise, initiate a "stepped care" approach to treatment, beginning with a single oral agent (see **Table 10F.2** and **Table 10G.3**):
- If fasting plasma glucose (FPG) is <240 mg/dL, sulfonylureas and metformin are usually the initial agents of choice as long as liver and kidney functions are normal.

- Sulfonylureas are recommended for both overweight and nonobese patients, and metformin if the patient is obese.
- Newly diagnosed individuals with the following characteristics should be considered for insulin therapy at the outset: lean individuals or those with severe weight loss, those with underlying renal or hepatic disease precluding use of oral agents, and those who are acutely ill or hospitalized (Powers 2001).
- Counsel women of childbearing age that they should use birth control measures if on an oral agent.
  - If they are planning to get pregnant, switch to insulin and attempt normal HgbA1c before they conceive. Refer to perinatologist for preconception counseling.
→ If target goals (FPG <126 mg/dL and HbA1c <7%) are not achieved after 8–12 weeks of monotherapy, consider combination therapy with another oral agent:
- Common combinations include the addition of metformin to sulfonylurea or sulfonylurea to metformin, sulfonylurea plus thiazolidinedione, and sulfonylurea plus α-glucosidase inhibitor (see **Table 10G.3**).
→ Insulin therapy is indicated if initial or ongoing FPG remains >240 mg/dL despite MNT, exercise, and maximum doses of 2 oral agents.
- Add evening intermediate-acting insulin to current oral regimen.
  - For patients with BMI <30, add NPH insulin at bedtime to control fasting hyperglycemia.
  - For patients with BMI >30, add 70/30 insulin at dinnertime to minimize postprandial hyperglycemia and control fasting glucose (Riddle 1997).
- In patients who do not achieve target goals with 1 injection plus 1 or more oral agents, discontinue oral agents and start primary insulin therapy.
  - Some patients with Type 2 DM may be managed on 2 injections per day consisting of NPH or lente as basal insulin in combination with regular insulin or lispro given at breakfast and dinner.
  - For those patients in whom target goals are not reached with twice daily injections, multiple flexible insulin therapy programs exist (see **Figure 10F.1, Idealized Insulin Effects of Several Insulin Regimens** in the **Type 1 Diabetes Mellitus** chapter). Approximately 40–50% of the total daily dose comprises the basal insulin component, and the remainder is divided among the mealtime doses. Examples of 3- and 4-injection-per-day regimens are as follows:
    - Three injections per day with NPH or lente as basal insulin: short-acting regular insulin or lispro and intermediate-acting insulin (NPH or lente) before breakfast, short-acting regular insulin or lispro before the evening meal, and intermediate-acting insulin at bedtime. The administration of NPH or lente at bedtime reduces nocturnal hypoglycemia, and serum insulin levels before breakfast are higher (Hirsch 1998).

- Three injections per day with ultralente as basal insulin: long-acting ultralente insulin divided equally in the morning and at dinner, with preprandial injections of short-acting regular insulin or lispro at each meal (Farkas-Hirsch 1998).
- Four injections per day with NPH or lente as basal insulin: small doses of NPH or lente in the morning, a larger dose at bedtime, and short-acting regular insulin or lispro at each mealtime.
- Institute "action plans" to adjust insulin dose, depending on self-monitoring of blood glucose (SMBG) results (see **Table 10F.4, Sample Plan for Premeal Short-Acting [Regular] Insulin Dosing** in the **Type 1 Diabetes Mellitus** chapter).
- Prescribe glucagon kit (per physician's consultation).
→ Initiate antihypertensive therapy if BP >130/80 mmHg.
- Current recommendations include ACE inhibitors as first-line therapy, in combination with selective beta-blockers, calcium channel antagonists, and low-dose diuretics if necessary (Prisant 2001).
→ Initiate ACE inhibitor therapy for all hypertensive Type 2 diabetics with microalbuminemia (ADA 2001).
→ Initiate lipid-lowering therapy with HMG-CoA reductase inhibitor (statins) in patients with LDL cholesterol ≥100mg/dL. Add resin if necessary to reach LDL goals (ADA 2001).
→ Initiate aspirin therapy (enteric-coated aspirin 81–325 mg/day) in patients with coexisting coronary heart disease (CHD) and peripheral vascular disease. If not contraindicated, consider as primary prevention in patients with CHD risk factors (ADA 2001).

CONSULTATION

→ Physician consultation for initiation and adjustment of oral agents or insulin
→ Physician referral for hospital management if HHNS is suspected
→ Physician consultation required during or after loss of consciousness due to hypoglycemia
→ Referral to nutritionist for instruction about medical nutrition therapy
→ Referral to appropriate specialist(s) when indicated (i.e., cardiologist, neurologist, nephrologist, ophthalmologist, podiatrist, perinatologist)
→ Referral to social services when appropriate

PATIENT EDUCATION

→ SMBG
- If patient is on diet alone, SMBG is up to the provider and patient's discretion. It may be an educational tool and motivating force for the patient to see the results of the diet and exercise program.
- Daily SMBG is important in patients on sulfonylurea or insulin therapy to monitor for and prevent asymptomatic hypoglycemia.

■ The optimal frequency of SMBG in patients with Type 2 diabetes should be determined by both patient and provider with the goal of achieving glycemic targets.

■ Frequency should be increased when making adjustments in diet, oral medications, or insulin regimens.

■ Instruct about use of the meter, including check strip, cleaning, and memory.
  • Advise the patient to bring her meter to all appointments. Recheck her technique at each visit.

■ Instruct about use of finger-sticking device and lancets.
  • Choose any finger.
    – Use sides of fingers and tips (avoid finger pads) and rotate sites.
  • Wash hands with soap and warm water.
    – Avoid using alcohol (unless in dirty environment) as it toughens skin.
  • Hang hand at side for 30–60 seconds to obtain blood sample more easily.

■ Teach the patient how to record blood glucose results in her record book.
  • Advise the patient to bring her record book to all appointments.
  • Advise the patient what her target blood sugar range should be.

→ Instruct the patient about insulin administration when indicated.

■ Instruct about insulin, including types, source, dose, onset, peak, and duration.

■ Instruct about technique for drawing, measuring, and injecting insulin.
  • Do not aspirate prior to injecting.

■ Instruct patient about site rotation.
  • Abdomen has best absorption, followed by arms, thighs, buttocks
  • Stay in the same region at the same time of day.
  • Change site by 1 inch each time.
  • Do not use same site more than once every 3–4 weeks.

■ Advise patient to re-use needles if patient has good personal hygiene, has no acute illness or ongoing problems with infection, and is physically capable of safely recapping a syringe. Needles may be re-used until they become dull or bent (ADA 2001).

■ Use a needle clipper device to dispose of needle. Discard syringe and lancets in a hard plastic or needle container.
  • Check local county policy for syringe take-back program.

■ Advise on insulin storage.
  • Keep bottles currently in use at room temperature, out of sunlight for up to 1 month, then discard. If stored, store in door of refrigerator and discard bottle after 3 months.

■ Review symptoms, causes, treatment, and prevention of hypoglycemia with the patient and her family. Instruct patient to carry at least 15 g of carbohydrate to be eaten or taken in liquid form in the event of a hypoglycemic reaction.

■ Advise the patient to obtain a medical alert bracelet and explain the bracelet's purpose.

■ Instruct the patient and her family members on use of glucagon kit.

■ Advise patient to call if blood sugar is <60 mg/dL on a daily or weekly basis.

→ Review symptoms, causes, treatment, and prevention of hyperglycemia.

→ Describe the importance of following prescribed meal plan to improve blood sugar control.

■ Encourage the patient to check blood sugars 1–2 hours after meals occasionally to see the effects of different foods on blood glucose.

→ Teach the patient about proper sick day management (e.g., colds, flu, infection):

■ Explain HHNS causes, treatment, and prevention.

■ Explain that illness, stress, or infection may raise blood sugar.

■ Advise patient never to stop taking medications, unless advised by her provider or if she is experiencing severe hypoglycemia.

■ Advise patient to check blood sugar every 4 hours.

■ Advise patient to call if blood sugar remains <300 mg/dL or <60 mg/dL

■ Advise patient to drink extra liquids, ½–¾ cup every ½–1 hour.

■ Advise patient to weigh herself daily and to call her provider if there is more than 5 lb. loss or gain.

■ Advise patient to check her temperature and to call if her temperature is greater than 101°F (38.3°C).

→ Advise the patient to have dilated retinal examination by an experienced ophthalmologist yearly.

→ Teach the patient about proper foot care.

→ Recommend a dental examination every 6 months.

→ Review local community resources. (See **Appendix 10F.1, Resources for Patients with Diabetes** in the **Type 1 Diabetes Mellitus** chapter.)

→ Instruct the patient regarding effects of smoking, alcohol, and drugs on diabetes. Counsel about lifestyle modification techniques when indicated.

→ Provide education for the patient's family about all aspects of diabetes care.

FOLLOW-UP

→ Number of visits will depend on blood glucose control, change in treatment program, and presence of complications.

→ May need to contact patient weekly to check on SMBG results.

→ See the patient within several weeks or 1 month if major changes in insulin dose are made.

→ See patient every 3–6 months if she is maintaining treatment goals (see **Table 10F.2**).

→ Per recommendations of the ADA (2001), the interim history should include:

■ Frequency, causes, and severity of hypoglycemia or hyperglycemia

- Results of regular glucose monitoring
- Adjustments by the patient of the therapeutic regimen
- Problems with adherence
- Symptoms suggesting development of the complications of diabetes
- Psychosocial status and lifestyle changes
- Other medical illnesses
- Current medications
- Tobacco and alcohol use

→ Physical examination should include:
- Yearly physical examination
- Check weight, blood pressure, and feet every visit, in addition to fundoscopic exam
- Dilated retinal examination by an experienced ophthalmologist yearly
- Women planning pregnancy should have an eye examination before pregnancy and during the first trimester. Referral to a perinatologist for prepregnancy counseling is strongly advised.

→ Diagnostic tests should include:
- HbA1c at least twice yearly if meeting treatment goals; quarterly if not meeting glycemic goals or there is a change in therapy
- Fasting cholesterol, HDL, triglycerides, and calculated LDL yearly
- Screen for microalbuminuria yearly by one of three methods (ADA 2001):
  - Albumin-to-creatinine ratio in random spot collection
  - 24-hour collection with creatinine
  - Timed (4-hour or overnight) collection

→ Patient education should include a review of:
- Diet—reasons for success or failure
- Exercise program—reasons for success or failure
- SMBG—technique and results; interpret results with patient
- Hypoglycemic/hyperglycemic problems, symptoms, treatment, causes, and prevention
- Medications
- Birth control and family planning issues
  - Advise 3 months of normal HgbA1c prior to conception
- Foot care, dental care (CDC 1991a)
- Habits: smoking, alcohol, drugs
- Psychological adjustment (CDC 1991a)
- Complications

→ See the "Treatment/Management" section.
→ Document in progress notes and on problem list.

BIBLIOGRAPHY

American Diabetes Association. 2001. Clinical practice recommendations. *Diabetes Care* 24(1):S1–S133.

Centers for Disease Control and Prevention (CDC). 1991a. *Take charge of your diabetes: a guide for patients.* Atlanta, Ga.: National Center for Chronic Disease Prevention and Health Promotion.

_____. 1991b. *The prevention and treatment of complications of diabetes mellitus, a guide for primary care practitioners.* Atlanta, Ga.: National Center for Chronic Disease Prevention and Health Promotion.

Conlon, P.C. 2001. A practical approach to Type 2 diabetes. *Nursing Clinics of North America* 36(2):193–202.

Eisenbarth, G.S., and Kahn, C.R. 1990. Etiology and pathogenesis of diabetes mellitus. In *Principles and practice of endocrinology and metabolism,* ed. K.L. Becker, pp. 1074–1084. Philadelphia: J.B. Lippincott.

Farkas-Hirsch, R. 1998. *Intensive diabetes management,* 2nd ed. Alexandria, Va.: American Diabetes Association.

Feinglos, M.N., and Bethel, M.A. 1998. Treatment of Type 2 diabetes mellitus. *Medical Clinics of North America* 82(4):757–790.

Florence, J.A., and Yeager, B.F. 1999. Treatment of Type 2 diabetes mellitus. *American Family Physician* 59(10): 2835–2844.

Genuth, S. 1998. DKA and HHNS in adults. In *Therapy for diabetes mellitus and related disorders,* 3rd ed., ed. H.E. Lebovitz, pp. 83–96. Alexandria, Va.: American Diabetes Association.

Goroll, A.H., and Mulley, A.G. 2000. *Primary care medicine: office evaluation and management of the adult patient,* 4th ed. Philadelphia: Lippincott Williams & Wilkins.

Groop, L.C., Groop. P.H., and Stenman, S. 1990. Combined insulin-sulfonylurea therapy in treatment of NIDDM. *Diabetes Care* 13 (Suppl. 3):47–52.

Haire-Joshu, D., ed. 1992. *Management of diabetes mellitus.* St. Louis, Mo.: Mosby.

Hirsch, I.B. 1998. Intensive treatment of Type 1 diabetes. *Medical Clinics of North America* 82(4): 689–719.

Horton, E.S. 1998. Exercise. In *Therapy for diabetes mellitus and related disorders,* 3rd ed., ed. H.E. Lebovitz, pp. 150–159. Alexandria, Va.: American Diabetes Association.

Karam, J.H. 1993. Diabetes mellitus and hypoglycemia. In *Current medical diagnoses and treatment,* ed. L.M. Tierney, pp. 912–948. Norwalk, Conn.: Appleton & Lange.

Lebovitz, H.E. 1998. Diagnosis and classification of diabetes mellitus. In *Therapy for diabetes mellitus and related disorders,* 3rd ed., ed. H.E. Lebovitz, pp. 5–7. Alexandria, Va.: American Diabetes Association.

Metzger, B.E., ed. 1991. Proceedings of the Third International Workshop Conference on Gestational Diabetes Mellitus. *Diabetes* 40 (Suppl. 2):1–201.

Peters, A.L., and Davidson, M.B. 1991. Insulin plus sulfonylurea agent for treating Type 2 diabetes. *Annals of Internal Medicine* 115:45–53.

Powers, A.C. 2001. Diabetes mellitus. In *Harrison's principles of internal medicine*, 15th ed., ed. E. Braunwald, pp. 2109–2137. New York: McGraw-Hill.

Prisant, L.M. 2001. Cardiovascular disease: how to reduce the risk in patients with diabetes. *Consultant* 41(3):461–470.

Quinn, L. 2001a. Type 2 diabetes: epidemiology, pathophysiology, and diagnosis. *Nursing Clinics of North America* 36(2):175–192.

_____. 2001b. Pharmacologic management of the patient with Type 2 diabetes. *Nursing Clinics of North America* 36(2):217–242.

Riddle, M.C. 1997. Tactics for Type 2 diabetes. *Endocrinology and Metabolism Clinics of North America* 26(3):659–677.

_____. 1999. Oral pharmacologic management of Type 2 diabetes. *American Family Physician* 60(9):2613–2620.

Schuman, C.R. 1988. Diabetes mellitus: definition, classification, and diagnosis. In *Diabetes mellitus*, 9th ed., eds. J.A. Galloway, J. Potvin, and C.R. Schuman, pp. 2–13. Indianapolis: Eli Lilly and Co.

Skyler, J.S. 1998. Insulin treatment. In *Therapy for diabetes mellitus and related disorders*, 3rd ed., ed. H.E. Lebovitz,

pp. 186–203. Alexandria, Va.: American Diabetes Association.

Sobel, D.S., and Ferguson, T. 1985. *The people's book of medical tests*. New York: Summit Books.

Star, W.L., and Murphy, J.R. 1999. Gestational diabetes. In *Ambulatory obstetrics: protocols for nurse practitioners/nurse-midwives*, 3rd ed., eds. W.L. Star, M.T. Shannon, L.L. Lommel et al. San Francisco: University of California-San Francisco Nursing Press.

United Kingdom Prospective Diabetes Study Group. 1998. Intensive blood-glucose control with sulphonylureas or insulin compared with conventional treatment and risk of complications in patients with Type 2 diabetes. *Lancet* 352(9131):837–853.

U.S. Department of Health and Human Services (USDHHS). 1999. *Diabetes statistics*. Washington, D.C.: the Author. Available at: http://www.niddk.nih.gov/health/diabetes/pubs/dmstats/dmstats.htm. Accessed on June, 6, 2001.

White, N.H., and Henry, D.N. 1992. Special issues in diabetes management. In *Management of diabetes mellitus*, ed. D. Haire-Joshu, pp. 249–309. St. Louis, Mo.: Mosby.

SECTION 11

Infectious Diseases

11-A	Diarrhea—Infectious	**11-2**
11-B	Hepatitis—Viral	**11-8**
11-C	Human Immunodeficiency Virus-1 Infection	**11-20**
11-D	Lyme Disease	**11-42**
11-E	Measles (Rubeola)	**11-49**
11-F	Mononucleosis	**11-52**
11-G	Mumps	**11-55**
11-H	Rubella	**11-57**
11-I	Tuberculosis	**11-60**
11-J	Varicella Zoster Virus	**11-69**

11-A

Diarrhea—Infectious

Infectious diarrhea is an increase in the frequency (i.e., two or more stools a day), fluidity (i.e., liquid stools), or volume of stools (i.e., more than 250 g per 24 hours) (Goodman et al. 1999, McQuaid 2002). Diarrhea is classified as acute if the symptoms last less than two weeks, persistent if they continue for more than two weeks, and chronic if they are present for more than a month (Ciesla et al. 2001). Generally, acute diarrhea is caused by viral or bacterial microorganisms, preformed toxins, or drugs. Persistent or chronic diarrhea is associated with parasites or noninfectious conditions (Ciesla et al. 2001, Jacobs 2002).

In the United States, approximately 70 million cases of diarrhea occur annually (Goodman et al. 1999). In 90% of individuals, these infections are self-limited and resolve without serious sequelae. However, complications, including severe dehydration, bacteremia/sepsis, renal failure, hypoglycemia, hypokalemia, hemorrhagic colitis, and disseminated intravascular coagulation, can occur. There are 5,000–10,000 deaths in the United States attributed to enteric infections each year, with most of these reported in young children and the elderly (Altekruse et al. 1997, Ciesla et al. 2001, Goodman et al. 1999).

Several types of pathogens can cause infectious diarrhea with varying incubation periods and symptoms. (See **Table 11A.1, Infectious Diarrhea, Selected Organisms**.) The mechanism by which the pathogen affects the gastrointestinal (GI) tract results in the clinical manifestations of the infection. Viral pathogens, including rotavirus, Norwalk-like viruses, and enteric adenoviruses, are the most common cause of infectious diarrhea in the United States (Aranda-Michel et al. 1999, Ciesla et al. 2001, Goodman et al. 1999). These infections often are associated with upper respiratory symptoms and the epidemics have a seasonal pattern.

Bacterial pathogens commonly associated with infectious diarrhea include *Escherichia coli*, *Staphylococcus aureus*, *Salmonella* species (*S. paratyphi*, *S. typhi*), *Shigella* species (*S. sonnei*, *S. flexneri*, *S. dysenteriae*), and *Campylobacter jejuni*. Bacterial infectious diarrhea is most frequently associated with ingestion of contaminated food or water (Ciesla et al. 2001, Goodman et al. 1999). Often there is a clustering of individuals

reporting similar symptoms; such epidemiological information contributes to the diagnosis.

In the United States, parasitic organisms are the least common cause of infectious diarrhea. *Giardia lamblia*, Cryptosporidia, and *Entamoeba histolytica* are the most frequently reported parasitic organisms, often causing mild clinical presentations in immunocompetent individuals.

Infectious diarrhea is categorized into two types: noninflammatory (Type I) and inflammatory (Type II). Noninflammatory diarrhea is characterized by watery stools usually of large volume; there is no fever, blood, or severe abdominal pain. Symptoms, which usually begin within a short period of time after exposure, result from alteration of the normal absorptive and secretory function of the small bowel due to an enterotoxin. The infection does not cause significant changes in the GI mucosa (Aranda-Michel et al. 1999, Goodman et al. 1999). Organisms associated with Type I infectious diarrhea include *S. aureus*, *G. lamblia*, and Cryptosporidia.

Inflammatory diarrhea is characterized by fever, bloody or mucoid stools of small volume, severe abdominal pain, tenesmus, and fecal urgency (Jacobs 2002). The pathogen invades the small or large bowel and causes an inflammatory reaction that results in leukocytes and often blood in the stool. The incubation period for Type II diarrhea is longer than that for Type I, usually 1–3 days (Aranda-Michel et al. 1999, Goodman et al. 1999, McQuaid 2002).

Certain variables have been noted to increase an individual's risk of experiencing infectious diarrhea, including her age, immune functioning, type(s) of exposure, and geographic regions where she lives or has visited. Transmission of the infectious pathogen occurs through fecal/oral spread (person to person) or through exposure to contaminated food or water.

DATABASE

SUBJECTIVE

→ Risk factors. The patient may (Aranda-Michel et al. 1999):
- Be elderly
- Be a day care center attendee

- Be a parent of a child with a history of diarrhea
- Be engaged in laboratory work involving exposure to pathogens
- Have a history of:
  - Recent travel to a foreign country in a region (e.g., Africa, Latin America, the Middle East, or Asia) where there is an increased likelihood of exposure to pathogens
  - Immunosuppression
  - Exposure via intimate contact with a partner who has infectious diarrhea
  - Exposure to a recent food-borne or water-borne outbreak
  - Recent ingestion of seafood, undercooked or raw meat or poultry, uncooked eggs, or improperly stored food
  - Recent hospitalization (e.g., within 30 days) and treatment with antibiotics (especially cephalosporins or clindamycin)

→ Symptoms may include (Aranda-Michel et al. 1999, Goodman et al. 1999, McQuaid 2002):
- Abrupt onset of one or more of the following symptoms, ranging from mild to severe intensity:
  - Fever
  - Rash
  - Malaise
  - Headache
  - Anorexia
  - Nausea
  - Vomiting
  - Abdominal cramping or pain that is often located in the right lower quadrant or periumbilical region
  - Increased flatulence that may be foul-smelling
  - Increased frequency of defecation
  - Watery, mucoid, slimy, or bloody stools
    NOTE: *Salmonella* and *Shigella* infections are associated with bloody, mucoid stools.
  - Foul-smelling stools
  - Fecal urgency
  - Rectal tenesmus
  - Weight loss
  - Lightheadedness, vertigo, syncope in patients with significant dehydration
  - Upper respiratory infection symptoms if the diarrhea is associated with a viral pathogen (e.g., rotavirus)

Table 11A.1.   INFECTIOUS DIARRHEA, SELECTED ORGANISMS

Noninflammatory Diarrhea	Inflammatory Diarrhea
Viral	Viral
Norwalk virus	Cytomegalovirus
Norwalk-like virus	
Rotavirus	
Protozoal	Protozoal
Giardia lamblia	*Entamoeba histolytica*
Crytosporidium	
	Bacterial
Bacterial	Cytotoxin production
Preformed enterotoxin production	Enterohemorrhagic
Staphylococcus aureus	*E. coli* O157:H7 (EHEC)
Bacillus cereus	*Vibrio parahaemolyticus*
Clostridium perfringens	*Clostridium difficile*
Enterotoxin production	Mucosal invasion
Enterotoxigenic	*Shigella*
E. coli (ETEC)	*Campylobacter jejuni*
Vibrio cholerae	*Salmonella*
	Enteroinvasive *E. coli* (EIEC)
	Aeromonas
	Plesiomonas
	Yersinia enterocolitica
	Chlamydia
	Neisseria gonorrhoeae
	Listeria monocytogenes

Source: Reprinted with permission from McQuaid, K.R. 2002. Alimentary tract. In *2002 current medical diagnosis & treatment*, 41st ed., eds. L.M. Tierney, Jr., S.J. McPhee, and M.A. Papadakis, p. 580. New York: Lange Medical Books/McGraw-Hill.

OBJECTIVE

→ Physical examination of the patient may be unremarkable or reveal any of the following findings (Aranda-Michel et al. 1999, Goodman et al. 1999, McQuaid 2002):

- Vital signs may be within normal limits (WNL) or may demonstrate an elevated pulse and temperature, and decreased weight
- Postural changes in the patient's pulse and blood pressure will be evident with significant dehydration.
- Tissue turgor will be poor if the patient is significantly dehydrated.
- Examination of the mouth may reveal dry mucosa with significant dehydration.
- Abdominal examination:
  - Auscultation may reveal hyperactive bowel sounds.
  - Percussion may demonstrate increased resonance.
  - Palpation may reveal tenderness, guarding, and rebound.
  NOTE: The presence of hypoactive bowel sounds and abdominal distention may indicate obstruction or toxic megacolon (Goodman et al. 1999).
- Rectal examination will be WNL or anal erythema and edema may be evident.

ASSESSMENT

→ Infectious diarrhea (viral, bacterial, parasitic)
→ R/O dehydration
→ R/O hemorrhagic colitis
→ R/O bacteremia/sepsis
→ R/O ischemic bowel
→ R/O acute abdomen (e.g., appendicitis, peritonitis, toxic megacolon)
→ R/O functional bowel disease (e.g., diverticulosis)
→ R/O drug toxicity (e.g., *Clostridium difficile*)
→ R/O pelvic inflammatory disease
→ R/O inflammatory bowel disease (e.g., ulcerative colitis)
→ R/O obstipation
→ R/O other causes of diarrhea

PLAN

DIAGNOSTIC TESTS

→ Because diagnostic testing for infectious diarrhea pathogens can be costly, with results often not available until after the patient's symptoms have resolved, diagnostic tests are not routinely ordered for patients with mild symptoms (e.g., no fever, abdominal pain, bloody stools, mucus in stools, or significant dehydration, and no exposure to unusual organisms, such as cholera) (Aranda-Michel et al. 1999, Goodman et al. 1999, McQuaid 2002). (See **Figure 11A.1, Evaluation of Acute Diarrhea**.)

→ For patients exhibiting moderate to severe symptoms or who have fever ($\geq 38.8°C/101.8°F$), bloody stools, or dehydration, the following tests can be ordered in consultation with a physician:

- Microscopic examination of fecal smears can be done in an office setting at minimal cost to the patient and can

help determine the need for additional testing. However, fecal smears require a fresh stool specimen for evaluation. Once a fecal sample is obtained, the following tests can be done (Aranda-Michel et al. 1999, Goodman et al. 1999, McQuaid 2002):

- Methylene blue stain:
  - Obtain a small fecal specimen with blood and mucus (if possible), mix with two drops of methylene blue stain, and place a coverslip over the specimen.
  - Evidence of increased polymorphonuclear cells suggests an invasive inflammatory process of the colon (e.g., *Shigella*, *Salmonella*, or *Campylobacter* infections or ulcerative colitis).
- Fecal lactoferrin latex agglutination assay:
  - A more sensitive assay to determine the presence of fecal leukocytes. Interpretation of findings is as above.
- Gram stain:
  - Standard Gram staining of a fecal smear may reveal an etiological organism such as *S. aureus* and may demonstrate increased leukocytes.
- Guaiac:
  - Standard guaiac testing will be positive if there is blood in the fecal specimen.

- Stool culture and sensitivity should be considered when a patient has evidence of leukocytes on microscopic evaluation of the fecal smear, has severe symptoms, or is immunosuppressed (Aranda-Michel et al. 1999).

- Collection of stool specimens on three separate days will increase the likelihood of identification of a pathogen.
- In many laboratories, clinicians must specifically request that evaluations for particular pathogens (e.g., *Campylobacter*) be performed.
- Positive results are almost always diagnostic of an etiological pathogen.
- Antibiotic sensitivities may be helpful in identifying resistant bacteria and in determining the most effective therapeutic agent.
- Negative results do not eliminate the possibility of a particular pathogen, as it is often difficult to obtain adequate stool specimens from some patients.

NOTE: One suggested way to obtain stool specimens is to have the patient place a sheet of plastic wrap under the toilet seat and pass the feces onto the plastic. The patient can then transfer the feces to the specimen cup. Advise the patient to prevent urine or water from touching the specimen.

- Specimens for ova and parasite determination also can be sent to the lab as indicated by the patient's history.
- Collection of a stool specimen on three separate days usually is necessary to obtain an adequate sampling.
- Because microscopic evaluation of such specimens requires experience on the part of the examiner, clinicians should send specimens for such tests to qualified laboratories.

- Cultures of food suspected to be contaminated with a pathogen (e.g., *S. aureus*)

- CBC may demonstrate leukocytosis with increased bands (i.e., left shift).
- Paired sera can be obtained and sent for hemagglutination titer with a fourfold rise in titer, specific to the pathogen suggestive of infection.
- Proctoscopy or sigmoidoscopy may be necessary to make a diagnosis in patients with bloody or mucoid diarrhea (usually ordered by the physician consultant).
- The string test (Entero-Test) can be done to identify parasites of the upper intestines (e.g., *G. lamblia*) but should be ordered by the physician consultant.
- Rectal swabs for sexually transmitted diseases should be sent if the patient reports a history of unprotected anal sexual activity (McQuaid 2002).

TREATMENT/MANAGEMENT

→ In most patients, infectious diarrhea is a self-limited illness that usually resolves within 2–5 days.
- Symptomatic treatment for infectious diarrhea includes (Aranda-Michel et al. 1999, Goodman et al. 1999, McQuaid 2002):
  - Avoidance of food for at least 24 hours or until the diarrhea substantially decreases or stops.
  - When food intake resumes, the patient should begin with easily digestible foods, such as toast, crackers, rice, broth-based soups, and decaffeinated tea.
    - The patient should avoid foods high in fat and protein (e.g., meat and eggs), as well as raw fruits and vegetables, until the symptoms are resolving.

Figure 11A.1. EVALUATION OF ACUTE DIARRHEA

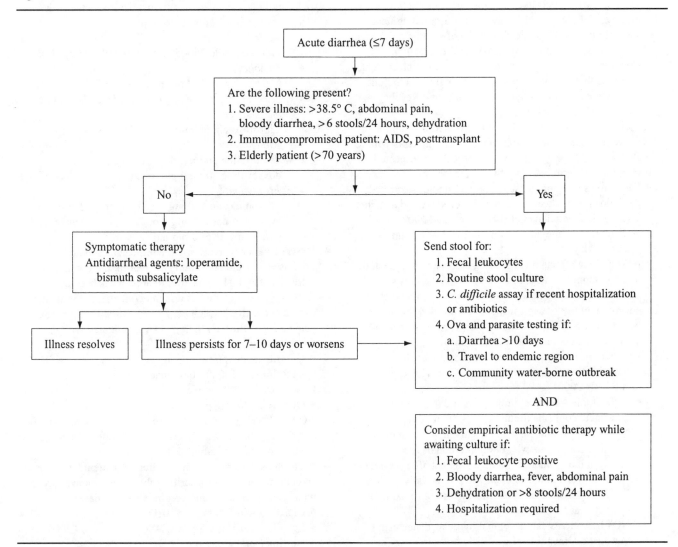

Source: Reprinted with permission from McQuaid, K.R. 2002. Alimentary tract. In *2002 current medical diagnosis & treatment*, 41st ed., eds. L.M. Tierney, Jr., S.J. McPhee, and M.A. Papadakis, p. 580. New York: Lange Medical Books/McGraw-Hill.

– Milk and milk products should not be resumed until after the acute phase of the illness because many patients develop a transient lactase deficiency that could aggravate the diarrhea.

■ Replacement of fluids and electrolytes is essential and should begin early in the illness with (Aranda-Michel et al. 1999, Goodman et al. 1999, McQuaid 2002):

  • Hourly ingestion of 8 ounces of fruit juice (apple or orange) mixed with a pinch of table salt and a teaspoon of honey or sugar

  OR

  • Decaffeinated, nondiet soda drinks that have lost their carbonation (leave the bottle of soda uncapped for several hours to eliminate carbonation)

  • An 8-ounce glass of water with ¼ teaspoon of baking soda also should be ingested.

■ Over-the-counter (OTC) oral replacement solutions should be initiated in patients with dehydration or large-volume diarrhea because these preparations contain glucose, sodium, and electrolytes in appropriate glucose-sodium ratios to facilitate absorption of sodium and water in the intestinal lumen (Aranda-Michel et al. 1999, Goodman et al. 1999, McQuaid 2002). Oral replacement solutions that are available as OTC preparations include Pedialyte RS®, Rehydralyte®, Ricelyte®, and Resol® (Aranda-Michel et al. 1999).

→ Antidiarrheal medications should be avoided if inflammatory bowel disease or invasive infections (e.g., patients with a high fever and bloody or mucoid diarrhea) are suspected because of an increased risk of toxic megacolon.

■ For patients in whom these conditions are not suspected, the following medications can be initiated (Aranda-Michel et al. 1999, Goodman et al. 1999, McQuaid 2002):

  • Bismuth subsalicylate 30 mL or 2 tablets p.o. up to 8 doses/day

  NOTE: Side effects include black stools and tongue and, less commonly, ringing in the ears. Also, patients should be advised that this drug contains salicylates and that the concomitant use of aspirin should be avoided. Pregnant women, patients with allergies to aspirin, or patients who are receiving certain other medications (e.g., anticoagulant therapy, methotrexate, or probenecid) should not use this medication (Centers for Disease Control and Prevention [CDC] 2000).

  • Loperamide 4 mg p.o. initially, then 2 mg after each unformed stool (maximum dose is 16 mg/day)

  NOTE: Discontinue use in patients in whom symptoms increase, in patients who develop blood or mucus in their stool, or if there is no improvement after 48 hours.

  • Diphenoxylate and atropine 5 mg p.o. initially, then 2.5–5.0 mg p.o. after each unformed stool (maximum 8 tablets/day)

  NOTE: Patients can develop drug dependence using this agent. Other side effects include central nervous system depression, headaches, confusion, intestinal obstruction, nausea, vomiting, and pancreatitis.

Atropine effects include possible increased intraocular pressure, urinary retention, tachycardia, flushing, and dry skin and mucous membranes. Contraindications for use include obstructive jaundice and pseudomembranous colitis.

→ Antimicrobial therapy in suspected or documented infectious diarrhea is controversial because most episodes are caused by viruses, are self-limited, and resolve without complications. However, antimicrobial therapy is indicated in patients in whom certain bacterial or parasitic pathogens are suspected, as treatment is associated with a decrease in both the duration of symptoms and serious sequelae. In addition, antibiotic therapy should be considered in patients, including the very young, elderly, or immunosuppressed, who are at increased risk of complications (McQuaid 2002).

■ If antimicrobial therapy is being considered, consultation with a physician is indicated.

■ The following antimicrobial agents can be prescribed depending on the patient's status, the suspected pathogen, and/or the results of diagnostic tests:

  • *C. difficile*:
    – Metronidazole 250–500 mg p.o. QID for 7–14 days

  • *G. lamblia*:
    – Metronidazole 250 mg p.o. TID for 7 days

  • *C. jejuni*, *S. typhi*, *Campylobacter*, *Shigella*, and *Salmonella* species:
    – Ciprofloxacin 500 mg p.o. BID for 3–5 days

  • *Vibrio cholerae*:
    – Tetracycline 500 mg p.o. QID for 3 days or doxycycline 300 mg p.o. once

  • *E. histolytica*:
    – Metronidazole 750 mg p.o. TID for 10 days followed by iodoquinol 650 mg p.o. TID for 20 days or paromomycin 500 mg p.o. TID for 7 days

  NOTE: Patients receiving metronidazole should be advised to avoid consuming alcohol for the duration of treatment and 24 hours after treatment has been completed.

→ Antimicrobial therapy has documented efficacy in treating traveler's diarrhea, which usually is caused by enterotoxigenic *E. coli*. Empiric therapy can be initiated with one of the following:

■ Ciprofloxacin 750 mg p.o. once

■ Levofloxacin 500 mg p.o. once

■ Norfloxacin 400 mg p.o. once

■ Ofloxacin 300 mg p.o. once

NOTE: *E. coli* resistance to trimethoprim-sulfamethoxazole and doxycycline is widely prevalent; therefore, these medications are not advised (CDC 2000).

→ If traveler's diarrhea continues after the patient has completed empiric therapy as described above, the following regimens can be initiated and continue for 3–5 days:

■ Ciprofloxacin 500 mg p.o. BID

■ Levofloxacin 500 mg p.o. QD

■ Norfloxacin 400 mg p.o. BID

■ Ofloxacin 300 mg p.o. BID

→ In addition to antimicrobial therapy, treatment of traveler's diarrhea with antimotility agents also is recommended as follows:

- Loperamide 4 mg p.o. initially followed by 2 mg p.o. after each unformed stool (not to exceed a maximum dose of 16 mg/day)

CONSULTATION

→ Consultation with a physician is indicated for any patient:

- With severe symptoms (e.g., dehydration, high fever, or bloody or mucoid stools)
- With symptoms that persist longer than 48 hours
- With conditions placing her at an increased risk of bacteremia/sepsis (e.g., the elderly and immunocompromised patients)
- If abdominal or rectal pain is reported
- If hemolytic-uremic syndrome is suspected (characterized by thrombocytopenia, hemolytic anemia, renal failure occurring 2–14 days after the onset of diarrhea) (Ciesla et al. 2001)

→ As needed for prescription(s).

PATIENT EDUCATION

→ Educate the patient about the cause of diarrhea, clinical course, plan of care, possible complications, possible side effects of medications, preventive measures (e.g., handwashing and proper food preparation), and the indicated follow-up.

→ If perianal discomfort is reported, review symptomatic relief measures, including sitz baths three times a day, witch hazel solution or pads to clean the perineal area, and use of soft tissue or absorbent cotton to dry the perineal area.

→ Educate the patient about ways to prevent further exposure and/or transmission of enteric pathogens through the proper handling and cooking of food, use of pasteurized milk, and handwashing with soap before and after handling food.

→ Educate the patient who is planning to travel to an area (e.g., Africa, Latin America, the Middle East, or Asia) where there is an increased risk of exposure to enteric pathogens associated with traveler's diarrhea about ways to reduce exposure. She should:

- Avoid ingesting raw vegetables, unpeeled fruits, ice or untreated water, and foods that are served uncooked or cold.
- Disinfect water by boiling it for at least 10 minutes (longer at higher altitudes), treat water chemically with commercially available disinfectants, or use a mixture of 5% chlorine bleach, 2 drops (0.1 mL) in a liter of water and set aside for 30 minutes at room temperature before using.
- Avoid purchasing and ingesting food from street vendors.
- Initiate pharmacologic therapy when symptoms begin:
  - Mild diarrhea (fewer than three loose stools/day without fever, pus, or blood): The patient can initiate therapy with loperamide (Imodium®) as described in "Treatment/Management," above.
  - Moderate diarrhea: Antimicrobial therapy can be start-

ed with regimens described in "Treatment/Management," above.

- Severe or persistent diarrhea with dehydration, fever, blood, and/or mucus in stools: The patient should seek medical evaluation (Jacobs 2002, McQuaid 2002).

→ Educate the patient about the importance of adequate hydration and self-repletion if she experiences diarrhea.

→ Educate patients who plan to travel abroad about preventive immunizations (e.g., *S. typhi* vaccination to prevent typhoid fever) that are recommended before they depart.

- Advice about preventive measures, possible therapeutic regimens, and recommended immunizations for international travelers can be obtained by calling the CDC at (404) 332-4559 or by visiting its Web site at www.cdc.gov/travel/diarrhea.htm.

FOLLOW-UP

→ See "Consultation," above.

→ Any patient who experiences persistent or worsening symptoms, or possible side effects associated with therapeutic interventions, should return as soon as possible for evaluation.

→ Many of the pathogens that cause infectious diarrhea (e.g., *Salmonella* and *Shigella*) are state-mandated, reportable diseases requiring a morbidity report to be filed with the department of public health. Contact the local department of public health for a complete list of pathogens that require such reports.

→ Document in progress notes and on problem list.

BIBLIOGRAPHY

Altekruse, S.F., Cohen, M.L., and Swerdlow, D.L. 1997. Emerging food-borne diseases. *Emerging Infectious Diseases* 3: 285–293.

Aranda-Michel, J., and Giannella, R.A. 1999. Acute diarrhea: a practical review. *American Journal of Medicine* 106:670–676.

Centers for Disease Control and Prevention (CDC). 2000. Traveler's diarrhea. Available at: http://www.cdc.gov/ncidod/dbmd/diseaseinfo/travelersdiarrhea_g.htm. Accessed on October 31, 2002.

Ciesla, W.P., and Guerrant, R.L. 2001. Infectious diarrhea. In *Current diagnosis & treatment in infectious diseases*, eds. W.R. Wilson and M.A. Sande, pp. 255–268. New York: Lange Medical Books/McGraw-Hill.

Goodman, L., and Segreti J. 1999. Infectious diarrhea. *Disease-A-Month* July:267–299.

Jacobs, R.A. 2002. General problems in infectious diseases. In *2002 current medical diagnosis & treatment*, 41st ed., eds. L.M. Tierney, Jr., S.J. McPhee, and M.A. Papadakis, pp. 1295–1321. New York: Lange Medical Books/McGraw-Hill.

McQuaid, K.R. 2002. Alimentary tract. In *2002 current medical diagnosis & treatment*, 41st ed., eds. L.M. Tierney, Jr., S.J. McPhee, and M.A. Papadakis, pp. 571–674. New York: Lange Medical Books/McGraw-Hill.

Lisa L. Lommel, R.N., C., F.N.P., M.S., M.P.H.
Jeanne R. Davis, R.N., F.N.P., M.P.H.

11-B

Hepatitis—Viral

Acute viral hepatitis is a systemic infection that predominantly affects the liver. It can be caused by any of five viral agents: hepatitis A virus (HAV), hepatitis B virus (HBV), hepatitis C virus (HCV), hepatitis D virus (HDV), or hepatitis E virus (HEV). Most cases of acute hepatitis are caused by HAV and HBV. Among all cases of newly diagnosed acute viral hepatitis reported in the United States, HAV accounts for 32%, HBV for 42%, and HCV for 20% (Holst et al. 2001). Most individuals with chronic viral hepatitis (illness lasting more than six months) are infected with HCV (85%), while 5% are infected with HBV (Holst et al. 2001).

Under most circumstances, none of the hepatitis viruses is known to directly damage hepatocytes. Liver damage and subsequent clinical symptoms associated with acute hepatitis are generally a result of the host's immune response to infection (Younossi 2000). Complications of viral hepatitis include acute (fulminant) liver failure, chronic hepatitis, cirrhosis, and hepatocellular carcinoma.

HAV

Hepatitis A is the most common cause of acute hepatitis in the United States (Cuthbert 2001). The principal modes of transmission are food or water contaminated with fecal material and contact with a person infected with hepatitis A (Centers for Disease Control and Prevention [CDC] 2002, Lauer et al. 2001, Younossi 2000). Individuals at risk for exposure to hepatitis A include those who work or are taken care of at day care centers or residential institutions, health care workers, deployed military personnel, individuals who engage in anal sexual contact, injection drug users, or individuals who travel to geographic regions where HAV is most prevalent (e.g. Africa, Asia, Latin America, Mexico, and South America) (Cuthbert 2001, Holst et al. 2001, Younossi 2000). Blood-borne transmission of hepatitis A is uncommon (CDC 2002, Holst et al. 2001). Maternal-neonatal transmission occurs but is infrequent and is often associated with HIV co-infection in the mother (Lauer et al. 2001). Casual household contact and contact with the saliva of infected individuals do not appear to be efficient modes of transmission (Lauer et al. 2001). Although the largest percentage of infected persons have no identifiable source of HAV infection, many or all of these cases are likely due to personal contact with an unidentified source shedding HAV (Cuthbert 2001).

HAV infection has an incubation period of 15–60 days (averaging 30 days) (CDC 2002, Holst et al. 2001, Younossi 2000). HAV replicates in the liver and is shed in high concentrations in feces from approximately two weeks before to approximately two weeks after the onset of clinical illness (CDC 2002, Holst et al. 2001). Rarely, fecal excretion can be prolonged, as determined by detection of viral nucleic acids for 3–11 months after infection (Cuthbert 2001).

Patients with hepatitis A have an excellent prognosis for complete recovery. HAV infection produces a self-limited disease that does not result in a carrier state and infection does not become chronic (CDC 2002, Holst et al. 2001, Malik et al. 2000, Younossi 2000). Antibody produced in response to HAV infection persists for life and confers protection against reinfection (CDC 2002, Holst et al. 2001). Normally, recovery occurs in 1–2 months (Younossi 2000).

However, 10–15% of patients with acute HAV infection may experience a relapse of symptoms during the six months after an apparent recovery from acute illness (CDC 2002). Acute liver failure from hepatitis A is rare (0.3% overall case-fatality rate) but occurs more frequently in people older than 50 years and in people with underlying chronic liver disease (CDC 2002). Cholestatic hepatitis is an uncommon variant of hepatitis A (Holst et al. 2001). Extrahepatic manifestations in patients with acute hepatitis A are rare but can include hemolysis, acalculous cholecystitis, acute renal failure, acute reactive arthritis, and pancreatitis (Cuthbert 2001).

HBV

Hepatitis B is the world's most common, blood-borne viral infection. In the United States, an estimated 1 million people have chronic HBV infection (Holst et al. 2001). The incidence of HBV infection in this country declined 60% between 1985 and 1995 largely due to improved screening of the blood supply (Holst et al. 2001). The disease is endemic almost everywhere in the world except the continental United States, Argentina, Australia, and parts of Europe. Five to 10% of all cases of HBV infection progress to chronic disease (Holst et al. 2001).

HBV is secreted and maintained in blood (which has the highest concentrations), saliva, semen, vaginal secretions, urine, and wound exudate of infected individuals (CDC 2002, Holst et al. 2001). HBV is efficiently transmitted by percutaneous or mucous membrane exposure to infectious body fluids. Behaviors that increase the risk of hepatitis B transmission include being sexually active with infected individuals, unsafe drug-injection practices, and unsafe tattooing and body-piercing practices (under nonsterile conditions). Travelers to endemic areas, military personnel, individuals with occupational exposure, adolescents, immigrants from endemic areas, persons from ethnic groups with high rates of HBV, and family members/partners of chronic hepatitis B carriers are also at increased risk of contracting the virus. Risk of perinatal transmission is as high as 90% if the mother is HbeAg-positive and approximately 10% if she is HbsAg-positive (Befeler et al. 2000). Nosocomial transmission of HBV to diabetic patients via a finger-stick device has been implicated in transmission. Transfusion-associated HBV has become rare in the United States since routine screening of blood and blood products has been in place.

The incubation period from time of exposure to onset of symptoms is approximately 50 days but can range from four weeks to six months (CDC 2002, Holst et al. 2001, Malik et al. 2000, Younossi 2000). In 90% of HBV cases, acute HBV infection is self-limited, with signs and symptoms lasting from days to weeks (Holst et al. 2001). In some patients with acute HBV infection, the clinical course is prolonged. Relapsing hepatitis can persist for as long as four months. Fulminant hepatitis develops in fewer than 1% of patients with acute HBV infection (Friedman 2002).

HBV infection becomes chronic in approximately 5–10% of patients (Holst et al. 2001). Chronic HBV infection is defined as persistence of HBsAg beyond six months. Two major factors influence the development of chronic infection: age at the time of infection and the immune status of the host (with a higher risk of chronicity in the immunocompromised host or after neonatal infection). Most patients with chronic HBV infection are asymptomatic carriers who are not at risk for liver damage. Chronic active hepatitis B, however, increases a patient's risk for developing cirrhosis and primary hepatocellular carcinoma.

Among persons with chronic HBV infection, the risk of death from cirrhosis or hepatocellular carcinoma is 15–25% (CDC 2002). Both acute and chronic HBV infection may be associated with extrahepatic manifestations. Glomerulonephritis and/or nephrotic syndrome are/is a rare complication of HBV infection occurring predominantly in children with active viral replication. Inflammatory arthritis may occur, particularly during acute infection. Polyarteritis nodosa is also a rare complication of HBV infection.

HCV

HCV accounts for approximately 20% of all cases of acute hepatitis and has emerged as one of the most important causes of chronic liver disease in the United States (Holst et al. 2001). More than two-thirds of all infected persons are younger than 50 years (CDC 2002). Acute infection is associated with an incubation period of 6–8 weeks, with a range of 2–26 weeks (Addesa et al. 2001, Bonkovsky et al. 2001, Lauer et al. 2001, Younossi 2000).

HCV is not efficiently cleared by the immune system after acute infection, and 75–85% of exposed individuals will progress to chronic infection after an acute infection (CDC 2002, Holst et al. 2001, Younossi 2000). An estimated 2.7 million individuals in the United States are chronically infected (CDC 2002). As those with chronic HCV infection are at increased risk of cirrhosis and hepatocellular carcinoma, the number of HCV-related deaths is expected to triple in the next 10–20 years (Holst et al. 2001). End-stage liver disease secondary to chronic HCV infection has become the leading indication for liver transplantation in the United States (Holst et al. 2001, Larson et al. 2001).

Direct percutaneous exposure is the most efficient way of transmitting HCV. The highest transmission rate, as well as prevalence, is among patients with repeated direct percutaneous exposure. These include intravenous drug users, persons with hemophilia treated with clotting factor concentrates produced before 1987, and recipients of transfusions from HCV-positive donors (CDC 2002, Holst et al. 2001). The risk of transfusion-associated HCV in the United States has decreased significantly in the last two decades. When HCV nucleic acid amplification testing is applied to pooled-donor plasma specimens, the risk of HCV transmission from donated blood is reduced from 1 in 100,000 to 1 in 500,000–1,000,000 per unit (Busch et al. 2000). Nucleic acid amplification testing enables the detection of the vast majority of blood donations that occur during the "window period" (i.e., when persons are infectious but show no evidence of infection in their blood by laboratory methods).

Other risk factors for transmission include past/present multiple sex partners (co-infection with HIV may increase the risk of sexual transmission of HCV), organ transplantation before 1992, and being a hemodialysis patient (Holst et al. 2001). The risk of transmission of HCV via sexual activity for patients with a steady partner appears to be very low; transmission by sexual or household exposures accounts for less than 10% of cases. Vertical transmission of HCV from a chronically infected mother to a neonate occurs at an average rate of 5–6% and appears to be most common when mothers have high titers of circulating HCV RNA (Larson et al. 2001). Studies evaluating transmission through breast-feeding have demonstrated an average rate of infection of about 4% in both breast-fed and bottle-fed infants of HCV-positive mothers; therefore, breast-feeding is not currently considered to be a route for HCV transmission. Sharing instruments to inhale substances ("straws") or body piercing or tattooing under nonsterile conditions are thought to be potential modes of transmission of hepatitis C; however, no epidemiological studies have demonstrated a clear link between these practices and the spread of HCV (Larson et al. 2001). Despite these known risk factors, 30–40% of patients with acute HCV deny knowledge of a specific exposure associated with acquiring the infection in the six months before onset of illness.

Approximately 15–20% of chronically infected patients progress to end-stage liver disease/cirrhosis over an average of 20 years (Addesa et al. 2001, Larson et al. 2001). A variety of factors may affect the rate of progression of disease, including age, gender, HIV infection, and extent of alcohol consumption (Younossi 2000). Alcohol abuse appears to have the most profound influence on progression of chronic hepatitis.

Patients with cirrhosis are at risk for ascites, gastrointestinal varices and bleeding, and hepatic decompensation. Hepatocellular carcinoma becomes a concern after 30 years of HCV infection and is more common in the presence of alcoholism, cirrhosis, and HBV co-infection. Patients with chronic hepatitis C may manifest extrahepatic syndromes, including arthritis, glomerulonephritis, lichen planus, cryoglobulinemia, porphyria cutanea tarda, leukocytoclastic vasculitis, keratoconjunctivitis sicca, Raynaud's syndrome, and systemic vasculitis. Fulminant hepatitis C is extremely rare.

HDV

Hepatitis D may be regarded as a complication of hepatitis B because HDV depends on infection with HBV. Modes of HDV transmission are similar to those of HBV. Percutaneous exposures are the most common form of transmission, mainly through intravenous drug abuse and blood transfusions. Sexual transmission is possible but less common.

Hepatitis D has infected more than 10 million people worldwide (Younossi 2000). In general, patients with hepatitis B and D are more likely to suffer from serious and progressive disease than are those with other forms of viral hepatitis. HDV superinfection (HDV infection acquired by a patient with pre-existing HBV infection) can transform mild hepatitis B into progressive chronic hepatitis B. Co-infection (acquisition of HDV and HBV at the same time) is self-limited in almost all patients (90%) and clinically indistinguishable from infection with hepatitis B alone. But it is associated with an increased likelihood of fulminant hepatitis in acute disease and has a more aggressive course in chronic disease (Holst et al. 2001, Malik et al. 2000).

HDV is endemic in Russia, Romania, southern Italy, Africa, and South America (Holst et al. 2001). The incubation period for HDV is 2–8 weeks. Fulminant hepatic failure can occur in 5–20% of cases of superinfection.

HEV

Hepatitis E virus is an acute, self-limited illness. It is spread by fecal-oral transmission and occurs endemically in developing countries that have inadequate sanitation. Water contamination is the major source of infection (Holst et al. 2001, Malik et al. 2000, Younossi 2000). Epidemics commonly follow periods of heavy rainfall and floods. Improved sanitation is critical for dis-

ease prevention. Direct person-to-person transmission is rare. Clinical occurrence rates are highest among young adults 15–40 years old (Malik et al. 2000, Younossi 2000). Although the mortality rate is usually low (0.07–0.6%), the illness may be particularly severe in pregnant women, in whom mortality rates from acute liver failure reach 15–25% (Malik et al. 2000, Younossi 2000). HEV is responsible for large epidemics of acute hepatitis and a proportion of sporadic hepatitis cases in southeast and central Asia, the southeast Pacific, the Middle East, parts of Africa, and Mexico.

Typically, the illness lasts 1–4 weeks. The incubation period for hepatitis E varies from 2–9 weeks (Holst et al. 2001, Younossi 2000). In a few patients, hepatitis E infection can lead to fulminant hepatic failure.

Hepatitis G

Hepatitis G (also referred to as GBV-C) is a blood-borne viral agent that has been detected in some patients with non-A, non-B, non-C, non-D, and non-E hepatitis. It is transmitted mainly through blood and blood products. It is closely related to HCV and is present in 10% of HCV-positive patients (Holst et al. 2001). Current data do not support a major role for this virus in causing liver disease (Friedman 2002, Younossi 2000). For this reason, hepatitis G virus will not be discussed further in this chapter.

DATABASE

SUBJECTIVE

→ Acute hepatitis is associated with a characteristic set of symptoms.
→ The symptoms caused by HAV, HBV, and HCV are indistinguishable, except that acute HCV infection is more frequently subclinical.
→ Prodromal phase:
  ▪ Onset may be abrupt or insidious.
  ▪ Prodromal symptoms of hepatitis frequently include anorexia, nausea, vomiting, malaise, flu-like symptoms (myalgias, fatigue, upper respiratory symptoms, mild fever), and aversion to smoking.
→ Icteric phase:
  ▪ Usually occurs 5–10 days after symptom onset, although it can occur concurrently.
  ▪ Most patients never develop clinical icterus.
  ▪ The patient may complain of clay-colored stools, dark or tea-colored urine, right upper quadrant (RUQ) or epigastric abdominal pain (which may be aggravated by jarring or exertion), or a skin rash or itching.
→ Convalescent phase:
  ▪ General symptoms in the convalescent phase may include the disappearance of jaundice, the return of appetite, resolving abdominal pain, and an increased sense of well-being.
→ If hepatitis is suspected, the patient's medical history should be reviewed for the risk factors described earlier in this chapter.

→ Assess for other possible risk factors of hepatitis—e.g., alcohol use, autoimmune disease, hemochromatosis, a history of Epstein-Barr infection, measles, exposure to hepatotoxic drugs, and drug hypersensitivity.

Hepatitis A

→ In adults, symptomatic infection is characteristic and jaundice common.
→ Onset is often abrupt.
→ Characteristic prodromal symptoms—anorexia, nausea, fatigue, and others—are followed within a few days to two weeks by dark urine and jaundice.
→ Nonspecific signs and symptoms parallel those of infectious mononucleosis and other viral syndromes.
→ The duration of the icteric phase varies, although complete resolution generally occurs within 3–6 months of onset of illness.
→ Rarely, when the disease follows a fulminant course, the patient may develop a cholestatic variant with striking jaundice that persists for months.

Hepatitis B

→ Onset of acute infection is symptomatic in half of patients (CDC 2002).
→ The prodromal period consists of nonspecific constitutional symptoms and may be followed by anorexia, myalgias, fatigue, jaundice, and RUQ abdominal pain.
→ A maculopapular rash, urticaria, arthralgias, and arthritis may occur.
→ Symptoms usually resolve within 2–3 months.
→ In adults, only 50% of acute HBV infections are symptomatic (CDC 2002).

Hepatitis C

→ As acute hepatitis C is usually anicteric and asymptomatic, HCV infection is infrequently diagnosed during the acute phase of infection.
→ Clinical manifestations, such as malaise, weakness, nausea, and anorexia, can occur (in 25–35% of patients), usually within 7–12 weeks after exposure to HCV (Holst et al. 2001).
→ In chronic hepatitis C, symptoms frequently are absent for many years (15–30) until liver disease becomes advanced; then, fatigue and malaise are common (Holst et al. 2001).

Hepatitis D

→ Illness onset is usually abrupt, with signs and symptoms resembling those of hepatitis B.

Hepatitis E

→ Signs and symptoms resemble those of other forms of viral hepatitis.
→ Only acute forms are recognized.
→ Asymptomatic and anicteric infections may occur in a significant number of cases.

OBJECTIVE
→ The patient may present with:
- Hepatomegaly
- An enlarged, soft, and tender liver
- Splenomegaly
- Jaundice
- Palatial petechiae
- Soft, enlarged lymph nodes (especially epitrochlear and cervical)
- Arthralgia with or without arthritis
- Skin revealing a diffuse, maculopapular, erythematous rash
- Signs of toxemia
- Hematuria

ASSESSMENT

→ Viral hepatitis
- Hepatitis A
- Hepatitis B
- Hepatitis C
- Hepatitis D
- Hepatitis E
→ R/O infectious mononucleosis
→ R/O cytomegalovirus
→ R/O herpes simplex virus infection
→ R/O drug-induced liver disease
→ R/O influenza
→ R/O upper respiratory tract infection
→ R/O biliary tract disease
→ R/O autoimmune hepatitis
→ R/O spirochetal diseases
→ R/O brucellosis
→ R/O rickettsial diseases
→ R/O collagen-vascular disease

PLAN

DIAGNOSTIC TESTS
→ The diagnosis of a viral hepatitis infection cannot be made on clinical grounds alone; it requires confirmatory serologic testing.

Hepatitis A

Antibody to Hepatitis A (Anti-HAV)
→ Appears early in the course of illness.
→ Both immunoglobulin M (IgM) anti-HAV and immunoglobulin G (IgG) anti-HAV are detectable in serum soon after the onset of illness.
- IgM anti-HAV:
  - An excellent test for diagnosing acute hepatitis A.
  - Total IgM levels often are elevated in acute hepatitis A infection, with titers peaking during the first week of clinical disease.
  - Can be detected for 3–6 months after acute infection.
- IgG anti-HAV:
  - Titers of IgG peak after one month of the disease.

- The IgG response to HAV persists for decades.
- The presence of IgG anti-HAV alone indicates previous exposure to HAV, recovery, noninfectivity, and immunity to reinfection.

Liver Enzymes

→ During the acute phase of illness, levels of alanine aminotransferase (ALT) and aspartate aminotransferase (AST) can show moderate to marked elevation, with either one ranging from 500–5,000 U/L.

→ Most adults having clinically apparent disease will recover, with restoration of normal aminotransferase values within six months.

Bilirubin

→ Bilirubin level can be normal or elevated.

→ Bilirubin concentrations are rarely >10 mg/dL, except in patients with acute liver failure and cholestatic hepatitis A.

→ Bilirubin values return to normal within six months.

Hepatitis B

→ Serologic markers for HBV infection are numerous.

→ The serologic diagnosis of HBV infection is established by detecting either antibodies and/or their respective antigens (i.e., HBsAg and anti-HBs, HBcAg and anti-HBc, or HBeAg and anti-HBe).

→ Monitoring an HBV infection and response to treatment can be performed using a combination of these tests. Typical test panels for specific situations include:
  - Diagnosis of acute viral hepatitis B by HBsAg (+) and anti-HBc (+)
  - Diagnosis of remote, prior HBV infection: HBsAg (-), total anti-HBc (+), and anti-HBs (+)
  - Monitoring ongoing HBV infection: HBsAg (+), total anti-HBc (+), anti-HBs ([-] if chronic infection), HBeAg (+ or -), anti-HBe (+ or -), and HBV DNA (+ if chronic)

→ See **Table 11B.1, Serologic and Molecular Tests for Hepatitis B.**

Hepatitis B Surface Antigen (HBsAg)

→ After acute infection, HBsAg is the first detectable virologic marker.

→ Detectable serum HBsAg usually precedes elevations in serum transaminases, as well as clinical symptoms, and remains detectable during the acute icteric period and beyond.

→ In most cases, the HBsAg becomes undetectable 1–2 months following onset of jaundice, rarely persisting beyond six months.

→ It is diagnostic for chronic persistent or active infection if present more than six months.

Antibody to HBsAg (Anti-HBs)

→ After HBsAg disappears, anti-HBs is produced and appears in serum following a resolved infection.

→ There may be a lag period (window) between the disappearance of HBsAg and the appearance of anti-HBs, during which time patients with HBV infection may not be identified by routine serologic testing.

→ Anti-HBs is the only HBV antibody marker present following immunization.

→ Anti-HBs is a marker of recovery and immunity.

Hepatitis B Core Antigen (HBcAg)

→ HBcAg is sequestered inside an HBsAg coat and is not usually detectable in the serum of HBV-infected patients.

→ Tests for HBcAg are generally limited to testing liver biopsy samples.

→ The presence of HBcAg in liver tissue indicates ongoing viral replication and can be interpreted as a measure of infectivity.

Antibodies to Hepatitis B Core Antigen (Anti-HBc)

→ The test of choice when performing prevaccination antibody screening in adult populations with a high prevalence of HBV infection.
  - Anti-HBc total:
    - Indicates current or previous infection; not associated with recovery or immunity.
  - IgM anti-HBc:
    - Appears shortly after HBsAg is detected; is diagnostic for acute HBV infection (first six months).
    - IgM anti-HBc may be detectable and can be used to identify acute HBV infection during the silent window period when patients have cleared HBsAg but do not yet have detectable anti-HBs.
  - IgG anti-HBc:
    - Appears during the acute phase; high titers persist for several months to one year.
    - Is positive for life and is positive in both recovered and chronic HBV infection.
    - Serves as a marker of prior hepatitis B infection.
    - Is not produced in individuals with postvaccine immunity.

Hepatitis B e antigen (HBeAg)

→ HBeAg is a viral protein secreted by HBV-infected cells and becomes detectable before the onset of clinical symptoms.

→ The presence of HBeAg indicates high levels of virus in the blood.

→ It is an indicator of the infectiousness of the carrier for both acute and chronic infection.

→ Persistence beyond 10 weeks indicates likely chronic liver disease, but the absence of this marker does not ensure absence of infection.

→ When negative in a person known to be HBsAg positive, it indicates low levels of virus in the blood or an "integrated phase" of HBV in which the virus is integrated into the host's DNA.

→ This test is often used to monitor the effectiveness of some HBV therapies, the goal of which is to convert an actively replicating state to an "e-antigen negative" state.

Anti-HBe

→ The disappearance of HBeAg often is followed by the appearance of anti-HBe, signifying diminished viral replication and decreased infectivity.

→ Conversion from HBeAg to anti-HBe usually indicates a benign outcome with no or low levels of viral replication and infectivity.

Liver Enzymes

→ Serum ALT and AST levels are typically mildly to moderately elevated in acute disease (into the 1,000 to several thousand U/L range, with ALT > AST) but may be normal in chronic infection.

Bilirubin

→ Serum bilirubin levels may be elevated in acute infection.

Liver Biopsy

→ Acute disease does not usually require a liver biopsy.

→ Biopsy should be performed in patients with suspected chronic hepatitis B in order to:

- Confirm the diagnosis of chronic hepatitis
- Grade the severity of liver damage
- Assess the stage (fibrosis or cirrhosis)
- Detect evidence of active viral replication

Hepatitis C

→ Two categories of virologic assays are used for diagnosing and managing HCV infection: serologic assays based on HCV immunologic characteristics and molecular-based assays based on the quantification and characterization of the HCV RNA (antibody tests and HCV RNA tests).

Antibodies to HCV (Anti-HCV)

→ The primary serologic screening assay for HCV infection is the enzyme immunoassay (EIA), of which there have been three consecutive versions, with a progressive increase in sensitivity.

→ The currently used enzyme immunoassays can detect antibodies within 4–10 weeks after infection.

→ The recombinant immunoblot assay (RIBA) has been used to confirm positive enzyme immunoassays.

→ Anti-HCV by EIA is recommended for routine testing of asymptomatic persons and can be detected 3–6 weeks following exposure.

→ Antibodies are measurable in 80% of patients within 15 weeks of exposure, in more than 90% within five months, and in more than 97% by six months after exposure.

→ Antibody tests are 97% specific but cannot identify an infection as acute, chronic, or resolved, as it remains positive with chronic infection and with clearance of the virus.

Table 11B.1.   SEROLOGIC AND MOLECULAR TESTS FOR HEPATITIS B

Test	Clinical Scenario		
Immunity	*Acute Infection*	*Chronic Infection*	*Resolution*
HBsAg	+	+	−
Anti-HBc			
IgM	+	−	−
IgG	+	+	+
Anti-HBs	−	−	+*
HBV DNA^	+	±	−
HBeAg^	+	±	−
Anti-HBe^	−	±	+

Anti-HBc: antibody to hepatitis B core antigen
Anti-HBe: antibody to hepatitis B e antigen
Anti-HBs: antibody to hepatitis B surface antigen
HBsAG: hepatitis B surface antigen
HBV DNA: hepatitis B virus DNA
HBeAG: hepatitis B e antigen

+ Positive findings
− Negative findings
± Inconclusive findings
* Confers immunity. Hepatitis B immunization results only in anti-HBs production.
^ Usually ordered in chronic infections only.

Source: Reprinted with permission from Saab, S., and Martin, P. 2000. Tests for acute and chronic viral hepatitis. *Postgraduate Medicine* 107(2):123–130. ©McGraw-Hill Companies.

HCV RNA

→ Assays based on the molecular detection of HCV RNA have been introduced in the last few years and can be categorized as qualitative and quantitative.

→ HCV RNA can be detected in serum or plasma within 1–2 weeks following exposure and weeks to months before elevation of serum ALT or the appearance of HCV antibody.

→ Qualitative tests for HCV RNA are the most sensitive assays for the presence of circulating virus and have become the gold standard for monitoring response to treatment.

→ The viral load (assays that detect quantitative HCV RNA) has been shown to be predictive of response to anti-HCV therapy but is not correlated with risk of disease progression or with disease severity.

Viral Genotyping

→ Helps predict the outcome of therapy.

→ Influences the choice and duration of therapeutic regimen.

→ Different methods are available for the genotyping of HCV.

Liver Enzymes

→ ALT level is useful for monitoring HCV infection and the efficacy of therapy in the intervals between molecular testing.

→ In persons with HCV infection, ALT levels may be normal or fluctuate. Neither a single normal value nor multiple normal values rules out active infection, progressive liver disease, or even cirrhosis.

→ Conversely, the normalization of ALT levels with antiviral therapy is not proof that therapy is successful.

Other Diagnostic Tests

→ Alkaline phosphatase and bilirubin may show slight increases.

→ Hypoalbuminemia and prolongation of prothrombin time are signs of advanced hepatic dysfunction.

→ Consider thyroid function tests, as autoimmune thyroid disease is a common autoimmune disorder in patients with chronic hepatitis C (Bonkovsky et al. 2001).

Liver Biopsy

→ Is the gold standard for determining the severity of HCV-related liver disease.

→ Biopsy generally is recommended for initially assessing persons with chronic HCV infection, although it is not mandatory.

→ The degree of fibrosis observed on liver biopsy appears to be the best means of predicting the risk of developing cirrhosis and, thus, the prognosis of individual patients with chronic HCV.

→ Biopsy also may rule out other, concurrent causes of liver disease.

Hepatitis D

→ Is necessary to establish a diagnosis of HBV by testing for HBV serologies.

→ The initial diagnosis of HDV is made serologically by detecting IgM antibody (anti-HDV IgM) to HDV antigen.

Anti-HDV

→ Indicates exposure.

■ IgM anti-HDV:
  • Indicates recent exposure.
  • If anti-HDV IgM is present with anti-HBc IgM, the patient has been co-infected with HDV.
  • If anti-HDV IgM is present but anti-HBc IgM is absent, HDV infection is a superinfection.

■ IgG anti-HDV:
  • Develops some weeks after primary infection and persists with chronic infection.
  • A high titer (>1:1,000) correlates well with ongoing chronic viral replication.
  • Low titers are associated with past infection.

HDV RNA

→ Indicates active infection.

Liver Biopsy

→ Liver biopsies also may be examined for the presence of HDV RNA.

Hepatitis E

Anti-HEV

→ Indicates exposure.

■ IgM anti-HEV:
  • Indicates current or recent infection.
  • Titers increase one month after infection, decline rapidly, and disappear over 4–5 months.

■ IgG anti-HEV:
  • Indicates previous infection and confers lifelong immunity.
  • Titers increase 6–8 weeks after infection.
  • Persists for at least several years.

HEV RNA

→ Indicates active infection.

Liver Enzymes

→ Elevations in serum ALT and AST occur in acute illness and 1–2 months after nonacute infection.

Bilirubin

→ May have variable degree of rise in serum bilirubin (predominantly conjugated).

Alkaline Phosphatase

→ A mild rise is possible.

Liver Biopsy

→ Not indicated.

TREATMENT/MANAGEMENT

General Principles of Hepatitis Treatment

The *Physicians' Desk Reference* (*PDR*) should be reviewed for indications, usage, contraindications, warnings, and adverse reactions regarding all pharmacologic agents discussed in this chapter.

→ The treatment of acute viral hepatitis is primarily symptomatic, regardless of the etiologic agent involved.

→ There is no confirmed benefit from pharmacologic therapies for acute hepatitis due to HAV, HBV, or HCV.

→ Most patients with acute hepatitis can be treated at home.

→ Hospital admission for acute hepatitis is only necessary when symptoms of nausea and vomiting preclude adequate nutrition and hydration, or when clinical and biochemical deterioration suggests progression to fulminant hepatic failure.

→ Symptomatic and supportive care is recommended and includes:

- The avoidance of hepatically metabolized drugs, particularly sedatives, although metoclopramide and phenothiazines may be given in the minimal effective doses for severe nausea, and oxazepam can be used if sedation is required

- Bed rest if the patient is frail or on an as-needed basis

- Minimal to moderate activity is recommended for all others (although activity strenuous enough to cause fatigue should be avoided)

- No dietary restrictions except for avoidance of alcohol and other potentially hepatotoxic agents

- Good caloric intake and maintenance of hydration

Pharmacologic Overview of Hepatitis Treatment

→ The primary goal of antiviral treatment is to suppress viral replication before there is irreversible liver damage.

→ Treatment options for chronic viral hepatitis are limited, consisting primarily of three drug classes:

- The interferons:
  - Synthetically produced versions of naturally occurring cytokine typically produced as part of the immune response to infection
  - Interfere with viral replication and possess immunoregulatory and anti-inflammatory properties

- Antiviral nucleoside analogues (ribavirin, lamivudine, and adefovir):
  - Act through interference with RNA (ribavirin) or DNA (lamivudine and adefovir) synthesis

- Non-nucleoside antiviral drugs (amantadine and rimantadine):
  - Are currently being investigated

Hepatitis A

→ No specific treatment exists for hepatitis A.

→ Patients usually require only supportive care, with no restriction on diet or activity.

→ Prevention:

- Improved sanitation

- Immune globulin following exposure (passive immunoprophylaxis) and/or vaccine (active immunoprophylaxis)

→ Hepatitis A vaccine:

- Two inactivated HAV vaccines (Havrix® and Vaqta®) are licensed for use in the United States. (See *PDR* for dosage regimens.)

- Active immunization with HAV vaccine generates

protective antibodies and appears to provide protection that lasts up to 10 or more years.

- Within 4 weeks after administration of either vaccine, antibodies to HAV are detectable in nearly 100% of vaccinated persons (Holst et al. 2001).

- While 1 booster is required after 6–12 months, immunosuppressed individuals may require additional boosters.

- Postvaccination serologic testing is not indicated.

- Hepatitis A vaccine is recommended for travelers to endemic areas, military personnel, users of illegal drugs (both injection and noninjection) or their partners, men who have sex with men, individuals with chronic liver disease (including people with chronic HBV and HCV infection), and workers with an occupational risk of infection (CDC 2002, Cuthbert 2001).

→ Immune globulin (IG):

- IG prophylaxis dosing for individuals who plan to travel in areas where hepatitis A is endemic:

Length of Stay	Dose Volume
<3 months	0.02 mL/kg
3+ months	0.06 mL/kg (can repeat every 4–6 months)

- A 2-mL dose prevents disease for 3–4 months.

- 5 mL protects for as long as 6 months.

- When administered IM before or within 2 weeks after exposure to HAV, IG is 85% or more effective in preventing hepatitis A (CDC 2002).

→ Postexposure prophylaxis:

- Persons who have not yet been vaccinated and are exposed to HAV (e.g., through household or sexual contact, by sharing illegal drugs with a person who has hepatitis A, or attendees of day-care centers where cases of hepatitis A have occurred) should be administered a single IM dose of IG (0.02 mL/kg) containing anti-HAV as soon as possible, preferably within 2 weeks after exposure (CDC 2002).

- Passive immunization with IG before exposure or within 2 weeks following HAV exposure protects against clinical disease in 70–90% of immunized individuals (Holst et al. 2001, Younossi 2000).

- Persons who have had 1 dose of hepatitis A vaccine at least 1 month before exposure to HAV do not need IG.

- If hepatitis A vaccine is recommended for a person receiving IG, it can be administered simultaneously at a separate anatomic injection site.

- The use of hepatitis A vaccine alone is not recommended for postexposure prophylaxis.

Hepatitis B

→ Acute HBV:

- Treatment of acute infection is largely supportive and antiviral therapy is not indicated.

→ Chronic HBV:

- Asymptomatic carriers of HBV without evidence of significant viral replication and without significant liver disease have an excellent long-term prognosis and do not require treatment.

- Therapy generally is indicated for HBV-infected patients with active viral replication, as evidenced by HBeAg positivity and significant HBV DNA levels, as well as active liver disease with serum ALT elevation and chronic hepatitis on liver histology.
- Treatment options for adult patients with well-compensated chronic HBV include interferons, lamivudine, and adefovir. Other nucleoside/nucleotide analogue agents are in clinical trials.
- Successful therapy is associated with a sustained loss of markers of viral replication (HBeAg) and HBV DNA, as well as by histologic improvement.

→ Drug therapy:
- Antiviral agents (interferon, lamivudine, or adefovir):
  - Interferon and lamivudine are the two best-studied agents for treating chronic HBV.
- Interferon:
  - Immediate beneficial effects in responders include biochemical improvement and loss of viral replication.
  - Sustained benefits include the potential for HBsAg clearance, improved histologic status, improved survival, and decreased incidence of hepatocellular carcinoma.
  - Remission is maintained in most patients who initially respond to interferon therapy, and additional seroconversion continues to occur after treatment is completed (Nguyen et al. 2001).
  - Interferon alpha-2b is recommended when screening reveals:
    - Persistent elevations in serum ALT levels
    - Detectable levels of serum HBsAg, HBeAg, and HBV DNA
    - Compensated liver disease
  - The recommended 4–6 month regimen for recombinant human interferon alfa-2b therapy is 30–35 million IU per week, administered subcutaneously or IM either as 5 million U daily or as 10 million IU 3 times/week.
  - Serum ALT concentrations should be measured every 2–4 weeks, and if values are not normal after 3 months of therapy, a beneficial response is unlikely and therapy should be discontinued.
  - Serum HBsAg, HBeAg, and HBV DNA should be measured at the end of therapy and 6 months post-treatment.
  - Adverse effects that may occur secondary to interferon are arthralgias, myalgias, fever/chills, headache, depression, malaise, and tachycardia. Long-term use is associated with alopecia, bone marrow suppression, cognitive changes, and mood changes. Severe adverse effects (cardiac/renal failure, severe depression with suicide risk, seizures, sepsis, retinopathy, and hearing impairment) occur in about 2% of patients.
- Lamivudine (nucleoside analogue):
  - Has emerged as another therapy for chronic hepatitis B and is a beneficial treatment option for patients with decompensated hepatitis B cirrhosis.
  - 100 mg p.o. QD may be used instead of interferon.

- Is effective in inducing HBeAg seroconversion.
- Has a good safety profile in the doses used to treat chronic HBV.
- Drug resistance is common with lamivudine (Davis 2002).
- Adefovir dipivoxil (nucleotide analogue):
  - Was recently approved by the FDA; minimal clinical experience.
  - Is administered as an oral 10 mg tablet.
  - Renal toxicity when used at higher doses for HIV.

→ Other therapies:
- Liver transplant:
  - Recommended for patients with end-stage chronic hepatitis, even though the new liver almost always becomes infected with HBV.

→ Prevention:
- Two products have been approved for hepatitis B prevention: hepatitis B vaccine and hepatitis B immune globulin (HBIG).
  - Hepatitis B vaccine provides protection from HBV infection when used for both pre-exposure immunization and postexposure prophylaxis in combination with HBIG.
  - The two available monovalent hepatitis B vaccines for use in adolescents and adults are Recombivax HB® and Engerix-B®.
  - The recommended vaccine dose varies by product and age of the recipient.
  - Vaccine should be administered IM in the deltoid muscle.
  - If the vaccination series is interrupted after the first or second dose of vaccine, the missed dose should be administered as soon as possible. The series does not need to be restarted if a dose has been missed.
  - Postvaccination serologic testing is advised for immunocompromised individuals and for health care workers. Nonresponders should be revaccinated.
  - See *PDR* for dosage regimens.

→ Postexposure prophylaxis after exposure to persons who have *acute* hepatitis B:
- Short-term immunity can be conferred by administering HBIG within 24 hours.
- The recommended dose of HBIG for children and adults is 0.06 mL/kg (CDC 2002).
- Sexual contacts:
  - Unvaccinated sex partners of persons with acute hepatitis B should receive postexposure immunization with HBIG and hepatitis B vaccine as soon as possible but at least within 14 days after the most recent sexual contact.
- Nonsexual household contacts:
  - These contacts of patients with acute hepatitis B are not at increased risk for infection unless they have other risk factors, but they should be encouraged to get vaccinated regardless (CDC 2002).
  - All household contacts of individuals with chronic hepatitis B should be vaccinated (CDC 2002).

→ Postexposure prophylaxis after exposure to persons who have *chronic* hepatitis B:

- Active postexposure prophylaxis with hepatitis B vaccine alone is recommended for sex or needle-sharing partners and nonsexual household contacts of persons with chronic HBV infection (CDC 2002).
- Special considerations:
  - Pregnancy and HIV infection are beyond the scope of this chapter.
  - Victims of sexual assault (CDC 2002):
    - If a victim is not fully vaccinated, completion of the vaccine series is recommended.
    - Unvaccinated persons should be administered active postexposure prophylaxis (i.e., vaccine alone) at the initial clinical evaluation.
    - Unless the offender is known to have active hepatitis B (i.e., is HbsAg-positive), HBIG is not required but may be administered if desired.

Hepatitis C

→ The efficacy of treating acute HCV infection is not known, as acute infection with HCV is usually asymptomatic and rarely recognized. Given the high rate of progression to, and the limited efficacy of therapy for, chronic infection, treatment of acute infection has been advocated. Because there have been few prospective, randomized, controlled trials assessing the efficacy of acute HCV infection treatment, an optimal therapeutic regimen and the best point at which to intervene have not yet been defined (Bonkovsky et al. 2001).

→ Treatment with interferon-alpha for 6–24 weeks in the setting of acute HCV appears to yield results comparable—and possibly superior—to results of using it for treating chronic HCV (Jaeckel et al. 2001).

→ The optimal therapeutic regimen and the best time to intervene in patients who have acute hepatitis C have not yet been defined. Risks and benefits should be assessed on an individual basis.

→ Treating all patients acutely infected with hepatitis C does incur risk. Drug toxicities will occur in 15% of patients who otherwise would have resolved the infection on their own (or who may have had a relatively benign clinical course with chronic infection).

→ Patients with decompensated liver disease are not candidates for antiviral therapy due to poor tolerability of the drug and the potential for increasing complications, such as life-threatening infections.

→ Chronic hepatitis C:

- The primary goal of therapy is HCV eradication.
- Secondary goals (when the primary goal is not possible) are preventing progression of liver disease and reducing the risk of hepatocellular carcinoma.
- The risks and benefits of treating patients with chronic HCV infection must be assessed on an individual basis.
- Only a subgroup of infected persons has a clear indication for therapy: those with detectable levels of HCV RNA and asymptomatic or compensated liver disease, and a liver biopsy showing fibrosis or at least moderate necrosis and inflammation.
- Persons with normal or elevated ALT levels and only minimal or mild necrotic and inflammatory changes also may be treated.
- Persons with persistently normal ALT levels and no histologic evidence of necrotic and inflammatory changes have an excellent prognosis without therapy and usually are not considered for therapy (except in controlled clinical trials).

→ Drug therapy:

- Interferon monotherapy or interferon plus ribavirin combination therapy:
  - Interferon monotherapy (Foster et al. 2000):
    - Commonly causes flu-like symptoms (which can be severe) during the first 2 weeks of therapy.
    - Patients receiving long-term treatment with interferon may notice fatigue and difficulties concentrating, which are reversible once treatment is discontinued.
    - The most feared complication of interferon therapy is suicidal depression. While most patients receiving interferon have mild depression, a small minority becomes severely depressed.
    - Interferon may cause bone marrow suppression.
  - Interferon and ribavirin combination therapy:
    - Interferon and ribavirin are the cornerstones of therapy for chronic HCV.
    - Combination therapy (interferon and ribavirin) is associated with a higher rate of sustained virological response and histological improvement compared to interferon monotherapy and seems to increase the rates of response in patients with cirrhosis (Davis 2000, Malik et al. 2000).
    - While interferon in combination with ribavirin is considered to be safe and effective, this combination may increase the risk of certain side effects, including insomnia, depression, irritability, a reversible hemolytic anemia, and more severe flu-like symptoms, than interferon alone (Davis 2000, Foster et al. 2000).
    - Ribavirin has been shown to be teratogenic (pregnancy category X) and pregnancy should be avoided for 6 months post-therapy.
  - The efficacy of interferon alone and in combination with ribavirin is strongly influenced by the genotype of HCV infection, the level of circulating virus, and the presence/absence of cirrhosis.
  - Persons infected with HCV genotype 1a or 1b (the most prevalent genotypes in the United States) benefit from the combination of interferon alfa and ribavirin.
    - Duration of treatment should be based on the HCV genotype and the pretreatment viral load (although tests for quantifying HCV RNA are not standardized and viral load fluctuates over time, so viral load is not always used for determining treatment regimen).
    - Patients infected with HCV genotype 2 or 3 and those with low viral loads before treatment usually

require only 24 weeks of treatment to achieve a sustained response.
- Patients infected with genotype 1 and those with a high viral load before treatment require a course of 48 weeks for an optimal outcome.
- Hepatitis C therapy dosages are usually prescribed by a specialist, as dose adjustments often are required to manage toxicity.
■ Pegylated interferons:
- When interferon is pegylated, its half-life is increased, the rate of drug clearance is decreased, and there are prolonged concentrations of interferon.
- At all doses, pegylated interferon alfa-2b is significantly more effective than nonpegylated interferon.
- The safety and tolerability of pegylated interferon are qualitatively similar to that of standard interferon.
- Persons who cannot be treated with ribavirin can be treated with pegylated interferon.
■ Pegylated interferon-alpha and ribavirin combination therapy:
- Pegylated interferon alpha-2a or alpha-2b in combination with ribavirin is currently the most effective regimen for treating chronic hepatitis C.
- Early reports of using pegylated interferon in conjunction with ribavirin show overall sustained response rates of up to 54% in patients with genotype 1 and higher response rates in those with genotypes 2 and 3 (Larson et al. 2001).
→ Other therapies:
■ Liver transplantation:
- It should be considered in patients with decompensated cirrhosis or early stage hepatocellular carcinoma.
- Although persistent viremia is universal following liver transplantation, the outcome of patients transplanted for HCV appears to be the same as that of patients who receive liver transplants for other conditions.
- Transplantation is the treatment of choice for patients with hepatocellular carcinoma confined to the liver.
→ Prevention:
■ A vaccine for hepatitis C is not available, and prophylaxis with IG is not effective in preventing HCV infection after exposure.
■ Only monitoring is recommended.

Hepatitis D
→ The only treatment for HDV is supportive.
→ A vaccine against and postexposure treatment for HDV are not available.
→ Because HDV depends entirely on HBV for replication, strategies aimed at eliminating HBV also will be effective in reducing HDV infection.

Hepatitis E
→ There is no treatment other than supportive care.
→ There is no vaccine for preventing hepatitis E and it is not known if IG prophylaxis is effective.

CONSULTATION
→ Consultation with and/or referral to a physician experienced in treating hepatitis should be considered in all cases of chronic hepatitis because advances in antiviral therapy and standards of practice for chronic hepatitis change rapidly.
→ Consultation especially should be considered in the following situations:
■ For patients who have cirrhosis and are therefore at dramatically increased risk of hepatocellular carcinoma.
■ When managing patients who have hepatitis during pregnancy or if the patient is otherwise at high risk. High-risk patients include the elderly and transplant recipients; those who have a difficult-to-manage, underlying chronic disorder, severe symptoms, or inadequate caloric/fluid intake; and those who are immunocompromised or abusing alcohol.
■ In cases of severe hepatitis with development of coagulopathy or any indication of hepatic encephalopathy.

PATIENT EDUCATION
→ The following recommendations are general guidelines that may be appropriate for all types of hepatitis:
■ Teach the parent and family about risk factors, pathophysiology, the management plan, the state of infectivity, and the availability of prophylactic hepatitis vaccines.
■ Advise the patient regarding transmission precautions until the period of infectivity has passed.
■ Patients in the carrier or chronic state should be advised to continue transmission precautions.
■ Teach the patient good personal hygiene.
■ Advise the patient not to prepare or serve food to others.
■ Advise the patient that intimate contact (sharing of bodily fluids) should be avoided.
■ Advise the patient to use barrier methods during sexual activity.
■ Persons who use illegal drugs or have multiple sex partners should be provided with information about substance abuse programs and how to get tested, how to reduce their risk of acquiring blood-borne and sexually transmitted infections, and how to avoid transmitting infectious agents to others.
■ Teach health care workers to observe universal precautions and sharps safety practices.
■ Advise the patient to encourage exposed contacts to consult their provider as soon as possible for prophylaxis and/or immunization if appropriate.
■ Advise the patient regarding a nutritious diet.
■ Advise the patient regarding supportive measures.
■ Advise the patient about regular physical activity as tolerated and to avoid becoming overtired.
■ Teach the patient to be aware of and omit hepatotoxic agents whenever possible—e.g., drugs and alcohol, hazardous environmental substances, and certain medications, such as acetaminophen and niacin.
■ Advise the patient to inform all health care providers of her hepatitis infection.

FOLLOW-UP

→ Patients with chronic hepatitis, especially those with chronic active hepatitis, should be followed by a physician.

→ Referral to a physician is recommended for persistent symptoms or abnormal laboratory values lasting longer than six months.

→ A public health nurse may assist the family with preventive care and teach the family in the home.

→ Referral to an alcohol or drug treatment program is recommended for patients with substance abuse problems.

→ Instruct the patient to return to the clinic as appropriate for follow-up laboratory testing, and discuss risks related to not complying with medical therapy.

→ If the patient has not been exposed to hepatitis A and/or B, recommend vaccination if she is at risk.

→ Advise/teach her regarding the American Cancer Society's recommendation for early detection of cancer in asymptomatic people (Zoorob et al. 2001):

- A fecal occult blood test yearly beginning at age 50 years
  AND
- A digital rectal exam and flexible sigmoidoscopy every 5 years beginning at age 50 years
  OR
- A digital rectal exam and colonoscopy every 10 years beginning at age 50 years
  OR
- A digital rectal exam and double contrast barium enema every 5–10 years beginning at age 50 years

→ If the patient has chronic HBV or HCV, advise her regarding screening for hepatocellular carcinoma and cirrhosis.

→ Document in progress notes and on problem list.

BIBLIOGRAPHY

Addesa, J.A., and Navarro, V.J. 2001. Concise review of the management of hepatitis C. *Comprehensive Therapy* 27(4): 277–283.

Befeler, A.S., and DiBisceglie, A.M. 2000. Hepatitis B. *Infectious Disease Clinics of North America* 14(3):617–632.

Bonkovsky, H.L., and Mehta, S. 2001. Hepatitis C: a review and update. *Journal of the American Academy of Dermatology* 44:159–179.

Busch, M.P., and Kleinman, S.H. 2000. Nucleic acid amplification testing of blood donors for transfusion-transmitted infectious diseases. *Transfusion* 40:143–159.

Centers for Disease Control and Prevention (CDC). 2002. Sexually transmitted diseases treatment guidelines 2002. *Morbidity and Mortality Weekly Report* 51(RR-6):59–66.

Cuthbert, J.A. 2001. Hepatitis A: old and new. *Clinical Microbiology Reviews* 14(1):38–58.

Davis, G.L. 2000. Current therapy for chronic hepatitis C. *Gastroenterology* 118:S104–S114.

_____. 2002. Update on the management of chronic hepatitis B. *Review of Gastroenterologic Disorders* 2(3):106–115.

Foster, G.R., and Thomas, H.C. 2000. Therapeutic options for HCV—management of the infected individual. *Bailliere's Clinical Gastroenterology* 14(2):255–264.

Friedman, L.S. 2002. Diseases of the Liver. In *Current medical diagnosis and treatment*, 41st ed., eds. L.M. Tierney, Jr., S.J. McPhee, and M.A. Papadakis, pp. 678–688. New York: Lange Medical Books/McGraw-Hill.

Holst, B., and Ritter, D. 2001. Managing viral hepatitis. *Clinician Reviews* 11(1):51–62.

Jaeckel, E., Cornberg, M., Wedemeyer, H. et al. 2001. Treatment of acute hepatitis C with interferon alfa-2b. *New England Journal of Medicine* 345(20):1452–1457.

Larson, A.M., and Carithers, R.L. 2001. Hepatitis C in clinical practice. *Journal of Internal Medicine* 249:111–120.

Lauer, G.M., and Walker, B.D. 2001. Medical progress: hepatitis C infection. *New England Journal of Medicine* 345(1): 41–52.

Malik, A.H., and Malet, P.F. 2000. Acute and chronic viral hepatitis. *Clinics in Family Practice* 2(1):35–57.

Nguyen, M.H., and Wright, T.L. 2001. Therapeutic advances in the management of hepatitis B and hepatitis C. *Current Opinion in Infectious Diseases* 14:593–601.

Saab, S., and Martin, P. 2000. Tests for acute and chronic viral hepatitis. *Postgraduate Medicine* 107(2):123–130.

Younossi, Z.M. 2000. Viral hepatitis guide for practicing physicians. *Cleveland Clinic Journal of Medicine* 67(Suppl. 1): SI:6–7.

Zoorob, R., Anderson, R., Cefalu, C. et al. 2001. Cancer screening guidelines. *American Family Physician* 63(6):1039–1040, 1042.

11-C

Human Immunodeficiency Virus-1 Infection

Human immunodeficiency virus-1 (HIV-1) infection is a complex infectious disease caused by a retrovirus that results in chronic immune dysfunction involving multiple organs and systems of the body. Most individuals infected with HIV-1 eventually develop *acquired immunodeficiency syndrome* (AIDS), a condition representing severe immune dysfunction and end-stage HIV disease.

It is estimated that 40 million people worldwide have HIV infection, most of whom live in developing countries. Globally, 48% (17.6 million) of adult HIV/AIDS cases occur in women (Joint United Nations Programme on HIV/AIDS 2001). The most current AIDS surveillance data for the United States indicate that as of June 2001, 793,026 persons had been diagnosed with AIDS (Centers for Disease Control and Prevention [CDC] 2002). These data also reveal a steady and dramatic increase in cases reported in women, from 7% in 1985 to 25% in 2001 (CDC 2002, Marlink et al. 2001). Black and Hispanic women are over-represented in this epidemic, with 77% of AIDS cases reported in these groups. AIDS is a leading cause of death for women age 25–44 years. Since the mid- to late 1990s, there has been a significant decline in AIDS cases and AIDS-associated deaths observed, primarily due to advances in HIV treatment and opportunistic infection prevention (Murphy et al. 2001). However, there is evidence that disparity exists between the rates at which men and women access medical care and HIV therapies, with women receiving fewer indicated therapeutic interventions compared to men (Cohn et al. 2001, Gardner et al. 2002, Marlink et al. 2001, Poundstone et al. 2001).

HIV transmission can occur through parenteral, sexual, or perinatal routes. Heterosexual transmission is now the leading mechanism for the acquisition of HIV by women in the United States (CDC 2002). Therefore, women with a history of unprotected sexual contact with a partner of unknown HIV status should be considered at risk for exposure. Furthermore, surveillance data indicate that young women are increasingly affected by this disease. In 2000, HIV confidential reporting from 34 regions in the United States indicated that 47% of new infections occurred in women younger than 25 years (CDC 2002). Factors associated with an increased risk of HIV transmission include the infectiousness of the patient (e.g., the viral load level in the HIV-infected person), susceptibility of the recipient (e.g., genetic factors, genital tract inflammation, cervical ectopy, other sexually transmitted diseases [STDs]), and viral properties (e.g., phenotypic characteristics, resistance to antiretroviral medications) (Hessol et al. 2001).

An in-depth presentation of the complex pathogenesis of HIV is beyond the scope of this chapter. However, a brief summary of HIV virology and the clinical progression of an infected individual will provide a basic understanding of the strategies for treating this disease.

HIV is a retrovirus consisting of a nucleoprotein core that is encapsulated by an outer lipid bilayer that contains envelope proteins. One of these surface envelope proteins, gp120, is responsible for HIV's binding to specific receptors on target cells, such as the CD4+ receptor site on T-helper lymphocyte cells. Additionally, co-receptors such as the CCR5 and CCXR4 chemokines also must be present on the target cell's surface for successful attachment of HIV to occur. Once the virus has attached to a target cell, it can enter the host cell through the action of another envelope protein, gp41. This transmembrane envelope protein helps fuse the HIV virion with the host cell's membrane and facilitates the transport of the viral nucleoproteins to the human immune cell's nucleus. It is at this point that the action of reverse transcriptase (RT) helps synthesize the HIV viral RNA genome into DNA. This DNA copy is then integrated into the host cell's chromosomal DNA, resulting in the formation of an HIV provirus. The assembly of the HIV virion continues as regulatory and structural HIV proteins are translated into the proviral particle. These synthesized viral protein fragments are structurally too long to allow completion of the assembly process, so the HIV enzyme protease is activated to shorten the protein fragments to the size required for completion of a new virion. After successfully being assembled, the HIV virion emerges through the host cell's membrane (a process called "budding") and is capable of attaching to and infecting other target cells in the body (Phillips et al. 2000).

The complex immune responses in the body require the proper functioning of CD4+ T-lymphocytes, one of the target cells for HIV. CD4+ T-lymphocytes actively participate in the immune response to foreign antigens and are responsible for the coordination of cell-mediated immunity. HIV viral replication in CD4+ T-lymphocytes eventually results in the host cell's death and, over a period of years, leads to the significant decline in immune functioning that characterizes HIV infection and AIDS. Other HIV-infected target cells, such as macrophages and lymphoid tissues, can have HIV viral replication occur without destruction of the host cell. Consequently, these cells function as reservoirs for HIV and remain capable of continuously producing infectious viral particles. An HIV-infected individual may remain asymptomatic for more than 10 years, but active and prolific viral replication is ongoing, with approximately 1 billion new virions produced every 24 hours (Ho et al. 1995, Pantaleo et al. 1993). This continual proliferation of new HIV virions, combined with the destruction of infected CD4+ T-lymphocytes, eventually renders the individual's immune system incapable of combating a variety of infections and neoplasms, and results in the development of conditions that are diagnostic of AIDS.

Knowledge of an infected individual's stage of HIV disease is necessary for developing a plan of care. The clinical manifestations of HIV infection vary depending on the level of immune deficiency the person is experiencing. Certain therapeutic interventions (e.g., antiretroviral therapy and opportunistic disease prophylaxis) are indicated at various stages of HIV disease in both symptomatic and asymptomatic patients. Consequently, it is important to monitor HIV disease progression through careful clinical assessments and laboratory tests.

Table 11C.1.   1993 REVISED CLASSIFICATION SYSTEM FOR HIV INFECTION AND EXPANDED SURVEILLANCE CASE DEFINITION FOR AIDS AMONG ADULTS AND ADOLESCENTS

CD4 Cell Category	Clinical Category A	Clinical Category B	Clinical Category C
1. 500 cells/mm^3	A1	B1	C1
2. 200–499 cells/mm^3	A2	B2	C2
3. <200 cells/mm^3	A3	B3	C3
	Category A Conditions	**Category B Conditions**	**Category C Conditions**
	• No symptoms • Acute HIV infection (resolves) • Generalized lymphadenopathy	• Bacillary angiomatosis • Oropharyngeal candidiasis • Vulvovaginal candidiasis: persistent, frequent, or poorly responsive to therapy • Cervical intraepithelial neoplasia II or III • Constitutional symptoms: fever, diarrhea >1 month, night sweats • Oral hairy leukoplakia • Herpes zoster: multiple episodes or involving >1 dermatome • Idiopathic thrombocytopenia purpura • Listeriosis • Pelvic inflammatory disease: particularly if complicated by tubo-ovarian abscess • Peripheral neuropathy	• Candidiasis of bronchi, trachea, lungs, or esophagus • Invasive cervical carcinoma • Coccidioidomycosis, disseminated or extrapulmonary • Cryptococcosis, extrapulmonary • Cryptosporidiosis (intestinal infection >1 month duration) • Cytomegalovirus disease (excluding liver, spleen, or lymph nodes) • HIV-related encephalopathy • Herpes simplex: chronic ulcer >1 month duration, or bronchitis, pneumonitis, or esophagitis • Histoplasmosis: disseminated or extrapulmonary • Isosporiasis: >1 month duration • Kaposi's sarcoma • Burkitt's lymphoma • Immunoblastic lymphoma • Primary lymphoma of the brain • *Mycobacterium avium* complex or *M. kansasii*: disseminated or extrapulmonary • *M. tuberculosis*: any site • Mycobacterium: other species or unknown species, disseminated or extrapulmonary • *Pneumocystis carinii* pneumonia • Recurrent bacterial pneumonia • Progressive multifocal leukoencephalopathy • *Salmonella* septicemia, recurrent • Toxoplasmosis of the brain • Wasting syndrome due to HIV

Source: Centers for Disease Control and Prevention (CDC). 1992. 1993 revised classification system for HIV infection and expanded surveillance case definition for AIDS among adolescents and adults. *Morbidity and Mortality Weekly Report* 41(RR-17):1–19.

Initially, a person infected with HIV may experience an acute retroviral syndrome that usually occurs 2–4 weeks after infection. Following this, a person may remain without symptoms of HIV disease for as long as 10 years. However, as the person's immune functioning continues to decline, clinical manifestations associated with opportunistic illnesses (OIs) (e.g., oral candidiasis and hairy leukoplakia) and AIDS-defining conditions are observed. (See **Table 11C.1, 1993 Revised Classification System for HIV Infection and Expanded Surveillance Case Definition for AIDS Among Adults and Adolescents.**)

As HIV infection progresses in women, an increased incidence of certain gynecological complications also is noted. The incidence of cervical dysplasia in HIV-infected women ranges between 11–60%, with recurrence rates after treatment higher in HIV-infected women than in uninfected women (Ellerbrock et al. 2000, Korn et al. 1995, Six et al. 1998). As a result, the CDC added invasive cervical carcinoma to the list of AIDS-defining conditions in January 1993 (CDC 1992). Despite this gender-specific category, AIDS surveillance data have not demonstrated an increase in the reports of invasive cervical cancer since this condition was added to the CDC AIDS-defining conditions. This is primarily attributed to the identification and aggressive treatment of cervical neoplasia in this population of women, as well as the beneficial effects of highly active antiretroviral therapy (HAART) on women's immune functioning resulting in alterations in the anticipated progression of cervical neoplasia (Robinson et al. 2002).

Recommended laboratory testing for HIV disease monitoring includes CD4+ T-lymphocyte cell counts and HIV viral load levels, and observing trends in these measurements over time. Because there is usually laboratory evidence of immune deterioration before there are physical manifestations of HIV disease progression, it is essential that these HIV disease laboratory markers are obtained at regular intervals (e.g., every 3–4 months) so that HAART and/or OI prophylaxis can be appropriately prescribed (Panel on the Clinical Practices for the Treatment of HIV Infection 2002). Absolute CD4+ T-lymphocyte cell counts >500 cells/mm^3 are considered to be normal. However, when the CD4+ T-lymphocyte count declines to <350 cells/mm^3, HIV-infected individuals often begin to have symptoms or physical signs of HIV disease progression (e.g., oral candidiasis and hairy leukoplakia). When a CD4+ T-lymphocyte cell count declines to <200 cells/mm^3, the HIV-infected individual is at significant risk for developing conditions that are diagnostic of AIDS (Bartlett et al. 2001, U.S. Public Health Service et al. 1999).

HIV viral load measurement has been clinically available since the mid-1990s. This test can quantify the number of HIV viral particles that exist outside infected cells in the blood, tissue, and other bodily fluids. High baseline viral load levels are associated with a shorter mean time to the diagnosis of AIDS and death (Mellors et al. 1997, Sterling et al. 2001). In women, there are data indicating that HIV disease progression may occur at lower viral load levels than in men (Gandhi et al. 2002; Kauf et al. 2001). The exact mechanism for this finding is unknown. However, there is concern that recommended guidelines for the initiation of HAART may not be addressing this discrepancy in disease progression for women at lower viral load levels compared to men, which could further contribute to more rapid advancement of HIV disease in women (Gandhi et al. 2002, Kauf et al. 2001).

Viral load measurements also are used to document an individual's response to HAART. Once an individual initiates HAART, there should be a significant decline in the baseline viral load measurement (i.e., a one log^{10} drop) demonstrated after 16–20 weeks. Undetectable viral load levels (i.e., those below the laboratory's level of detection) indicate suppression of viral replication (Panel on the Clinical Practices for the Treatment of HIV Infection 2002). A lack of significant decline or an increase in the viral load levels indicates ongoing viral replication with the associated destruction of CD4+ T-lymphocytes, infection of other target cells, and the possibility of viral resistance to the HAART medications.

An in-depth presentation of the plan of care for an HIV-infected woman throughout the course of this disease is beyond the scope of this chapter. However, the therapeutic options available to a woman during the asymptomatic phase of the disease, primary prophylaxis to prevent OIs, and therapeutic interventions for common minor OIs are presented with the understanding that current management strategies for HIV infection are changing continually. The rapid evolution of therapies and clinical trials available to HIV-infected women require that practitioners constantly update their knowledge regarding this disease, utilize infectious disease and/or HIV specialists as consultants, and make appropriate referrals so HIV-infected women receive timely and optimal therapy.

DATABASE

SUBJECTIVE

→ Risk factors may include:
- History of sexual contact with a person at increased risk of HIV infection, including:
  - History of injection drug use
  - History of bisexuality
  - Symptoms or diagnosis of HIV infection or AIDS
  - Hemophilia
  - Living in an area where HIV infection is endemic
  - Receipt of a blood transfusion, blood products, or tissue between the mid-1970s and June 1985
  - Sexual partner(s) at risk for HIV infection
- A sexual partner with unknown HIV serostatus
- History of injection drug use, needle-sharing behavior
- Receipt of a transfusion, blood product, or tissue between the mid-1970s and June 1985
- Living in an area where HIV infection is endemic (e.g., Central Africa)
- The patient's child(ren) has/have been diagnosed with HIV infection or AIDS
- Unscreened artificial insemination
- Occupational exposure to human blood or body fluids
- Clinical signs/symptoms associated with HIV infection
- Born to a woman with a history of or at risk for HIV/AIDS

→ Other factors that may be associated with HIV risk are:
- Drug use (e.g., alcohol, crack)
- Exchanging sex for money, drugs, food, shelter
- History of STDs
- Multiple sexual partners
- Sexual partner with a history of incarceration
  NOTE: Heterosexual transmission is now the leading route for the acquisition of HIV by women in the United States. Therefore, women with a history of unprotected sexual contact with a partner of unknown HIV status should be considered at risk.

→ Symptoms may include:

Acute HIV Retroviral Syndrome
(Panel on the Clinical Practices for the Treatment of HIV Infection 2002)
- Fever
- Sweats
- Rigors
- Malaise
- Sore throat
- Gastrointestinal symptoms, including anorexia, nausea, vomiting, and diarrhea
- Generalized rash
- Enlarged lymph nodes
- Headaches
- Oral ulcers
- Photophobia
- Altered mental status

Progressive HIV Infection
- HIV-infected individuals may remain asymptomatic for more than 10 years after seroconversion.
- Generalized manifestations may be reported, including:
  - Enlarged lymph nodes
  - Fatigue
  - Night sweats
  - Intermittent, low-grade fever
  - Weight loss
- Dermatological manifestations may be reported, including:
  - Dry skin (generalized)
  - Erythematous, scaly skin of the scalp, eyebrows, naso-labial folds, trunk, or groin (may indicate seborrheic dermatitis)
  - Grouped vesicles on the lips, genitalia, or perianal region that are usually painful and recurrent (may indicate herpes simplex virus [HSV] infection)
  - Painful eruption of blisters in a wide distribution (dermatomal pattern), usually unilateral and occurring on the trunk, head, or neck (may indicate herpes zoster)
  - Scaly patches with areas of central clearing (may indicate tinea infection)
  - Thick or crumbling fingernails or toenails (may indicate tinea infection)
  - Thick, erythematous, red plaques with well-defined margins; intermittently pruritic; usually reported at the site of trauma (may indicate psoriasis)
  - Erythematous, papular, pustular lesions at hair follicles of the face and/or trunk; may be tender and/or pruritic (may indicate folliculitis)
  - Oval nodules that become reddish purple; 1–2 cm; reported on back, trunk, legs, and hard palate of the oral cavity (may indicate Kaposi's sarcoma [KS], which rarely is reported in HIV-infected women)
  - Petechiae (may indicate thrombocytopenia)
- Ophthalmic manifestations may be reported, including:
  - Abrupt onset of small floating spots in the field of vision
  - Intermittent or persistent blurred vision
  - Intermittent flashes of light
  - Photophobia
  - Loss of vision
- Oral manifestations may be reported, including:
  - Aphthous ulcers of the tongue and buccal mucosa
  - Grouped vesicles or ulcers of the lips or buccal mucosa (may indicate HSV infection)
  - White patches on buccal mucosa and/or the tongue that may or may not scrape off (may indicate oral candidiasis or hairy leukoplakia)
  - Erythema, edema, bleeding of the gums (may indicate gingivitis)
  - Nodules that are reddish purple; usually reported on the hard palate (may indicate KS)
- Respiratory manifestations may be reported, including:
  - Dyspnea
    - May be mild to severe depending on the underlying condition
  - Shortness of breath
    - May be mild to severe
  - A persistent, dry, hacking cough (often noted in *Pneumocystis carinii* pneumonia)
  - Abrupt onset of a productive cough with minimal to copious amounts of purulent mucous (may indicate bacterial pneumonia; see the **Pneumonia** chapter in Section 5.)
- Gastrointestinal manifestations may be reported, including:
  - Chronic, intermittent diarrhea with or without bloating
  - Odynophagia
  - Dysphagia
  - Anorexia
  - Jaundice
  - Hematemesis, melena (rare).
- Neurological manifestations may be reported, including:
  - Memory lapses, mental confusion, inability to think clearly
  - Frequent or persistent headaches with or without fever
  - Dysesthesia of extremities
  - Headaches
  - Problems with coordination or balance
- Gynecological manifestations may be reported, including:

- Erythema and/or pruritis of vulvovaginal and/or perianal areas
- Vaginal discharge that is indicative of candidiasis, trichomonas, bacterial vaginosis, chlamydia, or gonor-rhea. (See the **Vaginitis** chapter in Section 12 and specific chapters in Section 13.)
- Recurrent, painful blister(s) or ulcer(s) in vulvovaginal and/or perianal regions (indicative of HSV; see the **Genital Herpes Simplex Virus** chapter in Section 13.)
- Verruciform lesions of the vulvovaginal, perineal, or anal regions that may be recurrent (indicative of condyloma)
- History or documented evidence of rapid, progressive development of squamous intraepithelial lesions (SILs)

OBJECTIVE

→ The physical examination may be within normal limits (WNL) or demonstrate significant pathological findings depending on the immune status of the patient and any concomitant conditions that may be present.

- General examination may reveal a thin, wasted body type.
- Vital signs are usually WNL but will change depending on any underlying illness (e.g., bacterial pneumonia) that may co-exist.
- Examination of the skin may reveal evidence of the following conditions:
  - Xerosis
  - Seborrheic dermatitis
  - Folliculitis
  - Psoriasis
  - Tinea infection
  - Herpes simplex or zoster
  - Molluscum contagiosum (see specific chapters for descriptions of these conditions)
  - Flat or elevated reddish purple nodule(s) or plaques varying in size from 1–2 cm (KS, rare in women)
- Examination of the eyes may reveal:
  - Cotton wool patches with or without evidence of hemorrhage (may indicate retinopathy)
  - Dry, granular, white retinal opacification with hemor-rhage (may indicate retinopathy)
  - Bright red, subconjunctival hemorrhage (may indicate KS or thrombocytopenia)
  - Visual field defects, optic atrophy, pupillary abnor-malities, cranial nerve palsies (may indicate neuro-ophthalmic signs of intracranial disease or other conditions)
- Examination of the oropharynx may reveal:
  - Erythema, edema, hypertrophy of gingiva (gingivitis)
  - Smooth, erythematous patches of the hard or soft palate, buccal mucosa, or dorsum of the tongue (atrophic candidiasis)
  - Raised white patches on the tongue or buccal mucosa that scrape off with a tongue blade. Patches may be on an erythematous base (candidiasis).

- Small, erythematous, eroded, or fissured lesions at the corners of the mouth (angular cheilitis)
- Reddish-purple-blue, flat or elevated, single or multiple lesions of the mouth (may indicate KS)
- Small vesicular or ulcerated, painful lesions of the lips, palate, or gingiva (may indicate HSV infection)
- Examination of the lungs will reveal findings consistent with any concomitant disease. (See Section 5, **Respirato-ry/Otorhinolaryngological Disorders**.)
  NOTE: Pulmonary problems in HIV-positive patients (e.g., *Pneumocystis carinii* pneumonia [PCP] and bacte-rial pneumonia) often present with physical-examination findings such as:
  - Tachypnea
  - Rales
  - Decreased breath sounds
- Cardiac examination is usually WNL. If significant dis-ease (e.g., endocarditis in patients who use injection drugs, or in cardiomyopathy) co-exists, the following symptoms may be evident:
  - Increased pulse rate
  - Murmur
  - S_3 gallop
- Abdominal examination may reveal an enlarged liver or spleen.
- Palpation of the patient's lymph nodes may reveal:
  - Enlarged, soft, mobile lymph nodes, most commonly noted in the occiput, anterior, and posterior cervical chains; axilla; the epitrochlear region; and inguinal, femoral, and popliteal regions with or without tenderness
  - Single or multiple, hard, enlarged node(s) (may indicate lymphoma)
- Neurological examination may reveal:
  - A flat affect
  - Diminished recent memory
  - Decreased fine and gross motor movements
  - Decreased proprioception
  - Abnormal and symmetrical or asymmetrical deep tendon reflexes
  - Decreased sensation in the extremities (the feet more so than the hands)
  - Paraparesis
  - Ataxia
- Musculoskeletal examination may reveal:
  - Decreased muscle tone, strength, mass
  - Muscle pain (may indicate myositis and/or mitochon-drial toxicity)
- Pelvic examination may reveal physical findings consistent with:
  - Vaginitis
  - Cervicitis
  - Condyloma acuminata
  - Molluscum contagiosum
  - HSV infection
  - Other STDs

- Vulvar/vaginal/cervical/anal intraepithelial neoplasia. (See specific chapters for descriptions of physical findings.)

ASSESSMENT

→ HIV-1 infection
→ R/O HIV-1 infection
→ R/O AIDS
→ R/O minor OIs (e.g., oral candidiasis)
→ R/O immune dysfunction from other causes (e.g., neoplasms and autoimmune disorders)
→ R/O STDs
→ R/O vaginal, cervical, anal dysplasia
→ R/O psychological disorders associated with chronic disease (e.g., depression)
→ Assess factors associated with increased risk of HIV infection

PLAN

DIAGNOSTIC TESTS

→ Verification of the HIV status of a new patient presenting for HIV-specific care is essential (either through obtaining a copy of previous test results or by repeat testing of the patient) before initiating any plan of care, particularly pharmacological interventions.
  - See "Patient Education," below, for information regarding informed consent and disclosure of HIV test results.
→ The following tests may be ordered to document the HIV status of a patient:
  - HIV-1 antibody tests usually demonstrate a positive result 3–12 weeks after infection with the virus (Feinberg et al. 2001).
    - However, in some individuals, it may take as long as six months to demonstrate detectable antibodies after infection with the virus.
    - The following tests can be performed:
      - The enzyme-linked immunosorbent assay (ELISA) test is a very sensitive but less specific antibody test used to initially screen for the presence of HIV antibodies.
        ➤ If the initial test is positive, the test usually is repeated on the same specimen.
        ➤ If the repeat ELISA test is positive, a confirmatory HIV test is done on the same specimen (e.g., Western Blot, immunofluorescence assay [IFA]).
      NOTE: The ELISA is only used as a screening test for HIV. A positive ELISA test result is not considered a positive HIV test; therefore, patients should not be told they are HIV-infected based on a positive ELISA test. Positive ELISA results require additional testing with more specific assays to detect HIV infection. If the confirmatory test(s) are positive, then a patient can be informed about her positive HIV serostatus.
      - IFA can be done to confirm the initial ELISA test. It involves a process whereby a fluorescein label is attached to HIV antibodies present in a specimen. This specimen is then evaluated under an ultraviolet microscope for the presence of bright spots of fluorescence, indicating a positive test.
        ➤ This test can be used to confirm positive ELISA results.
  - Western Blot is a confirmatory antibody test that uses protein electrophoresis to detect antibody responses to specific HIV viral proteins.
    ➤ It is a very sensitive and specific test with strict guidelines for interpreting findings. It is the preferred test for confirming positive ELISA results.
    ➤ A fully reactive Western Blot test confirms an HIV-seropositive ELISA result.
  NOTE: When both the ELISA and Western Blot test results are positive, the sensitivity and specificity are >99%, but the predictive value of the test depends on the seroprevalence of HIV in the population (Feinberg et al. 2001). In patients with indeterminate test results, repeat HIV-1 antibody testing should be performed at an interval appropriate to the last known HIV exposure (i.e., 6–12 weeks after the last exposure). Indeterminate results also can be caused by (Feinberg et al. 2001):
      * Advanced HIV infection with a decrease in p24 antibody titers
      * HIV-2 infection (more common in West Africa)
      * Autoantibodies due to autoimmune disease, collagen vascular disease, or malignancy
      * HIV subtype O or non-clade B strains
      * Cross-reaction with alloantibodies from pregnancy, blood transfusion, or organ transplantation
      * Previous receipt of an experimental HIV vaccine
    ➤ False-negative HIV-1 antibody tests can occur as a result of:
      * Being in the window period for antibody development after infection with HIV
      * Infection with HIV-1 subtype O
      * Agammaglobulinemia
- The following tests can be performed:
  - There are three rapid assays available—Single Use Diagnostic System (SUDS)®, Genic®, and Recombigen®—that can provide results in 10–30 minutes. Of these, only the SUDS® assay is FDA-approved for clinical use. The sensitivity and specificity of these assays are >99%; however, confirmation of rapid assay results is necessary with approved tests (e.g., IFA or Western Blot) (Feinberg et al. 2001).
  - Alternative tests that do not require phlebotomy include the OraSure® (saliva test) and Calypte HIV-1 urine enzyme immuno-assay. OraSure® has a sensitivity and specificity that are similar to those of standard HIV serology tests. Calypte testing can only be used for screening and must be performed by a physician. Positive results require confirmation

by standard assays (e.g., IFA or Western Blot) (Feinberg et al. 2001).

- Plasma HIV RNA can be measured by nucleic acid techniques that quantify the presence of viral particles in blood and bodily fluids. There are three commercially available assays that use different techniques to measure HIV viral particles outside of infected cells: reverse transcriptase polymerase chain reaction (RT-PCR), branched DNA (bDNA), and nucleic acid sequence-based amplification. These tests report the measurement of the viral particles in the number of copies per milliliter. The lower limits of the assays range from 20–50 copies/mL (ultrasensitive assays) to 400 copies/mL (standard assay). Although the three assays are considered to be reliable, they do not yield the same result when repeat testing is done on the same specimen. In addition, variations in results can occur at lower levels of viral particle quantification. Consequently, a patient should continue to have her viral load measured by the same assay whenever possible to minimize inter-assay variability.
  - The sensitivity is approximately 90–95%, but it increases when patients have CD4+ T cell counts <200/mm^3 (Rich et al. 1999).
  - The false-positive rate is 2–3% and is usually due to laboratory contamination (Rich et al. 1999). (See also **Table 11C.2, Indications for Plasma HIV RNA Testing** for additional information about viral load testing.)

- DNA polymerase chain reaction (DNA PCR) is a qualitative technique that amplifies the DNA of cells from a specimen to determine the presence of HIV within the cell (i.e., it is an intracellular assay). This test usually is performed to diagnose HIV infection in infants younger than 18 months or when there is an indeterminate serology (Feinberg et al. 2001).
  - It is very sensitive (>99%) and specific (98%), and provides results within a few days (Feinberg et al. 2001).
  - False-positive results are possible, as any trace of a DNA sequencing pattern similar to HIV may be interpreted as positive.
- HIV antigen (p24) is a measurement of the presence of HIV core protein in a specimen. In some countries, HIV viral load testing is unavailable or too costly.
  - When HIV replication is active, there is an increased concentration of this antigen in the patient's blood; however, during latency periods, p24 antigen may be undetectable. Therefore, this test may be negative in an infected patient and should not be used to determine HIV serostatus in the general population.
- HIV cultures can be performed on a number of body fluids and tissues, and may be positive depending on the concentration of the virus in the specimen. However, due to the accessibility of HIV viral load testing, this laboratory test is rarely used outside of research studies.

Table 11C.2. INDICATIONS FOR PLASMA HIV RNA TESTING*

Clinical Indication	Information	Use
Syndrome consistent with acute HIV infection	Establishes diagnosis when HIV antibody is negative or indeterminate	Diagnosis[†]
Initial evaluation of newly diagnosed HIV infection	Baseline viral load "set point"	Decision to start or defer therapy
Every 3–4 months in patients not on therapy	Changes in viral load	Decision to start therapy
2–8 weeks after initiation of antiretroviral therapy (ART)	Initial assessment of drug efficacy	Decision to continue or change therapy
3-4 months after initiation of ART	Maximal effect of therapy	Decision to continue or change therapy
Every 3–4 months in patients on ART	Durability of ART	Decision to continue or change therapy
Clinical event or significant decline in CD4+ T-cells	Association with changing or stable viral load	Decision to continue, initiate, or change therapy

* Acute illness (e.g., bacterial pneumonia, tuberculosis, HSV, PCP, etc.) and immunizations can cause an increase in plasma HIV RNA for 2–4 weeks; viral load testing should not be performed during this time. Plasma HIV RNA results should usually be verified with a repeat determination before starting or making changes in therapy.

† Diagnosis of HIV infection made by HIV RNA testing should be confirmed by standard methods such as Western Blot serology performed 2–4 months after the initial indeterminate or negative test.

Source: Panel on the Clinical Practices for the Treatment of HIV Infection, U.S. Department of Health and Human Services (DHHS); and the Henry J. Kaiser Family Foundation. 2002. *Guidelines for the use of antiretroviral agents in HIV-infected adults and adolescents.* Available at: http://www.aidsinfo.nih.gov/guidelines. Accessed on May 1, 2002.

- HIV cultures are expensive, the virus is difficult to grow, and meticulous laboratory procedures are essential to ensure accurate results.
- Erratic results can occur due to a number of factors (e.g., contamination of a specimen or low concentration of virus in the specimen). For these reasons, this process is not commonly used to determine HIV status.

→ CBC, differential, and platelet count should be obtained and may be WNL or reveal the following (Bartlett et al. 2001):
  - Anemia
  - Leukopenia
  - Lymphocytopenia
  - Decreased red blood cells (RBCs), hematocrit (Hct), or hemoglobin (Hgb)
  - Increased mean corpuscular volume to 105–110 fl in patients taking some antiretroviral medications (e.g., zidovudine [ZDV, AZT] or stavudine [d4T])
  - Thrombocytopenia

→ A complete T-lymphocyte count should be ordered and may reveal (Bartlett et al. 2001):
  - A decreased T-helper cell (CD4) count (a normal count is >500 cells/mm^3)
  - An increased T-suppressor cell (CD8) count
  - Inversion of the T-helper to T-suppressor ratio (normal is 2:1)

NOTE: There is considerable intra-laboratory and inter-laboratory variation in T-lymphocyte count results. Ideally, tests should be done at the same laboratory after being obtained at approximately the same time of day as a means of attaining some consistency in values. Furthermore, if possible, T-lymphocyte counts should be obtained four weeks after the patient recovers from any complication or illness, as intercurrent illness and complications can affect levels (Feinberg et al. 2001).

→ A chemistry panel should be performed and may be WNL or reveal the following in the presence of concomitant disease(s):
  - Elevated alanine aminotransferase (ALT) and aspartate aminotransferase (AST) (in the presence of hepatitis)
  - Elevated alkaline phosphatase (in the presence of liver or biliary disease)
  - Elevated lactate dehydrogenase (may be evidence of lymphoma or PCP if the CD4 count is <200 cells/mm^3)
  - Decreased serum cholesterol (may be depleted because of a chronic disease state with wasting)

→ A syphilis serology (e.g., VDRL or RPR) should be obtained with a confirmatory direct treponemal test if the serology is positive.

→ Hepatitis screening should be done and include hepatitis A, B, and C antibody testing. (See the **Hepatitis—Viral** chapter.)

→ Toxoplasmosis serology (IgG) should be done to determine the patient's serostatus. This is helpful to have documented if the patient develops symptoms of encephalitis in the future and a diagnosis of toxoplasmosis is being considered (Bartlett et al. 2001).

→ A varicella serology should be obtained in patients who are uncertain if they have had a varicella infection (Feinberg et al. 2001).

→ A cytomegalovirus (CMV) serology should be obtained in patients so that if transfusions are needed, CMV-negative blood products can be used (Feinberg et al. 2001).

→ G6PD level should be obtained, as patients with a deficiency of this enzyme may develop a hemolytic anemia when placed on some of the medications frequently used during the course of HIV disease (e.g., dapsone) (Feinberg et al. 2001).

→ Tuberculin skin testing should be done using a purified protein derivative (PPD).
  - An induration ≥5 mm at the site of the PPD is considered to be a positive tuberculin skin test in HIV-infected patients.
  - Patients with low CD4+ T-lymphocyte cell counts (e.g., <200 cells/mm^3) are usually anergic. Therefore, a chest x-ray should be done to eliminate the possibility of active tuberculosis infection in a patient with a history of exposure to or exhibiting symptoms suggestive of tuberculosis infection.

→ A chest x-ray should be done at baseline (e.g., upon diagnosis of HIV infection) and repeated as clinically indicated.

→ Cervical cytology should be performed on any patient who has not had one during the previous 6–12 months.
  - Guidelines regarding the frequency of Pap smears in HIV-positive women vary. However, the following schedules have been proposed (Anderson 2001):
    - Upon entry to care, women with early HIV infection without a history of any abnormal cervical cytology should have two Pap smears obtained six months apart.
      - If both results are benign, then annual Pap smear testing can be done.
    - Women should have a repeat Pap smear if there is no evidence of endocervical cells on their smears or after treatment for any cervical lesion or underlying inflammation.
    - Women without a history of abnormal cervical cytology who have symptomatic HIV disease or a CD4 count <200 should have Pap smear testing every six months.
    - Women with *any* abnormality noted on cervical cytology (including atypical squamous cells of undermined significance) or who have a history of untreated SILs should be referred for colposcopy with repeat evaluation(s) and Pap smear as recommended by the colposcopist.
    - Women should have appropriate cervical cultures to rule out the presence of STDs (e.g., *Chlamydia trachomatis*, gonorrhea, and HSV) as indicated.
    - A wet mount of vaginal secretions should be done to look for vaginal/cervical pathogens (e.g., candidiasis, trichomonas, bacterial vaginosis) requiring treatment.
    - In some practices, anal cytology specimens are obtained to look for anal SIL, due to reports of an increased incidence of this condition in HIV-infected individuals (Cardillo et al. 2001, Del Mistro et al. 2001). The long-term effects of this condition are

unknown but are being investigated in longitudinal, natural history studies of HIV-infected women and men.

→ Pregnancy testing should be considered in women of reproductive age when the possibility of conception is reported or suspected, especially before initiating systemic medications with known or unknown adverse fetal effects.

→ Routine follow-up tests of an HIV-positive patient should be done based on the patient's HIV disease progression and the therapeutic interventions in her plan of care.

- The following tests should be done every 3–4 months in all HIV-infected individuals (Panel on the Clinical Practices for the Treatment of HIV Infection 2002):
  - CD4+ T-lymphocyte cell count
    - If the result is <200/mm³, repeat one week after obtaining the initial low value (to determine whether or not to initiate OI prophylaxis).
  - Viral load level (see **Table 11C.2**) intervals and rationale
  - CBC
  - Chemistry panel (including BUN, creatinine, ALT, AST, and alkaline phosphatase)
  - Lipid panel (e.g., fasting cholesterol and triglyceride) if the patient is receiving HAART, to monitor for toxicities
- The following tests should be done according to current guidelines:
  - VDRL or RPR should be repeated annually or more frequently as indicated by the individual's history.
  - Chlamydia and gonorrhea cultures and vaginal/cervical

wet mounts should be repeated annually or more frequently, as indicated, in sexually active individuals.

- PPD should be done annually unless otherwise indicated. (See the **Tuberculosis** chapter.)
- Pap smear testing should be done according to the individual's history but at least annually in women without a history of abnormal Pap smear results or HPV (see above).

NOTE: Women who are taking certain HAART medications (e.g., nevirapine), have evidence of immune deterioration or increased viral activity, or have comorbidities (e.g., hepatitis C) may need more frequent monitoring of some of these laboratory tests.

- HIV drug resistance assays may be used to determine if a person's predominant viral strain has become resistant to antiretroviral medications. (See **Table 11C.3, Recommendations for the Use of Drug Resistance Assays**.) There are two types of resistance tests:
  - Genotyping determines mutations in the nucleotide sequencing of the viral genes that code for specific protease and RT enzymes (Feinberg et al. 2001).
  - Phenotyping determines the amount of antiretroviral medication necessary to inhibit HIV growth in culture (Feinberg et al. 2001).
- The benefit of these tests is that they can help tailor medication regimens for patients who have evidence of virologic breakthrough while on HAART. However, commercially available assays require a minimum level of

Table 11C.3.   RECOMMENDATIONS FOR THE USE OF DRUG RESISTANCE ASSAYS

Clinical Setting/Recommendation	Rationale
Recommended	
• Virologic failure during HAART	• Determine the role of resistance in drug failure and maximize the number of active drugs in the new regimen if indicated.
• Suboptimal suppression of viral load after initiation of antiretroviral therapy	• Determine the role of resistance and maximize the number of active drugs in the new regimen if indicated.
Consider	
• Acute HIV infection	• Determine if drug-resistant virus was transmitted and change regimen accordingly.
Not generally recommended	
• Chronic HIV infection before initiation of therapy	• Uncertain prevalence of resistant virus. Current assays may not detect minor drug-resistant species.
• After discontinuation of drugs	• Drug-resistant mutations may become minor species in the absence of selective drug pressure. Current assays may not detect minor drug-resistant species.
• Plasma viral load <1,000 HIV RNA copies/mL	• Resistance assays cannot be reliably performed because of low copy number of HIV RNA.

Source: Panel on the Clinical Practices for the Treatment of HIV Infection, U.S. Department of Health and Human Services (DHHS); and the Henry J. Kaiser Family Foundation. 2002. *Guidelines for the use of antiretroviral agents in HIV-infected adults and adolescents.* Available at: http://www.aidsinfo.nih.gov/guidelines. Accessed on May 1, 2002.

Table 11C.4. PROPHYLAXIS TO PREVENT FIRST EPISODE OF OPPORTUNISTIC DISEASE IN ADULTS AND ADOLESCENTS INFECTED WITH HUMAN IMMUNODEFICIENCY VIRUS

Pathogen	Indication	Prevention Regimens • First Choice	Alternatives
Strongly Recommended as Standard of Care			
*Pneumocystis carinii**	CD4+ count <200 µL or oropharyngeal candidiasis	Trimethoprim-sulfamethoxazole (TMP-SMZ), 1 DS p.o. QD (AI)	Dapsone 50 mg p.o. BID *or* 100 mg p.o. QD (BI); dapsone 50 mg p.o. QD *plus* pyrimethamine 50 mg p.o. QW *plus* leucovorin 25 mg p.o. QW (BI); dapsone 200 mg p.o. *plus* pyrimethamine 75 mg p.o. *plus* leucovorin 25 mg p.o. QW (BI); aerosolized pentamidine 300 mg QM via Respirgard II™ nebulizer (BI); atovaquone 1,500 mg p.o. QD (BI); TMP-SMZ 1 DS p.o. TIW (BI)
Mycobacterium tuberculosis (isoniazid-sensitive†)	TST reaction ≥5 mm *or* prior positive TST result without treatment *or* contact with a case of active TB	Isoniazid (INH) 300 mg p.o. *plus* pyridoxine 50 mg p.o. QD x 9 months (AII) or INH 900 mg p.o. *plus* pyridoxine 100 mg p.o. BIW x 9 months (BI); rifampin 600 mg p.o. *plus* pyrazinamide 20 mg/kg p.o. QD x 2 months (AI)	Rifabutin 300 mg p.o. QD plus pyrazinamide 20 mg/kg p.o. QD x 2 months (BIII); rifampin 600 mg p.o. QD x 4 months (BIII)
Mycobacterium tuberculosis (INH-resistant)	Same; high probability of exposure to INH-resistant TB	Rifampin 600 mg *plus* pyrazinamide 20 mg/kg p.o. QD x 2 months (AI)	Rifabutin 300 mg p.o. QD *plus* pyrazinamide 20 mg/kg p.o. QD x 2 months (BIII); rifampin 600 mg p.o. QD x 4 months (BIII); rifabutin 300 mg p.o. QD (CIII)
Mycobacterium tuberculosis (multidrug INH- and rifampin-resistant)	Same; high probability of exposure to multidrug-resistant TB	Choice of drugs requires consultation with public health authorities	None
Toxoplasma gondii§	IgG antibody to *Toxoplasma* and CD4+ count <100/µL	TMP-SMZ 1 DS p.o. QD (AII)	TMP-SMZ 1 SS p.o. QD (BIII); dapsone 50 mg p.o. QD *plus* pyrimethamine 50 mg p.o. QW *plus* leukovorin 25 mg p.o. QW (BI); atovaquone 1,500 mg p.o. with or without pyrimethamine 25 mg p.o. QD *plus* leukovorin 10 mg p.o. QD (CIII)
Mycobacterium avium complex¶	CD4+ count <50/µL	Azithromycin 1,200 mg p.o. QW (AI) or clarithromycin 500 mg p.o. BID (AI)	Rifabutin 300 mg p.o. QD (BI); azithromycin 1,200 mg p.o. QW *plus* rifabutin 300 mg p.o. QD
Varicella zoster virus (VZV)	Significant exposure to chickenpox or shingles for patients who have no history of either condition or, if available, negative antibody to VZV	Varicella zoster immune globulin (VZIG) 5 vials (1.25 mL per vial) IM administered 96 hours after exposure, ideally within 48 hours (AIII)	None
Generally Recommended			
*Streptococcus pneumoniae***	All patients	Pneumococcal vaccine 0.5 mL IM (CD4+ ≥200/µL) (BII); CD4+ <200/µL (CIII)— might re-immunize if initial immunization was given when CD4+ <200/µL and if CD4+ count increases to >200/µL on HAART (CIII)	None
Hepatitis B virus††	All susceptible (anti-HBc negative) patients	Hepatitis B vaccine: 3 doses (BII)	None
Influenza virus††	All patients (annually before influenza season)	Whole or split virus 0.5 mL IM per year (BIII)	Rimantadine 100 mg p.o. BID (CIII) or amantadine 100 mg p.o. BID (CIII)
Hepatitis A††	All susceptible (anti-HAV negative) patients with chronic hepatitis C	Hepatitis A vaccine: 2 doses (BIII)	None

(continued)

Table 11C.4. PROPHYLAXIS TO PREVENT FIRST EPISODE OF OPPORTUNISTIC DISEASE IN ADULTS AND ADOLESCENTS INFECTED WITH HUMAN IMMUNODEFICIENCY VIRUS *(continued)*

Pathogen	Indication	Prevention Regimens • First Choice	Alternatives
Not Routinely Indicated			
Bacteria	Neutropenia	Granulocyte-colony-stimulating factor (G-CSF) 5–10 µg/kg sub-q QD x 2–4 weeks or granulocyte-macrophage colony-stimulating factor (GM-CSF) 250 µg/m² IV over 2 hours QD x 2–4 weeks (CII)	None
Cryptococcus neoformans§§	CD4+ count <50/µL	Fluconazole 100–200 mg p.o. QD (CI)	Itraconazole 200 mg p.o. QD (CIII)
Histoplasma capsulatum§§	CD4+ count <100/µL in endemic geographic area	Itraconazole capsule 200 mg p.o. QD (CI)	None
Cytomegalovirus (CMV)¶¶	CD4+ count <50/µL and CMV antibody positivity	Oral ganciclovir 1 g p.o. TID (CI)	None

NOTE: Information included in these guidelines might not represent Food and Drug Administration (FDA) approval or approved labeling for the particular products or indications in question. Specifically, the terms "safe" and "effective" might not be synonymous with the FDA-defined legal standards for product approval. The Respirgard II™ nebulizer is manufactured by Marquest of Englewood, Colo.

Letters and Roman numerals in parentheses after regimens indicate the strength of the recommendation and the quality of evidence supporting it as follows:

Strength of the recommendation:

A = Strong evidence for efficacy and substantial clinical benefit support a recommendation for use (should always be offered)

B = Moderate evidence for efficacy—or strong evidence for efficacy but only limited clinical benefit—supports a recommendation for use (should generally be offered)

C = Evidence for efficacy is insufficient to support a recommendation for or against use, or evidence for efficacy might not outweigh adverse consequences (e.g., drug toxicity, drug interactions), the cost of the chemoprophylaxis, or alternative approaches (optional)

D = Moderate evidence for lack of efficacy or for adverse outcome supports a recommendation against use (should generally not be offered)

E = Good evidence for lack of efficacy or for adverse outcome supports a recommendation against use (should never be offered)

Quality of evidence supporting the recommendation:

I = Evidence from at least one properly randomized, controlled trial

II = Evidence from at least one well-designed clinical trial without randomization, from cohort or case-controlled analytic studies (preferably from more than one center); from multiple time-series studies; or dramatic results from uncontrolled experiments

III = Evidence from opinions of respected authorities based on clinical experience, descriptive studies, or reports of expert committees.

Anti-HBc = antibody to hepatitis B core antigen
BID = twice a day
BIW = twice a week
DS = double-strength tablet
HAART = highly active antiretroviral therapy
HAV = hepatitis A virus
HIV = human immunodeficiency virus
IM = intramuscular
IV = intravenous
p.o. = by mouth
QD= daily
QM = monthly
QW= weekly
SS = single-strength tablet
TIW = three times a week
sub-q = subcutaneous
TST = tuberculin skin test

* Prophylaxis also should be considered for persons with a CD4+ percentage of <14%, for persons with a history of an AIDS-defining illness, and possibly for those with CD4+ counts >200 but <250 cells/µL. TMP-SMZ also reduces the frequency of toxoplasmosis and some bacterial infections. Patients receiving dapsone should be tested for glucose-6 phosphate dehydrogenase deficiency (G6PD). A dosage of 50 mg QD is probably less effective than 100 mg QD. The efficacy of parenteral pentamidine (e.g., 4 mg/kg/month) is uncertain. Fansidar (sulfadoxine-

pyrimethamine) is rarely used because of severe hypersensitivity reactions. Patients who are being administered therapy for toxoplasmosis with sulfadiazine/pyrimethamine are protected against *Pneumocystis carinii* pneumonia (PCP) and do not need additional prophylaxis against PCP.

† Directly observed therapy is recommended for isoniazid (INH), 900 mg BIW; INH regimens should include pyridoxine to prevent peripheral neuropathy. Rifampin should not be administered concurrently with protease inhibitors or non-nucleoside reverse transcriptase inhibitors. There are reports of increased levels of hepatotoxicity (grade 3 or 4) observed in HIV-negative patients receiving combinations of rifampin and pyrazinamide for 2 months to treat latent TB infection (Jasmer et al. 2002, Stout et al. 2002). Therefore, liver enzymes should be measured routinely during treatment with these medications to monitor for and prevent progression of liver toxicity, if this combination is selected to treat latent TB infection. Rifabutin should not be given with hard-gel saquinavir or delavirdine; caution is also advised when the drug is co-administered with soft-gel saquinavir. Rifabutin may be administered at a reduced dose (150 mg QD) with indinavir, nelfinavir, or amprenavir; at a reduced dose of 150 mg QOD (or 150 mg 3 times weekly) with ritonavir; or at an increased dose (450 mg QD) with efavirenz; information is lacking regarding co-administration of rifabutin with nevirapine. Exposure to multidrug-resistant TB might require prophylaxis with two drugs; consult public health authorities. Possible regimens include pyrazinamide plus either ethambutol or a fluoroquinolone.

§ Protection against toxoplasmosis is provided by TMP-SMZ, dapsone plus pyrimethamine, and

(continued)

Table 11C.4. PROPHYLAXIS TO PREVENT FIRST EPISODE OF OPPORTUNISTIC DISEASE IN ADULTS AND ADOLESCENTS INFECTED WITH HUMAN IMMUNODEFICIENCY VIRUS *(continued)*

possibly by atovaquone. Atovaquone may be used with or without pyrimethamine. Pyrimethamine alone probably provides little, if any, protection.

¶ See footnote † regarding use of rifabutin with protease inhibitors or non-nucleoside reverse transcriptase inhibitors.

** Vaccination should be offered to persons who have a CD4+ T-lymphocyte count <200 cells/μL, although the efficacy might be diminished. Revaccination five years after the first dose or sooner if the initial immunization was given when the CD4+ count was <200 cells/μL and the CD4+ count has increased to >200 cells/μL on HAART is considered optional. Some authorities are concerned that immunizations might stimulate the replication of HIV. However, one study showed no adverse effect of pneumococcal vaccination on patient survival (McNaghten et al. 1999).

†† These immunizations or chemoprophylactic regimens do not target pathogens traditionally classified as opportunistic but should be

considered for use in HIV-infected patients as indicated. Data are inadequate concerning the clinical benefit of these vaccines in this population, although it is logical to assume that those patients who develop antibody responses will derive some protection. Some authorities are concerned that immunizations might stimulate HIV replication, although for influenza vaccination, a large observational study of HIV-infected persons in clinical care showed no adverse effect of this vaccine, including multiple doses, on patient survival (J. Ward, CDC, personal communication) or on viral load levels when patients have demonstrated, undetectable viral loads on HAART before immunization (Keller et al. 2000, Macias et al. 2001). Hepatitis B vaccine has been recommended for all children and adolescents and for all adults with risk factors for hepatitis B virus. Rimantadine and amantadine are appropriate during outbreaks of influenza A. Because of the theoretical concern that increases in HIV plasma RNA following vaccination during pregnancy might increase the risk of perinatal transmission of HIV, providers may wish to defer vacci-

nation until after antiretroviral therapy is initiated. For additional information regarding vaccination against hepatitis A and B and antiviral therapy against influenza, see CDC 1991, 1996, and 1999.

§§ In a few unusual occupational or other circumstances, prophylaxis should be considered; consult a specialist.

¶¶ Acyclovir is not protective against CMV. Valacyclovir is not recommended because of an unexplained trend toward increased mortality observed in persons with AIDS who were being administered this drug for prevention of CMV disease.

Source:Adapted from U.S. Public Health Service (USPHS) and Infectious Disease Society of America (IDSA). 1999. Guidelines for the prevention of opportunistic infections in persons infected with human immunodeficiency virus. *Morbidity and Mortality Weekly Report* 48(RR-10):3, 40–43.

---

measurable viral load (e.g., at least 1,000 copies) in order to have enough HIV genetic material available to perform the tests reliably. To increase the accuracy of the tests, the patient should already be on HAART when the sample is obtained (which is not the situation when a patient seroconverts or is newly diagnosed with HIV infection). This is necessary because a patient's current drug regimen exerts pressure on the HIV isolates and, if there is an increased viral load, the genotype or phenotype tests are better able to distinguish the mutations or isolates that are demonstrating potential or actual resistance in the presence of antiretroviral medications. Finally, these tests do not provide any information about the drug resistance of HIV isolates that may be present at very low levels (Kessler et al. 2000). Consequently, the interpretation of genotype and phenotype tests can be challenging and requires the expertise of providers with extensive experience using them in clinical situations.

TREATMENT/MANAGEMENT

→ The plan of care for an HIV-infected woman is based on her stage of HIV disease.
→ Women with early HIV disease and minimal or no immunosuppression should receive routine primary care and counseling about transmission risk reduction.
→ As HIV disease progresses to advanced immune dysfunc-

tion (CD4+ <200/mm³), the risk of developing a major OI or other condition associated with an AIDS diagnosis increases significantly. Prophylactic administration of a number of pharmacological agents may be indicated. (See **Table 11C.4, Prophylaxis to Prevent First Episode of Opportunistic Disease in Adults and Adolescents Infected with Human Immunodeficiency Virus**.)

- The management of patients who have progressed to this stage of HIV infection and/or who have a major OI or other AIDS-defining condition is beyond the scope of this chapter. Co-management with an HIV specialist is recommended.

→ The following therapeutic interventions are commonly recommended:

- An HIV-infected individual should be given the following immunizations after obtaining informed consent (see **Table 11C.4**):
  - Pneumococcal vaccination 0.5 mL IM. (See the **Pneumonia** chapter in Section 5 for additional information.)
  - Hepatitis B vaccination if she is at risk for hepatitis B infection (i.e., there is no evidence of hepatitis B immunity)
    - The series consists of 3 IM injections, each 0.5 mL, given at appropriate time intervals. (See the **Hepatitis—Viral** chapter for additional information.)
  - Hepatitis A vaccination if she is at risk for hepatitis A infection.

– The series consists of 2 IM injections, each 0.5 mL, given at appropriate time intervals. (See the **Hepatitis—Viral** chapter for additional information.)

- Influenza vaccination annually before the influenza season. (See the **Influenza** chapter in Section 5.)

■ Antiretroviral therapy should be offered according to current guidelines. (See **Table 11C.5, Indications for the Initiation of Antiretroviral Therapy in Chronically HIV-1 Infected Patients**; **Table 11C.6, Recommended Antiretroviral Agents for Initial Treatment of Established HIV Infection**; and **Table 11C.7, Characteristics of Antiretroviral Medications by Class**.)

■ Primary prophylaxis against opportunistic infections should be initiated based on a patient's disease stage and immunologic parameters.
NOTE: See **Table 11C.4.**

■ A patient with evidence of oral candidiasis and no clinical evidence of esophagitis (e.g., dysphagia, odynophagia, or retrosternal pain when swallowing) should be treated with one of the following:

- Clotrimazole oral troches: 1 troche 5 times a day for 1–2 weeks. (Advise the patient to suck, not swallow, the troche until it completely dissolves.)

- Nystatin 500,000 units (5 mL): Swish and swallow 5 times a day for 1–2 weeks.
NOTE: Nystatin is reportedly less effective than clotrimazole, ketoconazole, or fluconazole for treating oral candidiasis (Goldschmidt et al. 2001).

- Ketoconazole 200–400 mg p.o. every day for 1–2 weeks or fluconazole 100–200 mg p.o. for 1–2 weeks in recurrent or resistant cases of oral candidiasis.
NOTE: Ketoconazole requires gastric acid for absorption. Advise the patient to take this medication with orange juice. Because hepatotoxicity is a possible complication of ketoconazole and fluconazole use, appropriate monitoring of the patient's liver function tests is indicated when she uses these medications.

■ A patient with evidence of vaginitis, cervicitis, or other STDs should be treated as indicated. (See the **Vaginitis** chapter in Section 12 and chapters in Section 13.)

■ A patient with a positive tuberculin skin test should be treated according to current CDC recommendations. (See the **Tuberculosis** chapter.)

■ A patient with evidence of gingivitis and/or other dental disease should be referred for a dental examination and appropriate treatment.

Table 11C.5. INDICATIONS FOR THE INITIATION OF ANTIRETROVIRAL THERAPY IN CHRONICALLY HIV-1 INFECTED PATIENTS

The optimal time to initiate therapy in asymptomatic, nonpregnant individuals with >200 CD4+ T cells is not known. This table provides general guidelines, not absolute recommendations, for an individual patient who is not pregnant.

Clinical Category	CD4+ T Cell Count	Plasma HIV RNA	Recommendations
Symptomatic (AIDS, severe symptoms)	Any value	Any value	Treat
Asymptomatic, AIDS	CD4+ T cells <200/mm³	Any value	Treat
Asymptomatic	CD4+ T cells >200/mm³ but <350/mm³	Any value	Treatment generally should be offered, though controversy exists.*
Asymptomatic	CD4+ T cells >350/mm³	>55,000 (by bDNA or RT-PCR)§	Some experts would recommend initiating therapy, recognizing that the 3-year risk of developing AIDS in untreated patients is >30%, while some would defer therapy and monitor CD4+ T cell counts more frequently.
Asymptomatic	CD4+ T cells >350/mm³	<55,000 (by bDNA or RT-PCR)§	Many experts would defer therapy and observe, recognizing that the 3-year risk of developing AIDS in untreated patients is <15%.

* Clinical benefit has been demonstrated in controlled trials only for patients with CD4+ T cells <200/mm³. However, most experts would offer therapy at a CD4+ T cell threshold <350/mm³.

§ Although there was a 2.0–2.5 fold difference between RT-PCR and the first bDNA assay (version 2.0) used to determine viral load levels, with the current bDNA assay (version 3.0) values obtained by bDNA and RT-PCR are similar except for measurements at the lower end of the linear range (<1,500 copies/mL).

Source: Panel on the Clinical Practices for the Treatment of HIV Infection, U.S. Department of Health and Human Services (DHHS); and the Henry J. Kaiser Family Foundation. 2002. *Guidelines for the use of antiretroviral agents in HIV-infected adults and adolescents*, p. 37. Available at: http://www.aidsinfo.nih.gov/guidelines. Accessed on May 10, 2002.

Table 11C.6. RECOMMENDED ANTIRETROVIRAL AGENTS FOR INITIAL TREATMENT OF ESTABLISHED HIV INFECTION

This table provides a guide to the use of available treatment regimens for individuals with no prior or limited experience on HIV therapy. In accordance with the established goals of HIV therapy, priority is given to regimens for which clinical trials data suggest the following: sustained suppression of HIV plasma RNA (particularly in patients with a high baseline viral load) and sustained increase in CD4+ T cell count (in most cases, longer than 48 weeks), and favorable clinical outcome (i.e., delayed progression to AIDS and death). To be included in the "Strongly Recommended" category, particular emphasis is given to regimens that have been compared directly with other regimens that perform sufficiently well with regard to these parameters. Additional consideration is given to the regimen's pill burden, dosing frequency, food requirements, convenience, toxicity, and drug interaction profile compared with other regimens.

It is important to note that all antiretroviral agents, including those in the "Strongly Recommended" category, have potentially serious toxic and adverse side effects. The reader is strongly encouraged to consult the entire DHHS guideline (specifically Tables 13–19) and an HIV specialist while formulating an antiretroviral regimen.

Antiretroviral drug regimens comprise one choice each from columns A and B. Drugs are listed in alphabetical, not priority, order.

	Column A	Column B
Strongly Recommended	Efavirenz	Didanosine + lamivudine
	Indinavir	Stavudine + didanosine¶
	Nelfinavir	Stavudine + lamivudine
	Ritonavir + indinavir*†	Zidovudine + didanosine
	Ritonavir + lopinavir*‡	Zidovudine + lamivudine
	Ritonavir + saquinavir* (SGC§) or (HGC§)	

	Column A	Column B
Recommended as Alternatives	Abacavir	Zidovudine + zalcitabine
	Amprenavir	
	Delavirdine	
	Nelfinavir + saquinavir-SGC	
	Nevirapine	
	Ritonavir	
	Saquinavir-SGC	

No Recommendation; Insufficient Data#	Hydroxyurea in combination with antiretroviral drugs	
	Ritonavir + amprenavir*	
	Ritonavir + nelfinavir*	

Not Recommended	All monotherapies, whether from Column A or B**	

	Column A	Column B
Should Not Be Offered	Saquinavir-HGC††	Stavudine + zidovudine
		Zalcitabine + didanosine
		Zalcitabine + lamivudine
		Zalcitabine + stavudine

* Ritonavir increases plasma concentration of other protease inhibitors (PIs) by at least two mechanisms, including inhibition of gastrointestinal CYP450 during absorption and metabolic inhibition of hepatic CYP450. The 20-fold increase in saquinavir plasma concentrations with ritonavir co-administration is likely caused by inhibition of CYP450 at both sites and leads to a marked increase primarily in the saquinavir Cmax. For lopinavir, the addition of ritonavir increases both the peak concentration and the half-life (which subsequently results in a higher trough concentration). The result is a lopinavir area under the curve that is 100-fold higher compared to lopinavir alone. For other PIs, metabolism in the gastrointestinal tract plays a relatively minor role and the enhancement is primarily due to CYP450 inhibition in the liver. The addition of ritonavir to amprenavir, nelfinavir, or indinavir results in marked increases in half-life and trough levels, with a more moderate or minimal increase in the peak concentration.

† Based on expert opinion

†† Co-formulation as Kaletra

§ Saquinavir-SGC, soft-gel capsule (Fortovase®); saquinavir-HGC, hard-gel capsule (Invirase®)

¶ Pregnant women may be at an increased risk for lactic acidosis and liver damage when treated with the combination of stavudine and didanosine. This combination should be used in pregnant women only when the potential benefit clearly outweighs the potential risk.

This category includes drugs or combinations for which information is too limited to allow a recommendation for or against use.

** To prevent perinatal transmission, zidovudine monotherapy may be considered for prophylactic use in pregnant women who have a low viral load and high CD4+ T cell counts as discussed under "Considerations for Antiretroviral Therapy in the HIV-Infected Pregnant Woman" in this version of guidelines for antiretroviral therapy in adults and adolescents.

†† Use of saquinavir-HGC (Invirase®) is not recommended, except in combination with ritonavir.

Source: Panel on the Clinical Practices for the Treatment of HIV Infection, U.S. Department of Health and Human Services (DHHS); and the Henry J. Kaiser Family Foundation. 2002. *Guidelines for the use of antiretroviral agents in HIV-infected adults and adolescents*, p. 43. Available at: http://www.aidsinfo.nih.gov/guidelines. Accessed on May 10, 2002.

Table 11C.7.   CHARACTERISTICS OF ANTIRETROVIRAL MEDICATIONS BY CLASS

Name	FDA Pregnancy Category	Adult Dosing Recommendation	Administration	Oral Bioavailability	Metabolism and Elimination	Side Effects and Adverse Events*
Nucleoside and Nucleotide Reverse Transcriptase Inhibitors (NRTIs)						
Abacavir (Ziagen®, ABC)	C	300 mg p.o. BID	May take with or without meals (alcohol will ↑ ABC levels by 41%).	83%	Metabolized by glucuronyl transferase and alcohol dehydrogenase with 82% renal excretion of metabolites.	Hypersensitivity reaction that can be fatal (3% incidence). Symptoms include fever, rash, nausea, vomiting, fatigue, malaise, loss of appetite; respiratory symptoms that also may present include cough, shortness of breath, sore throat. **NOTE:** Patients who experience these symptoms should contact their clinician and have a medical evaluation immediately. If abacavir is stopped, it should not be reintroduced due to the possibility of life-threatening hypotension and death. See footnote regarding lactic acidosis risk with NRTIs.
Didanosine (Videx®, ddI)	B	**>60 kg:** 200 mg BID (buffered tablets), 250 mg (buffered powder), or 400 mg p.o. QD (EC capsule or buffered tablets) **<60 kg:** 125 mg p.o. BID (buffered tablets), 167 mg p.o. BID (buffered powder), or 250 mg p.o. QD (EC capsules or buffered tablets) **NOTE:** BID dosing is preferred, but QD dosing with EC ddI is an option for patients desiring simplified regimens.	Take ddI 30 minutes before or 2 hours after a meal (food intake will ↓ levels of ddI by 55%).	30–40%	Renal excretion (50%)	Peripheral neuropathy, nausea, diarrhea Pancreatitis: Both fatal and nonfatal cases of pancreatitis have been reported in patients who are treatment-naïve or treatment-experienced with ddI, and with ddI in combination with d4T or hydroxyurea. See footnote regarding lactic acidosis risk with NRTIs.
Lamivudine (Epivir®, 3TC)	C	150 mg p.o. BID	May take with or without meals.	86%	Renal excretion (unchanged)	Rare side effects: anemia, nausea, diarrhea, hair loss. See footnote regarding lactic acidosis risk with NRTIs.
Stavudine (Zerit®, d4T)	C	**>60 kg:** 40 mg p.o. BID **<60 kg:** 30 mg p.o. BID	May take with or without meals. Do not co-administer with zidovudine (AZT) due to antagonistic effect.	86%	Renal excretion (50%)	Peripheral neuropathy, anemia Pancreatitis (fatal and nonfatal cases) has been reported in patients who are treatment-naïve or treatment-experienced with ddI especially when used with d4T. See footnote regarding lactic acidosis risk with NRTIs.

*Lactic acidosis with hepatic steatosis is a rare but potentially fatal toxicity that has been reported with NRTI use. Pregnant women may be at an increased risk for lactic acidosis and liver damage when treated with ddI and d4T. This combination should be used in pregnant women only when the benefit outweighs the potential risk.

(continued)

Table 11C.7.   CHARACTERISTICS OF ANTIRETROVIRAL MEDICATIONS BY CLASS *(continued)*

Name	FDA Pregnancy Category	Adult Dosing Recommendation	Administration	Oral Bioavailability	Metabolism and Elimination	Side Effects and Adverse Events*
Tenofovir Disoproxil Fumarate (Viread®, TDF)	B	300 mg p.o. QD (NOT recommended for patients with creatinine clearance <60 mL/minute)	Bioavailability is increased with food intake.	39% with high fat meal, 25% in fasting state	Renal excretion via glomerular filtration and active tubular secretion.	Headache, nausea, vomiting, diarrhea, flatulence, asthenia. See footnote regarding lactic acidosis risk with NRTIs.
Zalcitabine (Hivid®, ddC)	C	0.75 mg p.o. TID	May take with or without meals.	85%	Renal excretion (70%)	Stomatitis, peripheral neuropathy. See footnote regarding lactic acidosis risk with NRTIs.
Zidovudine (Retrovir®, AZT, ZDV) **Combinations:** Combivir® (AZT and 3TC) Trizivir® (AZT, 3TC, and abacavir)	C	200 mg p.o. TID OR 300 mg p.o. BID **Combinations:** Combivir®: AZT 300 mg and 3TC 150 mg p.o. BID Trizivir®: AZT 300 mg, 3TC 150 mg, and abacavir 300 mg p.o. BID	May take with or without meals. Do not administer with stavudine (d4T) due to antagonistic effect.	60%	Metabolized to its glucuronide derivative, GAZT, with renal excretion of GAZT.	Bone marrow suppression (anemia, neutropenia), nausea, headache, asthenia, insomnia. See footnote regarding lactic acidosis risk with NRTIs.

Non-nucleoside Reverse Transcriptase Inhibitors (NNRTIs)

Name	FDA Pregnancy Category	Adult Dosing Recommendation	Administration	Oral Bioavailability	Metabolism and Elimination	Side Effects and Adverse Events*
Nevirapine (Viramune®, NVP)	C	200 mg p.o. QD for 14 days, then 200 mg p.o. BID	May take with or without meals.	>90%	Metabolized through the cytochrome P450 (3A inducer). 80% renal excretion (glucuronidated metabolites; <5% unchanged); 10% excretion in feces.	Rash†, ↑ transaminase levels, hepatitis
Delavirdine (Rescriptor®, DLV)	C	400 mg p.o. TID Can disperse 100 mg tablets in ≥3 ounces of water to produce a slurry. Requires acidic environment for absorption. Dosing with ddI or use of an antacid must be separated by 1 hour.	May take with or without meals.	85%	Metabolized through the cytochrome P450 (3A inhibitor). 51% renal excretion (<5% unchanged); 44% excretion in feces.	Rash†, ↑ transaminase levels, hepatitis, headaches

*Lactic acidosis with hepatic steatosis is a rare but potentially fatal toxicity that has been reported with NRTI use. Pregnant women may be at an increased risk for lactic acidosis and liver damage when treated with ddI and d4T. This combination should be used in pregnant women only when the benefit outweighs the potential risk.

†Rash has been reported in clinical trials investigating NNRTIs. In these studies, discontinuation of the drug due to rash occurred in 7% of patients taking nevirapine, 4.3% taking delavirdine, and 1.7% taking efavirenz. Although rare, Stevens-Johnson syndrome has been reported in patients using NNRTIs.

(continued)

Table 11C.7.   CHARACTERISTICS OF ANTIRETROVIRAL MEDICATIONS BY CLASS *(continued)*

Name	FDA Pregnancy Category	Adult Dosing Recommendation	Administration	Oral Bioavailability	Metabolism and Elimination	Side Effects and Adverse Events*
Efavirenz (Sustiva®, EFV)	C	600 mg p.o. qHS	High-fat meals can ↑ efavirenz levels by 50%. Avoid high-fat meals before dosing.	Data not available	Metabolized through the cytochrome P450 (mixed 3A inducer/inhibitor) pathway. 14–34% renal excretion (glucuronidated metabolites; <1% unchanged); 16–61% excretion in feces.	Rash†, ↑ transaminase levels, hepatitis, false-positive cannabinoid toxicology tests, CNS symptoms‡ Teratogenic in primates (anophthalmia, anencephaly, microophthalmia). **NOTE:** No data are available regarding the teratogenicity of other NNRTIs in nonhuman primates.
Protease Inhibitors (PIs)						
Amprenavir (Agenerase®, APV)	C	**>50 kg:** 1,200 mg p.o. BID **<50 kg:** 20 mg/kg p.o. BID (maximum 2,400 mg p.o. per day total dose) Combination of amprenavir 600 mg p.o. and ritonavir 100 mg p.o. can be used as an alternative.	High-fat meal ↓ levels by 21%. Should avoid high-fat meals before dosing.	Not determined in humans	Metabolized through the cytochrome P450 (3A4 inhibitor).	Nausea, diarrhea, vomiting, oral paresthesia, rash, fat redisposition, hyperglycemia, lipid abnormalities, ↑ liver function tests, possible ↑ in bleeding episodes in hemophiliac patients. **NOTE:** Agenerase oral solution is contraindicated in the following patients because it contains levels of propylene glycol that may be toxic: pregnant women, children <4 years old, patients with renal or hepatic failure, and patients receiving disulfiram or metronidazole.
Indinavir (Crixivan®, IDV)	C	800 mg p.o. every 8 hours Combination of indinavir 800 mg p.o. BID with ritonavir 100 mg or 200 mg p.o. BID is an alternative.	Take 1 hour before or 2 hours after a meal. Dosing with ddI must be separated by 1 hour. May take with or without meals.	65%	P450 cytochrome 3A4 inhibitor	Nephrolithiasis, nausea, gastrointestinal intolerance, metallic taste, headache, rash, asthenia, blurred vision, alopecia, fat redisposition, hyperglycemia, lipid abnormalities, ↓ platelet count, hyperbilirubinemia (inconsequential), possible ↑ in bleeding episodes in hemophiliac patients. **NOTE:** Patient should drink 8 glasses of water/day to reduce the risk of nephrolithiasis.

† Rash has been reported in clinical trials investigating NNRTIs. In these studies, discontinuation of the drug due to rash occurred in 7% of patients taking nevirapine, 4.3% taking delavirdine, and 1.7% taking efavirenz. Although rare, Stevens-Johnson syndrome has been reported in patients using NNRTIs.

‡ CNS symptoms include dizziness, insomnia, abnormal dreams, hallucinations, impaired concentration, amnesia, agitation, euphoria, somnolence, and depersonalization. The frequency of any of these symptoms has been reported to be 52% in patients taking efavirenz compared to 26% in controls. Symptoms usually diminish 4–6 weeks after discontinuation. Efavirenz should be used with caution in individuals with psychiatric conditions.

§ Poor glycemic control and ketoacidosis in patients with pre-existing and new-onset diabetes have been reported with the use of all protease inhibitors. In addition, fat redistribution and lipid abnormalities have been increasingly observed in patients receiving protease inhibitors. Patients with hyptertriglyceridemia or hypercholesterolemia should be evaluated for their risk of developing cardiovascular disease and pancreatitis with appropriate interventions initiated when abnormalities or increased risk of disease are determined.

(continued)

Table 11C.7. CHARACTERISTICS OF ANTIRETROVIRAL MEDICATIONS BY CLASS (continued)

Name	FDA Pregnancy Category	Adult Dosing Recommendation	Administration	Oral Bioavailability	Metabolism and Elimination	Side Effects and Adverse Events*
Lopinavir and Ritonavir (Kaletra®)	C	400 mg lopinavir and 100 mg ritonavir p.o. BID **NOTE:** Each capsule contains 133.3 mg of lopinavir and 33.3 mg of ritonavir. Oral solution contains 42% alcohol.	Moderate fat in meals can ↑ area under the curve levels by 48% (capsules) and 80% (solution). Take with food but avoid high-fat meals.	Data not available	P450 cytochrome 3A4 inhibitor	Gastrointestinal intolerance, nausea, asthesia, loss of strength, fat redisposition, hyperglycemia, lipid abnormalities, ↑ transaminase levels, possible ↑ in bleeding episodes in hemophiliac patients.
Nelfinavir (Viracept®, NLF)	B	750 mg p.o. TID OR 1,250 mg p.o. BID	Take with meal or snack to ↑ bioavailability.	20–80%	P450 cytochrome 3A4 inhibitor	Diarrhea, hyperglycemia, fat redisposition, lipid abnormalities, possible ↑ in bleeding episodes in hemophiliac patients.
Ritonavir (Norvir®, RTV)	B	600 mg p.o. every 12 hours **NOTE:** Dose escalation required as follows: Day 1–2 take 300 mg p.o. BID; Day 3–5 take 400 mg p.o. BID; Day 6–13 take 500 mg p.o. BID; Day 14 take 600 mg p.o. BID. Dosing with ddI must be separated by 2 hours. Combination with ritonavir 400 mg p.o. BID and saquinavir 400 mg p.o. BID is an alternative.	Taking with food may improve tolerability of medication (levels will ↑ by 15%).	Not determined	Potent P450 cytochrome 3A4 inhibitor	Nausea, vomiting, diarrhea, unpleasant taste, asthesia, paresthesias (circumoral, extremities), pancreatitis, hepatitis, fat redisposition, hyperglycemia, lipid abnormalities, ↑ triglycerides by >200%, ↑ transaminase levels, ↑ CPK, ↑ uric acid, possible ↑ in bleeding episodes in hemophiliac patients. **NOTE:** Multiple drug interactions can occur with ritonavir, resulting in an increase in side effects. Consult drug information or a clinical pharmacist regarding use of ritonavir with other medications.
Saquinavir Hard Gel (Invirase®, SQV HGC)	B	Saquinavir 400 mg p.o. and ritonavir 400 mg p.o. BID **NOTE:** Invirase should not be used without ritonavir to achieve adequate area under the curve levels.	May take with or without meals if dosed with ritonavir.	Hard gel capsule is erratic: 4%	Potent P450 cytochrome 3A4 inhibitor	Nausea, diarrhea, headache, fat redisposition, hyperglycemia, lipid abnormalities, ↑ transaminase levels, possible ↑ in bleeding episodes in hemophiliac patients.
Saquinavir Soft Gel (Fortovase®, SQV SGC)	B	1,200 mg p.o. TID	Take with large meal to improve bioavailability. Garlic supplements ↓ blood levels by 50%.	Soft gel capsule not determined	Potent P450 cytochrome 3A4 inhibitor	Nausea, dyspepsia, abdominal discomfort/pain, diarrhea, headache, fat redisposition, hyperglycemia, lipid abnormalities, ↑ transaminase levels, possible ↑ in bleeding episodes in patients with hemophilia.

§ Poor glycemic control and ketoacidosis in patients with pre-existing and new-onset diabetes have been reported with the use of all protease inhibitors. In addition, fat redistribution and lipid abnormalities have been increasingly observed in patients receiving protease inhibitors. Patients with hypertriglyceridemia or hypercholesterolemia should be evaluated for their risk of developing cardiovascular disease and pancreatitis with appropriate interventions initiated when abnormalities or increased risk of disease are determined.

Sources: Project Inform. 2002. *Drug interactions*. San Francisco: Project Inform; Panel on the Clinical Practices for the Treatment of HIV Infection, U.S. Department of Health and Human Services (DHHS); and the Henry J. Kaiser Family Foundation. 2002. *Guidelines for the use of antiretroviral agents in HIV-infected adults and adolescents*. Available at: http://www.aidsinfo.nih.gov/guidelines/adult/AAMay23.pdf. Accessed on May 10, 2002.

- The following agents can be used:
  - Hydrogen peroxide: Gargle for 30 seconds BID indefinitely.
  - Chlorhexidine gluconate oral rinse: 15 mL swished in the mouth for 30 seconds BID indefinitely.
  NOTE: Chlorhexidine gluconate can stain teeth.
  - A patient with any abnormality noted on cervical cytology should be evaluated and treated as indicated by an experienced colposcopist.

CONSULTATION

→ Physician consultation is indicated regarding the plan of care for any patient suspected of being HIV-infected or for whom there is documented evidence of an HIV-seropositive status with or without symptomatic disease.

→ Physician consultation is warranted in any HIV-infected patient for whom there is evidence of a major OI or AIDS-defining condition, lack of response to therapeutic interventions, or serious side effects or suspected toxicity to a medication, or who is being considered for OI maintenance therapy (e.g., ketoconazole for candidiasis) or prophylactic therapy (e.g., Septra DS® for PCP prophylaxis).

→ In clinical settings where physician consultation is limited or unavailable, current information regarding management of HIV disease is available from the HIV Telephone Consultation Service of the National HIV/AIDS Clinicians' Consultation Center: (800) 933-3413. In addition, clinicians can access several online resources to update their knowledge:
  - AIDS Treatment Information Service and HIV/AIDS Clinical Trials Information Service have merged into one Web site, AIDSinfo, which is accessible at www.aidsinfo.nih.gov. This site provides current national guidelines for treating HIV-infected individuals, as well as other information pertinent to their care.
  - The Body, www.thebody.com. It provides comprehensive information and resources regarding HIV.
  - CDC, www.cdc.gov. It provides several links to various topics related to HIV prevention, diagnosis, and treatment.
  - National Pediatric & Family HIV Resource Center, www.pedHIVAIDS.org. It provides comprehensive information and resources for clinicians who care for HIV-infected children and their families.

→ Psychological or psychiatric consultation is indicated for patients with evidence of moderate to severe psychiatric symptoms (e.g., anxiety or depression) or who may be exhibiting neuropsychiatric manifestations of HIV (e.g., HIV dementia).

→ As needed for prescription(s).

PATIENT EDUCATION

→ Educate the patient about HIV infection, including the clinical course (especially the chronicity of the disease), indicated diagnostic tests, therapeutic options available, modes of transmission, preventing HIV transmission to others, preventing further exposure to HIV and other STDs in sexually active women (see **Table 13A.2, Safer Sex Guidelines** in the **Chancroid** chapter in Section 13), symptoms of complications requiring immediate evaluation, and indicated follow-up.
  - A number of patient education materials are available from the CDC National AIDS Hotline, (800) 342-AIDS, as well as on the CDC Web site.

→ Discuss with the patient any referrals that are recommended and the importance of keeping such appointments.

→ Discuss with the patient the need for testing of individuals who may have been exposed by her through sexual contact or needle-sharing activities. If a women has children, assess the possible need for testing them based on the woman's history of exposure, date of first positive test result, and the ages of her children.

→ A patient who is continuing to inject drugs should be educated about the adverse effects on her health, the need to consider drug treatment, and the importance of avoiding sharing needles to prevent transmission of HIV and other infectious diseases (e.g., hepatitis B and C).

→ Before obtaining a patient's medical records, discuss with her the need for documentation and/or confirmation of her HIV status and how these can be obtained.
  - In many locations, a special consent for disclosure of HIV test results must be signed by the patient in addition to standard medical record release forms.
  - Furthermore, informed consent of a patient (in some states this is written consent) regarding HIV testing is required before performing such tests.
  - Initial disclosure of HIV test results should involve only the patient and the provider or counselor who ordered the test. However, the results should be disclosed to other providers directly involved in her care (if she consents).
  - Ideally, the patient should return to the provider or counselor to receive her results in person and to receive comprehensive follow-up counseling regarding the results (including the need for repeat testing in patients who have tested negative but who are continuing to participate in behaviors that place them at risk for exposure to HIV). During this session, appropriate psychosocial and medical referrals for the patient should be made as indicated.

→ Discuss and/or provide support for disclosure of a patient's HIV positive serostatus to her family and significant others. Assess her readiness for disclosure as well as her risk of psychological and physical abuse by her partner, family, or close friends if her serostatus is revealed. Make appropriate referrals for psychosocial assistance as indicated.

→ Advise the patient regarding any potential short-term or long-term side effects associated with medications and when immediate evaluation may be indicated.

→ Advise the patient that she should not donate blood products or consent to organ donation.

→ Advise the patient not to share personal hygiene implements that could be contaminated with blood (e.g., a toothbrush or razors).

→ Teach the patient ways to reduce the risk of becoming infected with toxoplasmosis, including properly cooking meat and, if she has a cat, recommending that another household member change the litter box.
■ If the patient lives alone and must change the litter box, she should use disposable gloves and wear a mask during the task, and thoroughly wash her hands when done.
→ Educate reproductive-age women who are sexually active and who want to postpone childbearing about the need to combine effective STD prevention and contraceptive methods.
■ There are limited data regarding the various contraceptive methods and their impact on HIV disease and/or transmission.
■ Most methods are acceptable if they are combined with effective STD prevention strategies.
• Intrauterine devices (IUDs) are not recommended because of the associated risk of uterine infections and the possibly higher risk of HIV transmission due to increased blood flow and foreign body inflammatory response possibly associated with IUD use (Anderson 2001).
■ Antiretroviral medications may alter the levels of hormonal contraceptives. Some of these medications significantly lower levels of ethinyl estradiol (e.g., lopinavir ↓ by 42%, nelfinavir ↓ by 47%, ritonavir ↓ by 40%, nevirapine ↓ by 29%) while others increase the levels (delavirdine ↑ by an unknown amount, efavirenz ↑ by 37%, indinavir ↑ by 24%) (Project Inform 2002). Consequently, clinicians prescribing hormonal agents to HIV-infected women who are receiving antiretrovirals should review current information about drug interactions among medications commonly used to treat HIV and, if possible, consult with a clinical pharmacist.
→ An HIV-infected woman considering pregnancy should be referred to a health care provider experienced in the care of HIV-infected pregnant women for an in-depth discussion of current information.
■ It is imperative to present current information regarding the effects of pregnancy on HIV disease progression, the effects of HIV infection on pregnancy outcome, perinatal transmission rates, interventions that reduce perinatal transmission rates (e.g., use of ZDV during antepartum, intrapartum, and neonatal periods), therapeutic interventions for the woman during pregnancy, care of an HIV-infected infant, and clinical trials available to the woman and her infant.
→ Women on HAART who suspect that they may be pregnant should contact their HIV care provider to discuss the risks versus benefits of continuing therapy during the first trimester. Voluntary surveillance program data do not demonstrate an increased rate of congenital anomalies in infants born to HIV-infected women receiving various antiretroviral medication regimens compared to the general population of pregnant women (Antiretroviral Pregnancy Registry Steering Committee 2002, Garcia et al. 2001).

Much of the data available through these programs address primarily the use of AZT or a combination of AZT and 3TC, with less information about other combinations of antiretroviral medications used during gestation. However, an increase in cranial deformities and a neural tube defect in primates born with in-utero exposure to efavirenz, a non-nucleoside reverse transcriptase inhibitor, have been documented. There was also a recent case study documenting a similar defect in an infant born to a woman who took efavirenz during the first trimester of her pregnancy (Fundaro et al. 2002).
→ Advise the woman regarding the need to disclose her HIV status to other medical providers so appropriate therapy for any illness or condition can be prescribed.
→ Educate the woman about community resources available to her for psychosocial support (e.g., HIV-specific women's groups, legal counseling, and financial aid).
→ Educate the woman about clinical trials that may be available to her.
■ For information about efficacy trials approved by the National Institutes of Health and the FDA, call the AIDS Clinical Trials Information Service at (800) TRIALS-A (874-2572) or visit the AIDSinfo Web site at www.aidsinfo.nih.gov.

FOLLOW-UP

→ See "Consultation," above.
→ Recommend follow-up evaluation of the asymptomatic, HIV-positive woman every 3–4 months for an HIV-specific evaluation (including laboratory tests).
■ See "Diagnostic Tests," above, for recommendations regarding additional follow-up tests and evaluations.
→ A woman with any symptoms of possible complications or side effects of a medication should return for evaluation as soon as possible.
→ An AIDS diagnosis is a reportable condition, with notification of the local public health department mandated by law. In some states, HIV infection also is a reportable condition. Contact the local public health department for the appropriate forms and procedure(s).
→ Document in progress notes and on problem list (as appropriate and without breaching patient confidentiality).

BIBLIOGRAPHY

Anderson J.R. 2001. HIV and reproduction. In *A guide to the clinical care of women with HIV*, ed. J.R. Anderson, pp. 213–274. Washington, D.C.: U.S. Department of Health and Human Services.

Antiretroviral Pregnancy Registry Steering Committee. 2002. *Antiretroviral Pregnancy Registry international interim report for 1 January 1989 through 31 July 2002.* Wilmington, N.C.: Registry Project Office.

Bartlett, J.G., and Gallant, J.E. 2001. *2001–2002 medical management of HIV infection.* Baltimore, Md.: John Hopkins University, Division of Infectious Diseases.

Cardillo, M., Hagan, R., Abadi, J. et al. 2001. CD4 T-cell count, viral load, and squamous intraepithelial lesions in women infected with the human immunodeficiency virus. *Cancer* 93(2):111–114.

Centers for Disease Control and Prevention (CDC). 1991. Hepatitis B virus: a comprehensive strategy for eliminating transmission in the United States through universal childhood vaccination. Recommendations of the Immunization Practices Advisory Committee (ACIP). *Morbidity and Mortality Weekly Report* 40(RR-13):1–19.

_____. 1992. 1993 revised classification system for HIV infection and expanded surveillance case definition for AIDS among adolescents and adults. *Morbidity and Mortality Weekly Report* 41(RR-17):1–19.

_____. 1996. Prevention of hepatitis A through active or passive immunization. Recommendations of the Immunization Practices Advisory Committee (ACIP). *Morbidity and Mortality Weekly Report* 45(RR-15):1–38.

_____. 1999. Prevention and control of influenza. Recommendations of the Immunization Practices Advisory Committee (ACIP). *Morbidity and Mortality Weekly Report* 48(RR-4): 1–49.

_____. 2002. *HIV/AIDS surveillance report—midyear edition* 14(1):1–41.

Cohn S.E., Berk, M.L., Berry, S.H. et al. 2001. The care of HIV-infected adults in rural areas of the United States. *Journal of Acquired Immune Deficiency Syndromes* 28(4):386–392.

Del Mistro, A., and Bianchi, L. 2001. HPV-related neoplasias in HIV-infected individuals. *European Journal of Cancer* 37(10):1227–1235.

Ellerbrock, T.V., Chiasson, M.A., Bush, T.J. et al. 2000. Incidence of cervical squamous intraepithelial lesions in HIV-infected women. *Journal of the American Medical Association* 283:1031–1037.

Feinberg, J., and Maenza, J. 2001. Primary medical care. In *A guide to the clinical care of women with HIV*, ed. J.R. Anderson, pp. 77–138. Washington, D.C.: U.S. Department of Health and Human Services.

Fundaro, C., Genovese, O., Rendeli, C. et al. 2002. Myelomeningocele in a child with intrauterine exposure to efavirenz. *AIDS* 16:299–300.

Gandhi, M., Bacchetti, P., Miotti, P. et al. 2002. Effect of gender/sex on viral load, pharmacokinetics and responses to antiretroviral therapy. 9th Conference on Retroviruses and Opportunistic Infections. Seattle, Wash., February 24–28, 2002. Available at: http://www.retroconference.org/2002/Abstract/13128.htm. Accessed on March 5, 2002.

Garcia, P.M., Beckerman, K., Watts, H. et al. 2001. Assessing the teratogenic potential of antiretroviral drugs: data from the Antiretroviral Pregnancy Registry (APR). Abstract I-1325. 41st Interscience Conference on Antimicrobial Agents and Chemotherapy. Chicago, Ill., December 16–19, 2001.

Gardner, L.I., Holmberg, S.D., Moore, J. et al. 2002. Use of highly active antiretroviral therapy in HIV-infected women: impact of HIV specialist care. *Journal of Acquired Immune Deficiency Syndromes* 29(1):69–75.

Goldschmidt, R.H., and Dong, B.J. 2001. Treatment of AIDS and HIV-related conditions: 2001. *Journal of the American Board of Family Practice* 14:283–309.

Hessol, N., and Greenblatt, R.M. 2001. Epidemiology and natural history of HIV infection in women. In *A guide to the clinical care of women with HIV*, ed. J.R. Anderson, pp. 1–32. Washington, D.C.: U.S. Department of Health and Human Services.

Ho, D., Neumann, A.U., Perelson, A.S. et al. 1995. Rapid turnover of plasma virions and CD4 lymphocytes in HIV-1 infection. *Nature* 373:123–126.

Jasmer, R.M., Saukkonen, J.J., Blumberg, H.M. et al. 2002. Short-course rifampin and pyrazinamide compared with isoniazid for latent tuberculosis infection: a multicenter clinical trial. *Annals of Internal Medicine* 137:693–695.

Joint United Nations Programme on HIV/AIDS (UNAIDS). 2001. *AIDS epidemic update. December 2001.* Geneva, Switzerland: UNAIDS.

Kauf, T.L., Gibbons, D.C., Kirkland, T.L. et al. 2001. Modeling the impact of revised DHHS HIV treatment guidelines on survival in women. Abstract I-1913. 41st Interscience Conference on Antimicrobial Agents and Chemotherapy. Chicago, Ill., December 16–19, 2001.

Keller, M., Deveikis, A., Cutillar-Garcia, M. et al. 2000. Pneumococcal and influenza immunization and human immunodeficiency virus load in children. *Pediatric Infectious Disease Journal* 19:613–618.

Kessler, H., Deeks, S.G., and Grant, R.M. 2000. *Understanding assays—guide to HIV resistance tests.* Atlanta, Ga.: Meditech Media.

Korn, A.P., and Landers, D.V. 1995. Gynecologic disease in women infected with human immunodeficiency virus type 1. *Journal of Acquired Immune Deficiency Syndrome and Human Retrovirology* 9:361–370.

Macias, J., Pineda, J.A., Leal, M. et al. 2001. HIV-1 plasma viremia not increased in patients receiving highly active antiretroviral therapy after influenza vaccination. *European Journal of Clinical Microbiology and Infectious Disease* 20:46–48.

Marlink, R., Kao, H., and Hsieh, E. 2001. Clinical care issues for women living with HIV and AIDS in the United States. *AIDS Research and Human Retroviruses* 17(1):1–33.

McNaghten, A.D., Hanson, D.L., Jones, J.L. et al. 1999. Effects of antiretroviral therapy and opportunistic illnesses primary chemoprophylaxis on survival after AIDS diagnosis. *AIDS* 13:1687–1695.

Mellors, J.W., Munoz, A., Giorgi, J.V. et al. 1997. Plasma viral load and CD4+ lymphocytes as prognostic markers of HIV-1 infection. *Annals of Internal Medicine* 128:946–954.

Murphy, E.L., Collier, A.C., Kalish, L.A. et al. 2001. Highly active antiretroviral therapy decreases mortality and morbidity in patients with advanced HIV disease. *Annals of Internal Medicine* 135(1):17–26.

Panel on the Clinical Practices for the Treatment of HIV Infection, U.S. Department of Health and Human Services (DHHS); and the Henry J. Kaiser Family Foundation. 2002.

Guidelines for the use of antiretroviral agents in HIV-infected adults and adolescents. Available at: http://www.aidsinfo.nih.gov/guidelines. Accessed on May 1, 2002.

Pantaleo, G., Graziosi, C., Demarest, J.F. et al. 1993. HIV infection is active and progressive in lymphoid tissue during the clinically latent stage of disease. *Nature* 362(6418):355–358.

Phillips, K.D., and Knox, M.L. 2000. HIV disease. In *Advanced pathophysiology. Application to clinical practice*, ed. M. Groer, pp. 410–447. Philadelphia: Lippincott Williams & Wilkins.

Poundstone, K.E., Chaisson, R.E., and Moore, R.D. 2001. Differences in HIV disease progression by injection drug use and by sex in the era of highly active antiretroviral therapy. *AIDS* 15(9):1115–1123.

Project Inform. 2002. *Drug interactions.* San Francisco: Project Inform.

Rich, J.D., Montaner, J., Conway, B. et al. 1999. Suppression of plasma viral load below 20 copies/mL is required to achieve a long-term response to therapy. *AIDS* 13:F23–28.

Robinson, W.R., and Freeman, D. 2002. Improved outcome of cervical neoplasia in HIV-infected women in the era of highly active antiretroviral therapy. *AIDS Patient Care and STDs* 16(2):61–65.

Six, C., Heard, I., Bergeron, C. et al. 1998. Comparative prevalence, incidence and short-term prognosis of cervical squamous intraepithelial lesions amongst HIV-positive and HIV-negative women. *AIDS* 12:1047–1056.

Sterling, T.R., Chaisson, R.E., and Moore, R.D. 2001. HIV-1 RNA, CD4 T-lymphocytes, and clinical response to highly active antiretroviral therapy. *AIDS* 12(17):2251–2257.

Stout, J.E., Engemann, J.J., Cheng, A.C. et al. 2002. Safety of 2 months of rifampin and pyrazinamide for treatment of latent tuberculosis. *American Journal of Respiratory and Critical Care Medicine.* Published ahead of print on November 21, 2002 as doi:10.1164/rccm.200209-998OC.

U.S. Public Health Service (USPHS) and Infectious Disease Society of America (IDSA). 1999. Guidelines for the prevention of opportunistic infections in persons infected with human immunodeficiency virus. *Morbidity and Mortality Weekly Report* 48(RR-10):1–66.

Maureen T. Shannon, C.N.M., F.N.P., M.S.

11-D

Lyme Disease

Lyme disease is a tick-borne systemic illness that can affect the skin, heart, joints, and nervous system, resulting in clinical manifestations that may persist for years. The disease was identified in 1977 in Lyme, Conn., when a cluster of children in the area were initially thought to have juvenile rheumatoid arthritis. Investigation into clusters of patients with similar symptoms revealed physical findings implicating an arthropod-borne infectious disease. The organism responsible for the illness was not identified until 1982. At that time, a previously unrecognized spirochete, now called *Borrelia burgdorferi*, was isolated and later recovered from patients with Lyme disease in the United States and patients with similar disorders in Europe (Steere 2001).

Since its identification, Lyme disease has been the leading vector-borne illness in the United States (Centers for Disease Control and Prevention [CDC] 1999, 2001a). The risk of acquiring infection varies depending on the geographic distribution, density, prevalence, and feeding habits of the vector ticks. In the United States, 90% of Lyme disease cases occur in 10 states: Connecticut, Rhode Island, New York, New Jersey, Delaware, Pennsylvania, Wisconsin, Maryland, Massachusetts, and Minnesota (CDC 2001b).

Ticks from the *Ixodes ricinus* complex are the vectors of Lyme disease, with various types responsible for transmission of the *B. burgdorferi* spirochete in different regions of the United States and Europe. In the United States, the eastern deer tick, *Ixodes scapularis* (also called *Ixodes dammini*), is the vector in the Northeast, Midwest, and Southeast. The western black-legged tick, *Ixodes pacificus*, is the vector along the West Coast. Infection rates among *Ixodes* ticks vary among geographic regions; knowledge of these rates can be beneficial when assessing the possibility of Lyme disease in a patient presenting with a tick bite. Ninety percent of Lyme disease cases reported to the CDC occur in 10 states in the Northeastern and Midwestern regions of the United States; cases are rarely reported in the Southeast (CDC 1999, Steere 2001).

The major host during the tick's larval and nymph stages is the white-footed mouse. The white-tailed deer serves as host during the tick's adult life. However, ticks have been found in several other types of wild animals and birds. Although clinical Lyme disease has been observed in domestic animals (e.g., dogs, cattle, and horses), pet ownership has not demonstrated any increased risk of infection (CDC 1999, Steere 2001).

The incidence of Lyme disease has a temporal pattern, with most cases reported during summer months, followed by spring and autumn months, respectively. This pattern is directly related to the two-year life cycle of the tick. During each stage of the life cycle (larval, nymph, and adult), the tick must feed once. The feeding times vary according to the tick's stage of development, with larvae feeding once between July and September, nymphs feeding during May to July, and adults feeding during autumn (Steere 2001). It is during these feedings that the tick acquires the spirochete from an infected host and may transmit the spirochete to uninfected hosts.

In vitro and animal studies have demonstrated that for the spirochete to be transmitted effectively from the infected tick to a host, the tick must remain attached for at least 24 hours (Steere 2001). Because larvae and nymphs are small and do not produce pain when biting a host (thereby remaining unnoticed), the highest incidence of transmission and reported cases of Lyme disease is noted during the months that the immature ticks, particularly nymphs, are feeding: spring through summer.

Asymptomatic infection is reportedly common (Steere 2001). However, in many instances, once a person has been bitten by an infected tick, a broad spectrum of clinical manifestations reflecting multisystem involvement can occur. As is common with other types of spirochetal diseases (e.g., syphilis), the complex, protean nature of Lyme disease has required classifying the disease process into various stages as a means of establishing guidelines for therapeutic interventions at each stage. (See **Table 11D.1, Lyme Disease Surveillance Case Definition [Revised]**.) The characteristic skin lesion associated with Lyme disease—erythema migrans—at the site of the tick's attachment usually develops in 80% of persons 3–30 days after the tick bite. This acute phase of infection is classified as *Stage 1 disease*. Regional lymphadenopathy and influenza-like symptoms also may be noted in Stage 1 disease (CDC 2001b, Steere 2001).

Table 11D.1. LYME DISEASE SURVEILLANCE CASE DEFINITION (REVISED)

Clinical Description

A systemic, tick-borne disease with protean manifestations, including dermatologic, rheumatologic, neurologic, and cardiac abnormalities. The best clinical marker for the disease is the initial skin lesion, erythema migrans, that occurs among 60–80% of patients.

Clinical Case Definition

* Erythema migrans

    OR

* At least one late manifestation, as defined below, and laboratory confirmation of infection

Laboratory Criteria for Diagnosis

* Isolation of *Borrelia burgdorferi* from clinical specimen

    OR

* Demonstration of diagnostic levels of IgM and IgG antibodies to the spirochete in serum or cerebral spinal fluid (CSF). A two-test approach using a sensitive enzyme immunoassay or immunofluorescence antibody followed by Western Blot is recommended.

Case Classification

Confirmed: a case that meets one of the clinical case definitions above

Comment: This surveillance case definition was developed for national reporting of Lyme disease; it is *not* appropriate for clinical diagnosis. Definition of terms used in the clinical description and case definition:

A. Erythema migrans (EM)

For purposes of surveillance, EM is defined as a skin lesion that typically begins as a red macule or papule and expands over a period of days to weeks to form a large round lesion, often with partial central clearing. A solitary lesion must reach at least 5 cm. Secondary lesions also may occur. Annular erythematous lesions occurring within several hours of a tick bite represent hypersensitivity reactions and do not qualify as EM. For most patients, the expanding EM lesion is accompanied by other acute symptoms, particularly fatigue, fever, headache, mild stiff neck, arthralgia, or myalgia. These symptoms are typically intermittent. The diagnosis of EM must be made by a physician. Laboratory confirmation is recommended for persons with no known exposure.

B. Late manifestations

Late manifestations include any of the following *when an alternate explanation is not found:*

■ **Musculoskeletal system**

Recurrent, brief attacks (weeks or months) of objective joint swelling in one or a few joints, *sometimes* followed by chronic arthritis in one or a few joints. Manifestations not considered as criteria for diagnosis include chronic progressive arthritis not preceded by brief attacks and chronic symmetrical polyarthritis. Additionally, arthralgia, myalgia, or fibromyalgia syndromes alone are not criteria for musculoskeletal involvement.

■ **Nervous system**

Any of the following, alone or in combination: lymphocytic meningitis; cranial neuritis, particularly facial palsy (may be bilateral); radiculoneuropathy; or, rarely, encephalomyelitis. Encephalomyelitis must be confirmed by showing antibody production against *B. burgdorferi* in the CSF, demonstrated by a higher titer of antibody in CSF than in serum. Headache, fatigue, paresthesia, or mild stiff neck alone are not criteria for neurologic involvement.

■ **Cardiovascular system**

Acute onset, high-grade (2nd or 3rd degree) atrioventricular conduction defects that resolve in days to weeks and are sometimes associated with myocarditis. Palpitations, bradycardia, bundle branch block, or myocarditis alone are not criteria for cardiovascular involvement.

(continued)

Table 11D.1.   LYME DISEASE SURVEILLANCE CASE DEFINITION (REVISED) *(continued)*

C. Exposure

Exposure is defined as having been in wooded, brushy, or grassy areas (potential tick habitats) in a county in which Lyme disease is endemic no more than 30 days before onset of EM. A history of tick bite is *not* required.

D. Disease endemic to county

A county in which Lyme disease is endemic is one in which at least two definite cases previously have been acquired or in which a known tick vector has been shown to be infected with *B. burgdorferi*.

E. Laboratory confirmation

As noted above, laboratory confirmation of infection with *B. burgdorferi* is established when a laboratory isolates the spirochete from tissue or body fluid, detects diagnostic levels of IgM or IgG antibodies to the spirochete in serum or CSF, or detects a significant change in antibody levels in paired acute- and convalescent-phase serum samples. States may determine the criteria for laboratory confirmation and diagnostic levels of antibody. Syphilis and other known causes of biologic false-positive serologic test results should be excluded when laboratory confirmation has been based on serologic testing alone.

Source: Centers for Disease Control and Prevention (CDC). 1997. Case definitions for infectious conditions under public health surveillance. *Morbidity and Mortality Weekly Report* 46(RR-10):1–55.

Stage 2 disease reflects the hematological and lymphatic spread of the spirochete, resulting in disseminated infection with clinical manifestations ranging from mild to severe multisystem problems. Symptoms can be musculoskeletal, dermatological, neurological, cardiac, lymphatic, ocular, gastrointestinal, genitourinary, or constitutional. Stage 2 disease usually occurs within a few days to weeks after inoculation of the spirochete (Chaparro et al. 2001).

Stage 3 disease indicates late, persistent infection with a range of symptoms developing months to several years after the initial stage of infection. The most common symptoms reported during this stage involve musculoskeletal problems (e.g., arthritis), neurological problems (e.g., chronic encephalomyelitis, chronic axonal polyradiculopathy), ocular problems (e.g., keratitis), dermatological problems (e.g., acrodermatitis chronica atrophicans), and generalized fatigue (Chaparro et al. 2001, Steere 2001).

Although very rare, congenital infection associated with adverse fatal/neonatal outcomes (e.g., congenital cardiac malformations, encephalitis) has been reported in women who acquired Lyme borreliosis during pregnancy (Schlesinger et al. 1985, Weber et al. 1988). The risk of acquiring infection through a blood transfusion is minimal and there is no risk of transmission via person-to-person contact. Despite the extensive morbidity associated with Lyme disease, there is a very low mortality rate (CDC 2001b, Steere, 2001).

DATABASE

SUBJECTIVE

→ Patients may be asymptomatic or report one or more of the following symptoms:

Stage 1 Disease

→ Symptoms usually occur 2–30 days after the tick bite and include (CDC 2001b, Chaparro et al. 2001, Steere 2001):

- Development of erythema migrans lesion ("bull's eye" lesion):
  - An erythematous (color ranging from pink to violaceous), annular plaque with a central area of clearing at the site of the tick bite (most commonly noted in the axilla, thigh, or groin).
  - Usually the lesion begins 3–30 days after the inoculation and resolves in 3–4 weeks.
  - It is observed in at least 80% of patients and is pathognomonic of Lyme disease.
  - Atypical presentations include vesicular, pruritic, or scaling lesions with indurated centers.

  NOTE: In order to be counted for surveillance purposes, a solitary lesion must be at least 5 cm.

- Fever
- Chills
- Malaise
- Myalgia

Stage 2 Disease

→ Symptoms may develop within days to weeks (range is from one week to two years) after the tick bite (Chaparro et al. 2001).

→ Constitutional symptoms include (CDC 2001b, Chaparro et al. 2001, Steere 2001):

- Severe fatigue
- Severe malaise

→ Dermatological manifestations include:
- Secondary annular lesions similar to the initial lesion but smaller
- Malar rash
- Diffuse erythema or urticaria
- Lymphocytoma:
  • A small, erythematous plaque or nodule that develops on the nipple in adults and on the ear in children
    - Very rare, occurring in only 1% of patients
    - Primarily seen in European populations

→ Neurological manifestations include:
- Headache (often intermittent)
- Stiff neck (usually mild)
- Bell's palsy symptoms—pain, paralysis of the face in cranial nerve VII or X
- Pain along spinal nerve distribution (radiculoneuritis)

→ Musculoskeletal manifestations include:
- Migratory pain in joints, tendons, muscles, bursae, or bones
- Swollen, red joints (usually episodes are transient and brief)

→ Lymphatic system manifestations include:
- Regional and/or generalized lymphadenopathy
- Splenomegaly

→ Cardiac manifestations include:
- Syncope or presyncope in patients with a conduction abnormality
- Shortness of breath and dyspnea or exertion in patients with myocarditis, pericarditis, or severe heart block
- Pleural pain—pericardial or substernal chest pain that may radiate to the neck, shoulders, back, or epigastrium

→ Ocular manifestations include:
- Conjunctival erythema and discharge
- Visual disturbances if there is severe ocular disease (e.g., in cases of iritis, retinal hemorrhage or detachment, or panophthalmitis)

→ Gastrointestinal manifestations include:
- Mild and/or recurrent signs and symptoms of hepatitis. (See the **Hepatitis—Viral** chapter.)

→ Respiratory manifestations include:
- Sore throat
- Nonproductive cough
- Signs and symptoms of respiratory distress in cases of adult respiratory distress syndrome (very rare)

Stage 3 Disease

→ Symptoms may appear months to several years after a tick bite (Chaparro et al. 2001, Steere 2001):
- Constitutional manifestations, including chronic fatigue
- Dermatological manifestations include:
  • Development of acrodermatitis chronica atrophicans lesions characterized by the gradual swelling and bluish-red to violaceous discoloration of a distal extremity
    - Later the lesions become atrophic and sclerotic.
- Musculoskeletal manifestations include:

• Swollen, erythematous, warm, painful joints (usually the knee) noted chronically or intermittently
- Neurological manifestations include:
  • Headache—mild to severe, episodic without associated auras
  • Hypersomnia
  • Problems with memory or thinking clearly
  • Tingling, burning, shooting pains in the extremities or trunk
  • Pain in the cervical, thoracic, or lumbosacral area of the spine
  • Progressive stiffness, weakness of the extremities
  • Urinary frequency, urgency, and incontinence

OBJECTIVE

→ The patient may exhibit one or more of the following physical findings depending on the stage of Lyme disease (Chaparro et al. 2001, Steere 2001):

Stage 1 Disease

- Temperature may be slightly elevated.
- Erythema migrans lesion may be observed at site of tick bite. (See "Subjective," above, for a description.)
- Palpable enlarged lymph node(s) in the area of the tick bite

Stage 2 Disease

- Vital signs may reflect an irregular heart rate (if there is a heart block) and an increased respiratory rate (if there is myocarditis, pericarditis, or pancarditis).
- Dermatological physical findings may be present and include:
  • Small, discrete, erythematous, annular, plaque-like lesions (similar to erythema migrans lesion) on the body
  • Small, reddish nodule or plaque on nipple (lymphocytoma)
  • Erythematous eruption over cheekbones
  • Diffuse erythema

→ Neurological physical findings may be present and include:
- Nuchal rigidity
- Diminished or absent facial movement in the distribution of cranial nerves VII and X
- Diminished sensation to light touch or pin prick in affected areas
- Hyperreflexia
- Unsteady or uneven gait
- Subtle evidence of memory problems

→ Musculoskeletal physical findings may be present and include:
- Muscle weakness
- Erythematous, edematous joint(s) that are warm and tender to palpation

→ Cardiac physical findings may be present and include:
- Irregular heart rate with the apical pulse rate greater than peripheral pulses (in atrioventricular nodal heart block)
- Tachycardia

- Gallop rhythm (in myocarditis)
- Pericardial friction rub (in pericarditis)
→ Ocular physical findings may be present and consistent with conjunctivitis, keratitis, iritis, or panophthalmitis. (See Section 2, **Ophthalmological Disorders**.)
→ Gastrointestinal physical findings may be present and consistent with hepatitis. (See the **Hepatitis—Viral** chapter.)
→ Respiratory physical findings may be present and include:
  - Tachypnea (if there is myocarditis, pericarditis, or pancarditis)
  - Auscultation of the lungs is usually within normal limits (WNL) but may reveal crackles at the bases if there is congestive heart failure associated with severe myocarditis.

Stage 3 Disease

→ Vital signs will be WNL.
→ Dermatological physical findings may include:
  - Evidence of acrodermatitis chronica atrophicans:
    - Edematous, doughy, bluish-red to violaceous colored extremities; or atrophic, sclerotic lesions of the extremities
→ Musculoskeletal physical findings may include:
  - Muscular weakness in affected extremities
  - Edematous, erythematous, tender joints (usually knee joints)
  - Evidence of subluxations inferior to lesions of acrodermatitis chronica atrophicans
→ Neurological physical findings may include:
  - Evidence of memory impairment upon neurological evaluation
  - Evidence of depression upon psychiatric evaluation
  - Diminished sensation to light touch or pin prick
  - Hyporeflexia or hyperreflexia with ankle clonus and Babinski signs
  - Mild weakness of the extremities
  - Unsteady or uneven gait
→ Ocular physical findings may be present and consistent with evidence of keratitis. (See the **Keratitis** chapter in Section 2.)

ASSESSMENT

→ Lyme disease (Stage 1, 2, or 3)
→ R/O chronic fatigue syndrome
→ R/O dermatological disease (e.g., nummular eczema)
→ R/O fibromyalgia
→ R/O other spirochetal diseases (e.g., syphilis, Rocky Mountain spotted fever)
→ R/O neurological disease (e.g., multiple sclerosis)
→ R/O autoimmune disease
→ R/O cardiac disease
→ R/O other infectious disease (e.g., HIV infection)

PLAN

DIAGNOSTIC TESTS

→ The diagnosis of Lyme disease is based *primarily* on clinical manifestations. Laboratory testing should only be performed if the clinical manifestations or epidemiologic features suggest Lyme disease and the test results would support the diagnosis (CDC 2001b, Chaparro et al. 2001).
→ Cultures:
  - Demonstration of the spirochete by culture is difficult except when biopsies of skin lesions are performed (CDC 2001b, Chaparro et al. 2001, Steere 2001). Rarely have cultures from plasma and cerebrospinal fluid demonstrated the spirochete (Steere 2001).
→ Polymerase chain reaction (PCR):
  - To identify spirochetal DNA in patient tissue and fluids. This test is useful for identifying *B. burgdorferi* in synovial fluid, but its sensitivity for use in other tissue and fluid samples has not been established (CDC 1999, Chaparro et al. 2001, Steere 2001).
→ Serology tests:
  - Antibody titers are the most practical approach to laboratory confirmation of Lyme disease (CDC 2001b, Chaparro et al. 2001, Steere 2001). However, even in successfully treated disease and in untreated disease that resolves, antibody titers may remain elevated for years. Consequently, interpretation of antibody titers must be within the context of the patient's history and clinical presentation, and not be based solely on seroreactivity to serologic tests (CDC 2001b).
  - Serum antibody titers:
    - IgM antibody begins to rise 2–4 weeks after the initial infection but has cross-reactivity with other spirochetal antigens (e.g., syphilis, Rocky Mountain spotted fever, autoimmune disease). IgM antibody peaks at 6–8 weeks and then begins to decline (Chaparro et al. 2001, Steere 2001). During the first few weeks of infection, only 20–30% of individuals demonstrate a positive IgM response (Steere 2001).
    - IgG antibody titer gradually increases 4–8 weeks after initial infection, peaks at approximately 4–6 months, and can remain measurable for months or years (CDC 2001b, Chaparro et al. 2001, Steere 2001).
    - A fourfold increase between an acute and convalescent titer indicates recent Lyme disease infection and is documented in approximately 70–80% of patients with infection, even after initiation of antibiotic therapy (Steere 2001).
  - Immunoblot testing (e.g., Western Blot):
    - Positive immunoblot testing after a positive or equivocal enzyme-linked immunoassay (ELISA) or immunofluorescent assay (IFA) result may be indicative of disease.
→ Antigen tests:
  - Lyme disease urine antigen testing is unreliable and should not be used to diagnose this infection (Steere 2001).
→ Other tests (e.g., electrophysiological, electrocardiogram) may be indicated depending on systemic manifestations of the disease. They should be ordered in consultation with a physician.

TREATMENT/MANAGEMENT

→ Essential to the treatment of the patient is the removal of the tick if it is still present. (Importantly, most ticks are immature and, therefore, smaller than adult ticks.)

  ▪ The best means of doing this is to remove the head of the tick using tweezers. (See "Patient Education," below.)

  ▪ If the tick is removed within 24 hours after attachment, the likelihood of spirochete transmission is significantly reduced.

→ A single prophylactic dose of doxycycline 200 mg p.o. administered within 72 hours of a tick bite that occurred in an endemic area reportedly reduces the incidence of Lyme disease in 87% of patients (Nadelman et al. 2001).

→ Antibiotic therapy is based on clinical manifestations and includes the use of oral and/or parenteral antibiotics.

  ▪ If parenteral therapy is indicated, the patient should be referred to a physician.

  ▪ The following are recommended regimens for treating Lyme disease at various stages (Chaparro et al. 2001, Steere 2001):

    • Early disease (e.g., erythema migrans) without systemic involvement:
      – Doxycycline 100 mg p.o. BID for 14–21 days
                        OR
      – Amoxicillin 500 mg p.o. TID for 14–21 days. If amoxicillin is indicated but the patient is allergic to penicillin, then she can be prescribed:
        ➤ Cefuroxime axetil 125 mg p.o. BID or 30 mg/kg in 2 divided doses for 14–21 days
                          OR
        ➤ Erythromycin 250 mg p.o. QID for 10–21 days (less effective than doxycycline or amoxicillin).

    • Cardiac disease:
      – First-degree heart block (PR interval <0.3 second):
        ➤ Same oral antibiotic regimens as listed under "Early disease," above.
      – Higher degree atrioventricular heart block (PR interval >0.3 second):
        ➤ Ceftriaxone 2 g IV every day for 14–28 days
                          OR
        ➤ Penicillin G sodium 3 million units IV every 4 hours for 14–28 days
                          OR
        ➤ Cefotaxime 2 g IV every 8 hours for 14–28 days

    • Neurological disease:
      – Bell's palsy without evidence of other neurological disease (e.g., meningitis)
        ➤ Oral antibiotic therapy with doxycycline or amoxicillin as listed above under "Early disease."
      – General neurological disease:
        ➤ Parenteral antibiotic therapy with ceftriaxone, penicillin G, or cefotaxime as listed above under "Cardiac disease."
        ➤ Alternative therapy, if the patient is allergic to ceftriaxone, penicillin, or cefotaxime, includes doxycy-

cline 100 mg p.o. TID for 30 days (may be ineffective for late-stage neurologic disease) (Steere 2001).

    • Lyme arthritis (intermittent or chronic):
      – Oral antibiotics listed under "Early disease," but therapy should continue for 30–60 days
                          OR
      – Intravenous antibiotics listed under "Cardiac disease," but therapy should continue for 14–28 days

  ▪ Pregnant women should avoid doxycycline for treating Lyme disease.

    • Tick bite in an endemic area:
      – Amoxicillin 500 mg p.o. TID for 10 days (Chaparro et al. 2001)

    • Early, localized infection:
      – Refer to early disease treatment.

    • Disseminated early disease or any manifestation of late disease:
      – Refer to the appropriate sections above.

    NOTE: Jarisch-Herxheimer reaction can occur in patients receiving antibiotic therapy for Lyme disease. (See the **Syphilis** chapter in Section 13 for a description of this reaction.)

→ Symptomatic treatment may be indicated and include the use of analgesics (i.e., nonsteroidal anti-inflammatory drugs) and bed rest at various stages of the disease. Corticosteroids are not recommended for treating Lyme disease.

→ A Lyme disease vaccine (LYMErix®) was approved in 1998 for use in patients 15–70 years old who reside, work, or recreate in areas of high or moderate risk of exposure to ticks that might harbor *B. burgdorferi* (CDC 1999). However, because of low demand, the manufacturer stopped producing the vaccine in February 2002.

CONSULTATION

→ Consultation with a physician is indicated in all cases of suspected disseminated or late-stage Lyme disease, for pregnant women, or for any patient with symptoms indicating the need for hospitalization.

→ As needed for prescription(s).

PATIENT EDUCATION

→ Educate the patient about Lyme disease, including its cause, clinical course, possible complications, treatment options, and indicated follow-up.

→ If the patient is pregnant, discuss possible perinatal complications, but reassure her these are extremely rare.

→ Instruct the patient about ways to reduce exposure to ticks, including:

  ▪ Avoiding tick habitats (e.g., tall grass, bushes, forests) during seasons when tick activity is at its peak

  ▪ Wearing clothing that reduces tick exposure (e.g., tightly woven, light-colored, long-sleeve shirts and long pants tucked into socks; hats; closed shoes)

  ▪ Using tick repellant as indicated. (Advise the patient to use as directed and to wash off the repellent as soon as possible after outdoor activity.)

- Clothing pesticide (e.g., permethrin) may be used on trouser legs and socks.
- If the patient has outdoor pet(s), advise her to inspect it/them frequently for ticks and to use antitick collars and baths as indicated.

→ Educate the patient about the importance of checking for and removing ticks immediately once they are discovered, as a means of reducing transmission of spirochetes.

- Instruct the patient how to properly remove ticks (by grasping the head of the tick, not the body, with tweezers and exerting steady upward pressure).
- Advise the patient not to attempt to burn or suffocate the tick before removal. Advise her to cleanse the area with soap and water once the tick is removed.

FOLLOW-UP

→ See "Consultation," above.
→ Document in progress notes and on problem list.

BIBLIOGRAPHY

Centers for Disease Control and Prevention (CDC). 1990. Case definitions for public health surveillance. *Morbidity and Mortality Weekly Report* 39(RR-13):1–39.

_____. 1995. Notice to readers. Recommendations for test performance and interpretation from the Second National Conference on Serologic Diagnosis of Lyme Disease. *Morbidity and Mortality Weekly Report* 44(31):590–591.

_____. 1997. Case definitions for infectious conditions under public health surveillance. *Morbidity and Mortality Weekly Report* 46(RR-10):1–55.

_____. 1999. Recommendations for the use of Lyme disease vaccine. Recommendations of the Advisory Committee on Immunization Practices (ACIP). *Morbidity and Mortality Weekly Report* 48(RR-7):1–17.

_____. 2001a. Lyme disease—United States, 1999. *Morbidity and Mortality Weekly Report* 50(10):181–185.

_____. 2001b. Lyme disease. Available at: http://www.cdc.gov/ncidod/dvbid/lyme/diagnosis.htm. Accessed on December 10, 2001.

Chaparro, S., and Montoya, J.G. 2001. Borrelia and leptospira species. In *Current diagnosis & treatment in infectious diseases*, eds. W.R. Wilson and M.A. Sande, pp. 680–689. New York: Lange Medical Books/McGraw-Hill.

Nadelman, R.B., Nowakowski, J., Fish, D. et al. 2001. Prophylaxis with single-dose doxycycline for the prevention of Lyme disease after an *Ixodes scapularis* tick bite. *New England Journal of Medicine* 345(2):79–84.

Schlesinger, P.A., Duray, P.H., Burke, B.A. et al. 1985. Maternal-fetal transmission of the Lyme disease spirochete, *Borrelia burgdorferi*. *Annals of Internal Medicine* 103:67–68.

Steere, A.C. 2001. Lyme disease. *New England Journal of Medicine* 345(2):115–125.

Weber, K., Bratzke, H.J., Neubert, U. et al. 1988. *Borrelia burgdorferi* in a newborn despite oral penicillin for Lyme *borreliosis* during pregnancy. *Pediatric Infectious Disease Journal* 7:286–289.

11-E

Measles (Rubeola)

Measles (*rubeola*) is an acute systemic illness caused by one of the paramyxoviruses. It usually occurs in preschool-age children, but outbreaks in adolescent and adult populations have been documented. From 1989 to 1991, a major increase in measles cases was reported in the United States (Centers for Disease Control and Prevention [CDC] 1992). However, more recent surveillance data indicate a significant decline in measles cases in the United States, with a record low number of cases reported in 1999 (CDC 2000).

Measles infection is most often associated with a lack of or incomplete immunization, although a small percentage of cases has been reported in patients with apparently adequate immunization histories (CDC 1992, 1999). An atypical measles syndrome has been reported in adults and adolescents who received inactivated measles vaccine or live measles vaccine before 1 year of age. These individuals develop a hypersensitivity rather than protective immunity to measles and, when infected by the measles virus, experience a severe systemic illness that can be fatal (Bouckenooghe et al. 2002, Sonnen et al. 2001).

Measles is transmitted by direct exposure to infectious droplets or, less frequently, by airborne spread, and is contagious 3–5 days before the eruption of the acute exanthem (Committee on Infectious Diseases 2000). Patients remain contagious for four days after the appearance of the exanthem; however, immunocompromised patients may remain contagious for the duration of the illness due to the prolonged viral excretion in respiratory droplets (Committee on Infectious Diseases 2000). The incubation period is 8–12 days from exposure to the onset of prodromal symptoms.

Complications associated with measles infection include cervical adenitis, otitis media, pneumonia, encephalitis, and death (0.6% among children in the United States) (Bouckenooghe et al. 2002, Committee on Infectious Diseases 2000, Sonnen et al. 2001). The highest complication rates are reported in children younger than 5 years old, but complications have been noted in adolescents and adults as well. An extremely rare complication of measles infection is subacute sclerosing panencephalitis. SSPE is a progressive, degenerative, central nervous system disease resulting from persistent measles virus infection. It is characterized by intellectual and behavioral deterioration and convulsions. SSPE usually develops several years after the initial measles infection and is not contagious. In immunosuppressed individuals, measles infection is associated with an increased risk of morbidity and mortality (Bouckenooghe et al. 2002, Committee on Infectious Diseases 2000). Subacute measles encephalitis characterized by seizures, neurologic deficits, stupor, and death has been reported in this population (Bouckenooghe et al. 2002).

Measles occurring during pregnancy has been associated with an increased rate of spontaneous abortion and preterm birth. In addition, pregnant women experiencing measles are at an increased risk of developing pneumonia and measles-related death. There is no association between measles infection during pregnancy and an increased risk of congenital anomalies (Signore 2001).

DATABASE

SUBJECTIVE

→ Prodrome symptoms may include (Bouckenooghe et al. 2002, Signore 2001):
  - Fever (often 40° C/104° F or higher)
  - Cough (nonproductive, persistent)
  - Pharyngitis
  - Rhinorrhea, nasal congestion, sneezing
  - Eye discharge, erythema
  - Photosensitivity
→ Symptoms may include (Bouckenooghe et al. 2002, Signore 2001):
  - Koplik's spots (pathognomonic of measles):
    • Tiny, white crystal-like lesions on the buccal mucosa, inner conjunctiva, or vagina occurring approximately two days before the rash and remaining for 1–4 days.
  - Eruption of a confluent, erythematous, irregular, maculopapular rash beginning on the face and extending to the trunk and then the extremities; develops 3–4 days after the onset of prodrome symptoms.

- In atypical measles, patients report a high fever, arthralgias, headache, abdominal pain, a rash without Koplik's spots, and a history of measles vaccination.

OBJECTIVE

Classic Measles

→ Physical findings include (Bouckenooghe et al. 2002, Committee on Infectious Diseases 2000, Signore 2001):
- Elevated temperature (may be 40° C/104° F or higher)
- Erythematous conjunctiva with or without discharge
- Pharyngeal edema
- Tonsillar exudate (usually yellow)
- White coating on the dorsum of tongue with erythema of the margins and tip
- Koplik's spots on buccal mucosa, inner conjunctival folds
- Generalized lymphadenopathy
- Erythematous, irregular, maculopapular rash with a distinctive eruptive pattern:
  - On the first day, a rash begins on the face; on the second day, facial eruption begins to coalesce and eruption begins on the trunk; on the third day, the facial rash fades, trunk eruption coalesces, and a rash begins on extremities.
  - After the third day, the rash continues to fade, reversing the pattern in which it appeared, with slight desquamation often observed.
- After the rash subsides, hyperpigmentation is observed in severe cases or in fair-skinned patients.

Atypical Measles (Bouckenooghe et al. 2002)

→ The patient may present with:
- Elevated temperature
- Maculopapular, hemorrhagic rash that may become vesicular
  - May be confluent
  - Usually starts on the palms and soles of the feet and progresses to the trunk
- Absence of Koplik's spots
- Tenderness to abdominal palpation may be present
- Decreased breath sounds (if there is co-existent pleural effusion)

ASSESSMENT

→ Measles (rubeola)
→ R/O atypical measles
→ R/O rubella
→ R/O mononucleosis
→ R/O scarlet fever (group A beta-hemolytic *Streptococcus*)
→ R/O drug reaction

PLAN

DIAGNOSTIC TESTS

→ The following diagnostic tests may be ordered to support or confirm the diagnosis (Bouckenooghe et al. 2002,

Committee on Infectious Diseases 2000, Signore 2001):
- Complete blood count with differential may reveal leukopenia.
- Urinalysis may reveal proteinuria.
- Immunoglobulin testing (acute and convalescent serum antibody titers):
  - Acute sera should be obtained for IgG titers four days after appearance of the rash, and the convalescent titer 2–4 weeks later.
    - Usually a fourfold increase in titer is observed.
  - A single specimen can be obtained for measles-specific IgM antibody. The specimen should be obtained 3–30 days after the onset of the rash.
    - If specimens are obtained within two days or after 30 days of rash onset, a false-negative IgM result will occur.
→ SSPE: High titers of measles antibody may be demonstrated in cerebrospinal fluid and serum.
→ The presence of measles in a culture of blood, urine, conjunctiva, or nasopharyngeal washings taken during the febrile phase of the disease is diagnostic; however, viral isolation is technically difficult to perform (Signore 2001).
→ Chest x-ray may reveal evidence of pneumonia or pleural effusion in patients with these complications.

TREATMENT/MANAGEMENT

→ Respiratory isolation of the patient for 7 days after the onset of the rash will reduce transmission to other susceptible individuals (Bouckenooghe et al. 2002, Committee on Infectious Diseases 2000).
→ Bed rest, increased fluids, and acetaminophen as needed should be recommended for relief of fever and malaise.
→ In children, young adults with severe disease, and immuno-compromised patients, vitamin A 400,000 units p.o. once, repeated 24 hours and 4 weeks after the initial dose, may reduce the morbidity associated with measles infection. It maintains respiratory and gastrointestinal mucosa, and enhances immune functioning (Committee on Infectious Diseases 2000, Sonnen et al. 2001).
→ No antiviral medication is available for treating measles infection.
→ Initiate appropriate antibiotic therapy for specific secondary bacterial infections (e.g., otitis media or pneumonia; see appropriate chapters for specific treatments).
→ Treatment of neurological complications (e.g., encephalitis or SSPE) requires hospitalization and is managed by the consulting physician.
→ In susceptible individuals who are known to have been exposed to measles, administration of the live-virus vaccine within 5 days of exposure can provide protection.
- Obtain informed consent before immunization.
- If susceptible individuals report an exposure beyond 5 days but within 6 days of contact, immunoglobulin 0.25 mg/kg can help prevent clinical illness.
  - Active immunization with live measles-virus vaccine is

recommended 3 months later (Bouckenooghe et al. 2002, Committee on Infectious Diseases 2000).

NOTE: If susceptible individuals have not received immunizations for mumps or rubella, consider vaccinating them with measles, mumps, and rubella live vaccine (MMR) (0.5 mL) unless they are persons in whom vaccination is contraindicated (i.e., pregnant women and women who are considering pregnancy within 3 months after vaccination). Live measles vaccine should not be given to patients who are significantly immunocompromised. MMR may be given to asymptomatic HIV-infected patients. (See the **Human Immunodeficiency Virus-1 Infection** chapter.) Mumps vaccine is contraindicated in patients with a history of anaphylaxis to eggs or neomycin.

CONSULTATION

→ Indicated for patients suspected of having atypical measles infection and/or patients with possible serious complications (e.g., pneumonia or encephalitis).
→ As needed for prescription(s).

PATIENT EDUCATION

→ Discuss the communicability, symptomatic treatment, need for isolation (when appropriate), and possible complications of measles infection. Advise the patient to call or return to the office if signs/symptoms of complications develop.
→ Educate the patient about the possible need for immunizing family members and/or close contacts.
  ▪ Determining susceptible close contacts and appropriate interventions can reduce infection and/or clinical illness.

FOLLOW-UP

→ At three months, immunize with live measles-virus vaccine those susceptible patients who received IgG after exposure to measles.
→ If confirmation of a measles diagnosis is desired, patients should undergo a measles-specific IgM antibody test 3–30 days after the onset of the rash.
→ Document in progress notes and on problem list.

BIBLIOGRAPHY

Bouckenooghe, A.R., and Shandera, W.X. 2002. Infectious diseases: viral and rickettsial. In *2002 current medical diagnosis & treatment*, 41st ed., eds. L.M. Tierney, Jr., S.J. McPhee, and M.A. Papadakis, pp. 1366–1368. New York: Lange Medical Books/McGraw-Hill.

Centers for Disease Control and Prevention (CDC). 1992. Measles surveillance—United States, 1991. *Morbidity and Mortality Weekly Report* 41(SS-6):1–12.

_____. 1999. Transmission of measles among a highly vaccinated school population—Anchorage, Alaska, 1998. *Morbidity and Mortality Weekly Report* 47:1109–1111.

_____. 2000. Measles—United States, 1999. *Morbidity and Mortality Weekly Report* 49(25):557–560.

Committee on Infectious Diseases. *Red book 2000. Report of the Committee on Infectious Diseases*, 25th ed., pp. 385–396. Elk Grove Village, Ill.: American Academy of Pediatrics.

Signore, C. 2001. Rubeola. *Primary Care Update for OB/GYNs* 8(4):138–140.

Sonnen, G., and Henry, N.H. 2001. Measles. In *Current diagnosis & treatment in infectious diseases*, eds. W.R. Wilson and M.A. Sande, pp. 1318–1320. New York: Lange Medical Books/McGraw-Hill.

11-F

Mokonucleosis

Infectious mononucleosis is an acute infectious disease caused by herpes viruses, specifically Epstein-Barr virus (EBV) and cytomegalovirus (CMV). In most instances, EBV is the cause of infectious mononucleosis. Most EBV and CMV infections occur during childhood, are asymptomatic, and do not result in manifestations of mononucleosis. However, the chance of developing infectious mononucleosis after EBV exposure increases with age. In the United States, it is usually observed in individuals 10–35 years old, with a peak incidence in those 15–19 years old (Godshall et al. 2000).

Transmission usually requires close contact with a person shedding the virus, probably through infectious oropharyngeal secretions. A person with infectious mononucleosis can have viral shedding for several months after the acute clinical phase of the disease. The incubation period is estimated to be 4–7 weeks after the initial exposure to EBV (Moffat 2001).

The clinical manifestations of infectious mononucleosis are extremely variable, ranging from asymptomatic infection to severe infection, which can result in death. Ninety-five percent of patients recover without complications, although recovery from the acute infection may take from three weeks to two months. Complication rates range from 2.5–5% in some populations and include splenic rupture, hemolytic anemia, immune thrombocytopenia, cardiac complications (e.g., heart block, pericarditis), pneumonia, encephalitis, meningitis, Guillain-Barré syndrome, and depression (Drew 2001, Godshall et al. 2000, Jenson 2000, Katon et al. 1999, Moffat 2001).

A rare syndrome called *chronic active mononucleosis* also has been reported. It is characterized by persistent or recurrent fatigue, fever, headache, hepatitis, pharyngitis, and depression. A patient with this syndrome must have experienced these symptoms for at least one year and have a history of infectious mononucleosis and an absence of other underlying causes of chronic infection (Maia et al. 2000).

DATABASE

SUBJECTIVE

→ The patient may be asymptomatic or may report one or more of the following (Godshall et al. 2000, Moffat 2001):
  - Exposure to a person with mononucleosis
  - Fever
  - Pharyngitis
  - Malaise
  - Headache
  - Nausea
  - Rash
  - Vomiting
  - Anorexia
  - Myalgia
  - Lymphadenopathy
  - Abdominal pain (if hepatomegaly and/or splenomegaly are/is present)
  - Jaundice

→ If there is myocardial involvement, the patient may report chest pain or dyspnea.

→ In CNS involvement, the patient may report photophobia, stiff neck, or neuritis.

OBJECTIVE

→ Physical examination may reveal one or more of the following (Auwaerter 1999, Godshall et al. 2000, Moffat 2001):
  - Elevated temperature (usually <39° C in most patients)
  - Palpable lymph nodes, particularly in the posterior cervical chain
  - Erythematous posterior pharynx/tonsils with or without exudate.
  - Palatal petechiae
  - Palpebral edema
  - Maculopapular or petechial rash (noted in 10% of patients with mononucleosis, and in up to 90% of adolescents and adults with mononucleosis who take ampicillin during the infection)

- Jaundice (if there is hepatitis)
- Hepatosplenomegaly
- Nuchal rigidity, photosensitivity in patients with CNS involvement (approximately 1–5% of patients)

ASSESSMENT

→ Acute infectious mononucleosis (EBV)
→ R/O CMV infection
→ R/O acute pharyngitis
→ R/O acute hepatitis
→ R/O thrombocytopenia
→ R/O rubella
→ R/O toxoplasmosis
→ R/O hemolytic anemia
→ R/O pneumonia
→ R/O encephalitis, meningitis
→ R/O myocarditis
→ R/O influenza
→ R/O other viral syndromes

PLAN

DIAGNOSTIC TESTS

→ The following laboratory tests may be ordered if indicated (Moffat 2001, Okano 2000):
- Complete blood count (CBC):
  - Decreased hematocrit if anti-i antibodies are present
- Differential:
  - Increased leukocytes, increased lymphocytes with many atypical lymphocytes noted, increased monocytes
  - Decreased granulocytes
- Platelet count:
  - Decreased if there is associated thrombocytopenia
- Mononucleosis heterophile antibody (Monospot) test:
  - Can be positive by the end of the first week but usually becomes positive by the third or fourth week after clinical manifestations.
  - In approximately 5–15% of patients with EBV-associated mononucleosis, this test will be negative.
  - If heterophile antibody test is negative, consider testing for other viral pathogens (e.g., CMV).
- Serum EBV-specific antibody testing:
  - A rise in IgM antibody against viral capsid antigen (VCA) is observed during acute illness.
  - IgG antibody to VCA (anti-VCA IgG) titers rise rapidly early after the onset of infection and remain elevated for long periods. Because of this, paired sera for anti-VCA IgG may not be helpful in determining acute mononucleosis infection.
  - A rise in antibody titer against early antigens (anti-D or anti-R) can be demonstrated in some patients. The anti-D subset indicates recent EBV infection; however, up to 30% of acutely infected patients do not demonstrate this antibody. In addition, cross-reaction with other herpes viruses can occur occasionally (Drew 2001, Moffat 2001).

- Antibody against EBV nuclear antigen (EBNA) is not detected until 4–12 weeks after the onset of infection and excludes recent infection when present. This antibody persists throughout life.
- Liver function tests (e.g., ALT, AST) will be elevated when hepatitis is present.
- Cerebrospinal fluid will demonstrate increased pressure, abnormal lymphocytes, and protein if there is CNS involvement.
- Electrocardiogram may demonstrate abnormal T-waves and prolonged PR intervals if there is myocardial involvement.
- Ten percent of patients will have a false-positive VDRL or RPR test result if these tests are obtained during acute infection.

TREATMENT/MANAGEMENT

→ Symptomatic treatment of infectious mononucleosis includes rest and the use of analgesics and antipyretics (e.g., acetaminophen, nonsteroidal anti-inflammatory drugs) as needed for relief of fever, myalgia, and pharyngitis.
- Warm saline gargles (1 tsp. salt in 8 oz. warm water) TID-QID may further relieve pharyngitis symptoms.
→ Corticosteroid therapy can be initiated in severely ill patients who have enlarged lymphoid tissue (threatening airway obstruction), severe thrombocytopenia, or autoimmune hemolytic anemia.
- Consultation with a physician is indicated in such cases.
→ Clinicians should avoid frequently palpating the spleen, to reduce the possibility of rupture.
→ Isolation of patients with mononucleosis is not necessary, as it is not highly contagious.

CONSULTATION

→ Physician consultation and management are indicated for patients with severe complications associated with mononucleosis (e.g., severe thrombocytopenia, myocardial involvement, CNS involvement).
→ As needed for prescription(s).

PATIENT EDUCATION

→ Educate the patient about infectious mononucleosis, including the cause, clinical course, treatment, possible method of transmission and infectivity, and possible complications. Reassure the patient that isolation is not necessary.
→ Advise the patient to avoid lifting heavy objects or exercising for one month after the symptoms resolve, to reduce the possibility of splenic rupture (Moffat 2001).
→ Advise the patient not to donate blood for several months after infection because of the possibility of transmission via blood transfusions.

FOLLOW-UP

→ In complicated cases, follow-up is on the recommendation of the consulting physician.

→ Document in progress notes and on problem list.

BIBLIOGRAPHY

Auwaerter, P.G. 1999. Infectious mononucleosis in middle age. *Journal of the American Medical Association* 281(5):454–459.

Drew, W.L. 2001. Herpes viruses. In *Current diagnosis & treatment in infectious diseases*, eds. W.R. Wilson and M.A. Sande, pp. 408–410. New York: Lange Medical Books/McGraw-Hill.

Godshall, S.E., and Kirchner, J.T. 2000. Infectious mononucleosis. Complexities of a common syndrome. *Postgraduate Medicine* 107(7):175–186.

Jenson, H.B. 2000. Acute complications of Epstein-Barr virus infectious mononucleosis. *Current Opinion in Pediatrics* 12:263–268.

Katon, W., Russo, J., Ashley, R.L. et al. 1999. Infectious mononucleosis: psychological symptoms during acute and subacute phases of illness. *General Hospital Psychiatry* 21:21–29.

Maia, D.M., and Peace-Brewer, A.L. 2000. Chronic, active Epstein-Barr virus infection. *Current Opinion in Hematology* 7:59–63.

Moffat, L.E. 2001. Infectious mononucleosis. *Primary Care Update for OB/GYNs* 8(2):73–77.

Okano, M. 2000. Haematological associations of Epstein-Barr virus infection. *Bailliere's Clinical Haematology* 13(2):199–214.

11-G

Mumps

Mumps, an infectious disease caused by a paramyxovirus, results in inflammation of the salivary glands. With the introduction of live mumps vaccine in 1977, reported cases have declined steadily in the United States. In recent years, however, reported mumps cases have increased nationally. Most mumps infections occur in children 5–14 years old, although older adolescents and adults can be infected (Buxton et al. 1999).

Mumps outbreaks usually occur during the late winter and early spring months. The disease is transmitted through infected respiratory droplets and has a usual incubation period of 14–21 days, although some cases have occurred in individuals exposed 12–25 days before symptom onset. Patients are most infectious 1–2 days before and up to nine days after parotid gland swelling (Committee on Infectious Diseases 2000, McQuone 1999, Sonnen et al. 2001). Although most persons with mumps experience painful salivary gland inflammation, 30% may have a subclinical infection (Committee on Infectious Diseases 2000). Both acute and subclinical mumps infections provide lifelong immunity.

Mumps is usually a self-limited disease that resolves within 7–9 days. However, mumps infection may result in serious complications, including meningoencephalitis, deafness (rare), thyroiditis, hepatitis, thrombocytopenia, nephritis, pancreatitis, oophoritis, and orchitis in postpubertal males (Bouckenooghe et al. 2002). Overall mortality rates associated with mumps infection are low; however, the highest rates of mumps-associated deaths have been reported in persons 19 years old or older (Committee on Infectious Diseases 2000). Although mumps infection during pregnancy has not been associated with an increased rate of congenital malformations, there is an increased rate of spontaneous abortions reported in women who are infected with mumps during the first trimester (Committee on Infectious Diseases 2000, Sonnen et al. 2001).

DATABASE

SUBJECTIVE

→ The patient may report:
- No immunization for mumps
- Exposure to a person with mumps infection

→ Symptoms may include (Committee on Infectious Diseases 2000, Sonnen et al. 2001):
- Fever (may be high if associated with meningitis)
- Malaise
- Painful swelling of one or both salivary glands
- Headache, lethargy, stiff neck (if there is associated meningitis)
- Nausea, vomiting, upper abdominal pain (if there is associated pancreatitis)

OBJECTIVE

→ The patient may present with (Bouckenooghe et al. 2002, Committee on Infectious Diseases 2000, Sonnen et al. 2001):
- Elevated temperature (may be high if associated with meningitis or pancreatitis)
- Tender, enlarged parotid gland(s) (in 70% of mumps infections)
- Enlarged, tender, submaxillary and sublingual lymph glands
- Erythema, edema of Stensen's duct
- Meningitis/encephalitis-associated symptoms—nuchal rigidity, photophobia, confusion
  - Meningeal signs have been reported in up to 30% of mumps cases.
- Pancreatitis-associated symptoms:
  - Upper abdomen tender to palpation usually without guarding, rebound, or rigidity; abdomen may be distended
- Oophoritis-associated symptoms:
  - Lower abdominal/pelvic pain, ovarian enlargement
- Diminished hearing if there is eighth cranial nerve damage (rare)

ASSESSMENT

→ Mumps
→ R/O parotitis from other causes (e.g., bacteria, other viruses, drug reaction)

→ R/O cervical adenitis
→ R/O parotid gland calculi
→ R/O meningitis/encephalitis
→ R/O oophoritis
→ R/O eighth cranial nerve neuritis (deafness rare)
→ R/O pancreatitis

PLAN

DIAGNOSTIC TESTS

→ The diagnosis of mumps is usually based on the clinical presentation of the patient. However, the following tests may be ordered if indicated (Committee on Infectious Diseases 2000):
  ▪ Complete blood count (CBC) with differential:
    • Lymphocytosis is present.
  ▪ Serum amylase:
    • Often is elevated even without pancreatitis.
  ▪ Culture of saliva and cerebrospinal fluid samples:
    • Will demonstrate mumps virus.
  ▪ Paired sera complement fixation testing:
    • Will demonstrate a fourfold increase in mumps antibody titers.
  ▪ Cerebrospinal fluid:
    • Lymphocytic pleocytosis
    • Glucose level normal to low (present with meningitis)
  ▪ Audiometry tests may demonstrate decreased hearing.

TREATMENT/MANAGEMENT

→ Treatment of patients with mumps infection depends on symptoms.
  ▪ Bed rest is advised during the febrile phase.
  ▪ Acetaminophen with or without codeine may be necessary for analgesia.
  ▪ Alkaline mouthwashes may reduce some discomfort.
  ▪ Adequate hydration (i.e., force fluids) should be recommended.
→ Isolation of the patient until nine days after the onset of symptoms is necessary to reduce possible transmission.
→ Hospitalization is indicated for patients with serious sequelae (e.g., meningitis/encephalitis, severe pancreatitis).
→ Mumps immune globulin has proved ineffective in treating susceptible patients exposed to mumps and is no longer available (Committee on Infectious Diseases 2000).
→ Live mumps vaccine given to susceptible persons exposed to mumps infection has not been effective in preventing illness.
  ▪ However, immunization at this time can protect such individuals from future mumps infection.
  ▪ No increased risk of reactions or complications has been associated with live mumps vaccination when administered to a patient during the incubation phase of the infection or to a person already immune to mumps (Committee on Infectious Diseases 2000).
  ▪ If susceptible individuals have not received immunizations for measles or rubella, consider vaccinating them with mumps-measles-rubella (MMR) vaccine, 0.5 mL, unless contraindicated.

• MMR should not be given to a pregnant woman or a woman who is considering becoming pregnant within 3 months of vaccination.

NOTE: Mumps vaccine is contraindicated in persons with a history of anaphylaxis reaction to eggs or neomycin, an immunodeficiency disease, or those who are receiving immunosuppressive therapy or large doses of corticosteroids, antimetabolites, radiation, or alkylating agents (Committee on Infectious Diseases 2000). Patients with asymptomatic HIV infection may receive MMR vaccine. (See the **Human Immunodeficiency Virus-1 Infection** chapter.)

CONSULTATION

→ Physician consultation is warranted for patients suspected of having serious complications (e.g., meningitis, encephalitis, pancreatitis).
→ As needed for prescription(s).

PATIENT EDUCATION

→ Educate the patient about the course of the illness, symptomatic relief measures, symptoms of complications, and the need for isolation until parotid gland swelling resolves.
→ Educate the patient about the need for future immunization with measles-rubella vaccine if the patient was born after 1957 and cannot document vaccination against or actual infection with measles or rubella.

FOLLOW-UP

→ See "Consultation," above.
→ Follow-up evaluation is not necessary in uncomplicated mumps infection.
→ Document in progress notes and on problem list.

BIBLIOGRAPHY

Bouckenooghe, A.R., and Shandera, W.X. 2002. Infectious diseases: viral and rickettsial. In *2002 current medical diagnosis & treatment*, 41st ed., eds. L.M. Tierney, Jr., S.J. McPhee, and M.A. Papadakis, pp. 1368–1370. New York: Lange Medical Books/McGraw-Hill.

Buxton, J., Craig, C., Daly, P. et al. 1999. An outbreak of mumps among young adults in Vancouver, British Columbia, associated with "rave" parties. *Canadian Journal of Public Health* 90(3):160–163.

Committee on Infectious Diseases. 2000. *Red book 2000. Report of the Committee on Infectious Diseases*, 25th ed., pp. 405–408. Elk Grove Village, Ill.: American Academy of Pediatrics.

McQuone, S.J. 1999. Acute viral and bacterial infections of the salivary glands. *Otolaryngology Clinics of North America* 32(5):793–811.

Sonnen, G., and Henry, N.H. 2001. Measles. In *Current diagnosis & treatment in infectious diseases*, eds. W.R. Wilson and M.A. Sande, pp. 418–420. New York: Lange Medical Books/McGraw-Hill.

11-H

Rubella

Rubella infection is a systemic illness caused by a togavirus transmitted by inhalation of infectious nasophyngeal secretions. The period of communicability is from a few days before to seven days after the onset of the rash (Committee on Infectious Diseases 2000). The incubation period is 14–21 days. Generally, rubella is a mild infection and may be asymptomatic in 50% of patients (Committee on Infectious Diseases 2000).

Encephalitis and thrombocytopenia are complications associated with rubella infection that are observed more frequently in school-age children. Polyarthritis may occur during acute infection and persist for weeks after resolution of symptoms in some adult patients (Bouckenooghe et al. 2002). Rarely, adults may experience myocarditis, encephalitis, erythema multiforme, or orchitis as a result of rubella infection (Bouckenooghe et al. 2002, Sonnen et al. 2001).

The greatest morbidity and mortality rates associated with rubella result from exposure during pregnancy. Rubella infection occurring during pregnancy is associated with spontaneous abortion, stillbirth, or congenital rubella in the neonate. Congenital rubella syndrome (CRS) is a constellation of abnormalities, including ophthalmic anomalies, cardiac anomalies (e.g., atrial or ventricular septal defects, patent ductus arteriosus), neurological problems (e.g., mental retardation, microcephaly), sensorineural deafness, and other complications such as growth retardation, thrombocytopenia, and jaundice (Committee on Infectious Diseases 2000, Signore 2001). The risk of CRS is highest during the first trimester, with an incidence of up to 80% in exposed fetuses. Maternal rubella infection during 13–16 weeks of gestation has a reported CRS incidence of 45–50%, but the incidence declines significantly after this point in gestation to 6% at 17–20 weeks and to less than 1% in exposures occurring after 20 weeks of pregnancy (Ghidini et al. 1993, Signore 2001). However, fetal infection without CRS sequelae is possible, especially if maternal infection occurs after 36 weeks of gestation (Signore 2001).

Although rubella immunization has dramatically reduced the incidence of both postnatal rubella infection and CRS in the United States, a fivefold increased incidence was reported in 1988, with more than 50% of cases occurring among individuals 15 years old or older (Centers for Disease Control and Prevention [CDC] 1991). Clustered outbreaks continue to occur in populations that do not have adequate immunizations (Danovaro-Holliday et al. 2000). An estimated 10% of young adults in the United States remain susceptible to rubella infection (Committee on Infectious Diseases 2000, Sonnen et al. 2001).

DATABASE

SUBJECTIVE

→ The patient may be asymptomatic or report any of the following symptoms (Bouckenooghe et al. 2002, Committee on Infectious Diseases 2000, Signore 2001):

■ A history of exposure to a person with rubella infection during the previous three weeks

■ Prodromal symptoms (usually seven days before rash eruption), including:
  • Low-grade fever
  • Headache
  • Malaise
  • Anorexia
  • Sore throat
  • Mild conjunctivitis
  • Rhinitis
  • Nonproductive cough
  • Suboccipital, postauricular, and/or cervical lymph node enlargement

■ Eruption of a fine rash beginning on the face and neck, and progressing to the trunk and extremities within 2–3 days after the facial rash appears. The patient may report rapid disappearance of the rash (usually within one day after the rash is noted on regions of the body).

■ Joint pain in 25% of adults, which may continue for one week or longer

OBJECTIVE

→ The patient may present with (Signore 2001, Sonnen et al. 2001):

- Temperature slightly elevated but usually within normal limits
- Fine, pink, discrete, maculopapular rash on the face, neck, trunk, and/or extremities
- Postauricular, occipital, and/or cervical lymphadenopathy
- Erythema of the palate and posterior pharynx
- Evidence of swollen joints in a symmetrical pattern

ASSESSMENT

→ Rubella infection
→ R/O measles (rubeola)
→ R/O atypical measles
→ R/O infectious mononucleosis
→ R/O drug reaction
→ R/O enterovirus infection
→ R/O scarlet fever

PLAN

DIAGNOSTIC TESTS

→ Diagnostic tests usually are done only if confirmation of a rubella diagnosis is indicated (e.g., in pregnant women). The following tests may be ordered if indicated (Committee on Infectious Diseases 2000, Signore 2001, Sonnen et al. 2001):
  - Consider a urine or serum pregnancy test for any woman of reproductive age presenting with suspected rubella and a history of no contraception and/or unprotected coitus (unless she has just completed her menses).
→ Culture for rubella virus can be done with specimens obtained from throat swabs, blood, urine, and cerebrospinal fluid (as clinically indicated) and will be positive.
→ Acute and convalescent serum specimens can be obtained and sent for rubella virus hemagglutination inhibition (HI) testing.
  - If a patient has a recent infection, a fourfold or higher increase in HI titer will be reported (Committee on Infectious Diseases 2000).
→ Recently, more sensitive tests for rubella have become available. They include fluorescent immunoassays, latex agglutination tests, passive hemagglutination tests, enzyme immunoassay tests, and hemolysis-in-gel tests.
  - These tests have demonstrated positive results in patients who did not demonstrate immunity using the HI tests.
  - It is advisable to consult the laboratory that will be performing diagnostic tests for rubella to determine which tests it can perform and what the sensitivity is for each one.
→ The presence of rubella-specific IgM antibody (serum testing) indicates recent acute infection.
→ CBC may demonstrate leukopenia in early infection.
→ Platelet count may be decreased if thrombocytopenia is present.

→ Tests for rheumatoid factor will be negative in patients with rubella-associated arthritis.

TREATMENT/MANAGEMENT

→ Supportive treatment consists of bed rest while febrile, analgesics for arthritis/arthralgia, and antipyretics (e.g., acetaminophen) as needed.
→ Isolation of the patient from susceptible individuals is indicated until 1 week after the initial eruption of the rash.
NOTE: An estimated 10% of postpubertal populations in the United States lack evidence of rubella immunity and are susceptible to infection if exposed.

CONSULTATION

→ Patients with suspected encephalitis should be referred to a physician for further evaluation and treatment as indicated.
→ Pregnant women with suspected rubella infection should be referred to an obstetrician/perinatalogist for further evaluation, counseling, and follow-up.

PATIENT EDUCATION

→ Educate the patient about rubella infection, duration of symptoms, infectivity, possible complications, and symptomatic treatment options.
→ Educate the patient about the need to avoid contact with susceptible individuals until one week after initial eruption of the rash.
→ If the patient is pregnant, discuss perinatal risks associated with acute rubella infection.
→ In postpubertal patients without documented evidence of rubella vaccination or rubella immunity, immunization with rubella vaccine (0.5 mL) or in combination with measles vaccine or mumps-measles-rubella (MMR) vaccine should be considered.
  - Rubella vaccine is contraindicated in pregnant women due to the theoretical risk of congenital rubella.
  - Nonpregnant women of childbearing age who receive rubella vaccine should be advised not to become pregnant until three months after the immunization.
  - Rubella vaccine is a live virus vaccine and is contraindicated in patients with immunodeficiency diseases, those who are receiving immunosuppresive therapy, or those who are receiving large doses of corticosteroids, antimetabolites, radiation, or akylating agents (Committee on Infectious Diseases 2000).
  - Patients with asymptomatic HIV infection may receive an MMR. (See the **Human Immunodeficiency Virus-1 Infection** chapter.)

FOLLOW-UP

→ See "Consultation," above.
→ Document in progress notes and on problem list.

BIBLIOGRAPHY

Bouckenooghe, A.R., and Shandera, W.X. 2002. Infectious diseases: viral and rickettsial. In *2002 current medical diagnosis & treatment*, 41st ed., eds. L.M. Tierney, Jr., S.J. McPhee, and M.A. Papadakis, pp. 1371–1373. New York: Lange Medical Books/McGraw-Hill.

Centers for Disease Control and Prevention (CDC). 1991. Update on adult immunization recommendations of the Immunization Practices Advisory Committee (ACIP). *Morbidity and Mortality Weekly Report* 40(RR-12):24–26.

Committee on Infectious Diseases. 2000. *Red book 2000. Report of the Committee on Infectious Diseases*, 25th ed., pp. 495–500. Elk Grove Village, Ill.: American Academy of Pediatrics.

Danovaro-Holliday, M.C., Le Baron, C.W., Allensworth, C. et al. 2000. A large rubella outbreak with spread from the workplace to the community. *Journal of the American Medical Association* 284(21):2733–2739.

Ghidini, A., and Lynch, L. 1993. Prenatal diagnosis and significance of fetal infections. *Western Journal of Medicine* 159(3):366–373.

Signore, C. 2001. Rubella. *Primary Care Update for OB/GYNs* 8(4):133–137.

Sonnen, G., and Henry, N.H. 2001. Measles. In *Current diagnosis & treatment in infectious diseases*, eds. W.R. Wilson and M.A. Sande, pp. 1318–1320. New York: Lange Medical Books/McGraw-Hill.

11-1

Tuberculosis

Tuberculosis is an infection caused by a member of the *Mycobacterium* genus that includes *Mycobacterium tuberculosis*, *Mycobacterium bovis*, and *Mycobacterium africanum* (Geiter 2000). Although illness in humans as a result of infection with *M. bovis* and *M. africanum* has been reported, such instances are rare. Most illnesses associated with mycobacteria are a result of infection with *M. tuberculosis*.

M. tuberculosis is an aerobic, nonmotile, non-spore-forming, slow-growing bacterium that is an obligate parasite. Though it infects humans primarily, other primates and mammalian species in close and fairly constant contact with humans (e.g., cats and dogs) can be infected, though these species are not reservoirs of the organism.

Almost every case of tuberculosis infection occurs through inhalation of small (1–5 μm), infected respiratory droplets. Usually, prolonged exposure to an infectious person or environment is necessary for effective transmission to occur. However, there is epidemiologic evidence of transmission through more casual contact (e.g., church or classroom gatherings) (Geiter 2000). Factors facilitating transmission include decreased natural resistance to the organism and crowded living conditions favoring airborne spread of *M. tuberculosis* (Geiter 2000).

Tuberculosis remains a major health problem worldwide: 15 million new cases are reported each year and the disease is responsible for 3 million deaths annually (Chesnutt et al. 2002). In the United States, it is estimated that 15 million individuals have latent tuberculosis infection (Chesnutt et al. 2002). Specific factors that reportedly increase the risk of tuberculosis infection within a population include lower socioeconomic status, non-Caucasian race, recent immigration from countries with a high prevalence of tuberculosis, injection drug use, alcoholism, HIV infection, end-stage renal disease, homelessness, and residence in a long-term health care or correctional facility (Centers for Disease Control and Prevention [CDC] 2000a, Geiter 2000, Small et al. 2001). In addition, people in certain age groups are more likely to develop active disease when they are infected with tuberculosis—specifically, children younger than 5 years, adolescents, young adults, and the elderly (CDC 2000a).

The pathological features of tuberculosis result from the host's degree of hypersensitivity and the local concentration of the antigen. Once *M. tuberculosis* is inhaled, it is transmitted to the terminal airspaces where the organism is ingested by macrophages. At this point, the organism either dies or remains viable and multiplies.

The site of infection is usually in lung segments where greater airflow facilitates the deposition of the inhaled bacilli. The most commonly affected sites are the anterior segment of the upper lobes, and the middle lobe, lingula, and the lower division of the lower lobes. Dissemination of the organism also can occur as a result of lymphohematogenous spread from the primary pulmonary site to extrapulmonary sites, including the kidneys, bones, bone marrow, liver, spleen, ovaries, endometrium, and brain (Geiter 2000).

In most individuals infected with tuberculosis, the cell-mediated immune response is adequate to limit multiplication of the bacilli; effective encapsulation and calcification of the organism occurs. This is categorized as *latent tuberculosis infection* (LTBI) (CDC 2000a, Small et al. 2001). However, 10% of persons with LTBI cannot contain the organism effectively. These persons eventually will develop pulmonary or extrapulmonary clinical disease. In half of these patients, active disease occurs within two years after LTBI; the remainder develop clinical disease at some later time in their lives (CDC 2000a, Geiter 2000). In HIV-infected populations, the risk of developing clinical disease is 10% per year after LTBI (CDC 1998).

Multidrug-resistant tuberculosis (MDR-TB) is a problem in several areas of the world, especially in regions of China, Russia, and Eastern Europe (Espinal et al. 2001). In the United States, MDR-TB was reported in 1.2% of patients with newly diagnosed tuberculosis, compared to 5.6% among previously treated patients in a survey conducted by the World Health Organization between 1996 and 1999 (Espinal et al. 2001). Approximately 15% of patients with tuberculosis in the United States are resistant to at least one of the antituberculosis drugs (Chesnutt et al. 2002). Factors associated with MDR-TB include unsuccessful tuberculosis therapy, patient noncompliance with medications, immigration from a country where there is a high prevalence of MDR-TB, and prolonged exposure to a patient infected with MDR-TB (Chesnutt et al. 2002). The case-fatality rate associated with MDR-TB is reportedly high. MDR-TB outbreaks in hospitals and prisons in Florida and New York were associated with a 70–90% mortality rate (Chesnutt et al. 2002).

DATABASE

SUBJECTIVE

→ High-risk factors include (CDC 2000a):

- History of close contact (e.g., sharing the same household or enclosed environments) with a person who has or is suspected of having tuberculosis
- Persons with medical risk factors associated with an increased risk of active tuberculosis. If infection occurs, these patients include those with a history of:
  - Silicosis
  - Gastrectomy
  - Jejunoileal bypass
  - Loss of 10% or more of ideal body weight
  - Chronic renal failure
  - Conditions requiring prolonged, high-dose corticosteroid therapy and/or other immunosuppressive therapy
  - Particular hematological disorders (e.g., leukemia, lymphoma)
  - Malignancies
  - Persons with HIV infection
  - Persons with abnormal chest x-ray demonstrating fibrotic lesions consistent with old, healed tuberculosis
  - Positive tuberculin skin test within two years without evaluation for preventive therapy

→ Patients infected with tuberculosis may be asymptomatic (latent infection) or may report one or more of the following symptoms (Chesnutt et al. 2002, Geiter 2000, Small et al. 2001):

- Cough that may be productive of mucopurulent sputum; sputum may be slightly blood-tinged.
- Fever, often remittent and occurring in the early afternoon
- Night sweats
- Malaise
- Keratitis or conjunctivitis
- Erythema nodosum—painful red nodules commonly appearing on the anterior aspects of the legs
- Hemoptysis (rare)
- Anorexia
- Weight loss
- Intermittent chills
- Chest pain secondary to extension of infection into the pleura
- Pharyngeal and mouth ulcers (rare)
- Hoarseness (rare, associated with laryngeal involvement)
- Dysphagia (rare, associated with laryngeal involvement)
- Enlarged, firm, tender cervical or supraclavicular lymph nodes that may soften, slough, and drain
- If there is co-existent meningitis, possible CNS symptoms

varying in intensity (e.g., headache, change in mentation, nuchal rigidity, confusion)

- If skeletal tuberculosis develops, the patient may have red, painful joints (usually monoarticular, weight-bearing) or bony point tenderness, with symptoms starting after a traumatic event.
- Dysuria, gross hematuria, and flank pain if there is renal involvement (70% of patients with renal tuberculosis report such symptoms)
- Pelvic pain, abdominal pain, and/or menstrual disorders are possible in women with genital tuberculosis infection.

NOTE: In immunocompromised (e.g., HIV-infected) and elderly patients, the symptoms of tuberculosis may be subtle and often are atypical.

OBJECTIVE

→ Physical examination may be unremarkable or may reveal one or more of the following findings, depending on the extent of the infection and the immune status of the patient (Chesnutt et al. 2002, Geiter 2000, Small et al. 2001):

- Vital signs:
  - Within normal limits (WNL) or
  - Possibly an elevated temperature (>37.7° C/100° F), pulse, and respiratory rate, depending on the status of the patient
- The patient's weight may be less than the 10th percentile of ideal body weight for height.
- Skin:
  - May be pale if the patient has moderate to severe anemia (secondary to hematologic abnormalities associated with miliary tuberculosis).
  - Elevated, tender, erythematous nodules of the anterior aspect of the legs may be noted in cases of erythema nodosum.
- Eyes:
  - May be evidence of keratitis or conjunctivitis. (See the **Conjunctivitis** and **Keratitis** chapters in Section 2.)
- Mouth:
  - May be ulcerations.
- Lymphadenopathy:
  - Usually palpation of a single, firm, enlarged, tender cervical or supraclavicular node (although, over time, the node may soften, slough, and produce drainage).
- Palpation of the chest wall may reveal:
  - Decreased tactile fremitus in the presence of pleural thickening or fluid.
- Dullness to percussion of the chest wall
- Auscultation of the lungs may reveal:
  - Increased tubular breath sounds and whispered pectoriloquy
  - Post-tussive rales (elicited after the patient takes several short coughs)
  - Distant, hollow breath sounds ("amphoric" sounds noted over tuberculosis cavities)
  - Rubs (with pleural effusion)

- Abdominal examination may reveal:
  - Splenomegaly
- Examination of the extremities may reveal:
  - Erythema nodosum and/or a single erythematous, tender, weight-bearing joint
- Neurological examination may reveal:
  - Confusion
  - Nuchal rigidity (with meningeal involvement)
  - Photosensitivity
- Pelvic examination may reveal:
  - Granulomatous, ulcerating cervical mass and/or
  - Enlarged, tender ovaries or uterus

ASSESSMENT

→ Tuberculosis infection (latent, active)
→ R/O MDR-TB
→ R/O meningitis
→ R/O pneumonia
→ R/O cancer
→ R/O encephalitis
→ R/O immune deficiency (e.g., HIV infection)

PLAN

DIAGNOSTIC TESTS

→ Tuberculin skin tests (TSTs):
  - Though they are an important screening tool, TSTs do not distinguish between past infection or current disease. Currently it is recommended that TSTs be targeted to those groups of individuals at high risk for exposure to tuberculosis (CDC 2000a, Geiter 2000, Small et al. 2001).
  - There are two types of TSTs: the Mantoux test and multiple puncture devices.
    - The Mantoux test is the best screening test and is recommended for detecting tuberculosis. It consists of an intradermal injection of 0.1 mL solution containing 5 tuberculin units of purified protein derivative (PPD) using a #26 or #27 needle on the volar aspect of the patient's forearm.
      - If the PPD is placed correctly, a raised, blanched wheal will occur.
      - Injections deeper than the subdermal layer may result in the "washing out" of the PPD solution by vascular flow, thereby reducing the amount of antigen administered to the patient.
      - The test should be read 48–72 hours after placement for any evidence of induration (not erythema) at the skin test site.
      - The transverse diameter of the induration should be measured in millimeters. A test is positive if the induration reaches the size required for specific risk groups, as indicated below (CDC 2000a, Chesnutt et al. 2002, Small et al. 2001):
        ➤ A reaction ≥5 mm is considered positive if the patient is HIV-positive, is an organ transplant recipient or is immunosuppressed and receiving

the equivalent of ≥15 mg/day of prednisone for ≥1 month, is a close contact of a person with tuberculosis, or has evidence of old, healed tuberculosis (e.g., fibrotic changes) on chest x-ray.
➤ A reaction ≥10 mm is considered positive if the patient:
  * Has immigrated within the last five years from a country with a high incidence of tuberculosis
  * Is an injection drug user
  * Works in a mycobacterial laboratory
  * Lives or works in a high-risk congregate setting such as a correctional facility, hospital or other health care facility, long-term care facility (e.g., a nursing home), homeless shelter, or residential facility for patients with acquired immune deficiency syndrome (AIDS) (CDC 2002)
  * Reports a history of medical conditions associated with an increased risk of active tuberculosis, including silicosis, weight 10% or more below ideal body weight, chronic renal failure, diabetes mellitus, gastrectomy, jejunoileal bypass, certain malignancies (e.g., carcinoma of the head, neck, lung), or certain hematological disorders (e.g., leukemia, lymphoma)
  * Children 4 years old or younger
  * Children and adolescents exposed to high-risk adults
  * A reaction ≥15 mm is considered positive in all other patients.

NOTE: When induration does occur, the amount of the reaction correlates with the likelihood of infection (e.g., a reaction ≥20 mm is highly indicative of infection) (CDC 2000a, Small et al. 2001).

– The sensitivity of the PPD is reportedly 100%. However, a negative PPD does not eliminate the possibility of tuberculosis infection. It takes 2–10 weeks after infection for the tissue hypersensitivity response of a positive test reaction to occur. False-negative results can occur in persons with active tuberculosis infection and may be a result of malnutrition, general illness (e.g., intercurrent viral illnesses), corticosteroid therapy, or other causes of anergy (e.g., advanced HIV infection). False-positive results can occur if there is infection with a nontuberculosis mycobacterium (e.g., *M. bovis*). There is also a higher likelihood of a false-positive result in geographic areas with a low prevalence of tuberculosis (CDC 2000a, Small et al. 2001).

– Patients vaccinated with Calmette-Guerin bacillus (BCG) will have a positive tuberculin test that is either in response to the vaccination or evidence of tuberculosis infection. In the United States, a patient with a history of BCG vaccination and a positive tuberculin test is considered to have tuberculosis infection and should be evaluated further to exclude the possibility of active infection (CDC 2000a).

→ Sputum specimens for diagnostic testing should be taken to confirm active pulmonary tuberculosis infection.

■ Sputum specimen collection for acid-fast bacilli (AFB) stain and culture should be done early in the morning.

• Sputum acid-fast stain: Evidence of acid-fast bacilli provides a presumptive diagnosis of infection and indicates that the patient is highly infectious (CDC 2000a, Small et al. 2001). Acid-fast stains will be positive in up to 80% of patients with pulmonary tuberculosis (Chesnutt et al. 2002). However, acid-fast stains do not provide a definitive diagnosis of tuberculosis, as saprophytic, nontuberculous mycobacteria can colonize airways (Chesnutt et al. 2002).

• Sputum for AFB culture: A positive result provides a definitive diagnosis of tuberculosis infection and can reveal organisms resistant to antituberculosis drugs (CDC 2000a, Small et al. 2001).

■ Three early-morning, daily collections should be sufficient to obtain an adequate sample.

■ Other options for obtaining specimens for AFB smear or culture include sputum induction, bronchoscopy, and aspiration of gastric contents (Chesnutt et al. 2002). The latter is rarely done because of the success of sputum induction techniques.

→ Nucleic acid (DNA or RNA) amplification can be done on sputum specimens but should be interpreted within the context of the patient's signs and symptoms, and the laboratory's experience with these tests (CDC 2000b). The CDC has developed specific criteria for the use and interpretation of these tests by clinicians (CDC 2000b). Consultation with an infectious disease specialist is advised when ordering these tests.

→ DNA fingerprinting can be done to identify specific strains of *M. tuberculosis* in certain circumstances, such as person-to-person transmission or cross-contamination in the laboratory (Chesnutt et al. 2002).

→ Blood cultures can be performed and may be positive if there is co-existent mycobacteremia.

→ CBC may be WNL or may reveal a decreased hemoglobin/hematocrit, an increased leukocyte count (10,000–15,000 cells/mm^3), decreased platelets, and an increased monocyte count (in 10% of patients).

→ A serum chemistry panel should be ordered to rule out hepatic and/or kidney involvement. It may reveal:

■ Hyponatremia in advanced disease or if associated with Addison's disease

■ Elevated liver function tests (ALT, AST) when there is hepatic involvement or in association with other medical conditions (e.g., substance abuse)

→ If there is associated renal involvement, a urinalysis may reveal pyuria, hematuria, and albuminuria (a rare finding usually associated with amyloidosis).

→ Chest x-ray should be ordered when a patient has a positive PPD, has signs and symptoms suggestive of tuberculosis infection, and/or before initiation of antituberculosis medications.

■ Certain chest x-ray findings are suggestive of pulmonary tuberculosis. The following may be evident (CDC 2000a, Chesnutt et al. 2002, Small et al. 2001):

• Patchy, nodular infiltrate in the apical or subapical posterior regions of the upper lobes or superior segment of the lower lobes

• Areas of cavitation

• Air-fluid levels are commonly noted in lower-lobe cavities, but are uncommon in upper-lobe tuberculosis.

• Evidence of bronchogenic spread may be demonstrated when multiple, discrete infiltrates adjacent to a cavity are observed.

• Granulomatous and exudative lesions, fibrotic scars, and caseation may be noted.

• Evidence of a pneumonic lesion with enlarged hilar nodes in any lobe of the lung is suggestive of primary tuberculosis infection.

• Presence of a miliary infiltrate may be evident.

• In some patients, pleural effusion may be the only x-ray finding.

NOTE: In HIV-positive patients, chest x-ray findings may be subtle and atypical and can result in misdiagnosis.

→ Analysis of cerebrospinal fluid (CSF) in patients suspected of CNS involvement will reveal increased lymphocytes and polymorphonuclear cells, increased protein, and a decreased glucose level.

■ AFB stain of CSF may be positive. CSF culture for AFB often is positive, but it takes a number of weeks before results are obtained. Negative AFB stain and/or culture results do not rule out CNS disease.

→ If genital tuberculosis is suspected, AFB smears and cultures of tissue obtained during surgery, cervical biopsy, or endometrial scraping may be positive (Des Prez et al. 1990).

→ Computer tomography scan or magnetic resonance imaging may demonstrate focal lesions, basilar arachnoid meningitis, cerebral infarction, and/or hydrocephalus in patients with CNS involvement (Des Prez et al. 1990).

TREATMENT/MANAGEMENT

→ The treatment options presented in this section are limited to patients with LTBI. The goal is to prevent the development of active tuberculosis disease. Consultation with an expert in the treatment of active tuberculosis disease (e.g., a pulmonologist or an infectious disease specialist) is advised, as improper treatment can result in serious consequences for the patient and her close contacts. Updated information about the current recommendations for treating tuberculosis is available online at the CDC's Web site: ww.cdc.gov/nchstp/tb/pubs/corecurr.

→ Treatment of LTBI is recommended for patients who do not have evidence of active pulmonary or extrapulmonary disease but who have positive TST reactions. There is no uniform definition of a positive TST reaction for all individuals. What defines a positive TST reaction for a given individual depends on the competency of her immune system. Positive TST reactions are defined as follows (CDC 2002):

- TST reaction ≥5 mm induration:
  - HIV-positive persons and persons with risk factors for HIV infection whose HIV status is unknown but who are suspected of being infected
  - Recent contact with a TB case
  - Patients with fibrotic lesions on chest x-ray consistent with old TB
  - Patients with organ transplants, and other immunosuppressed patients receiving the equivalent of ≥15 mg/day of prednisone for ≥1 month
- A TST reaction ≥10 mm induration:
  - Recent arrivals (within five years) from high-prevalence countries
  - Intravenous drug user known to be HIV-negative
  - Patients with medical conditions associated with an increased risk of active tuberculosis. (See the high-risk factors under "Subjective," above.)
  - Individuals who live or work in high-risk congregate settings (e.g., correctional facilities, hospitals, or long-term care facilities)
  - Children younger than 4 years
  - Children and adolescents exposed to adults in high-risk categories
  - Mycobacteriology laboratory personnel
- A TST reaction ≥15 mm induration:
  - Patients with no known risk factors for TB may be considered for LTBI treatment.
- Some patients with an initial negative TST (reaction <5 mm induration) who have been close contacts of infectious persons should be considered for LTBI therapy until a negative repeat tuberculin test is done at 10–12 weeks after the last documented contact with the infectious person. These patients include:
  - Children younger than 4 years
  - Immunosuppressed patients
  - Any other patient who may develop active disease quickly after becoming infected with TB
  NOTE: For patients known or suspected of being HIV-infected and for other immunocompromised patients, treatment for LTBI should be initiated and completed regardless of the magnitude of their skin test reactions (CDC 2002).
→ Information about the first-line medications used to treat LTBI, their side effects, recommended laboratory monitoring, and contraindications is presented in **Table 11I.1, First-Line Antituberculosis Medications**. The regimens that can be considered for treating LTBI in HIV-negative and HIV-infected patients are presented in **Table 11I.2, Regimen Options for Treatment of Latent Tuberculosis Infection in HIV-Negative Adults**, and **Table 11I.3, Regimen Options for Treatment of Latent Tuberculosis Infection in HIV-Infected Adults**, respectively.
  - Isoniazid (INH) is the recommended agent for treating LBTI and has proven to be more than 90% effective in preventing the development of active tuberculosis when taken as prescribed.

- The recommended regimen for INH preventive therapy is (CDC 2002):
  - 5 mg/kg (maximum dose = 300 mg) p.o. every day for 9 months in immunocompetent and immunosuppressed (e.g., HIV-infected) patients
  NOTE: INH therapy for 6 months is acceptable but is considered by most authors to be inferior to 9 months of therapy (CDC 2000a, CDC 2002, Geiter 2000, Small et al. 2001). Six-month INH therapy is estimated to be 70% effective in preventing the development of active tuberculosis when taken as prescribed (CDC 2002).
  - 15 mg/kg (maximum = 900 mg) p.o. twice a week for 9 months may be considered for patients for whom compliance may be a concern (e.g., homeless and substance-abusing patients); however, the medication should be administered via directly observed therapy (DOT) (CDC 2002). Such regimens have been successful, with minimal toxicity and no increase in drug resistance reported thus far (CDC 2000a, Small et al. 2001).
  NOTE: Hepatotoxicity is a concern with INH therapy, especially in elderly patients, patients with liver disorders (e.g., chronic hepatitis, regular alcohol use), cancer patients, uremic patients, and pregnant women. However, such toxicity is rarely observed in healthy patients younger than 20 years. Transient increases in transaminase levels are reported in 10–20% of patients using INH (CDC 2002, Small et al. 2001). Active hepatitis and end-stage liver disease are relative contraindications for using INH to treat LTBI (CDC 2002). In addition to hepatotoxicity, INH has been associated with peripheral neuropathy and it can lower the seizure threshold in patients with a history of seizure disorders. The addition of vitamin B-6 (pyridoxine), 10–50 mg p.o. daily, can prevent or ameliorate these problems.
- Rifampin (RIF) 10 mg/kg (maximum 600 mg) p.o. daily for 4 months can be an alternative to the longer INH regimens cited above regarding HIV-negative patients. Less-frequent dosing regimens (e.g., twice weekly DOT) are not recommended when using RIF for LTBI.
- RIF 10 mg/kg (maximum 600 mg) and pyrazinamide (PZA) 15–20 mg/kg (maximum 2 g) daily for 2 months to treat LTBI in HIV-infected patients have been documented to be as effective as INH for longer durations (CDC 1998, Small et al. 2001). This combination can be administered on a twice-weekly DOT schedule if indicated, with adjustments in the PZA dose based on the patient's weight. This regimen has not been studied in HIV-negative patients and should be used only when other effective therapies cannot be administered (CDC 2002).
  NOTE: There is recent evidence of increased hepatotoxicity and mortality associated with the use of this combination in HIV-negative patients (CDC 2001). Therefore, patients for whom this combination is being considered should be under the clinical care of an infectious disease and/or tuberculosis specialist. In addition, patients receiving this regimen

Table 11.1.   FIRST-LINE ANTITUBERCULOSIS MEDICATIONS

Drug	Route	Adult Daily Dose in Mg/Kg (Maximum Dose)	Adult Twice Weekly in Mg/Kg (Maximum Dose)*	Adult Three Times a Week in Mg/Kg (Maximum Dose)*	Adverse Reactions	Monitoring	Comments
Isoniazid (INH)	p.o. or IM	5 (300 mg)	15 (900 mg)	15 (900 mg)	Rash, hepatic enzyme elevation, hepatitis, peripheral neuropathy, mild CNS effects, drug interactions resulting in increased phenytoin or disulfiram levels	Baseline measurement of hepatic enzymes for adults. Repeat measurements if: - baseline results are abnormal - patient is at high risk for adverse reactions - patient has symptoms of adverse reactions	Hepatitis risk increases with age and alcohol consumption. Pyridoxine may prevent peripheral neuropathy and CNS effects.
Rifampin (RIF)	p.o. or IV	10 (600 mg)	10 (600 mg)	10 (600 mg)	Gastrointestinal (GI) upset, drug interactions, hepatitis, bleeding problems, flu-like symptoms, rash, renal failure, fever	Baseline measurement of complete blood count (CBC), platelets, and hepatic enzymes. Repeat measurements if: - baseline results are abnormal - patient has symptoms of adverse reactions	Significant interactions with methadone, birth control hormones, and many other drugs. Contraindicated or should be used with caution when administered with protease inhibitors (PIs) and non-nucleoside reverse transcriptase inhibitors (NNRTIs). Colors body fluids orange and may permanently discolor contact lenses.
Rifabutin (RFB)†	p.o. or IV	5 (300 mg) or (150 mg)§ or (450 mg)¶	5 (300 mg) or 5§ (300 mg) or (450 mg)¶	Not known; Not known; Not known	Rash, hepatitis, fever, thrombocytopenia. With increased levels of RFB: - severe arthralgias - uveitis - leukopenia	Baseline measurements of CBC, platelets, and hepatic enzymes. Repeat measurements if: - baseline results are abnormal - patient has symptoms of adverse reactions. Use adjusted daily dose of RFB and monitor for decreased antiretroviral activity and for RFB toxicity if RFB is taken concurrently with PIs or NNRTIs.	Reduces levels of many drugs (e.g., PIs, NNRTIs, methadone, dapsone, hormonal contraceptives, ketaconazole, etc.). Colors body fluids orange and may permanently discolor contact lenses.
Pyrazinamide (PZA)	p.o.	15–30 (2 g)	50–70 (4 g)	50–70 (3 g)	Hepatitis, rash, GI upset, joint aches, hyperuricemia, gout (rare)	Baseline measurements of uric acid and hepatic enzymes. Repeat measurements if: - baseline results are abnormal - patient has symptoms of adverse reactions	Treat hyperuricemia only if patient has symptoms. May make glucose control more difficult in diabetics.
Ethambutol (EMB)#	p.o.	15–25	50	25–50	Optic neuritis, rash	Baseline and monthly tests of visual acuity and color vision	Optic neuritis may be unilateral; therefore, check each eye separately.
Streptomycin (SM)	IM or IV	15 (1 g)	25–30 (1.5 g)	25–30 (1.5 g)	Ototoxicity (hearing loss or vestibular dysfunction), renal toxicity	Baseline hearing and renal function tests; repeat as needed.	Ultrasound and warm compresses to injection site may reduce pain. Avoid or reduce the dose in adults ≥60 years old.

NOTE: Consult product insert for detailed information about these medications. Adjust weight-based dosages as weight changes.

*Administration of all intermittent dosing regimens should be directly observed.

†The concurrent administration of rifabutin with hard-gel saquinavir and delavirdine is contraindicated. An alternative is rifabutin with indinavir, nelfinavir, amprenavir, ritonavir, efavirenz, or possibly soft-gel saquinavir and nevirapine. Caution is advised when using rifabutin with soft-gel saquinavir and nevirapine because data regarding the use of rifabutin with these medications are limited.

§If nelfinavir, indinavir, amprenavir, or ritonavir is administered with rifabutin, blood concentrations of rifabutin increase. Thus, when rifabutin is combined with these medications, the daily dose of rifabutin is reduced from 300 mg to 150 mg when used with nelfinavir, indinavir, or amprenavir, and to 150 mg 2 or 3 times a week when used with ritonavir.

¶If efavirenz is administered with rifabutin, blood concentrations of rifabutin decrease. Thus, when rifabutin is used with efavirenz, the daily dose of rifabutin should be increased from 300 mg to 450 mg or 600 mg.

#No maximum dosages for ethambutol are available, but in obese patients the dosage should be calculated based on lean body weight.

Source: Centers for Disease Control and Prevention (CDC). 2002. Core curriculum on tuberculosis. Available at: http://www.cdc.gov/nchstp/tb/pubs/corecurr. Accessed on December 1, 2002.

should only be given prescriptions for a two-week supply of the medications so they will return for clinical evaluations before obtaining a refill.

■ Because the use of RIF is contraindicated in HIV-infected patients receiving certain anti-HIV medications (e.g., some protease inhibitors and non-nucleoside reverse transcriptase inhibitors), rifabutin (RFB) can be substituted for RIF and used in combination with PZA daily for 2 months. The dose of RFB may require adjustment based on the type of antiretroviral medication an HIV-infected patient may be taking. (See **Table 11I.1**.)

CONSULTATION

→ Consultation with a physician is indicated for any patient who has or is suspected of having active tuberculosis.

→ Consultation with a physician specializing in the evaluation and treatment of tuberculosis is indicated for any patient

with HIV infection, evidence of concomitant debilitating disease, exposure to suspected drug-resistant tuberculosis, pregnancy, symptoms of toxicity associated with therapeutic agents, or suspected noncompliance with treatment regimens.

→ As needed for prescription(s).

PATIENT EDUCATION

→ Educate patients about tuberculosis infection—the cause, transmission, clinical manifestations, clinical course, diagnostic tests, treatment options, need for strict compliance with treatment regimens, possible side effects/toxicity of therapeutic agents, interactions between antituberculosis medications and other drugs, prognosis, and the importance of follow-up evaluations.

→ Educate patients about symptoms of active tuberculosis disease and adverse effects of their therapy (e.g., hepatitis),

Table 11I.2. REGIMEN OPTIONS FOR TREATMENT OF LATENT TUBERCULOSIS INFECTION IN HIV-NEGATIVE ADULTS

Drug	Duration: Daily Regimen	Duration: Twice Weekly Directly Observed Treatment (DOT) Regimen	Comments
Isoniazid (INH)	9 months	9 months	Minimum of 270 doses administered within 12 months. Twice-weekly regimens should consist of at least 76 doses administered within 12 months. Recommended regimen for pregnant women. Contraindicated for persons who have active hepatitis and end-stage liver disease.
INH	6 months	6 months	Minimum of 180 doses administered within 9 months. Twice-weekly regimens should consist of at least 52 doses administered within 9 months. Recommended regimen for pregnant women. Six-month regimen not recommended for those patients with fibrotic lesions on chest radiographs. Contraindicated for persons who have active hepatitis and end-stage liver disease.
Rifampin (RIF) and Pyrazinamide (PZA)	2 months	2 or 3 months	Minimum of 60 doses to be administered within 3 months. Twice-weekly regimens should consist of at least 16 doses to be administered for 2 months or 24 doses to be administered for 3 months. May be used for INH-intolerant patients. Avoid pyrazinamide for pregnant women because of the risk of adverse effects on the fetus. This regimen has not been evaluated in HIV-negative persons. Contraindicated for persons who have active hepatitis and end-stage liver disease.
RIF	4 months	Not recommended	Minimum of 120 doses administered within 6 months. For persons who are contacts of patients with INH-resistant, RIF-susceptible tuberculosis. May be used for patients who cannot tolerate INH or PZA.

Source: Centers for Disease Control and Prevention (CDC). 2002. Core curriculum on tuberculosis. Available at: http://www.cdc.gov/nchstp/tb/pubs/corecurr. Accessed on December 1, 2002.

Table 11I.3. **REGIMEN OPTIONS FOR TREATMENT OF LATENT TUBERCULOSIS INFECTION IN HIV-INFECTED ADULTS**

Drug	Duration: Daily Treatment	Duration: Twice Weekly Directly Observed Treatment (DOT)	Comments	Contraindications
Isoniazid (INH)	9 months	9 months	Minimum of 270 doses administered within 12 months. Twice-weekly regimens should consist of at least 76 doses administered within 12 months. INH can be administered concurrently with nucleoside reverse transcriptase inhibitors (NRTIs), protease inhibitors (PIs), or non-nucleoside reverse transcriptase inhibitors (NNRTIs).	History of an INH-induced reaction including hepatitis, skin or other allergic reactions, or neuropathy Known exposure to a person who has INH-resistant TB Chronic, severe liver disease
Rifampin (RIF) and Pyrazinamide (PZA)*	2 months	2–3 months	Minimum of 60 doses to be administered within 3 months. Twice-weekly regimens should consist of at least 16 doses to be administered for 2 months or 24 doses to be administered for 3 months. Dose adjustments, alternative therapies, or other precautions might be necessary when rifamycins are used (e.g., patients using hormonal contraception should be advised to use a barrier method as a back-up; patients receiving methadone may require dose adjustments). PIs or NNRTIs generally should not be administered concurrently with rifampin. In this situation, an alternative is rifabutin and PZA.	History of a rifamycin-induced reaction, including hepatic, skin, or other allergic reactions, or thrombocytopenia Pregnancy Chronic, severe liver disease Chronic, severe hyperuricemia
Rifabutin (RFB)† and PZA*	2 months	2–3 months	Minimum of 60 doses to be administered within 3 months. Twice-weekly regimens should consist of at least 16 doses to be administered for 2 months or 24 doses to be administered for 3 months. Dose adjustments, alternative therapies, or other precautions might be necessary when rifamycins are used (e.g., patients using hormonal contraception should be advised to use a barrier method as a back-up; patients receiving methadone may require dose adjustments).	History of a rifamycin-induced reaction, including hepatic, skin, or other allergic reactions, or thrombocytopenia Pregnancy Chronic, severe liver disease Chronic, severe hyperuricemia

NOTE: For patients whose organisms are resistant to one or more drugs, consultation with a TB medical expert is advised, as therapy will require at least two drugs to which there is demonstrated susceptibility. Clinicians should review the drug-susceptibility pattern of the TB strain isolated from the infecting source-patient before choosing a preventive therapy regimen.

*For patients with intolerance to PZA, some experts recommend a rifamycin (rifampin or rifabutin) alone for preventive treatment. Most experts agree that available data support the recommendation that this treatment can be administered for as short a duration as 4 months, although some experts would treat for 6 months.

†The concurrent administration of rifabutin with hard-gel saquinavir and delavirdine is contraindicated. An alternative is rifabutin with indinavir, nelfinavir, amprenavir, ritonavir, efavirenz, or possibly soft-gel saquinavir and nevirapine. Caution is advised when using rifabutin with soft-gel saquinavir and nevirapine because data regarding the use of rifabutin with these medications are limited.

Source: Centers for Disease Control and Prevention (CDC). 2002. Core curriculum on tuberculosis. Available at: http://www.cdc.gov/nchstp/tb/pubs/corecurr. Accessed on December 1, 2002.

and advise them to return for an immediate evaluation if they experience any of these.

→ Educate patients about the importance of avoiding concurrent use of alcohol while receiving antituberculosis medication(s) due to the risk of increased hepatotoxicity.

→ Inform patients with LTBI that they are not infectious and do not pose a danger of transmitting TB to others unless they develop active pulmonary disease.

→ Educate patients about the increased risk of active tuberculosis in individuals with HIV infection. If a patient has not been tested previously, counsel and refer her for HIV testing.

FOLLOW-UP

→ Patients being managed by an infectious disease and/or tuberculosis specialist should have follow-up as recommended by that clinician.

→ Clinical monitoring of patients on antituberculosis medications should be done at least monthly. Patients receiving RIF and PZA should be clinically monitored at 2, 4, 6, and 8 weeks after therapy begins.

→ The patient's adherence to her antituberculosis regimen should be assessed at least once a month if she is not receiving her medications through a DOT program. For patients receiving the shorter duration therapy of RIF and PZA, adherence evaluations should take place at 2, 4, 6, and 8 weeks.

→ Baseline laboratory evaluations (e.g., AST, ALT, bilirubin) should be obtained for all patients before antituberculosis therapy begins. Periodic monitoring throughout the course of treatment is indicated if there are any abnormal baseline test results or if the patent is at an increased risk for adverse side effects (e.g., patients with chronic liver disease, pregnant women, and HIV-infected patients). (**See Table 11I.1.**)

→ Tuberculosis is a CDC-reportable disease. Notification of the local public health department is mandated by law when a patient is diagnosed with tuberculosis.

→ Document in progress notes and on problem list.

BIBLIOGRAPHY

Centers for Disease Control and Prevention (CDC). 1998. Prevention and treatment of tuberculosis among patients infected with human immunodeficiency virus: principles of therapy and revised recommendations. *Morbidity and Mortality Weekly Report* 47(RR-20):1–58.

_____. 2000a. Targeted tuberculin testing and treatment of latent tuberculosis infection. *Morbidity and Mortality Weekly Report* 49(RR-6):1–51.

_____. 2000b. Update: nucleic acid amplification tests for tuberculosis. *Morbidity and Mortality Weekly Report* 49(26):593–594, 603.

_____. 2000c. Updated guidelines for the use of rifabutin or rifampin for the treatment and prevention of tuberculosis among HIV-infected patients taking protease inhibitors or nonnucleoside reverse transcriptase inhibitors. *Morbidity and Mortality Weekly Report* 49(9):185–189.

_____. 2001. Update: fatal and severe liver injuries associated with rifampin and pyrazinamide for latent tuberculosis infection, and revisions in American Thoracic Society/CDC recommendations—United States, 2001. *Morbidity and Mortality Weekly Report* 50:733–735.

_____. 2002. Core curriculum on tuberculosis. Available at: http://www.cdc.gov/nchstp/tb/pubs/corecurr. Accessed on December 1, 2002.

Chesnutt, M.S., and Prendergast, T.J. 2002. Lung. In *2002 current medical diagnosis & treatment*, 41st ed., eds. L.M. Tierney, Jr., S.J. McPhee, and M.A. Papadakis, pp. 309–316. New York: Lange Medical Books/McGraw-Hill.

Des Prez, R.M., and Heim, C.R. 1990. Mycobacteria disease. In *Principles and practice of infectious diseases*, 3rd ed., eds. G.L. Mandell, R.G. Douglas, Jr., and J.E. Bennett, pp. 1877–1906. New York: Churchill Livingstone.

Espinal, M.A., Laszlo, A., Simonsen, L. et al. 2001. Global trends in resistance to antituberculosis drugs. *New England Journal of Medicine* 344(17):1294–1303.

Geiter, L., ed. 2000. *Ending neglect. The elimination of tuberculosis in the United States*. Washington, D.C.: National Academy Press.

Small, P.M., and Fujiwara, P.I. 2001. Management of tuberculosis in the United States. *New England Journal of Medicine* 345:189–200.

11-J

Varicella Zoster Virus

Varicella zoster virus (VZV) is a member of the herpes virus family (human herpes virus 3) and causes infection and its sequelae only in humans. It is responsible for two distinct illnesses: *primary varicella zoster virus* infection (chickenpox) and reactivation of *latent varicella zoster virus* (herpes zoster or shingles). Because these illnesses have different clinical manifestations and treatments, each is presented individually.

Varicella Zoster Virus Infection (Chickenpox)

Before the availability of the varicella vaccine in 1995, 4 million cases of primary VZV infection (chickenpox) were reported each year in the United States (Centers for Disease Control and Prevention [CDC] 1999). Most chickenpox infections occur in children younger than 10 years old. Approximately 90% of adults with unknown or unreliable histories of chickenpox exposure or infection have serologic evidence of VZV immunity (CDC 1999, Committee on Infectious Diseases 2000, Liesegang 1999). However, infection in adolescents and adults is of concern, as 5–10% of healthy young adults in the United States remain susceptible to chickenpox (McCrary et al. 1999). There are increased rates of chickenpox-associated complications and deaths reported in infants, adolescents, pregnant women, adults, and immunocompromised persons (CDC 1999). Complications associated with chickenpox have resulted in up to 11,000 hospitalizations and 100 deaths per year (CDC 1999).

Chickenpox is highly contagious. It is spread by inhalation of infectious respiratory droplets or by direct contact with varicella lesions. The incubation period is usually 14–16 days, but the range is 8–21 days. Shorter incubation periods have been reported in immunocompromised patients and longer incubation periods (up to 28 days) have been noted in patients who receive varicella zoster immune globulin (VZIG) (Committee on Infectious Diseases 2000). Patients are contagious 1–2 days before the onset of varicella lesions and remain infectious until all lesions have crusted (Committee on Infectious Diseases 2000, McCrary et al. 1999). The duration of varicella from the prodro-

mal phase to the disappearance of all lesions is usually less than two weeks (Bouckenooghe et al. 2002).

Although rare, asymptomatic primary infection has been reported. An episode of varicella usually provides lifelong immunity against subsequent outbreaks, although reinfections have been reported (Committee on Infectious Diseases 2000, Cohen et al. 1999).

VZV-related viral pneumonia is responsible for most hospitalizations and deaths in adults; however, the incidence of group A beta-hemolytic streptococcal infections complicating chickenpox has increased in recent years (Bouckenooghe et al. 2002, Cohen et al. 1999). Other complications associated with varicella include encephalitis, hepatitis, thrombocytopenia, arthritis, conjunctivitis, carditis, nephritis, herpes zoster (shingles), vasculitis, and neurological disorders such as transverse myelitis, aseptic meningitis, and Guillain-Barré syndrome (Bouckenooghe et al. 2002, Cohen et al. 1999, McCrary et al. 1999, Uhoda et al. 2000). Reye syndrome is a complication associated with the administration of aspirin during chickenpox that affects children, but it is rarely reported in adults.

VZV primary infection during pregnancy is associated with a number of maternal, fetal, and neonatal complications. Pregnant women are at an increased risk for VZV-related pneumonia. If varicella occurs during the first or second trimester, there is an increased chance of fetal malformations, including limb atrophy, growth retardation, chorioretinitis, cataracts, scarring of the skin, deafness, and cortical atrophy (Committee on Infectious Diseases 2000). Maternal VZV primary infection occurring between five days before and two days after delivery is associated with severe neonatal varicella and an increased risk of neonatal mortality (Committee on Infectious Diseases 2000). Both in utero and neonatal varicella can result in herpes zoster during infancy and childhood (Committee on Infectious Diseases 2000).

It is anticipated that the incidence of VZV primary infection and its associated complications will decrease significantly with more widespread immunization of susceptible individuals. A live-attenuated varicella zoster vaccine (Oka strain) was developed in Japan in 1970. In 1995, this vaccine (VARIVAX®) was approved for use in the United States to prevent primary infection in all high-risk susceptible persons older than 1 year (CDC 1999, Gershon 2001). High-risk susceptible persons include those who work or live in environments where exposure to VZV is likely (e.g., teachers of young children, child care staff, and residents and staff members in institutional settings), persons who work or live in environments where VZV transmission may occur (e.g., college students, prison inmates, and military personnel), adults and adolescents living in households with children, nonpregnant women of childbearing age, and international travelers (CDC 1999, Committee on Infectious Diseases 2000).

In 85–90% of vaccinees, VZV antibody titers have persisted for several years after the initial immunization. Immunization with the varicella zoster vaccine reduces the risk of acquiring wild-type VZV infection by 70–90% (CDC 1999, Cohen et al. 1999). The most common side effects are slight erythema and mild pain at the injection site (in up to 20% of vaccinees), mild fever (in up to 10% of vaccinees), and the development of a mild rash at the injection site or more generalized (in 5% of vaccinees) (CDC 1999, Gershon 2001). In clinical trials of the vaccine, most persons who developed VZV infection after the immunization were infected with wild-type VZV and did not have virologic evidence of vaccine-associated infection. The development of vaccine-related zoster is rare (CDC 1999, Gershon 2001).

Transmission of vaccine-type virus from vaccinees to susceptible immunocompetent persons is extremely rare. When this has occurred, the persons with vaccine-type virus infection experienced mild disease without complications (CDC 1999). Vaccine-type virus transmission has not been observed unless the vaccinee develops a rash. Immunocompromised vaccinees that develop a postimmunization rash are more likely to transmit vaccine-type virus than are healthy vaccinees (Gershon 2001).

The varicella vaccine is not licensed for use in persons with leukemia, blood dyscrasias, lymphoma, or other malignancies affecting the lymphatic or hematopoietic systems. Also, it should not be administered to pregnant women, persons receiving high-dose systemic steroids or undergoing immunosuppressive therapy, or persons with hypogammaglobulinemia, dysgammaglobulinemia, or cellular immunodeficiencies (e.g., congenital T-cell abnormalities, human immunodeficiency virus syndrome [HIV], etc.). A recent study indicated that the vaccine is safe, immunogenic, and effective in children with HIV infection who are asymptomatic (CDC Class 1) and have CD4+ T-lymphocyte measurements of 25% or greater. In this population, there is a substantial benefit to immunization: reduced morbidity and mortality associated with wild-type VZV infection. Therefore, immunosuppressed children may receive varicella vaccine (Committee on Infectious Diseases 2000).

DATABASE

SUBJECTIVE

→ The patient may report one or more of the following (Committee on Infectious Diseases 2000, Bouckenooghe et al. 2002, McCrary et al. 1999):

- Exposure to chickenpox or suspected chickenpox during the previous three weeks
- Prodromal symptoms of fever, headache, myalgia, arthralgia, or anorexia (may occur 24 hours before eruption of the rash)
- Pruritic rash with discrete lesions ranging from macular to papular to vesicular to crusted. The vesicular lesions have been described as resembling "dewdrops on a rose petal" (Bouckenooghe et al. 2002, p. 1359).
- Centripetal (extremities to trunk) distribution of rash
- If varicella pneumonia is present, the patient may report the development of fever, dry cough, dyspnea, and possible pleuritic chest pain and/or hemoptysis approximately 1–6 days after the eruption of the rash.
- If encephalitis is present, the patient may report seizures, altered sensorium, headache, and/or ataxia.
- If severe thrombocytopenia is present, the patient may report unexplained bruising.

OBJECTIVE

→ Temperature may be elevated.
→ The patient presents with evidence of macular, papular, vesicular, and crusted lesions on her body, including scalp and mucous membranes. Various types of lesions are present simultaneously.
→ If pneumonia co-exists, physical findings may be minimal and include an increased respiratory rate and presence of crackles on auscultation of the lungs.
→ If encephalitis co-exists, the patient may demonstrate ataxia, nystagmus, nuchal rigidity, and/or altered mental status.
→ If thrombocytopenia co-exists, the patient may demonstrate petechiae and ecchymosis.

ASSESSMENT

→ Primary varicella zoster virus infection (chickenpox)
→ R/O disseminated zoster
→ R/O disseminated herpes simplex virus (HSV) infection
→ R/O eczema vaccinia
→ R/O generalized vaccinia
→ R/O atypical measles
→ R/O rickettsial pox
→ R/O thrombocytopenia
→ R/O other vesicular eruptions (e.g., poison oak)

PLAN

DIAGNOSTIC TESTS

→ Diagnosis is usually made on clinical findings. However, adjunctive laboratory tests may be ordered if a definitive diagnosis is required (Bouckenooghe et al. 2002, Cohen et al. 1999, Committee on Infectious Diseases 2000).
→ Complete blood count (CBC) may reveal leukopenia and/or thrombocytopenia.
→ Cultures of scrapings from the base of the vesicles can reveal evidence of VZV in 30–60% of infected individuals. The sample must be obtained within the first 3–4 days after

the onset of the rash for optimum results. Cultures from other sites (e.g., respiratory secretions) rarely produce a positive result (Cohen et al. 1999, Committee on Infectious Diseases 2000). Growth of the virus in culture usually requires 3–5 days (Liesegang 1999). Viral cultures are less sensitive in identifying VZV than DNA detection by polymerase chain reaction (PCR) or antigen detection by direct immunofluorescence (Liesegang 1999).

→ PCR of body fluid or tissue for determination of VZV DNA is very sensitive and can distinguish between wild-type virus and vaccine strains (Committee on Infectious Diseases 2000, Liesegang 1999).

→ Direct fluorescent antigen (DFA) detection from a vesicle scraping can distinguish between VZV and HSV. It is more sensitive and rapid than cultures (Committee on Infectious Diseases 2000, Liesegang 1999).

→ Tzanck smear can be done if a rapid result is necessary. Biopsies or scrapings of early skin lesions are stained and may reveal multinucleated giant cells, epithelial cells with acidophilic intranuclear inclusions, or homogenization of nuclear chromatin, each of which is diagnostic of HSV infection (Liesegang 1999). However, this test cannot distinguish between VZV and HSV infections (Liesegang 1999, McCrary et al. 1999).

→ Fluorescent antibody to membrane antigen (FAMA) test of smear obtained from a lesion will be positive. Although considered to be highly sensitive and specific, this test is not widely available because of the cost and technical elements required to perform it (Committee on Infectious Diseases 2000).

→ Enzyme-immunoassay (EIA) of acute and convalescent serum samples for IgG can be done to determine which individuals are susceptible to VZV and which have had the infection in the past (Liesegang 1999). This test may not be sensitive enough to demonstrate an immune response to varicella vaccination (Committee on Infectious Diseases 2000).

→ Latex agglutination (LA) of acute and convalescent serum samples for IgG can be done. This test is more sensitive and can be done more rapidly than the EIA (Committee on Infectious Diseases 2000).

→ Complement-fixation test of acute and convalescent serum samples for IgG may be positive. Complement-fixation tests are not useful for determining immune status because antibody levels diminish with time; therefore, the sensitivity of this test is poor (Committee on Infectious Diseases 2000).

→ Chest x-ray of a patient suspected of having pneumonia may reveal findings consistent with pulmonary inflammation and infiltration.

TREATMENT/MANAGEMENT

→ Respiratory and contact isolation of the patient is recommended until primary crusts have disappeared. Lesions should be kept clean.

→ Bed rest should be maintained while the patient is febrile.
  ▪ Acetaminophen should be used for analgesia and fever

because aspirin has been associated with an increased risk of Reye syndrome, although it is rare in adults.

→ Topical therapy for relief of pruritus may include the application of calamine lotion to lesions and/or colloidal oatmeal baths as needed.
  ▪ If necessary, systemic antihistamines, such as diphenhydramine 25 mg capsule p.o. once every 4–6 hours, can be recommended.
    ● Advise patients taking antihistamines about the possible side effects (e.g., drowsiness) and the need to avoid activities requiring concentration (e.g., driving).

→ If secondary bacterial infection of the lesions occurs, topical antibiotic creams such as mupirocin 2% ointment can be applied TID-QID (Bouckenooghe et al. 2002).
  ▪ If extensive bacterial infection is evident, consider prescribing antistaphylococcal oral antibiotics such as dicloxacillin 250 mg p.o. QID for 10 days (Bouckenooghe et al. 2002).

→ For patients with varicella infection who are at high risk for complications (e.g., immunocompromised persons and pregnant women), intravenous antiviral therapy with acyclovir 30 mg/kg/day in 3 divided doses for 7 days should be initiated as soon as possible to decrease the risk of serious sequelae (Bouckenooghe et al. 2002).
  ▪ Intravenous antiviral therapy also is indicated in immunocompetent patients with severe varicella-associated complications (e.g., pneumonitis or corneal involvement) (Bouckenooghe et al. 2002). The dose and administration are the same as for patients at high-risk for VZV-associated complications.
  ▪ Oral antiviral therapy initiated within 48 hours after the onset of VZV rash has been documented to reduce fever and extensive skin lesions, and may be prescribed for healthy adults older than 18 years as follows (Bouckenooghe et al. 2002, Cohen et al. 1999):
    ● Acyclovir 800 mg p.o. 5 times a day for 5 days
    NOTE: Famciclovir and valacyclovir are two other antiviral medications that require less frequent dosing and may be recommended by some infectious disease specialists; however, these agents are not approved by the Food and Drug Administration for this use.

→ VZIG 125 units/10 kg body weight (up to a total dose of 625 units) IM should be given to susceptible persons at *high risk* of developing progressive varicella disease (see **Table 11J.1, Types of Exposure to Varicella or Zoster for which VZIG Is Indicated for Susceptible Persons** and **Table 11J.2, Candidates for VZIG, Provided Significant Exposure Has Occurred**) (Committee on Infectious Diseases 2000).
  ▪ VZIG must be administered within 96 hours of exposure to varicella to be effective. The duration of the protective effect of VZIG is unknown.
  ▪ If an individual continues to be exposed to a patient with varicella, a second injection should be administered 3 weeks after the initial dose.
  ▪ Because asymptomatic varicella is known to occur, laboratory tests for varicella immune status in high-risk,

susceptible individuals can be done before administering VZIG if performing such tests will not delay VZIG administration beyond 96 hours after exposure.
NOTE: VZIG is not recommended for low-risk, susceptible individuals.
→ Varicella zoster vaccine: In healthy, susceptible, nonpregnant persons exposed to VZV, administering varicella vaccine within 72 hours after exposure may prevent or decrease symptoms associated with wild-type varicella infection (CDC 1999, Cohen et al. 1999, Committee on Infectious Diseases 2000, Gershon 2001, McCrary et al. 1999).

CONSULTATION

→ Consultation with a physician is recommended for all patients at increased risk of serious sequelae (e.g., pregnant women, immunosuppressed patients) or patients with clinical evidence of severe disease (e.g., pneumonia, encephalitis) who require hospitalization.
→ As needed for prescription(s).

PATIENT EDUCATION

→ Educate the patient about varicella, including transmission, infectivity, clinical course, treatment(s), signs and symptoms of possible complications, and when further evaluation may be needed.
→ Assess the possible need to administer varicella vaccine to any low-risk, susceptible person in close contact with the patient.
→ Assess the possible need to administer VZIG to any high-risk, susceptible person in close contact with the patient.
→ If hospitalization is indicated (e.g., in case of pneumonia or encephalitis), the physician responsible for the patient's care

Table 11J.1. **TYPES OF EXPOSURE TO VARICELLA OR ZOSTER FOR WHICH VZIG IS INDICATED FOR SUSCEPTIBLE PERSONS***

Household	Residing in the same household
Playmate	Face-to-face± indoor play
Hospital	Varicella: In same room with 2–4 beds or adjacent beds in a large ward, face-to-face contact with an infectious staff member or patient, or a visit by a person considered to be infectious
	Zoster: Intimate contact (e.g., touching or hugging) with a person considered to be infectious
Newborn Infant	Onset of varicella in the mother within 5 days before delivery or within 48 hours after delivery. Varicella zoster immune globulin (VZIG) is not indicated if the mother has zoster.

* Patients should meet the criteria of both significant exposure and candidacy for receiving VZIG, as provided in Table 11J.2.
± Experts differ about the duration of face-to-face contact that warrants administration of VZIG. However, the contact should be nontransient. Some experts consider contact of 5 or more minutes as constituting significant exposure; others define it as more than 1 hour.

Source: Committee on Infectious Diseases. 2000. *Red book 2000. Report of the Committee on Infectious Diseases*, 25th ed., p. 630. Elk Grove Village, Ill.: American Academy of Pediatrics. Reprinted with permission from the American Academy of Pediatrics.

Table 11J.2. **CANDIDATES FOR VZIG*, PROVIDED SIGNIFICANT EXPOSURE HAS OCCURRED**

• Immunocompromised individuals, including those with human immunodeficiency virus infection or those receiving chronic immunosuppressive therapy

• Susceptible pregnant women

• A newborn infant whose mother had onset within 5 days before delivery or within 48 hours after delivery

• A hospitalized premature infant (≥28 weeks gestation) whose mother lacks a reliable history of chickenpox or serologic evidence of protection against varicella

• A hospitalized premature infant (<28 weeks gestation or weighing ≤1,000 g) regardless of maternal history of varicella or varicella zoster virus serostatus

*Varicella zoster immune globulin

Source: Committee on Infectious Diseases. 2000. *Red book 2000. Report of the Committee on Infectious Diseases*, 25th ed., p. 630. Elk Grove Village, Ill.: American Academy of Pediatrics. Reprinted with permission from the American Academy of Pediatrics.

should discuss this decision, as well as indicated treatment(s), with her.

→ If the patient is pregnant, discuss the possible perinatal risks associated with varicella infection and administer appropriate antiviral therapy.

→ Educate patients who are at high risk for VZV exposure and infection about the availability of varicella vaccine (VARIVAX®) to prevent VZV infection. The dose and administration of the vaccine are as follows (CDC 1999, Committee on Infectious Diseases 2000, Gershon 2001):

- 0.5 mL subcutaneously, although IM administration has demonstrated similar immune results
- In healthy children ages 12 months through 12 years, a single immunization is adequate to develop cell-mediated and humoral immune responses to VZV. However, in persons 13 years old or older, two doses of the vaccine should be administered to attain optimal immune responses to VZV. The second dose of varicella vaccine should be given 1–2 months after the initial dose.
- Eligible HIV-infected children require two doses of the vaccine within three months of each other and should be monitored closely for evidence of postimmunization rash.
- Children and adolescents who receive the vaccine should not take aspirin for six weeks after the immunization to reduce the possibility of Reye syndrome.
- Because up to 90% of persons 18 years old or older with an unreliable history of varicella infection have serologic evidence of VZV immunity, it may be helpful and cost effective to obtain serologic tests in this population before administering the vaccine.
- Women of childbearing age who receive varicella vaccine should be advised to avoid pregnancy for at least three months afterward (CDC 1996). If a woman is pregnant or conceives within three months of receipt of the vaccine, clinicians are requested to contact the VARIVAX® Pregnancy Registry at (800) 986-8999.
- Pregnant mothers or other household members do not constitute a contraindication for the immunization of children and other high-risk, VZV-susceptible persons. Transmission of vaccine-type virus from immunized healthy children to mothers is rare and immunization of a child will afford significant protection for the mother against exposure to and infection with wild-type varicella virus.

FOLLOW-UP

→ Follow-up visits will be based on the clinical presentation or determined by the managing physician.

→ Document in progress notes and on problem list.

Herpes Zoster (Shingles)

Herpes zoster (shingles) is a reactivation of latent varicella zoster virus infection, reportedly experienced by 10–20% of the population (Liesegang 1999, McCrary et al. 1999). Generally, it is thought to result from decline in cell-mediated immunity usually associated with advanced aging, immunosuppression, and

certain malignancies, although herpes zoster can occur in otherwise healthy persons. The characteristic eruption of cutaneous herpes zoster is a painful vesicular → pustular → crusted and confluent rash along single or multiple dermatomes. The rash usually resolves in 10 days but may require one month for complete resolution (Cohen et al. 1999, Landow 2000). The patient usually reports a history of chickenpox.

The most frequent complication associated with herpes zoster is postherpetic neuralgia (pain that lasts more than one month after zoster). This complication is increasingly more prevalent in older patients. Postherpetic neuralgia usually resolves within two months in 50% of patients and within one year after the onset of pain in 70–80% of patients (Cohen et al. 1999, McCrary et al. 1999).

The Ramsay Hunt syndrome is a complication noted in some patients, entailing cutaneous lesions in the external auditory canal, facial palsy, vertigo, and tinnitus. It is associated with diminished hearing (McCrary et al. 1999). Other complications include cutaneous scarring; cellulitis; encephalitis; myelitis; motor neuropathies (in 5% of herpes zoster patients, usually transient); Guillain-Barré syndrome; cerebrovasculopathy (15% mortality rate), usually associated with ophthalmic zoster; ocular inflammation (e.g., optic neuritis, keratitis, conjunctivitis, optic atrophy, second-degree glaucoma); vasculopathy (e.g., thrombosis); pneumonia; enterocolitis; myocarditis; pancreatitis; and esophagitis (Bouckenooghe et al. 2002, Cohen et al. 1999, McCrary et al. 1999).

The more severe complications associated with herpes zoster are usually reported in immunosuppressed patients or are due to disseminated disease. Disseminated herpes zoster is defined as more than 20 cutaneous lesions noted outside of the primary and immediately adjacent dermatomes (Cohen et al. 1999, McCrary et al. 1999). It is uncommon for immunocompetent patients to have disseminated disease; however, this reportedly occurs in up to 40% of immunosuppressed patients diagnosed with herpes zoster. This condition is associated with visceral organ involvement in approximately 10% of patients (Cohen et al. 1999, McCrary et al. 1999).

DATABASE

SUBJECTIVE

→ The patient may report one or more of the following (Landow 2000):

- A history of chickenpox, immunosuppression, previous herpes zoster episode
- Prodromal symptoms of fever, headache, dysesthesia(s), malaise 1–4 days before eruption of lesions
- Eruption of painful vesicles in a dermatome pattern
- Evolution of blisters into pustules 3–4 days after initial eruption, with crusting usually occurring 7–10 days after initial eruption
- Symptoms specific to nerve involvement (e.g., facial weakness if there is trigeminal involvement, peripheral motor weakness if motor neuropathies co-exist)
- Symptoms associated with complications (e.g., headache,

stiff neck, problems with coordination, altered mental status if encephalitis/meningoencephalitis co-exist)
- Dyspnea if pneumonia co-exists
- Symptoms of visual disturbance and pain if ocular complications co-exist

OBJECTIVE

→ Vital signs are usually within normal limits unless a complication such as encephalitis or pneumonitis co-exists.
- If such complications occur, there may be an elevated temperature, heart rate, and respiratory rate.
→ Examination of the skin will reveal vesicular → pustular → crusted and grouped lesions, usually along a single dermatome (most often thoracic and lumbar nerve root distributions; trigeminal and cervical distribution is less common).
- The presence of vesicles on the lateral and superior aspect of the nose is called Hutchinson's sign and indicates involvement of the nasociliary division of the ophthalmic nerve (McCrary et al. 1999).
→ In disseminated herpes zoster, there will be evidence of 20 lesions or more outside the primary and adjacent dermatome(s), usually appearing 4–11 days after eruption of the lesions in the primary dermatome (Cohen et al. 1999, Landow 2000, McCrary et al. 1999).
→ If there is co-existent pneumonia, pulmonary symptoms, including increased respiratory rate and crackles, will be evident.
→ If encephalitis or meningoencephalitis co-exists, examination may reveal associated symptoms of nuchal rigidity, nystagmus, evidence of ataxia, and mental status changes.
→ If there are co-existent motor neuropathies, examination may reveal evidence of abnormalities in the area of nerve distribution (e.g., facial palsy if there is trigeminal nerve involvement).
→ If there is co-existent ocular involvement, examination may reveal evidence of abnormalities (e.g., conjunctivitis, keratitis) suggestive of pathology specific to a site in the eye. (See specific chapters in Section 2, **Ophthalmological Disorders**, for physical findings and treatment.)
→ If there is co-existent Ramsay Hunt syndrome, examination may reveal evidence of lesion in the external auditory canal and the tympanic membrane, with facial palsy and diminished hearing.

ASSESSMENT

→ Herpes zoster (shingles)
→ R/O disseminated herpes zoster
→ R/O zosteriform HSV infection
→ R/O cellulitis
→ R/O encephalitis/meningoencephalitis
→ R/O pneumonia
→ R/O herpes zoster-associated neuropathies
→ R/O herpes zoster ocular complications
→ R/O immunosuppression
→ R/O other vesicular eruptions

PLAN

DIAGNOSTIC TESTS

→ The classic dermatome eruption characterizing herpes zoster is usually sufficient to diagnose this condition. (See "Primary Varicella Zoster Infection" under "Diagnostic Tests" for information about available laboratory tests for VZV.)
→ If disseminated herpes zoster or severe complications of herpes zoster occurs in a patient without a history of immunosuppression, consider diagnostic tests (e.g., HIV antibody testing, evaluation for possible malignancy) as indicated to identify possible cause(s) of immunosuppression.

TREATMENT/MANAGEMENT

→ Isolation of the patient from varicella-susceptible individuals in the household or hospital is indicated whenever possible.
→ Because virus can be recovered from vesicular fluid, precautions should be taken by any varicella-susceptible individuals who may be caring for a patient with herpes zoster (e.g., they should use gloves when in contact with lesions).
→ Symptomatic treatment of discomfort associated with herpes zoster includes acetaminophen or more potent prescription medications as indicated.
→ To reduce the likelihood of secondary bacterial infection, the lesions should be kept clean through gentle cleansing and drying of involved areas. If secondary bacterial infection occurs, antibiotic therapy specifically effective against staphylococci and streptococci is indicated.
→ Antiviral therapy for herpes zoster infection is based on the immune status of the patient and the severity of the illness (e.g., dermatomal versus disseminated herpes zoster, the presence of pneumonia or encephalitis, or ophthalmic complications).
- To be effective, acyclovir should be started as soon as possible after symptom onset (preferably within 72 hours) or while lesions are still forming (Cohen et al. 1999).
- The following are antiviral treatment recommendations (Cohen et al. 1999, Landow 2000, Liesegang 1999, McCrary et al. 1999):
  - Dermatomal herpes zoster:
    - Immunocompetent patient:
      ➤ Acyclovir 800 mg p.o. 5 times a day for 7 days
      OR
      ➤ Valacyclovir 1,000 mg p.o. every 8 hours for 7 days
      OR
      ➤ Famciclovir 500 mg p.o. every 8 hours for 7 days
    - Immunosuppressed patient:
      ➤ The oral antiviral regimens listed above, but the duration of therapy is 7–10 days.
      NOTE: For patients with immunosuppression due to HIV infection, hematologic or solid organ malignancies, or organ transplantation, intravenous acyclovir may be administered, 10 mg/kg every 8 hours for 7–10 days (Cohen et al. 1999).

- Ophthalmic zoster:
  - Immunocompetent patient:
    - ➤ Same antivirals, doses, and route as for derma-tomal zoster; however, ophthalmology consultation is warranted.
  - Immunosuppressed patient:
    - ➤ Acyclovir 10 mg/kg IV every 8 hours for 10 days. Ophthalmology consultation is warranted.
- Disseminated herpes zoster, herpes zoster pneumonia, visceral and neurological complications:
  - Immunocompetent and immunosuppressed patient:
    - ➤ Acyclovir 10 mg/kg IV every 8 hours for 10 days

NOTE: Patients with severe disease or complications should be hospitalized. Antiviral treatment should be determined by the physician responsible for the patient's care.
→ Symptomatic treatment of discomfort associated with herpes zoster includes acetaminophen or more potent prescription medications as indicated. Several topical therapies have been studied, but there is no substantial evidence to support their use.
→ Systemic steroid therapy to decrease the duration of associated pain and possibly to reduce the incidence of postherpetic neuralgia is controversial (Bouckenooghe et al. 2002, Committee on Infectious Diseases 2000, McCrary et al. 1999). According to some authors, there may be some benefit in prescribing systemic steroids to adults 50 years old or older (Cohen et al. 1999). If systemic steroid therapy is being considered for a patient, consultation with a physician is indicated.
→ Tricyclic antidepressants have been shown to decrease neuropathic pain associated with herpes zoster in up to 50% of patients in some studies (McCrary et al. 1999). Use of these medications, especially in elderly patients, should be closely monitored because of their anticholinergic side effects.

CONSULTATION

→ Physician consultation is warranted for patients with severe disease (e.g., disseminated herpes zoster), zoster-associated complications, or immunosuppression, or if systemic steroid therapy is being considered.
→ As needed for prescription(s).

PATIENT EDUCATION

→ Educate the patient about the cause of herpes zoster, its duration, possible complications, treatment options including any side effects, and the possibility of recurrence (approximately 5%) (Cohen et al. 1999).
→ Educate the patient about the infectivity of the vesicular fluid and the need to have varicella-susceptible individuals (e.g., household members) avoid contact with the lesions until they crust over. Varicella-susceptible household contacts should consult their primary care provider to discuss the possibility of prophylaxis. If a varicella-susceptible household contact is immunosuppressed, they should seek immediate medical evaluation.
→ If there is evidence of disseminated herpes zoster or complications, educate the patient about the possible need for further evaluation to rule out underlying immunosuppressive conditions (e.g., HIV infection, malignancy).
→ Advise the patient to avoid direct sun exposure of affected area(s) to prevent hyperpigmentation of skin.

FOLLOW-UP

→ A patient hospitalized and managed by a physician should return for follow-up as recommended by the physician.
→ In uncomplicated, dermatomal herpes zoster, the patient should return for evaluation if any complications (including postherpetic neuralgia) develop.
→ Document in progress notes and on problem list.

BIBLIOGRAPHY

Bouckenooghe, A.R., and Shandera, W.X. 2002. In *2002 current medical diagnosis & treatment*, 41st ed., eds. L.M. Tierney, Jr., S.J. McPhee, and M.A. Papadakis, pp. 1359–1363. New York: Lange Medical Books/McGraw-Hill.
Centers for Disease Control and Prevention (CDC). 1996. Notice to readers. Establishment of VARIVAX {registered} pregnancy registry. *Morbidity and Mortality Weekly Report* 45(11):239.
_____. 1999. Prevention of varicella. Updated recommendations of the Advisory Committee on Immunization Practices (ACIP). *Morbidity and Mortality Weekly Report* 48(RR06):1–5.
Cohen, J.I., Brunell, P.A., Straus, S.E. et al. 1999. Recent advances in varicella-zoster virus infection. *Annals of Internal Medicine* 130(11):922–932.
Committee on Infectious Diseases. 2000. *Red book 2000. Report of the Committee on Infectious Diseases*, 25th ed., pp. 624–638. Elk Grove Village, Ill.: American Academy of Pediatrics.
Gershon, A.A. 2001. Live-attenuated varicella vaccine. *Infectious Disease Clinics of North America* 15(1):65–81.
Landow, K. 2000. Acute and chronic herpes zoster. An ancient scourge yields to timely therapy. *Postgraduate Medicine* 107(7):107–118.
Liesegang, T.J. 1999. Varicella zoster viral disease. *Mayo Clinic Proceedings* 74:938–998.
McCrary, M.L., Severson, J., and Tyring, S.K. 1999. Varicella zoster virus. *Journal of the American Academy of Dermatology* 41:1–14.
Uhoda, I., Pierard-Franchimont, C., and Pierard, G.E. 2000. Varicella-zoster virus vasculitis: a case of recurrent varicella without epidermal involvement. *Dermatology 2000* 200:173–175.

SECTION 12

Genitourinary Disorders

12-A Abnormal Uterine Bleeding **12-3**
12-B Abnormal Cervical Cytology **12-13**
12-C Amenorrhea—Secondary **12-24**
12-D Dysmenorrhea **12-37**
12-E Ectopic Pregnancy **12-42**
12-F Endometriosis. **12-48**
12-G Hirsutism **12-53**
12-H Infertility **12-62**
      12-HA Clomiphene Citrate **12-76**
12-I Pelvic Inflammatory Disease. **12-81**
12-J Pelvic Masses. **12-87**
      → Fibroids and Adenomyosis **12-87**
      → Ovarian/Adnexal Masses. **12-89**
12-K Pelvic Pain—Acute **12-96**
12-L Pelvic Pain—Chronic **12-100**
12-M Perimenopausal and Menopausal Symptoms
and Hormone Therapy. **12-109**
12-N Polyps—Cervical and Endometrial **12-121**
12-O Premenstrual Syndrome and Premenstrual
Dysphoric Disorder **12-124**
12-P Sexual Dysfunction **12-132**
12-Q Toxic Shock Syndrome **12-146**
12-R Urinary Tract Disorders **12-151**
      12-RA Urinary Tract Infection **12-151**
      12-RB Female Urinary Incontinence **12-157**
      12-RC Overactive Bladder **12-161**
      12-RD Interstitial Cystitis **12-164**
12-S Vaginitis **12-167**
      12-SA Atrophic Vaginitis **12-167**
      12-SB Bacterial Vaginosis **12-170**
      12-SC Candidal Vulvovaginitis **12-174**
      12-SD Cytolytic Vaginitis **12-180**
      12-SE *Trichomonas vaginalis* Vaginitis. **12-182**
      12-SF Table 12SF.1. Vaginal Infections **12-186**
      12-SG Vaginitis Bibliography. **12-187**

12-T Vulvar Disease **12-189**

    12-TA Red Lesions of the Vulva **12-189**

        → Cutaneous Candidiasis **12-189**

        → Contact Dermatitis (Reactive Vulvitis) **12-191**

        → Paget's Disease **12-193**

    12-TB White Lesions of the Vulva **12-195**

        → Lichen Sclerosus **12-195**

        → Squamous Cell Hyperplasia **12-197**

    12-TC Dark Lesions of the Vulva **12-200**

        → Lentigo **12-200**

        → Nevi **12-200**

        → Seborrheic Keratosis **12-201**

        → Melanoma **12-202**

    12-TD Small Lesions of the Vulva **12-205**

        → Epidermal Cysts **12-205**

        → Acrochordons **12-206**

        → Hidradenitis Suppurativa **12-206**

        → Hemangiomas **12-208**

        → Caruncle (Urethral) **12-209**

        → Fox-Fordyce Disease **12-209**

    12-TE Large Lesions of the Vulva **12-211**

        → Bartholin's Cyst/Abscess **12-211**

        → Verrucous Carcinoma **12-214**

    12-TF Ulcerative Lesions of the Vulva **12-216**

        → Squamous Cell Carcinoma **12-216**

        → Basal Cell Carcinoma **12-219**

    12-TG Vulvar Intraepithelial Neoplasia **12-221**

    12-TH Vulvodynia **12-224**

12-U Vaginal Intraepithelial Neoplasia **12-233**

Winifred L. Star, R.N., C., N.P., M.S.
Joan Y. Okasako, R.N., C.S., F.N.P., M.S.

12-A

Abnormal Uterine Bleeding

Abnormal uterine bleeding is a common and often debilitating condition that may account for 15% of clinic visits and almost 25% of gynecological operations (Goudas et al. 1997). Alterations in the female menstrual cycle are health concerns frequently encountered by clinicians in gynecological practice. Menstrual bleeding is considered abnormal if it occurs more frequently than every 21 days (polymenorrhea), exceeds a total blood loss of 80 mL (menorrhagia), and persists for longer than seven days (hypermenorrhea) (Sheth et al. 1999). In addition, infrequent menstrual bleeding with intervals of 35 days to three months (oligomenorrhea) and an absence of menstrual bleeding for three consecutive cycles or up to six months (amenorrhea) are abnormal bleeding patterns (Policar 2001).

The etiology of abnormal uterine bleeding may be attributable to organic causes, which include complications of pregnancy, benign and malignant genital tract and pelvic abnormalities, systemic illnesses, endocrinological disorders, and iatrogenic and extragenital causes (March et al. 1997). (See **Table 12A.1, Classification of Abnormal Uterine Bleeding**.)

Systemic causes of abnormal uterine bleeding may include hereditary disorders of coagulation, the most common of which is von Willebrand's disease (Lusher 1999). It is estimated that von Willebrand's disease affects 1% of the world's population and occurs in all racial and ethnic groups (Ellis et al. 1999, Lusher et al. 1996). Studies have shown that von Willebrand's disease is found in 10.7% of patients presenting with menorrhagia (Dilley et al. 2001). The etiology of abnormal uterine bleeding may also include acquired causes of coagulation dysfunction resulting from liver disease, myeloproliferative disorders, severe sepsis, idiopathic thrombocytopenic purpura, hypersplenism, and uremia (Herbst 2001, Lusher 1999). Other systemic causes include liver disease and renal disease, which result in impaired metabolism and excretion of estrogens, respectively (Kim 2000).

Endocrinological disorders contributing to abnormal uterine bleeding may include hypothyroidism and hyperthyroidism (Speroff et al. 1999). In addition, hyperprolactinemia, Cushing's disease, Addison's disease, and polycystic ovary syndrome (PCOS) may also result in abnormal uterine bleeding (Bravender et al. 1999).

Abnormal uterine bleeding may be attributed to pelvic pathologies including fibroids, cervical or endometrial polyps, cervical lesions, ovarian tumors, neoplasia, endometriosis, and adenomyosis (Shaw et al. 1999). In addition, the presence of genital tract injury or foreign objects and/or infection should be investigated (Speroff et al. 1999).

Iatrogenic causes of organic bleeding include exposure to certain medications, such as corticosteroids, anticoagulants, β-lactam antibiotics, phenothiazines, monoamine oxidase inhibitors, digoxin, tricyclic antidepressants, sex steroids, phenytoin, and medicated or nonmedicated intrauterine devices (IUDs) (Lusher 1999, Motashaw 1999, Sheth et al. 1999). Herbal remedies such as ginseng may be associated with estrogenic activity and abnormal bleeding (Speroff et al. 1999). Lifestyle factors such as stress, eating disorders, and vigorous exercise may also contribute (Motashaw 1999).

Dysfunctional uterine bleeding (DUB) is defined as abnormal uterine bleeding with no demonstrable organic cause and, therefore, is a diagnosis of exclusion. DUB accounts for the majority of cases of abnormal uterine bleeding, may occur at any time between menarche and menopause, and is usually the result of anovulation. Less frequently, ovulatory cycles are involved (Chen et al. 1998). It is estimated that 50% of women with DUB are 40–50 years old, whereas 20% of cases occur in adolescents (March et al. 1997).

The most common cause of DUB is anovulation, which results from a disturbance of the feedback mechanism of the hypothalamic-pituitary-ovarian axis (HPO-axis) or from declining ovarian hormonal function (March et al. 1997). Normal ovulatory cycles are the result of an intact HPO-axis that stimulates the sequential exposure of the endometrium to estrogen, followed by progesterone and estrogen, and finally by a decline in levels of both ovarian hormones resulting in the cyclic proliferation, secretion, and synchronized shedding characteristic of a normal menstrual cycle (American College of Obstetricians and Gynecologists [ACOG] 2000).

During an anovulatory cycle, a corpus luteum is not produced and the ovary fails to secrete progesterone while continuing to produce estrogen. The continuous exposure of the endometrium to estrogen without the stabilizing influence of progesterone results in a fragile, thickened endometrium that may shed in an asynchronous manner, resulting in various abnormal bleeding patterns—i.e., menorrhagia, polymenorrhea, metrorrhagia, etc. (ACOG 2000). Continuous exposure of the endometrium to unopposed estrogen may result in endometrial hyperplasia with cellular atypia, which is a precursor to adenocarcinoma (ACOG 2000, Speroff et al. 1999).

Anovulatory bleeding also may be associated with changes in the production of endometrial prostaglandins that influence vasoconstriction and blood loss (ACOG 2000). Lower levels of PGF-2α result in abnormal vasoconstriction and increased menstrual blood loss (Smith et al. 1982).

Although less common, DUB associated with ovulatory cycles may be caused by local biochemical events that result in a loss of local endometrial hemostasis (Livingstone et al. 2002, Munro 2001). Ovulatory DUB occurs predominantly after

Table 12A.1. CLASSIFICATION OF ABNORMAL UTERINE BLEEDING

Organic Causes

Local Pelvic Factors
Leiomyomas
Polyps
Endometriosis
Adenomyosis
Pelvic inflammatory disease
Endometritis
Salpingitis
Tubo-ovarian mass
Ovarian tumors
Abortion
Trophoblastic disease
Ectopic pregnancy
Retained products of conception
Intrauterine device
Traumatic lesions
Foreign body
Atrophic vaginitis
Malignant lesions of the vulva, vagina, cervix, endometrium,
    fallopian tube, or ovary
Endometrial hyperplasia
Tuberculosis
Other genital lesions: anatomical, benign masses, inflammatory,
    infection, sexually transmitted disease

Endocrinological Disorders
Thyroid dysfunction
Diabetes mellitus
Hypothalamic disorders: psychogenic, organic disease, eating
    disorders, polycystic ovary syndrome
Pituitary diseases: hyperprolactinemia, acromegaly
Adrenal diseases: Cushing's syndrome, Addison's disease, tumors,
    congenital adrenal hyperplasia

Systemic Disease
Coagulation disorders: von Willebrand's disease, idiopathic
    thrombocytopenia purpura, Factor V, VII, VIII, IX, X, XI
    deficiencies, platelet function defects, dysfibrinogenemias
Increased endometrial fibrinolysins
Hepatic disease
Renal disease
Hypersplenism
Vitamin K deficiency
HIV-related thrombocytopenia
Systemic lupus erythematosus
Leukemia
Aplastic anemia
Sepsis

Iatrogenic Factors
Oral, subdermal, or injectable hormones (estrogen or progesterone)
Corticosteroids
Digitalis
Phenytoin
Propranolol
Phenothiazines
Butyrophenones
Aspirin
Tranquilizers
Tricyclic antidepressants
Chemotherapeutic agents
Tamoxifen
Herbs: ginseng

Extragenital Factors
Urinary tract
Gastrointestinal tract

Lifestyle Factors
Stress
Eating disorders
Vigorous exercise

Dysfunctional Causes

Anovulatory: HPO axis disturbances, declining ovarian function
Ovulatory: Persistent corpus luteum, luteal phase deficiency, decreased estrogen at midcycle, increased endometrial fibrinolysins

Source: Adapted with permission from Benjamin, F., and Seltzer, V.L. 1987. Excessive menstrual bleeding, menorrhagia, and dysfunctional uterine bleeding. In *Gynecology principles and practice*, eds. Z. Rosenwaks, F. Benjamin, and M.L. Stone. New York: Macmillan.

adolescence and before the perimenopause and has been reported in up to 10% of ovulatory women (Herbst 2001). The etiology of ovulatory DUB may be multifactorial: Studies have shown that endometrial lysosomal enzyme activity is increased (Fraser et al. 1996) and levels of vasodilating prostaglandins in the endometrial stroma may be altered (Makarainen et al. 1986, Smith et al. 1981). Nitric oxide, a potent vasodilator and inhibitor of platelet aggregation, may also be involved in ovulatory DUB (Cameron et al. 1998, Munro 2001).

Menorrhagia, one of most frequently encountered patterns of ovulatory DUB, may be the result of increased fibrinolysis and altered prostaglandin production resulting in the inhibition of platelet aggregation and the promotion of vasodilatation (Van Eijkeren et al. 1992). Polymenorrhea may result from a short follicular phase or inadequate luteal phase. In addition, oligomenorrhea may be caused by a prolonged follicular phase during the menstrual cycle (Oriel et al. 1999).

DATABASE

SUBJECTIVE

→ Normal uterine bleeding is described as menstrual cycles that are 28 ± 7 days in duration, have a menstrual flow of 4 ± 2 days, and involve a blood loss of 40 ± 20 mL. The average menstrual iron loss is 16 mg (March et al. 1997).

■ Menstrual blood loss may be difficult to quantify. Studies have shown that women's subjective assessment of menstruation does not correlate with the actual blood loss (Hallberg et al. 1964, Shaw et al. 1999).

• Women exhibiting menstrual blood loss >80 mL characterized their periods as "light" (34%), whereas 47% of the women who described their periods as "heavy" did not have a menstrual blood loss >80 mL (Chimbira et al. 1980, Shaw et al. 1999).

• The number of sanitary pads or tampons used may not be a reliable indicator of menstrual blood loss because there may be considerable variability in the absorption capacities of sanitary products and individual hygiene practices.

→ A patient with abnormal bleeding may present with any of the following bleeding patterns (March et al. 1997, Sheth et al. 1999, Speroff et al. 1999):

■ Menorrhagia: uterine bleeding lasting longer than seven days or a blood loss >80 mL, occurring at regular intervals. Etiologies may include:
• Myomas
• Endometrial polyps
• Adenomyosis
• Infection
• Intrauterine contraceptive devices
• Chronic liver failure
• Inherited clotting deficiencies
• Thrombocytopenia
• Hypothyroidism
• HPO-axis disturbances
• PCOS

• Obesity
• Endometrial hyperplasia
• Endometrial adenocarcinoma
• Ovarian neoplasms
• Warfarin therapy
• Ateriovenous malformation of the uterine wall (rare)

■ Metrorrhagia: uterine bleeding of variable amounts occurring at irregular but frequent intervals. Etiologies may include:
• Copper-containing intrauterine contraceptive devices
• Exogenous or endogenous unopposed estrogen
• Thyroid disease
• Coagulopathies
• Benign or malignant genital lesions
• Trauma or foreign bodies
• Cervical lesions
• Infections
• Polyps
• Myomas
• Functional ovarian cysts
• Ovarian tumors
• Endometriosis
• Luteal phase defect

■ Menometrorrhagia: uterine bleeding that is prolonged and occurs at irregular intervals.
• See the previously listed etiologies for menorrhagia and metrorrhagia.

■ Polymenorrhea: menstrual cycles occurring at regular intervals of fewer than 21 days.
• Etiologies may include immature HPO-axis; systemic, endocrine, or metabolic disorders; or psychogenic causes.

■ Oligomenorrhea: menstrual cycles occurring at intervals of more than 35 days. Etiologies include HPO-axis dysfunction, eating disorders, systemic disease, drug abuse, and endocrine disorders.

■ Hypomenorrhea: an abnormally small amount of menstrual bleeding. Etiologies include Asherman's syndrome, Cushing's syndrome, levonorgestrel-containing IUDs, and congenital obstruction of the outflow tract.

■ Amenorrhea: in previously menstruating woman, the absence of periods for six months or at least three of the previous menstrual cycles.

■ Postmenopausal bleeding: uterine bleeding occurring six months after the last menstrual cycle. Etiologies may include hormone replacement therapy, atrophic vaginitis, infection, hyperplasia or carcinoma of the endometrium, malignancies of the reproductive tract, polyps, urethral caruncle, and trauma.

■ Postcoital bleeding: bleeding occurring after intercourse. Etiologies include cervical neoplasia, infection with human papillomavirus or other organisms, cancer, polyps, and trauma.

■ Intermenstrual bleeding: bleeding occurring between regular menses.

■ Premenstrual spotting: spotting occurring up to one week before a regular period.

- Postmenstrual spotting: spotting occurring up to one week after regular menses.

→ History: Assessment of a patient presenting with abnormal uterine bleeding requires a complete medical history and may include evaluation of the following entities:

■ Menstrual cycle and obstetrical/gynecological history:
  • Age at menarche/menopause
  • Gravidity and parity
  • Last normal menstrual period
  • Previous normal menstrual periods (ideally the last three)
  • Usual cycle length, duration of flow, presence of clots
  • Onset/change in menstrual cycle (i.e., gradual or sudden)
  • Number of pads or tampons used during normal and abnormal bleeding
    – Frequency of use and degree of saturation
  • Impact of bleeding on lifestyle (i.e., lost time at work, soiled clothing, etc.)
  • Precipitating factors associated with abnormal bleeding (i.e., exercise, intercourse, trauma, douching, pessary use, etc.)
  • Prior episodes of abnormal bleeding and/or diagnoses of gynecological disorders including treatment
  • Associated physical symptoms:
    – Bloating
    – Cramping
    – Irritability
    – Breast tenderness
    – Abdominal or pelvic pain
    – Dyspareunia
    – Pain during defecation, blood in urine or stool
    – Mittelschmerz
    – Abnormal vaginal discharge, odor or itching, blood-tinged discharge, leukorrhea
    – Urinary frequency, urgency or dysuria
    – Fever, chills, nausea or vomiting
    – Diarrhea or constipation
    – General weakness, backache, leg cramps
  • Infertility
  • Dates and complications of past pregnancies
  • Number of spontaneous and therapeutic abortions
  • History of ectopic pregnancy
  • Current breast-feeding status
  • Pap smear history
  • History of sexually transmitted disease (STD) or pelvic inflammatory disease

■ Sexual history:
  • Sexual preference, number of partners, sex practices, date of last coitus, sexual partner history

■ Contraceptive history:
  • Types of methods used
  • Desire for future fertility

■ Medical history:
  • Current general health, complete history of medical problems, including treatment
  • Previous surgeries
  • Medications

■ Habits: use of tobacco, alcohol, and drugs; exercise training schedule

■ Nutritional status: dietary habits and weight fluctuations

■ Environmental/occupational hazards

■ Review of systems:
  • Weight gain/loss
  • Hair loss
  • Unwanted hair growth
  • Appetite changes
  • Petechiae
  • Bruising
  • Bleeding from the gums
  • Prolonged bleeding after minor cuts or dental surgery
  • Hot flashes
  • Hot/cold sensitivity
  • Night sweats
  • Fatigability or weakness
  • Headaches
  • Galactorrhea
  • Vaginal dryness
  • Recent illness
  • Any other symptoms of systemic, endocrine, or metabolic disease, and/or genitourinary or gastrointestinal disorders

■ Family history: uterine or ovarian malignancies in first degree relatives, tuberculosis, menorrhagia, endometriosis, bleeding disorders, DES exposure

■ Social history: education/occupation, situational life stress, marital/domestic/social support status, anxiety level, general life satisfaction, cultural barriers

---

OBJECTIVE

→ The evaluation of women with abnormal uterine bleeding should include a complete physical examination with an assessment of the following (March et al. 1997):

■ Vital signs:
  • Heart rate and blood pressure in the sitting and reclining positions, and temperature
  NOTE: Patients who are hypotensive and/or who demonstrate orthostatic hypotension are clinically unstable and should be treated accordingly in an emergency care setting.

■ General:
  • Height
  • Weight
  • Skin pallor
  • Stature
  • Habitus
  • Posture
  • Motor activity
  • Gait
  • Dress
  • Grooming
  • Personal hygiene
  • Manner

- Mood
- Affect
- Developmental state of secondary sex characteristics
- Evidence of systemic or endocrine disorders
■ Hair: texture, loss of axillary/pubic or scalp hair, hirsutism
■ Eyes, ears: stare, lid lag, exophthalmos, gross auditory defects, auditory acuity, fundoscopic changes
■ Neck: thyroid nodules or enlargement, lymph nodes, buffalo hump
■ Skin:
  - Pallor
  - Jaundice
  - Petechiae
  - Ecchymoses
  - Hematomas
  - Palmar erythema
  - Spider hemaniomata
  - Dry
  - Moist
  - Warm
  - Cold
  - Rough
  - Acne
  - Lesions
  - Nail bed color
  - Acanthosis nigricans
■ Deep tendon reflexes
■ Extremities: edema, perfusion, wasting, tremors
■ Heart/lungs: general evaluation
■ Breasts: striae, masses, nipple discharge, dimpling, tenderness
■ Abdomen: striae, ascites, hepatomegaly, splenomegaly, tenderness, pulses, inguinal nodes
■ Pelvis:
  - External genitalia, Bartholin's/urethral/Skene's glands:
    – Hair distribution, lesions, edema, cysts, clitoral hypertrophy
  - Vagina:
    – Traumatic lesions, erythema, foreign bodies, abnormal discharge, atrophy
  - Cervix:
    – Lesions, purulent discharge, polyps, eversions, inflammation, atrophy, Chadwick's sign
  - Uterus:
    – Enlargement, irregularity, masses, tenderness, sensation of increased warmth, fixation of pelvic organs, Hegar's sign
  - Adnexae:
    – Masses, tenderness
  - Rectum:
    – Masses, bleeding

ASSESSMENT

→ Abnormal uterine bleeding (organic causes)
→ Dysfunctional uterine bleeding (anovulatory or ovulatory)
→ R/O complication of pregnancy in reproductive-age women

PLAN

DIAGNOSTIC TESTS

→ The patient's age, reproductive status, and specific information from the history and physical examination will determine the type of diagnostic/laboratory tests. Consultation with a physician may be necessary.
→ A pregnancy test (qualitative β-hCG) should be performed on all patients of reproductive age. If it is positive, serial serum quantitative β-hCG testing may help diagnose specific pregnancy disorders (March et al. 1997, Munro 2001).
→ A CBC as indicated will rule out significant anemia.
→ Menstrual calendars may be utilized to establish specific bleeding patterns if the history is unclear.
→ The reported number of tampons/pads may not accurately assess menstrual blood loss.
→ The alkaline hematin method, the gold standard for assessing menstrual blood loss, is time-consuming and impractical for routine clinical use (Chen et al. 1998).
→ Pap smear: cervical cytology that adequately samples the ectocervix and endocervical canal as indicated (March et al. 1997).
→ Endocervical samples for *Neisseria gonorrhoeae* and *Chlamydia trachomatis* testing as indicated.
→ Wet mount with normal saline and KOH as indicated.
→ Biopsy of any suspicious vulvar, vaginal, or cervical lesion. Consult with a physician.
→ Basal body temperature measurements and cervical mucous charting, the use of ovulation prediction indicators, and Day 21 progesterone levels may differentiate between ovulatory and anovulatory cycles.
→ Endometrial biopsy may be performed in women who are:
  ■ 35 years old or older
  ■ Obese
  ■ 30 years old or older with a significant history of anovulation or oligoovulation
  ■ Postmenopausal but not on hormone replacement therapy
  ■ Postmenopausal, currently on hormone replacement therapy, and exhibiting unscheduled bleeding episodes (Long 1996)
→ Transvaginal ultrasonography of the pelvis may be indicated for:
  ■ Detection of endometrial polyps or submucosal fibroids
  ■ Measurement of endometrial thickness
  ■ Evaluation of pregnancy complications
  ■ Evaluation of ovarian masses (Long 1996)
→ Magnetic resonance imaging and computerized tomography scan may be used in diagnosing adnexal masses, adenomyosis, and leiomyomas (Sheth et al. 1999).
→ Hysteroscopy remains the gold standard for evaluating the endometrium; however, other technologies are emerging (Oriel et al. 1999). Consult with a physician. Hysteroscopy allows for:
  ■ Visualization of intrauterine adhesions
  ■ Evaluation and removal of submucosal leiomyomas and endometrial polyps

- Visualization and removal of embedded IUDs
- Endometrial biopsy for diagnosis of carcinoma (March 1997)
→ Hysterosalpingography (HSG) allows radiographic visualization of the endometrial cavity and may be used to evaluate the caliber and patency of the fallopian tubes. Consult with a physician.
  - Use of HSG in evaluating DUB may facilitate the diagnosis of:
    - Submucosal leiomyomas
    - Endometrial polyps
    - Asherman's syndrome
    - Endometrial tuberculosis
    - Endometrial hyperplasia (Richmond 1997)
→ Dilatation and curettage (D&C) is generally reserved for acute bleeding episodes resulting in hypovolemia and for older women for whom the suspicion for malignancy is high (March et al. 1997).
  - Other indications for D&C include the presence of endometrial polyps and, if an endometrial sampling was inadequate, to establish a histologic diagnosis.
→ Additional laboratory tests may include:
  - Ferritin level (if anemia is present)
  - ESR
  - Coagulation profile:
    - Peripheral blood smear
    - Prothrombin time
    - Partial thomboplastin time
    - Bleeding time
    - Ristocetin cofactor assay for the von Willebrand's factor
  - ANA, DNA binding, and lupus inhibitor
  - Hormone levels:
    - FSH
    - LH
    - Estradiol
    - Progesterone
    - Prolactin
    - Testosterone and DHEAS if hirsutism and virilizing symptoms are present
  - Thyroid function tests: TSH; T3, T4, and FTI if TSH is abnormal
  - Liver/renal function tests: creatinine, BUN, serum transaminases
  - Adrenal function testing: fasting a.m. serum cortisol, 17-hydroxyprogesterone
  - FBS, hemoglobin A1C, glucose tolerance testing

TREATMENT/MANAGEMENT

→ See "Diagnostic Tests."
→ Assessment for the clinical signs of orthostatic hypotension will identify hemodynamically unstable women who require an immediate referral to the emergency department (March et al. 1997).

Acute Hemorrhagic Bleeding

→ The patient should be managed by a physician in an emergency care setting. A comprehensive discussion of clinical management is beyond the scope of this chapter.

Acute, Heavy Bleeding

→ Drug options may include the following regimens:
  - Conjugated estrogens (CE) or estradiol: conjugated estrogen 1.25 mg p.o. or estradiol 2 mg p.o. every 4 hours for 24 hours followed by CE 1.25 mg p.o. or estradiol 2 mg p.o. per day for 7–10 days (Speroff et al. 1999). **NOTE:** Estrogen therapy must be followed by progestin coverage and a withdrawal bleed (Speroff et al. 1999).
  - Low-dose, monophasic, combined oral contraceptive BID for 5–7 days. The patient should be advised to expect heavy withdrawal bleeding 2–4 days after stopping therapy. Then initiate a low-dose, monophasic, combined oral contraceptive on the fifth day of menstrual flow (or on a Sunday start) in the standard 21/7 day cycle pattern (Speroff et al. 1999).
    - An alternative to the standard 21/7 cycle pattern is a monophasic, continuous 84/7 regimen—i.e., 84 days of continuous pill use with a 7-day placebo or pill-free interval (Kaunitz et al. 2002). **NOTE:** High-dose estrogen therapy—i.e., multiple doses of oral contraceptives within a 24-hour period—may precipitate a thrombotic event. This therapy may be contraindicated in women with a history of thrombosis or a family history of idiopathic venous thromboembolism (Speroff et al. 1999). Antiemetics may be indicated with multiple estrogen doses (Bravender et al. 1999).

Chronic Anovulatory Bleeding

→ Endometrial assessment to exclude endometrial carcinoma is indicated in the following circumstances:
  - 35 years old or older
  - Obese women under age 35
  - Women with a history of chronic anovulation
  - Women who do not respond to medical therapy (ACOG, 2000)
  NOTE: Other risk factors for endometrial carcinoma include nulliparity, late menopause (older than 52 years), diabetes, hypertension, PCOS, feminizing ovarian tumors, and tamoxifen therapy for longer than 2 years (Herbst 2001).
→ Drug options may include the following regimens:
  - Low-dose, combined oral contraceptives for women of reproductive age and nonsmoking women older than 35 years without evidence of vascular disease (ACOG 2000, Bravender et al. 1999, Chuong et al. 1996)
  - Medroxyprogesterone acetate (MPA): 10 mg p.o. per day for at least 10–14 days per month for 3–6 cycles (Bravender et al. 1999, Shwayder 2000, Speroff et al. 1999)
  - Norethindrone acetate: 5–10 mg p.o. QD–TID for 10–14 days per month (Bravender et al. 1999, Chuong et al. 1996). Progestin therapy may be extended for 14–21 days

per month for recalcitrant anovulatory DUB (Chuong et al. 1996, Munro 2001).

- Micronized progesterone: 200 mg p.o. BID for 10–14 days per month (Forstein 2000, Policar 2001)

NOTE: Withdrawal bleeding will occur 2–7 days after the last pill of each progestin or progesterone cycle.

- Depot-medroxyprogesterone acetate (Depo-Provera®): 150 mg IM every 12 weeks (Speroff et al. 1999)
- For *perimenopausal women*, options include:
  - Cyclic CE: 0.625–1.25 mg p.o. per day for 25 days with MPA 10 mg p.o. added on Days 15–25 (Chuong et al. 1996)
  - Low-dose, combined oral contraceptives for nonsmokers without evidence of vascular disease (Chuong et al. 1996, Kaunitz 2002)
  - Newer combination hormonal contraceptives may be appropriate in certain cases—e.g., a monthly contraceptive injection containing MPA 25 mg/estradiol cypionate 5 mg, a weekly transdermal contraceptive patch releasing norelgestromin 150 μg/ethinyl estradiol 20 μg daily, or a 3-week contraceptive vaginal ring releasing etonogestrel 120 μg/ethinyl estradiol 15 μg daily (Kaunitz 2002). Consult with a physician.
  - Any of the previously mentioned progestin or progesterone regimens.

Metrorrhagia

→ See "Diagnostic Tests" regarding indications for endometrial biopsy.

→ Hysteroscopy, hysterosalpingography, sonohysterogram, pelvic ultrasound as indicated. Consult with a physician.

→ Appropriate laboratory tests as indicated. See "Diagnostic Tests."

→ Observation alone may suffice if no organic pathology is identified.

- Recommend a menstrual calendar.
- Basal body temperature and mucus charting also may be recommended to document ovulation.

→ Identified organic pathology should be treated appropriately. Consult with a physician as indicated.

→ Premenstrual spotting may be treated with cyclic progestins if pregnancy is not desired and there is no evidence of pathology: MPA 10 mg p.o. per day for 7–12 days beginning on Day 15 of the menstrual cycle (Field 1988).

→ Midcycle spotting may be treated with estrogen if pregnancy is not desired and there is no evidence of pathology: CE 1.25–2.5 mg p.o. per day or ethinyl estradiol 10–20 μg p.o. per day beginning 1–3 days before ovulation and continuing until 2–4 days after ovulation (Field 1988).

→ Midcycle or premenstrual/postmenstrual spotting or bleeding may be treated with low-dose oral contraceptives if pregnancy is not desired and there is no evidence of pathology (Field 1988).

→ Treatment may also include nonsteroidal anti-inflammatory drugs (NSAIDs) such as ibuprofen 400–800 mg p.o. TID for 5 days (Diaz et al. 1990, Nutley et al. 1997).

Menorrhagia

→ Combined, low-dose oral contraceptives may induce endometrial atrophy and reduce menstrual blood loss (Fraser et al. 1991, Shaw et al. 1999).

→ Progestin-releasing intrauterine devices, such as the levonorgestrel intrauterine system (Mirena®), may prevent endometrial proliferation and reduce menstrual blood loss.

- Studies have shown that menstrual blood loss may be reduced by 95% after 6 months and patients may experience oligomenorrhea or amenorrhea (Munro 2001, Tang et al. 1995).

→ Long-acting depo-medroxyprogesterone acetate (Depo-Provera®): 150 mg IM every 12 weeks may induce endometrial atrophy and reduce menstrual blood loss (Shaw et al. l999).

→ NSAIDs reduce prostaglandin levels and may reduce menstrual blood loss by 20–30% in women with menorrhagia (Chen et al. 1998).

- Ibuprofen: 400 mg p.o. TID for the first 3 days of menses or the duration of menstrual bleeding (Chuong et al. 1996, Herbst 2001, March et al. 1997). Some patients may require higher dosages or more frequent dosing schedules (e.g., 400–800 mg p.o. every 4–6 hours). Consult with a physician.
- Naproxen sodium: 275 mg p.o. QID after a loading dose of 550 mg p.o. Continue treatment for the first 3 days of menses or for the duration of menstrual bleeding (March et al. 1997).
- Mefenamic acid: 500 mg p.o. TID for the first 3 days of menses or for the duration of menstrual bleeding

→ Long-cycle progestins: norethindrone 5 mg p.o. TID on Days 5–26 of the menstrual cycle for treating ovulatory menorrhagia (Munro 2000)

→ Danazol: 200–400 mg p.o. per day for 3 cycles

- May inhibit ovulation, cause lower serum estrogen levels, and induce endometrial atrophy (Shaw et al. 1999).
- Side effects may include:
  - Weight gain (2–4 kg)
  - Acne
  - Seborrhea
  - Hirsutism
  - Hot flashes
  - Mood changes including depression
  - Unfavorable lipid profiles
- Consultation with a physician is advised.

→ GnRH-agonist compounds: depot leuprolide 3.75 mg IM monthly or nafarelin 0.2–0.4 mg intranasally BID

- These agents bind with greater affinity to receptor sites on the anterior pituitary gland, resulting in lower circulating levels of estrogen and, therefore, endometrial atrophy (Gardner et al. l990, MacKay 2002).
- Side effects may include hot flashes and bone density loss.
- Consultation with a physician is advised.

→ Antifibrinolytic agents such as ε-aminocaproic acid and tranexamic acid have been shown to reduce menstrual blood loss, although side effects such as nausea, dizziness, diarrhea, and headaches may limit their use (March et al. 1997).

- Tranexamic acid 1 g p.o. every 6 hours for the first 4 days of the menstrual cycle may be used to treat ovulatory DUB (Munro 2001).
  - Contraindicated in patients with a history of renal failure or thrombolytic events.
→ Surgical options:
- D&C should be reserved for women with acute bleeding episodes that result in hypovolemia and for women for whom the suspicion for malignancy is high (March et al. 1997).
- Endometrial ablation with laser, electrocautery, or photovaporization under hysteroscopic visualization may be performed by a physician skilled in operative hysteroscopy (Chuong et al. 1996).
  - Endometrial ablation also may be accomplished by a thermal balloon containing a 5% dextrose solution heated to 92°C (Neuwirth et al. 1994, Stabinsky et al. 1999).
  - Ablative therapies usually are preceded by 4–6 weeks of danazol or GnRH agonists that may induce endometrial atrophy and increase treatment efficacy (Fraser et al. 1996).
  - An endometrial biopsy to rule out malignancy must be performed before any ablative therapies are initiated.
- Hysterectomy is generally reserved for patients in whom all treatment has failed and there is no desire for future fertility. Hysterectomy is definitive treatment for menorrhagia; some women may prefer this option as their first choice.

Postmenopausal Bleeding

→ Endometrial assessment (endometrial biopsy or D&C) to exclude endometrial carcinoma is indicated in women older than 35 years. Transvaginal ultrasonography may be used to assess endometrial thickness (<5 mm indicates atrophy) (MacKay 2002).
→ If endometrial biopsy results indicate simple hyperplasia without atypia, treat with cyclic progestin: MPA 10 mg p.o. per day or norethindrone 5 mg p.o. per day for 21 days/month for 3 months. Cyclic progestin therapy is followed by a repeat endometrial biopsy or D&C to reassess endometrial tissue (MacKay 2002). Consult with a physician.
→ Patients with moderate to severe hyperplasia (and for whom hysterectomy is medically inadvisable) may be treated with megestrol acetate: 40–160 mg p.o. per day (Herbst 2001). Patients require periodic endometrial sampling and physician consultation is mandated.
→ Endometrial biopsy results indicating hyperplasia with atypia or carcinoma may require hysterectomy. Physician consultation is mandated (Herbst 2001).
→ Postmenopausal women receiving hormone replacement therapy may benefit from a dose adjustment after excluding endometrial pathology. (See the **Perimenopausal and Menopausal Symptoms and Hormone Therapy** chapter for information on drugs and dosages.)

Additional Considerations

→ Iron supplementation therapy as indicated (Munro 2001).
→ An appropriate evaluation and treatment of any identified systemic disorder (i.e., liver disease, renal disease, coagulation disorder, etc.) should be performed. Refer the patient to an appropriate health care provider as indicated.
→ Further investigation is warranted if abnormal bleeding is persistent or recurrent after hormonal treatment (Speroff et al. 1999).
→ One must keep in mind that anovulatory bleeding may occur in women with leiomyomata who otherwise may be asymptomatic; management should proceed accordingly (Munro 2001).

CONSULTATION

→ Consultation with a physician is advised for all cases of abnormal bleeding and for endometrial or genital tract biopsies as indicated.
→ Patients with acute heavy bleeding should be managed by a physician.

PATIENT EDUCATION

→ Advise the patient to maintain a menstrual calendar and to monitor the quantity of pads or tampons used per day.
→ Explain the etiologies of abnormal bleeding, essential laboratory and diagnostic tests, and possible treatment options.
- Patient education handouts may be beneficial.
→ Discuss treatment options (i.e., medical versus surgical) and initiate a physician referral if warranted. Include the patient in the decision-making process.
→ For hormonal therapy, discuss the risks and benefits of the therapy and side effects of all medications. In addition, discuss the expected effects (i.e., heavy withdrawal bleeding after progestin therapy) and the parameters for follow-up.
→ Address issues of weight management, eating disorders, inadequate or excessive physical exercise, stress management, and abuse of drugs, alcohol, and tobacco as indicated.

FOLLOW-UP

→ Patients with acute bleeding should return promptly for further evaluation if therapy is ineffective in abating the bleeding episode.
→ Scheduled follow-up visits will vary according to the etiology of and treatment for abnormal uterine bleeding. Assess the patient at regular intervals—i.e., 3–6 months or as needed.
→ Assess the growth of all leiomyomas as indicated.
→ Review all laboratory and diagnostic test results with the patient and document the course of treatment in the progress notes.
→ Refer the patient to the appropriate specialist as indicated.
→ Annual visits should include an evaluation of all gynecological or medical issues and a thorough physical examination.

BIBLIOGRAPHY

Agarwal, N., and Kriplani, A. 2002. Medical management of dysfunctional uterine bleeding. *International Journal of Gynecology and Obstetrics* 75(2):199–201.

American College of Obstetricians and Gynecologists (ACOG). 2000. *Management of anovulatory bleeding. Practice Bulletin No. 14.* Washington, D.C.: the Author.

Bravender, T., and Emans, S.J. 1999. Menstrual disorders: dysfunctional uterine bleeding. Adolescent gynecology, part 1: common disorders. *Pediatric Clinics of North America* 46(3):545–553.

Cameron, I.T., and Campbell, S. 1998. Nitric oxide in the endometrium. *Human Reproduction Update* 4:565–569.

Chen, B.H., and Giudice, L.C. 1998. Dysfunctional uterine bleeding. *Western Journal of Medicine* 169(5):280–284.

Chimbira, T.H., Anderson, A.B.M., and Turnbull, A.C. 1980. Relation between measured menstrual blood loss and patients' subjective assessment of loss, duration of bleeding, number of sanitary towels used, uterine weight and endometrial surface area. *British Journal of Obstetrics and Gynaecology* 87:603–609.

Chuong, C.J., and Brenner, P.F. 1996. Management of abnormal uterine bleeding. *American Journal of Obstetrics and Gynecology* 175(3):787–792.

Diaz, S., Croxatto, H.B., Pavez, M. et al. 1990. Clinical assessment of treatments for prolonged bleeding in users of Norplant® implants. *Contraception* 42(1):97–109.

Dilley, A., Drews, C., Miller, C. et al. 2001. Von Willebrand's disease and other inherited bleeding disorders in women with diagnosed menorrhagia. *Obstetrics and Gynecology* 97(4):630–636.

Ellis, M.H., and Beyth, Y. 1999. Abnormal vaginal bleeding in adolescence as the presenting symptom of a bleeding diathesis. *Journal of Pediatric and Adolescent Gynecology* 12(3):127–131.

Field, C.S. 1988. Dysfunctional uterine bleeding. *Primary Care* 15(3):561–575.

Fornstein, D.A. 2000. Managing common problems in perimenopausal women. *Journal of the American Osteopathic Association* 100(10):S17–S22.

Fraser, I.S., Healy, D.L., Torode, H. et al. 1996. Depot goserelin and danazol pre-treatment before rollerball endometrial ablation for menorrhagia. *Obstetrics and Gynecology* 87:544–550.

Fraser, I.S., Hickey, M., and Song, J.Y. 1996. A comparison of mechanisms underlying disturbances of bleeding caused by spontaneous dysfunctional uterine bleeding or hormonal contraception. *Human Reproduction* 11(2):165–178.

Fraser, I.S., and McCarron, G. 1991. Randomized trial of 2 hormonal and 2 prostaglandin-inhibiting agents in women with a complaint of menorrhagia. *Australian and New Zealand Journal of Obstetrics and Gynecology* 31:66–70.

Gardner, R.L., and Shaw, R.W. 1990. LHRH analogues in the treatment of menorrhagia. In *Dysfunctional uterine bleeding*, ed. R.W. Shaw, pp. 149–159. Carnforth, United Kingdom: Parthenon Press.

Goudas, V.T., and Dumesic, D.A. 1997. Polycystic ovary syndrome. *Endocrinology and Metabolic Clinics of North America* 26:893–912.

Hallberg, L., and Nilsson, L. 1964. Determination of menstrual blood loss. *Scandinavian Journal of Clinical Laboratory Investigation* 16:244–248.

Herbst, A. 2001. Neoplastic diseases of the uterus. In *Comprehensive gynecology*, 4th ed., eds. M.A. Stenchever, W. Droegemueller, A.L. Herbst et al., pp. 919–954. St. Louis, Mo.: Mosby.

Kaunitz, A.M. 2002. Abnormal uterine bleeding in the perimenopausal patient. *Contemporary OB/GYN* 47(4):69–88.

Kaunitz, A.M., Westhoff, C., and Leonhardt, K.K. 2002. Therapeutic options to reduce or halt menstruation. *Female Patient* April suppl:12–16.

Kim, M.H. 2000. Dysfunctional uterine bleeding. In *Textbook of gynecology*, 2nd ed., eds. L.J. Copeland and J.F. Jarrell, pp. 533–540. Philadelphia: W.B. Saunders.

Livingstone, M., and Fraser, I.S. 2002. Mechanisms of abnormal uterine bleeding. *Human Reproduction Update* 8(1):60–67.

Long, C.A. 1996. Evaluation of patients with abnormal uterine bleeding. *American Journal of Obstetrics and Gynecology* 175(3):784–786.

Lusher, J.M. 1999. Systemic causes of excessive uterine bleeding. *Seminars in Hematology* 36(3):10–20.

Lusher, J.M., and Sarnaik, S. 1996. Hematology. *Journal of the American Medical Association* 275:1814–1815.

MacKay, H.T. 2002. Gynecology. In *Current medical diagnosis and treatment*, eds. L.M. Tierney, S.J. McPhee, and M.A. Papadakis, pp. 745–779. New York: McGraw-Hill.

Makarainen, L., and Ylikorala, O. 1986. Primary and myoma-associated menorrhagia: role of prostaglandins and effects of ibuprofen. *British Journal of Obstetrics and Gynaecology* 93:974–978.

March, C.M. 1997. Hysteroscopy and the uterine factor in infertility. In *Infertility, contraception, and reproductive endocrinology*, 4th ed., eds. R.A. Lobo, D.R. Mishell, R.J. Paulson et al., pp. 580–603. Malden, Mass.: Blackwell Science.

March, C.M., and Brenner, P.F. 1997. Dysfunctional uterine bleeding. In *Infertility, contraception, and reproductive endocrinology*, 4th ed., eds. R.A. Lobo, D.R. Mishell, R.J. Paulson et al., pp. 384–402. Malden, Mass.: Blackwell Science.

Mishell, D.R. 2001. Abnormal uterine bleeding. In *Comprehensive gynecology*, 4th ed., eds. M.A. Stenchever, W. Droegemueller, A.L. Herbst et al., pp. 1079–1097. St. Louis, Mo.: Mosby.

Motashaw, N.D. 1999. Management of the pubertal patient. In *Menorrhagia*, eds. S. Sheth and C. Sulton, pp. 73–77. Oxford, United Kingdom: Isis Medical Media.

Munro, M.G. 2000. Medical management of abnormal uterine bleeding. *Obstetrics and Gynecology Clinics of North America* 27(2):287–305.

_____. 2001. Dysfunctional uterine bleeding: advances in diagnosis and treatment. *Current Opinion in Obstetrics and Gynecology* 13(5):475–489.

Neuwirth, R.S., Duran, A.A., Singer, A. et al. 1994. The endometrial ablator: a new instrument. *Obstetrics and Gynecology* 83:792–796.

Nutley, T., and Dunson, T.R. 1997. Treatment of bleeding problems associated with progestin-only contraceptives: survey results. *Advances in Contraception* 13:419–428.

Oriel, K.A., and Schrager, S. 1999. Abnormal uterine bleeding. *American Family Physician* 60(5):1371–1380.

Policar, M. 2001. Contraceptive technology audiocassette No. 530. *Amenorrhea and dysfunctional bleeding in teens through menopause.* San Francisco: Contemporary Forums.

Richmond, J.A. 1997. Hysterosalpingography. In *Infertility, contraception, and reproductive endocrinology*, 4th ed., eds. R.A. Lobo, D.R. Mishell, R.J. Paulson et al., pp. 567–579. Malden, Mass.: Blackwell Science.

Shaw, R.W., and Duckitt, K. 1999. Management of menorrhagia in women of childbearing age. In *Menorrhagia*, eds. S. Sheth and C. Sulton, pp. 79–97. Oxford, United Kingdom: Isis Medical Media.

Sheth, S.S., and Allahbadia, G.N. 1999. Diagnosis of dysfunctional uterine bleeding. In *Menorrhagia*, eds. S. Sheth and C. Sulton, pp. 23–42. Oxford, United Kingdom: Isis Medical Media.

Shwayder, J.M. 2000. Pathophysiology of abnormal uterine bleeding. *Obstetrics and Gynecology Clinics of North America* 27(2):219–235.

Smith, S.K., Abel, M.H., Kelly, R.W. et al. 1981. Prostaglandin synthesis in the endometrium of women with ovular dysfunctional uterine bleeding. *British Journal of Obstetrics and Gynaecology* 88:434–442.

_____. 1982. The synthesis of prostaglandins from persistent proliferative endometrium. *Journal of Clinical Endocrinology and Metabolism* 55:284–289.

Speroff, L., Glass, R.H., and Kase, N.G. 1999. Dysfunctional uterine bleeding. In *Clinical gynecologic endocrinology and infertility*, 6th ed., eds. L. Speroff, R.H. Glass, and N.G. Kase, pp. 575–593. Baltimore, Md.: Lippincott Williams & Wilkins.

Stabinsky, S.A., Einstein, M., and Breen, J.L. 1999. Modern treatments of menorrhagia attributable to dysfunctional uterine bleeding. *Obstetrical and Gynecological Survey* 54(1):61–72.

Tang, G.W., and Lo, S.S. 1995. Levonorgestrel-releasing intrauterine device in the treatment of menorrhagia. *Contraception* 51:231–235.

Van Eijkeren, M.A., Christiaens, G.C.M.L., Scholten, P.C. et al. 1992. Menorrhagia: current drug treatment concepts. *Drugs* 43(2):201–209.

12-B
Abnormal Cervical Cytology

The most widely accepted classification system for cervical cytology is the NCI Bethesda System, which was revised in 2001 (Solomon et al. 2002) and is found in **Table 12B.1, The 2001 Bethesda System (Abridged)**.

The Bethesda System provides detailed descriptive information and recommendations for follow-up of abnormal findings. It includes these components:
→ A statement of the specimen type
→ A statement of the adequacy of the specimen
→ A general categorization (optional)
→ The use of automated review
→ The use of ancillary testing
→ Interpretation/result

Specimen Type

Specimen type specifies whether sampling has been obtained in the conventional method or with the newer, liquid-based cytology methods. In liquid-based cytology, cells are collected from the cervix as in a conventional Pap smear but are then placed in a preservative solution instead of on a slide. The solution is processed, and red and white blood cells, mucus, and debris are separated out. A layer of randomized, representative cells is evenly distributed on a slide in a monolayer. This process minimizes obscuring cells, improves specimen adequacy, and may decrease the reporting of atypical cells while increasing the detection of squamous intraepithelial lesions (Biscotti et al. 2002). An additional advantage of liquid-based cytology is that the residual solution can be used for HPV DNA testing (ancillary testing).

Specimen Adequacy

Adequacy of the specimen may be compromised by obscuring blood or inflammation, or scarce cellularity, which may necessitate repeat screening. The revised Bethesda System has retained the two categories "satisfactory" and "unsatisfactory" but has eliminated "satisfactory but limited by" to reduce confusion about the need to repeat sampling. Absence of endocervical cells may be noted in the report but is no longer considered an absolute indication for repeat sampling.

General Categorization

The "general categorization" component separates the diagnosis into "negative for intraepithelial lesion or malignancy" and "epithelial cell abnormality," thus simplifying triage of cytology reports. "Other" refers to cytologically normal cells whose presence may represent disease.

Interpretation/Result

The "interpretation/result" component of the report provides more detail for each category. Infection, reactive changes, and other non-neoplastic changes are found under the "negative for intraepithelial lesion or malignancy" category. Cytological abnormalities representing the spectrum—from squamous and glandular atypia to premalignancy to carcinoma—are reported under the category "epithelial cell abnormalities." The main changes brought about at the 2001 Bethesda conference include two new categories for atypical cells: ASC-US (atypical squamous cells of undetermined significance) and ASC-H (atypical squamous cells, cannot exclude high-grade squamous intraepithelial lesion). Terminology for low-grade squamous intraepithelial lesion (LSIL) and high-grade squamous intraepithelial lesion (HSIL) remains the same. Atypical glandular cells (AGC) have been divided into three new categories: AGC (specify endocervical, endometrial, or not otherwise specified [NOS]); AGC, favor neoplastic (specify endocervical or NOS); and endocervical adenocarcinoma in situ (AIS).

Most cervical cancer and its precursors are induced by certain types of human papillomavirus (HPV), which are sexually transmitted (Richart 1987). There are more than 125 types of HPV, of which forty affect the human genitalia. Genital HPV is further divided into low risk, intermediate risk, and high risk types, which can be detected by commercially available DNA tests. HPV also is associated with malignant transformation in the vagina, vulva, and anus (Spitzer et al. 1989). Many HPV infections resolve in 1–2 years after initial exposure.

Atypia of undetermined significance (i.e., ASC-US) may represent an early lesion with progressive potential or may occur as a result of a benign process, such as vaginitis, tampon use, intercourse, or spermicide use. Forty percent to 50% of ASC-US reports are associated with HPV (Cox 2001). Recent studies suggest that HPV DNA testing is a viable option for secondary screening of ASC-US results (Solomon et al. 2001). Those patients who test positive for high-risk DNA types are then referred for colposcopy.

ASC-US may be followed by qualifiers such as "favor reactive/reparative changes" or "suggestive of LSIL." However, "atypical squamous cells, cannot exclude HSIL (ASC-H)," forms a separate category based on the higher rate of histologic HSIL associated with this diagnosis.

Squamous intraepithelial lesion (SIL) is disordered cell proliferation resulting from a cellular response to HPV infection.

LSIL combines older terms—koilocytic atypia, condyloma, cervical intraepithelial neoplasia 1 (CIN 1), and mild dysplasia. Certain low-risk types of HPV (types 6, 11, and 42) as well as high-risk types are associated with LSIL (Lorincz et al. 1992). Rates of regression of LSIL are high, especially in young females (Moscicki 2001). HSIL includes abnormalities previously graded as moderate to severe dysplasia and carcinoma-in-situ (CIN 2–3). Certain high-risk types of HPV (types 16, 18, 31, 33, 35, 39, 45, 51, 52, 56, 58, 59, and 68) are commonly found in HSIL and their persistence over time is associated with the development of invasive cancer (Lorincz et al.1992). HSIL has a low rate of spontaneous regression and is considered an indication for treatment.

AGC is an uncommon diagnosis (0.1–0.3% of all cytologic samples) (Korn et al. 1998) but is ominous for invasive cancer of either the cervix or the endometrium and requires aggressive evaluation. Ten percent to 30% of patients with AGC will have high-grade disease on histology (Solomon et al. 2002). Unfortu-

---

Table 12B.1.   THE 2001 BETHESDA SYSTEM (ABRIDGED)

Specimen Adequacy
  Satisfactory for evaluation (*note presence/absence of endocervical/transformation zone component*)
  Unsatisfactory for evaluation… (*specify reason*)
    Specimen rejected/not processed (*specify reason*)
    Specimen processed and examined, but unsatisfactory for evaluation of epithelial abnormality because of (*specify reason*)

General Categorization (Optional)
  Negative for intraepithelial lesion or malignancy
  Epithelial cell abnormality
  Other

Interpretation/Result
  Negative for Intraepithelial Lesion or Malignancy
    Organisms
      Trichomonas vaginalis
      Fungal organisms morphologically consistent with *Candida* species
      Shift in flora suggestive of bacterial vaginosis
      Bacteria morphologically consistent with *Actinomyces* species
      Cellular changes consistent with herpes simplex virus
    Other non-neoplastic findings (*Optional to report; list not comprehensive*)
      Reactive cellular changes associated with
        inflammation (includes typical repair)
        radiation
        intrauterine contraceptive device
      Glandular cells status posthysterectomy
      Atrophy

Interpretation/Result (continued)
  Epithelial Cell Abnormalities
    Squamous cell
      Atypical squamous cells (ASC)
        of undetermined significance (ASC-US)
        cannot exclude HSIL (ASC-H)
      Low-grade squamous intraepithelial lesion (LSIL) encompassing: human papillomavirus/mild dysplasia/cervical intraepithelial neoplasia (CIN) 1
      High-grade squamous intraepithelial lesion (HSIL) encompassing: moderate and severe dysplasia, carcinoma in situ; CIN 2 and CIN 3
    Squamous cell carcinoma
    Glandular cell
      Atypical glandular cells (AGC) (*specify endocervical, endometrial, or not otherwise specified*)
      Atypical glandular cells, favor neoplastic (*specify endocervical or not otherwise specified*)
      Endocervical adenocarcinoma in situ (AIS)
      Adenocarcinoma
    Other (*List not comprehensive*)
      Endometrial cells in a woman ≥40 years of age

AUTOMATED REVIEW AND ANCILLARY TESTING
(*Include as appropriate*)

EDUCATIONAL NOTES AND SUGGESTIONS
(*Optional*)

Source: Reprinted with permission from Solomon, D., Davey, D., Kurman, R. et al. 2002. The 2001 Bethesda System: terminology for reporting results of cervical cytology. *Journal of the American Medical Association* 287(16):2114–2119.

nately, cervical cytology is not as sensitive in screening for glandular abnormalities as it is for squamous abnormalities.

The "Other" category has been modified from the 1988 version of the Bethesda System to include the reporting of endometrial cells in women 40 years old or older, regardless of the last menstrual date and status.

Cofactors

Many cofactors contribute to the etiology of squamous cell carcinoma of the cervix. These include multiple sexual partners, early age at first intercourse, cigarette smoking, immunosuppression, and genetic susceptibility. Oral contraceptive use has been shown in different studies to be both contributory and protective (Moreno et al. 2002, Moscicki 2001).

Diagnosis

Because of the high prevalence of HPV, the sexually active female population should have cervical cytology screening every 1–3 years beginning at the onset of sexual activity. In women who are immunosuppressed, cytology screening should be performed annually. Proper technique is essential to reduce false-negative sampling errors. (See **Table 12B.2, Obtaining a Cytological Sample**.)

The DNA hybridization techniques that detect and type the papillomavirus are widely available, and may help to triage certain patients into low-risk and high-risk categories. Appropriate patients for HPV typing are those with ASC-US cytology; they need to be tested only for high-risk types. Those with ASC-H, LSIL, HSIL, or AGC already are considered at higher risk and

Figure 12B.1.   MANAGEMENT OF WOMEN WITH ATYPICAL SQUAMOUS CELLS OF UNDETERMINED SIGNIFICANCE (ASC-US)

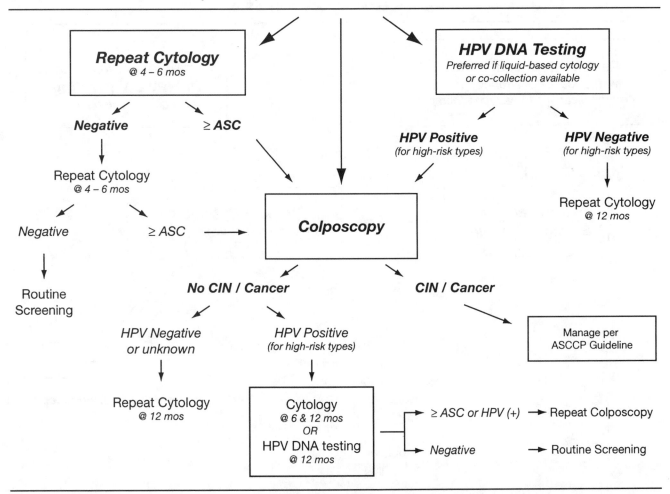

Source: The Consensus Guidelines algorithms originally appeared in and are reprinted from *The Journal of Lower Genital Tract Disease* Vol. 6 Issue 2 and are reprinted with the permission of ASCCP © American Society for Colposcopy and Cervical Pathology 2002. No copies of the algorithms may be made without the prior consent of ASCCP.

Table 12B.2. OBTAINING A CYTOLOGICAL SAMPLE

An endocervical brush and plastic spatula are the ideal materials for obtaining a cervical sample. A single slide for both ectocervical and endocervical sampling may be used. Vaginal pool sampling has a high false-negative rate and should be avoided. The following steps are recommended in sampling the cervix:

- A speculum moistened with water and not lubricant (which may contaminate the specimen) should be inserted into the vagina. Bimanual examination should be performed after the cytological smear is obtained.
- Excessive amounts of cervical or vaginal discharge should be gently removed with a cotton swab, with care taken to avoid scraping the cervical epithelium. Cervical cultures should be performed after the cytological sampling.
- Cytological sampling should be avoided during times of heavy menstrual bleeding. If bleeding is minimal, the sample may be taken and will usually be adequate for evaluation.
- The ectocervix should be sampled first by scraping the entire cervical portio with a plastic spatula.
- The endocervical canal is sampled by inserting the brush gently until resistance is met, then turning the brush only one-quarter turn to prevent excessive bleeding. When both samples have been obtained, they should rapidly be applied to the slide in a uniform fashion and be fixed (ideally within 4 seconds). Spray fixatives should be held at least 10 inches from the slide to prevent distortion of the cells.

©L. Hanson, 2003

Figure 12B.2. MANAGEMENT OF WOMEN WITH ATYPICAL SQUAMOUS CELLS OF UNDETERMINED SIGNIFICANCE (ASC-US) IN SPECIAL CIRCUMSTANCES

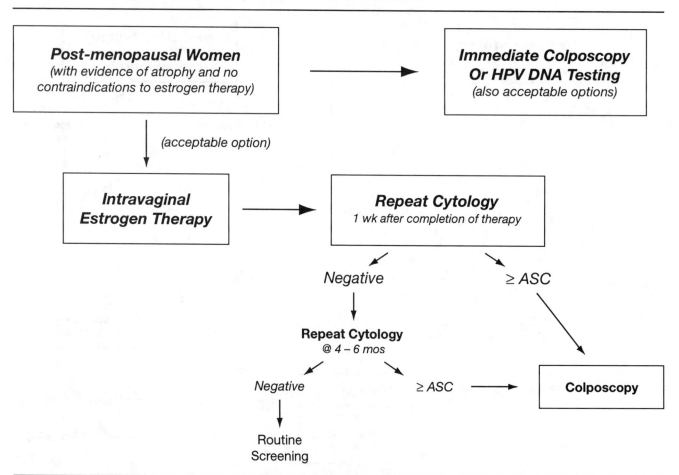

should not have reflex HPV typing. HPV typing is acceptable as a 12-month follow-up screen in women with ASC-H and LSIL when no CIN has been found, as many HPV infections will resolve over time. HPV typing should not be used as an additional screen in those patients with normal cervical cytology.

Colposcopy and directed biopsy are methods for evaluating patients who have abnormal cervical cytology results. Clinicians with specialized training may perform colposcopic examinations and therapeutic procedures in certain settings. While it is not the intent of this chapter to serve as a guide for colposcopy, aspects of the colposcopic examination and therapeutic options will be mentioned. Clinicians who perform colposcopy should refer to site-specific guidelines and protocols.

Colposcopy and directed biopsy allow the clinician to rule out the presence of invasive carcinoma and to select the best method of treatment by determining the location and extent of pre-invasive lesions. Three percent to 5% acetic acid is applied to the cervix, which is then viewed under magnification with the colposcope. The location of the squamocolumnar junction is noted; it may appear on the cervical portio or may be located in the endocervical canal. The squamocolumnar junction marks the inner border of the transformation zone, an area where abnormalities are likely to arise. Its location will influence treatment decisions.

Abnormal lesions may be represented by acetowhite epithelium, punctation, mosaic patterns, and/or atypical blood vessels. Directed biopsy of these lesions allows for histologic confirmation of colposcopic findings. An endocervical curettage is often performed to determine if abnormal tissue is present in the endocervical canal. Colposcopic evaluation of the vaginal and vulvar surfaces is indicated to assess for multifocal genital tract lesions. (See the **Human Papillomavirus** chapter in Section 13.) After application of acetic acid, Schiller's or Lugol's solution also may be applied to the cervix and vaginal tissues. These iodine solutions stain mature squamous epithelium, which is high in glycogen, a deep mahogany brown. Columnar epithelium and dysplastic epithelium are nonglycogenated and do not stain with iodine.

Figure 12B.3. MANAGEMENT OF WOMEN WITH ATYPICAL SQUAMOUS CELLS: CANNOT EXCLUDE HIGH-GRADE SIL (ASC-H)

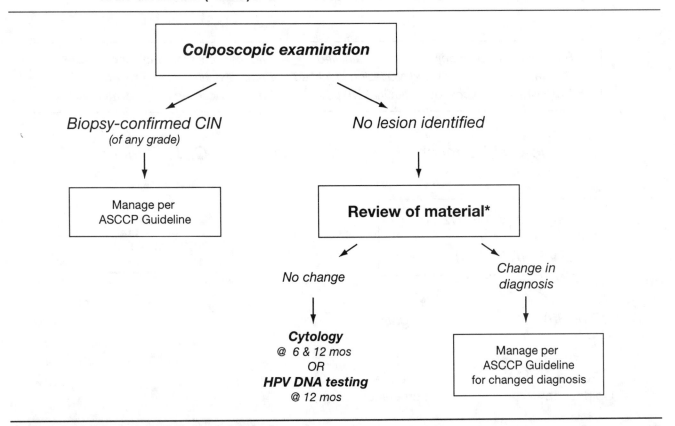

* Includes referral cytology, colposcopic findings, and all biopsies
Source: The Consensus Guidelines algorithms originally appeared in and are reprinted from *The Journal of Lower Genital Tract Disease* Vol. 6 Issue 2 and are reprinted with the permission of ASCCP © American Society for Colposcopy and Cervical Pathology 2002. No copies of the algorithms may be made without the prior consent of ASCCP.

Management

After cytology, HPV DNA type, histology, and/or colposcopic findings are compared and evaluated, management decisions can be made. A consensus conference of experts sponsored by the American Society for Colposcopy and Cervical Pathology (ASCCP) met in 2001 and developed evidence-based guidelines for managing abnormal cervical cytology (Wright et al. 2002). (See **Figures 12B.1–12B.8**.) All guidelines will likely be revised over time as new technologies are developed and/or refined. Separate consensus guidelines for managing women with cervical histological abnormalities will be published at a later date. The reader is directed to future ASCCP guidelines and publications.

In many settings, LSIL is followed by expectant management—i.e., by colposcopy and cervical cytology at four- to six-month intervals. Treatment is initiated if LSIL persists, if the diagnosis progresses to HSIL, if the patient desires therapy, or if she is unreliable or unlikely to return for follow-up. Patients with AGC that represents neoplasia are always treated. Treatment may include local destructive methods, such as cryotherapy, laser ablation, chemical ablation (with 5-fluorouracil in cream), excisional biopsy, loop electrosurgical excision procedure (LEEP), and conization (laser or cold knife).

DATABASE

SUBJECTIVE

→ Risk factors may include:
- History of HPV infection
- Multiple sexual partners
- Early age at first intercourse
- Sexual partner with HPV or a history of HPV exposure
- Drug, alcohol, and/or tobacco use
- Poor health habits, including infrequent Pap smears

Figure 12B.4. MANAGEMENT OF WOMEN WITH LOW-GRADE SQUAMOUS INTRAEPITHELIAL LESIONS (LSIL)*

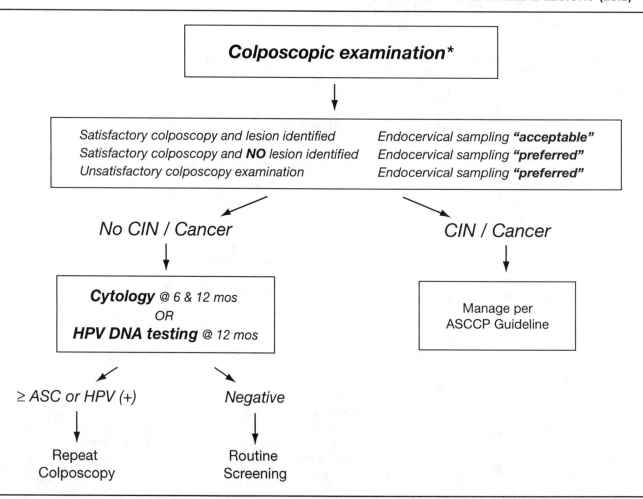

---

* Management options may vary if the woman is pregnant, postmenopausal, or an adolescent (see text)

Source: The Consensus Guidelines algorithms originally appeared in and are reprinted from *The Journal of Lower Genital Tract Disease* Vol. 6 Issue 2 and are reprinted with the permission of ASCCP © American Society for Colposcopy and Cervical Pathology 2002. No copies of the algorithms may be made without the prior consent of ASCCP.

- Immunosuppressive disease or therapy
→ Symptoms may include:
  - Vaginal discharge, odor, intermenstrual or postcoital bleeding (sometimes seen with cervical malignancy)
  - Weight loss, fatigue (late signs of cervical carcinoma)
→ History to include:
  - Age
  - Age at first intercourse
  - Number of sexual partners
  - Birth control method, use of barrier method
  - History of HPV or other sexually transmitted infections in the patient or partner(s)
  - Date of last Pap smear and result
  - Prior abnormal cervical cytology
  - History of diethylstilbestrol (DES) exposure in utero
  - History of drug, alcohol, or tobacco abuse
  - History of medical condition (including HIV status) or therapies that alter the function of the immune system

- Menstrual history, including the date of the last menstrual period; current pregnancy, unexplained vaginal bleeding, menopause

---

OBJECTIVE

NOTE: Colposcopic evaluation and directed biopsy should be performed only by clinicians with special training. Aspects of this examination have been italicized below to emphasize this distinction.

→ *External genitalia may exhibit erythema, atrophy, discharge, or gross lesions (including condylomata or leukoplakia). Acetowhite lesions with or without vessels may be present after application of 3–5% acetic acid, suggesting a subclinical HPV infection or vulvar intraepithelial neoplasia* (data indicate that some acetowhite lesions represent a benign, non-HPV entity) (Bergeron et al. 1990).

→ *Speculum examination may reveal discharge, erythema, or atrophy of the cervix and/or vagina, and gross lesions*

Figure 12B.5.   MANAGEMENT OF WOMEN WITH LOW-GRADE SQUAMOUS INTRAEPITHELIAL LESIONS IN SPECIAL CIRCUMSTANCES

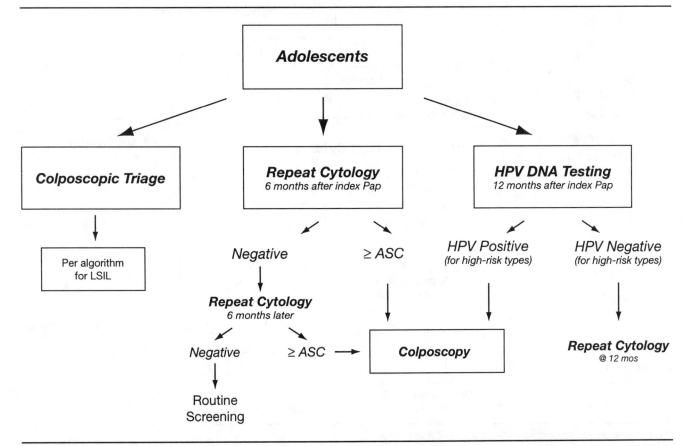

Source: The Consensus Guidelines algorithms originally appeared in and are reprinted from *The Journal of Lower Genital Tract Disease* Vol. 6 Issue 2 and are reprinted with the permission of ASCCP © American Society for Colposcopy and Cervical Pathology 2002. No copies of the algorithms may be made without the prior consent of ASCCP.

including condylomata and leukoplakia. Cervical carcinoma may present as an ulceration, a raised friable lesion, or necrosis, or it may appear as normal cervical tissue. Classic DES changes (cervical sulcus, collar) may be noted.

→ Wet smear may indicate fungal, bacterial, or trichomonal infection.

→ Cervical cultures may indicate chlamydia, gonorrhea, herpes, or other infections.

→ *Colposcopic examination (after application of 3–5% acetic acid) may reveal acetowhite lesions of the vulva, vagina, and cervix with or without the presence of abnormal vessels (punctations, mosaicism, atypical vessels). The squamocolumnar junction should be located.*

→ Nonstaining cervical and vaginal tissue may be observed after application of an iodine solution (Schiller's or Lugol's solution).

→ Bimanual examination may reveal a hard, enlarged, and fixed cervix (in late cervical carcinoma).

→ See the **Human Papillomavirus** chapter in Section 13.

ASSESSMENT

→ Cytologic diagnosis

→ HPV DNA diagnosis

→ R/O condylomata acuminata

→ R/O vaginitis/cervicitis

→ R/O atrophic vaginitis

→ R/O concomitant sexually transmitted diseases (STDs)

→ *Assess the presence of colposcopic vulvar, vaginal, and/or cervical lesion(s), including the location, extent, and characteristics of lesions.*

→ *Assess the location of the squamocolumnar junction.*

Figure 12B.6.   MANAGEMENT OF WOMEN WITH LOW-GRADE SQUAMOUS INTRAEPITHELIAL LESIONS IN SPECIAL CIRCUMSTANCES

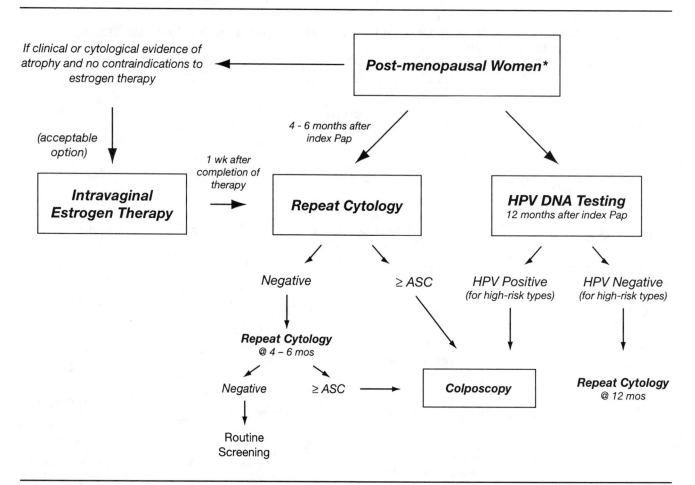

* For low-risk, post-menopausal women with a history of negative screening

PLAN

DIAGNOSTIC TESTS

→ Pap smear may be repeated. (See **Figures 12B.1–12B.8** for interval.)

→ HPV DNA typing as indicated. (See **Figures 12B.1–12B.8** for indication and interval.)

→ Wet mount as indicated to assess for vaginitis

→ Appropriate testing to rule out STDs

→ *Cervical, vaginal, and/or vulvar biopsies as indicated by site-specific guidelines and protocols*

TREATMENT/MANAGEMENT

→ Negative for intraepithelial lesion or malignancy
  - Organisms:
    - Treat with an appropriate agent if the patient is symptomatic or as indicated.
  - Other non-neoplastic findings (reactive changes, atrophy, no endocervical cells):
    - No need to treat or repeat.

- Other:
  - Endometrial biopsy may be indicated in a woman 40 years old or older who has endometrial cells on Pap smear. The decision may be influenced by risk factors, such as obesity, diabetes, abnormal bleeding pattern, and phase of the menstrual cycle (endometrial cells are normal in the first 10–12 days of the cycle) (The Permanente Medical Group 2001).

→ ASC-US. (See **Figure 12B.1, Management of Women with Atypical Squamous Cells of Undetermined Significance [ASC-US].**)

→ ASC-US in postmenopausal women. (See **Figure 12B.2, Management of Women with Atypical Squamous Cells of Undetermined Significance [ASC-US] in Special Circumstances.**)

→ ASC-H. (See **Figure 12B.3, Management of Women with Atypical Squamous Cells: Cannot Exclude High Grade SIL [ASC-H].**)

→ LSIL. (See **Figure 12B.4, Management of Women with Low-Grade Squamous Intraepithelial Lesions [LSIL].**)

Figure 12B.7.   MANAGEMENT OF WOMEN WITH HIGH-GRADE SQUAMOUS INTRAEPITHELIAL LESIONS (HSIL)*

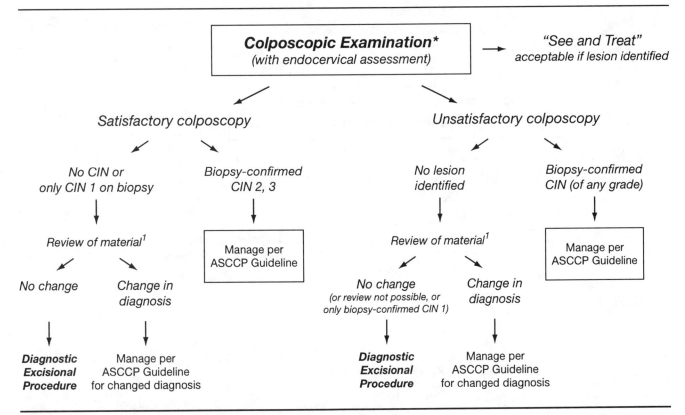

* Management options may vary if the woman is pregnant, postmenopausal, or an adolescent

1 Includes referral cytology, colposcopic findings, and all biopsies

Source: The Consensus Guidelines algorithms originally appeared in and are reprinted from *The Journal of Lower Genital Tract Disease* Vol. 6 Issue 2 and are reprinted with the permission of ASCCP © American Society for Colposcopy and Cervical Pathology 2002. No copies of the algorithms may be made without the prior consent of ASCCP.

→ LSIL in adolescents. (See **Figure 12B.5, Management of Women with Low-Grade Squamous Intraepithelial Lesions in Special Circumstances**.)

→ LSIL in postmenopausal women. (See **Figure 12B.6, Management of Women with Low-Grade Squamous Intraepithelial Lesions in Special Circumstances**.)

→ HSIL. (See **Figure 12B.7, Management of Women with High-Grade Squamous Intraepithelial Lesions [HSIL]**.)

→ AGC, AGC, favor neoplastic, AIS. (See **Figure 12B.8, Management of Women with Atypical Glandular Cells [AGC]**.)

→ Adenocarcinoma
 ■ Refer to a physician for evaluation and definitive therapy.

→ Malignant cells
 ■ Refer to a physician for evaluation and definitive therapy.

CONSULTATION

→ As indicated by cytology and clinical findings. This may include consultation with the cytopathologist for clarification or review of findings.

→ Referral to a physician as indicated for colposcopy and/or definitive therapy. See "Treatment/Management," above.

→ Depending on site-specific policy, referral to a physician for colposcopy may be required if the patient has HSIL on cervical cytology.

→ Depending on site-specific policy, referral to a physician for colposcopy may be required if the patient is pregnant and has abnormal cytology.

→ Referral to a physician is mandatory if cytology or clinical findings indicate malignancy.

PATIENT EDUCATION

→ Discuss the concept of cervical cancer and its precursors being related to infection by a sexually transmitted agent (i.e., HPV).

Figure 12B.8.   **MANAGEMENT OF WOMEN WITH ATYPICAL GLANDULAR CELLS (AGC)**

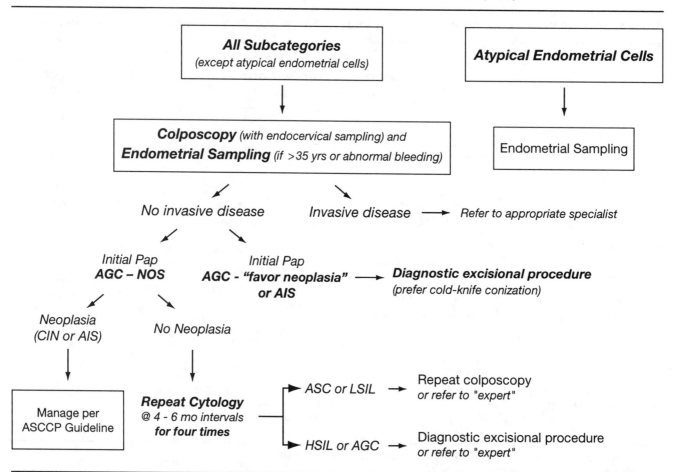

Source: The Consensus Guidelines algorithms originally appeared in and are reprinted from *The Journal of Lower Genital Tract Disease* Vol. 6 Issue 2 and are reprinted with the permission of ASCCP © American Society for Colposcopy and Cervical Pathology 2002. No copies of the algorithms may be made without the prior consent of ASCCP.

- Advise regarding sexual transmission of HPV and methods to prevent spread and re-infection. (See **Table 13A.2, Safer Sex Practices** in the **Chancroid** chapter in Section 13, and **Table 12I.1, Recommendations for Individuals to Prevent STD/PID** in the **Pelvic Inflammatory Disease** chapter.)
→ Discuss the possible premalignant nature of cervical intraepithelial neoplasia and the need for close and continuous follow-up.
→ Discuss the emotional effect of an abnormal cytological finding on the patient's self-esteem, body image, and sexuality.
  - Refer for counseling when indicated.
→ Discuss the possible relationship of cigarette smoking as a co-carcinogen. (See the **Human Papillomavirus** chapter in Section 13.)

FOLLOW-UP

NOTE: Site-specific practices for follow-up vary.
→ Patient treated for LGSIL/HGSIL:
  - Cytology every 4–6 months for one year (colposcopy and endocervical sampling often are done on the first visit), then every 6 months for at least one more year.
→ See also **Figures 12B.1–12B.8**.

BIBLIOGRAPHY

Bergeron, C., Ferenczy, A., Richart, R.M. et al. 1990. Micropapillomatosis labialis appears unrelated to human papillomavirus. *Obstetrics and Gynecology* 76(2):281–286.

Bernard-Pearl, L., and Smith-McCune, K. 2001. Controversies in the management of ASCUS and AGCUS: two very different beasts. *Obstetrics, Gynecology and Fertility* 24(1):7–23.

Biscotti, C.V., O'Brien, D.L., Gero, T.L. et al. 2002. *Journal of Reproductive Medicine* 47(1):9–13.

Coppelson, M., Pixley E., and Reid, B. 1986. *Colposcopy*, 3rd ed. Springfield, Ill.: Charles C. Thomas.

Cox, J.T. 2001. Understanding an ASCUS Pap result. *HPV News* 11(2):2–4.

Korn, A., Judson, P., and Zaloudek, C. 1998. Importance of atypical glandular cells of uncertain significance in cervical cytologic smears. *Journal of Reproductive Medicine* 43:774–778.

Lorincz, A.T., Reid, R., Jenson A.B. et al. 1992. Human papillomavirus infection of the cervix: relative risk associations of 15 common anogenital types. *Obstetrics and Gynecology* 79:328–337.

Moreno, V., Bosch, F.X., Munoz, N. et al. 2002. Effects of oral contraceptives on risk of cervical cancer in women with human papillomavirus infection: the IARC multicentric case-control study. *Lancet* 359(3):1085–1092.

Moscicki, A.B. 2001. Risks for incident human papillomavirus infection and low-grade squamous intraepithelial lesion development in young females. *Journal of the American Medical Association* 285(23):2995–3002.

Nelson, J.H., Averette, H.E., and Richart, R.M. 1984. Dysplasia, carcinoma in situ, and early invasive cervical carcinoma. *CA-A Cancer Journal for Clinicians* 34:306–327.

The Permanente Medical Group. 2001. *Cervical cancer screening.*

Richart, R.M. 1987. Causes and management of cervical intraepithelial neoplasia. *Cancer* 60(8):1951–1959.

Solomon, D., Davey, D., Kurman, R. et al. 2002. The 2001 Bethesda System: terminology for reporting results of cervical cytology. *Journal of the American Medical Association* 287(16):2114–2119.

Solomon, D., Shiffman, M., and Tarone, R. 2001. Comparison of three management strategies for patients with atypical squamous cells of undetermined significance; baseline results from a randomized trial. *Journal of the National Cancer Institute* 93(4):293–299.

Spitzer, M., Krumholz, B.A., and Seltzer, V.L. 1989. The multicentric nature of disease related to human papillomavirus infection of the female lower genital tract. *Obstetrics and Gynecology* 73(3):303–307.

Wright, T., Cox, J.T., Massad, L.S. et al. 2002. 2001 consensus guidelines for the management of women with cervical cytological abnormalities. *Journal of the American Medical Association* 267(16):2120–2129.

12-C

Amenorrhea—Secondary

Secondary amenorrhea is defined as the absence of menses for six months or a length of time equal to at least three of the previous menstrual cycles (Speroff et al. 1999). For women with prior *oligomenorrhea*, the diagnosis necessitates up to 12 months without menses or at least six cycle intervals (McIver et al. 1997). Cyclic menstrual bleeding requires a uterus with a responsive endometrium, an unobstructed outflow tract, normally functioning ovaries, and an intact hypothalamic-pituitary-ovarian axis (Kiningham et al. 1996). Once pregnancy has been eliminated as a cause of missed menses, the approach to evaluating the amenorrheic patient can be broken down into four "compartments" where pathology may be encountered (Speroff et al. 1999), which are reviewed below.

In addition, this chapter will review *anovulation* associated with *polycystic ovary syndrome* and "postpill amenorrhea."

Compartment 1:
Disorders of the Uterus (Outflow Tract)

Destruction of the endometrium as a result of curettage, uterine surgery, or infection may result in *intrauterine adhesions* (IUAs) or synechiae (*Asherman's syndrome*) and produce secondary amenorrhea. Infectious causes include tuberculosis and schistosomiasis, which are rare; intrauterine device (IUD)-related endometritis; and severe generalized pelvic infection. IUAs may partially or completely obliterate the endometrial cavity, the internal cervical os, the cervical canal, or combinations of these areas. Extensive uterine scarring may be associated with such complications as reproductive failure, premature labor, placenta accreta/previa, and/or postpartum hemorrhage (Mishell, Jr. 1997, Speroff et al. 1999).

Compartment 2:
Disorders of the Ovary

Ovarian failure (*hypergonadotrophic hypogonadism*) normally presents at the time of menopause, which occurs, on average, at age 50–51 years. *Premature ovarian failure* (POF) is a condition that causes amenorrhea, hypoestrogenism, and elevated gonadotropins before the age of 40 years (Anasti 1998). In women with secondary amenorrhea, POF occurs in 4–18% (Anasti 1998). Although POF was once thought to be permanent, a very small number of patients will experience spontaneous remission with a return of normal ovarian function and a remote possibility of future pregnancy (Anasti 1998, Speroff et al. 1999).

The causes of POF may be idiopathic, autoimmune, or due to radiotherapy or cytotoxic drugs. In most cases, the etiology is unknown. Autoimmune ovarian failure occurs in other organ-specific autoimmune diseases (e.g., autoimmune thyroid disease, Addison's disease, and Type 1 diabetes mellitus) (McIver et al. 1997). Other conditions associated with POF include myasthenia gravis, Crohn's disease, rheumatoid arthritis, idiopathic thrombocytopenia purpura, vitiligo, galactosemia, systemic lupus erythematosus, and autoimmune hemolytic anemia (Anasti 1998, Speroff et al. 1999). Occasionally, infection or surgery may precipitate POF. The condition occurs in association with mumps and in women who have had ovarian cystectomies (usually bilateral) for removal of benign ovarian cysts (e.g., dermoid cysts or endometriomas) (Warren 1996).

Ovarian (or adrenal) tumors and ovarian stromal hyperthecosis, conditions that may secrete androgens autonomously, can also result in secondary amenorrhea and pronounced virilization. (See the **Hirsutism** chapter.)

Compartment 3:
Disorders of the Anterior Pituitary

Hyperprolactinemia is the most common endocrine disorder of the hypothalamic-pituitary axis. Causes may be physiologic, pathologic, or pharmacologic. Elevated prolactin produces amenorrhea by affecting the frequency/amplitude of pulses of gonadotropin-releasing hormone (GnRH), probably through changes in dopamine release. In addition, hyperprolactinemia may interfere with ovulation and normal corpus luteum formation by acting directly on the ovary (Biller 1999, Luciano 1999, Shoupe et al. 1997, Speroff et al. 1999). A significant metabolic consequence of chronic hyperprolactinemia is osteopenia/osteoporosis, which is associated with prolonged hypoestrogenism caused by hyperprolactinemia-induced hypogonadism (Luciano 1999).

The most common tumor of the pituitary is the *prolactin-secreting adenoma*, which is thought to cause dysfunction by suppressing GnRH secretion and inhibiting the release of luteinizing hormone (LH) and follicle-stimulating hormone (FSH), and by affecting ovarian secretion of androgens (Warren 1996). Prolactin-secreting adenomas <1 cm in diameter are referred to as *microadenomas*; tumors >1 cm are referred to as *macroadenomas* (Speroff et al. 1999). As many as one-third of patients with secondary amenorrhea will have a pituitary adenoma, and if galactorrhea is present, half will have an abnormal sella turcica.

Suspicion of a pituitary tumor may be increased if the patient has signs of acromegaly or Cushing's disease with excessive secretion of growth hormone and adrenocorticotropic hormone (ACTH). Rarely, a tumor that secretes thyroid-stimulating hormone (TSH) (fewer than 1–3% of pituitary tumors) causes secondary hyperthyroidism and disruption of menstrual cycles (Speroff et al. 1999, Warren 1996). Other rare tumors include craniopharyngiomas (hypothalamic-pituitary lesion), meningiomas, gliomas, metastatic tumors, and chordomas. Malignant tumors of the pituitary are quite rare (Speroff et al. 1999).

Non-neoplastic lesions, which can cause pituitary compression leading to hypogonadotrophic amenorrhea, include cysts, tuberculosis, sarcoidosis, and fat deposits (Speroff et al. 1999). *Pituitary insufficiency* can be a result of *Sheehan's syndrome* (ischemia and infarction of the pituitary as late sequelae to obstetrical hemorrhage/hypotension) or radiation, surgery, or trauma to the pituitary gland (Gomel et al. 1990).

The *empty sella syndrome* is another, mostly benign entity that may be associated with galactorrhea and normal or elevated prolactin. This condition is characterized by herniation of the subarachnoid membrane into the sella turcica due to a congenital defect or incompetence of the sellar diaphragm (Shoupe et al. 1997, Speroff et al. 1999). Compression of the pituitary gland causing hyperprolactinemia or galactorrhea may ensue; a prolactin-secreting adenoma also may coexist (Speroff et al. 1999).

Pharmacologic causes of hyperprolactinemia and secondary amenorrhea include drugs that interfere with dopamine metabolism or action. Examples of such drugs are antipsychotics (phenothiazine derivatives), antidepressants (tricyclics, monoamine oxidase inhibitors), antihypertensive agents (calcium channel blockers, methyldopa, reserpine), narcotics, and oral contraceptives (Kiningham et al. 1996, Luciano 1999, Mishell, Jr. 1997, Shoupe et al. 1997).

A variety of *pathologic factors* can affect prolactin production. They include renal failure, cirrhosis, neurogenic factors such as chest wall lesions or spinal cord lesions, chronic chest wall irritation or chest trauma, and herpes zoster (Shoupe et al. 1997). An indirect pituitary effect that causes amenorrhea is *hypothyroidism*. Primary hypothyroidism (usually *Hashimoto's thyroiditis*) is responsible for about 3–5% of cases of galactorrhea/hyperprolactinemia. The disease is characterized by low serum thyroxine (T4) and decreased negative feedback on the hypothalamic-pituitary axis, resulting in increased secretion of thyrotropin-releasing hormone and increased levels of both TSH and prolactin (Shoupe et al. 1997).

Lastly, there is a *physiological factor* that affects prolactin: lactation. Throughout breast-feeding, prolactin levels remain elevated, although their patterns or values do not predict the postpartum duration of amenorrhea or infertility (Speroff et al. 1999). (See also "Diagnostic Tests," below.)

Compartment 4: Disorders of the Central Nervous System (Hypothalamus)

Hypothalamic amenorrhea (hypogonadotropic hypogonadism) is usually diagnosed by excluding pituitary lesions (Speroff et al. 1999). Hypothalamic problems are the most common category of hypogonadotrophic amenorrhea and are frequently associated with a stressful life situation (e.g., death in the family, divorce, or school/work stress). In addition, women with eating disorders, those who are underweight, or those who exercise strenuously can develop hypothalamic amenorrhea (Mishell, Jr. 1997, Speroff et al. 1999). The prevalence of menstrual dysfunction in athletic women varies with the level of competition and degree of concomitant psychological stress (Reid 2000). Simple weight loss also may trigger hypothalamic amenorrhea.

The mechanisms believed to be responsible for stress and exercise-related hypothalamic amenorrhea appear to be related to increases in endogenous opioids and dopamine, which result in the alteration of GnRH pulsatile secretion. That, in turn, inhibits LH and FSH release. Weight loss-associated amenorrhea appears to be mainly attributable to failure of normal GnRH release and possibly a pituitary disorder when weight loss is severe (Mishell, Jr. 1997, Speroff et al. 1999). Estradiol levels depend on the degree of hypothalamic suppression and, in some cases, may be quite low (e.g., in cases of exercise-induced amenorrhea or anorexia nervosa). Because osteoporosis is a concern in amenorrheic women with low estradiol levels, they may need hormone therapy if the hypothalamic dysfunction is longstanding.

In 1992, the American College of Sports Medicine coined the term "the female athlete triad," a syndrome comprising three interrelated components: disordered eating, amenorrhea, and osteoporosis. Many female athletes are at risk of one or more of these patterns, which, alone or in combination, can reduce physical performance and cause morbidity and mortality. Clinicians should become aware of this triad and incorporate strategies to recognize, prevent, and treat these problems in physically active women (Fagan 1998, Otis et al. 1997, West 1998).

Uncommon hypothalamic lesions associated with amenorrhea may include craniopharyngiomas, granulomatous disease (tuberculosis and sarcoidosis), and sequelae of encephalitis (Mishell, Jr. 1997). Severe and debilitating systemic illness also may cause hypothalamic amenorrhea.

Polycystic Ovary Syndrome

Polycystic ovary syndrome (PCOS) is a multilevel abnormality characterized by ovarian dysfunction (oligomenorrhea, anovulation, infertility), androgen excess (hirsutism, acne), and morphological abnormalities of the ovaries (cystic enlargement, stromal expansion) (Norman et al. 2001). Clinical expression of PCOS is quite heterogeneous, however, and the above-mentioned features may not be consistently present. No single factor is responsible for the abnormalities associated with this syndrome and, to date, there is no accepted theory about its pathogenesis (Guzick 1998, Hunter et al. 2000, Lobo et al. 1997). In addition to the major features of the disorder, insulin resistance and compensatory hyperinsulinemia are intrinsic to PCOS, along with an increased prevalence of features of the *metabolic syndrome* (i.e., glucose intolerance, Type 2 diabetes mellitus, and hyperlipidemia) (Iuorno et al. 2001, Norman et al. 2001). Diversity in the expression of the syndrome may be explained by genetic as well as environmental modulation (Lobo et al. 1997).

It is postulated that PCOS arises from a variety of causes, and once established, the condition has a chronic and self-perpetuating nature (Lobo et al. 1997). Defects may occur in the hypothalamic compartment (dopamine, opioids), the pituitary (LH sensitivity), and the adrenal gland (hyperandrogenism) (Lobo et al. 1997). Activation of the hypothalamic-pituitary axis causes LH stimulation of ovarian androgen excess (i.e., increased amounts of testosterone, androstenedione, and dehydroepiandrosterone [DHEA], although these may not be consistently elevated on testing) (Lobo et al. 1997). Hyperestrogenism due to unopposed estrogen, a major endocrine feature of PCOS, may contribute to the characteristic gonadotropin abnormalities. Hyperinsulinemia contributes to ovarian and adrenal hyperandrogenism (Lobo et al. 1997). Mild increases in prolactin occur in some women.

The chronic anovulatory state of PCOS, with the long-term effects of unopposed estrogen, places women at risk for endometrial hyperplasia, endometrial cancer, and possibly breast cancer (Hunter et al. 2000). Risk for coronary artery disease also may exist secondary to abnormal lipoprotein profiles (i.e., elevated levels of cholesterol, triglyceride, and low-density lipoprotein cholesterol, and low levels of high-density lipoprotein cholesterol and Apo A1 levels) (Carmina et al. 1999, Lobo et al. 1997). As noted above, the insulin resistance associated with PCOS presents increased risk for glucose intolerance or Type 2 diabetes mellitus (Carmina et al. 1999, Hunter et al. 2000, Lobo et al. 1997). When present, obesity accentuates the endocrine disturbance and the long-term consequences and risks (Carmina et al. 1999, Lobo et al. 1997).

Adrenal abnormalities resulting in excessive androgen production, such as late-onset (i.e., adult-onset or nonclassic) congenital adrenal hyperplasia (CAH), can mimic PCOS and must be ruled out in patients with hirsutism or other virilizing signs. (See the **Hirsutism** chapter.)

Postpill Amenorrhea

It was postulated that a specific syndrome of secondary amenorrhea after discontinuation of oral contraceptives (OCs) affected some women due to the suppressive effects of the hormone on the hypothalamic-pituitary-ovarian axis—the so-called "postpill amenorrhea." More recent work indicates that the incidence of secondary amenorrhea following OC discontinuation is no greater than the incidence that occurs spontaneously in the population at large (Reid 2000). Investigation should be pursued if a patient remains amenorrheic six months after discontinuing the pill (or 12 months after discontinuing Depo-Provera®) (Speroff et al. 1999).

DATABASE

SUBJECTIVE

→ Symptoms are variable and depend on the compartment affected. Patients typically present with hypomenorrhea, oligomenorrhea, amenorrhea (at times with terminal menorrhagia), and/or galactorrhea.
  ■ A number of systems may be affected as described previously.
→ Stress, exercise, malnutrition, and obesity are commonly associated factors.
→ Certain medications, listed previously, may be involved.
→ History of the patient with amenorrhea/galactorrhea requires systematic consideration of the many possible etiologies. Thorough history-taking will include:
  ■ Menstrual cycle and obstetrical/gynecological/ history:
    • Age at menarche, pubertal development
    • Gravidity, parity
    • Number/date of abortions (spontaneous/induced) and complications thereof
    • Previous menstrual pattern: usual cycle interval, duration, and amount of flow; onset and type of change in menstrual cycle characteristics; events surrounding onset of amenorrhea
    • Date of last normal menstrual period and prior menstrual periods (ideally the last three)
    • Molimina: bloating, cramping
    • Irritability, breast tenderness, mittelschmerz, etc.
    • Associated physical symptoms
    • Diagnosis of other gynecological disorders and how they were managed
    • Obstetric and/or gynecologic surgery/procedures
    • Outcomes and complications of pregnancy or delivery, date of last delivery
    • Current breast-feeding status
    • Pap smear and history of sexually transmitted disease
  ■ Sexual history
  ■ Contraceptive history, desire for future fertility
  ■ Medical history:
    • General health
    • Present and past major medical disorders/serious illnesses (systemic, endocrine, metabolic, etc.) and how they were managed
    • Childhood illnesses, particularly mumps
  ■ Environmental/occupational hazards
  ■ Hospitalizations
  ■ Surgeries

- Trauma—particularly chest wall trauma, chronic chest wall irritation
- Radiation therapy/exposure, chemotherapy
- Medications
- Habits—tobacco, drugs, alcohol, exercise/athletic training
- Nutritional status—dieting, anorexia, bulimia
- Review of systems:
  - Weight gain or loss, appetite changes.
    NOTE: Normal body fat in adult women is 26%. A 15% loss of weight can decrease the percentage of body fat from 26% to 17%, often resulting in amenorrhea (Shoupe 1997).
  - Bruisability
  - Hot flashes
  - Night sweats
  - Hot/cold sensitivity
  - Fatigability
  - Muscle wasting
  - Weakness
  - Increased hair growth, hair loss
  - Headaches (associated with pituitary adenomas—usually bifrontal, retro-orbital, or bitemporal)
  - Visual changes, possibly with associated visual field defects
  - Galactorrhea (about one-third of women with galactorrhea have normal menses)
  - Defeminizing signs (loss of female body contour, decrease in breast size)
  - Signs of virilization (temporal baldness, hirsutism, deepening of voice, clitoromegaly)
  - Vaginal dryness
  - Libido changes
  - Changes in mental status (e.g., depression)
  - Recent illness
  - Other symptoms of systemic, endocrine, or metabolic disease
- Psychosocial history:
  - Education/occupation, marital/partner status, social support, environmental/psychological stressors, anxiety level, life satisfaction, etc.
- Family history:
  - Age of mother and sister(s) at menarche and menopause, history of menstrual dysfunction/amenorrhea, PCOS, infertility, genetic problems, autoimmune disorders, endocrinopathies

---

OBJECTIVE

→ Pay attention to the stigmata of thyroid disease, adrenal disease, signs of virilization, and pregnancy.
→ Perform a thorough physical examination. Important components to assess may include, but are not limited to (Clark-Coller 1991, Lichtman et al. 1990):
- Vital signs (usually within normal limits)
- General:
  - Height, weight, stature, habitus

NOTE: Waist circumference >90 cm (about 35 inches) is predictive of abnormal endocrinologic and metabolic function and is associated with increased risk of cardiovascular disease (Speroff et al. 1999). A waist-to-hip girth ratio of >0.85 (upper body obesity) is often associated with insulin resistance and hyperandrogenism (Reid 2000).
  - Posture, motor activity, gait
  - Dress, grooming, personal hygiene
  - Manner, mood, affect
  - Developmental stage of secondary sex characteristics
  - Stigmata of systemic or endocrine disease
- Hair:
  - Loss of axillary/pubic hair, hirsutism
- Eyes:
  - Stare, lid lag, exophthalmus, visual field defects, fundoscopic changes
- Neck:
  - Thyroid masses/enlargement, lymph nodes, "buffalo hump"
- Skin:
  - Dry, moist, warm, cold, rough, acne, facial plethora, palmar erythema, acanthosis nigricans
- Deep tendon reflexes
- Extremities:
  - Edema, wasting
- Heart/lungs:
  - General assessment
- Breasts:
  - Striae, tenderness, masses, and galactorrhea, which exists in only one-third of women with increased prolactin levels
- Abdomen:
  - Striae, organomegaly, masses, tenderness, inguinal nodes, pulses
- Pelvis:
  - Complete assessment of mons pubis, vulva, vagina, cervix, uterus, adnexa, and rectum, noting any abnormalities and all pertinent findings.
    - Note any virilizing signs (e.g., clitoromegaly), signs of estrogen deficiency, and indications of pregnancy (e.g., Chadwick's/Hegar's signs, enlarged uterus).
- Other:
  - Calculation of body mass index (BMI). Normal is 20–25. BMI = weight [kg]/height squared [m²] (Eden 1991).
  - Breast secretions may be examined microscopically for evidence of fat, which confirms milk.
  - Formal visual field testing by an ophthalmologist may be indicated when the patient has headaches/visual changes, which could be evidence of a pituitary macroadenoma or suprasellar extension of a pituitary lesion (American College of Obstetricians and Gynecologists [ACOG] 1989, Speroff et al. 1989, Zacur et al. 1989).

ASSESSMENT

→ Amenorrhea—secondary
→ R/O pregnancy
→ R/O thyroid disease
→ R/O galactorrhea
→ Attempt to establish etiological diagnosis within compartments 1–4.

PLAN

DIAGNOSTIC TESTS

(ACOG 1989; Kiningham et al. 1996; Mandel, S., personal communication, January 2002; McIcver et al. 1997; Reid 2000; Speroff et al. 1999):

→ The diagnostic protocol may vary according to the case presentation, site-specific procedures, and consultation with the physician. (See **Figure 12C.1, Algorithm for Secondary Amenorrhea**.)

Figure 12C.1. ALGORITHM FOR SECONDARY AMENORRHEA

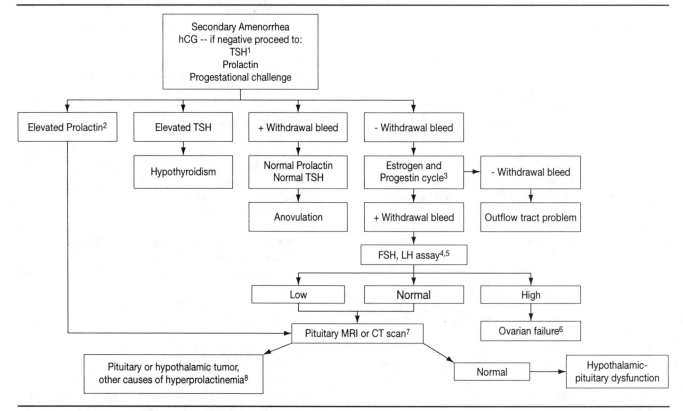

[1] May also order T3, T4, FTI if patient has signs of hyperthyroidism; may order FSH, LH, estradiol at outset or later as shown; may order testosterone, DHEA-S, 17-OHP if signs of androgen excess.

[2] Cut-off levels vary. Check laboratory norms.

[3] May be omitted in patient with normal pelvic exam and no history of curettage.

[4] Wait 2 weeks to assay if exogenous estrogen was used.

[5] May order estradiol.

[6] If under age 30 years, may order the following to rule out autoimmune disease: thyroid antibodies, a.m. cortisol, calcium, phosphorus, CBC, sedimentation rate, total protein, albumin:globulin ratio, rheumatoid factor, antinuclear antibody. Order a karyotype if POF diagnosed under age 30 years.

[7] Coned-down view of sella turcica may be substituted if cost is a factor. However, if coned-down view is abnormal, prolactin is >100 ng/mL, or the patient has a history of visual problems or headaches, proceed to MRI or CT.

[8] May include hypothyroidism, empty sella syndrome, renal disease, acromegaly. See text for further discussion.

Source: Adapted with permission from Speroff, L., Glass, R.H., and Kase, N.G. 1999. *Clinical gynecologic endocrinology and infertility*, 6th ed. Philadelphia: Lippincott Williams & Wilkins.
Additional sources: Mishell, D.R., Jr. 1997. Secondary amenorrhea without galactorrhea or androgen excess. In *Mishell's textbook of infertility, contraception, and reproductive endocrinology*, 4th ed., eds. R.A. Lobo, D.R. Mishell, Jr., R.J. Paulson et al., pp. 311–322. Malden, Mass.: Blackwell Science. Shoupe, D., and Mishell, D.R., Jr. 1997. Hyperprolactinemia: diagnosis and treatment. In *Mishell's textbook of infertility, contraception, and reproductive endocrinology*, 4th ed., eds. R.A. Lobo, D.R. Mishell, Jr., R.J. Paulson et al., pp. 323–341. Malden, Mass.: Blackwell Science.

Step 1

→ Rule out pregnancy, thyroid disease, and hyperprolactinemia (see note below).

→ Administer a *progestational challenge* to assess endogenous estrogen level and outflow tract competence. Clinical practice varies regarding medication types, dosages, and duration of use. Consult with a physician. Examples may include:

■ Medroxyprogesterone acetate 5–10 mg p.o./day for 5–10 days

OR

■ Micronized progesterone 200–300 mg p.o./day at HS for 5–7 days

OR

■ Progesterone in oil 100–200 mg IM

NOTE: This product contains peanut oil. Do not administer to women who are allergic to peanuts.

● Withdrawal bleeding: The patient may bleed within 2–14 days. "Bleeding in any amount beyond a few spots is considered a positive withdrawal response" (Speroff et al. 1999, p. 426). Only a few spots implies marginal levels of endogenous estrogen—follow the patient closely and re-evaluate periodically (Speroff et al. 1999). Positive withdrawal bleeding, absence of galactorrhea, and a normal prolactin rule out the presence of a significant pituitary tumor (Speroff et al. 1999).

NOTE: Ideally, serum prolactin should be drawn between 8:00 a.m. and 12:00 p.m. Normal values will vary depending on the laboratory. Repeat sampling of the patient while fasting is suggested if results are elevated or ambiguous (Biller et al. 1999). If the clinical presentation is strongly suggestive of a hyperprolactinemic state but the prolactin level is WNL or only mildly elevated, ask the lab to repeat the test using serial dilutions (Biller et al. 1999). Bear in mind the physiological causes of elevated prolactin (Shoupe et al. 1997):

– Early morning hours
– Sleep
– High-protein, high-fat meal at lunch
– Stress (physical/psychological)
– Pregnancy/suckling
– Breast/bimanual pelvic examination (neither produces a *significant* prolactin increase in most women)
– Coitus
– Exercise
– Late follicular phase of menstrual cycle

Step 2

→ *Estrogen and progestin cycle:* Purpose is to challenge Compartment 1 capacity with exogenous estrogen if there is a negative withdrawal bleed after the progestational challenge. Administer:

■ Conjugated estrogen 1.25 mg/day p.o. for 21 days

OR

■ Estradiol 2 mg/day p.o. for 21 days

PLUS

■ Medroxyprogesterone acetate 5–10 mg/day p.o. on the last 5 days

● A second course of the above estrogen and progestin cycle may be used if no withdrawal bleeding occurs after the first cycle (ACOG 1989, Speroff et al. 1999).

NOTE: Compartment 1 abnormalities are not commonly encountered. Thus, from a practical standpoint and in the absence of a reason to suspect a problem, Step 2—the estrogen and progestin cycle—may be omitted (Speroff et al. 1999).

Step 3

→ *Gonadotropin assay* (FSH and LH): Purpose is to determine the cause of estrogen deficiency as either a follicular (Compartment 2) or a CNS-pituitary (Compartment 3–4) defect. FSH and LH results will be as follows:

■ Abnormally high—hypergonadotrophic state: postmenopausal, castrate, or ovarian failure.

NOTE: Women younger than 30 years with premature ovarian failure (POF) on the basis of elevated gonadotropins must have a karyotype performed to establish the presence of mosaicism (Speroff et al. 1999).

■ Abnormally low—hypogonadotrophic state: hypothalamic or pituitary dysfunction.

■ Normal range—normal adult female (Speroff et al. 1999).

NOTE: Wait two weeks to assay FSH and LH after administering estrogen and progestin in Step 2.

Step 4

→ If the gonadotropin assay is abnormally low or in the normal range, imaging of the sella turcica is performed to assess for signs of abnormal change. Imaging evaluation is also done in the presence of hyperprolactinemia. (See **Figure 12C.1.**)

Additional Testing

→ Based on the clinical picture and/or initial laboratory tests, additional laboratory tests may include, but are not limited to (ACOG 1989, Mishell, Jr., 1997, Speroff et al. 1999):

■ To R/O autoimmune disease in cases of POF: CBC, ESR, FBS, free T4, TSH, ANA, RF, total protein, albumin: globulin ratio, calcium, phosphorus, and a.m. cortisol.

■ To assess hypoestrogenic states: serum estradiol.

■ For hirsutism: testosterone, DHEAS, 17 alpha-hydroxyprogesterone (17-OHP).

■ For suspicion of Cushing's disease: 24-hour urinary levels of free cortisol, ACTH levels, dexamethasone suppression test.

■ For suspected congenital adrenal hyperplasia: 17-OHP.

■ For suspected acromegaly: measurement of growth hormone during oral glucose tolerance test, insulin-like growth factor-I (IGF-I). IGF-I also should be measured in all patients who have macroadenomas.

NOTE: Consultation with a physician is recommended regarding ordering laboratory tests. Consult with a physician and refer the patient to an endocrinologist if there is suspicion of a virilizing tumor, Cushing's syndrome, adult-onset CAH, or acromegaly. Patients with signs of these disorders will require specialized tests (as cited above) to make the diagnosis. (See also the **Hirsutism** chapter.)

→ Additional diagnostic considerations may include, but are not limited to:

- Simple evaluation of ovulation, undertaken by the patient with basal body temperature charting, observation of cervical mucus changes, and attention to secondary fertility signs such as mittelschmerz, menstrual molimina, etc.
- LH kits may be used when pregnancy is desired. (See the **Infertility** chapter.)
- Assessment for insulin resistance and glucose tolerance should be considered in all anovulatory, hyperandrogenic women. Tests may include:
  - Fasting plasma glucose:
    - Normal = <110 mg/dL
    - Impaired fasting glucose = 100–125 mg/dL
    - Diabetes = ≥126 mg/dL
  - Fasting glucose:insulin ratio:
    - Ratio <4.5 is consistent with insulin resistance
  - 2-hour glucose screen after 75 g glucose load:
    - Normal = <140 mg/dL
    - Impaired glucose tolerance = 140–199 mg/dL
    - Diabetes = ≥200 mg/dL (Lebovitz 1998, Speroff 1999). (See the **Diabetes** chapters in Section 10 for more information.)
- Lipoprotein analysis in PCOS patients for determining cardiovascular risk. (See the **Hyperlipidemia** chapter in Section 6 for further information.)
- Microscopic evaluation of breast fluid—fat globules confirm the presence of milk.
- Endometrial biopsy may be performed to rule out hyperplasia/cancer when history is consistent with chronic oligoovulation or anovulation. Consult with a physician.
- Ultrasound imaging of the ovaries has been used to help diagnose PCOS.
  - Findings may include enlarged ovaries with an increased number of follicles (2–10 mm diameter) arranged peripherally around increased mass of stroma (Lobo et al. 1997).
  NOTE: "Polycystic ovaries" are frequently seen in other endocrine disturbances (including hypothalamic amenorrhea), may be encountered in up to 23% of normal women, and may not be present in women with PCOS (Lobo et al. 1997). Thus, the presence of polycystic ovaries should not be used as a criterion for diagnosis (Hunter et al. 2000, Lobo et al. 1997).
- Hysterography or hysteroscopy may be used to evaluate Asherman's syndrome; a typical pattern of multiple synechiae is seen.
  NOTE: Hysteroscopy is more accurate because it will detect minimal adhesions (Speroff et al. 1999).

- Visual field testing by an ophthalmologist to assess optic nerve compression may be indicated when the patient has visual symptoms/headaches, evidence of a macroadenoma, or suprasellar extension of the prolactinoma (ACOG 1989, Zacur et al. 1989).
- Consider bone mineral density (BMD) testing in individuals who have evidence of hypoestrogenism (i.e., serum estradiol <30 pg/mL) (Zacur et al. 1989).

TREATMENT/MANAGEMENT

→ A diagnostic work-up will attempt to establish etiology.
→ Ongoing treatment/management will be determined by the location of the identified pathology of amenorrhea and the fertility goals of the patient.

Compartment 1: Disorders of the Uterus (Outflow Tract)

→ Asherman's syndrome:

- Refer to a physician. Therapy will vary according to the physician responsible for the patient's care.
- The patient is usually evaluated with hysteroscopy or hysterosalpinography. Hysteroscopic lysis of synechiae/adhesions may be attempted.
- A broad-spectrum antibiotic is started preoperatively and continued for 10 days; postoperatively, a pediatric Foley catheter with 3 mL of fluid is placed inside the uterus (to prevent adhesions) and removed after 7 days. Some physicians place an IUD postoperatively to prevent agglutination of the uterine cavity.
  - Additionally prescribed is 2 months worth of high stimulatory doses of estrogen: conjugated estrogens 2.5 mg/day p.o., 3 out of 4 weeks with medroxyprogesterone acetate 10 mg/day p.o. added during the third week.
    - Antiprostaglandin medications may be given if cramping is present (ACOG 1989, Speroff et al. 1999).

Compartment 2: Disorders of the Ovary

→ Premature ovarian failure:

- If the patient is younger than 35 years, consider autoimmune disease as a cause. Refer to a specialist.
- In consultation with a physician, order selected blood tests for autoimmune disease. (See the diagnostic algorithm in **Figure 12C.1.**)
- If the patient is younger than 30 years, order a karyotype and refer to a physician if it is abnormal.
  - Mosaicism with a Y chromosome is associated with a significant chance of malignant tumor formation within the gonad. Therefore, excision of the gonadal areas is required. Refer the patient to a physician.
  - If the karyotype is normal, as an added precaution perform an annual pelvic examination on patients with POF (Speroff et al. 1999).
- Offer hormonal therapy to prevent osteoporosis in patients with POF. (See the **Perimenopausal and Menopausal Symptoms and Hormone Therapy** chapter.)

■ Contraception is advised for women with POF while on hormone therapy if pregnancy is not desired (a very remote possibility). These patients may be recipients of oocyte donation and embryo transfer if childbearing is desired (ACOG 1989).

→ Suspected androgen-producing ovarian (or adrenal) tumors:
■ The patient will present with rapidly progressing signs of androgen excess. Refer to a specialist. (See the **Hirsutism** chapter.)

Compartment 3:
Disorders of the Anterior Pituitary

→ Hyperprolactinemia/pituitary tumors:
■ The goals of therapy include establishing normal estrogen secretion and menstrual cycles, eliminating galactorrhea, treating prolactin-secreting macroadenomas and some microadenomas, correcting hypothyroidism if detected, and/or inducing ovulation if desired.
  • Management may include periodic observation, hormone replacement, dopamine agonist therapy, ovulation induction, surgery, or radiation (Shoupe et al. 1997).
  • The patient usually is referred to a physician if care is anticipated to be long-term or when treating pituitary adenomas. In some settings, the primary care provider may co-manage the patient in close consultation with the specialist.
■ Periodic observation:
  • Appropriate in the following instances: regular ovulatory cycles, microadenomas without bothersome galactorrhea, normal/slightly elevated prolactin levels, and when fertility is not an issue (Shoupe et al. 1997, Speroff et al. 1999).
    – Order prolactin level yearly.
    – Refer to a specialist as indicated if there are infertility concerns.
    – If anovulation with unopposed estrogen secretion occurs, cyclic progestins or OCs should be offered to induce regular uterine bleeding (Shoupe et al. 1997). (See the PCOS section below.)
■ Hormone replacement:
  • For hyperprolactinemia with associated hypoestrogenism (Shoupe et al. 1997):
    – OCs or hormone replacement therapy (HRT).
    – Calcium supplementation is also advised. (See the Compartment 4 treatment/management section below and the **Perimenopausal and Menopausal Symptoms and Hormone Therapy** chapter for drug regimens. See also the **Osteoporosis** chapter in Section 8 and **General Nutrition Guidelines**, Section 16.)
■ Dopamine agonists:
  • Indicated for treatment of macroadenomas and when microadenomas are associated with bothersome galactorrhea and infertility. The patient should be managed and followed by a physician. Drug options include:

    – Bromocriptine 2.5 mg p.o. BID (see side effects, below)
    – Slow-release bromocriptine 5–15 mg p.o. daily
    – Depo-bromocriptine 50–75 mg IM monthly (faster response, advantageous when there are large tumors associated with visual field impairment) (Speroff et al. 1999).
      ➤ Side effects of bromocriptine include nausea, vomiting, abdominal cramps, fatigue, headaches, nasal congestion, and dizziness. These effects can be minimized by slowly building tolerance toward the usual 2.5 mg BID dose. Initially, start treatment with a 2.5 mg dose at bedtime (with a snack). If intolerance occurs with this initial dose, the tablet may be cut in half and a slower program followed. Usually after 1 week, the second 2.5 mg dose can be added at breakfast or lunch. Extremely sensitive patients may divide the tablets and devise their own schedule of increasing the dosage in order to achieve tolerance. Vaginal administration of 2.5 mg/day avoids many side effects (Shoupe et al. 1997, Speroff et al. 1999).
      NOTE: Macroadenoma shrinkage may require larger doses of bromocriptine (e.g., 5–10 mg/day). Once shrinkage has occurred, progressively lower the dose until the lowest maintenance dose is achieved. Prolactins are checked every 3 months until stable; an MRI is repeated after 1 year of treatment. Treatment is usually long-term/indefinite (Speroff et al. 1999). Refer the patient to a physician for management.
    – Cabergoline 0.5–3 mg p.o. once weekly (may be given twice weekly if necessary).
      ➤ Low rate of side effects (headache is most common), can be administered vaginally if necessary. "The low rate of side effects and the once weekly dosage make cabergoline an attractive choice of initial treatment, replacing bromocriptine" (Speroff et al. 1999, p. 455).
    – Pergolide 50–150 p.o. daily.
      ➤ More potent, longer-lasting, better tolerated; may be effective in bromocriptine-resistant patients (Speroff et al. 1999).
    – Quinagolide 75–300 mg at HS.
      ➤ Long-acting, higher affinity for dopamine receptor, may be used for bromocriptine-resistant tumors, reduced side effects, antidepressant properties (Speroff et al. 1999).
■ Ovulation induction:
  • Refer the patient to a physician as indicated. (See the **Infertility** chapter.)
■ Surgery: transsphenoidal resection of pituitary adenomas may be employed in certain cases:
  • Complete or partial failure of medical therapy
  • Supracellar extension of tumor

- Persistent visual-field impairment after dopamine agonist therapy
- Poor compliance/intolerance of medical regimen (Shoupe et al. 1997, Speroff et al. 1999)
- Best results are in women with prolactins in the 150–500 ng/mL range (Speroff et al. 1999)
- Surgery may be considered as a debulking procedure for very large tumors (with or without invasion) before long-term dopamine agonist therapy (Speroff et al. 1999).
- Follow-up for postsurgical patients with persistent/recurrent amenorrhea/oligomenorrhea and hyperprolactinemia includes:
  - ➤ Prolactin levels every 6 months and pituitary imaging every few years
  - ➤ Dopamine agonist therapy in the event of tumor regrowth or for induction of ovulation (Speroff et al. 1999)
- ▪ Radiation: may arrest the progressive growth of a pituitary adenoma. However, it is not advised except for rare patients who fail to respond to medical/surgical management (Shoupe et al. 1997).
  - All patients require ongoing surveillance for hypopituitarism after radiation. Physician management is required.

Additional Considerations:
- ▪ Conception may occur in sexually active women who are hyperprolactinemic. Advise the patient regarding birth control methods if she does not desire pregnancy.
- ▪ For galactorrhea developing when the patient is taking a prescribed medication (e.g., a major tranquilizer or antihypertensive):
  - If unable to stop the medication, assess prolactin:
    - If <100 ng/mL, no intervention is necessary except for yearly follow-up of prolactin (Shoupe et al. 1997). If estradiol levels are low, treat with OCs or HRT.
    - If >100 ng/mL, proceed with pituitary evaluation—i.e., coned down view of sella turica, MRI, or CT scan (Shoupe et al. 1997).
- → Empty sella syndrome:
  - ▪ MRI or CT will establish a definitive diagnosis.
  - ▪ Advise the patient that the prognosis usually is benign and endocrine abnormalities are unlikely.
  - ▪ May follow with yearly prolactin levels
  - ▪ Consult with a physician
- → Other pituitary lesions:
  - ▪ Patients with radiographic evidence of rare pituitary tumors or a history suggestive of Sheehan's syndrome should be followed by a physician.
- → Primary hypothyroidism:
  - ▪ When established as the cause of hyperprolactinemia, thyroxine replacement therapy is indicated. (See the **Thyroid Disorders** chapter in Section 10.) Refer the patient to a physician as indicated.

Compartment 4: Disorders of the Central Nervous System (Hypothalamus)

→ Hypothalamic dysfunction:
- ▪ Attempt to ameliorate the underlying cause of hypothalamic dysfunction.
- ▪ Undertake nutritional counseling and discussion regarding exercise patterns, weight loss, and stress management techniques. Refer to a nutritionist as indicated.
- ▪ Refer to a psychiatrist or other mental health provider, and physician as indicated, for patients with anorexia nervosa or bulimia, especially in severe cases.
- ▪ Advise regarding hormone therapy for patients with hypothalamic dysfunction who are hypoestrogenic. Options include (Speroff et al. 1999):
  - OCs if the patient wants effective contraception
    OR
  - HRT:
    - Conjugated estrogens 0.3–0.625 mg
      OR
    - Estradiol 0.5–1 mg/day p.o.
      PLUS
    - Medroxyprogesterone acetate 5 mg p.o. for 12–14 days every month (or equivalents) (Speroff et al. 1999)

  NOTE: Women who want to avoid monthly bleeding can be given the daily combined approach to HRT: conjugated estrogens 0.3–0.625 mg/day p.o. PLUS medroxyprogesterone acetate 2.5 mg/day p.o. (Speroff et al. 1999).
  - A daily intake of calcium in the range of 1,000–1,500 mg (dietary or supplemental) is strongly encouraged (Speroff et al. 1999). (See also the **Perimenopausal and Menopausal Symptoms and Hormone Therapy** chapter and Section 16, **General Nutrition Guidelines**.)
- ▪ BMD assessment of the spine and hip is suggested in patients who have been amenorrheic for longer than 2 years (Smith et al. 1986). Periodic measurements of bone density are worthwhile to assess adequacy of hormonal treatment in patients with hypothalamic/hyperprolactinemic amenorrhea.
- ▪ Refer patients with infertility to a specialist as indicated.
→ Polycystic ovary syndrome (PCOS):
- ▪ Treatment goals include maintaining a normal endometrium, reducing insulin resistance and avoiding the effects of hyperinsulinemia, lowering the risks of cardiovascular disease and diabetes, antagonizing the action of androgens on target tissues, and correcting anovulation (Hunter et al. 2000, Speroff et al. 1999). (See specific chapters for treatment/management of associated problems of hirsutism, infertility, and/or dysfunctional uterine bleeding.)
- ▪ First-line treatment strategies include lifestyle modifications—weight reduction, a healthy diet, and regular exercise.
  - Studies indicate that weight loss may lower the degree of hyperinsulinemia and lead to amelioration of insulin resistance (Tan et al. 2001).

- Long-term screening for diabetes and lipoprotein abnormalities is appropriate. Yearly laboratory testing may be undertaken for women who are obese.
- Pharmacologic options to avoid abnormal endometrial proliferation include (Hunter et al. 2000, Speroff et al. 1999):
  - Medroxyprogesterone acetate 5–10 mg/day p.o. for 12–14 days every month (or equivalent progestin)

    OR
  - OCs: the ideal choice when reliable contraception is essential (they have a favorable effect on lipoprotein and androgen production).
- Oral insulin-sensitizing agents (**NOTE:** These drugs are not FDA-approved for use in PCOS. Caution is advised when using them—see below. The patient should be managed by a physician and a current literature review is advised):
  - Primary use is for treating Type 2 diabetes mellitus.
  - They target various aspects of insulin resistance syndrome and may correct certain metabolic abnormalities associated with PCOS (Parulkar et al. 2001).
  - They have been shown to improve insulin sensitivity and reduce LH and free testosterone levels in PCOS patients.
  - They may improve dyslipidemia and reduce risk for cardiovascular disease.
  - They may improve ovulatory function and fertility; have been used in anovulatory women who are resistant to clomiphene.
  - They may be useful as primary or adjunctive treatment of PCOS. However, their use in this disorder is relatively new. Ongoing study with controlled trials regarding their safety and effectiveness is necessary to support a recommendation for use (Hunter et al. 2000, Parulkar et al. 2001, Sood et al. 2000, Speroff et al. 1999, Tan et al. 2001). Options include:
    - Metformin (biguanide): 500 mg p.o. QD for 1 week, increasing to 500 mg BID for the second week, then 500 mg TID by the third week (Hock et al. 2000, Kolodziejczyk et al. 2000. See also the review by Iuorno et al. 2001).
      - ➤ A 3-month therapeutic trial may be useful in determining efficacy (Hock et al. 2000).
      - ➤ Side effects are mostly gastrointestinal—nausea, vomiting, diarrhea. There is a risk of lactic acidosis, especially in patients with renal insufficiency. Do not use if creatinine is >1.4 mg/dL or with risk of renal dysfunction. (See *Physicians' Desk Reference* [*PDR*] or drug package insert for additional information.)
    - Pioglitazone (thiazolidinedione): doses for use in PCOS are not established; 15 mg p.o. BID has been used in some clinical settings.
      - ➤ Side effects may include increased water retention, edema, weight gain, hypoglycemia, and increased plasma volume associated with nonclinically significant drops in hemoglobin/hematocrit (Lawrence et al. 2000).
      - ➤ Contraindicated in patients with cardiac failure or history of cardiac failure (New York Heart Association [NYHA] stages I–IV) and/or hepatic impairment (Pioglitazone Summary Sheet 2002, Woolworton 2002).
      - ➤ Regular monitoring of liver function tests is necessary. (See *PDR* or drug package insert for additional information.)
    - Rosiglitazone (thiazolidinedione): doses in PCOS patients are not established; 4 mg p.o. QD for 5 months has been used (Cataldo et al. 2001).
      - ➤ Side effects may include increased water retention, edema, weight gain, hypoglycemia, and increased plasma volume associated with nonclinically significant drops in hemoglobin/hematocrit (Lawrence et al. 2000).
      - ➤ Contraindicated in patients with acute liver disease, cardiac failure, or a history of cardiac failure (NYHA stages I–IV) (Rosiglitazone Summary Sheet 2002, Woolworton 2002).
      - ➤ Idiosyncratic hepatotoxicity has been reported with this drug (Al-Salman et al. 2000, Forman et al. 2000, Ravinuthala et al. 2000, Sood et al. 2000). Regular monitoring of liver function tests is necessary. (See *PDR* or drug package insert for additional information.)

        NOTE: Insulin sensitizing agents may induce ovulation. Discuss contraceptive options if pregnancy is not desired. Pioglitazone and rosiglitazone are Category C drugs (have been demonstrated to retard fetal development in animal studies) (Iuorno et al. 2001).
    - D-chiro-inositol: moiety of an inositol glycan mediator of insulin action. It still is under investigation, entering phase III clinical trials.
- For infertile patients with PCOS:
  - Weight reduction, improved diet, exercise
  - Ovulation induction, insulin sensitizing agents, gonadotropins, assisted reproductive technologies, surgical procedures (e.g., laparoscopic ovarian electrocautery). Refer to a specialist.

→ Postpill amenorrhea:
- Work-up for amenorrhea is warranted if a woman does not menstruate within 6 months of discontinuing OCs or 12 months after discontinuing Depo-Provera®.
  - Proceed as detailed under "Diagnostic Tests," above.
  - Advise the patient to use contraception if pregnancy is not desired.

CONSULTATION

→ Consultation with a physician is suggested for all patients with amenorrhea and may be indicated to determine necessary diagnostic tests.
→ Refer patients with Asherman's syndrome, endocrinopathies, autoimmune disorders, pituitary or hypothalamic lesions,

galactorrhea, infertility, or anorexia nervosa or bulimia to a specialist (e.g., a gynecologist, endocrinologist, or reproductive endocrinologist, rheumatologist, or psychiatrist) for medical management. Depending on the policies of the practice setting, certain patients may be co-managed with the physician.

→ As needed for endometrial biopsy in cases of PCOS with long-standing amenorrhea.

→ Refer the patient to a physician when insulin-sensitizing agents are being considered for use in PCOS.

→ As needed for prescription(s).

PATIENT EDUCATION

→ When the patient is referred to a specialist, the physician should detail the specific diagnostic and therapeutic modalities. Co-managed patients should be cared for with a comprehensive plan in mind. The primary care provider will complement and supplement the specialist's care and ensure that the patient's goals and objectives are considered.

→ Specific patient education will depend on the etiology of the amenorrhea. Discuss diagnostic tests and procedures in terms that the patient will understand. Patient-education materials are a useful adjunct to teaching. Highlights are presented here.

→ Asherman's syndrome:
  ■ Review treatment modalities. The physician will detail the particulars.

→ POF:
  ■ Patients need psychological support if loss of fertility is a major issue. Direct patients to the appropriate resources if there is an interest in pursuing pregnancy via oocyte donation or embryo transfer.
  ■ Discuss the need for contraception if the patient is on HRT.
  ■ OCs are an option if pregnancy is not desired.

→ Hyperprolactinemia/galactorrhea:
  ■ Advise patients treated with dopamine agonists that the average time to restoration of menses is 5–6 weeks; galactorrhea may take 6–12 weeks to resolve. Upon discontinuing treatment, amenorrhea and galactorrhea usually recur in about 4–6 weeks (Speroff 1999).
  ■ Discuss the side effects of treatment. (See "Treatment/Management.")

→ Hypothalamic amenorrhea:
  ■ Discuss the mechanism of dysfunction. Discuss with athletes the "female athlete triad" of disordered eating, amenorrhea, and osteoporosis.
    • A change in lifestyle (e.g., moderation of exercise and weight gain) will be appropriate for some amenorrheic athletes. A reduction in exercise plus an optimal diet are often enough to restore a normal menstrual cycle (Genazzani et al. 1991).
  ■ Discuss healthy eating patterns and adequacy of calcium intake. (See Section 16.)
  ■ For women placed on OCs/HRT for long-standing amenorrhea, advise regarding use and potential side effects.

• Alert patients that they will have regular withdrawal bleeding while on OCs or cyclic HRT, but that upon discontinuing therapy, amenorrhea is likely to recur.
  ■ Encourage women who decline hormonal therapy to have BMD evaluation if their estradiol levels are low.
  ■ Women with anorexia nervosa or bulimia usually require psychological counseling about the disorder. (See the **Eating Disorders** chapter in Section 14.)

→ PCOS:
  ■ Discuss the increased risk for lipoprotein abnormalities, diabetes mellitus, and glucose intolerance in pregnancy. Other pregnancy complications include an increased risk for spontaneous abortion (may be as high as 40%).
  ■ Counsel regarding a low-fat/low-cholesterol diet. (See Section 16.) If obesity is a factor for the PCOS patient, she may benefit from joining a weight-loss program.
    • Weight loss improves hyperinsulinemia and hyperandrogenism. Only a small percentage of weight (i.e., 5–10%) needs to be lost to have a beneficial impact on insulin resistance and cardiovascular function (Pasquali et al. 2000, Speroff et al. 1999).
  ■ Address the potential for hyperplastic endometrial change with chronic anovulation and discuss the importance of periodic progestins or combined OCs.
    • Alert women who are placed on OCs for cycle control to the potential for irregular menses/oligomenorrhea/amenorrhea when or if the pills are discontinued.
  ■ When fertility is desired, ovulation induction often is indicated. Discuss the need for referral to a gynecologist or infertility specialist.

→ "Post-pill amenorrhea":
  ■ Advise that there is no long-term effect on fertility. Normal menstrual cycles should resume within six months of OC discontinuation and within 12 months after discontinuation of Depo-Provera®.
  ■ Discuss contraceptive options. Despite amenorrhea, spontaneous ovulation may occur.

FOLLOW-UP

→ Follow-up of amenorrheic patients varies and depends on the identified underlying condition. Establish a plan of care with a consultant as indicated, including ongoing surveillance. (See "Treatment/Management" for particulars.)

→ Document the diagnosis of secondary amenorrhea, anovulation, and/or galactorrhea in the progress notes and on the problem list. Specify the underlying etiologies.

BIBLIOGRAPHY

Al-Salman, J., Arjomand, H., Kemp, D.G. et al. 2000. Hepatocellular injury in a patient receiving rosiglitazone. A case report. *Annals of Internal Medicine* 132:121–124.

American College of Obstetricians and Gynecologists (ACOG). 1989. *Amenorrhea*. Technical Bulletin No. 128. Washington, D.C.: the Author.

Anasti, J.N. 1998. Premature ovarian failure: an update. *Fertility and Sterility* 70(1):1–15.

Biller, B.M.K. 1999. Hyperprolactinemia. *International Journal of Infertility* 44(2):74–77.

Biller, B.M.K., and Luciano, A. 1999. Guidelines for the diagnosis and treatment of hyperprolactinemia. *Journal of Reproductive Medicine* 44(12):1075–1084.

Carmina, E., and Lobo, R.A. 1999. Polycystic ovary syndrome (PCOS): Arguably the most common endocrinopathy is associated with significant morbidity in women. *Journal of Clinical Endocrinology and Metabolism* 84(6):1897–1899.

Cataldo, N.A., Abbasi, F., McLaughlin, T.L. et al. 2001. Improvement in insulin sensitivity followed by ovulation and pregnancy in a woman with polycystic ovary syndrome who was treated with rosiglitazone. *Fertility and Sterility* 76(5):1057–1059.

Clark-Coller, T. 1991. Dysfunctional uterine bleeding and amenorrhea. *Journal of Nurse-Midwifery* 36(1):49–62.

Eden, J.A. 1991. The hazards of amenorrhea. *Medical Journal of Australia* 154:536–542.

Fagan, K.M. 1998. Pharmacologic management of athletic amenorrhea. *Sports Pharmacology* 17(2):327–341.

Forman, L.M., Simmons, D.A., and Diamond, R.H. 2000. Hepatic failure in a patient taking rosiglitazone. *Annals of Internal Medicine* 132:118–121.

Genazzani, A.R., Petraglia, F., De Ramundo, B.M. et al. 1991. Neuroendocrine correlates of stress-related amenorrhea. *Annals of the New York Academy of Sciences* 626:125–129.

Gomel, V., Munro, M.G., and Rowe, T.C. 1990. *Gynecology: a practical approach.* Baltimore, Md.: Williams & Wilkins.

Guzick, D. 1998. Polycystic ovary syndrome: symptomatology, pathophysiology, and epidemiology. *American Journal of Obstetrics and Gynecology* 179(6, Part 2):S89–S93.

Hock, D.L., and Seifer, D.B. 2000. New treatments of hyperandrogenism and hirsutism. *Obstetrics and Gynecology Clinics of North America* 27(3):567–581.

Hunter, M., and Sterrett, J.J. 2000. Polycystic ovary syndrome: It's not just infertility. *American Family Physician* 62(5):1079–1089.

Iuorno, M.J., and Nestler, J.E. 2001. Insulin-lowering drugs in polycystic ovary syndrome. *Obstetrics and Gynecology Clinics of North America* 28(1):153–164.

Kiningham, R.B., Apgar, B., and Schwenk, T.L. 1996. Evaluation of amenorrhea. *American Family Physician* 53(4):1185–1194.

Kolodziejczyk, B., Duleba, A.J., Spaczynski, R.Z. et al. 2000. Metformin therapy decreases hyperandrogenism and hyperinsulinemia in women with polycystic ovary syndrome. *Fertility and Sterility* 73(6):1149–1154.

Lawrence, J.M., and Reckless, J.P.D. 2000. Pioglitazone. *International Journal of Clinical Practice* 54(9):614–618.

Lebovitz, H.E. 1998. Diagnosis and classification of diabetes mellitus. In *Therapy for diabetes and related disorders*, 3rd ed., ed. H.E. Lebovitz, p. 6. Alexandria, Va.: American Diabetes Association.

Lichtman, R., and Papera, S. 1990. *Gynecology: Well-woman care.* Norwalk, Conn.: Appleton & Lange.

Lobo, R.A., and Carmina, E. 1997. *Polycystic ovary syndrome,* 4th ed., eds. R.A. Lobo, D.R. Mishell, Jr., R.J. Paulson et al., pp. 363–383. Malden, Mass.: Blackwell Science.

Luciano, A.A. 1999. Clinical presentation of hyperprolactinemia. *Journal of Reproductive Medicine* 44:1085–1090.

McIver, B., Romanski, S.A. , and Nippoldt, T.B. 1997. Evaluation and management of amenorrhea. *Mayo Clinic Proceedings* 72:1161–1169.

Mishell, D.R., Jr. 1997. Secondary amenorrhea without hyperprolactinemia or hyperandrogenism. In *Infertility, contraception, and reproductive endocrinology,* 3rd ed., eds. R.A. Lobo, D.R. Mishell, Jr., R.J. Paulson et al., pp. 311–322. Malden, Mass.: Blackwell Science.

Nestler, J.E., Jakubowicz, D.J., Reamer, P. et al. 1999. Ovulatory and metabolic effects of D-chiro-inositol in the polycystic ovary syndrome. *New England Journal of Medicine* 340:1314–1320.

Norman, R.J., Kidson, W.J., Cuneo, R.C. et al. 2001. Metformin and intervention in polycystic ovary syndrome. *Medical Journal of Australia* 174(11):554–555.

Otis, C.L., Drinkwater, B., Johnson, M. et al. 1997. The female athlete triad. *Official Journal of the American College of Sports Medicine* 29(5):i–ix.

Parulkar, A.A., Pendergrass, M.L., Granda-Ayala, R. et al. 2001. Nonhypoglycemic effects of thiazolidinediones. *Annals of Internal Medicine* 134(1):61–71.

Pasquali, R., Gambineri, A., Biscotti, D. et al. 2000. Effect of long-term treatment with metformin added to hypocaloric diet on body composition, fat distribution, and androgen and insulin levels in abdominally obese women with and without the polycystic ovary syndrome. *Journal of Clinical Endocrinology and Metabolism* 85(8):2767–2774.

Pioglitazone Summary Sheet. Available at: http://www.keele. ac.uk/depts/mm/MTRAC/ProductInfo/summaries/P/ PIOGLITAZONEs.html. Accessed on April 11, 2002.

Ravinuthala, R.S., and Nori, U. 2000. Rosiglitazone toxicity. *Annals of Internal Medicine* 133(8):658.

Reid, R.L. 2000 Amenorrhea. In *Textbook of gynecology,* 2nd ed., ed. L.J Copeland, pp. 541–569. Philadelphia: W.B. Saunders.

Rosiglitazone Summary Sheet. Available at: http://www.keele. ac.uk/depts/mm/MTRAC/ProductInfo/summaries/R/ ROSIGLITAZONEs.html. Accessed on April 30, 2002.

Shoupe, D. 1997. Effects of nutrition, stress, and exercise on reproductive function. In *Infertility, contraception, and reproductive endocrinology,* 3rd ed., eds. R.A. Lobo, D.R. Mishell, Jr., R.J. Paulson et al., pp. 449–463. Malden, Mass.: Blackwell Science.

Shoupe, D., and Mishell, D.R., Jr. 1997. Hyperprolactinemia: diagnosis and treatment. In *Infertility, contraception, and reproductive endocrinology,* 3rd ed., eds. R.A. Lobo, D.R. Mishell, Jr., R.J. Paulson et al., pp. 323–341. Malden, Mass.: Blackwell Science.

Smith, E.L., and Zook, S.K. 1986. Exercise can reduce bone loss. *Contemporary OB/GYN* 28:53–61.

Sood, V., Colleran, K., and Burge, M.R. 2000. Thiazolidinediones: a comparative review of approved uses. *Diabetes Technology and Therapeutics* 2(3):429–440.

Speroff, L., Glass, R.H., and Kase, N.G. 1989. *Clinical gynecologic endocrinology and infertility*, 4th ed. Baltimore, Md.: Lippincott Williams & Wilkins.

_____. 1999. *Clinical gynecologic endocrinology and infertility*, 6th ed. Baltimore, Md.: Lippincott Williams & Wilkins.

Tan, W.C., Yap, C., and Tan, A.S.A. 2001. Clinical management of PCOS. *Acta Obstetricia et Gynecologica Scandinavica* 80:689–696.

Warren, M.P. 1996. Evaluation of secondary amenorrhea. *Journal of Clinical Endocrinology and Metabolism* 81(2):437–442.

West, R.V. 1998. The female athlete. *Sports Medicine* 26 (2):63–71.

Woolworton, E. 2002. Rosiglitazone (Avandia) and pioglitazone (Actos) and heart failure. *Canadian Medical Association Journal* 166(2):219.

Zacur, H.A., and Seibel, M.M. 1989. Steps in diagnosing prolactin-related disorders. *Contemporary OB/GYN* 34(3):84–96.

Ann M. Brennan, R.N., M.S., A.N.P., P.N.P.
Joan R. Murphy, R.N., C., M.S., N.P., C.N.S.

12-D

Dysmenorrhea

Dysmenorrhea, described as painful menstruation, is one of the most frequently encountered gynecological disorders in menstruating women. Roughly half of women of childbearing age experience some degree of dysmenorrhea, causing considerable disruption in their lives (Wolf et al. 1999). Approximately 10% of these women have dysmenorrhea severe enough to render them incapacitated for 1–3 days each month, resulting in increased absenteeism and economic loss, which in turn lowers the productivity of both the individual and society (Hillen et al. 1999).

Dysmenorrhea often follows a typical cyclic pattern, presenting a few days before to a few days after the start of menstrual flow. It is characterized by mild to severe cramping in the lower abdomen but may present as pain in the back or down the thighs. It also may be accompanied by systemic symptoms, such as gastrointestinal upset, diarrhea, nausea, low backache, headache, syncope, and fatigue (Dawood et al. 1990, Granot et al. 2001).

Dysmenorrhea is classified as primary or secondary based on the etiology of presenting symptoms. *Primary dysmenorrhea* is defined as painful menstruation in the absence of specific pelvic pathology. *Secondary dysmenorrhea* involves underlying pelvic pathology that produces painful menstrual cramping. When dysmenorrhea does not respond to standard medical management or when it occurs for more than two or three days or throughout the menstrual cycle, secondary dysmenorrhea should be considered (Dawood et al. 1990, Schroeder et al. 1999). Differential diagnosis may need to be based on more than history alone, as symptoms can be similar. However, management of primary and secondary dysmenorrhea differs significantly and is directed at the specific etiology (Smith 1997).

Primary dysmenorrhea occurs mainly in women in their teens and early twenties. The rate tends to decrease with age, especially after age 35. Pregnancy and vaginal delivery do not necessarily resolve symptoms but may provide some relief owing to a reduction of α-adrenergic receptors in the uterine wall that occurs during pregnancy (Smith 1997). Some epidemiological studies have indicated that the severity of primary dysmenorrhea can be associated with duration of menstrual flow,

cigarette smoking, obesity, and alcohol consumption that may prompt some women to adopt healthier lifestyles (Coco 1999). Dysmenorrhea also tends to run in families; however, it is unclear if this is primarily due to genetic predisposition or is anticipated based on family history (Smith 1997).

Primary dysmenorrhea presents as cyclic lower abdominal discomfort ranging from mild to severe. The cause of this discomfort is not fully understood but is believed to be linked to the action of uterine prostaglandins, specifically PGF2α (prostaglandin factor) (Coco 1999). Just before and during early menstruation, PGF2α production is increased by disintegrating endometrial cells. This stimulates myometrial contractions and sloughing of the endometrial lining. There is strong clinical evidence indicating that women with higher levels of PFG2α in menstrual fluid have more severe dysmenorrhea (Coco 1999). Furthermore, women with primary dysmenorrhea produce 8–13 times more prostaglandins in general than do nondysmenorrhic women, and produce prostaglandins seven times faster. The increased pain experienced during the first 48–72 hours of menstruation correlates well with the increased production and release of prostaglandins that occur during this period, which further contributes to symptoms (Smith 1997).

The pain experienced with primary dysmenorrhea is characteristically suprapubic, crampy, spasmodic, and may be labor-like in nature or may be described as a dull ache or a stabbing feeling. It generally starts at or soon after menarche (6–12 months) when ovulatory cycles are established (Schroeder et al. 1999). Menstrual pain usually lasts 48–72 hours and can begin as early as a few hours before or just after the onset of bleeding. It is most severe during the first or second day of menses. Systemic symptoms occur in approximately 50% of patients. Physical examination is primarily based on ruling out secondary causes of dysmenorrhea, such as pelvic or ovarian masses (Coco 1999). Pain is typically not reproducible during the bimanual exam. Therefore, the physical exam in patients experiencing primary dysmenorrhea will most likely be within normal limits. A rectal exam should be a routine part of the assessment to rule out pathology, but it is generally negative (Schroeder et al. 1999).

Secondary dysmenorrhea should be considered with later onset of symptoms and in women experiencing ovulatory cycles. The specific pathologic condition acts directly or indirectly on pelvic anatomy causing pain that can also be influenced by normal physiological changes during menstruation (Smith 1997). Often the history will reveal possible causative factors and aid in further evaluation. Secondary dysmenorrhea should be considered when there is a history of recurrent pelvic inflammatory disease (PID), irregular menstrual cycles, menorrhagia, use of an intrauterine device (IUD), or infertility (Dawood et al. 1990).

The etiology of secondary dysmenorrhea can be classified as intrauterine or extrauterine. Intrauterine pathology may include adenomyosis, congenital abnormalities, infection, myomas, polyps, and cervical stenosis (Smith 1997). Cervical stenosis may cause secondary dysmenorrhea by impeding menstrual flow through the cervical canal with subsequent increased intrauterine pressure. A history of scant menstrual flow and severe cramping throughout the menstrual period should alert the clinician to the possibility of cervical stenosis.

Extrauterine causes of secondary dysmenorrhea include endometriosis; functional ovarian cysts; inflammation; scarring; musculoskeletal, gastrointestinal, and urinary pathology; and benign or malignant tumors (Smith 1997). Endometriosis should be considered if dysmenorrhea becomes more severe as menses progress.

DATABASE

SUBJECTIVE

Primary Dysmenorrhea

→ Onset is usually within three years of menarche.
→ The patient describes cramping as:
- Suprapubic
- Intermittent
- Sharp/colicky
- Possibly radiating to inner thighs, back, groin, sacrum
- Beginning within hours of onset of menses
- Diminishing within 24–48 hours
→ Associated symptoms may include:
- Nausea
- Diarrhea
- Headache
- Fatigue
- Bloating
- Breast tenderness
- Flushing
- Anxiety
- Palpitations
→ Risk factors may include:
- Single
- Delayed childbearing
- Overweight
- Smoking
- Positive family history
- Higher socioeconomic status
- Retroflexed uterus

Secondary Dysmenorrhea

→ Onset of dysmenorrhea is generally in adulthood with a probable history of previous, pain-free menstrual cycles.
→ Signs and symptoms are often nonspecific and may be more associated with the underlying pathology.
→ Pain may be described as dull, starting earlier and lasting longer than cramping associated with primary dysmenorrhea, or it may be similar to pain experienced with primary dysmenorrhea.
→ The patient may complain of pelvic pain for more than 2–3 days or throughout the menstrual cycle.
→ Pain may occur during ovulation and with intercourse, and may increase with age.
→ The patient may have a history of PID, irregular menstrual cycles, menorrhagia, IUD use, or infertility.

Primary and Secondary Dysmenorrhea

→ History to include:
- Description of usual menstrual pattern
- Detailed sexual history
- Age at menarche
- Description of menstrual pain:
  • Should include onset, character, duration, severity, timing during the menstrual cycle, and age when it started.
- History of analgesic use, palliative measures, efficacy of treatment
- Associated symptoms
- A thorough obstetrical and gynecological history, which is usually sufficient to make a diagnosis of primary dysmenorrhea (Coco 1999)

OBJECTIVE

Primary Dysmenorrhea

→ Pelvic and abdominal examination is usually within normal limits. If some pain is elicited, it should be limited to midline and is generally nonspecific (Coco 1999).

Secondary Dysmenorrhea

→ May find pelvic pathology on pelvic or abdominal examination, sonogram, laparoscopy, hysterosalpingogram, or hysteroscopy.

ASSESSMENT

Dysmenorrhea (Primary or Secondary)

→ R/O possible causes of secondary dysmenorrhea:
- Endometriosis
- PID
- Other pelvic infection
- Fibroids
- Adenomyosis
- Cervical stenosis and polyps
- Fibroids, myomas
- Inflammation, scarring

- Congenital abnormalities
- Presence of an IUD
- Chronic pelvic pain
- Functional ovarian cysts
- Benign or malignant tumors
- Musculoskeletal, gastrointestinal, and urinary pathology
- Intrauterine adhesions (Asherman's syndrome)
- Inflammatory bowel disease

PLAN

DIAGNOSTIC TESTS

Primary Dysmenorrhea

→ None specifically

Secondary Dysmenorrhea

→ Tests may include:
- Sonogram
- Laparoscopy
- Hysteroscopy
- Hysterosalpingogram
- Laboratory tests as indicated. These may include CBC, RPR, pregnancy test, cervical screening for *Neisseria gonorrhoeae* and *Chlamydia trachomatis*, and Pap smear.

TREATMENT/MANAGEMENT

Primary Dysmenorrhea

→ Pharmacological agents useful in treatment may include:
- Oral contraceptives:
  - The drug of choice if the patient also desires birth control pills as method of contraception (Coco 1999).
  - Several studies indicate the use of combined oral contraceptives as the most effective treatment for primary dysmenorrhea when birth control is also desired (Davis et al. 2001).
  - Mechanism:
    - Decreased menstrual fluid volume secondary to suppression of endometrial growth
    - Suppression of ovulation, resulting in low levels of prostaglandins
  - Effective in up to 90% or more cases of dysmenorrhea (Coco 1999)
  - A trial of oral contraceptives for 3–4 months is reasonable for evaluating effectiveness.
    - Oral contraceptives and nonsteroidal anti-inflammatory drugs (NSAIDs) work through different mechanisms; therefore, a combination may be more effective for refractory symptoms (Coco 1999).
→ NSAIDs, also known as prostaglandin synthetase inhibitors:
- Most appropriate, first-line option when oral contraceptives are not the birth control method of choice (Coco 1999).
- Mechanism:
  - Inhibit prostaglandin synthesis and release in endometrial tissue, which results in suppression of menstrual fluid prostaglandins.

- Also have direct analgesic properties and act as anti-thrombotic agents (Schroeder et al. 1999).
- Various studies have demonstrated pain relief in 64–100% of subjects (Coco 1999).
- Advantages over oral contraceptives:
  - Taken only 2–3 days of the menstrual cycle.
  - Do not suppress the pituitary-gonadal axis.
  - Oral-contraceptive-related metabolic effects are not present (Dawood 1984, 1985, 1990).
- The patient should start taking an NSAID as soon as menstrual pain begins or at the onset of menstruation.
- Options: Within the NSAIDs classification of carboxylic acids, four major subgroups have been shown to be effective in the treatment of dysmenorrhea:
  - Salicylic acids (aspirin, diflunisal). Initial dose is 1,000 mg, subsequent dose is 500 mg every 12 hours (Dolobid®) (Schroeder et al. 1999, Smith 1997)
    - Low potency for reducing prostaglandin synthesis in the uterus, slow onset of action
  - Indoleacetic acids (indomethacin). Initial dose is 25 mg, subsequent dose is 25 mg TID (Indocin®) (Schroeder et al. 1999, Smith 1997). *[handwritten: NSAIDs]*
    - Side effects limit use of drugs in this group. *[handwritten: Ponstel NSAID]*
  - Fenamates (mefenamic acid). Initial dose is 500 mg, subsequent dose is 250 mg every 4–6 hours (Ponstel®) (Schroeder et al. 1999, Smith 1997).
  - Arylpropionic acids (Schroeder et al. 1999, Smith 1997):
    - Ibuprofen: Initial dose is 600 mg, subsequent dose is 600 mg every 4 hours (Motrin®).
    - Naproxen: Initial dose is 500 mg, subsequent dose is 250 mg every 4–6 hours (Naprosyn®).
    - Naproxen sodium: Initial dose is 550 mg, subsequent dose is 275 mg every 6–8 hours (Anaprox®).
    - Ketoprofen. Initial dose is 75 mg, subsequent dose is 75 mg TID (Orudis®).

  NOTE: The drug of choice is either arylpropionic acids or a fenamate. Research favors fenamates over the propionic acids (Smith 1997).
- Another classification of NSAID is enolic acids:
  - Oxicams (piroxicam): Initial dose is 20 mg, subsequent dose is 20 mg QD (Feldene®) (Schroeder et al. 1999).
    - Not shown to be as effective as carboxylic acids.
- Treatment:
  - Continue NSAID treatment through the first 48–72 hours of menstrual flow rather than on an as-needed basis. Rationale:
    - Corrects the biochemical derangement caused by excessive production and release of prostaglandins (Dawood et al. 1990).
    - Maximal prostaglandin release is during the first 48 hours of the menstrual flow (Dawood et al. 1990).
- If dysmenorrhea persists during the first few hours after the NSAID is taken, increase the starting dose by 50% or double it at the onset of the next cycle while keeping the maintenance dose essentially the same.

- A trial of up to 2–4 menstrual cycles is needed to determine effectiveness. If therapy is unsuccessful, try an NSAID from a different group (Smith 1997).
- Contraindications for NSAIDs:
  - Aspirin-sensitive asthma, gastrointestinal ulcers, inflammatory bowel disease (Smith 1997).
- Side effects of NSAIDs:
  - Uncommon and generally mild but serious side effects are possible (Smith 1997).
  - Gastrointestinal side effects can be reduced if an NSAID is taken with food or an antacid. (See *Physicians' Desk Reference.*)
  NOTE: Side effects of NSAIDs may include nephrotoxicity, hepatotoxicity, and platelet dysfunction/blood dyscrasias.
→ Nondrug therapies:
  - Exercise:
    - Suppresses prostaglandin release.
    - Releases beta endorphins that decrease pain perception.
    - Shunts blood away from the uterus (Treybig 1989).
  - Dietary changes:
    - Restriction of salt, sugar, caffeine (Fankhauser 1996).
    - Vitamin E (200–600 IU/d) (Fankhauser 1996):
      - A mild prostaglandin inhibitor that improves circulation to the uterus secondary to its ability to reduce arteriolar spasm (Treybig 1989).
    - Magnesium (50–100 mg BID) (Fankhauser 1996):
      - Up to an 84% decrease in pain symptoms, mostly Days 2 and 3 of cycle (Coco 1999).
  - Sexual activity:
    - Sexual excitement and orgasm may decrease dysmenorrhea secondary to uterine arteriolar vasodilation (Treybig 1989).
  - Pregnancy:
    - Reduces the number of adrenergic nerves that only partially regenerate after delivery. This may result in a decrease or absence of pain (Treybig 1989).
  - Application of local heat with a heating pad or hot-water bottle:
    - Studies suggest a central analgesia effect and a direct effect of the activity on the uterus when heat is used in combination with ibuprofen (Akin et al. 2001).
    - Increases blood flow and decreases muscle spasm (Treybig 1989).
  - Acupuncture:
    - One study indicated an improvement in pain symptoms of up to 91% and a 41% decrease in the use of analgesics (Coco 1999).
  - Transcutaneous electrical nerve stimulation:
    - May be useful for:
      - Patients who have contraindications or have experienced side effects with oral contraceptives or NSAIDs.
      - Patients who do not get adequate pain relief from NSAIDs.
  - May not be widely available or affordable.
  - Mechanism:
    - Inhibits propagation of pain-related impulses (the "gate control" theory).
    - Increases the release of endorphins, with subsequent pain relief (Dawood 1990, Dawood et al. 1990).

Secondary Dysmenorrhea

→ Specific therapy should be aimed at correcting the underlying cause of the condition. There may be some temporary relief achieved with analgesics, antispasmodics, or oral contraceptives. However, only resolving the underlying condition will be successful (Smith 1997).
→ See the chapters **Pelvic Pain—Acute**, **Pelvic Pain—Chronic**, **Endometriosis**, **Pelvic Masses**, **Pelvic Inflammatory Disease**, and **Abnormal Uterine Bleeding**.
→ Stress relief, hypnosis, psychotherapy may be helpful.
→ Referral to a support group may be indicated.
→ Record keeping: The patient should keep a diary of symptomatology and basal body temperatures for the first 2–4 months of treatment.
  - Useful for assessing the characteristics of the pain, associated symptoms, and efficacy of treatment (Treybig 1989).

CONSULTATION

→ For evaluation of possible causes of secondary dysmenorrhea, if suspected.
→ As needed for prescription(s).

PATIENT EDUCATION

→ Explain the process of menstruation and the etiology of dysmenorrhea. Patients with primary dysmenorrhea should be reassured that their condition is not caused by pelvic pathology.
→ Review daily living modifications.
→ Advise the patient to initiate NSAIDs at the first sign of menses.
→ Instruct the patient about proper use of oral contraception and NSAIDs, including potential side effects.
→ Discuss diary-keeping.
→ Encourage regular exercise and proper nutrition.
→ Encourage follow-up visits.

FOLLOW-UP

→ Re-evaluation after one month is recommended to assess treatment efficacy.
→ Document in progress notes and on problem list.

BIBLIOGRAPHY

Akin, M.D., Weingand, K.W., Hengehold, D.A. et al. 2001. Continuous low-level topical heat in the treatment of dysmenorrhea. *Obstetrics and Gynecology* 97(3):343–349.

Coco, A.S. 1999. Primary dysmenorrhea. *American Family Physician* 60(2):489–496.

Davis, A., and Westhoff, C. 2001. Primary dysmenorrhea in adolescent girls and treatment with oral contraceptives. *Journal of Pediatric Adolescent Gynecology* 14:3–8.

Dawood, Y.M. 1984. Ibuprofen and dysmenorrhea. *American Journal of Medicine* 77:87–94.

_____. 1985. Dysmenorrhea. *Journal of Reproductive Medicine* 30(3):154–167.

_____. 1988. Nonsteroidal anti-inflammatory drugs and changing attitudes toward dysmenorrhea. *Clinical Obstetrics and Gynecology* 33(1):168–178.

_____. 1990. Dysmenorrhea. *Clinical Obstetrics and Gynecology* 33(1):168–178.

Dawood, Y.M., and Ramos, J. 1990. Transcutaneous electrical nerve stimulation (TENS) for the treatment of primary dysmenorrhea: a randomized crossover comparison with placebo TENS and ibuprofen. *Obstetrics and Gynecology* 75:656–660.

Fankhauser, M. 1996. Treatment of dysmenorrhea and premenstrual syndrome. *Journal of the American Pharmaceutical Association* NS36(8):503–513.

Granot, M., Yarnitsky, D., Itskovitz-Eldor, J. et al. 2001. Pain perception in women with dysmenorrhea. *Obstetrics and Gynecology* 98(3):407–411.

Hillen, T., Grbavac, S., Johnston, P. et al. 1999. Primary dysmenorrhea in young Western Australian women: prevalence, impact, and knowledge of treatment. *Journal of Adolescent Health* 25(1):40–45.

Hoffman, P.G. 1988. Primary dysmenorrhea and the premenstrual syndrome. In *Office gynecology*, 3rd ed., ed. R.H. Glass, pp. 209–229. Baltimore, Md.: Williams & Wilkins.

Pernoll, M.L., and Benson, R.C. 1987. Complications of menstruation, abnormal uterine bleeding. In *Current obstetric and gynecologic diagnosis and treatment*, pp. 613–614. Norwalk, Conn.: Appleton & Lange.

Schroeder, B., and Sanfilippo, J.S. 1999. Dysmenorrhea and pelvic pain in adolescents. *Pediatric Clinics of North America* 46(3):555–571.

Smith, R.P. 1997. Menstrual pain. In *Gynecology in primary care*, pp. 389–404. Baltimore, Md.: Williams & Wilkins.

Sullivan, N. 1990. Dysmenorrhea. In *Gynecology: well-woman care*, eds. R. Lichtman and S. Papera, pp. 345–353. Norwalk, Conn.: Appleton & Lange.

Sundell, G., Milsom, J., and Andersch, B. 1990. Factors influencing the prevalence and severity of dysmenorrhea in young women. *British Journal of Obstetrics and Gynaecology* 97:588–594.

Treybig, M. 1989. Primary dysmenorrhea or endometriosis? *Nurse Practitioner* 14(5):8–18.

Wolf, L., and Schumann, L. 1999. Dysmenorrhea. *Journal of the American Academy of Nurse Practitioners* 11(3):125–130.

Women's Primary Care Program. 1989. Dysmenorrhea/premenstrual syndrome. Lecture presented at the University of California-San Francisco School of Nursing.

12-E
Ectopic Pregnancy

Ectopic pregnancy is a pregnancy that occurs outside of normal implantation sites within the uterine cavity. The fallopian tubes are the most frequent sites of ectopic pregnancy (Tenore 2000). Other, less common extrauterine sites of implantation include the cervix, ovaries, and abdominal cavity. In addition, *heterotopic pregnancies* (simultaneous intrauterine and extrauterine pregnancy) can occur. Although heterotopic pregnancies are rare (approximately 1 in 10,000–50,000 pregnancies), there is an increased risk of up to 1 in 100 in women undergoing assisted reproductive procedures (Habana et al. 2000, Lemus 2000). There also have been rare case reports of bilateral ectopic pregnancies occurring in women who have received gonadotropin releasing hormone (GnRH) agonists and undergone in vitro fertilization (Dean et al. 1998, Hugues et al. 1995, Klipstein et al. 2000).

Annually, ectopic pregnancy occurs in 2% of all pregnancies in the United States (Barnhart et al. 2000, Tenore 2000). A sixfold increase in the incidence of ectopic pregnancies has been noted since the 1970s (Tenore 2000). Multiple factors have been implicated in this increased incidence, including and increase in sexually transmitted diseases (STDs), assisted reproduction (e.g., ovulation induction, in vitro fertilization, gamete intrafallopian transfer [GIFT]), and earlier diagnosis of ectopic pregnancies due to improved technology and provider awareness (Carr et al. 2000, Tenore 2000).

Ectopic pregnancy is the leading cause of maternal death during the first trimester in the United States (Carr et al. 2000). Most maternal deaths are attributed to a delay in diagnosis, either because patients failed to seek evaluations and treatment or providers failed to diagnose and treat the condition in a timely manner. However, the fatality rate associated with ectopic pregnancy has declined significantly since 1970, from 35.5/10,000 to 3.8/10,000 in 1989 (Goldman et al. 1993). Presumably this is because of earlier detection and intervention as a result of improved technology, a higher index of suspicion on the part of clinicians, and the more conservative treatment options currently available.

A number of pathophysiological mechanisms have been cited as probable causes of ectopic pregnancies. Tubal ectopic pregnancies are a result of inhibition or prevention of normal tubal transport of an embryo because of damage to the mucosal lining of the fimbria and/or fallopian tube. The etiology of such damage may be secondary to infection (e.g., pelvic inflammatory disease [PID]), inflammation (e.g., chronic salpingitis or tubal diverticula), tubal/uterine surgery, and exposure to diethyl stilbestrol (DES).

Other possible risk factors that may contribute to ectopic pregnancies include ovum defects (e.g., premature or delayed ovulation, or postmature ovum), hormonal dysfunction (e.g., hyperestrogenism), use of GnRH agonists, cigarette smoking, mechanical interference with implantation (e.g., intrauterine devices [IUDs]), sterilization failure, and older maternal age (Barnhart et al. 2000, Bouyer et al. 2000, Dean et al. 1998, Lemus 2000, Philips et al. 1992).

Complications associated with an ectopic pregnancy can be severe and life-threatening. They are related to the length of gestation, site of implantation, any delay or failure to diagnose the condition, and method of treatment. The most emergent complication is excessive blood loss due to tubal rupture or development of a pelvic hematocele. Such blood loss may result in anemia, the need for transfusions, and, rarely, the development of disseminated intravascular coagulopathy or death. Regardless of the therapeutic intervention chosen in the management of a patient with an ectopic pregnancy, careful monitoring for any evidence of acute or chronic blood loss is essential.

An increased incidence of repeated ectopic pregnancy is another complication reported in the literature. Recurrence rates of 9–15% have been documented. Women with a history of predisposing conditions involving tubal damage are more likely to have repeated ectopic pregnancies (Carr et al. 2000, Kjellberg et al. 2000, Strobelt et al. 2000). In addition, the type of therapeutic intervention chosen can have an impact on recurrence rates. The incidence of repeat ectopic pregnancies is less with conservative treatments (e.g., expectant management, medical management, and conservative surgical procedures) compared to more extensive surgical procedures and procedures involving more manipulation of the fallopian tube(s) (e.g., "milking" the tube to remove the products of conception [POCs]) (Carr et al. 2000, Kjellberg et al. 2000, Lipscomb et al. 2000, Morlock et al. 2000, Strobelt et al. 2000).

Persistent ectopic pregnancy can occur when retained trophoblastic tissue continues to proliferate at the site of implantation. This complication has been reported in up to 8% of women undergoing salpingostomy (Carr et al. 2000). Persistent ectopic pregnancy can result in hemorrhage, continued tubal destruction, and, rarely, the development of choriocarcinoma. Clinicians should consider this possible complication in any patient with persistent elevation of serum human chronic gonadotropin (hCG) levels after therapy for an ectopic pregnancy (Carr et al. 2000).

DATABASE

SUBJECTIVE

→ Risk factors may include (Carr et al. 2000, Dean et al. 1998, Klipstein et al. 2000, Lemus 2000, Philips et al. 1992, Tenore 2000):
  - A history of one or more of the following:
    - PID
    - Prior ectopic pregnancy
    - Tubal or uterine surgery
    - Infertility or infertility treatment
    - Current or past use of an IUD (as a result of IUD prevention of intrauterine pregnancy but not extrauterine pregnancy)
    - Cigarette smoking
    - Factors associated with uterine or tubal anatomic abnormalities (e.g., DES exposure, salpingitis, and isthmica nodosa)
    - Hormones used to induce ovulation or down-regulation of a cycle with a GnRH agonist
    - Assisted reproduction (e.g., GIFT and in vitro fertilization)
    - Prior therapeutic abortion with complications (i.e., endometritis or retained POCs)

  NOTE: Although several risk factors associated with ectopic pregnancy have been reported in the literature, in many instances women do not have an identifiable risk factor.

→ Symptoms may include one of more of the following (Carr et al. 2000, Klipstein et al. 2000, Lemus 2000, Philips et al. 1992, Tenore 2000):
  - Abdominal pain, which is reported by approximately 75% of women experiencing an ectopic pregnancy
    - Pain may range in intensity and character from a mild, dull, cramp-like sensation to a severe, sharp pain.
    - Women experiencing acute blood loss associated with tubal rupture usually report the sudden onset of severe, lower quadrant abdominal pain that may be intermittent and associated with backache, dizziness, and fainting.
    - Women experiencing chronic blood loss from "minor" tubal ruptures may report less severe abdominal symptoms.
  - Amenorrhea

  - Abnormal vaginal bleeding, which may vary from slight intermenstrual spotting to profuse vaginal bleeding
  - Associated symptoms of pregnancy (e.g., nausea, vomiting, and breast tenderness/enlargement) may or may not be reported depending on the gestation of the pregnancy (i.e., after eight weeks gestation, the patient may not notice any associated symptoms)
  - Significant blood loss, lightheadedness, vertigo, and/or syncopal episodes
  - Shoulder pain, which may be reported by patients experiencing hemorrhage as blood pools under the diaphragm
  - In addition to abdominal pain, a patient with an abdominal pregnancy may report persistent nausea and vomiting, general malaise, painful fetal movements, fetal movements high in the abdominal cavity, and decreased fetal movements.

OBJECTIVE

→ Physical examination may reveal one or more of the following findings (Carr et al. 2000, Klipstein et al. 2000, Lemus 2000, Philips et al. 1992, Tenore 2000):
  - Vital signs are within normal limits (WNL) or they may demonstrate changes associated with significant blood loss (e.g., decreased blood pressure, rapid/therapy pulse, rapid respirations, and orthostatic changes).
  - The patient may appear to be in no distress, may be anxious, or may be unconscious (depending on symptoms and blood loss).
  - Skin pallor may be observed in patients with significant blood loss.
  - Upon abdominal examination:
    - Decreased bowel sounds may be noted if a mild paralytic ileus has occurred (may be noted in patients with chronic abdominal blood loss).
    - If hemoperitoneum is present, tenderness to palpation with or without rebound, guarding.
    - Cullen's sign (bluish discoloration of the umbilical area) may be noted and is associated with hemoperitoneum.
    - If there is an abdominal pregnancy, uterine size is smaller than dates, a distinct mass may be observed outside the uterus, fetal parts may be easily palpated, and fetal activity may be noted high within the abdomen.
  - Upon pelvic examination:
    - A speculum may reveal varying amounts of blood (minimal to profuse) at the introitus, in the vaginal vault, and/or coming from the cervical os.
    - Bimanual may be WNL if the pregnancy is in an early stage of gestation or there is an adnexal mass with or without tenderness to palpation.
      - There may be a doughy sensation when the pouch of Douglas is palpated (posterior vaginal wall) due to the accumulation of blood in this area secondary to a hemoperitoneum.

ASSESSMENT

→ Ectopic pregnancy (tubal, cervical, ovarian, or abdominal)
→ R/O appendicitis
→ R/O spontaneous abortion
→ R/O gestational trophoblastic neoplasia
→ R/O ruptured corpus luteum cyst
→ R/O intrauterine gestation earlier than suggested by menstrual dates
→ R/O intrauterine pregnancy with corpus luteum cyst
→ R/O PID
→ R/O urinary calculi

PLAN

DIAGNOSTIC TESTS

→ Most ectopic pregnancies are diagnosed by a number of tests and procedures ordered depending on the patient's status (i.e., stable versus in shock) as well as the point in gestation when the patient presents for an evaluation.

- Because a patient with a suspected ectopic pregnancy is at risk for significant morbidity and mortality due to hemorrhage, physician management of such patients is warranted and any diagnostic tests should be ordered in consultation with the physician.
- Complete blood count may reveal a decreased erythrocyte count, hemoglobin, and hematocrit consistent with acute or chronic blood loss, as well as a mild leukocytosis.

→ Pregnancy tests:

- Quantitative serum beta-human chorionic gonadotropin (ß-hCG) radioimmunoassay:
  - Currently, this is considered the gold standard for evaluating patients with a possible ectopic pregnancy.
    - A positive result can be obtained 7–10 days after conception and is highly sensitive (99%).
    - In normal, early intrauterine pregnancies, a doubling of this hormone level is expected every 1.5 days until seven weeks, then every 3.5 days (Carr et al. 2000).
    - Although abnormal results do not confirm the existence of an ectopic pregnancy, they may help the clinician formulate a plan of care when an ectopic pregnancy is suspected.
    - Serial testing can be done every 48 hours to determine if a normal or abnormal pregnancy is occurring.
  - ß-hCG levels that demonstrate an increase of <66% increase over 48 hours are associated with ectopic pregnancies or a spontaneous abortion of intrauterine pregnancies in 85% of patients.
  - In abdominal pregnancies, the ß-hCG may be abnormally elevated for the stage of gestation.
  - The discriminatory zone of ß-hCG: ß-hCG levels can be used with ultrasonography to determine the presence of an early ectopic pregnancy (especially at a gestational stage [i.e., less than 10 weeks gestation] when tubal rupture is less likely to occur).
    - Discriminatory zones of ß-hCG levels are the levels at which an intrauterine gestational sac should be reliably visible by ultrasound.
    - When the ß-hCG is 6,000–6,500 IU/L (International Reference Preparation), an intrauterine gestational sac should be visible by transabdominal ultrasound in more than 90% of pregnant patients (Carr et al. 2000).
    - When an ultrasound is done using a vaginal transducer, the discriminatory zone for ß-hCG is reportedly in the range of 1,500–2,000 IU/L (International Reference Preparation) (Carr et al. 2000, Lemus 2000, Tulandi et al. 2000).
      - ➤ At these levels, if an intrauterine gestational sac is not visible, the pregnancy may not be viable or it may be an ectopic implantation. However, the presence of an intrauterine gestational sac does not absolutely eliminate the possibility of an ectopic pregnancy, as heterotopic pregnancy, although rare, can occur (Carr et al. 2000, Lemus 2000).

  NOTE: Individual institutions should establish specific discriminatory zone ranges based on their quality of ultrasonography, the ß-hCG radioimmunoassay techniques utilized, and the reference standard for quantifying the ß-hCG level. Clinicians must know the discriminatory zones currently used in their institutions in order to evaluate patients properly.

  - Urine hCG tests: Several rapid, ultrasensitive monoclonal antibody urine tests are available to assess ß-hCG levels (e.g., Tandem Icon II® and First Response®).
    - These tests can reliably detect pregnancy 7–10 days after conception and can offer rapid screening of women for ectopic pregnancy; however, additional testing with serum ß-hCG and ultrasonography also may be indicated.
    - The reported false-negative rate of rapid urine hCG tests is 1%.

- Serum progesterone levels:
  - Low levels of progesterone have been associated with abnormal pregnancies, including spontaneous abortions and ectopic pregnancies (Carr et al. 2000, Lemus 2000, Perkins et al. 2000).
  - A single serum progesterone level does not confirm the existence of an ectopic pregnancy; however, a low level can alert the clinician to the possibility of a potentially abnormal pregnancy requiring further evaluation and testing (Perkins et al. 2000).

- Ultrasonography (Atri et al. 2001, Thoma 2000):
  - Both transabdominal and transvaginal ultrasonography can be used to evaluate a patient suspected of having an ectopic pregnancy, either by ruling out the presence of an intrauterine pregnancy or demonstrating the presence of a gestational sac outside of the uterus.
  - The accuracy of ultrasound results in determining an ectopic pregnancy is based on the stage of gestation, the implantation site, the type of ultrasound being performed, and the capabilities of the sonographer.

- Abdominal ultrasound:
  - The absence of an intrauterine gestational sac six weeks from the patient's last menstrual period or the absence of a fetal pole seven weeks from the last menstrual period may indicate an ectopic pregnancy, especially if serum ß-hCG levels are 6,000–6,500 IU/L.
  - The presence of a gestational sac and fetal pole does not eliminate the possibility of an ectopic pregnancy in all patients, as heterotopic pregnancy can occur.
  - Evidence of a gestational sac or fetus outside of the uterine cavity (e.g., in the interstitial portion of the fallopian tube, in the abdomen, or in the ovary) confirms the diagnosis of an ectopic pregnancy at these sites.
  - The presence of an intrauterine gestational sac-like structure (i.e., a "pseudogestational sac") may be observed in an ectopic pregnancy and can be confused with an intrauterine gestational sac.

  NOTE: A pseudogestational sac can result from accumulation of blood in the uterine cavity, the development of the decidual lining without a trophoblastic rim, or the development of a thick, proliferative endometrium (Thoma 2000).
  - Transvaginal ultrasound (Atri et al. 2001, Carr et al. 2000, Lemus 2000, Thoma 2000):
    - The use of transvaginal ultrasound in evaluating ectopic pregnancy has been documented in several studies and is reportedly more accurate than abdominal ultrasound in locating early-gestation ectopic pregnancies and determining the size of the gestational sac.
      - ➤ Evidence of extrauterine fetal cardiac pulsations indicates an ectopic pregnancy.
      - ➤ Visualization of a sac-like adnexal ring is indicative of an ectopic pregnancy.
      - ➤ Visualization of echogenic fluid may indicate an ectopic pregnancy. This finding also correlates with a hemoperitoneum in many patients.
      - ➤ Evidence of fluid in the cul-de-sac may indicate an ectopic pregnancy.
  - Culdocentesis:
    - Aspiration of unclotted blood indicates intraperitoneal bleeding and an ectopic pregnancy in patients with signs and symptoms associated with this condition.
    - Absence of fluid from the cul-de-sac does not eliminate the possibility of an ectopic pregnancy.
  - If the patient has had a recent therapeutic abortion, the pathology report on the POCs may be able to confirm and an intrauterine pregnancy, in which case the likelihood of a simultaneous ectopic pregnancy is remote.
  - Laparoscopy often is performed when confirmation and further intervention are indicated.
    - This procedure can locate the site of an extrauterine pregnancy, assess bleeding, and, if indicated, accomplish removal of the ectopic contents in some patients.

TREATMENT/MANAGEMENT

→ A patient suspected of having an ectopic pregnancy should be cared for by a physician qualified to manage this condition.
  - Therapeutic options and interventions are determined by the physician based on the patient's status, symptoms, site of implantation, stage of gestation, and desire to maintain fertility.
  - The decision-making regarding the various treatment options is beyond the scope of this chapter. However, a brief presentation of these therapeutic interventions will be presented.
→ Expectant management:
  - Spontaneous resolution of extrauterine pregnancies is reportedly as high as 80% (Buster et al. 2000, Carr et al. 2000, Lemus 2000, Tenore 2000, Tulandi et al. 2000).
    - Expectant management involving close observation without the use of medical or surgical interventions has been studied in a very select group of patients with ectopic pregnancies. The inclusion criteria for entry into the studies were (Atri et al. 2001, Carr et al. 2000, Lemus 2000, Lipscomb et al. 2000, Strobelt et al. 2000, Tenore 2000, Tulandi et al. 2000):
      - An initial serum ß-hCG level of ≤1,500 IU/L
      - A consistent decline in hCG level
      - No intrauterine sac identified by ultrasound
      - Ectopic pregnancy with greatest dimension <3.5 cm
      - No symptoms reported by the patient
      - No evidence of tubal rupture or bleeding (by ultrasound and/or laparoscopy)
      - Patient compliance with required serial testing and follow-up visits
        - ➤ Complications associated with this treatment plan included an increase in abdominal pain (self-limited), formation of a hematoma, late tubal rupture, hemorrhage, and persistent ectopic pregnancy.
        - ➤ Tubal patency and return of reproductive performance in patients involved in expectant management strategies were higher than what have been observed in patients undergoing surgical interventions. However, due to possible complications, this expectant management approach generally is not recommended.
→ Medical interventions:
  - The use of pharmacological agents for treating ectopic pregnancies has been studied. The various success rates depend on the type of agent used, the method of administration (i.e., systemic versus local injection), patient tolerance of the agent, stage of gestation of the pregnancy, and size of the gestational sac (Buster et al. 2000, Carr et al. 2000, Lemus 2000, Tenore 2000, Tulandi et al. 2000).
    - The highest efficacy rates are reported in patients who receive single or repeated systemic methotrexate (Hajenius et al. 2001, Lipscomb et al. 2000, Morlock et al. 2000).

- However, other agents, such as systemic RU-486 (mifepristone) and local injections of prostaglandins, actinomycin D, and potassium chloride, have been studied; efficacy rates varied (Hajenius et al. 2001).
- Complications associated with this plan of care include possible adverse effects of the pharmacological agent(s), tubal rupture, bleeding, and persistent ectopic pregnancy.
  - Women who are Rh negative and antibody screen (Du) negative should be given Rh immune globulin (RhIG) in the following recommended doses:
    - 50 µg of RhIG (Micro RhoGam®) IM if the ectopic gestation is <13 weeks
    - 300 µg of RhIG (RhoGam®) IM if the gestation is >13 weeks (American College of Obstetricians and Gynecologists 1998)

→ Surgical interventions:
  - Various types are used to manage ectopic pregnancies.
  - Decisions regarding which surgical procedure is indicated are based on the status of the patient, the threat or evidence of rupture, bleeding, the size of the gestational sac, the accessibility of the ectopic pregnancy, the desire of the patient to maintain fertility, the skill of the surgeon, and the availability of various laparoscopic instruments.
  - Surgical procedures that may be performed include (Carr et al. 2000, Lemus 2000, Tenore 2000):
    - Laparoscopy with removal of the POC and/or oviduct
    - Linear salpingostomy
    - Segmental resection of the fallopian tube
    - Salpingectomy
    - Laparotomy
    - Hysteroscopy
  - The more conservative surgical interventions are less life-threatening and have a higher likelihood of maintaining tubal patency than more extensive procedures.
  - Complications associated with the surgical procedures include:
    - Hemorrhage
    - Infection
    - Anesthesia complications
    - Persistent ectopic pregnancy (primarily associated with conservative surgical procedures)
    - Decreased tubal patency
    - Decreased reproductive performance
    - Death

CONSULTATION

→ Consultation with a physician is warranted for any patient suspected of having an ectopic pregnancy.
  - The evaluation and management of the woman should be by the consulting physician.
→ Consultation with a psychologist or psychiatrist may be indicated for patients and their partners who are experiencing prolonged, severe depression associated with pregnancy loss.
  - This may be especially important for women or couples who have undergone assisted reproduction procedures (e.g., GIFT or in vitro fertilization) and are facing the loss of a desired pregnancy and the possibility of further reduction in fertility as a result of this condition.
  - In addition, the threat of death may precipitate a psychological crisis for the woman and/or her partner, requiring crisis intervention.

PATIENT EDUCATION

→ Education of the patient with a suspected or documented ectopic pregnancy should include information about the condition, diagnostic tests that will be ordered, treatment options, possible complications associated with the condition and treatment(s), and indicated follow-up.
  - Ideally, such discussions should occur between the patient and the physician responsible for her care.
  - In situations where the patient's condition is unstable, the physician, the patient, and a patient's relative or partner should discuss the plan of care whenever possible.
→ Women undergoing outpatient therapy (e.g., expectant or medical management) should be educated about the possibility of sudden rupture of an ectopic pregnancy and the rapid blood loss associated with this condition.
  - The patient should receive a thorough review of signs and symptoms that occur.
  - The patient should be advised not to operate motor vehicles or be involved in similar activities that require concentration because of the possibility of syncopal episodes that can occur with tubal rupture and significant blood loss.
  - The patient should have a plan for immediate access to medical treatment if any signs and/or symptoms associated with tubal rupture and hemorrhage develop (e.g., someone should be immediately available to drive her to the hospital).
→ Referral of the patient and her partner to community resources that provide support as they work through the loss of a pregnancy may be necessary.
→ Education of all sexually active women of reproductive age regarding ways to prevent STDs will help prevent and eventually reduce the incidence of ectopic pregnancies (especially tubal pregnancies).
→ If a woman with risk factors is contemplating pregnancy, she should be educated about the possibility of an ectopic pregnancy and the need to obtain an evaluation as soon as possible after conception so her pregnancy can be carefully monitored for evidence of extrauterine implantation.
→ After a woman has completed therapy for an ectopic pregnancy, she should be counseled about the need to postpone conception for three months to allow complete recovery of the ectopic implantation site.
  - Contraception should be provided after a discussion of available methods.

FOLLOW-UP

→ Follow-up evaluation of the patient with an ectopic pregnancy is by the physician or clinician responsible for her care.

→ Serum ß-hCG levels should be monitored in a woman who has had an ectopic pregnancy to determine if the condition has been resolved.
- The frequency of testing is based on the gestation of the pregnancy and the type of treatment the woman is undergoing.
- Testing should be recommended by the physician or clinician managing the woman's care.
- A consistent decline in ß-hCG levels should be observed. A level that plateaus or increases warrants further evaluation and possibly a change in therapy (Carr et al. 2000, Tenore 2000).

→ Women being treated for an ectopic pregnancy without evidence of immunity to rubella should be considered for rubella immunization during the follow-up period.
- Thorough counseling regarding the need to postpone conception until at least three months after immunization, as well as provision of an effective contraceptive method during this period, is essential.
- Document in progress notes and on problem list.

BIBLIOGRAPHY

American College of Obstetricians and Gynecologists (ACOG). 1998. *Medical management of tubal pregnancy. Clinical management guidelines for obstetrician-gynecologists.* ACOG Practice Bulletin No. 3. Washington, D.C.: the Author.

Atri, M., Chow, C.M., Kintzen, G. et al. 2001. Expectant treatment of ectopic pregnancies: clinical and sonographic predictors. *American Journal of Roentgenology* 176:123–127.

Barnhart, K., Esposito, M., and Coutifaris, C. 2000. An update on the medical treatment of ectopic pregnancy. *Obstetrics and Gynecology Clinics of North America* 27(3):653–667.

Bouyer, J., Rachou, E., Germain, E. et al. 2000. Risk factors for extrauterine pregnancy in women using an intrauterine device. *Fertility and Sterility* 74(5):899–908.

Buster, J.E., and Heard, M.J. 2000. Current issues in medical management of ectopic pregnancy. *Current Opinion in Obstetrics and Gynecology* 12:525–527.

Carr, R.J., and Evans, P. 2000. Ectopic pregnancy. *Primary Care* 27(1):169–183.

Dean, N., and Tan, S.L. 1998. An ectopic pregnancy masked by follicular initiation of gonadotropin-releasing hormone agonist for pituitary desensitization prior to in vitro fertilization. *Journal of Assisted Reproduction and Genetics* 15:161–163.

Goldman, E.E., Lawson, H.W., Xia, Z. et al. 1993. Surveillance for ectopic pregnancy—United States, 1970–1989. *MMWR CDC Surveillance Summary* 42:73–85.

Habana, A., Dokras, A., Giraldo, J.L. et al. 2000. Cornual heterotopic pregnancy: contemporary management options. *American Journal of Obstetrics and Gynecology* 182(5): 1264–1270.

Hajenius, P.J., Mol, B.W.J., Bossuyt, P.M.M. et al. 2001. Interventions for tubal ectopic pregnancy (Cochrane Review). *Cochrane Library* 3:1–81.

Hugues, J.M., Olszewska, B., Dauvergne, P. et al. 1995. Two-step diagnosis of bilateral ectopic pregnancy following in vitro fertilization. *Journal of Assisted Reproduction and Genetics* 12:460–462.

Kjellberg, L., Lalos, A., and Lalos, O. 2000. Reproductive outcome after surgical treatment of ectopic pregnancy. *Gynecologic and Obstetric Investigation* 49:227–230.

Klipstein, S., and Oskowitz, S.P. 2000. Bilateral ectopic pregnancy after transfer of two embryos. *Fertility and Sterility* 74(5):887–888.

Lemus, J.F. 2000. Ectopic pregnancy: an update. *Current Opinion in Obstetrics and Gynecology* 12:369–375.

Lipscomb, G.H., Stovall, T.G., and Ling, F.W. 2000. Nonsurgical treatment of ectopic pregnancy. *New England Journal of Medicine* 343(18):1325–1329.

Morlock, R.J., Lafata, J.E., and Eisenstein, D. 2000. Cost-effectiveness of single-dose methotrexate compared with laparoscopic treatment of ectopic pregnancy. *Obstetrics and Gynecology* 95(3):407–412.

Perkins, S.L., Al-Ramahi, M., and Claman, P. 2000. Comparison of serum progesterone as an indicator of pregnancy nonviability in spontaneous pregnant emergency room and infertility clinic patient populations. *Fertility and Sterility* 73(3):499–504.

Philips, R.S., Tuomala, R.E., Feidblum, P.J. et al. 1992. The effect of cigarette smoking, *Chlamydia trachomatis* infection, and vaginal douching on ectopic pregnancy. *Obstetrics and Gynecology* 79:85–90.

Strobelt, N., Mariani, E., Ferrari, L. et al. 2000. Fertility after ectopic pregnancy. Effects of surgery and expectant management. *Journal of Reproductive Medicine* 45(10): 803–807.

Tenore, J.L. 2000. Ectopic pregnancy. *American Family Physician* 61(4):1080–1088.

Thoma, M.E. 2000. Early detection of ectopic pregnancy visualizing the presence of a tubal ring with ultrasonography performed by emergency physicians. *American Journal of Emergency Medicine* 18:444–448.

Tulandi, T., and Sammour, A. 2000. Evidence-based management of ectopic pregnancy. *Current Opinion in Obstetrics and Gynecology* 12:289–292.

Kim K. O'Hair, R.N.P., M.S.N.

12-F

Endometriosis

Endometriosis is the presence of glandular and stromal endometria in ectopic sites. It is described as a continuum of change that begins at the cellular level and may be expressed in chronic pelvic pain and infertility, or it may be totally without symptoms (Eskenazi et al. 1997). Although its prevalence is unknown, endometriosis may affect 2–15% of women of reproductive age, including an estimated 5 million women in the United States. It is believed to affect 20–40% of infertile women (Mahmood et al. 1990) and 4.5–32% (mean 18.8%) of patients with chronic pelvic pain (Duleba 1997). Endometriosis usually occurs in the pelvis, with the most common sites being the ovaries, the posterior cul-de-sac, and the uterosacral ligaments (Gerbie et al. 1988). Endometrial tissue has been found in such obscure sites as the stomach, gall bladder, lungs, kidneys, and brain. It also has been found in men undergoing hormonal therapy to treat prostate cancer (Eskenazi et al. 1997).

The usual age of onset is in the middle twenties; however, girls as young as 12–13 years old, occasionally before menarche, have been diagnosed with endometriosis. The highest incidence is found in women 40–44 years old (Corwin 1997). There is a decline in the number of women affected at approximately 45 years of age, which is thought to be related to waning estrogen levels in the perimenopausal period (Eskenazi et al. 1997). While *de novo* cases of endometriosis in menopause are quite uncommon, it has been identified in approximately 5% of menopausal women on estrogen replacement therapy (Corwin 1997). Although endometriosis is considered a benign condition, 105 cases of malignant neoplasms arising from it have been reported since 1925 (Heaps et al. 1990).

Endometriosis is one of the most common causes of pelvic pain and infertility among women. While 20–40% of women with infertility are found to have endometriosis, the exact nature of this relationship is unclear (Mahmood et al. 1990, Zreik et al. 1997). In moderate or severe cases of endometriosis, anatomical defects (e.g., pelvic adhesions, fibrosis, distal fimbrial agglutination, ovarian scarring) may interfere with ovulation, ovum pick-up, or embryo transport. In the absence of an anatomical alteration, however, there is no clear explanation for the infertility. Factors under consideration include ovulatory dysfunction, hormonal abnormalities, autoimmunity, a "hostile" pelvic environment, and an increased risk of spontaneous abortion. The possibility exists that delayed childbearing or infertility may actually predispose a woman to endometriosis and not the converse (Mahmood et al. 1990, Zreik et al. 1997). Moderate to severe endometriosis has been more often associated with problems of infertility, but any woman experiencing unexplained infertility should be considered for an evaluation for endometriosis (Wellbery 1999).

While a great deal of research has been done on the etiologies, diagnostic evaluations, and treatments proposed for this disease, very little is known about the psychological and emotional impact it has on a woman and her family. Patients with chronic pelvic pain from various sources, including endometriosis, have been observed to have psychological profiles that may include depression, dysfunctional family interactions, or childhood sexual or physical abuse (Zreik et al. 1997). Depression is not an uncommon response in women experiencing chronic pain nor is it uncommon in infertile women desiring conception. In addition, lost work time, reduced productivity, and other economic and social costs have not been completely evaluated (Eskenazi et al. 1997).

Although endometriosis was first described in the 1880s and has been studied extensively, uncertainty persists regarding its etiology, pathogenesis, natural history, and relationship to infertility diagnosis and management. Etiological theories include celomic metaplasia, embryonic cell rest, transportation of endometrial implants by the lymph or hematologic system, and transportation by retrograde menstruation.

The theory of celomic metaplasia refers to the ability of the peritoneal mesothelium to undergo metaplasia and produce ectopic endometrium as a response to chronic inflammation or chemical changes from refluxed menstrual blood. Embryonic cell rest theory is based on the assumption that cells of Muellerian origin may develop into functioning endometrium (Wellbery 1999). Neither theory is well supported by evidence (Metzger et al. 1989, Wellbery 1999).

The theories of hematologic or lymphatic transport of endometrial tissue to ectopic areas may provide an explanation for endometrial implants in sites as diverse as the lungs and brain. Retrograde menstruation through the fallopian tubes into the peritoneum has been identified on laparoscopy and is estimated to occur in as many as 90% of all women (Hill 1997). Once retrograde menstrual blood is present in the peritoneum, it is potentially available for transport via either transport system.

In women without endometriosis, presumably endometrial tissue, debris, and blood are destroyed before they can be implanted in the pelvis. In women with endometriosis, the tissue does have an opportunity to implant and can begin to proliferate (Wellbery 1999). Eventually, the endometrial tissue develops an independent vascular supply and responds to the alterations of the menstrual cycle hormones, growing and shedding tissue that may then again disseminate throughout the peritoneum (Corwin 1997). It has been proposed that an aberrant autoimmune process may reduce immune responsiveness or perhaps an inflammatory process may also play a role in endometrial implantation and proliferation (Hill 1997).

Aside from the confusion regarding the pathophysiology of endometriosis, one of the predominant complaints of the patient is pelvic pain. The inflammatory response to the presence of endometrial implants leads to localized production of several types of inflammatory mediators, especially prostaglandins, cytokines, and complement proteins. The prostaglandins in particular are active in the severe dysmenorrhea experienced by these women (Corwin 1997). The tissue damage caused by the inflammatory response to the endometrial implants can result in extensive fibrosis and adhesions (Zreik et al. 1997). Adhesions can provoke a pain response by direct neuronal damage, by tissue ischemia, or by secondary damage to the vascular supply to the affected area (Zreik et al. 1997). Endometriosis presents a diagnostic challenge because the extent of endometriotic lesions may bear no relationship to the extent of pain (Duleba 1997).

DATABASE

SUBJECTIVE

→ Risk factors: Numerous studies have identified several risk factors for endometriosis, but results often have been confusing and contradictory. In their review of well-designed analytic epidemiologic studies, Eskenazi et al. (1997) observed the following:
  ▪ Sociodemographic characteristics:
    • Age: There is a positive relationship between age and endometriosis.
    • Race: Some studies have shown Japanese and other Asian women to be at greater risk than other women, but this may reflect selection biases and small study populations. Endometriosis has been noted in all races.
    • Socioeconomic status: Endometriosis has been identified in all socioeconomic classes.
  ▪ Reproductive health factors:
    • Several risk factors for endometriosis have been identified (Corwin 1997, Duleba 1997, Eskenazi et al. 1997):
      – Shorter cycle length: less than 28 days
      – Longer duration of flow: more than seven days
      – Menorrhagia, metrorrhagia
      – History of obstruction of menstrual flow
      – Increased peripheral body fat
      – History of sexually transmitted disease or pelvic inflammatory disease
    • Factors that reduce risk include:
      – Use of oral contraceptives (risk may increase after discontinuation of use)
      – Greater and earlier parity
  ▪ Lifestyle factors:
    • Smoking: An inverse relationship to endometriosis has been noted in some studies.
    • Caffeine: A positive relationship has been found between higher caffeine intake (more than 1–2 cups per day) and endometriosis.
    • Alcohol: A positive relationship has been found in some studies between more than one serving of alcohol per week and endometriosis, but it is not considered very significant.
    • Exercise: An inverse relationship to endometriosis has been reported.

→ History:
  ▪ Medical history:
    • Gastrointestinal diseases and conditions (bowel obstruction, irritable bowel syndrome, etc.), renal disease, bladder diseases (interstitial cystitis, recurrent urinary tract infection)
  ▪ Family history:
    • Endometriosis and infertility may involve familial or genetic factors.
  ▪ Medication history:
    • Pain control, contraception, antidepressants
  ▪ Psychosocial history:
    • Psychological support systems, assessment for childhood sexual or physical abuse, coping/stress management skills

→ Symptoms (Duleba 1997, Shaw 1991, Wellbery 1999):
  ▪ Dysmenorrhea, especially with increasing severity, gradually extending into the premenstrual and/or postmenstrual phases of the menstrual cycle
  ▪ Dyspareunia, especially on deep penetration, often positional and aggravated by proximity to menses
  ▪ Pelvic pain
  ▪ Abnormal uterine bleeding, rectal bleeding, or cyclic hemoptysis of the lungs
  ▪ Rectal pain, painful defecation, diarrhea, constipation, or bowel obstruction
  ▪ Dysuria, hematuria, or ureteral obstruction
  ▪ Severity of symptoms does not correlate with the extent of disease, but it may correlate with the depth or site of the lesion (Duleba 1997).

OBJECTIVE

→ A complete abdominal, pelvic, and rectal examination should be performed. Examination at the time of menses may provide greater detail and an opportunity to palpate nodularity.

- Abdomen:
  - Observe for diffuse or focal tenderness. On occasion, a post-cesarean section scar may develop into endometriosis.
- Pelvis:
  - For many women with endometriosis, the pelvic examination may be completely normal.
  - External genitalia, the vagina, and cervix should be examined for red, blue, or hemorrhagic nodules.
  - The uterus should be examined for tenderness, mobility, masses, fixed retroversion, or nodules.
  - Adnexae may be enlarged or fixed or have reduced mobility, tenderness, or nodularity.
  - Rectovaginal: nodularity or focal tenderness in the cul-de-sac, rectovaginal septum, or uterosacral ligaments.
→ Laparoscopy of the pelvis, conducted by a physician, allows for a definitive diagnosis by direct visualization of endometrial implants and provides an opportunity for biopsy confirmation. As the findings on pelvic examination often are completely normal, diagnosis and assessment can only be made by surgical observation of the pelvis.
  - In many cases, confirmation of endometriosis by laparoscopy will be necessary before therapy.
  - Visualization at the time of surgery allows for staging the degree of endometriosis using criteria developed by the American Society for Reproductive Medicine.
    - This classification system is useful but controversial regarding the development of treatment plans for infertility or pain management (Corwin 1997).
  - Laparoscopy may be deferred in younger women who are not immediately concerned with fertility; treatment is initiated based on symptom management.

ASSESSMENT

→ R/O endometriosis
→ R/O dysmenorrhea
→ R/O endometritis
→ R/O intrauterine or ectopic pregnancy
→ R/O pelvic inflammatory disease
→ R/O tuboovarian abscess
→ R/O uterine fibroids
→ R/O ovarian cysts
→ R/O appendicitis
→ R/O inflammatory bowel disease (Crohn's disease, ulcerative colitis) or obstruction
→ R/O cancer (cervical, uterine, ovarian)
→ R/O urinary tract infection, pyelonephritis, kidney stones
→ R/O ruptured endometrioma (a rare occurrence that may lead to generalized peritonitis [Lichtman et al. 1990])
→ See these chapters: **Abnormal Uterine Bleeding, Pelvic Pain—Acute, Pelvic Pain—Chronic, Infertility, Sexual Dysfunction, Dysmenorrhea, Pelvic Masses**, and **Ectopic Pregnancy**. In Section 7, see the **Abdominal Pain** chapter.

PLAN

DIAGNOSTIC TESTS

→ Laboratory evaluations of serum markers have been limited. CA-125 evaluations lack the sensitivity and specificity required of a reliable diagnostic or screening test and are not recommended, but they may prove helpful in monitoring the response to medical or surgical intervention (Duleba 1997).
→ Diagnostic imaging studies may identify patients with endometriosis.
  - Transvaginal ultrasonography is of limited effectiveness except in cases of endometriomas and other ovarian lesions.
  - Magnetic resonance imaging can detect pigmented hemorrhagic lesions, but it is not universally used in diagnosing endometriosis (Duleba 1997).
→ Appropriate tests to rule out other conditions may include, but are not limited to:
  - Pregnancy test
  - Screening for gonorrhea/chlamydia
  - Urine culture and sensitivity
  - CBC

TREATMENT/MANAGEMENT

→ Treatment should be individualized and based on the following:
  - Age
  - Severity of symptoms
  - Extent of disease
  - Wishes of the patient
  - The desire for pregnancy
  - Duration of infertility
  - Associated pelvic pathology
→ Expectant management, conservative surgical treatment, or pharmacologic therapy may be most appropriate for the woman who wishes to retain her reproductive function. Superovulation therapies such as in vitro fertilization and gamete intrafallopian tube transfer may be utilized for infertile women.
  - Expectant management is appropriate for women with mild or moderate endometriosis who present with infertility.
  - Conservative surgical treatment:
    - Various procedures can be done with laparoscopic electrocautery, excision, or laser surgery. Conservative therapy is indicated (Adamson et al. 1997, Corwin 1997):
      - To confirm the diagnosis
      - When an anatomical alteration (e.g., adhesions) may be interfering with conception
      - For chocolate cysts, endometriomas, or other lesions of the ovary
      - When medical therapy fails to result in conception or the relief of symptoms. Surgical intervention for infertile women with endometriosis has been observed to be more efficacious than pharmacotherapy in achieving conception (Corwin 1997).
→ Definitive surgical treatment (Adamson et al. 1997):

- Total hysterectomy and bilateral salpingo-oophorectomy with excision of implants is an option when all other medical and surgical interventions have failed and the woman no longer wishes to maintain reproductive function.

→ Pharmacologic therapy:
- Drugs of choice:
  - GnRH agonists reduce endogenous estrogen production resulting in shrinkage of endometrial tissue. A disadvantage of these drugs is the development of mild osteopenia; however, "add-back" therapies with low-dose estrogen or progesterone can provide protection against bone loss (Corwin 1997, Kettel et al. 1997).
  - Pain and symptom relief may be considerable with the use of GnRH agonists, but pain and symptoms may recur in up to 25% of women with mild endometriosis and in 70% of women with severe disease (Kettel et al. 1997).
    - Nafarelin:
      ➤ Usual dose is one spray (200 µg) intranasally twice a day, alternating nares.
      ➤ Dosage may be increased to 800 µg if menses persist after 2 months of treatment.
      ➤ Initiate therapy within 2–4 days of menses.
        * Pregnancy risk category X. Avoid pregnancy; barrier methods recommended (*Physicians' Desk Reference* [*PDR*] 2002).
    - Leuprolide acetate:
      ➤ Recommended dosage is a single 3.75 mg IM injection every 4 weeks, not to exceed 6 months.
      ➤ Initiate therapy within first 2 weeks of menses.
        * Pregnancy risk category X. Avoid pregnancy; barrier methods recommended (*PDR* 2002).
    - Goserelin:
      ➤ Recommended dosage is 3.6 mg subcutaneous depot to the anterior abdomen every 4 weeks for 6 months.
  - Non-GnRH agonists
    - Danazol: Suppresses estrogen production, resulting in endometrial tissue shrinkage.
      ➤ Initial dose is 400 mg p.o. per day for 6–9 months.
      ➤ May need to be titrated up to 800 mg p.o. per day if menses persist during initial treatment cycles.
      ➤ Adverse effects include headache, flushing, sweating, mood swings, and atrophic vaginitis. Hirsutism, virilization, acne, changes in libido, reduction of breast size, weight gain, and voice deepening also may occur (Saltiel et al. 1991).
      ➤ Pain relief after treatment is quite high initially (95%), but recurrence rates are variable—up to 38%, with the highest rates among women who have more severe disease (Kettel et al. 1997, Wellbery 1999).
      ➤ Barrier methods of contraception are recommended due to teratogenicity.
        * Pregnancy risk category X. Avoid pregnancy (*PDR* 2002).

- Progestational compounds:
  - Medroxyprogesterone acetate: 30 mg p.o. per day for 3 or more months
- Continuous oral contraceptives suppress ovulation and reduce symptoms of pain and dysmenorrhea. They often have been used after surgery or other medical treatment for women who do not desire conception (Corwin 1999). Recurrence of pain after therapy is common.
  - A low-dose combination oral contraceptive with 20–30 µg of ethinyl estradiol and a progestin.
  - Usual dose is 1 pill per day. Increase to 2 pills if breakthrough bleeding occurs. When breakthrough bleeding stops, return to 1 pill each day.
  - If symptom control is unsuccessful after 3 months, consider GnRH agonist therapy.

→ Pain management:
- Pain management, especially management of chronic pain, is challenging for all practitioners.
  - Chronic pain can delay the healing processes, alter immune response, increase stress levels, and result in depression, anxiety, and other psychological distress (Stege 1998).
  - For the woman with mild symptoms, treatment may be limited to nonsteroidal anti-inflammatory drugs.
  - Other pain management modalities, such as massage therapy, pelvic floor rehabilitation, and/or biofeedback, also may be efficacious.
  - For specific medications and treatments, see the **Pelvic Pain—Chronic** and **Dysmenorrhea** chapters.

CONSULTATION

→ Physician consultation should be considered in all suspected cases and is required in cases where more conservative measures do not provide relief of symptoms or conception cannot be achieved.
→ Consultation with pain management specialists, physical therapists skilled in managing pelvic pain, reproductive endocrinologists, gynecologic surgeons, and mental health providers may be necessary.

PATIENT EDUCATION

→ Discuss proposed etiologic theories regarding endometriosis.
→ Provide patient education regarding risks/benefits of surgical and drug therapies to aid in decision-making. Drug regimens vary considerably in terms of cost, and patients should be informed of the expense involved.
→ Advise patients that the natural history of endometriosis is unknown and that response to treatments may be unpredictable (Candiani et al. 1991).
→ Inform patients of alternative/complementary forms of symptom management, including herbal teas, prostaglandin inhibitors, heat, massage, and vitamin E supplements.
→ Advise patients to contact the National Endometriosis Association at (800) 992-ENDO or online at www.endometriosisassn.org for information. Another helpful Web site has

been provided by the National Institutes of Health at www. nichd.nih.gov/publications/pubs/endometriosis/index.htm

→ Encourage exercise both for stress management and antidepressive effects, especially for patients using danazol therapy, as exercise has been shown to reduce side effects.

→ Encourage stress management and development of coping skills. Endometriosis is a chronic progressive disease, and patients benefit from support groups and mental health support as needed.

FOLLOW-UP

→ Follow-up evaluations should be individualized according to treatment choices and patient needs.

→ Ongoing psychological support is an important component of care.

→ Follow up on any abnormal findings.

→ Document in progress notes and on problem list.

BIBLIOGRAPHY

Adamson, G.D., and Nelson, H.P. 1997. Surgical treatment of endometriosis. *Obstetrics and Gynecology Clinics of North America* 24(2):375–405.

Candiani, G.B., Vercelli, P., Fedela, L. et al. 1991. Mild endometriosis and infertility: a critical review of epidemiologic data, diagnostic pitfalls, and classification limits. *Obstetrical and Gynecological Survey* 46(6):374–378.

Corwin, E.J. 1997. Endometriosis: pathophysiology, diagnosis, and treatment. *Nurse Practitioner* 22(10):35–55.

Duleba, A.J. 1997. Diagnosis of endometriosis. *Obstetrics and Gynecology Clinics of North America* 24(2):331–344.

Eskenazi, B., and Warner, M.L. 1997. Epidemiology of endometriosis. *Obstetrics and Gynecology Clinics of North America* 24(2):235–257.

Gerbie, A.B., and Merrill, J.A. 1988. Pathology of endometriosis. *Clinical Obstetrics and Gynecology* 31(4):779–786.

Heaps, J.M., Nieberg, R.K., and Berek, J.S. 1990. Malignant neoplasms arising in endometriosis. *Obstetrics and Gynecology* 75(6):1023–1028.

Hill, J.A. 1997. Immunology and endometriosis: fact, artifact, or epiphenomenon? *Obstetrics and Gynecology Clinics of North America* 24(2):291–302.

Kettel, L.M., and Hummel, W.P. 1997. Modern medical management of endometriosis. *Obstetrics and Gynecology Clinics of North America* 24(2):361–373.

Lichtman, R., and Smith, S.M. 1990. Multiorgan disorders. In *Gynecology: well-woman care*, eds. R. Lichtman and S. Papera. Norwalk, Conn.: Appleton & Lange.

Mahmood, T.A., and Templeton, A. 1990. Pathophysiology of mild endometriosis: review of the literature. *Human Reproduction* 5(7):765–784.

Metzger, D.A., and Haney, E.F. 1989 Etiology of endometriosis. *Obstetrics and Gynecology Clinics of North America* 16(1):1–14.

Physicians' desk reference. 2002. Montvale, N.J.: Medical Economics.

Saltiel, E., and Garabedian-Ruffalo, S.M. 1991. Pharmacologic management of endometriosis. *Clinical Pharmacy* 10(7): 518–531.

Shaw, R.W. 1991. Endometriosis: the next ten years. *British Journal of Clinical Practice* 72(Suppl.):59–63.

Stege, J.F. 1998. Basic philosophy of the integrated approach: overcoming the mind-body split. In *Chronic pelvic pain*, eds. J.F. Stege, D.A. Metzger, and B.S. Levy. Philadelphia: W.B. Saunders.

Wellbery, C. 1999. Diagnosis and treatment of endometriosis. *American Family Physician* 60(6):1753–1999.

Zreik, T.G., and Olive, D.L. 1997. Pathophysiology: the biological principles of disease. *Obstetrics and Gynecology Clinics of North America* 24(2):259–267.

Winifred L. Star, R.N., C., N.P., M.S.
Joan Y. Okasako, R.N., C.S., F.N.P., M.S.

12-G

Hirsutism

Hirsutism is defined as the presence of androgen-stimulated excessive growth of bodily hair in locations where hair is not commonly found in women. It should not be confused with *hypertrichosis*, which implies a generalized increase in body hair of the relatively fine (vellus) type that does not grow in a male pattern of distribution (American College of Obstetricians and Gynecologists [ACOG] 1995, Conn et al. 1998, Lobo et al. 1997). In particular, hirsutism refers to "midline hair"—on the cheeks (sideburns), above the upper lip (mustache), and on the chin (beard); on the chest and intermammary region; on the inner thighs; along the midline lower back entering the intergluteal area; or as a male escutcheon (Lobo et al. 1997). In most women, this excessive hair growth occurs in response to abnormally increased levels of circulating androgens.

Virilization, a more pronounced form of androgenization, is hirsutism accompanied by temporal balding, deepening of the voice, increased muscle mass, enlargement of the clitoris, decreased breast size, and/or loss of female body contour (ACOG 1995, Lobo et al. 1997). Virilization should arouse suspicion for adrenal hyperplasia or androgen-producing tumors of adrenal or ovarian origin (Speroff et al. 1999).

Idiopathic hirsutism (also referred to as *simple* or *peripheral hirsutism*) is a term that should be used only to refer to hirsute women with normal ovulatory function and normal circulating androgens (Azziz et al. 2000).

Ethnicity, age, race, and other genetic factors greatly influence the characteristics and distribution of body hair. For instance, Asians, Native Americans, light-skinned Caucasians, and some Africans have less hair while women of Mediterranean descent commonly have coarse hair on the upper lip, arms, and legs. Elderly women may have increased facial hair but diminished pubic/axillary hair (Lobo et al. 1997, Nestler 1989). Cultural and societal attitudes, as well as psychology, affect individual perception regarding bodily hair. Approximately 2–10% of the population manifest some evidence of hirsutism (Azziz et al. 2000, Plouffe 2000).

A basic endocrinology review helps further understand hirsutism. Androgens are secreted by both the ovary and adrenal gland in response to the pituitary-derived trophic hormones, leuteinizing hormone (LH), and adrenocorticotropic hormone (ACTH). The main androgenic hormones are testosterone, dehydroepiandrosterone (DHEA), dehydroepiandrosterone sulfate (DHEAS), and androstenedione. Testosterone comes from three sources: the ovary, adrenal gland, and peripheral conversion (in the liver, skin, and fat). In women, about 50% of testosterone comes from peripheral conversion of androstenedione, and 50% is secreted by the adrenal gland and ovary in equal amounts (except at midcycle, when ovarian contribution increases by 10–15%) (Speroff et al. 1999). DHEAS is derived almost exclusively from the adrenal gland and 90% of DHEA is adrenal in origin (Speroff et al. 1999). After testosterone is secreted into the circulation, its biologic response is modified by serum binding, the cyclic growth process of hair, and the level of 5-alpha-reductase activity in skin (Lobo et al. 1997).

The cyclic phases of hair growth are (1) anagen, the growing phase (85–90% of the life cycle); (2) catogen, the rapid involution phase; and (3) telogen, the quiescent phase. The second and third phases constitute 10–15% of the cycle (Plouffe 2000, Speroff et al. 1999). Two types of body hair occur: *vellus* hair (short, fine, nonpigmented) and *terminal* hair (long, coarse, pigmented). The latter is responsive to circulating reproductive hormones. Increased androgen levels associated with puberty cause the pilosebaceous units (PSUs) on the axilla, pubis, back, face, chest, abdomen, and extremities to differentiate into an androgen-sensitive end-unit, either a terminal hair follicle or a sebaceous follicle (Deplewski et al. 2000, Ehrmann et al. 1990). Local conversion of testosterone to its 5-alpha-reduced product, dihydrotestosterone (DHT), is necessary for normal growth of androgen-dependent hair. Hirsutism is a reflection of increased 5-alpha-reductase activity that produces more DHT, leading to the stimulation of hair growth (Speroff et al. 1999). Although androgens serve as the main regulators of 5-alpha-reductase in skin, additional factors modulate the effects of androgens on 5-alpha-reductase activity (e.g., genetic expression of 5-alpha-reductase, insulin-like growth factor-I, and transforming growth factor-ß) (Deplewski et al. 2000, Lobo et al. 1997). Thus, the sum of endocrinologic factors that influence the PSUs include the rate and amount of androgen secretion, the concentration of sex hormone-binding globulin (SHBG), the metabolism of androgens, and the sensitivity of the PSUs to androgens (ACOG 1995).

Considering the factors that control hair growth, the etiology of hirsutism can be attributed to altered androgen metabolism, increased androgen production, decreased androgen binding, and exogenous androgen ingestion (ACOG 1995).

Altered Androgen Metabolism

Idiopathic hirsutism is among the most common types of hirsutism. The pathophysiology is presumed to be a primary increase in skin 5-alpha-reductase activity and possibly an alteration in androgen receptor function. The prevalence varies widely according to the ethnic or racial group studied. Generally, fewer than 20% of all hirsute women carry this diagnosis (Azziz et al. 2000).

Increased Androgen Production

→ Polycystic ovary syndrome (PCOS). This condition probably constitutes the most common cause of hirsutism. PCOS consists of a combination of hyperandrogenism and chronic anovulation manifested by a constellation of findings that may include hirsutism, oligomenorrhea, amenorrhea, dysfunctional uterine bleeding, acne, obesity, infertility, and polycystic ovaries (Kalve et al. 1996, Lobo et al. 1997, Lobo et al. 2000). Evidence suggests that the principal underlying disorder is one of insulin resistance, with resultant hyperinsulinemia and excess ovarian androgen production (Hunter et al. 2000). Women with PCOS are at increased risk for impaired glucose tolerance, Type 2 diabetes mellitus, hypertension, lipid abnormalities (i.e., increased total cholesterol, LDL-C, and triglycerides, and decreased HDL-C), cardiovascular disease, endometrial hyperplasia and endometrial cancer, and perhaps breast cancer (Creatsas et al. 2000, Hunter et al. 2000, Lobo et al. 2000).

→ Ovarian stromal hyperthecosis, a condition that results from differentiation of ovarian interstitial cells into testosterone-producing luteinized stromal calls, also can cause hyperandrogenism. The history reveals a long-lasting pattern of anovulation or amenorrhea and a slow, progressive form of androgen excess. Serum testosterone levels are markedly elevated, above those commonly found in PCOS. Ultrasound may distinguish this disorder from PCOS, based on the finding of bilateral enlarged ovaries—more solid, with little cystic activity (Lobo et al. 1997).

→ Adrenal abnormalities resulting in excessive androgen production are relatively uncommon. They include congenital adrenal hyperplasia (CAH), Cushing's syndrome, and androgen-secreting neoplasias.

- Late-onset (also called adult-onset or nonclassic) CAH is generally caused by deficiencies in the adrenal enzymes that are used to synthesize glucocorticoids: an enzymatic

21-hydroxylase deficiency (21-OHD), which constitutes 90% of cases and is now recognized as the most common autosomal recessive disorder); *11ß-hydroxylase deficiency* (11ß-OHD), which is more rare; or *3ß-hydroxysteroid dehydrogenase deficiency* (3ß-HSD), which is quite subtle. The net result of 21-OHD and 11-OHD is increased adrenal production of cortisol precursors and androgens. Hirsutism involving 3ß-HSD is probably due to target tissue conversion of the increased secretion of androgen precursors, as this enzyme defect precludes significant androgen production (Deaton et al. 1999, Speroff et al. 1999). The clinical presentation of late-onset 21-OHD is identical to that of PCOS. Its prevalence varies according to ethnic background—higher in Ashkenazi Jews and women of Southern European ancestry (Lobo et al. 1997).

- Cushing's syndrome arises from the persistent oversecretion of cortisol. It develops due to pituitary ACTH overproduction (Cushing's disease); ectopic ACTH overproduction by tumors; autonomous cortisol secretion by the adrenal gland or, very rarely, ovarian tumors; or the secretion of corticotropin-releasing hormone by a tumor, which is extremely rare (Speroff et al. 1999).

- Androgen-secreting neoplasias:
  - Androgen-producing adrenal tumors: adenomas and carcinomas
  - Androgen-producing ovarian tumors: Sertoli-Leydig cell tumors, hilus cell tumors, lipoid cell tumors, granulosa-theca tumors, cystadenomas, cystadeno-carcinomas, Brenner tumors, and Krukenberg tumors (Lobo et al. 1997). Functioning androgen-secreting ovarian tumors are rare and represent only 1% of all ovarian tumors (Barth 1997).

Decreased Androgen Binding

Androgens are bound to SHBG or albumin. SHBG is decreased by insulin, and increased by estrogens and thyroid hormone; thus, binding capacity is increased in hyperthyroidism, in pregnancy, and by estrogen-containing medication. In hirsutism, SHBG is depressed by excess androgen (and, when present, by hyperinsulinemia). The percent free and active testosterone is elevated as is the metabolic clearance rate of testosterone (ACOG 1995, Speroff et al. 1999).

Exogenous Androgens

Exogenous causes may include medications such as anabolic steroids, synthetic progestins, methyltestosterone, testosterone-containing creams, cyclosporine, danazol, minoxidil, diazoxide, phenytoin, glucocorticoids, DHEA (available as a food supplement), and penicillamine (ACOG 1995, Davis 1999, Sakiyama 1996, Speroff et al. 1999).

An in-depth discussion of all the etiologies associated with hirsutism is beyond the scope of this chapter. Refer to the "Bibliography" for additional information.

DATABASE

SUBJECTIVE

→ The patient may present with the following features:
- Increased hair growth
- Acne
- Weight gain, obesity
- Infertility
- Menstrual irregularities: oligomenorrhea or amenorrhea, menorrhagia, or menometrorrhagia
- Pelvic pain, pressure
- Increased abdominal girth
- Progressive or rapid virilization: alopecia, temporal balding, deepening of the voice, increased muscle mass, enlargement of the clitoris, decreased breast size, and/or loss of female body contour

→ Features associated with Cushing's syndrome that may be present are:
- Hypertension
- Fine hair on face, back, extremities
- Moon facies, plethora
- Centripetal obesity
- Abdominal striae
- Supraclavicular and dorsal neck fat pads
- Muscle wasting, weakness
- Thin skin, easy/spontaneous bruising
- Amenorrhea
- Symptoms of latent/overt diabetes
- Osteoporosis
- Psychosis

→ Features associated with CAH that may be present are:
- Shortened stature
- Severe acne, pronounced hirsutism
- Amenorrhea, oligomenorrhea, infertility
- Frequent illness

→ Features of thyroid disease may be present. (See the **Thyroid Disorders** chapter in Section 10.)

→ History to include:
- Race, ethnicity
- Height, weight
- Age at onset of pubertal development
- Age at onset and rate of progression of hirsutism
- Menstrual cycle history
- History of increased libido, clitoromegaly, and/or other signs of virilization
- Environmental factors
- Medication and drug history
- Pregnancy symptoms
- Signs/symptoms associated with Cushing's syndrome, CAH, and/or thyroid disease (See above and the **Thyroid Disorders** chapter in Section 10.)
- Complete medical and surgical history
- Additional review of systems
- Family history
- Psychosocial impact of hirsutism, emotional response to hair growth

OBJECTIVE

→ Ideally, a complete physical examination is performed with attention to the following:
- Height, weight, blood pressure
- Skin for oiliness, acne; acanthosis nigricans—brown to black and velvety hyperpigmentation on the skin around the neck, axilla, groin, umbilicus, or intertriginous areas—associated with insulin resistance
- Body habitus (pattern of body fat distribution)
  - A waist-to-hip measurement ratio of >0.85 or a waist circumference >90 cm (about 35 inches) indicates android obesity, which is predictive of abnormal endocrinologic and metabolic function and is associated with increased risk for cardiovascular disease (Hunter et al. 2000, Speroff et al. 1999).
- Hair growth on face, chest, breasts, abdomen, lower back, arms, and legs.
  NOTE: A hirsutism scoring scale by Ferriman et al. (1961) has been utilized to quantify the degree of hirsutism. (See **Figure 12G.1, Hirsutism Scoring**.) A total score of ≥8 signifies hirsutism; however, it is important to interpret the findings in relation to the ethnic background of the patient.
- Excessive vellus hair growth (hypertrichosis)
- Signs of virilization: alopecia, frontal/temporal baldness, deepened voice, breast involution, increased muscle mass
  NOTE: Rapidly progressing virilization should always suggest the presence of an androgen-producing tumor (Lobo et al. 1997).
- Breasts for galactorrhea
- Abdominal/pelvic masses.
- Clitoromegaly (clitoral index 100 mm^2 or clitoral shaft diameter >1 cm)
  NOTE: The clitoral index is obtained by multiplying the vertical and horizontal dimensions of the clitoris; normal size is ≤35 mm^2 (Nestler 1989).
- Features associated with Cushing's syndrome, CAH, and/or thyroid disease. (See "Subjective," above, and the **Thyroid Disorders** chapter in Section 10.)

ASSESSMENT

→ Hirsutism
→ R/O hypertrichosis
→ Assess for specific etiologies of hirsutism: idiopathic, exogenous/iatrogenic factors, ovarian causes (PCO, ovarian tumors), adrenal causes (adrenal tumors, Cushing's syndrome, adult-onset CAH).
→ R/O hyperprolactinemia
→ R/O thyroid disease

PLAN

DIAGNOSTIC TESTS

→ A history and physical exam are the best predictors of ovarian and adrenal androgen-secreting tumors (Azziz 2002).

Figure 12G.1.   HIRSUTISM SCORING

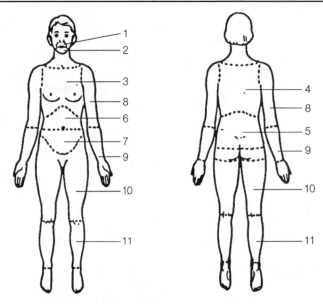

(Grade 0 at all sites indicates absence of terminal hair.)

Site	Grade	Definition
1. Upper Lip	1	A few hairs at outer margin
	2	A small moustache at outer margin
	3	A moustache extending half way from outer margin
	4	A moustache extending to midline
2. Chin	1	A few scattered hairs
	2	Scattered hairs with small concentrations
	3 & 4	Complete coverage, light and heavy
3. Chest	1	Circumareolar hairs
	2	With midline hair in addition
	3	Fusion of these areas, with three-quarters coverage
	4	Complete coverage
4. Upper Back	1	A few scattered hairs
	2	Rather more, still scattered
	3 & 4	Complete coverage, light and heavy
5. Lower Back	1	A sacral tuft of hair
	2	With some lateral extension
	3	Three-quarters coverage
	4	Complete coverage
6. Upper Abdomen	1	A few midline hairs
	2	Rather more, still midline
	3 & 4	Half and full coverage
7. Lower Abdomen	1	A few midline hairs
	2	A midline streak of hair
	3	A midline band of hair
	4	An inverted, V-shaped growth
8. Arm	1	Sparse growth affecting not more than a quarter of the limb surface
	2	More than this; coverage still incomplete
	3 & 4	Complete coverage, light and heavy
9. Forearm	1, 2, 3, 4	Complete coverage of dorsal surface; 2 grades of light and 2 of heavy growth
10. Thigh	1, 2, 3, 4	As for arm
11. Leg	1, 2, 3, 4	As for arm

NOTE: Scores in each area are added. Total score ≥8 indicates hirsutism.

Source: Reprinted with permission from Ferriman, D., and Gallwey, J.D. 1961. Clinical assessment of body hair growth in women. *Journal of Clinical Endocrinology and Metabolism* 21:1440. ©The Endocrine Society.

→ The goal of laboratory testing is to identify uncommon but serious disease. Patients with mild hirsutism and no menstrual disturbance do not necessarily require evaluation. Confer with a physician regarding recommended testing.

→ The three following screening tests are commonly ordered. Site-specific practices will dictate their use. Check with the laboratory for regional normal values:

■ Serum total testosterone:
  • Normal range = 20–80 ng/dL.
  • Values >200 ng/dL require further investigation for an androgen-producing tumor.
  NOTE: It is not necessary to measure free testosterone; routine total testosterone adequately screens for testosterone-secreting tumors. Patients presenting with rapid virilization require full evaluation for androgen-producing tumors even if the total testosterone level is within normal limits. Total testosterone may be in the normal range in a hirsute woman (Speroff et al. 1999). Refer all patients with markedly elevated levels to a physician for further testing/management.

■ Serum DHEAS:
  • Upper limit of normal = 350 μg/dL in most labs.
  • Value >700 μg /dL is a marker for abnormal adrenal function.
  NOTE: Markedly elevated levels are rare. In evaluating hirsute women, DHEAS measurement has a very low yield unless the serum testosterone is elevated. DHEAS levels often are slightly elevated in hirsute women, and in association with hyperprolactinemia. Levels show an inverse relationship with age: Peaks occur around age 25–35 and decrease 10–20% per decade (Kaiser Permanente Clinical Laboratory 2001). Refer all patients with elevated levels to a physician for further testing/management.

■ 17-alpha-hydroxyprogesterone (17-OHP):
  • Baseline level = <200 ng/dL. It should be measured in the early morning and in the follicular phase (within 8–10 days of the beginning of menstruation or a progestin-induced withdrawal bleed) (Azziz 2002).
  • Levels from 200–799 ng/dL require ACTH testing (discussion of which is beyond the scope of this chapter).
  • Levels >800 ng/dL are virtually diagnostic of 21-OHD (Speroff et al. 1999). Refer all patients with elevated levels to a physician for further testing/management.

→ Evaluation of suspected Cushing's syndrome should be carried out by a physician. It includes measurements of 24-hour urinary free cortisol excretion and late evening plasma cortisol levels.

■ Initial screening is done via a single-dose overnight dexamethasone suppression test: 1 mg of dexamethasone given orally at 11:00 p.m., with plasma cortisol measurement at 8:00 a.m. the following day.
  • Plasma cortisol value <5 μg /dl rules out Cushing's syndrome.
  • Cushing's syndrome is unlikely with intermediate values between 5–10 μg/dL.
  • Value >10 μg/dL is diagnostic of adrenal

hyperfunction. Obese women may have up to a 13% false positive rate (Speroff et al. 1999).

■ If the single-dose overnight test is abnormal, establish the diagnosis by measuring 24-hour urinary free cortisol.
  • 24-hour urinary free cortisol >250 μg is virtually diagnostic of Cushing's syndrome (Speroff et al. 1999).

■ Final confirmation is provided by a low dose, 2-day dexamethasone suppression test (Speroff et al. 1999):
  • Dexamethasone 0.5 mg p.o. every 6 hours is administered for 2 consecutive days after 2 days of baseline 24-hour urinary 17-hydroxysteroid and free cortisol measurements.
  • Cushing's syndrome patients will not lower urinary 17-hydroxysteroids below 2.5 mg/day and free cortisol below 10 μg on the second day of dexamethasone suppression (Speroff et al. 1999).

■ The etiology of Cushing's syndrome can be established by combining a high dose dexamethasone suppression test with ACTH measurement. Discussion of the test is beyond the scope of this chapter; refer the patient to a physician.

→ Patients presenting with rapid virilization, an abdominal/pelvic mass, and/or very high levels of testosterone or DHEAS should be evaluated for an adrenal/ovarian tumor. Confer with a physician about ordering appropriate diagnostic tests; refer the patient to a physician for definitive management.

■ Diagnostic assessments may include ultrasonography, computed tomography, magnetic resonance imaging, angiography, and ovarian/adrenal vein catheterization.

→ Evaluate anovulatory, hyperandrogenic women for insulin resistance and glucose tolerance (Lebovitz 1998, Speroff et al. 1999). Tests may include:

■ Fasting plasma glucose:
  • Normal = <110 mg/dL.
  • Impaired fasting glucose = 100–125 mg/dL.
  • Diabetes = ≥126 mg/dL.

■ Fasting glucose:insulin ratio
  • A ratio <4.5 is consistent with insulin resistance.

■ A 2-hour glucose screen after 75 g glucose load:
  • Normal = <140 mg/dL.
  • Impaired = 140–199 mg/dL.
  • Diabetes = ≥200 mg/dL.

→ Order a prolactin level in anovulatory women.

→ Additional laboratory tests/diagnostic procedures will depend on the clinical presentation and may include but are not limited to: pregnancy test, LH, FSH, estradiol, TSH, thyroid function tests, lipid panel (fasting total cholesterol, HDL-C, LDL-C, triglycerides), endometrial biopsy, and mammography.

TREATMENT/MANAGEMENT

→ The wishes of the patient play an important part in hirsutism treatment strategies. Some women may wish to simply camouflage facial hair with heavy make up or bleaching agents. In cases of mild hirsutism without evidence of ovulatory dysfunction, no treatment is required and reassurance may be all that is needed.

→ Undertake medical management approaches in consultation with a physician (see below). When possible, discontinue drugs that cause hirsutism.

■ Mechanical methods:

• Procedural or cosmetic means of controlling, removing, or destroying hair complement medical management. Most physical and chemical methods of hair removal are temporary; they do not have an effect on the hair-growth process (Bergfeld 2000, Washenik 2001). Options include:

– Plucking (tweezing): May cause a post epilation pustule or scar.

– Waxing: A certain hair length is necessary. Use with caution to prevent thermal burns. May be done professionally.

– Shaving: one of oldest, safest methods of hair depilation. It will not increase the rate of growth or the coarseness or darkness of subsequent hair growth.

NOTE: All of the above methods may irritate skin or result in folliculitis and/or ingrown hairs (Azziz et al. 2000).

– Sugaring

– Bleaching

– Chemical depilatory agents (e.g., calcium thioglycolates)

➤ A mild topical corticosteroid or skin moisturizer may be applied after use to prevent irritant contact dermatitis. (See **Table 12TB.1, Potency Ranking of Some Commonly Used Topical Corticosteroids** in the **White Lesions of the Vulva** chapter.)

– Hair-removing gloves of fine sandpaper or pumice stone.

• Epilation or permanent hair removal: electrolysis, thermolysis, photothermolysis (laser or nonlaser light sources). Must be performed by certified/licensed trained professionals (Dierickx 2000, Wheeland 1997).

– Side effects include pain, perifollicular edema and erythema, hypo/hyperpigmentation (usually transient), infection (low risk), herpes simplex outbreaks (uncommon), and scarring (rare) (Dierickx 2000, Dierickx et al. 1999).

• Photodynamic therapy: still under investigation as a treatment option for hirsutism (Dierickx 2000, Ort et al. 1999).

■ Medical methods:

• Medical treatment of hirsutism is aimed at ovarian suppression, adrenal suppression, enzyme inhibition, and/or peripheral inhibition of androgens (Azziz 2002, Falcone et al. 1993). Consult with physician regarding drug treatment regimens. Options may include:

– Eflornithine hydrochloride cream 13.9% (Vaniqua®): FDA-approved for unwanted facial hair growth. It does not remove hair but rather interferes with an enzyme, L-ornithine decarboxylase, that affects the rate of hair regrowth (Azziz 2002).

➤ Apply a thin layer to affected areas of the face and adjacent involved areas under the chin BID (at least 8 hours apart); rub in thoroughly. Areas should not be washed for at least 4 hours. Refer to drug package insert.

➤ Improvement may be visible in 4–8 weeks. After discontinuing treatment, hair growth will rapidly return; thus, continued use of this medication is required to suppress hair growth (Azziz 2002).

NOTE: Should be used in conjunction with other hair removal procedures (e.g., electrolysis or laser).

➤ Side effects may include skin irritation, redness, tingling or burning sensations, rash, and folliculitis (http://Vaniqua.com/2001).

– Combined low-dose oral contraceptive (OC): inhibits ovarian and adrenal androgen production. It is the initial treatment of choice for anovulatory women with hirsutism (Speroff et al. 1999).

➤ Theoretically, the best formulations are drospirenone, desogestrel, gestodene, or norgestimate, which are associated with greater increases in SHBG and decreases in free testosterone. However, all low-dose formulations likely produce similar clinical responses (Speroff et al. 1999).

➤ Six months of treatment usually are necessary before results are obtained. Combined treatment with electrolysis, laser, or nonlaser light source technologies is not recommended until hormonal suppression has been used for at least 6 months.

➤ OC treatment may be continued for 1–2 years, when therapy may be stopped to observe the patient for ovulatory cycles (Speroff et al. 1999).

➤ If the patient is not responding well to the OC, add an antiandrogen—preferably spironolactone or finasteride. (See the respective sections below.)

– Oral or depo forms of medroxyprogesterone acetate: may be used when OCs are contraindicated or undesired. Dosages are:

➤ 10–20 mg p.o. every day

OR

➤ 150 mg IM every 3 months (Speroff et al. 1999)

– Spironolactone 50–200 mg p.o. daily. Treatment may be commenced at 50 mg BID and increased to 100 mg BID if no response is noted after 3 months (Rittmaster 1999, Sakiyama 1996). Response is slow—maximal effect is demonstrated only after 6 months; after a period of time, a maintenance dose of 25–50 mg/day may be utilized (Speroff et al. 1999).

➤ Spironolactone is an aldosterone-antagonist diuretic that inhibits ovarian and adrenal synthesis of androgens, and 5-alpha-reductase activity. It may be tried when an OC is unacceptable or ineffective. Combined with a low-dose OC, it may provide better clinical response as well as a means of contraception and cycle control (Speroff et al. 1999).

➤ Side effects may include fatigue, headache, poly-menorrhea, gastrointestinal disturbance, breast tenderness, diuresis, hyperkalemia, and hypotension.

NOTE: Spironolactone should be used with an effective method of contraception; theoretically, its interference with testosterone action could result in feminization of a male fetus. (See the *Physicians' Desk Reference* [*PDR*] or drug package insert for additional information.)

- Spironolactone cream 2–5% may be used to treat acne. There is no systemic absorption or side effects (Speroff et al. 1999).
- Finasteride 5 mg p.o. daily. Lower doses can be used and the pills can be cut into quarters (Rittmaster 1999, Speroff et al. 1999).
  ➤ Inhibits 5-alpha-reductase activity. Improvement is noted after 6 months of therapy. The main advantage of its use is a lack of side effects (Lobo et al. 1997, Speroff et al. 1999). Finasteride is used in the United States for treating men who have androgenetic alopecia and benign prostatic hypertrophy (Azziz et al. 2000).

NOTE: Finasteride should be used with an effective method of contraception, as its action may interfere with normal development of a male fetus. (See the *PDR* or drug package insert for additional information.)

- Flutamide 250 mg p.o. daily (Speroff et al. 1999)
  ➤ A nonsteroidal antiandrogen that directly inhibits hair growth and blocks androgen receptors.
  ➤ Side effects include dry skin, increased appetite, decreased libido, amenorrhea, nausea/vomiting, and greenish tint to urine (Azziz et al. 2000, Conn et al. 1997, Deplewski et al. 2000, Rittmaster 1999). (See the *PDR* or drug package insert for additional information.)

NOTE: Flutamide should be used with an effective method of contraception, as its action may interfere with normal development of a male fetus. Not used extensively as a treatment option due to its expense and potential for hepatotoxicity.

- Cyproterone acetate (may not be currently available in the United States): a potent progestational agent that inhibits gonadotropin secretion and blocks androgen action by binding to androgen receptor (Speroff et al. 1999).
  ➤ Dose is 50–100 mg p.o. daily on Days 5–14, combined with 30 µg or 50 µg of ethinyl estradiol on Days 5–25 (the "reversed sequential regimen") (Speroff et al. 1999).
  ➤ Improvement is seen by the third month of treatment.
  ➤ Side effects include fatigue, edema, loss of libido, weight gain, and mastalgia (Speroff et al. 1999).

NOTE: Cyproterone is available in many parts of the world as an oral contraceptive "Diane" (2 mg cyproterone acetate and 50 µg ethinyl estradiol) or "Dianette" (2 mg cyproterone acetate and 35 µg ethinyl estradiol) (Speroff et al. 1999).

- GnRH agonists:
  ➤ Leuprolide acetate 3.75 mg IM, monthly injection

  OR

  ➤ Nafarelin acetate intranasal spray 400 µg BID (Sakiyama 1996)
  ➤ GnRH agonist therapy markedly suppresses gonadotropin secretion, ovarian androgen, and estrogen (Azziz 1992). It is a complicated, expensive treatment regimen reserved for more severe cases of ovarian hyperandrogenism due to significant hyperthecosis and marked hyperinsulinemia (Speroff et al. 1999).

NOTE: Long-term use of GnRH agonists often leads to hypoestrogenic side effects (e.g., hot flashes, osteoporosis, urogenital atrophy), so estrogen-progestin add-back therapy should be initiated after the GnRH maintenance dose has been established (Sakiyama 1996, Speroff et al. 1999). Add-back therapy consists of:

  ∗ 0.625 mg conjugated estrogen or
    1.0 mg estradiol per day *combined with*
    2.5 mg medroxyprogesterone acetate or
    0.35 mg norethindrone daily

    OR

  ∗ An oral contraceptive (preferable) (Speroff et al. 1999).

- Other agents used to treat hirsutism include (Falcone et al. 1993, Lobo et al. 1997, Speroff et al. 1999):
  ➤ Cimetidine 300 mg p.o. QID, which has had a disappointing clinical response
  ➤ Progesterone skin cream (frequent application required, concentrated action at point of application)
  ➤ Corticosteroids suppress ACTH secretion. They are used for patients with adrenal enzyme deficiency (e.g., CAH) to suppress adrenal androgen production. Refer to a physician for management. Regimens include:

  ∗ Dexamethasone 0.5 mg p.o. daily

    OR

  ∗ Prednisone 5–7.5 mg p.o. daily (Speroff et al. 1999).

NOTE: Women with CAH may need higher doses to normalize steroid levels; alternate-day therapy may be used with higher doses. For these patients, consider adding an OC or antiandrogen (Speroff et al. 1999).

  ➤ Ketoconazole: A dose of 400 mg/day blocks androgen synthesis by inhibiting cytochrome P450-dependent enzyme pathways.

NOTE: This is the agent of last resort because it is hepatotoxic. There is a high incidence of side effects, and chronic treatment may suppress adrenal corticosteroid production.

→ PCOS patients may be managed with insulin-sensitizing pharmacologic agents that lower insulin levels, LH, and free testosterone, thus leading to improved clinical manifestations of hyperandrogenism (Kolodziejczyk et al. 2000). Consult with a physician regarding indications, dosage, and duration of use. (See the **Amenorrhea—Secondary** chapter for additional information.)

→ Patients with suspected Cushing's syndrome, CAH, stromal hyperthecosis, or androgen-producing tumors of the ovaries or adrenals should be managed by a physician.

→ Hyperprolactinemic patients should be treated appropriately. (See the **Amenorrhea—Secondary** chapter.)

→ If oligomenorrhea, amenorrhea, or dysfunctional bleeding is a problem, cyclic progestins or oral contraceptives may be used. (See the **Amenorrhea—Secondary** and **Abnormal Uterine Bleeding** chapters.)

→ If infertility is an issue, ovulation induction may be indicated. (Refer to the **Infertility** chapter.)

→ Surgery does not play a role in the treatment of hirsutism unless a tumor is present (Conn et al. 1998).

→ Address nutritional aspects of obesity. Refer to a nutritionist as indicated.
 ▪ The patient may be referred to a weight loss program.
 ▪ Encourage a regular exercise program. (See Section 16, **General Nutrition Guidelines**.)

CONSULTATION

→ The scope of practice regarding evaluation/management of hirsute women will vary depending on site-specific policies.

→ Consult with a physician regarding ordering diagnostic tests.

→ Consultation with a physician (preferably an endocrinologist or reproductive endocrinologist) is recommended in all cases of severe hirsutism. Drug therapy should be undertaken in consultation with a physician.

→ Evaluation and management of patients with suspected Cushing's syndrome, CAH, or androgen-producing tumors of the ovaries or adrenals should be undertaken by a physician, ideally an endocrinologist or reproductive endocrinologist.

PATIENT EDUCATION

→ Discuss the etiologies of hirsutism, usual treatment/management modalities, physical methods of depilation, and permanent methods of hair removal.

→ When the patient is on a systemic drug, review side effects. Consult the *PDR* or drug package insert.
 ▪ With antiandrogens (e.g., spironolactone, finasteride, flutamide), alert the patient to the possibility of feminization of a male fetus if pregnancy occurs. Adequate contraception is therefore advisable.

→ Be sure the patient understands that diminution of the hirsute condition may not occur until after six months of drug therapy because of the physiology of hair growth.
 ▪ Temporary methods of depilation may be used during this time, but electrolysis or other permanent methods of hair

removal should not be used until after six months of hormonal suppression.
 ▪ The best response to treatment occurs in a woman who has had a short duration of hirsutism. The usual response to treatment is initial reduction of new hair followed by thinning/softening of existing terminal hair and less frequent need for depilation (Leshin 1987).

→ If the patient is diagnosed with PCOS, educate her regarding the long-term implications of diabetes, hypertension, lipid abnormalities, cardiovascular disease, endometrial hyperplasia/cancer, and possibly breast cancer. Stress healthy eating patterns and exercise. Referral to a nutritionist may be indicated. (See the **Amenorrhea—Secondary** chapter.)

→ Psychosocial implications of hirsutism may be a factor for some women. Ensure that the patient has some form of social support and utilize appropriate referral sources as indicated.

FOLLOW-UP

→ Encourage patients to continue medical therapy for one or two years. It is reasonable to stop therapy after this time to re-evaluate the patient's condition. In some cases, hirsutism will not recur; in others, therapy will need to be reinstituted. Ultimately, clinical response and patient desires will dictate when medical therapy should be discontinued.

→ Serial photography of the hirsute patient's response to therapy may be helpful to both the clinician and patient. A woman's subjective assessment regarding the change in frequency of mechanical means of hair removal is another way to measure the success of therapy.

→ Follow-up also will depend on the specific drug therapy.
 ▪ Failure of drug therapy to suppress hair growth after 6–12 months should arouse suspicion of adrenal disease or an ovarian tumor (Speroff et al. 1999).
 ▪ Electrolytes (especially potassium) and blood pressure should be assessed within the first two weeks at each dose level of spironolactone (Lobo et al. 1997).
 ▪ Frequent monitoring of liver enzymes is necessary if flutamide or ketoconazole is used (Hock et al. 2000).
 ▪ Monitoring testosterone levels is advised when GnRH agonists are used (goal is <40 ng/dL) (Speroff et al. 1999).
 ▪ When corticosteroids are used, if the treatment regimen suppresses the morning cortisol level below 2.0 µg/dL, the dose should be reduced to avoid inability to react to stress (Speroff et al. 1999).

→ PCOS patients should have long-term follow-up and screening for diabetes and cardiovascular disease. Yearly screening may be appropriate in women who are obese.

→ Offer genetic counseling to women with 21-hydroxylase deficiency.

→ Ongoing psychological support of the hirsute woman is important.

→ Document in progress notes and problem list.

BIBLIOGRAPHY

American College of Obstetricians and Gynecologists (ACOG). 1995. Evaluation and treatment of hirsute women. *Technical Bulletin No. 203*. Washington, D.C.: the Author.

Azziz, R. 1992. Treating hirsutism with GnRH agonists. *Contemporary OB/GYN* 37(6):33–48.

_____. 2002. Advances in the evaluation and treatment of unwanted hair growth. *Contemporary OB/GYN* 47(2):98–106.

Azziz, R., Carmina, E., and Sawaya, M.E. 2000. Idiopathic hirsutism. *Endocrine Reviews* 21(4):347–362.

Barnes, R.B. 1991. Adrenal dysfunction and hirsutism. *Clinical Obstetrics and Gynecology* 34(4):827–834.

Barth, J.H. 1997. Investigations in the assessment and management of patients with hirsutism. *Current Opinions in Obstetrics and Gynecology* 10:187–192.

Bergfeld, W. 2000. Hirsutism in women. *Postgraduate Medicine* 107(7):93–104.

Carmina, E., and Lobo, R. 1997. Dynamic tests for hormone evaluation. In *Infertility, contraception, and reproductive endocrinology*, 4th ed., eds. R.A. Lobo, D.R. Mishell, Jr., R.J. Paulson et al., pp. 471–483. Malden, Mass.: Blackwell Science.

Conn, J.J., and Jacobs, H.S. 1997. The clinical management of hirsutism. *European Journal of Endocrinology* 136:339–348.

_____. 1998. Managing hirsutism in gynaecological practice. *British Journal of Obstetrics and Gynaecology* 105:687–696.

Creatsas, G., Koliopoulos, C., and Mastorakos, G. 2000. Combined oral contraceptive treatment of adolescent girls with polycystic ovary syndrome. *Annals of the New York Academy of Sciences* 900:245–252.

Davis, S. 1999. Syndromes of hyperandrogenism in women. *Australian Family Physician* 28(5):447–451.

Deaton, M.A., Glorioso, J.E., and McLean, D.B. 1999. Congenital adrenal hyperplasia: not really a zebra. *American Family Physician* 59(5):1190–1197.

Deplewski, D., and Rosenfield, R.L. 2000. Role of hormones in pilosebaceous unit development. *Endocrine Reviews* 21(4):363–392.

Dierickx, C.C. 2000. Hair removal by lasers and intense pulsed light sources. *Seminars in Cutaneous Medicine and Surgery* 19(4):267–275.

Dierickx, C., Alora, B., and Dover, J.S. 1999. A clinical overview of hair removal using lasers and light sources. *Dermatology Clinics* 17(2):357–366.

Ehrmann, D.A., and Rosenfield, R.L. 1990. An endocrinologic approach to the patient with hirsutism. *Journal of Clinical Endocrinology and Metabolism* 71(1):1–4.

Falcone, T., Bourque, J., Granger, L. et al. 1993. Polycystic ovarian syndrome. *Current Problems in Obstetrics, Gynecology, and Fertility* 16(2):65–95.

Ferriman, D., and Gallwey, J.D. 1961. Clinical assessment of body hair growth in women. *Journal of Clinical Endocrinology and Metabolism* 21:1440.

Hock, D.L., and Seifer, D.B. 2000. New treatments of hyperandrogenism and hirsutism. *Obstetrics and Gynecology Clinics of North America* 27(3):567–581.

Hunter, M.H., and Sterrett, J.J. 2000. Polycystic ovary syndrome: It's not just infertility. *American Family Physician* 62(5):1079–1089.

Kaiser Permanente Clinical Laboratory 2001. Available at: http://clinical-library.ca.kp.org/clib/lab/manual/ri900100.htr. Accessed June 28, 2001.

Kalve, E., and Klein, J.F. 1996. Evaluation of women with hirsutism. *American Family Physician* 54(1):117–124.

Kolodziejczyk, B., Duleba, A.J., Spaczynski, R.Z. et al. 2000. Metformin therapy decreases hyperandrogenism and hyperinsulinemia in women with polycystic ovary syndrome. *Fertility and Sterility* 73(6):1149–1154.

Lebovitz, H.E. 1998. Diagnosis and classification of diabetes mellitus. In *Therapy for diabetes and related disorders*, 3rd ed., ed. H.E. Lebovitz, p. 6. Alexandria, Va.: American Diabetes Association.

Leshin, M. 1987. Southwestern internal medicine conference: hirsutism. *American Journal of the Medical Sciences* 284(5):369–383.

Lobo, R.A., and Carmina, E. 1997. Androgen excess. In *Infertility, contraception, and reproductive endocrinology*, 4th ed., eds. R.A. Lobo, D.R. Mishell, Jr., R.J. Paulson et al., pp. 342–362. Malden, Mass.: Blackwell Science.

_____. 2000. The importance of diagnosing the polycystic ovary syndrome. *Annals of Internal Medicine* 132:989–993.

Lobo, R.A., and Kletzky, O.A. 1991. Dynamics of hormone testing. In *Infertility, contraception, and reproductive endocrinology*, 3rd ed., eds. D.R. Mishell, Jr., V. Davajan, and R.A. Lobo, pp. 518–534. Malden, Mass.: Blackwell Science.

Nestler, J.E. 1989. Evaluation and treatment of the hirsute woman. *Virginia Medical*: 310–315.

Nestler, J.E., Jakubowicz, D.J., Reamer, P. et al. 1999. Ovulatory and metabolic effects of D-chiro-inositol in the polycystic ovary syndrome. *New England Journal of Medicine* 340:1314–1320.

Ort, R.J., and Anderson, R. 1999. Optical hair removal. *Seminars in Cutaneous Medicine and Surgery* 18(2):149–158.

Plouffe, L., 2000. Disorders of excessive hair growth in the adolescent. *Adolescent Gynecology* 27(1):79–99.

Rittmaster, R.S. 1999. Antiandrogenic treatment of polycystic ovary syndrome. *Endocrinology and Metabolism Clinics of North America* 28(2):409–421.

Sakiyama, R. 1996. Approach to patients with hirsutism. *Western Journal of Medicine* 165(6):386–391.

Speroff, L., Glass, R.H., and Kase, N.G. 1999. *Clinical gynecologic endocrinology and infertility*, 6th ed., pp. 524–556. Baltimore, Md.: Lippincott Williams & Wilkins.

Untitled entry. Available at: http://www.Vaniqua.com/2001. Accessed March 26, 2001.

Washenik, K. (moderator). 2001. The stigma of unwanted facial hair. *Medical Crossfire* 2(1):2–14.

Wheeland, R.G. 1997. Laser-assisted hair removal. *Dermatology Clinics* 15(3):469–477.

Anita Levine-Goldberg, R.N., N.P., M.S.
Lori M. Weseman, R.N., M.S., N.P.

12-H
Infertility

Infertility is defined as the inability or diminished ability to produce offspring (Bernstein et al. 1982). Statistically, approximately 25% of women under the age of 35 years conceive in the first cycle of unprotected intercourse, 60% within six months, 80% within nine months, and 85% within one year.

Infertility is a shared concern for a couple. The problems of infertility are distributed equally between the male and female. Approximately 20% of problems are with the male partner and 35% with the female partner. Thirty-five percent of infertility problems are due to combined male/female factors and approximately 10% are of undetermined etiology. Limiting the evaluation to one member of a couple would be incomplete and may result in a delay of diagnosis and treatment.

Generally, the diagnosis of infertility is not made unless the couple has been sexually active for one year without the use of contraception. Exceptions to this one-year period include advanced maternal age (35 years or older), irregular or absent menses, previously diagnosed infertility problems, exposure to diethylstilbestrol (DES) in utero of either the male or female, abnormal development of sex organs, known or suspected uterine/tubal disease or endometriosis, or a partner who is known to be subfertile. The goal of the primary care provider is to provide the couple with an accurate diagnosis, information, and treatment resulting in a positive outcome—ideally, a pregnancy or, at least, a decision to pursue alternative avenues or to accept no further treatment.

Infertility represents a very real loss to the couple. Loss of self-esteem and of feminine and masculine identities, mutual marital goals unfulfilled, and, especially, the inability to conceive are keenly felt by the couple, particularly with the onset of menses. The media, fertile friends, and overbearing family members add to the feelings of loss and frustration. The infertility evaluation can be very trying for the couple due to the cost, loss of privacy, and invasiveness of testing. The primary care provider should recognize that infertility represents a life crisis for couples and be aware of the intensity and variety of emotional responses that couples may manifest. Counseling may be indicated.

Upon completion of the infertility evaluation, the couple will fall into one or more of the following categories:
→ Male-factor infertility
→ Pelvic-factor infertility
→ Endocrine-factor infertility
→ Immunological infertility
→ Unexplained infertility
→ Age-related infertility
→ Other factors

The primary care provider should then focus treatment of the couple to minimize or remedy the infertility factor(s).

Male-Factor Infertility

The male partner is recognized as a contributor to infertility in approximately 30–40% of infertile couples (Berkowitz 1986). Although therapy for treatment of male-factor infertility is limited, early evaluation of the male is important.

Findings of complete male infertility are made with at least two abnormal semen analyses. (See **Table 12H.1, Normal Semen Analysis**.) The full evaluation should include a complete medical and reproductive history and a physical exam by a urologist.

Anatomic Defects of the Penis, Testicles, or Excretory Ducts (e.g., Varicocele)

A varicocele, or enlarged veins within the scrotum, results from dilation of the spermatic vein and can cause oligospermia. In all likelihood, it does that by raising testicular temperature (Howards 1992). Varicoceles are found in about 15% of the normal male population and in about 40% of men with infertility.

Antisperm Antibodies

Autoimmunity to sperm can result in decreased fertility. Assays such as the immunobead test and mixed agglutination reaction (SpermMar™) look for sperm-bound antibodies. Evaluation of female serum or cervical mucus for antibodies using immunobead techniques also is necessary.

Sperm Penetration Disorders

For several years, a mixed gamete penetration assay has been utilized by Overstreet (Overstreet et al. 1980). This test evaluates the spermatozoa's ability to penetrate the zona pellucida of the human egg. The most commonly used test for predicting the fertilizing capacity of the human sperm is the sperm penetration assay. The test is performed by co-incubation of prepared human sperm with fresh human eggs retrieved from hysterectomy specimens or with denuded hamster eggs. Further investigation is needed to show that the test is an absolute predictor of infertility (Grunfeld 1989). Clinically, the test may be useful in identifying abnormalities of sperm not evident by its count, motility, or morphology, especially in cases of unexplained infertility.

Infections of the Genital Tract

Infection can play a role in infertility. Epididymal or prostatic infections with *Neisseria gonorrhoeae*, *Chlamydia trachomatis*, or Gram-negative organisms can cause ductal obstruction or orchitis (Grunfeld 1989).

Treatment of other organisms, such as T *mycoplasma* (*Ureaplasma urealyticum*), is more controversial. Rehewy et al. (1978) did not find improvement in the pregnancy rate with eradication of the organism, while Toth et al. (1983) found a substantially higher pregnancy rate in organism-free groups. The value of treating T mycoplasma still needs to be determined.

Low Semen Volume

Low semen volume may be due to retrograde ejaculation, ductal obstruction, or decreased production from the male accessory glands.

Abnormal Liquefaction

Semen liquefaction usually occurs 20–30 minutes after ejaculation. Semen that does not undergo normal liquidation and is associated with a poor postcoital test may be a factor in infertility.

Low Sperm Count (Concentration)

Low sperm count may be due to illness or temperature variations.

Decreased Motility

Decreased sperm motility may be related to trauma, infection, or exposure.

Decreased Normal Morphology

Decreased normal morphology may be a consequence of toxic exposure or neoplasm. Intrauterine insemination is the treatment of choice for many of the diagnoses associated with male-factor infertility. (See **Appendix 12H.1, Indications for Intrauterine Insemination**.) Donor inseminations and intracytoplasmic sperm injection (ICSI) are other options.

Pelvic-Factor Infertility

Pelvic-factor infertility includes Asherman's syndrome, cervical factor, endometriosis, and tubal disease or obstruction.

Asherman's Syndrome

In this disorder, ovulation may occur normally, but there is no lush endometrial lining on which the embryo can implant. This syndrome results from adhesions that have occurred following surgery or a procedure. Patients may present with amenorrhea because there is no uterine lining to shed. However, regular bleeding has been documented in women presenting with Asherman's syndrome (Reid et al. 1992). Diagnosis is confirmed by either hysterosalpingogram or hysteroscopy.

Cervical Factor

For approximately 10–15% of women with infertility problems, a poor sperm-transport mechanism is the etiology. The causes may include, but are not limited to, cervical stenosis, poor quality or quantity of cervical mucus, and varicosities of the endo-

---

Table 12H.1. NORMAL SEMEN ANALYSIS

Ejaculate volume	2.0 mL or more
Sperm concentration	20 million/mL or more
Motility	50% or more with forward progression or
	25% or more with rapid progression within 60 minutes of ejaculation
Morphology	30% or more normal forms
White blood cells	Fewer than 1 million/mL
Immunobead test	Fewer than 20% spermatozoa with adherent particles
SpermMar™ test	Fewer than 10% spermatozoa with adherent particles

Source: World Health Organization. 1992. *Laboratory manual for the examination of human semen and sperm cervical mucus interaction.* Cambridge, United Kingdom: Cambridge University Press.

cervical canal. As seen through the colposcope, the endocervical canal will have a poorly developed columnar epithelium with prominent superficial varicosities, which may respond to cryosurgery or laser cautery. Postcoital testing can be done to assess for cervical factor infertility.

Endometriosis

Endometriosis is the presence of endometrial tissue outside of the endometrial cavity and most commonly on the peritoneal cavity, fallopian tubes, ovaries, bladder, and bowel. It is theorized that there is a reflux of endometrial tissue during menses and/or vascular or lymphatic transport of endometrial fragments that enables the tissue to "implant" onto pelvic organs (Ishimaru et al. 1991). These implantations, called endometriomas, may continue to "leak" endometrial tissue to the surrounding pelvic organs.

In the general population, there is a 7–8% incidence of endometriosis, while in the infertile population the incidence may be as high as 25–35% (Olive et al. 1993). Symptoms may include dysmenorrhea, dyspareunia, and chronic pelvic pain. The diagnosis of endometriosis can be made only after direct visualization by laparoscopy or during pelvic surgery. The condition is then classified depending on the extent of the disease, utilizing the system set forth by the American Fertility Society that stages the disease from Stage I to Stage IV based on a numerical scoring system. Classification of the disease is necessary to determine the best treatment modality.

The underlying mechanism that causes infertility in women with severe endometriosis is scarring and adhesion formation following the inflammatory process of the disease. These adhesions can interfere with tubal-ovarian interaction, preventing fertilization. However, in patients with minimal endometriosis, the causative factor is not as clear. Theories include altered smooth-muscle contractility of the fallopian tube secondary to increased prostaglandin production by the disease, uterine irritability, or altered ovarian steroidogenesis also due to increased prostaglandin production (Older 1983). (See the **Endometriosis** chapter.)

Tubal Disease/Obstruction

Tubal disease and/or obstruction can be the result of adhesion formation from pelvic surgery, trauma (e.g., from an intrauterine device [IUD]), or disease such as pelvic inflammatory disease (PID) or endometriosis. Tubal patency also may be damaged due to a previous ectopic pregnancy or surgical alteration, as in the case of an elective tubal ligation for sterilization.

Adhesion formation secondary to PID is usually the result of a previous infection or multiple infections, with *N. gonorrhoeae* and *C. trachomatis* being the causative agents. An inflammatory response follows sexual transmission of the agent; patients with fulminant PID often present with high fever, severe pelvic pain, and mucopurulent vaginal discharge. These patients are treated with antibiotics, though damage to the fallopian tubes may have already occurred.

Patients may also contract a sexually transmitted disease (STD) with ensuing PID and damage to the fallopian tubes without experiencing any symptoms. PID may also result from a septic abortion or IUD use. Patients with a history of ectopic pregnancy, PID, tubal surgery, septic abortion, or ruptured appendix should be evaluated early in the infertility work-up for tubal integrity. (See also the **Pelvic Inflammatory Disease** chapter and Section 13.)

Endocrine-Factor Infertility

Primary Amenorrhea

Women presenting with primary amenorrhea (no spontaneous uterine bleeding by age 17 years) must be evaluated for chromosomal abnormalities, congenital absence of the uterus, or androgen-insensitivity syndrome. Management of primary amenorrhea is beyond the scope of this chapter.

Hypothalamic Factors

Hypothalamic dysfunction/failure may result from stress, excessive exercise (e.g., long-distance running or ballet), and/or severe weight loss resulting from eating disorders (anorexia/bulimia). All of these conditions have an effect on estrogen production and the pulsatility of gonadotropin releasing hormone (GnRH) (Berga et al. 1991). Ovulatory cycles generally resume when stress is reduced and there is a return to normal weight and exercise patterns, though this may be delayed for up to a year.

A vast number of milder, even subclinical forms of hypothalamic dysfunction may also result in anovulation. The ovulatory disorder may be treated relatively easily, while the underlying etiology of the disturbance may be more difficult to treat.

Pituitary Factors

Increased circulating prolactin (PRL) is recognized as a common cause of amenorrhea, anovulation, and other defects of the hypothalamic-pituitary-ovarian axis. Women with hyperprolactinemia may present with galactorrhea, polymenorrhea, oligomenorrhea, amenorrhea, decreased libido, and infertility. Hyperprolactinemia may be due to hypothyroidism or, secondarily, to medications such as antihistamines, tranquilizers, antidepressants, antihypertensives, antiemetics, or oral contraceptives.

The most common cause of hyperprolactinemia is a prolactin-secreting adenoma (prolactinoma). Hyperprolactinemia also has been found to be associated with luteal-phase deficiency due to defective folliculogenesis and inhibition of progesterone secretion caused by higher concentrations of PRL (100 ng/mL) (Jones 1989). Chronic anovulation may be due to hyperprolactinemia in 38% of women (Jones 1989). It appears that increased PRL secretion inhibits hypothalamic GnRH release, resulting in decreased circulating luteinizing hormone (LH) and follicle stimulating hormone (FSH).

Sheehan's syndrome is pituitary failure resulting from a disturbance of pituitary circulation immediately following childbirth. In this rare condition, the pituitary shuts down LH and FSH production; consequently, the follicles do not develop.

Thyroid Factors

Disorders affecting thyroid function are common in women of reproductive age. Menorrhagia, anovulation, oligomenorrhea, and amenorrhea may be associated with hypofunction and hyperfunction of the thyroid. (See the **Thyroid Disorders** chapter in Section 10.) Hypothyroidism is a causative factor in infertility due to hyperprolactinemia. There are myriad clinical presentations of abnormal thyroid function; therefore, a high level of suspicion is advised.

Adrenal Factors

Dysfunction of the adrenal glands or ovaries can result in increased androgen levels, which in turn result in abnormal estrogen levels that interfere with FSH and LH feedback systems (as in polycystic ovary syndrome, or PCOS). The three principal androgens in women are testosterone, androstenedione, and dehydroepiandrosterone sulfate (DHEAS). Hyperandrogenism describes an elevation of the circulating level of testosterone, DHEAS, and/or androstenedione.

The pathophysiological consequences of hyperandrogenism in women may include virilization, hirsutism, acne, diminished breast size, dysfunctional uterine bleeding, and anovulation (Marut 1989). Androgen-secreting tumors of the ovary or adrenals are rare but should always be ruled out when androgen levels are high. (See the **Hirsutism** chapter.)

Polycystic Ovary Syndrome

PCOS is the most common cause of ovarian dysfunction. An excess of ovarian androgen production results in chronic anovulation. Decreased FSH stimulation results in impaired follicle development, and the increased androgen production causes elevated LH, which interferes with GnRH. Often, patients with PCOS have ovaries that are encapsulated in a smooth, pearly white capsule. The end result is an ovary that contains multiple follicles in various stages of development and persistent anovulation. Patients with PCOS often present with amenorrhea, obesity, hirsutism, and acne. Lab data reveal an elevated LH to FSH ratio (at least 2:1) and increased testosterone (>70 ng/dL) and DHEAS levels. PCOS is considered a problem of persistent anovulation with a spectrum of etiologies and clinical manifestations, including insulin resistance, hyperinsulinemia, and hyperandrogenism (Speroff et al. 1999).

Premature Ovarian Failure

In this condition, oocytes are "used up" before the age of 40 years. Patients with this condition will present with amenorrhea and, possibly, menopausal symptoms. Clinically, early follicular FSH and LH levels are >20 mIU/mL on more than one occasion. Irradiation for Hodgkin's disease may cause this condition, though the cause is usually unclear.

Luteinized Unruptured Follicle

In patients with this syndrome, ovulation may appear to have occurred according to hormonal laboratory data, but the ovum is not released from the follicular cavity. This may be caused by inadequate follicular development, premature LH surge, or progesterone release, and is difficult to diagnose consistently. Diagnosis is by visualization of the ovary using ultrasound or laparoscopy. The syndrome may occur normally in all women intermittently.

Immunological Infertility

Controversy exists about the relationship between positive sperm antibodies and infertility. The serum immunoglobulins IgG, IgM, and IgA have been evaluated by modifications of the direct and indirect Combs assay and some correlation with infertility has been established. In addition, immunoglobulins have been detected on the surface of sperm with use of an immunobead test. (See "Antisperm Antibodies" under "Male-Factor Infertility," above.) Antibodies against the sperm surface become harmful due to phagocytosis and complement-mediated cytotoxicity (Serafini et al. 1989). Antisperm antibodies (ASAs) found on the surface of sperm by direct testing are more significant than ASAs found in the serum or seminal plasma by indirect testing. Postcoital testing in immunologically affected couples usually reveals no cervical spermatozoa in a woman whose partner is known to have sperm, in contrast to what was previously thought to be an absence of sperm motility. ASA testing should also be considered when there is sperm agglutination or unexplained infertility. Testing is not needed if intracytoplasmic sperm injection (ICSI) will be performed.

Unexplained Infertility

Ten percent to 15% of infertile couples who undergo a thorough evaluation will be "diagnosed" with unexplained or idiopathic infertility. It is a diagnosis of exclusion. Infertility evaluation and treatment is not an exact science. It is possible that the cause of couples' infertility is still unknown.

Age-Related Infertility

Diminished Ovarian Reserve

This term describes ovaries that no longer contain eggs that can reliably produce a successful pregnancy.

A measurable decline in fertility is associated with aging in the female (i.e., 35 years old or older). Other reasons include chemotherapy, radiation therapy, autoimmune diseases, and certain genetic conditions. This is especially significant when considering assisted reproductive technology procedures. According to the "1999 Assisted Reproductive Technology Success Rates," live birth rates per in vitro fertilization (IVF) cycle were approximately 5% in women 43 years old or older (Centers for Disease Control and Prevention 2001). Women older than 39 years experience more luteal-phase abnormalities. The rate of miscarriage is 50% or higher in women who are 44 years old or older. Diagnosis is made using a combination of tests considered singly or together. Abnormal FSH or estradiol on Day 2 or 3 or an abnormal value on a clomiphene citrate challenge test

(CCCT) predicts that a successful pregnancy will be achieved about 5% of the time (Scott et al. 1995). (See the **Clomiphene Citrate** chapter for details about CCCT.)

Other Factors

Repeated Pregnancy Loss

Two categories of patients who have experienced repeated pregnancy loss are those with:

→ Three or more consecutive pregnancy losses at any gestational age, and

→ An unexplained second trimester loss and any number of subsequent pregnancy losses at any gestational age.

The risk of another miscarriage after three consecutive losses is 30–45% (Speroff et al. 1999). Causes can include age, genetics, uterine abnormalities, cervical abnormalities, hormonal imbalances, infection, and immunologic issues.

Luteal-Phase Deficiencies

The luteal-phase defect or inadequate luteal phase is believed to be caused by insufficient FSH and/or LH release and stimulation, which causes suboptimal corpus luteum development. This results in inadequate progesterone production. Consequently, the endometrial lining develops inadequately and implantation of the fertilized ovum is unsuccessful. This defect also may be caused by a lack of cellular receptors for progesterone in the endometrium (Serafini et al. 1989).

A short luteal phase is when the time interval between the LH peak and the onset of menses is less than 11 days due to insufficient duration of progesterone production. The short luteal phase is confirmed by basal body temperature (BBT) readings during at least 2–3 cycles.

A histological diagnosis of inadequate luteal phase is based on an endometrial biopsy that shows a lag of two or more days in two different menstrual cycles (Witten et al. 1985). Normally fertile women may, on occasion, have an out-of-phase endometrial biopsy. Daily luteal-phase progesterone levels in women with luteal-phase defect are generally lower than in normal women, though the difference may be minimal.

DATABASE

SUBJECTIVE

→ A review of health history should include:

- The age of both members of the couple
- The approximate date the couple stopped using contraception
- History and outcome of any previous pregnancies involving both partners:
  - Couples with a history of three or more spontaneous pregnancy losses should be referred for further evaluation, including genetic karotyping.
- The length and regularity of the menstrual cycle, magnitude of flow, and age at menarche
- Symptoms and treatment of dysmenorrhea or dyspareunia
- History and treatment of abnormal bleeding

- Symptoms of ovulation—e.g., breast tenderness, acne, mittelschmerz, mood changes, spotting, changes in libido, and increased midcycle vaginal discharge
- Frequency of coitus, use of lubricants, and the couple's perception of whether or not ejaculation occurs in the vagina
- Religious practices that may relate to intercourse or fertility
- Duration of amenorrhea, if any
- The presence of physical or emotional stress, weight fluctuation, or medication taken before cessation of menses
- The presence or history of galactorrhea
- History of STD or PID; treatment and/or sequellae
- Previous pelvic or other surgery, and complications, if any
- Review of any previous infertility evaluation and treatment
- Pertinent medical history suggestive of an endocrine disorder
- History of serious medical illnesses
- DES exposure
- History of IUD use and sequellae, if any
- History of oral contraceptive or Depo-Provera® use
- Previous abnormal Pap smear and subsequent treatment
- Social history: use of alcohol, prescription drugs, OTC drugs (e.g., laxatives or antihistamines), recreational drugs, and herbal preparations; smoking
- Eating habits suggestive of eating disorders
- Exercise history and habits
- Family history with attention to endocrine, genetic, or reproductive abnormalities
- History of exposure to radiation or toxic chemicals
- Use of saunas or hot tubs

→ Investigation of a woman with repeated pregnancy loss should include:

- A review of systems with attention to systemic diseases, including:
  - Diabetes
  - Collagen vascular disorders
  - Thyroid dysfunction
  - History of thromboembolic events (e.g., stroke, deep vein thrombosis, pulmonary emboli)
- A description of the patient's work environment with attention to possible toxic exposures
- Surgical history
- History of cervical treatment or disease
- Obstetrical history, including whether previous losses were associated with curettage
- Obstetrical history with attention to possible curettage for retained products
- Family history of inborn errors of metabolism (e.g., Tay-Sachs disease, chromosomal anomalies, stillborns, early infant deaths, pregnancy loss)
- Medication history
- DES exposure
- Social history, including smoking, alcohol and caffeine consumption, and use of illicit drugs

OBJECTIVE

→ A comprehensive physical examination should be conducted, with special attention to:
- Vital signs
- Height and weight:
  - Assess desirable body weight. (See **General Nutrition Guidelines**, Section 16.)
- Signs of hyperandrogenism: acne, oily skin, hirsutism, etc.
- Thyroid examination:
  - Assess for masses.
  - Note if the patient has any signs of hypothyroidism or hyperthyroidism. (See the **Thyroid Disorders** chapter in Section 10.)
- Abdominal examination:
  - Assess for scars, masses, and tenderness.
- Breast examination:
  - Assess for galactorrhea.
- Pelvic, rectal examination. Assess for:
  - Normal hair distribution
  - Signs of clitoromegaly
  - Signs of vaginal/cervical infection or abnormality
  - Cervical mucus relative to time of menstrual cycle
  - Uterine or adnexal abnormalities
  - Nodularity of the uterosacral ligaments or cul-de-sac
  - Rectal masses
- See the **Hirsutism** chapter.

ASSESSMENT

→ Infertility: primary or secondary
→ R/O male-factor infertility
→ R/O pelvic factor infertility
→ R/O endocrine infertility
→ R/O immunological infertility
→ R/O unexplained infertility
→ R/O diminished ovarian reserve
→ R/O repeated pregnancy loss
→ R/O luteal-phase insufficiency

PLAN

DIAGNOSTIC TESTS

→ Tests should proceed from simpler, less invasive to more complicated and invasive.
→ Routine laboratory tests (values may vary by laboratory) may include:
- Rubella titer
- VDRL or RPR
- FSH, estradiol (Day 2–3 of cycle)
  - FSH >12 mIU/mL or estradiol >80 pg/mL (diminished ovarian reserve)
- If amenorrhea, then FSH and LH
  - FSH and LH <5 mIU/mL (hypothalamic-pituitary dysfunction or failure)
  - FSH >20 mIU/mL in the follicular phase during two separate cycles (premature ovarian failure)

- High LH with low or normal FSH (ratio of 3:1 or higher) (PCOS)
  NOTE: While a 3:1 or higher ratio is typical of PCOS, this condition should not be ruled out if the ratio is less than 3:1.
- Prolactin—early to mid-morning; no breast stimulation 24 hours before test (normal = <20 ng/mL in most labs [Speroff et al. 1999])
- Progesterone (mid-luteal should be >10 ng/mL)
- Fasting glucose (normal = <110 mg/dL)
- TSH (normal = 0.2–3.2 μU/mL)
- Pap smear, gonorrhea, chlamydia testing
- *T mycoplasma* culture
  NOTE: T mycoplasma, now referred to as *Ureaplasma urealyticum*, has been reported as a possible factor in cases of infertility with unknown etiology. This is controversial; studies comparing colonization in fertile and infertile populations are plagued by conflicting results and poor controls (Grunfeld 1989).

If indicated:
- Testosterone (normal = <70 ng/dL total)
- DHEAS (normal = 15–17 years old: 35–535 μg/dL; 18–30 years old: 29–781 μg/dL; 31–50 years old: 12–379 μg/dL)
- Fasting insulin levels (normal = <10–20 U/mL)

→ Specific infertility tests and procedures:
NOTE: The primary care provider can order tests, interpret results in consultation with a physician, and provide couples with information regarding tests and procedures. Tests listed here should be done in the order suggested.
- BBT charting:
  - Two to three cycles of BBT monitoring are sufficient to suggest that ovulation has occurred.
  - BBT readings also are used to guide woman about:
    - When to start using LH predictor kits
    - Scheduling of postcoital testing
    - Timing of intrauterine insemination (IUI)
- Urine LH (ovulation predictor) kits:
  - LH surge ovulation predictor kits detect the normal preovulatory surge of LH and translate the surge as an abrupt color change from the colorless readings before the surge.
  - LH kits available over the counter:
    - Used daily by women, starting 2–3 days before expected ovulation until an obvious color change is seen, signaling that ovulation will occur in the next 24–26 hours.
  - LH kit readings now are used routinely by primary care providers for optimal timing of postcoital testing and IUI, and for timing of coitus during peak ovulation.
  - The LH kit *predicts* ovulation, whereas ovulatory readings are *retrospective* based on BBT readings.
  - If a woman's history strongly suggests anovulation, kits should not be used because of their cost.

- LH kit readings should not be used as a diagnostic tool without confirmation by laboratory and clinical data.
■ Mid-luteal phase serum progesterone:
  - Should be obtained 7 days after presumed ovulation as determined by an LH predictor kit.
  - Normal = 10–15 ng/mL as an indirect indicator of ovulation; higher values are expected in the clomiphene citrate cycle.
  - A false negative result is possible if the sample is obtained too early or too late in the luteal phase due to normal pulsatile variations of serum progesterone.
■ Sonography/serum estradiol:
  - Pre-ovulatory sonography is highly useful for evaluating adequate follicular development.
  - A sector scanner with high resolution is easily used in the practice setting; a vaginal transducer provides a sonographically improved image of ovarian follicles.
  - Potential ovulation is defined as follicles measuring ≥16–18 mm.
  - Serum estradiol drawn at the time that follicles measure ≥16–18 mm should show a level of 400 pg/mL (site-specific values vary).
■ Examination of semen:
  - Semen analysis should be obtained early in the infertility evaluation.
  - Values for the same individual will fluctuate over time; one abnormal result is not sufficient to make a diagnosis.
  - At least 2–3 abnormal semen analyses done over 2–3 months are necessary before classifying male-factor infertility.
  - In the event of abnormal findings, referral the patient to a urologist specializing in male-factor infertility.
  - See **Table 12H.1, Normal Semen Analysis** and **Appendix 12H.2, Collection of Sample for Semen Analysis**.
■ Immune tests:
  - Detect the presence of sperm-bound antibodies by binding a marker substance, which is coated with antibodies directed against human immunoglobulin to sperm; assessed with a microscope.
  - Binding requires motile sperm for detection; these tests are useless when motility or sperm count is very low.
    – Immunobead test:
      ➤ Uses washed sperm.
      ➤ The only test that can localize the specific site of antibody binding on the sperm (i.e., head, tail, midpiece).
    – Mixed agglutination test (SpermMar™):
      ➤ Can use unprepared semen.
      ➤ Binding to the sperm is detected by the presence of latex particles.
    NOTE: "Because both unexplained infertility and immunologic infertility are treated with intrauterine inseminations, the usefulness of sperm antibody testing is limited" (Speroff et al. 1999, p. 1084).
■ Sperm penetration assay:

- Evaluates spermatozoa's ability to penetrate the zona pellucida of a human egg.
- Fresh human eggs retrieved from hysterectomy specimens are ideal, if available; if not, denuded hamster eggs can be used.
- There are many variations of this test. Its value depends on the experience of the lab. It is considered a useful tool for predicting successful fertilization in IVF cycles versus who would benefit from ICSI.
■ Postcoital test:
  - A postcoital (or Sims-Hühner) test evaluates sperm survival in cervical mucus.
  - It is performed just before ovulation as determined by a color change on the LH predictor. Because the technique, timing, and interpretation of the test are controversial, its utility and predictive value have been questioned. Treatments such as IUI and assisted reproductive technology (ART) have effectively negated unrecognized cervical factors. Routine postcoital testing is unnecessary.
■ Endometrial biopsy:
  - Confirms ovulation or diagnoses luteal-phase defects.
  - A specimen is obtained several days before the expected onset of menses (between cycle Days 24–26 in a 28- to 30-day cycle).
  - Results should reveal histological evidence that the endometrium appears as expected for the stated post-ovulatory day on which the biopsy was taken.
  - A single abnormal result is common and not indicative of pathology unless it is confirmed by a second biopsy.
  - The provider should do a urine pregnancy test first. The patient may choose to abstain from sexual intercourse during that month.
■ Ultrasound:
  - Used to diagnose significant uterine pathology—i.e. myomas and adenomyosis.
■ Sonohysteroscopy:
  - Transvaginal ultrasound with an injection of sterile water or saline to document the size and shape of the uterus, polyps, submucosal myomas, or synechiae.
■ Hysterosalpingogram (HSG):
  - Should generally precede diagnostic laparoscopy and hysteroscopy.
  - Performed by a physician; findings are interpreted by a radiologist and gynecologist.
  - Involves injection of water or oil-based dye into the uterine cavity to evaluate fallopian-tube patency and uterine abnormalities.
  - Done under fluoroscopy shortly after menses in the follicular phase (Day 7–10) before anticipated ovulation.
  - Many providers prescribe doxycycline 100 mg p.o. BID for 5 days, starting the day before the HSG, as a prophylactic.
  - Studies have reported an improved pregnancy rate following the use of HSG with an oil-based dye, indicating that there may be some therapeutic value to HSG.

- Clomiphene citrate challenge test:
  - Recommended for unexplained infertility or age-related infertility. An abnormal response indicates a poor prognosis regardless of the woman's age (Scott 1995).
  - FSH and estradiol are drawn on Day 3, followed by 100 mg of clomiphene citrate (2, 50-mg tablets) on Days 5–9. On Day 10, an FSH is drawn.
  - If any of the three blood tests is abnormal, the whole test is considered abnormal.
- Laparoscopy:
  - Performed by a physician at the end of an infertility evaluation unless there is a history of major pelvic pathology, strong suspicion of endometriosis, or significant tubal disease.
  - In many instances, laparoscopy is not needed if the patient plans to go to ART.
  - Performed under general anesthesia during the follicular phase of the cycle to prevent possible disruption of early pregnancy.
  - HSG is commonly performed again during laparoscopy to evaluate tubal patency by directly observing dye spilled from fimbriated ends of the fallopian tube.
- Hysteroscopy:
  - Often done at the time of laparoscopy or alone in the office.
  - Involves direct visualization of the uterine cavity for adhesions, tumors, or anomalies such as endometrial and endocervical polyps and fibroids.

→ Test procedures for women with repeated pregnancy loss:
- Maternal and paternal karyotype
- Karyotype of abortus material also may be appropriate by advance arrangement with a genetics laboratory.
- FSH cycle Day 2 or 3
- TSH
- Prolactin
- Antinuclear antibody
- Prothrombin time, platelets
- Lupus anticoagulant
- Anticardiolipin antibody
- Mid-luteal serum progesterone
- Chlamydia, gonorrhea tests
- Mycoplasma culture (or empiric treatment of the couple with doxycycline, 100 mg p.o. BID for 10 days)
- Endometrial biopsy 7 days after ovulation and before the onset of menses
- A study of the uterine cavity with sonography, hysterosalpingogram, hysteroscopy

TREATMENT/MANAGEMENT

→ Diagnostic evaluation as outlined above.
→ Specific therapy based on the patient's history and findings of diagnostic evaluation.

Male-Factor Infertility

→ Treatment of male-factor infertility focuses on intrauterine insemination. (**See Table 12H.1, Normal Semen Analysis** and **Appendix 12H.3, Timing of Intrauterine Insemination**.)
→ Additional male infertility problems and treatment may include:
- Varicocele—surgical repair (varicocelectomy) or percutaneous embolization
  - Most studies have shown improvement in fertility after varicocele treatment.
- Pyospermia—empiric therapy:
  - Doxycycline 100 mg p.o. BID for 3 weeks for the male partner (prostate poorly vascularized, seminiferous tubules sheltered by blood-testes barrier)
  - Doxycycline 100 mg p.o. BID for 10–14 days for the female partner (to coincide with the last 2 weeks of the male's therapy)
- Antisperm antibodies—intrauterine insemination (IUI). (See **Appendix 12H.3, Timing of Intrauterine Insemination**.)
  - If unsuccessful after 6 cycles of IUI, may progress to IVF. (See **Appendix 12H.4, Assisted Reproductive Technology**.)
  - Steroid therapy may be considered, though there is concern regarding reactions to glucocorticoids.
- A poor semen analysis with poor sperm penetration assay results—donor sperm or ICSI
- Infections of the genital tract:
  - Antibiotic therapy for the couple.
  - Repeat semen analysis after 2 months; if leukospermia (>8 white blood cells per high-power field) persists, semen should be cultured.
    - Refer to a urologist.
- Low semen volume:
  - Refer to a urologist for complete evaluation.
  - Use multiple ejaculations IUI.
- Abnormal liquidation:
  - Refer to a urologist for evaluation of prostate and seminal vesicles.
- Low sperm count:
  - If persistent or azoospermic, refer to a urologist for complete evaluation.
- Decreased motility:
  - Refer to a urologist.
- Decreased normal morphology:
  - Refer to a urologist.

Pelvic-Factor Infertility

→ Asherman's syndrome:
- Lysis of adhesions by hysteroscopy (performed by a physician).
- Hormone administration may be utilized after surgical intervention to prevent recurrence of scarring.
  - Regimen: conjugated estrogens 2.5 mg p.o. for 3 of 4

weeks plus medroxyprogesterone acetate 10 mg daily added to the third week (Speroff et al. 1999)

→ Cervical-factor infertility.
  ▪ IUI is now the treatment of choice. (See **Appendix 12H.1, Indications for Intrauterine Insemination** and **Appendix 12H.3, Timing of Intrauterine Insemination**.)
  ▪ Refer for ART as necessary. (See **Appendix 12H.4, Assisted Reproductive Technology**.)

→ Endometriosis:
  ▪ See the **Endometriosis** chapter.
  ▪ Consider referral for ART.

→ Tubal disease/obstruction:
  ▪ Refer for IVF.
  ▪ Fallopian tube recanalization:
    • For evaluating proximal tubal occlusion and possibly correcting it.
      – Operative laparoscopy is more cost-effective than laparotomy.
      – Involves traumatic instrumentation, tissue handling, and various methods of adhesion prevention.
      – The prognosis for pregnancy following surgery for bilateral tubal disease is very poor. If pregnancy has not occurred within 18 months after extensive surgery and the woman is younger than 35 years, consider repeating the procedure. If the woman reaches her 35th birthday, refer her for ART. (See **Appendix 12H.4, Assisted Reproductive Technology**.)
  ▪ Tubal ligation reversal:
    • The ability to reverse sterilization procedures is determined by the amount of tubal damage incurred at the time of sterilization, the length of the remaining tubes for reanastomosis, and the type of surgical technique used.

Endocrine Infertility

→ Primary amenorrhea:
  ▪ Refer to an endocrinologist.

→ Hypothalamic factors.
  ▪ Refer for treatment of an eating disorder as necessary. (See the **Eating Disorders** chapter in Section 14.)
  ▪ A return to ovulatory status may require a change in exercise habits.
    • Counsel or refer as necessary.
  ▪ Ovulation induction by administration of clomiphene citrate. (See the **Clomiphene Citrate** chapter.)
  ▪ May require ovulation induction by "superovulation therapy" (human gonadotropins).
  ▪ Refer for ART as necessary if the woman fails to conceive by means of ovulation induction therapy.
  ▪ See also the **Amenorrhea—Secondary** chapter.

→ Pituitary factors:
  ▪ A prolactin level >100 ng/mL is highly suggestive of a pituitary-secreting adenoma.
    • Refer the woman for MRI or CT and treatment by an endocrinologist.

▪ Administer a dopamine agonist to normalize the prolactin level (Speroff et al. 1999):
  • Bromocriptine mesylate 2.5 mg p.o. BID (can start with an initial dose of 2.5 mg at HS to minimize side effects)
                        OR
  • Cabergoline tablets 2.5 mg p.o. twice a week or 0.5–3 mg once a week. (See the **Clomiphene Citrate** chapter.) Consult with a physician.
▪ In the event of hyperprolactinemia due to hypothyroidism, begin thyroid hormone replacement. (See the **Thyroid Disorders** chapter in Section 10.)
  • See also the **Amenorrhea—Secondary** chapter.
▪ Sheehan's syndrome:
  • Refer the patient to a reproductive endocrinologist for treatment.
▪ Hypothyroidism:
  • See the **Thyroid Disorders** chapter in Section 10.
  • Maintain TSH in the normal range by administering thyroid hormone 0.1–0.15 mg per day (site policies may vary).
    – Consult with a physician.
  • Refer to an endocrinologist for treatment of other thyroid disorders.
▪ Adrenal factors:
  • Androgen-secreting tumors of the ovary or adrenals are rare but should be ruled out when androgen levels are high.
  • Women with abnormal levels should be referred to an endocrinologist.
  • See the **Hirsutism** chapter.
  • Abnormal (low) testosterone level:
    – Treat with dexamethasone 0.5 mg p.o. at bedtime to decrease nighttime adrenocorticotropic hormone production (Speroff et al. 1999). A low testosterone reflects low ovarian output, so these women may respond poorly to ovulation induction therapy without the addition of dexamethasone.
    – Consult with a physician.
▪ Polycystic ovary syndrome:
  • Referral to a safe, structured, weight-loss program is recommended for the obese PCOS woman, though the parameters of weight-loss success and return to normal ovulatory status are hard to measure.
  • Induce ovulation by administering clomiphene citrate (CC). (See the **Clomiphene Citrate** chapter.)
    – If a woman fails to conceive after 3–6 ovulatory cycles on CC therapy or does not ovulate on 150 mg clomiphene, refer her for more aggressive therapy.
  • If the fasting glucose/fasting insulin ratio is less than 4.5, consider treating with metformin HCL.
    – First evaluate creatinine and SGPT levels and repeat again 2 months after treatment. Start metformin 500 mg p.o. QD for 1 week, then increase to BID for 1 week and then 500 mg TID for 3 weeks. Experience dictates starting slowly and increasing gradually (Speroff et al. 1999).

– If spontaneous ovulation does not occur in 3 months, retreat with CC 100 mg. If ovulation does not occur, refer the patient for ART.
- Administration of human gonadotropins (superovulation):
  – Refer the patient for ART if she is not responsive to CC or to CC and a dopamine agonist. Injectable gonadotropins can be used with or without IVF.
- Surgery:
  – Refer PCOS patients to a physician for possible ovarian stromal cautery. Punctures are made with a needle into the cysts during laparoscopy.
- Premature ovarian failure:
  - Refer the patient for ART.
  - Donor oocytes or use of the GnRH pump to attempt to induce ovulation offers limited success.
  - Estrogen replacement for protection of bones.
  - Therapy will be patient- and site-specific.
  - See also the **Perimenopausal and Menopausal Symptoms and Hormone Therapy** chapter.
  - Refer the couple with premature ovarian failure for crisis counseling, as this diagnosis is naturally quite devastating.
  - Counsel couples to consider options—adoption, surrogacy (check state laws), and child-free living.
- Luteinized unruptured follicle (LUF):
  - Administer human chorionic gonadotropin (HCG) by injection.
    – Acts like an LH surge to induce ovulation, which should occur 24–36 hours after the injection.
    – Consult with a physician.
    – The couple is instructed to have intercourse on the day of injection and every other day thereafter until follicle rupture is evidenced by ultrasound.
    – See the **Clomiphene Citrate** chapter for a description of ultrasound evidence of ovulation.
  - CC therapy and HCG, or gonadotropin therapy and HCG, also are used as a treatment for LUF in some practices.

Immunological Infertility

→ Suppressive steroid therapy has had limited success.
→ Use IUI to attempt to bypass immobilizing antibodies secreted in cervical mucus.
→ Refer the patient for ART if pregnancy does not occur after six IUI cycles or sooner, depending on the woman's age.
→ Counsel the couple to consider options—adoption, surrogacy, or child-free living.

Unexplained Infertility

→ Treat the couple empirically for mycoplasma.
- Doxycycline 100 mg p.o. BID for a minimum of 10 days (site-specific policies vary).
→ Ovulation induction (see the **Clomiphene Citrate** chapter) combined with ultrasound monitoring and IUI for six ovulatory cycles.

- If unsuccessful, refer the patient for gonadotropin/IUI therapy.
→ Refer the patient for ART as appropriate.
→ Counsel the couple, keep them actively involved in decision-making, help them to "let go" when all avenues of therapy have been exhausted, and encourage them to explore adoption, surrogacy, and child-free living.

Age-Related Infertility

Diminished Ovarian Reserve

→ Counsel couples that empiric therapy beyond age 43 is not efficacious or cost-effective.
→ Counsel them regarding donor oocytes, adoption, surrogacy, and child-free living.
→ In the event of age-related, luteal-phase abnormalities, treatment includes CC therapy with support of the luteal phase by administering micronized progesterone vaginally, 100 mg every 12 hours until 10 weeks of pregnancy.
→ If the patient is older than 40 years, do a clomiphene challenge test and refer for ART.

Other Factors

Repeated Pregnancy Loss

NOTE: Treatment depends on the causative factor.
→ Müllerian anomalies or fibroids impinging on the uterine cavity:
- Refer to a physician for appropriate surgery (e.g., hysteroscopic resection of the uterine septum).
→ Karyotypic abnormalities:
- Refer for genetic counseling; possibly refer for ART with donor gametes.
→ Intrauterine synechiae:
- Refer for appropriate surgery.
→ Age 44 years or older:
- The spontaneous abortion rate is greater than 50%; treatment generally is not successful.
→ DES exposure:
- No specific treatment.
- Refer for colposcopic examination.
- Counsel regarding the risk of pathology secondary to DES exposure to cervix.
- Counsel to consider adoption, surrogacy, or child-free living.
→ History of thrombosis/embolic events or abnormality in bleeding times and positive anticardiolipin autoantibodies:
- Administer low-dose aspirin, 60–80 mg p.o. per day (1 "baby aspirin").
- Consult with a physician.
- Immediately refer to a perinatologist upon documentation of pregnancy by appropriately rising hCG titers, as these pregnancies are at high risk for sudden fetal loss.
→ Isolated abnormal immune tests of low titer (e.g., ANA 1:80 or low positive IgC anticardiolipin antibody).
- Administer aspirin, 60–80 mg p.o. per day empirically.

■ Refer to a perinatologist upon documentation of pregnancy viability.

→ Unexplained early losses for women with well-documented luteal-phase deficiency:

■ Luteal-phase support or CC and luteal-phase support with micronized progesterone.

■ Review and advise against illicit drug use, smoking, or chronic alcohol use.

■ Advise appropriate counseling.

Luteal-Phase Defect

→ Administer micronized progesterone vaginal suppositories, 100 mg twice daily in the luteal phase until onset of menses. In the event of a pregnancy, continue this regimen until around 10 weeks of pregnancy, at which time it is presumed that placental production of progesterone is adequate.

■ Consult with a physician.

→ CC and HCG 10,000 units IM (see the **Clomiphene Citrate** chapter):

■ Consult with a physician.

■ Measure serum progesterone level 7 days following administration of HCG (15–30 ng/mL is normal in a CC-enhanced cycle).

■ Refer to BBT charting to monitor the length of the luteal phase and assess the efficacy of treatment.

CONSULTATION

→ Refer the patient to a physician for consultation regarding abnormal clinical findings and for discussion of treatment modalities.

→ Refer to specialists as indicated (e.g., a reproductive endocrinologist, urologist, or counselor).

→ Refer to support groups/counseling (e.g., RESOLVE peer-support group).

→ Hold ongoing discussions with the infertility team to ensure that the woman's treatment is up-to-date.

→ As needed for prescription(s).

PATIENT EDUCATION

→ Provide information regarding basic anatomy and physiology, with an emphasis on the normal menstrual cycle, ovulation, frequency, and timing of and positions for intercourse.

→ Advise against the use of lubricants and douches. Explain the effects of drugs, heat, and excessive alcohol consumption on spermatogenesis.

→ Describe for the couple the infertility evaluation, risks, expected overall cost, and time involved, and thoroughly discuss their expectations.

→ Refer the couple to the office manager or accountant to discuss insurance reimbursement and the cost of individual tests.

→ Discuss laparoscopy/hysteroscopy:

■ Classified as same-day surgery. Postoperative patients may resume normal activities in 1–3 days.

■ Common after-effects may include:

• Generalized stiffness
• Sore throat
• Shoulder pain (referred pain secondary to carbon dioxide application to abdomen for insertion and visualization with a laparoscope)
• Bloating of the abdomen
• Abdominal wall tenderness

■ Evaluate the couple's coping skills and whether additional counseling is needed.

→ Infertility counseling is based on brief psychotherapy or a crisis-intervention model:

■ In some cases, the infertility experience triggers responses that are linked to past losses, unresolved grief, or poor self-esteem (Mahlstedt 1985).

■ Several important features should be kept in mind when counseling couples:

• They need information about their medical situation and options so they have a sense of control.
• They need to identify feelings that have resulted directly from the infertility.
• They may need help restoring their self-esteem.
• They need to discuss and explore the feelings of loss and guilt before resolution is possible.
• They may need help with decision-making in terms of treatment modalities.

FOLLOW-UP

→ Careful interpretation and explanation of all laboratory data or clinical findings are necessary. Institute necessary treatment modalities.

→ Specific treatment follow-up should assess the management plan and possible side effects of drug therapies and changes in physical status. Test for pregnancy following any treatment regimen.

→ The patient may need assurance that the infertility evaluation is progressing in a thorough, timely manner and that tests are being done properly. She may need assistance with scheduling of tests or treatments.

→ Ongoing consultation with the infertility team regarding the patient's clinical data, treatment modalities, and emotional status is necessary.

→ Offer the patient pertinent referrals to specialists in the event of unusual findings.

→ Pertinent counseling and ongoing assessment of a couple's emotional status are recommended. Refer them to a counselor experienced with infertility.

■ A referral list should include a variety of specialists from varying religious backgrounds.

■ Refer the couple to adoption resources.

→ Refer the couple to an endometriosis support group in the area as indicated.

■ The Endometriosis Association (8585 North 76th Place, Milwaukee, Wis. 53223) has many regional chapters and publishes a newsletter.

→ Refer the couple to a RESOLVE infertility peer-support

group (1310 Broadway, Somerville, Mass. 02144, www.resolve.org).

→ Document in progress notes and on problem list.

BIBLIOGRAPHY

Berga, S.L., Loucks, A.B., Rossmanith, W.G. et al. 1991. Acceleration of luteinizing hormone pulse frequency in functional hypothalamic amenorrhea by dopaminergic blockade. *Journal of Clinical Endocrinology and Metabolism* 72:151–153.

Berkowitz, G.S. 1986. Epidemiology of infertility and early pregnancy wastage. *Reproductive failure*. London: Churchill Livingstone.

Bernstein, J., and Mattox, J.H. 1982. An overview of infertility. *Journal of Obstetric, Gynecologic and Neonatal Nursing* 11(5):309–314.

Centers for Disease Control and Prevention, American Society for Reproductive Medicine, Society for Assisted Reproductive Technology. 2001. RESOLVE. *1999 assisted reproductive success rates*. Atlanta, Ga.: Centers for Disease Control and Prevention.

Grunfeld, L. 1989. Workup for male infertility. *Journal of Reproductive Medicine* 34(2):143–149.

Henzl, M. 1989. Role of nafarelin in the management of endometriosis. *Journal of Reproductive Medicine* 34(12): 1021–1024.

Howards, S.S. 1992. Varicocele. *Infertility and Reproductive Medicine Clinics of North America* 3:429.

Ishimaru, T., and Masuzaki, H. 1991. Peritoneal endometriosis: endometrial tissue implantation as its primary etiologic mechanism. *American Journal of Obstetrics and Gynecology* 165:210–211.

Jones, E. 1989. Hyperprolactinemia and female infertility. *Journal of Reproductive Medicine* 34(2):117–125.

Mahlstedt, P.P. 1985. The psychological component of infertility. *Fertility and Sterility* 43(3):635–638.

Marsman, J.W.P. 1987. Clinical versus subclinical variococeles: venographic findings and improvement of fertility after embolization. *Radiology* 155(3):635–638.

Marut, E.L. 1989. Polycystic ovary syndrome. *Journal of Reproductive Medicine* 34(1):104–107.

Mazor, M., and Simons, H. 1983. *Infertility: medical, emotional, and social considerations*. New York: Human Science Press.

Older, J. 1983. *Endometriosis*. New York: Scribner.

Olive, D.L., and Schwartz, L.B. 1993. Endometriosis. *New England Journal of Medicine* 328:1759.

Olivier, S., Lesser, C., and Bell, K. 1984. Providing infertility care. *Journal of Obstetric, Gynecologic and Neonatal Nursing* March–April:415.

Overstreet, J.W., Yanagimachi, R., Katz, D.F. et al. 1980. Penetration of human spermatozoa into the human zona pellucida and the zonafree hamster egg: a study of fertile donors and infertile patients. *Fertility and Sterility* 33(5):534–542.

Rehewy, M.S.E., Thomas, A.J., Hafez, E.S.E. et al. 1978. *Ureaplasma urealyticum* (T mycoplasma) in seminal plasma and spermatozoa from infertile and fertile volunteers. *European Journal of Obstetrics and Gynecologic Reproductive Biology* 8(5):247-251.

Reid, P.C., Thurrell, W., Smith, J.H. et al. 1992. YAG laser endometrial ablation: histological aspects of uterine healing. *International Journal of Gynecological Pathology* 11(3): 174–179.

Scott, Jr., R.T., and Hofmann, G.E. 1995. Prognostic assessment of ovarian reserve. *Fertility and Sterility* 63:1.

Scott, Jr., R.T., Opsahl, M.S., Leonardi, M.R. et al. 1995. Life table analysis of pregnancy rates in a general infertility population relative to ovarian reserve and patient age. *Human Reproduction* 10:1706–1710.

Serafini, P., and Batzofin, J. 1989. Diagnosis of female infertility: a comprehensive approach. *Journal of Reproductive Medicine* 34(1):29–37.

Speroff, L., Glass, R.H., and Kase, N. 1999. *Clinical gynecologic endocrinology and infertility*, 6th ed. Baltimore, Md.: Lippincott Williams & Wilkins.

Thatcher, S. 1989. Anovulatory infertility causes and cures. *Journal of Reproductive Medicine* 34(1):17–24.

Toth, A., Lesser, M.L, Brooke, A. et al. 1983. Subsequent pregnancies among 161 couples treated for T mycoplasma genital tract infection. *New England Journal of Medicine* 308(9):505–507.

Witten, B.I., and Martin, S.A. 1985. The endometrial biopsy as a guide to the management of luteal phase defect. *Fertility and Sterility* 44(4):460–465.

World Health Organization. 1992. *Laboratory manual for the examination of human semen and sperm cervical mucus interaction*. Cambridge, United Kingdom: Cambridge University Press.

APPENDIX 12H.1.

Indications for Intrauterine Insemination

Indications for simple sperm wash without swim-up:	Indications for IUI with swim-up and various column techniques:
Coital dysfunction	Antisperm antibodies (male and female)
Retrograde ejaculation	Donor insemination
Cervical mucus abnormalities	Low semen volume (collect and combine multiple ejaculates over 1–4 hour period)
Anatomical defects of genital organs	Oligoasthenospermia
	Seminal fluid liquefaction defect
	Teratospermia
	Vasectomy reversal
	Unexplained infertility
	In conjunction with ovulation induction

APPENDIX 12H.2.

Collection of Sample for Semen Analysis

- Abstinence before specimen collection should be 2–3 days.
- Specimen is obtained by masturbation into a clear container (usually provided by the laboratory).
- The couple is advised not to use lubrication.
- A Milex sheath (a condom that is nontoxic to sperm) may be used if religious practices prohibit masturbation.
- Deliver the specimen to the laboratory within 1 hour from time of collection.
- The specimen is to be kept warm in transit (next to the body is usually adequate).

APPENDIX 12H.3.

Timing of Intrauterine Insemination

Natural cycles or frozen specimens   Inseminate the day following positive results from an ovulation predictor kit

Ovulation-induced cycles   Inseminate 36 hours after HCG injection

APPENDIX 12H.4.

Assisted Reproductive Technology

Type	Acronym	Indications
In vitro fertilization	IVF	Tubal disease, unexplained infertility, male-factor infertility, endometriosis, immunological infertility, DES exposure, cervical-factor infertility, possibly resistant anovulation
Gamete intrafallopian transfer	GIFT	Unexplained infertility, male-factor infertility, mild endometriosis, possibly immunological infertility, DES exposure, cervical-factor infertility, possibly resistant anovulation
Zygote intrafallopian transfer	ZIFT	Unexplained infertility
Tubal embryo transfer	TET	IVF failure when poor sperm is involved
Peritoneal oocyte and sperm transfer	POST	Unexplained infertility
Subzonal insertion of sperm by microinjection	SUZI	Male-factor infertility
Intracytoplasmic sperm injection	ICSI	Male-factor infertility

Anita Levine-Goldberg, R.N., N.P., M.S.
Lori M. Weseman, R.N., M.S., N.P.

12-HA Infertility
Clomiphene Citrate

As many as 30% of women with infertility have some form of ovulatory dysfunction secondary to a variety of endocrine factors. Clomiphene citrate (CC) is first-time pharmacological therapy for induction of ovulation in women with evidence of endogenous estrogen production. CC is a nonsteroidal agent with estrogenic and anti-estrogenic properties, and supports events that occur in normal ovulatory cycles. Secretion of gonadotropin releasing hormone (GnRH) occurs first under the influence of CC, causing increased pulse frequency of luteinizing hormone (LH) and follicle stimulating hormone (FSH). Simply put, because the body is tricked into thinking there is a lack of estrogen, an increased production of LH and FSH ensues.

Recently, CC has been combined with bromocriptine mesylate or cabergoline in patients who have galactorrhea and/or hyperprolactinemia. Patients with increased prolactin secretion (prolactin-secreting adenomas should be ruled out) and a positive progesterone withdrawal bleed may be treated with either drug or in combination with CC to decrease prolactin concentration and allow ovulation to occur. Bromocriptine mesylate and cabergoline are dopamine receptor agonists used in women with idiopathic hyperprolactinemia when anovulation is the causative factor (Colao et al. 1997, Jones 1989).

The exact mechanism of prolactin-induced anovulation is unclear; evidence suggests that prolactinemic inhibition of normal ovulation occurs at the level of the hypothalamus. A disturbance in amplitude and frequency of LH pulsations occurs in women with hyperprolactinemia, and patients may present clinically with galactorrhea, menstrual dysfunction, hirsutism, diminished libido, or unexplained infertility.

Hyperprolactinemia also has been found in association with a shortened luteal phase and deficient luteal function due to effects on ovarian steroidogenesis and folliculogenesis. Higher concentrations (100 ng/mL) of prolactin appear to inhibit progesterone secretion (Check et al. 1989). Certain metabolic disturbances—in particular, hypothyroidism—also may be associated with hyperprolactinemia. Treatment of the causative disorder may result in a return to normal prolactin level; however, CC and bromocriptine mesylate or cabergoline is an effective treatment option for many infertile women.

Among women treated with CC, ovulation is achieved in an average of 75–80% of well-selected patients, with a pregnancy rate of 35–40%. Patients with hypothalamic pituitary failure do not respond to CC therapy. Pregnancy occurs at a higher rate in the first three ovulatory cycles—up to 85% in the first three cycles, down to 7% in the fourth cycle, and down to approximately 5% at six cycles or more (Hammond et al. 1983). Clearly, extending CC therapy beyond 3–6 ovulatory cycles is not as effective and may place considerable stress on the couple.

DATABASE

SUBJECTIVE

→ A review of health history should include:

- Age of both members of the couple
- Approximate date the couple stopped using contraception
- History and outcome of any previous pregnancies for both partners; length of time to conceive in previous pregnancies
- Length and regularity of the menstrual cycle, magnitude of flow, age at menarche
- Symptoms, treatment of dysmenorrhea or dyspareunia
- History of abnormal bleeding; treatment
- Symptoms of ovulation—i.e., breast tenderness, acne, mittelschmerz, mood changes, spotting, changes in libido, increased midcycle vaginal discharge
- Frequency of coitus, use of lubricants, perception of the couple as to whether or not ejaculation is completed in the vagina
- Religious practices that may relate to intercourse or infertility
- Duration of amenorrhea, if any
  - Presence of physical or emotional stress, weight fluctuation, or medication taken before cessation of menses
- Presence or history of galactorrhea
- History of sexually transmitted diseases, pelvic inflammatory disease; treatment and/or sequellae

- Previous pelvic or other surgery; complications, if any
- Review of any previous infertility evaluation and treatment
- Pertinent medical history suggestive of an endocrine disorder
- History of serious medical illnesses
- Exposure to diethylstilbestrol (DES)
- History of intrauterine device use; sequellae if any
- History of oral contraceptive use
- Social history:
  - Use of alcohol; prescription drugs, over-the-counter drugs (e.g., laxatives, antihistamines), or recreational drugs; herbal remedies; caffeine
  - Smoking history
- Eating habits: any that are suggestive of an eating disorder
- Exercise history, habits
- Family history with attention to endocrine, genetic, or reproductive abnormalities
- History of exposure to radiation or toxic chemicals
- Use of saunas or hot tubs

OBJECTIVE

→ See the **Infertility** chapter.

ASSESSMENT

→ Ovulatory dysfunction requiring ovulation induction by administration of CC
→ R/O endocrine infertility
  - R/O hypothalamic-pituitary dysfunction/failure
  - R/O polycystic ovary syndrome (PCOS)
  - R/O androgen abnormalities
→ R/O unexplained infertility
→ R/O luteal-phase infertility

PLAN

DIAGNOSTIC TESTS

→ Normal values will vary by laboratory.
→ Rubella titer is indicated.
→ VDRL or RPR is indicated.
→ Chlamydia and gonorrhea testing is recommended.
→ Laboratory tests to evaluate dysovulation are directed at evaluation of the hypothalamic-pituitary-ovarian axis.
  - Fasting prolactin (no breast stimulation 24 hours before the test).
  - Thyroid stimulating hormone (TSH)
  - FSH, LH, and estradiol—Day 2–3 of cycle
    - FSH and LH <5 mIU/mL (hypothalamic-pituitary dysfunction or failure)
    - FSH >20 mIU/mL in the follicular phase during two separate cycles (premature ovarian failure)
    - FSH >10–12 mIU/mL or estradiol >80 pg/mL should be referred for a clomiphene citrate challenge test (CCCT)
      – The CCCT, a test of ovarian reserve, is performed by measuring Day 3 FSH and estradiol, administering CC 100 mg p.o. daily on cycle Days 5–9, and then

measuring FSH again on Day 10. The test is considered abnormal if either the Day 3 or the Day 10 FSH, or the estradiol, is above the threshold value for the laboratory (lab values may vary) (American Society for Reproductive Medicine 2002).
- High LH with low or normal FSH (ratio of 3:1 or higher) in PCOS
  NOTE: While a 3:1 or higher ratio is typical of PCOS, it should not be ruled out if the ratio is less than 3:1.
- Mid-luteal phase progesterone
- Dehydroepiandrosterone sulfate (DHEAS)
- Testosterone:
  - Clinical signs of excess androgen include hirsutism and acne.
  - An elevated DHEAS indicates overactive adrenal contribution to circulating androgens.
  - Highly elevated testosterone levels may be indicative of an androgen-secreting neoplasm in the ovary.
  - In the presence of high normal values, especially of DHEAS, patients may respond poorly to CC without the addition of dexamethasone 0.5 mg at bedtime to decrease nighttime adrenocorticotropic hormone production (Speroff et al. 1999).
- Two to three months of basal body temperature (BBT) readings are helpful in assessing the woman's menstrual cycle; not necessary for women with infrequent, spontaneous menses.
- LH predictor kits are recommended for use in women with regular menses.
- Consider an endometrial biopsy in women with longstanding (longer than 3 months) amenorrhea to rule out hyperplasia; otherwise, not necessary as a pre-CC evaluation.
- Progesterone withdrawal/challenge:
  - Rule out pregnancy by ß-hCG assay before challenge.
  - Progesterone administered orally (medroxyprogesterone acetate 10 mg p.o. daily for 5–10 days or IM progesterone in oil 100–150 mg—1 dose) to determine the existence of endogenous estrogen production. (Site-specific policies may vary.) Use 10 mg for 12–14 days for patients with longstanding amenorrhea to achieve full conversion of endometrium.
  - Optimal candidates for CC therapy are those who have a withdrawal bleed following progesterone administration.
    – Bleeding is evidence of an intact hypothalamic-pituitary-ovarian axis.
  - Those who do not respond may have premature ovarian failure or hypothalamic-pituitary failure and will not respond to CC. These patients should be referred for assisted reproductive technology (see Appendix **12H.4, Assisted Reproductive Technology** in the **Infertility** chapter) and/or counseling.
  - Semen analysis is necessary before CC administration to rule out male-factor infertility. (See **Table 12H.1, Normal Semen Analysis** in the **Infertility** chapter.)

TREATMENT/MANAGEMENT

→ Contraindications to CC therapy include:
- Primary pituitary or ovarian failure
- Thyroid or adrenal disease (these conditions may be treated first, followed by CC administration if it still is necessary)
- Abnormal uterine bleeding of undetermined origin
- Liver disease or dysfunction (check liver function tests before initiating CC in women with a positive history)
- Ovarian enlargement or ovarian cysts (>6 cm)
- Pregnancy

→ Dosage/administration of CC (Speroff et al. 1999):
- The recommended initial dose is 50 mg/day p.o. for 5 consecutive days beginning on cycle Day 2, 3, 4, or 5.
- If ovulation is not achieved with the 50 mg dose, increase the dose in steps by 50-mg increments each month (to a maximum of 200–250 mg for 5 days).
- The dosage is the same when treating patients who have luteal-phase defects or PCOS. (See the **Infertility** chapter.)
- The initial dose for unexplained infertility is often 100 mg. **NOTE:** CC acts negatively on cervical mucus, especially at doses of 150–200 mg. Treatment with conjugated estrogens 0.625 mg/day p.o. for 1 week after the last CC pill may improve the cervical mucus. Intrauterine insemination (IUI) is also an option in patients with compromised cervical mucus. (See the **Infertility** chapter for a discussion of IUI.)
- Once ovulation is achieved, continue CC therapy at an effective dose until the woman conceives or until termination of treatment. Most clinicians recommend 3 months of clomid, then a 1-month break before resuming another 3 months of treatment.
  - The prognosis is poor if conception does not occur after 6 months of well-timed intercourse/IUI.
- Ovulation is anticipated approximately 5–10 days after stopping CC treatment.
- Progesterone levels will be drawn 1 week after ovulation.
- CC cycles can be longer than spontaneous cycles; 30–33 day cycles are not unusual.
- Intercourse is recommended every other day from Day 15 until a rise on the BBT chart occurs.
- An LH predictor kit can be useful.
- Menstruation is expected 14 days after ovulation.
- Rule out pregnancy if spontaneous menstruation does not occur, especially if the temperature on the BBT chart remains elevated.
- If the regular CC protocol fails and all other infertility factors have been ruled out or are being managed, may use extended CC protocol, though it is controversial.
  - Use 250 mg CC for 8 days plus 10,000 units human chorionic gonadotropin for injection 6 days later (Speroff et al. 1999).
  - Most clinicians now recommend gonadotropins for CC therapy failure.

- If the history suggests oligo-ovulation as the sole cause of infertility, treat with CC for 3 cycles.
  - If no response, do a further work-up.
  - See the **Infertility** chapter.

→ Gonadotropins:
- Gonadotropins or menotropins are a mixture of FSH and LH. They are administered by IM injection.
- Menotropins act directly on the ovaries to stimulate growth of follicles. They bypass the hypothalamic-pituitary axis.
- Ovarian function must be present to ensure that follicles are capable of being stimulated by FSH and LH.
- Gonadotropins do not trigger ovulation.
  - HCG must be administered after gonadotropin therapy to mimic the endogenous LH surge and thus stimulate ovulation.
- Gonadotropins and HCG given in a sequential manner are indicated for inducing ovulation:
  - As first-line therapy for anovulatory, infertile women with low to normal levels of FSH and LH or age-related infertility issues with a normal CCCT.
  - As second-line therapy in women who fail to ovulate or conceive after optimal doses of CC.
  - For unexplained infertility.
  NOTE: Induction of ovulation with gonadotropins requires advanced training of health care providers as well as constant monitoring and follow-up. The primary care provider should refer the woman requiring gonadotropin therapy to a clinician experienced in superovulation therapy.

→ CC and dopamine agonists:
- CC has been combined with bromocriptine mesylate or cabergoline in patients who show evidence of increased prolactin secretion.
  - First-line therapy is a dopamine agonist. Add CC if a dopamine agonist alone does not restore ovulatory function.
    - Bromocriptine mesylate: 2.5 mg p.o. BID to normalize prolactin levels
                    OR
    - Cabergoline: 2.5 mg p.o. twice a week or 0.5–3 mg once a week (Speroff et al. 1999)
  NOTE: Women with luteal-phase defects on CC and dopamine agonist therapy may require micronized progesterone 100 mg vaginally BID.
- Discontinue CC and the dopamine agonist when pregnancy is confirmed.
- Side effects of bromocriptine mesylate:
  - Nausea, vomiting, dizziness, syncope
    - Give small, divided doses with meals or at bedtime, gradually increasing the dosage to a therapeutic dosage to ameliorate side effects.
- Side effects of cabergoline: in general, less severe than with bromocriptine mesylate; the most common complaint is headache.

→ Complications associated with CC therapy:
- Ovarian hyperstimulation/enlargement (rare):
  - Ovaries are significantly enlarged, tender, and fragile with hyperstimulation.
  - Pelvic examinations, transvaginal sonogram are contraindicated if this is suspected.
  - CC therapy should be discontinued for 1–2 cycles if symptoms do not abate spontaneously.
- Rupture of ovarian cyst:
  - Ovarian hyperstimulation followed by rupture of ovarian cysts can cause internal bleeding, low blood pressure, and severe dizziness, necessitating hospital-ization and/or surgery.
    - Patients complaining of pelvic pain after receiving CC should be evaluated carefully.
  - If enlargement (>6 cm) of the ovary occurs, CC is to be discontinued until the ovaries return to pretreatment size. Dosage should be reduced for the next cycle.
  - A cyst <6 cm rarely ruptures. It is safe to continue under these conditions.
- Congenital malformations/spontaneous abortion:
  - Several large, long-term studies have shown that rates of congenital malformations and spontaneous abortions in CC pregnancies are not greater than in spontaneous pregnancies (Shoham et al. 1991).
- Multiple gestation:
  - Most commonly twins—occurs in 3–5% of CC pregnancies.
  - Less than 1% result in triplets or more.
  - Starting CC on cycle Day 3 instead of Day 5 recruits more follicles and is associated with a higher multiple gestation rate.

→ Monitoring ovulation during CC:
- BBT charts:
  - Ovulation is presumed if BBT rises by 1° F.
- Home ovulation predictor kits:
  - Used by the patient to pinpoint ovulation, timing of coitus, postcoital test, or IUI.
- Postcoital test:
  - Anti-estrogenic properties of CC may cause cervical mucus to become thick, tenacious, and cellular, impairing sperm transport and survival.
  - A postcoital test at midcycle can be used to assess for anti-estrogenic effects.
  - IUI in conjunction with CC therapy should be consid-ered if cervical mucus quality is compromised.
  - May also treat with conjugated estrogens 0.625 mg p.o. for 1 week after the last CC pill (Speroff et al. 1999).
- Serum estradiol levels:
  - Preovulatory estradiol levels should be >200–300 pg/mL.
- Ultrasound:
  - Using a vaginal transducer, ultrasound should be performed starting around Day 10, then every other day until the dominant follicle measures 14 mm, then daily until it measures 16–18 mm (the follicle grows 1–3 mm/day).

- HCG is administered when there is no response to maximum dose or there is a short luteal phase. Timing of the administration of HCG is calculated with the use of ultrasound measurements.
- Ultrasound evidence of ovulation (presumptive) includes:
  - Disappearance of the dominant follicle with or without fluid in the cul-de-sac
  - Cystic change in the dominant follicle with created border
  - "Filling in" of the dominant follicle (appears "cob-webby")
  - Collapse of the follicle (emergence of corpus luteum)
- Endometrial biopsy:
  - Obtained 2 days before expected menstruation.
  - Results should indicate a proper secretory endometrium (not more than 2 days out of phase).
  - Serum ß-hCG before the biopsy should be drawn to rule out pregnancy, though patients can be reassured that the risk of the biopsy interrupting an early pregnancy is extremely low.
- Mid-luteal progesterone:
  - Progesterone level should be drawn around 7 days after expected ovulation to determine whether ovulation has occurred and what the potential is for a normal luteal phase.
  - Normal = 12–30 ng/mL in a CC-enhanced cycle.
  - Support of the luteal phase with administration of micronized progesterone per vagina (100 mg QD–BID) is suggested by many infertility practitioners.

CONSULTATION

→ Physician consultation is recommended regarding labora-tory data, clinical findings, and correct administration of ovu-lation induction therapy.
→ Referral to a specialist is indicated in the event of unusual laboratory data or clinical findings (e.g., abnormal androgen levels or ovarian failure).
→ Referral to a physician for second-line therapy (i.e., gonad-otropins) is recommended if the patient fails to achieve ovulation or pregnancy on CC therapy.
→ Ongoing discussion with the infertility care team is recom-mended to ensure that the patient's care continues to be up-to-date and effective.
→ Referral for counseling and treatment of eating disorders or to a weight loss program, as necessary.
→ As needed for prescription(s).

PATIENT EDUCATION

→ Discussion and explanation should include:
- A normal reproductive cycle
- Factors contributing to the patient's specific dysovulation diagnosis (e.g., excessive exercise, PCOS).
- The recommended treatment regimen, action of CC, and realistic chances for ovulation and conception.

- Ovulation occurs in 75–80% of well-selected patients with pregnancy rate of 10%.
- Correct medication administration—amount, days of the cycle, duration of the therapy (5 days).
- When ovulation is expected, when intercourse should take place; possible physical signs of ovulation, though many patients experience no symptoms and need to be reassured.
- A thorough description of potential side effects, especially those that should be reported to the office immediately (e.g., visual disturbance or abdominal or pelvic pain).
  - Side effects of CC therapy may include, but are not limited to:
    - Vasomotor flushes
    - Insomnia
    - Bloating
    - Breast tenderness
    - Fatigue
    - Mild mood alterations—lability, irritability, or depression
    - Nausea
    - Dizziness, headaches
    - Abdominal or pelvic pain (mild to severe)
    - Visual disturbances—blurring, spots, flashes of light
  - Less frequent side effects may include:
    - Abnormal uterine bleeding
    - Increased urination
    - Urticaria and allergic dermatitis
    - Weight gain
    - Reversible hair loss
- Monitoring techniques, timing of tests (e.g., BBT instruction, home ovulation predictor kits, biopsies, ultrasonography, postcoital testing, blood tests).
- Additional treatment options in the event that the patient does not achieve ovulation or pregnancy with CC therapy.
→ Reassure the patient that side effects generally resolve spontaneously with discontinuation of CC.
→ The patient also needs to be aware of any adverse reactions to CC therapy (discussed previously in this chapter).
→ Offer educational handouts regarding the correct administration of medication, schedule of tests, side effects, and when to call the office.

FOLLOW-UP

→ Rule out pregnancy if there are no menses after the CC cycle or if there is abnormal bleeding; refer for prenatal care as needed.
→ Interpret laboratory data and clinical findings pertaining to documentation of ovulation.
  - If ovulation has occurred, instruct the woman to continue the same dose during the next cycle.

- If there is no evidence of ovulation, increase the dose by 50 mg.
→ Advise the woman to return to the office in the event of moderate to severe pain.
  - Discontinue CC until the ovaries are of normal size and nontender.
  - Refer to a physician as necessary.
→ Hold ongoing discussions with the woman regarding CC therapy, dose changes, side effects, and emotional status. Telephone follow-up is often adequate.
→ Hold ongoing discussions with the physician/infertility team regarding ovulation status, medication changes, and the patient's condition.
→ If the patient is ovulating well with the proper dose, continue for 3 months. Take a one-month break and then continue for another 3 months with IUI.
→ Refer as necessary for second-line therapy (i.e., gonadotropins or in vitro fertilization).
→ Encourage the woman to take a 1–2 month break from treatment if she appears overwhelmed.
→ Refer to a specialist if the woman has a medical problem beyond the scope of the primary care provider.
→ Refer to a counselor/support group as necessary.
→ Document in progress notes and on problem list.

BIBLIOGRAPHY

American Society for Reproductive Medicine. 2002. A practice committee report. *Aging and infertility in women.* Available at: http://www.asrm.org/Media/Practice/ageandinfertility.pdf. Accessed on July 1, 2003.

Check, J., Wu, C., and Adelson, H. 1989. Bromocriptine versus progesterone therapy for infertility related to luteal-phase defects in hyperprolactinemic patients. *International Journal of Fertility* 34(3):209–214.

Colao, A., DiSarno, A., Sarnacchiaro F. et al. 1997. Prolactinomas resistant to standard dopamine agonists respond to chronic cabergoline treatment. *Drugs* 49:255.

Hammond, M.G., Halme, J.K., and Talbert, L.M. 1983. Factors affecting the pregnancy rate in clomiphene citrate induction of ovulation. *Obstetrics and Gynecology* 62(2):196–202.

Jones, E. 1989. Hyperprolactinemia and female infertility. *Journal of Reproductive Medicine* 34(2):117–125.

Shoham, Z., Zosmer, A., and Insler, V. 1991. Early miscarriage and fetal malformations after induction of ovulation (by clomiphene citrate and/or human menotropins), in vitro fertilization, and gamete intrafallopian transfer. *Fertility and Sterility* 55(1):1–11.

Speroff, L., Glass, R.H., and Kase, N.G. 1999. *Clinical gynecologic endocrinology and infertility,* 6th ed. Baltimore, Md.: Lippincott Williams & Wilkins.

Talbert, L.M. 1983. Clomiphene citrate induction of ovulation. *Fertility and Sterility* 39(6):742–743.

Winifred L. Star, R.N., C., N.P., M.S.
Melanie Deal, R.N., C., N.P., M.S.

12-1

Pelvic Inflammatory Disease

Pelvic inflammatory disease (PID) encompasses a range of upper genital tract inflammatory disorders that include endometritis, salpingitis, pelvic peritonitis, tubo-ovarian abscess (TOA), and perihepatitis (Centers for Disease Control and Prevention [CDC] 2002). PID originates from the ascent of microorganisms from the lower to the upper genital tract (Westrom et al. 1999). In the United States, more than 1 million women are treated each year for PID, with direct medical costs reaching a staggering $1.88 billion in 1998 (Rein et al. 2000).

Two major groups of microorganisms are responsible for the disease. One group includes sexually transmitted agents—*Chlamydia trachomatis* and *Neisseria gonorrhoeae*. The second group includes a wide variety of anaerobic, aerobic, and mycoplasma organisms of the lower genital tract (including the bacteria involved in bacterial vaginosis): *Escherichia coli*, *Haemophilus influenzae*, *Bacteroides*, *Gardnerella vaginalis*, *Peptostreptococcus*, *Staphylococcus*, *Actinomyces*, and *Mycoplasma hominis* (CDC 2002, Walker et al. 1999). Although viruses and protozoa have been isolated from the upper genital tract, the causative role of herpes simplex virus, cytomegalovirus, or *Trichomonas vaginalis* in PID remains unproven (Clarke et al. 1997, Westrom et al. 1999).

Chlamydia and gonorrhea are important causative agents of PID (Westrom et al. 1999). Fifty percent to 80% of patients hospitalized with PID are infected with *N. gonorrhoeae* or *C. trachomatis* (Sweet et al. 2002). However, the relative distribution of these agents recovered from the upper genital tract in women with PID varies greatly depending on the prevalences of chlamydia and gonorrhea within a given population (Paavonen 1998). Moreover, a significant proportion of chlamydia-associated PID is subclinical and, therefore, may be underestimated.

Authorities now believe that bacterial vaginosis (BV) plays a causative role in acute PID (Paavonen 1998). Invasive diagnostic and therapeutic procedures, such as dilatation and curettage, induced abortion, insertion of an intrauterine device (IUD), and hysterosalpingography, also may result in PID (Westrom et al. 1999).

Theories regarding the mechanisms for transport of bacteria to the upper genital tract include vector transmission via sperm or trichomonads, canalicular spread, passive transport of particulate matter, uterine contractions, movement by menstrual reflux or an IUD string, and hematogenous or lymphatic spread (Walker et al. 1999). *N. gonorrhoeae* and *C. trachomatis* may pave the way for some cases of PID that are ultimately caused by secondary invasion of endogenous organisms (Westrom et al. 1999). Sexually transmitted disease (STD) pathogens more often are isolated from women with milder, short-standing infection, whereas endogenous organisms are associated with more advanced disease (Walker et al. 1999, Westrom et al. 1999).

Because of the wide variation in signs and symptoms of PID among women, clinical diagnosis is difficult and imprecise. A broad clinical spectrum exists, including subclinical ("silent" or atypical PID); mild, moderate, and severe PID; and chronic PID (CDC 1991, Westrom et al. 1999). Mild symptoms and vague, subtle signs are not easily recognized as PID, and many cases go undiagnosed (CDC 1991, 2002). Recently, there has been increasing evidence of an epidemic of silent, asymptomatic infection; however, the magnitude of this problem has yet to be defined (Westrom et al. 1999).

Periappendicitis and perihepatitis—or Fitz-Hugh-Curtis (FHC) syndrome—are extrapelvic manifestations of disseminated PID. Both *N. gonorrhoeae* and *C. trachomatis* are causative agents. Progressive perihepatitis causes "violin-string" adhesions between the abdominal wall and liver.

Sequelae of PID are significant and include ectopic pregnancy, involuntary infertility, pelvic adhesions, TOA, chronic pelvic pain, recurrent infection, and depression. Delay in diagnosis and treatment probably contributes to inflammatory sequelae in the upper reproductive tract (CDC 2002).

After only one episode of PID, ectopic pregnancy risk increases sevenfold. Twelve percent of women are infertile after a single episode, 25% after two episodes, and more than 50% after three or more episodes of PID (CDC 1991). Chronic pelvic pain is reported in 24–75% of women after one episode of PID (Paavonen 1998). Thus, prevention of PID is of paramount importance. Health care providers can play a major role by maintaining up-to-date knowledge, providing appropriate preventive services—including medical management and risk-reduction counseling—and promoting sex-partner evaluation (CDC 1991).

DATABASE

SUBJECTIVE

→ Risk factors include:
- Age younger than 25 years
- New/multiple sexual partners (especially within the previous 30 days)
- A partner with penile discharge/urethral symptoms/STD
- Gonorrhea or chlamydia
- Previous PID
- BV
- Menses (within seven days of onset for STD-related PID)
- Cervical ectopy (eversion)
- Recent, invasive, gynecological medical procedure
- Pelvic surgery
- Impairment of local/systemic defense mechanisms:
  - Congenital/acquired immunodeficiency syndromes
  - Systemic diseases
  - Immunosuppressive drugs
  - Local defense mechanisms: iatrogenic injuries, immature local immune system
- Douching
- IUD use (primarily in the first few months after insertion; may not be STD-related)
- No/nonbarrier method of contraception
  NOTE: Combined oral contraceptives are associated with a *decreased* risk of PID.
- Lower socioeconomic status
- Never married; divorced or separated
- Smoking
- Behavioral factors: risk-taking, poor health-seeking behaviors (i.e., poor motivation/compliance with diagnosis/treatment/follow-up)

→ Symptoms may include:
- Bilateral lower abdominal or pelvic pain (most common symptom)
  - Pain is subacute at onset, nonradiating, dull, and unrelieved by position change.
- Increase or change in vaginal discharge
- Dysuria, frequency, urgency
- Deep dyspareunia
- Dysmenorrhea
- Irregular bleeding: menorrhagia, menometrorrhagia, oligomenorrhea, amenorrhea, postcoital bleeding
- Rectal symptoms: frequent stools, passage of mucus, tenesmus
- Fever, chills, malaise, nausea, vomiting in severe cases
- Right upper quadrant pain with FHC syndrome
- Complaints associated with silent or atypical infection.
  - May consist only of metrorrhagia, abnormal vaginal discharge, or urinary tract symptoms.
- STD-related PID is more often associated with the follicular phase of the menstrual cycle (Westrom et al. 1999).

NOTE: No symptom is pathognomonic for PID. All symptoms standing alone have low positive and negative predictive values (Westrom et al. 1999). In some cases, the patient may be asymptomatic.

→ History:
- Menstrual cycle
- Contraceptive use
- Description of symptoms:
  - Onset, duration, quality/quantity, frequency, course, aggravating/relieving factors, associated symptoms
- History of same/similar problem
- STD history (including dates, treatment)
- Sensitive questioning regarding recent sexual activity (including date of last exposure, sex practices, sites of exposure, number and gender of partners in the last 1–2 months, and use of condoms/spermicides)
- Sex partner history (including travel, drug use)
- General health, including acute/chronic illness
- Surgery
- Medications
- Allergies
- Habits (including travel and use of illegal drugs, both injection and noninjection)
- Laboratory tests for syphilis, hepatitis B, HIV
- Review of systems

OBJECTIVE

NOTE: Traditional clinical criteria used in assessing/diagnosing PID can be insensitive and nonspecific. A low threshold for diagnosis is recommended (CDC 2002). (See also "Diagnostic Tests/Diagnostic Criteria," below.)

→ The patient may appear ill or, in severe cases, distressed.

→ Physical examination may reveal the following:
- Vital signs:
  - Fever is present in fewer than 50% of cases (>100.4° F or >38° C).
  - Assess for orthostatic changes in blood pressure and pulse as indicated.
- Abdominal examination:
  - Decreased bowel sounds, tenderness, rebound tenderness/guarding
  - Right upper quadrant tenderness may be present in FHC syndrome.
- Pelvic examination:
  - Vagina: profuse, abnormal discharge
  - Cervix: mucopurulent discharge
    - See details under "Diagnostic Tests" in the *Chlamydia trachomatis* chapter in Section 13.
    - Cervical motion tenderness is common.
    - Cervical contact bleeding and/or erythema/edema in the zone of ectopy.
  - Uterus: usually tender. Assess size, shape, consistency, and mobility.
  - Adnexa: usually tender bilaterally. Fullness or masses may be present.

- Recto/vaginal: may be tender. Fullness/masses in cul-de-sac may be palpable.
  NOTE: Pay attention to a mucopurulent discharge and/or subtle signs of uterine/adnexal tenderness. Silent or atypical PID or subclinical endometritis may be present. Acute disease is more often associated with *N. gonorrhoeae*, while silent disease is more often associated with *C. trachomatis* (Westrom et al. 1999).
→ Additional findings:
  - Gram stain of endocervical mucus may reveal ≥ 10–30 white blood cells (WBCs)/oil immersion field and/or Gram-negative, intracellular diplococci (gonorrhea).
  - Wet mounts of vaginal discharge may reveal clue cells/amines (indicative of BV).
    - More than three WBCs/high power field has been associated with mucopurulent cervicitis and PID (lower predictive value in a high-STD-risk population).
    - An absence of WBCs has a high negative predictive value in excluding PID as the diagnosis (Westrom et al. 1999).
  - Tests for *N. gonorrhoeae* and/or *C. trachomatis* may be positive.
  - WBC count may be >10,000/mm³ (two-thirds of cases).
  - Erythrocyte sedimentation rate (ESR) may be >15 mm/hr (nonspecific finding).
  - C-reactive protein may be >2 mg/dL (70–93% sensitivity; 67–90% specificity; more sensitive and specific than ESR).
  - Serological chlamydia antibodies may be present and are indicative of either past or present infection (in 20–40 % of women with a history of PID [CDC 1991]). Not recommended for routine diagnostic work-up.
  - Serum levels of CA-125 are elevated in 25–35% of patients with PID. This test is investigational and not recommended for routine diagnostic work-up.

ASSESSMENT

→ PID
→ R/O chlamydia and/or gonorrhea
→ R/O complications of pregnancy
→ R/O appendicitis
→ R/O tubo-ovarian abscess
→ R/O other gynecological conditions/disorders:
  - Ovarian cyst
  - Endometriosis
  - Dysmenorrhea
  - Mittelschmerz
  - Hemorrhagic ovarian cyst
  - Ovarian torsion
  - Ovarian tumor
  - Polycystic ovaries
  - Leiomyomata
  - Threatened abortion
  - Pelvic congestion
  - Pelvic adhesions
→ R/O gastrointestinal disorders:

- Mesenteric lymphadenitis
- Regional ileitis
- Enteritis
- Irritable bowel disorder
- Constipation
- Gastroenteritis
- Diverticulitis
- Inflammatory bowel disease
→ R/O cystitis, pyelonephritis, nephrolithiasis
→ R/O FHC syndrome

PLAN

DIAGNOSTIC TESTS/DIAGNOSTIC CRITERIA

→ See also "Objective," above.
  - Clinical diagnosis of PID is imprecise. No single historical, physical, or laboratory finding is both sensitive and specific for diagnosis (CDC 2002).
→ Health care providers should maintain a low threshold of diagnosis for PID (CDC 2002).
→ Minimum diagnostic criteria (and no other cause can be identified):
  - Uterine/adnexal tenderness
                OR
  - Cervical motion tenderness (CDC 2002)
→ Additional diagnostic criteria used to increase the specificity of diagnosis include (CDC 2002):
  - Oral temperature >101° F (>38.3° C)
  - Abnormal cervical or vaginal discharge
  - Presence of WBCs on wet mount of vaginal secretions
  - Elevated ESR
  - Elevated C-reactive protein
  - Laboratory documentation of cervical infection with *N. gonorrhoeae* or *C. trachomatis*
→ The most specific criteria for diagnosis include (CDC 2002):
  - Histopathological evidence of endometritis on endometrial biopsy
  - Transvaginal sonography or magnetic resonance imaging showing thickened, fluid-filled tubes with or without free pelvic fluid or tubo-ovarian complex
  - Laparoscopic abnormalities consistent with PID.
  NOTE: Diagnostic evaluation that includes some of these more extensive studies may be warranted in certain cases. Physician evaluation and management are necessary.
→ Additional considerations:
  - Serial quantitative ß-hCGs as indicated to rule out ectopic pregnancy.
  - Sensitive testing for *C. trachomatis* and *N. gonorrhoeae* should be performed.
  - Serological HIV testing should be offered.
  - Culdocentesis may be performed by a physician to provide culture material and to assist in ruling out an ectopic pregnancy or hemorrhagic ovarian cyst.
  - Additional laboratory tests may include but are not limited to: Pap smear, VDRL or RPR, urinalysis, urine culture and sensitivities, liver enzymes, total bilirubin, alkaline phosphatase, amylase, and hepatitis B screen.

TREATMENT/MANAGEMENT

→ The goals of therapy are to preserve fertility, prevent the risk of a future ectopic pregnancy, and reduce long-term sequelae (Sweet et al. 2002). Thus, it is important to make an accurate diagnosis and to treat promptly.

- The minimum criteria for pelvic inflammation, as detailed above, should be used to initiate empiric treatment in the absence of other established causes (CDC 2002).

→ Hospitalization should be considered in the following instances (CDC 2002):

- Surgical emergencies (e.g., appendicitis) cannot be excluded.
- Patient is pregnant.
- Patient has nausea and vomiting, high fever, or is otherwise severely ill.
- Patient has a TOA.
- Patient is unable to follow or tolerate an outpatient regimen.
- Patient does not respond clinically to oral antimicrobial therapy.

NOTE: Discussion of inpatient therapy is beyond the scope of this chapter. Refer to the CDC 2002 citation in the bibliography.

→ The choice of treatment regimen may be influenced by its availability and cost, patient acceptance, and antimicrobial susceptibility (CDC 2002).

→ Antimicrobial options should be broad-spectrum to include coverage for *N. gonorrhoeae*, *C. trachomatis*, Gram-negative facultative bacteria, streptococci, and anaerobes (CDC 2002).

→ Outpatient treatment:

- Regimen A (CDC 2002):
  - Ofloxacin 400 mg p.o. BID for 14 days
    OR
  - Levofloxacin 500 mg p.o. once daily for 14 days
    WITH OR WITHOUT
  - Metronidazole 500 mg p.o. BID for 14 days
    NOTE: The addition of metronidazole provides anaerobic coverage, which is not adequately ensured by the fluoroquinolones alone (CDC 2002). Fluoroquinolone resistance to gonorrhea is significant in some geographic areas. (See the **Gonorrhea** chapter in Section 13.) In those areas, a test-of-cure for gonorrhea-documented PID should be performed in patients receiving a fluoroquinolone regimen (Bolan 2002).
- Regimen B (CDC 2002):
  - Ceftriaxone 250 mg IM in a single dose
    OR
  - Cefoxitin 2 g IM in a single dose and probenecid 1 g p.o. administered concurrently in a single dose
    OR
  - Another parenteral, third-generation cephalosporin— e.g., ceftizoxime or cefotaxime
    PLUS

- Doxycycline 100 mg p.o. BID for 14 days
  WITH OR WITHOUT
- Metronidazole 500 mg p.o. BID for 14 days
  NOTE: Anerobic coverage is improved with the addition of metronidazole (CDC 2002). Refer to the *Physicians' Desk Reference* regarding contraindications for and adverse reactions to the above medications.

→ Additional considerations:

- IUD wearers should have the device removed and anti-microbial therapy initiated promptly.
  - Discuss alternative options for contraception.
- A large TOA or a TOA that fails to respond to antibiotics or ruptures will require surgery (transvaginal or laparoscopic drainage) (Westrom et al. 1999).
- Pregnant women with PID (or suspicion thereof) should be hospitalized and treated with parenteral antibiotics (CDC 2002).

→ Partner therapy:

- Evaluation and treatment of sex partners is imperative.
  - Partners should be treated empirically with regimens effective against *N. gonorrhoeae* and *C. trachomatis* (CDC 2002).
  - Provide referrals to a provider/facility that offers appropriate STD care as indicated.

CONSULTATION

→ Consultation is recommended in all cases of PID. Co-management with a physician is appropriate for patients undergoing outpatient therapy. Cases of severe PID should be referred to a physician for management.

→ Referral to a physician is indicated when considering invasive diagnostic procedures (e.g., endometrial biopsy, culdocentesis) or surgery.

→ When alternate diagnoses are suspected (e.g., ectopic pregnancy, appendicitis), refer the patient to a physician.

→ If the patient fails to respond to outpatient therapy, refer her to a physician for further management.

PATIENT EDUCATION

→ Discuss the etiology, course, treatment, follow-up, and potential sequelae of PID and the importance of partner treatment.

- Patient-education materials are a helpful adjunct to teaching. Written materials may be obtained from:
  - CDC National Prevention Information Network
    P.O. Box 6003
    Rockville, Md. 20849-6003
    (800) 458-5231, www.cdcnpin.org
  - American Social Health Association
    P.O. Box 13827
    Research Triangle Park, N.C. 27709
    (919) 361-8400, www.ashastd.org
- Additional resources for patients are:
  - National STD Hotline: (800) 227-8922 or (800) 342-2437, en Español: (800) 344-7432
  - www.iwannaknow.org (for adolescents)

→ Advise the patient to finish the full course of medication and return for follow-up. Advise abstinence from intercourse until both patient and partner complete the prescribed medication.

→ Advise pelvic rest and adequate sleep, hydration, and nutrition. Analgesics may be taken (e.g., acetaminophen) as needed.

▪ If symptoms worsen or recur, the patient should return for re-evaluation promptly.

→ Additional recommendations for all patients (especially adolescents) include healthy sexual behaviors, appropriate health-seeking behaviors, risk-reduction behaviors, and use of barrier methods of contraception and spermicides. (See **Table 12I.1, Recommendations for Individuals to Prevent STD/PID** and **Table 13A.2, Safer Sex Practices** in the **Chancroid** chapter in Section 13.)

→ Routine screening for STDs in high-risk groups is advised. These groups include adolescents and people in whom STDs are highly prevalent, such as women with multiple partners, prostitutes, illicit drug users, and individuals trading sex for drugs (CDC 1991). Individuals residing in jail and those presenting to emergency rooms should have STD testing when a gynecological examination is performed.

→ Allow the patient to vent her feelings of surprise, shame, fear, or anger regarding diagnosis of an STD as indicated. Psychological support may be important in helping the patient gain control over her sexual situation and prevent future STDs.

FOLLOW-UP

→ The patient should for return for reassessment within 72 hours.

▪ Criteria for clinical improvement include defervescence, a reduction in abdominal tenderness (direct or rebound), and a reduction in uterine, adnexal, and cervical motion tenderness (CDC 2002).

▪ Patients who do not respond to therapy (or who worsen) within 72 hours usually require hospitalization, additional diagnostic tests, and surgical intervention (CDC 2002). Physician consultation is mandatory.

▪ Symptoms that persist 2–14 days after outpatient treatment should arouse suspicion of an alternate diagnosis (e.g., appendicitis, endometriosis, ruptured ovarian cyst, or adnexal torsion). Laparoscopy may be considered in such cases (Morgan 1991).

→ In patients receiving a fluoroquinolone regimen, a test-of-cure should be performed if gonorrhea was documented and the patient lives in a fluoroquinolone-resistant geographic area. Ideally, the test-of-cure should be both a culture and a nucleic acid amplification test. If only a nonculture test is used, positive results should be followed up with a culture

Table 12I.1. RECOMMENDATIONS FOR INDIVIDUALS TO PREVENT STD/PID

General Preventive Measures	Specific Recommendations
Maintain healthy sexual behavior	Postpone initiation of sexual intercourse until at least 2–3 years after menarche. Limit the number of sex partners. Avoid casual sex and sex with high-risk partners. Ask potential sex partners about STDs and inspect their genitals for lesions/discharge. Avoid sex with infected partners. Abstain from sex if STD symptoms appear.
Use barrier methods of contraception	Use condoms, diaphragms, and/or vaginal spermicides for STD protection and use consistently and correctly throughout all sex.
Adopt healthy medical-care-seeking behaviors	Seek medical evaluation promptly after having unprotected sex with someone who is suspected of having an STD. Seek medical care immediately when genital lesions/discharge appear. Seek routine check-ups for STDs if not in mutually monogamous relationship, even if there are no symptoms.
Comply with management instructions	Take all medications as directed, regardless of symptoms. Return for follow-up evaluation as instructed. Abstain from sex until symptoms resolve and patient and partner treatment is completed.
Ensure partner evaluation	Notify all sex partners when diagnosed with an STD. Tell them to seek evaluation and treatment. If preferred, assist health care provider in identifying partner.

Source: Adapted from the Centers for Disease Control and Prevention. 1991. Pelvic inflammatory disease: guidelines for prevention and management. *Morbidity and Mortality Weekly Report* 40(RR–5):1–25.

and susceptibility testing before the patient receives alternative treatment (Bolan 2002).

→ Rescreening for both *C. trachomatis* and *N. gonorrhoeae* may be performed 4–6 weeks after completing therapy (CDC 2002).

→ History on follow-up of ambulatory patients should include symptom status, medication compliance, drug reaction/side effects, partner therapy, sexual exposure, and use of condoms.

→ Follow up on all laboratory tests ordered. Treat all concomitant STDs and other identified conditions.

→ Negative HIV tests may be repeated in three months. Continue to encourage safer sex.

→ HIV-positive results should be conveyed in person and by a provider who has received training in the complexities of test disclosure.

  ■ HIV-positive persons should be referred to the appropriate provider/agency for early intervention services.

  ■ HIV-infected women with PID may be at increased risk for a complicated clinical course and should be followed closely.

→ Offer the hepatitis A vaccine to women at risk for sexual transmission of this virus (e.g., users of injection and noninjection illegal drugs). (See the **Hepatitis—Viral** chapter in Section 11.)

→ Offer the hepatitis B vaccine to all women seeking treatment for an STD who have not been previously vaccinated. (See the **Hepatitis—Viral** chapter for further information.)

→ Newly diagnosed hepatitis B antigen-positive individuals should have liver function tests and receive counseling regarding the implication of their positive status and the need for immunoprophylaxis of sex partners and household members.

  ■ See the **Hepatitis—Viral** chapter.

→ PID is a reportable communicable disease in some states.

→ Gonorrhea and chlamydia are reportable communicable diseases in all states.

→ Document in progress notes and on problem list.

BIBLIOGRAPHY

Bolan, G. 2002. New 2002 STD treatment guidelines. *Medical Board of California Action Report* 82:10–14.

Centers for Disease Control and Prevention (CDC). 1991. Pelvic inflammatory disease: guidelines for prevention and management. *Morbidity and Mortality Weekly Report* 40 (RR–5):1–25.

_____. 2002. Sexually transmitted disease treatment guidelines 2002. *Morbidity and Mortality Weekly Report* 51(RR–6): 48–51.

Clarke, L.M., Duerr, A., Yeung, K.A. et al. 1997. Recovery of cytomegalovirus and herpes simplex virus from upper and lower genital tract specimens obtained from women with pelvic inflammatory disease. *Journal of Infectious Diseases* 176:286–288.

Physician's desk reference. 2002. 56th ed. Montvale, N.J.: Medical Economics.

Morgan, R.J. 1991. Clinical aspects of pelvic inflammatory disease. *American Family Physician* 43(5):1725–1732.

Paavonen, J. 1998. Pelvic inflammatory disease: from diagnosis to prevention. *Dermatologic Clinics* 16(4):747–756.

Rein, D.B., Kassler, W.J., Irwin, K.L. et al. 2000. Direct medical cost of pelvic inflammatory disease and its sequelae: decreasing, but still substantial. *Obstetrics and Gynecology* 95(3):397–402.

Sweet, R.L., and Gibbs, R.S. 2002. *Infectious diseases of the female genital tract,* 4th ed. Philadelphia: Lippincott Williams & Wilkins.

Walker, C.K., Workowski, K.A., Washington, A.E. et al. 1999. Anaerobes in pelvic inflammatory disease: implications for the Centers for Disease Control and Prevention's guidelines for treatment of sexually transmitted diseases. *Clinical Infectious Diseases* 29(Suppl 1):S29–S36.

Westrom, L., and Eschenbach, D. 1999. Pelvic inflammatory disease. In *Sexually transmitted diseases,* 3rd ed., eds. K.K. Holmes, P.F. Sparling, P.-A. Mårdh et al., pp. 783–809. New York: McGraw-Hill.

Winifred L. Star, R.N., C., N.P., M.S.
Ann-Marie McNamara, R.N., C., N.P., M.S.

12-J

Pelvic Masses

Patients with pelvic masses may present with various signs and symptoms or they may be completely asymptomatic with a mass found on examination. The etiologies of pelvic masses are quite varied and may stem from the genital tract, gastrointestinal (GI) tract, or urinary tract. (See **Table 12J.1, Pelvic Masses—Differential Diagnoses**.) Management of pelvic masses depends, to a large extent, on the age of the patient, the size and nature of the mass, and symptoms. Common types of pelvic masses by age group will be highlighted.

Adolescence

During adolescence, an imperforate hymen, vaginal agenesis, or a vaginal septum may give rise to a hematocolpos or hematometrium with secondary pelvic or abdominal masses. The most common adnexal masses in this age group are functional ovarian cysts and dermoid cysts. Of genital tract malignancies during adolescence, more than two-thirds arise from germ cells. Other neoplastic tumors are of the epithelial and stromal cell type (DiSaia et al. 2002, Lovvorn et al. 1998, Pfeifer et al. 1999). The differential diagnoses for this age group also include ectopic pregnancy, torsion, endometrioma, tubo-ovarian abscess (TOA), hydrosalpinx, Mülerian anomaly, appendiceal abscess, paraovarian cyst, paratubal cyst, and peritoneal inclusion cyst (Pfeifer et al. 1999). Rarely, leiomyomata of the uterus may arise.

Reproductive Years and Menopause

Most pelvic masses occur during the reproductive years, with both benign and malignant lesions presenting; most, however, are benign. Masses seen in women during this time may develop from the uterus, cervix, adnexa, and other organ systems. Findings include ectopic pregnancy, myomas, and a variety of adnexal masses of gynecological origin, including functional ovarian cysts, ovarian neoplasms, and endometriosis (DiSaia et al. 2002). On occasion, extragenital masses are found, including peritoneal and omental cysts, retroperitoneal lesions, and diseases of the GI tract (DiSaia et al. 2002).

In the perimenopause and menopause, the chance of malignancy associated with a pelvic mass increases. Sex-cord stromal tumors may occur at any age but are found predominantly during menopause. Ovarian endometriomas, especially in women on hormone replacement therapy, also should be considered.

The pelvic masses detailed in this chapter are representative of some of the more commonly encountered gynecological pathologies in women's primary care.

Fibroids and Adenomyosis

Leiomyomata uteri, commonly known as fibroids, are estrogen-sensitive, benign, muscle cell tumors of the uterus. They are the most frequently encountered tumors of the pelvis, with the highest incidence in a woman's fifth decade of life. The etiology is unknown; however, a genetic predisposition is suspected (Grabo et al. 1999). The prevalence is estimated to be between 20–40% of all women, with African American women at 3.2 times greater risk than Caucasian women (Meisler 1999).

Myomas are classified by subgroups according to their anatomic location. (See "Objective," below.) Complications arising from fibroids may include abnormal bleeding, anemia, pelvic pain, activity limitation, fatigue, urinary and bowel problems, infertility, spontaneous abortion, and preterm labor (Daya 2000, Moorehead et al. 2001). After menopause, fibroids generally regress secondary to reduced estrogen stimulation.

Adenomyosis is a result of the aberrant growth of endometrial glands and stroma from the basalis layer of the endometrium into the myometrium. The stimulus for this benign invasion is unknown, although hyperestrogenemia, myometrial weakness, increased expression of receptors of human chorionic gonadotropin/luteinizing hormones, and tenascin in inhibiting cell attachment are suspected (Tafazoli et al. 1999). The reported incidence has varied widely over the years, from a low of 5.7% in uteri removed for leiomyomata to a high of 69.6% of unselected hysterectomy specimens (Guarnaccia et al. 2000). The diagnosis commonly is made incidentally by the pathologist at hysterectomy or autopsy. Other pelvic pathology such as

Table 12J.1.   PELVIC MASSES—DIFFERENTIAL DIAGNOSES

Vaginal

Developmental anomalies
· imperforate hymen
· vaginal septum
Relaxation
· cystocele
· rectocele
· enterocele

Foreign body
Bartholin's/Gartner's duct cyst
Neoplasm
· sarcoma botryoides
· vaginal cancer
· benign lesions

Cervical

Nabothian cyst
Fibroid

Ectopic
Carcinoma

Uterine

Pregnancy
· cornual
· cervical
Displacement
· retro
· lateral
Fibroids
Adenomyosis
Round ligament tumors
Malignancies
· endometrial adenocarcinoma
· adenosquamous carcinoma
· sarcoma

Rare tumors
· hemangiopericytoma
Congenital anomalies
· defects in Müllerian fusion
· associated urinary tract
  anomalies
Hematometra/pyometra
· transverse vaginal septum
· vaginal atresia
· cervical stenosis
· cervical cancer

Tubal

Mesonephric duct remnants
· paraovarian cyst
· hydatid of Morgagni
Ectopic
Acute salpingitis
· pyosalpinx
· tubo-ovarian abscess
Chronic salpingitis
· hydrosalpinx

Tuberculosis
Other chronic granulomas
Benign neoplasms
· fibroids/fibromas
· teratomas
· rare lipomas, hemangiomas,
  adenoid tumors
· salpingitis isthmica nodosa
Tubal carcinoma

Ovarian*

Epithelial stromal tumors
· serous
· mucinous
· endometroid
· clear cell
· Brenner
· mixed
· undifferentiated carcinoma
· squamous tumors
Germ cell tumors
· dysgerminoma
· endodermal sinus tumor
· embryonal carcinoma
· polyembryoma
· choriocarcinoma
· teratoma
· mixed forms
Sex-cord stromal tumors
· granulosa-stromal
· androblastomas: Sertoli-
  Leydig
· gynandroblastoma
· unclassified
Sex-cord tumor with annular
  tubules
Steroid (lipid) cell tumors
Gonadoblastoma
· pure
· mixed
Soft tissue tumors
Unclassified tumors

Secondary (metastatic) tumors
Tumor-like conditions
· pregnancy luteoma
· hyperplasia of ovarian
  stroma, hyperthecosis
· massive edema
· follicle cyst
· corpus luteum cyst
· polycystic ovaries
· luteinized follicle cysts
  and/or corpora lutea
· endometriosis
· simple cysts
· inflammatory lesions
· ectopic
· fibromatosis
Tumors of rete ovarii
· adenoma
· adenocarcinoma
Mesothelial tumors
· adenomatoid tumor
· mesothelioma
Tumors of uncertain origin
· small cell carcinoma
· tumor of Wolffian origin
· hepatoid carcinoma
· myxoma
Gestational trophoblastic
  diseases
Malignant lymphomas,
  leukaemias, plasmacytoma

Extragenital

Endometriosis
Inflammatory
· appendicitis
· diverticulitis
· perirectal abscess
Hematocele
Ascites
Urological
· bladder
· urachael cysts
· pelvic kidney
· transplant
· tumor
Gastrointestinal
· inflammatory
· tumor
· stool/gas

Retroperitoneal
· teratoma
· meningomyelocele
· presacral chordoma
· lymphocyst
· lymphoma
· sarcoma group
Abdominal wall lesions
· hematoma
· muscle tumor
· abscess
· lipoma
· scar implants
Foreign body

Sources: Gates, E. 1990. Pelvic masses. Lecture notes. University of California-San Francisco.
*Adapted with permission from Scully, R.E., and Sobin, L.H. 1999. Histological typing of ovarian tumours. In *International histological classification of ovarian tumours*, 2nd ed. Berlin: Springer. ©Springer-Verlag GmbH & Co. KG, 1999.

endometriosis and uterine leiomyomas may coexist with adenomyosis (Rapkin 1996).

Ovarian/Adnexal Masses

The finding of an enlarged ovary may be indicative of a non-neoplastic functional cyst or the presence of a benign or malignant cystic or solid neoplasm. There is a wide range of types and patterns of ovarian tumors. The tumors are difficult to define because they overlap and because the pathological terminology is imprecise (Young et al. 2001). (See **Table 12J.1**.) Within each category of ovarian tumor, a designation is made regarding its nature: benign, borderline malignant potential, or malignant (Berek et al. 1996). Only 20% of all ovarian neoplasms are malignant (DiSaia et al. 2002).

Treatment of ovarian masses depends on the etiology of the tumor and the age of the patient. In the premenarchal and postmenopausal female, ovarian masses must be considered highly suspect for malignancy and promptly investigated (DiSaia et al. 2002). A select group of ovarian and adnexal masses is discussed below.

Among the most frequently encountered ovarian masses are *functional cysts*. A follicular cyst may form if the dominant follicle fails to ovulate or when other follicles fail to undergo normal atresia (Neinstein 1996). Estrogen may be produced by the cyst and cause menstrual irregularity. Normally, these cysts resolve spontaneously within a few days to two weeks but can persist longer. On clinical grounds alone, a functional cyst cannot be readily distinguished from a true ovarian neoplasm (DiSaia et al. 2002).

Corpus luteum cysts are less common. They occur after ovulation when limited spontaneous bleeding fills the central cavity of the corpus luteum with blood. Subsequently, the blood is reabsorbed and a cystic space remains. If bleeding is excessive, the corpus luteum may rupture and precipitate a surgical emergency. Corpus luteum cysts are more likely than follicular cysts to produce menstrual irregularities. Smaller corpus luteum cysts often resolve spontaneously.

Other physiological ovarian cysts, such as *theca lutein cysts*, may be associated with hydatidiform mole, choriocarcinoma, multiple gestation, diabetes, Rh sensitization, clomiphene citrate and human menopausal gonadotropin/human chorionic gonadotropin ovulation induction, and the use of gonadotropin-releasing hormone (GnRH) analogs (Hillard 1996). *Simple cysts* frequently occur in postmenopause.

Mature benign cystic teratomas (dermoids) are unique germ cell tumors (usually multicystic) that contain hair, sebaceous debris, and occasionally, teeth, cartilage, or bone. Teratomas account for approximately 15% of all ovarian tumors and are the most common ovarian neoplasms in women in the second and third decades of life (DiSaia et al. 2002). Complications of teratomas include torsion, rupture, and hemorrhage. An association with autoimmune hemolytic anemia may occur (Buchwalter et al. 2001).

Serous and mucinous cystadenomas are other common benign cystic neoplasms. Cystadenomas may vary in size (the average is 5–20 cm). The serous type is more common than the mucinous one. Bilaterality of serous cystadenomas occurs in as many as 10% of cases, in contrast with mucinous cystadenoma, for which there is no significant incidence of bilaterality. Mucinous cystadenomas may become huge—some reportedly weighing more than 300 pounds. Whether cystadenomas and benign cystic teratomas are precursors of malignancy is as yet unknown (DiSaia et al. 2002).

Ovarian *fibromas* make up about 3% of all benign tumors. Most are unilateral and found in the left ovary (Adelson et al. 2000). They usually occur in later reproductive years. *Endometriomas* are another common cause of ovarian enlargement. (See the **Endometriosis** chapter for further discussion.)

Torsion of the ovary (or tube and ovary) is an uncommon but important cause of pelvic pain associated with a pelvic mass. Most torsions occur with benign ovarian masses of 5–10 cm. Pregnancy and enlarged ovaries due to ovulation induction are predisposing factors. The relative risk of torsion also increases with dermoids, paraovarian cysts, solid benign tumors, and serous cysts. Most often, the right ovary is involved; in 10% of cases, the contralateral adnexa may torse at a future time (Herbst et al. 1992).

Fallopian tube neoplasms are rare. More commonly, adnexal masses due to tubal disease are inflammatory or represent an ectopic pregnancy (DiSaia et al. 2002).

Sex-cord stromal tumors account for about 5% of ovarian neoplasms. Some of these tumors will produce hirsutism and other signs of virilization (Rice et al. 1995).

Malignant neoplasms of the ovary account for 5% of all cancers among women. Ovarian cancer will develop in approximately 12 of every 1,000 women in the United States older than 40 years and is the leading cause of death from gynecological cancer. Incidence rates increase dramatically with age; the largest number of patients are in the 60–64 year age group. Unfortunately, this type of cancer does not often cause symptoms or the symptoms are vague, until metastasis has occurred (two-thirds of cases). The endometrium, GI tract, and breast are the most frequent sites of origin of tumors metastatic to the ovary (Berek et al. 1996, DiSaia et al. 2002).

DATABASE

SUBJECTIVE

→ History should include a thorough evaluation of the menstrual cycle characteristics, last normal and previous normal menstrual periods, signs/symptoms of pregnancy, questions regarding the nature of pain and other associated symptoms, sexual/contraceptive history, medical history, medication history, and family history of cancer.

Fibroids

→ Presentation may include the following:
- Most women asymptomatic
- Abnormal bleeding (30% of women)
- Menorrhagia, hypermenorrhea, metrorrhagia. Severity of bleeding and other symptoms depend upon the location, size, and number of fibroids.

- Pelvic pressure, pelvic pain/dull ache/heaviness, dysmenorrhea, urinary urgency/frequency/incontinence, constipation, or other lower GI tract or rectal symptoms
- Increased abdominal girth without appreciable weight change
- Infertility, spontaneous abortion (rarely)
- Dyspnea
- Symptoms of anemia. (See the **Anemia** chapter in Section 10.)
- Severe, acute pelvic pain may be associated with sudden degeneration or torsion of fibroid.

Adenomyosis

→ Presentation may include the following:
- The woman is usually multiparous; onset between the ages of 35–50 years.
- Secondary dysmenorrhea
- Menorrhagia, hypermenorrhea, polymenorrhea, or premenstrual spotting
- Dyspareunia occasionally—deep, midline pelvis
- Uterine tenderness before and during menstruation
- Increasing symptom severity in untreated cases
- Associated leiomyomas in 50% of cases; signs and symptoms may mimic fibroids.

Ovarian/Adnexal Masses

→ Most ovarian neoplasms are asymptomatic unless rupture or torsion occurs, in which case sudden, severe, unilateral pain in the lower abdomen and pelvis may ensue as well as intraperitoneal hemorrhage and signs of shock. Internal bleeding from a corpus luteum cyst may follow coitus, trauma, exercise, or a pelvic examination.
→ Symptoms usually are not specific to the type of tumor. In some cases, specific symptoms may depend on the size and location of the tumor. Complaints may include:
- Mild, lower-abdominal or pelvic discomfort, ache, pain, pressure, heaviness, or unilateral cramping
- Pain referred to the iliac or inguinal area; inner, upper thigh; or vulva
- Dyspareunia
- Increased abdominal girth or a mass
→ Additional symptoms may include:
- Irregularity of the menstrual cycle—e.g., delayed flow; irregular/intermittent spotting; menorrhagia; oligomenorrhea; amenorrhea
- Urinary frequency/retention/incontinence
- Anorexia, nausea, vomiting; eructation; flatulence, constipation, or other alteration in bowel habits
- Edema/varicosities of the lower extremities
- Dyspnea
- Symptoms/signs of feminization or virilization
- Symptoms/signs of Cushing's syndrome or hyperthyroidism
- Symptoms of pregnancy
NOTE: Moderate anorexia, nausea, vague abdominal or pelvic discomfort, abdominal enlargement or distention,

increased flatulence or bloating, and/or indigestion should arouse suspicion for ovarian cancer. Colicky pain, melena, altered bowel habits, or diminution of stool caliber is associated with sigmoid cancer.
→ Postulated risk factors for ovarian cancer include nulliparity, nonuse of oral contraceptives, infertility, early menarche, late menopause, prior history of malignancy (especially breast and colon), familial ovarian cancer, and environmental factors (DiSaia et al. 2002, Morrow et al. 1998).

OBJECTIVE

→ Vital signs as indicated.
- Temperature may be elevated if there is pelvic infection; hypotension/tachycardia may be present in cases of rupture/hemorrhage.
→ A complete abdominal examination, including inspection, auscultation, percussion, and palpation, and a complete pelvic and rectovaginal examination are mandatory in evaluating pelvic masses. A rectovaginal examination allows the examiner to fully palpate the surface of a mass in the posterior cul-de-sac and assess nodularity of the uterosacral ligaments.
- The patient should void before examination. Ideally, the bowel should be empty to avoid misdiagnosis of fecal material as an adnexal mass (DiSaia et al. 2002).
NOTE: A pelvic examination should be performed gingerly so an adnexal mass is not inadvertently ruptured.
→ Peripheral lymph nodes should be carefully assessed. A breast examination also should be performed.

Fibroids

→ Findings typically include a firm, irregular, mobile, nontender, enlarged uterus. Uterine size generally is described in gestational weeks—e.g., 10 weeks' size.
NOTE: The adnexa may be difficult to palpate secondary to the enlarged or laterally displaced uterus.
→ A normal retroverted uterus may mimic a posterior-wall myoma projecting into the cul-de-sac; a pedunculated fibroid may be confused with an ovarian tumor.
→ Degenerating myomas may result in the uterus becoming softer and more cystic.
→ Uterine fixation or tenderness may indicate infection or endometriosis.
→ A menopausal woman's fibroids should regress in size.
- An enlarging uterus after menopause should arouse suspicion for sarcomatous degeneration or possibly an ovarian neoplasm.
→ Anatomical location and characteristics of fibroids (Adelson et al. 2000, Herbst et al. 1992, Lichtman et al. 1990):
- *Interstitial* (intramural): most common; within the myometrium, rounded shape.
- *Submucosal*: beneath the endometrium, protruding into uterine cavity; 5–10% of all myomas; associated with bleeding problems, infertility, spontaneous abortion; growth may lead to pedunculation.

- *Subserosal* (subperitoneal): bulging though outer uterine wall
- *Interligamentous*: within broad ligament
- *Pedunculated*: myoma with thin pedicle attached to uterus; difficult to distinguish from ovarian masses
- *Parasitic*: extruding from uterus with accessory blood supply; may grow laterally into broad ligament and produce hydroureter; difficult to distinguish from ovarian masses
- *Cervical*: 3–8% of myomas; most small, asymptomatic; may become pedunculated and protrude through external os leading to ulceration/infection

Adenomyosis

→ In adenomyosis, the uterus is diffusely enlarged, globular with a finely nodular surface, and possibly tender. Usually it is 2–3 times the normal size but often not greater than 14-weeks' size unless there are concomitant fibroids.

Ovarian/Adnexal Masses

NOTE: It is not possible on physical examination to determine with certainty whether an ovarian mass is benign or malignant (Morrow et al. 1998). See below for characteristics of certain masses.

→ Note the location of the mass with respect to the uterus, and its mobility, consistency, contour, size, and bilaterality.

- Most ovarian neoplasms are lateral or posterior to the uterus (an exception is the dermoid, which is usually anterior to the broad ligament).

→ Dullness over the mass, tympany in the flanks, and no tone difference with position change is characteristic of a cyst. Shifting dullness in the flanks is characteristic of ascites. Lower abdominal veins may be distended in the presence of large ovarian cysts.

→ Abdominal rigidity with local/rebound tenderness may be present if an ovarian cyst or TOA has ruptured. (See the **Pelvic Inflammatory Disease** chapter for additional information.)

→ Benign tumor characteristics:

- Commonly smooth-walled, cystic, mobile, unilateral, and <8 cm (DiSaia et al. 2002).
- *Follicular cysts* may be from a few millimeters to 15 cm (the average is 2.5–3 cm) and solitary or multiple. Corpus luteum cysts range from 3–10 cm (the average is 4 cm).
- *Dermoids* range from a few millimeters to 25 cm. Most are less than 10 cm. They may be single or multiple and may occur bilaterally in 10–15% of cases.
- *Cystadenomas* may vary in size (the average is 5–20 cm, but some are larger).
  - Serous cystadenomas are more common than the mucinous type. Bilaterality of serous cystadenomas occurs in as many as 10% of cases.
  - Mucinous cystadenomas may become huge (some reportedly weigh more than 300 pounds). No significant incidence of bilaterality (DiSaia et al. 2002).

- *Fibromas* range in size from small nodules to 50-pound tumors (the average diameter is 6 cm). Most are unilateral.

→ Malignant tumor characteristics:

- Usually solid (or semisolid), bilateral, irregular, fixed, and associated with nodules in the cul-de-sac. There may be associated ascites (DiSaia et al. 2002).
  - Cul-de-sac or uterosacral, ligamentous nodularity also may be associated with endometriosis.

NOTE: A palpable ovary in a postmenopausal female suggests the possibility of malignancy. Bilateral ovarian findings in any age group also may be indicative of malignancy.

→ Ascites and hydrothorax may occur with ovarian tumors (Meigs' syndrome).

→ Additional features observed on physical examination include pleural effusion, leg edema, and the stigmata of abnormal hormone production (Morrow et al. 1998).

ASSESSMENT

→ Uterine mass
- R/O pregnancy
- R/O uterine fibroid(s), also known as myoma(s), leiomyoma(s), fibromyoma(s)
  - R/O leiomyosarcoma
  - R/O endometrial carcinoma
- R/O adenomyosis
  - R/O endometriosis
  - R/O multiple leiomyomas
  - R/O salpingitis isthmica nodosa
  - R/O idiopathic uterine hypertrophy of multiparity (fibrosis uteri)
  - R/O pelvic congestion syndrome
- R/O ovarian/bowel tumors
- R/O anemia
- R/O uterine/urinary tract infection
- R/O endometrial hyperplasia/cancer

→ Ovarian/adnexal mass
- R/O ectopic pregnancy
- R/O rupture/torsion
- R/O pyosalpinx, hydrosalpinx, TOA
- R/O benign versus malignant lesion
- R/O conditions mimicking ovarian neoplasms: pedunculated fibroid; low-lying, distended cecum; redundant sigmoid colon; appendiceal abscess; impacted feces; carcinoma of the sigmoid colon; diverticulitis; hematoma of rectus muscle; urachal cyst; retroperitoneal neoplasm/abscess; pelvic kidney

→ R/O abdominal pathology, such as appendicitis, cholecystitis, or peptic ulcer disease or other GI disturbance

PLAN

DIAGNOSTIC TESTS

Fibroids and Adenomyosis

→ A presumptive diagnosis usually is made on abdominal and bimanual pelvic examination.

→ Pelvic ultrasound may be ordered for confirmation, baseline assessment, and clinical follow-up of fibroid-size progression.
  ▪ Sonography also may be utilized in cases where symptoms are suggestive of fibroids but none is palpable.
  ▪ Ultrasonography will be useful in distinguishing fibroids from the most common misdiagnosis of ovarian neoplasm.
→ MRI has been used to assess the number, size, and location of fibroids, to distinguish other pathological disease states, and to evaluate fibroid size progression and response to therapy. Consult with a physician.
→ Abdominal x-ray may be less commonly used to identify concentric uterine calcifications. Generally, it is not a clinically useful test to rule out fibroids; however, fibroids may be diagnosed incidentally by x-ray when x-ray is ordered for other reasons.
→ Hysterosalpingography, endovaginal sonography, and MRI may be used to establish a diagnosis of adenomyosis. Consult with a physician.
→ An endometrial biopsy should be performed to rule out endometrial adenocarcinoma in a woman with suspected adenomyosis. Consult with a physician. (See the **Abnormal Uterine Bleeding** chapter for additional information.)
→ A definitive diagnosis of adenomyosis can be made only by histopathology of the lesion.
→ Additional tests may include, but are not limited to, the following as indicated: pregnancy test, Pap smear, CBC, ESR, urinalysis, urine culture and sensitivities, sexually transmitted disease (STD) screening, hysteroscopy, and intravenous pyelogram. Consult with a physician as indicated regarding ordering of specific tests.

Ovarian/Adnexal Masses

→ Preliminary diagnosis is made on bimanual pelvic and rectovaginal examination. If the bowel is filled with fecal material and the examination is difficult or inconclusive, a cathartic or enema may be prescribed. Re-examination should be performed after the patient's bowel has been evacuated.
→ Abdominal or transvaginal ultrasound, color Doppler ultrasonography, CT scanning, MRI, and x-ray are all techniques used to evaluate and diagnose ovarian neoplasms. Consult with a physician regarding ordering these tests.
→ Culdocentesis performed by a physician may be used in acute cases when intraperitoneal bleeding or hemorrhage is suspected.
→ Pap smears may pick up transmigrating ovarian carcinoma cells on rare occasions.
→ Endoscopy is indicated if there has been GI bleeding or there is a suggestion of rectosigmoid disease. Contrast studies of the GI tract also may be indicated. Refer the patient to a physician.
→ Liver function studies should be ordered in the presence of ascites or when malignancy is suspected. Refer the patient to a physician.

→ The need for surgery to evaluate an adnexal mass will be determined by the gynecologist in charge of the patient's care. Definitive diagnosis of tumor type is made by histologic evaluation.
→ Additional tests may include, but are not limited to, the following as indicated (consult with a physician regarding ordering specific tests):
  ▪ Pregnancy test
  ▪ CBC
  ▪ ESR
  ▪ STD screening
  ▪ Specific ovarian and GI tumor markers (e.g., CA-125, ß-hCG, lactate dehydrogenase, alpha-fetoprotein, carcinoembryonic antigen level)
  ▪ Testosterone
  ▪ Dehydroepiandrosterone sulfate
  ▪ Urinalysis
  ▪ Urine culture and sensitivities
  ▪ Stool for occult blood
  ▪ Liver function studies
  ▪ Renal function studies
  ▪ Electrolytes
  ▪ Chest x-ray
  ▪ Colposcopy
  ▪ Endometrial biopsy
  ▪ Endocervical curettage

NOTE: Serum CA-125 measurement is of limited benefit in identifying ovarian malignancy in premenopausal women because elevations can be associated with endometriosis, adenomyosis, leiomyomata, pregnancy, and pelvic inflammatory disease (Morrow et al. 1998). Elevated CA-125 levels in women younger than 50 years is associated with malignancy less than 25% of the time. In women older than 50 years, an elevated CA-125 is associated with a malignant mass 80% of the time (DiSaia et al. 2002). Nongynecologic inflammatory processes also may increase CA-125 (e.g., acute hepatitis/pancreatitis, chronic liver disease, colitis, diverticulitis, congestive heart failure, and pneumonia) (DiSaia et al. 2002).

→ See the chapters on **Endometriosis**, **Ectopic Pregnancy**, **Amenorrhea—Secondary** (for polycystic ovary syndrome), and **Pelvic Inflammatory Disease** (for TOA) for additional diagnostic tests.

TREATMENT/MANAGEMENT

Fibroids

→ Expectant management is all that is required for an asymptomatic woman. Re-examination after confirmation of fibroids (or suspicion of adenomyosis) is tailored to the individual.
→ Indications for definitive treatment include abnormal bleeding, pain, urinary or bowel disorders, infertility problems, recurrent spontaneous abortion, rapidly enlarging fibroids, and anemia.

→ More aggressive treatment modalities are tailored to the individual patient based on age, severity of symptoms, plans for childbearing, and the desire to retain the uterus.

→ Surgical options may include:
- Hysteroscopic resection
- Hysteroscopic myomectomy via laser
- Uterine artery embolization
- Abdominal myomectomy
- Hysterectomy
  - Indications for hysterectomy include (McDonald 2000):
    - Large fibroids causing pelvic pain, pelvic pressure, bladder urgency, rectal pressure, or ureteral obstruction
    - Menorrhagia and anemia uncorrectable by curettage and progestins
    - Rapidly enlarging fibroids

→ Medical management may include:
- GnRH agonists may be employed to induce a hypogonadotrophic, hypogonadal state. The patient is managed by a physician.
  - Presurgical treatment with these agents facilitates myomectomy by reducing the size and vascularity of fibroids. In addition, surgery may be avoided altogether or the proposed route of surgery may change based on fibroid shrinkage.
  - Reduction in fibroid volume appears to depend on the level of estrogen suppression, with the greatest reduction usually achieved within the first 12 weeks. After therapy is discontinued, regrowth to pretreatment size (or beyond) occurs within 2–6 months in 40% of patients (Daya 2000).
  - Fibroid size reduction during therapy can be monitored by pelvic examination.
  - Side effects of GnRH therapy are varied and may include:
    - Hot flushes
    - Vaginal dryness
    - Weight gain
    - Amenorrhea
    - Loss of bone density
    - Decreased libido/breast size
    - Depression
    - Fatigue
    - Headaches
    - Insomnia
    - Arthralgias/myalgias
    - Adverse effects on lipid metabolism
      - To counter some of these effects, "add-back" estrogen/progestin therapy may be used.
  - See Scialli et al. 2000 for additional information regarding GnRH therapy.
- Depo-medroxyprogesterone acetate (Depo-Provera®) also may be used for medical management. Consult with a physician.

→ Iron-deficiency anemia must be treated. (See the **Anemia** chapter in Section 10.)

Adenomyosis

→ Treatment depends on the severity of the disease.
- The uterine-conserving procedures—endometrial ablation, laparoscopic myometrial electrocoagulation, and excision—are effective in more than 50% of patients.
- Oral contraceptives or prostaglandin synthetase inhibitors may be tried.
- Hysterectomy remains the definitive therapy and is indicated in severe cases (Tafazoli et al. 1999).

Ovarian/Adnexal Masses

→ The goals of management include (Berek et al. 1996):
- Establishing the origin of the mass
- Distinguishing between physiological cysts and neoplastic cysts/tumors
- Determining if the mass is benign or malignant
- Removing/treating the primary cancer if the mass is malignant
- If possible, removing/treating all metastatic disease

→ In consultation with a physician, set up appropriate diagnostic testing.

→ Patients in whom ruptured cysts/masses are suspected require prompt intervention and immediate referral to an emergency facility.

→ When an ovarian malignancy is suspected, immediate referral to a physician is warranted. Further management will be undertaken by the physician. The details of managing cancer patients are beyond the scope of this chapter.

→ Indications for surgical intervention include (DiSaia et al. 2002):
- An ovarian cystic structure >5 cm that has been observed 6–8 weeks without regression
- Any solid ovarian lesion
- Any ovarian lesion with papillary vegetation on the cyst wall
- Any ovarian mass >10 cm in diameter
- Ascites
- A palpable adnexal mass in a premenarchal or postmenopausal patient
- If torsion or rupture is suspected

NOTE: Prompt referral to a physician is required if any of the above criteria exists or if the patient has significant pain.

→ In premenopausal women, most cystic masses <7 cm resolve within 6–8 weeks (DiSaia et al. 2002). Functional ovarian cysts may be treated conservatively.
- Perform a pelvic examination every 3–4 weeks. Oral contraceptives may be employed to suppress ovulation (provided no contraindications exist).
- Cysts >10 cm or those >5 cm that persist longer than 6–8 weeks without regression require surgery (DiSaia et al. 2002, Drake 1998).

→ Corpus luteum cysts may be managed expectantly, provided there is no active intraperitoneal bleeding; most regress spontaneously.

→ Treatment of benign cystic teratomas is surgical.

→ Treatment of suspected malignancy is laparotomy, usually including total hysterectomy and bilateral salpingo-oophorectomy.

→ Unilocular cystic masses <5 cm in a postmenopausal woman are usually benign. These patients generally are managed by a physician.

  ▪ In some settings, these patients may be conservatively managed with utilization of serial transvaginal ultrasound, possibly in conjunction with CA-125 levels.

  ▪ Pelvic washings obtained by laparoscope also may be sent for cytological evaluation.

→ See the chapters on **Endometriosis**, **Ectopic Pregnancy**, **Amenorrhea—Secondary** (for polycystic ovary syndrome) and **Pelvic Inflammatory Disease** (for TOA) regarding additional management.

CONSULTATION

→ Advised for all newly diagnosed pelvic masses.

→ For a rapidly enlarging uterus or if a malignancy in the pelvis is suspected, refer the patient to a physician promptly.

→ When considering endometrial biopsy, consult with a physician.

→ For medical management with GnRH agonists and Depo-Provera®, the patient generally is managed by a physician. This depends, however, on the practice setting.

→ Patients with severe anemia, infertility, or recurrent pregnancy loss should be referred to a specialist.

→ Patients with suspected rupture/torsion or TOA require emergency intervention.

PATIENT EDUCATION

→ Discuss the nature of uterine fibroids or adenomyosis if it is suspected.

  ▪ Informative patient-education pamphlets with good illustrations are a useful adjunct to teaching. The American College of Obstetricians and Gynecologists has a useful pamphlet on fibroids.

→ Reassure the patient regarding the benign nature of fibroids.

→ Alert the patient to the signs and symptoms of an enlarging uterus.

→ Discuss the need for regular follow-up and the various treatment options for fibroids and/or adenomyosis.

→ Ascertain the patient's desire regarding contraception and childbearing, and discuss appropriate contraception.

  ▪ Oral contraceptives are options. Follow the patient for potential fibroid growth secondary to hormonal stimulation (unlikely with a low-dose contraceptive).

  ▪ Intrauterine devices (IUDs) are acceptable if the uterine cavity is normal. Levonorgestrel-containing IUDs may improve associated symptoms of menorrhagia.

  ▪ A diaphragm may be used if it does not exacerbate symptoms.

→ Women with infertility or recurrent pregnancy loss require psychological support throughout the investigation. Refer the patient to an infertility specialist as indicated.

→ When a suspected ovarian mass is encountered, discuss the physical findings with the patient and outline possible treatment options. Definitive management in many cases will be carried out by the physician, who should fully discuss the treatment approaches with the patient. Benign ovarian tumors have an excellent prognosis.

→ If ovarian malignancy is suspected, try not to alarm the patient. Utilize appropriate resources and refer to a physician promptly.

  ▪ Suggest that a support person accompany the patient to the doctor's appointment.

  ▪ Set up appropriate diagnostic tests in consultation with the physician and ensure the patient understands the importance of follow-up.

FOLLOW-UP

→ After initial discovery of fibroids, uterine reassessment is tailored to the individual. Long-term interval follow-up will depend on the stability of the fibroids and patient symptomatology.

→ Utilization of pelvic ultrasound or MRI may be indicated in difficult cases to follow myoma progression, determine the response to medical therapy, or as an adjunct to routine, intermittent assessment of the pelvis.

→ Monitoring for worsening of dysmenorrhea is warranted for a patient with adenomyosis who is taking oral contraceptives.

→ Follow-up of ovarian masses will depend on the case presentation and in many cases will be handled by the physician. (See "Treatment/Management," above.)

→ If cancer is diagnosed, supportive care for the patient and her family is paramount to the recovery process.

  ▪ The prognosis for ovarian cancer depends on the cell type, stage, and grade.

  ▪ Body image and sexuality issues need to be addressed.

  ▪ Patients will be closely followed by a gynecological oncologist and possibly an oncological clinical nurse specialist if available.

→ Advise all women regarding the American Cancer Society's Guidelines for mammography. (See Section 4, **Breast Disorders**.)

→ Documentation in progress notes regarding pelvic masses should include onset, nature of the mass, progression, rapidity/stability of growth, timing/results of monitoring modalities, and definitive therapy as indicated. Update the problem list periodically.

BIBLIOGRAPHY

Adelson, M.D., and Adelson, K.L. 2000. Miscellaneous benign disorders of the upper genital tract. In *Textbook of gynecology*, 2nd ed., ed. L.J. Copeland, pp. 723–739. Philadelphia: W.B. Saunders.

Berek, J.S., Fu, Y.S., and Hacker, N.F. 1996. Ovarian cancer. In *Novak's gynecology*, eds. J.S. Berek, E.Y. Adashi, and P.A. Hillard. Baltimore, Md.: Williams & Wilkins.

Buchwalter, C.L., Miller, D., and Jenison, F.L. 2001. Hemolytic anemia and benign pelvic tumors. A case report. *Journal of Reproductive Medicine* 46(4):401–404.

Daya, A. 2000. Habitual abortion. In *Textbook of gynecology*, 2nd ed., ed. L.J. Copeland, pp. 227–271. Philadelphia: W.B. Saunders.

DiSaia, P.J., and Creasman, W.T. 2002. *Clinical gynecologic oncology*, 6th ed. St. Louis, Mo.: C.V. Mosby.

Drake, J. 1998. Diagnosis and management of the adnexal mass. *American Family Physician* 57(10):2471–2476.

Gates, E. 1990. *Pelvic masses*. Lecture notes. University of California-San Francisco.

Grabo, T.N., Fahs, P.S., Nataupsky, L.G. et al. 1999. Uterine myomas: treatment options. *Journal of Obstetric, Gynecologic, and Neonatal Nursing* 28:23–31.

Guarnaccia, M.M., Silverberg, K., and Olive, D.L. 2000. Endometriosis and adenomyosis. In *Textbook of gynecology*, 2nd ed., ed. L.J. Copeland, pp. 687–722. Philadelphia: W.B. Saunders.

Herbst, A.L., Mishell, D.R., Stenchever, M.A. et al. 1992. *Comprehensive gynecology*, 2nd ed. St. Louis, Mo.: Mosby Year Book.

Hillard, P.A. 1996. Benign diseases of the female reproductive tract: symptoms and signs. In *Novak's gynecology*, eds. J.S. Berek, E.Y. Adashi, and P.A. Hillard. Baltimore, Md.: Williams & Wilkins.

Lichtman, R., and Papera, S. 1990. *Gynecology. Well-woman care*. Norwalk, Conn.: Appleton & Lange.

Lovvorn, H.N., Tucci, L.A., and Stafford, P.W. 1998. Ovarian masses in the pediatric population. *AORN Journal* 67(3): 568–576.

McDonald, T.W. 2000. Hysterectomy. In *Textbook of gynecology*, 2nd ed., ed. L.J. Copeland, pp. 1023–1051. Philadelphia: W.B. Saunders.

Meisler, J.G. 1999. Conversation with the experts. Toward optimal health: the experts respond to fibroids. *Journal of Women's Health and Gender-Based Medicine* 8(7):879–883.

Moorehead, M.E., and Conard, C.J. 2001. Uterine leiomyoma. A treatable condition. *Annals of the New York Academy of Sciences* 948:121–129.

Morrow, C.P., and Curtin, J.P. 1998. *Synopsis of gynecologic oncology*, 5th ed. New York: Churchill Livingstone.

Muto, M.G., and Friedman, A.J. 1995. The uterine corpus. In *Kistner's gynecology. Principles and practice*, eds. K.J. Ryan, R.S. Berkowitz and R.L. Barbarieri. St. Louis, Mo.: Mosby.

Neinstein, L.S. 1996. *Adolescent health care. A practical guide*, 3rd ed. Baltimore, Md.: Williams & Wilkins.

Pfeifer, S.M., and Gosman, G.G. 1999. Evaluation of adnexal masses in adolescents. *Pediatric Clinics of North America* 46(3):573–592.

Rapkin, A.J. 1996. Pelvic pain and dysmenorrhea. In *Novak's gynecology*, eds. J.S. Berek, E.Y. Adashi and P.A. Hillard. Baltimore, Md.: Williams & Wilkins.

Rice, L.W., and Barbieri, R.L. 1995. The ovary. In *Kistner's gynecology. Principles and practice*, eds. K.J. Ryan, R.S. Berkowitz and R.L. Barbarieri, St. Louis, Mo.: Mosby.

Scialli, A.R., and Levi, A.J. 2000. Intermittent leuprolide acetate for the nonsurgical management of women with leiomyomata uteri. *Fertility and Sterility* 74(3):540–546.

Scully, R.E., and Sobin, L.H. 1999. Histological typing of ovarian tumours. In *International histological classification of ovarian tumours*, 2nd ed. Berlin: Springer.

Tafazoli, F., and Reinhold, C. 1999. Uterine adenomyosis: current concepts in imaging. *Seminars in Ultrasound, CT, and MRI* 20(4):267–277.

Young, R.H., and Scully, R.E. 2001. Differential diagnosis of ovarian tumors based primarily on their patterns and cell types. *Seminars in Diagnostic Pathology* 18(3):161–235.

Winifred L. Star, R.N., C., N.P., M.S.
Jenna A. Lewis, M.S.N., W.H.N.P., A.N.P.

12-K

Pelvic Pain—Acute

Pelvic pain is one of the most common symptoms for which women seek medical care. The focus of this chapter is acute pain; the following chapter discusses chronic pelvic pain. *Acute pelvic pain* is defined as pain that has been present for hours or days. Inadequately treated acute pelvic pain may inadvertently lead to serious short-term sequelae (hemorrhage or shock) and long-term consequences (infertility). Therefore, the clinician's first task is to determine whether the condition requires emergency treatment or immediate physician referral.

Although pelvic pain has many causes, a careful history and physical exam can help the clinician rule out all but a few diagnoses. (See **Table 12K.1, Causes of Acute Pelvic Pain**.)

Gynecologic-Related Pain

Pelvic inflammatory disease (PID) is infection of the upper reproductive tract. Anatomically, inflammation may be found in the endometrium, fallopian tubes, ovaries, or peritoneum. Therefore, PID encompasses endometritis, salpingitis, tubo-ovarian abscess, and pelvic peritonitis. The most common pathogens are *Chlamydia trachomatis*, *Neisseria gonorrhoeae*, and anaerobic and facultative anaerobic bacteria. *Ovarian cysts* and *masses* can cause acute pain when they stretch surrounding tissue, torse, or rupture. Often, the whole adnexa will be involved. *Mittleschmerz* is pain caused by ovulation. The pain occurs midcycle, is unilateral, and generally lasts no longer than 24–36 hours.

Obstetric-Related Pain

Ectopic pregnancy is defined as any pregnancy that does not occur in the endometrial cavity of the uterus. All heterosexually active women of reproductive age are at risk for ectopic pregnancy, but the risk increases when a woman has a history of PID, an intrauterine device in place, or a history of tubal ligation or infertility treatment.

Spontaneous abortion sometimes causes acute pain, typically cramping. Pain is associated with abnormal bleeding as the contents of the uterus are expelled. A threatened abortion causes a similar pain profile, but it is accompanied by light bleeding without evidence of passed tissue.

Urologic-Related Pain

Infection, the most common source of urinary pain, can cause acute suprapubic pressure or a "pulling" sensation that increases with urination. *Urolithiasis* (urinary stones) may also cause acute pain.

Gastrointestinal-Related Pain

Gastrointestinal illness may present as pelvic pain. *Gastroenteritis* is the most likely etiology, but *appendicitis* and *bowel obstruction* also must be considered.

Musculoskeletal-Related Pain

Acute trauma leading to *muscle strain*, *fracture* of a bone, or *separation of the pubic symphysis* can all cause pelvic pain.

Table 12K.1.   CAUSES OF ACUTE PELVIC PAIN

More Common
Ectopic pregnancy
Spontaneous, incomplete, or threatened abortion
Ovarian/adnexal cyst or mass
Urinary tract infection
Gastroenteritis
Appendicitis
Less Common
Degenerating/torsing fibroid
Ureteral obstruction
Intestinal obstruction
Diverticulitis
Herpes zoster

DATABASE

SUBJECTIVE

→ Obtain a complete description of the pain, including the onset, location, radiation, character, intensity, duration, aggravating and alleviating factors, and relationship to the menstrual cycle and coitus. (See **Table 12K.2, Evaluation of Acute Pelvic Pain**.)

- Onset:
  - Sudden onset suggests a mechanical cause. Consider an ovarian origin such as torsion or ruptured cyst, ectopic pregnancy, a degenerating fibroid, or urinary blockage.
  - Insidious onset suggests pelvic inflammatory disease.
- Location:
  - Unilateral pain suggests a tubo-ovarian process, including ectopic pregnancy.
  - Pain in the low central pelvis suggests PID. However, PID also may present with unilateral pain when a fallopian tube or ovary is involved.
  - Epigastrium pain suggests appendicitis, which is heralded by discomfort starting in the epigastrium, moving to the umbilicus, and then localizing to the right lower quadrant.
  - Flank pain suggests cholecystitis.
  - Suprapubic pain suggests cystitis. When it is accompanied by costovertebral pain, consider pyelonephritis.
- Character:
  - Constant, steadily increasing pain suggests rupture of an ectopic pregnancy or a tubo-ovarian abscess.
  - Crampy, intermittent pain is characteristic of contractions of hollow, muscular viscous—for example, the uterus and bowel. Therefore, threatened abortion and bowel obstruction should be considered.
  - Dull, aching pain that radiates to the lower back or thighs often is associated with PID or urinary tract infection.
- Duration:
  - Severe pain lasting more than four hours indicates a condition that likely requires surgical evaluation or concentrated medical management.
  - PID, ectopic pregnancy, and appendicitis also can present more insidiously, despite their emergent nature.
  - Urinary tract infections may be of abrupt onset or discomfort may be present for days.
- Radiation:
  - Kidney-stone pain radiates down the involved flank and into the pelvis.
  - Appendicitis pain initially is periumbilical, then shifts to the right lower quadrant in several hours.
  - Musculoskeletal pain may involve the lower back and cause pain to radiate down one or both legs.
  - Dysmenorrhea and endometriosis pain may radiate to the lower back or down the legs (associated rectal pain in endometriosis may be referred from another organ or be secondary to perirectal lesions).
- Relationship to menstrual cycle:
  - Pain or bleeding that occurs after a missed menses may indicate a spontaneous abortion or an ectopic pregnancy. It is important to determine if the previous menstrual period was normal in flow and duration and if any intermenstrual bleeding occurred.
  - Pain during menses is most typically dysmenorrhea.
  - Midcycle pain may be due to mittelschmerz (ovulatory pain).
- Associated symptoms:
  - Fever, chills, and malaise indicate infection from any source.
  - Lightheadedness, dizziness, fainting, and shoulder tip pain may be associated with intraperitoneal bleeding.
  - Urinary urgency, frequency, dysuria, or hematuria suggests urinary tract infection.
  - Nausea, vomiting, diarrhea, constipation, melena, or changes in pain associated with meals indicates a gastrointestinal source.

→ For further information, also see the "Subjective" portion of the **Abdominal Pain** chapter in Section 7, and the "Subjective" portion of the following chapters in Section 12: **Urinary Tract Infection**, **Interstitial Cystitis**, **Pelvic Inflammatory Disease**, **Vaginitis**, and **Abnormal Uterine Bleeding**. Also see Section 8, **Musculoskeletal Disorders**, and Section 13, **Sexually Transmitted Diseases**.

OBJECTIVE

→ Perform a complete abdominal, pelvic, and rectal examination. (See **Table 12K.2, Evaluation of Acute Pelvic Pain** and **Table 12K.3, Physical Examination Features in the Woman with Acute Pelvic Pain**.)

- The abdominal examination should include:
  - Inspection for distension, visible peristalsis, scarring, and masses.
  - Auscultation for altered bowel signs.
  - Percussion to delineate masses and free air.
  - Palpation for hepatosplenomegaly, guarding, rebound tenderness, site of maximal tenderness, masses, and costovertebral angle tenderness.
- The pelvic examination should include:
  - Inspection of external genitalia for lesions, discharge, and bleeding.
  - Speculum examination for vaginal or cervical lesions, discharge, or bleeding.
  - Bimanual examination to assess for cervical motion tenderness, and palpation for masses, tenderness, fullness, and fixation.
- The rectovaginal examination should include:
  - Assessment of masses, tenderness, nodularity in the cul-de-sac or rectum, and the presence or absence and consistency of stool.

→ Also assess vital signs, as fever may be present in inflammatory and infectious states and orthostatic changes in pulse and blood pressure may be indicative of intraperitoneal bleeding.

Table 12K.2. EVALUATION OF ACUTE PELVIC PAIN

Cause	Subjective Findings	Objective Findings	Diagnostic Tests
Ectopic Pregnancy	Mild to severe pain, may be unilateral or specific, with or without bleeding	Adnexal tenderness; if ruptured, may have orthostatic hypotension or tachycardia; blood in the vagina	Positive hCG; abnormal rising of ß-hCG; ultrasound shows empty uterus and possibly adnexal mass
Spontaneous Abortion	Abnormal bleeding; cramping pelvic pain	Blood or tissue in vagina; enlarged uterus	Positive hCG; abnormal rising of ß-hCG; ultrasound may show intrauterine pregnancy or tissue
Adnexal Mass or Cyst	Unilateral pain	Adnexal tenderness and fullness or mass; if ruptured, may have orthostatic hypotension or tachycardia	Normal or elevated WBC; normal or elevated ESR; ultrasound shows mass or cyst
Pelvic Inflammatory Disease	Diffuse pelvic pain; may be unilateral if it involves tubo-ovarian abscess; vaginal discharge; fever and chills	Normal or elevated temperature; vaginal discharge; diffuse pain, cervical motion tenderness, or adnexal pain	Normal or elevated WBC; normal or elevated ESR; increased WBC on microscopic exam; tests positive for *C. trachomatis* or *N. gonorrhoeae*
Urinary Tract Infection	Pain with urination; increased frequency; urgency; flank or midback pain	Normal exam or suprapubic tenderness; CVA tenderness	Urinalysis significant for nitrites, bacteria, protein, RBC, casts
Appendicitis	Epigastric or periumbilical pain, localizing to RLQ; diffuse abdominal pain; anorexia, nausea, vomiting	Normal or elevated temperature; RLQ tenderness	Normal or increased WBC

Source: Adapted with permission from Carlson, K.J., and Eisenstat, S.A. 1995. *Primary care of women.* St. Louis, Mo.: Mosby.

Table 12K.3. PHYSICAL EXAMINATION FEATURES IN THE WOMAN WITH ACUTE PELVIC PAIN

General

Appearance

Vital signs

Abdominal Exam

Appearance: distension, masses, and scarring

Auscultation: altered bowel sounds

Percussion: masses and free air

Palpation: hepatosplenomegaly, guarding, rebound tenderness, site of maximal tenderness, masses, and costovertebral angle tenderness

Pelvic Pain

External genitalia: appearance, tenderness, lesions, discharge, and bleeding

Vagina: appearance, tenderness, discharge, and bleeding

Cervix: appearance, discharge, and cervical motion tenderness

Uterus: size, shape, consistency, mobility, and tenderness

Adnexa: mass, tenderness, fullness, and fixation

Rectal: masses, uterosacral ligament nodularity or tenderness, and stool for color, mucus, and the presence of blood

NOTE: A patient with an acute abdomen due to ruptured ectopic pregnancy, tubo-ovarian abscess, or appendicitis urgently requires immediate referral for emergency care.

→ Objective findings associated with these conditions may include:

- Fever and orthostatic changes in pulse and blood pressure
- Extreme cervical motion and pelvic tenderness
- Rigid abdomen
- Guarding
- Rebound tenderness
- Pelvic mass
- Adnexal induration or fixation
- Positive pregnancy test, decreased Hgb/Hct, increased WBC and ESR
- Pelvic ultrasound showing a complex adnexal mass, and possibly culdocentesis revealing nonclotting blood or pus.

→ Gastrointestinal and musculoskeletal disorders may manifest with acute abdominal pain and multiple signs and symptoms. For further discussion, see the **Abdominal Pain** chapter in Section 7 and specific chapters in Section 8.

ASSESSMENT

→ See **Table 12K.1** and **Table 12K.2**.

PLAN

DIAGNOSTIC TESTS

→ The following initial laboratory studies are warranted for the patient experiencing severe acute pain: ß-hCG, CBC, ESR, liver enzymes, total bilirubin, alkaline phosphatase, amylase, electrolytes, urinalysis, urine culture and sensitivities, and endocervical samples for *C. trachomatis* and *N. gonorrhoeae*.

→ Imaging studies may include pelvic ultrasound, flat and upright x-rays of the abdomen (including the diaphragm), IVP, CT scan, and diagnostic laparoscopy.

→ Laboratory evaluation of stable patients depends upon diagnostic considerations and may include the following: sensitive pregnancy test, CBC, ESR, urinalysis, urine culture and sensitivities, endocervical samples for *C. trachomatis* and *N. gonorrhoeae*, liver enzymes, total bilirubin, alkaline phosphatase, amylase, and electrolytes.

→ See also **Table 12K.2** and "Diagnostic Tests" in specific chapters.

TREATMENT/MANAGEMENT

→ Patients with evidence of peritoneal irritation, rupture, or obstruction should be referred to an emergency facility immediately.

→ Specific treatment/management will depend on the underlying identified problem. (See specific chapters.)

→ When the diagnosis is uncertain, repeated histories and physical examinations may produce new data and allow for appropriate diagnosis, referral, and treatment.

CONSULTATION

→ Consultation is suggested for all patients with suspected or confirmed ectopic pregnancy, rupture, fulminating PID including tubo-ovarian abscess, and pyelonephritis.

→ Patients with acute, severe pain should be referred to a physician immediately.

→ Referral to a mental health provider is warranted when psychosomatic pain is suspected or there is depression, neurosis, or hysteria.

PATIENT EDUCATION

→ Patient education will depend on the underlying disorder. Refer to the appropriate chapters. Encourage compliance with therapeutic regimens and follow-up care.

FOLLOW-UP

→ Follow-up will depend on patient presentation, diagnosis, and treatment/management modalities.

→ When the diagnosis is uncertain, reassessment is indicated. A pain diary, menstrual calendar, and perimenstrual-symptoms calendar may help clarify the diagnosis.

→ Document significant pelvic pathology on the problem list. Thorough progress notes are important.

BIBLIOGRAPHY

American College of Obstetricians and Gynecologists. 1989. *Chronic pelvic pain*. Technical Bulletin No. 12. Washington, D.C.: the Author.

_____. 1997. *Diagnostic laparoscopy for acute pelvic pain*. Technical Bulletin No. 25. Washington, D.C.: the Author.

Carlson, K.J., and Eisenstat, S.A. 1995. *Primary care of women*. St. Louis, Mo.: Mosby.

Dornbrand, L., Hoole, A.J., and Fletcher, R.H. 1997. *Manual of clinical problems in adult ambulatory care*. Philadelphia: Lippincott-Raven.

Economy, K.E., and Laufer, M.R. 1999. Pelvic pain. *Adolescent Medicine* 10(2):291–304.

Hewitt, G.D., and Brown, R.T. 2000. Acute and chronic pelvic pain in female adolescents. *Medical Clinics of North America* 84(4):1009–1025.

Howard, F.M., and Perry, C.P. 2000. *Pelvic pain diagnosis and management*. Philadelphia: Lippincott Williams & Wilkins.

Kresch, A.J. 1992. *Kresch pain analysis and mapping*. Palo Alto, Calif.: Fertility and Gynecology Center of Northern California.

Jenna A. Lewis, M.S.N., W.H.N.P., A.N.P.
Winifred L. Star, R.N., C., N.P., M.S.

12-L

Pelvic Pain—Chronic

Chronic pelvic pain (CPP) is defined as pain in the lower abdomen or pelvis of at least 3–6 months duration. It is a common problem, occurring in 15% of all adult women in the United States (Mathias et al. 1996). Of the more than 9 million women with chronic pelvic pain, approximately 10% consult a gynecologist. The remainder consult health care providers in other specialties, and 75% do not seek care at all. Chronic pelvic pain is the indication for 25–35% of laparoscopies and 10–15% of hysterectomies performed in the United States (Reiter 1998).

Although chronic pelvic pain is common, its pathophysiology still is not well understood. The traditional medical model postulates a direct relationship between tissue damage, stimulation of nociceptors, and pain. In general, this model explains acute pain well but falls short when applied to chronic pelvic pain. When using the traditional model, diagnosis and treatment of CPP can be highly frustrating for both the patient and the clinician. Often, a woman is seen for repeated visits by multiple clinicians, ultimately to be told that there is nothing wrong. Her providers are equally disappointed by their inability to adequately alleviate her pain. Rather than trying to categorize pain as "real" when it is associated with physical findings versus "not real" when it occurs in the absence of objective injuries, it may be more helpful to consider an integrative model.

An integrated pain model recognizes that—in addition to physical factors—emotional, environmental, and cultural factors affect pain perception. Mood, general health status, beliefs about pain, anxiety, social and familial support, and employment status all can influence how a woman perceives and manages pain. When chronic pelvic pain is seen as a biopsychosocial problem, both the patient and the clinician are better able to recognize all of the contributing factors, which ultimately leads to more successful treatment.

The differential diagnosis of chronic pelvic pain is lengthy and includes conditions originating in the gynecological, gastrointestinal, genitourinary, neurological, musculoskeletal, and psychological systems. (See **Table 12L.1, Causes of Chronic Pelvic Pain**.) However, a careful evaluation usually results in successful diagnosis and management of the pain in many women. This chapter outlines the major causes of CPP. Most often, the woman in pain chooses a practitioner based on her impression of which organ system is involved. However, it is important to keep in mind that CPP may arise from any structure in or related to the pelvis.

Gynecologic-Related Pain

Endometriosis is the presence of endometrial glands and stromal tissue located outside the endometrial cavity. Classic symptoms are dysmenorrhea and dyspareunia. Typically, pain builds up toward the menses and gradually declines during menstruation. Many women have some degree of pain throughout the cycle but describe a great variation in severity over the course of the month. Physical findings are usually nonexistent, but when they are present, they classically include nodular, tender, uterosacral ligaments.

The relationship of endometriosis to chronic pain is unclear. Endometriosis is a common finding on laparoscopy, even among women who do not experience pain. In one prospective study involving 100 patients undergoing laparoscopy for infertility, chronic pelvic pain, or tubal sterilization, similar rates of both macroscopic and microscopic endometriosis were found in all three groups (Balasch et al. 1996). Also confounding is evidence that there is no clear correlation between severity of the disease and degree of pain (Matorras et al. 1996). While it is likely that many women with endometriosis are pain-free, when women do experience chronic pelvic pain, endometriosis is often to blame (Moore et al. 2000).

Adhesions are fibrous tissues that form following a peritoneal wound, usually surgery or infection. Adhesions abnormally join anatomic structures to one another. The two most common procedures likely to produce adhesions in women are appendectomy and laparotomy (Howard et al. 2000). *Pelvic inflammatory disease* (PID) also may lead to the formation of adhesions (see discussion below). Like endometriosis, adhesions and chronic pelvic pain appear to be linked in some women, while other women with adhesions remain asymptomatic. Pain due to adhesions usually increases with stretching movements or organ distension.

Chronic PID refers to either recurrent episodes of upper genital tract infection or the residual damage caused by past episodes of pelvic infection. This damage may take the form of adhesions or perhaps an alteration in the behavior of the nerves themselves, due to the effects of products released by microorganisms or the immune system (Moore et al. 2000).

Ovarian remnant syndrome and *trapped ovary syndrome* are both related to adhesion formation. In the former condition, dense adhesions form around a remnant of ovarian tissue left behind following oophorectomy. In the latter condition, pain occurs when adhesions form around one or both ovaries that have been conserved during hysterectomy. In both cases, the pain is cyclical and may be associated with postcoital ache. Ovarian suppression or removal should eliminate the pain.

Fibroids can produce pelvic pain, although most fibroids are asymptomatic. Classic fibroid-related symptoms are menorrhagia, dysmenorrhea, and pressure-type pain that may extend from the pelvis to the low back, the kidneys, or the bowel. A pedunculated fibroid can undergo intermittent torsion, causing recurrent sharp pain (Howard et al. 2000).

Bowel-Related Pain

Irritable bowel syndrome (IBS) is the most common cause of pain arising from the bowel in women of reproductive age, affecting 10–20% of the general population and approximately 30% of chronic-pelvic-pain sufferers (Gelbaya et al. 2001, Moore et al. 2000). IBS is distinguished from inflammatory bowel disease and malignancy by several criteria. Most importantly, the patient does not experience weight loss or bloody stool. Instead, classic symptoms include pain relieved by bowel movement and alteration of stool frequency and form. Patients may feel bloated and they may pass mucus. Note that some women with IBS symptoms are actually lactose intolerant; it may be helpful for them to try a dairy-free diet to assess how it affects pain.

Bladder-Related Pain

Urethral syndrome and *interstitial cystitis* are the most common causes of bladder-related chronic pelvic pain. Both are associated with urgency, frequency, and suprapubic pain. In contrast to acute cystitis, the urine culture will be negative.

Unlike urethral syndrome, interstitial cystitis is an inflammatory process. As a result, patients with interstitial cystitis have increased pain as the bladder fills, followed by relief upon voiding. For the same reason, interstitial cystitis generally causes nocturia as the bladder fills, whereas urethral syndrome does not. Interstitial cystitis can be diagnosed on cystoscopy by finding petechial, submucosal hemorrhages called *glomerulations*. Rarely, a Hunner's ulcer is found, which is diagnostic. Urethral syndrome sufferers will have a negative cystoscopy (Howard et al. 2000).

Table 12L.1.   CAUSES OF CHRONIC PELVIC PAIN

Gynecological	Gastrointestinal	Urinary
More Common	*More Common*	*More Common*
Endometriosis	Irritable bowel syndrome	Interstitial cystitis
Adhesions	Lactose intolerance	Urethral syndrome
Less Common	Constipation	*Less Common*
Adenomyosis	*Less Common*	Neoplasm
Chronic pelvic inflammatory disease	Inflammatory bowel disease	Urethral diverticulitis
Degenerating fibroids	Diverticulitis	
Neoplasm	Neoplasm	
Ovarian remnant syndrome		

Musculoskeletal	Psychiatric	Neurologic
		Nerve entrapment syndrome
More Common	*More Common*	
Muscular strain	Depression	
Less Common	Physical or sexual abuse	
Myofascial syndrome (trigger points)	Somatization	
Degenerative joint disease	*Less Common*	
Disc disease	Opioid seeking	
Fibromyalgia	Hypochondriasis	

Musculoskeletal-Related Pain

Separation of the pubic symphysis or other *sacroiliac dysfunction* can occur following pregnancy or trauma (Moore et al. 2000). Often, a woman is aware that her symptoms began after a particular event, but sometimes the original insult occurred many years previously and it comes to light only when an additional factor arises, such as deconditioning as a result of reduced exercise or strain from repeated heavy lifting.

Whether *myofascial pain syndromes* exist is controversial, but there is growing emphasis on their role in causing chronic abdominal and pelvic pain (Howard et al. 2000). The most commonly reported condition is pain associated with trigger points (Reiter 1998). A trigger point is a tender nodule located in a palpable band of muscle fibers. Associated pain is usually constant and reproducible, and it does not follow a dermatomal or nerve root distribution. Palpation of the affected muscle by applying sustained deep pressure is the method used most frequently to diagnose trigger points.

Fibromyalgia is chronic, diffuse, muscular pain often associated with chronic fatigue and depressed mood. The American College of Rheumatology criteria for fibromyalgia include a history of widespread pain and at least eleven specific tender points on exam. Women with fibromyalgia commonly have chronic pelvic pain. (See the **Fibromyalgia** chapter in Section 8.)

Psychologic-Related Pain

Depression is the most common psychological cause of chronic pelvic pain. There are a number of theories regarding the link between mental distress and its physical manifestation. Some research suggests that certain personality traits, coping mechanisms, or health beliefs may predispose a person to the development of chronic pain (Moore et al. 2000). Factors that correlate with chronic pain include a tendency to "catastrophize," use of negative coping strategies, a feeling of no control over pain, and a belief that pain represents ongoing tissue damage. Social and cultural factors such as job security, demands on a woman's time, and family roles also may contribute. Other research suggests that depression is more likely a consequence than a cause of chronic pain (McGowan et al. 1998). These studies emphasize that pain compromises quality of life and thus leads to depression.

Trauma such as *domestic violence* and *sexual abuse* also can cause physical and mental illness that manifests as chronic pelvic pain. Some women have had experiences so overwhelming that the experiences may be unspeakable and cannot be processed consciously. When the level of a traumatic experience exceeds a woman's coping mechanisms, she can express the trauma as physical pain. For this reason, always consider past and present history of domestic violence, sexual abuse, and other forms of trauma when a woman presents with chronic pelvic pain.

DATABASE

SUBJECTIVE

→ The most important component in the evaluation of a woman with chronic pelvic pain is the history and physical examination. It is unlikely that a complete evaluation can be performed in one 15-minute office visit. When limited time is available at the first visit, the clinician should establish a

---

Table 12L.2.   OBTAINING A COMPLETE HISTORY OF CHRONIC PELVIC PAIN

General	Gastrointestinal	Musculoskeletal
Past medical history	Constipation	Low back pain
Past surgical history	Diarrhea	Sciatica
Prior evaluations for pelvic pain	Blood in stool	Relation of pain to movement and posture
Medications	Mucus in stool	History of physical trauma
History of chemical dependency	Changes in caliber of stool	
	Increased pain with certain foods, particularly dairy, chocolate, and spices	**Psychosocial**
Pain	Weight loss	Symptoms of depression or anxiety
Character		Suicidal ideation
Severity	**Urinary**	History of physical, sexual, or emotional abuse
Onset	Dysuria	Impact of pain on lifestyle and interpersonal relationships
Location	Urgency	Woman's perception of the cause of the pain
Alleviating and aggravating factors	Frequency	
	Suprapubic pain	
Gynecologic	Costovertebral angle pain	
Relation to menses	Hematuria	
Relation to sexual activity		
New sexual partners		
If heterosexual, method of birth control		

---

relationship with the patient, begin the evaluation, and also set expectations by explaining that because chronic pain is complex, multiple visits may be required. Usually, patients do not mind returning for further appointments if they are told that their problem is not simple and that it is important to allow adequate time for a thorough work-up.

→ Elicit a description of the pain—its character, severity, onset, and modifying factors. Take time to complete a thorough review of systems, focusing especially on the gynecologic, gastrointestinal, urinary, musculoskeletal, and psychiatric systems. (See **Table 12L.2, Obtaining a Complete History of Chronic Pelvic Pain**.)

→ It may be helpful to have patients fill out a health history and pelvic pain questionnaire before their visit if it is known they are coming in for a pelvic pain evaluation. (See **Figure 12L.1, Pain Questionnaire**.) Also useful are pain maps that allow patients to mark the location of their pain. (See **Figure 12L.2, Pain Map**.)

OBJECTIVE

→ As with eliciting a history, the physical examination should focus not just on the gynecologic system, but also on any other systems that may be involved. In particular, consider a woman's affect, examine the abdomen and pelvis, perform a musculoskeletal exam, and check for point-specific tenderness of the abdominal wall. (See **Table 12L.3, Physical Examination Features in the Woman with Chronic Pelvic Pain**.)

ASSESSMENT

→ See the differential diagnoses in the introduction and **Table 12L.1**.

PLAN

DIAGNOSTIC TESTS

→ Laboratory studies:
  ■ The history and physical examination are the most important components of the evaluation. Only a few laboratory studies are recommended for all women with chronic pelvic pain. (See **Table 12L.4, Laboratory Studies Used in the Evaluation of Chronic Pelvic Pain**.) These strongly recommended tests are most useful in identifying inflammatory or infectious conditions that are suspected based on history and physical exam findings. Performing these labs also may provide reassurance.

→ Imaging studies and procedures:
  ■ Many clinicians consider pelvic ultrasound to be an essential component in the evaluation of chronic pelvic pain, while others utilize ultrasonography more selectively, such as when body size limits the physical exam.
    • Ultrasound is a key tool in diagnosing a mass. It occasionally suggests endometriosis.
    • Most diseases that cause chronic pelvic pain will yield a negative ultrasound. Endometriosis and pelvic adhesions require surgery for definitive diagnosis. Irritable bowel syndrome, interstitial cystitis, urethral

---

Table 12L.3.   PHYSICAL EXAMINATION FEATURES IN THE WOMAN WITH CHRONIC PELVIC PAIN

General	Pelvic Exam
Appearance	External genitalia: appearance and tenderness
Affect	Vagina: appearance, discharge, and tenderness
Back	Urethra: discharge, tenderness
Range of motion	Cervix: appearance, discharge, and cervical motion tenderness
Point tenderness (spine, trigger points)	Uterus: size, shape, consistency, and mobility
Costovertebral tenderness	Adnexa: mass, ovarian size, and tenderness
Chest Wall	Rectal: mass, uterosacral ligament nodularity or tenderness, stool (color, mucus, blood)
Point tenderness (trigger points)	**Extremities**
Abdomen	Leg length
Appearance	Tenderness with straight-leg raising or hip abduction
Tenderness	Strength and sensation
Organ enlargement	Gait
Masses	
Bowel sounds	
Bruits	

Source: Adapted with permission from Scialli, A.R. 1999. Evaluating chronic pelvic pain. A consensus recommendation. *Journal of Reproductive Medicine* 44(11):945–952.

syndrome, myofascial trigger points, and depression all will produce negative ultrasound findings.

- Sometimes ultrasound reassures the patient and thus is helpful in coping with chronic pain. On the other hand, clinicians must take care not to communicate that a negative ultrasound invalidates the woman's pain experience.

■ Other imaging studies and procedures may be useful if the history and exam indicate potential pathology in a specific organ system. They include:

- Upper GI series
- Barium enema
- Sigmoidoscopy
- Cystoscopy
- Magnetic resonance imaging
- Hysterosalpingogram

■ Historically, laparoscopy has been considered the gold standard for diagnosing chronic pelvic pain, but its role is somewhat controversial. (See the **Endometriosis** chapter.)

- Although laparoscopy may be helpful in diagnosing endometriosis, many other causes of chronic pain, including musculoskeletal, bladder, and bowel-related syndromes, will produce negative laparoscopic findings.
- Chronic pelvic pain experts increasingly endorse the use of empiric treatment first, followed by laparoscopy only if empiric therapy fails (Peters et al. 1991, Scialli 1999).

Table 12L.4.   LABORATORY STUDIES USED IN THE EVALUATION OF CHRONIC PELVIC PAIN

Strongly recommended tests

CBC including differential

Urinalysis

N. gonorrhoeae and C. trachomatis testing

Tests that may be indicated based on history and exam findings

Vaginal wet smear

Sedimentation rate

Antinuclear antibody, rheumatoid factor, and other tests for auto-antibodies

Stool culture for infectious agents

Stool guaiac

Endometrial biopsy

Source: Adapted with permission from Scialli, A.R. 1999. Evaluating chronic pelvic pain. A consensus recommendation. *Journal of Reproductive Medicine* 44(11):945–952.

TREATMENT/MANAGEMENT

→ If the history, physical, and imaging studies do not suggest a cause of chronic pelvic pain, the primary goal is to relieve suffering and to improve quality of life. Toward this end, empiric therapy should be initiated.

■ Nonsteroidal anti-inflammatory agents (NSAIDs):

- Empiric therapy usually begins with NSAIDs to alleviate pain.
- NSAIDs given on a regular basis at an appropriate dose are typically effective within a few days in women who are going to respond. It is important to dose the medication on a schedule rather than as needed, usually beginning one day before the expected onset of pain. (See the **Dysmenorrhea** chapter.)

■ Hormones: oral and injectable contraceptives and progestin-only methods:

- If antiprostaglandins are insufficient, prescribe a hormonal method to suppress the ovarian cycle.
- First-line agents are oral contraceptives and the progestin-only, injectable contraceptive depo-medroxy-progesterone acetate (DMPA). Between these two choices, it is appropriate to allow patient preference to dictate treatment because there is no proven benefit of one option over the other in treating chronic pelvic pain (Reiter 1998, Schroeder et al. 1999).
  - Endometriosis implants are stimulated by estrogen whereas androgens result in atrophy. Therefore, choose a progestin-dominant, moderately androgenic oral contraceptive.
  - Monophasic pills are preferable to tricyclics. They may be dosed for a withdrawal bleed every 21 days or in a continuous fashion.
    ➤ If symptoms do not improve within 3 months on oral contraceptives, initiate another intervention.
  - The most useful synthetic progestin is DMPA, 150 mg every 3 months. An oral alternative is medroxy-progesterone acetate used as a continuous regimen, 10–30 mg daily.

■ Gonadotropin releasing hormone therapy agonists (GnRHa):

- Women who are not diagnosed after a complete evaluation and who fail to respond to NSAIDs, oral contraceptives, and perhaps antibiotics (see below) should be considered highly likely to have endometriosis or adenomyosis (Scialli 1999).
- Nearly all women with endometriosis will experience dramatic improvement with GnRHa therapy. Therefore, some experts recommend prescribing GnRHa empirically to make a presumptive diagnosis of endometriosis or adenomyosis. The most common regimens are depo-leuprolide acetate 3.75 mg IM every 4 weeks or 11.25 mg IM every 12 weeks (Schroeder et al. 1999). Other experts prefer to confirm a diagnosis of endometriosis before initiating therapy. In either case, physician consultation is warranted.

Figure 12L.1.   PAIN QUESTIONNAIRE

Date:_____   Name: _____

Age: _____   G: _____   P: _____   LMP: _____   Cycle Day: _____

1. Pain Location (List each different location and number it)	2. Date First Noticed	3. Events Preceding Pain	4. Pain Description (Adjectives to describe typical pain; list cycle days)	5. Pain Intensity (Rate each pain)
PAIN LOCATION	ONSET	EVENTS PRECEDING	DESCRIPTION	RATE PAIN FROM 0-10

6. Overall interference of pain with life (0–10)

Work   School   Social activities   Child care   Sports and exercise   Relationships   Other

_____   _____   _____   _____   _____   _____   _____

7. Description of things that:

INCREASE PAIN			**DECREASE PAIN**		
Intercourse	Yes	No	Lying down	Yes	No
Bowel movement	Yes	No	Heating pad	Yes	No
Urination	Yes	No	Hot bath	Yes	No
Physical activities	Yes	No	Medication	Yes	No
Other:	Yes	No	Other:	Yes	No

8. Prior treatment or medical workup:

Surgeries: Date: Diagnosis:
GI Studies: Date: Diagnosis:
Other:

9. Use of Medication:

DATES: **EFFECTIVENESS:**
A.
B.
C.
D.

10. Current symptoms other than pain:

A. Bleeding
B. Bowel probems / nausea
C. Headache
D. Fatigue
E. Other

Source: Reprinted with permission from Carter, J.E. 1996. *Chronic pelvic pain: diagnosis and treatment*, p. 30. Arvada, Colo.: Medical Education Collaborative.

- The side-effect profile for GnRHa reduces its use as a long-term treatment option for most women. The agonist creates a hypoestrogenic environment, causing a pseudo-menopause with effects such as hot flushes and vaginal dryness. In addition, GnRHa carries the risk of trabecular bone loss. To minimize these effects, using an "add back" therapy with an estrogen agent is often recommended (Hornstein et al. 1998, Schroeder et al. 1999).
- Antibiotics:
  - Antibiotics are rarely recommended for chronic pelvic pain because the incidence of infection is not high enough to justify presumptive treatment.
  - Antibiotics are warranted when a woman with chronic pelvic pain and uterine tenderness does not meet standard clinical criteria for endometritis or salpingitis, but she has a positive cervical test for *Neisseria gonorrhoeae* or *Chlamydia trachomatis*, or when she has an endometrial biopsy suggesting chronic endometritis. (For treatment regimen, see the **Pelvic Inflammatory Disease** chapter.)

- Narcotics:
  - Narcotic analgesics are not recommended for treating chronic pelvic pain because there is no proof they provide long-term relief and they have high abuse and addiction potential.
  - These agents have a smooth muscle effect that may exacerbate functional dysmotility disorders.
  - They have a sedating effect that alters cognition and may limit restoration of normal function.
- Oral fiber supplementation and antispasmotics:
  - These may be helpful for dysmotility disorders, including irritable bowel syndrome and constipation. (See Section 7, **Gastrointestinal Disorders**.)
  - Oral fiber supplementation increases stool bulk and water content and decreases transit time, relieving pain and constipation. Most constipation sufferers benefit from 20–30 g of fiber daily. Synthetic fiber such as methylcellulose and psyllium are more water soluble than natural fiber and may cause less gas and bloating.
  - Antispasmodic agents such as dicyclomine (10–20 mg

FIGURE 12L.2.   PAIN MAP

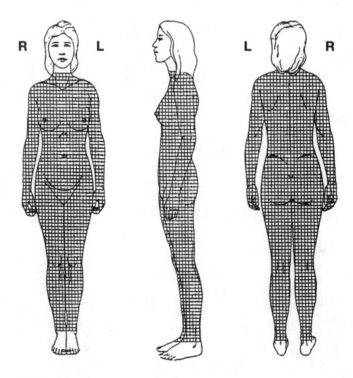

Source: Reprinted with permission from Carter, J.E. 1996. *Chronic pelvic pain: diagnosis and treatment*, p. 31. Arvada, Colo.: Medical Education Collaborative.

p.o. TID to QID initially—may be increased to 40 mg QID if tolerated) help reduce sigmoid motility in response to fat and decrease postprandial pain, gas, and bloating. Of the antispasmotics, dicyclomine is the most selective agent and has the fewest side effects.

- Antidepressants:
  - Antidepressants have been shown to reduce depressive symptoms related to chronic pain syndromes.
  - The tricyclic antidepressants imipramine and amitriptyline generally are considered first-line among antidepressants for treating chronic pain because they have been shown to improve pain tolerance, restore normal sleep, and reduce depression associated with chronic pain (Reiter 1998).
  - Selective serotonin reuptake inhibitors are less well studied in relationship to chronic pelvic pain, but they are commonly used as first-line therapy for depression and may be useful for chronic pain sufferers who have associated depression.
  - For further discussion of antidepressants and their use, see Section 14, **Behavioral Disorders**.
- Treatments for *myofascial syndrome*:
  - Abdominal wall trigger points are amenable to treatment with a variety of modalities, including transcutaneous electric nerve stimulation, acupuncture, and local anesthetic injections.
  - Musculoskeletal pain also may respond to physical therapy and to stretch-and-release massage techniques. Refer to a specialist.
- Cognitive-behavioral therapy and psychotherapy:
  - Many different modalities may be helpful in addressing the psychosocial component of chronic pelvic pain.
  - Classes focusing on relaxation, stress management, and coping with pain may help some women, whereas others benefit more from individual psychotherapy. Therapy should involve concrete goal-setting and behavioral modification techniques.
  - Early childhood issues, past abuses, and any unresolved grief issues may need to be dealt with.

PATIENT EDUCATION

→ The rapport between the clinician and the woman with chronic pain is a key element in successful treatment. Rapport relies on continuous, open communication and education.

- Set realistic expectations.
  - Inform the patient that a complete work-up for chronic pain likely will require more than one visit.
  - Outline a diagnosis and treatment plan, including the history and physical exam, diagnostic tests, and management options so the patient is included as a partner in her care and has realistic expectations.
- After the diagnosis, focus on pain relief.
  - If an underlying condition is not diagnosed, the goal of treatment is to alleviate pain and disability.

- Explain to the patient that in some cases, there may never be a clear diagnosis, but that a high degree of pain relief is possible.
- Attend to psychosocial issues.
  - If psychosocial issues play a major role in the chronic pain, support and encourage the patient to follow through with behavioral and psychological assessment and validate her bravery in confronting depression, abuse, or trauma.
- Consult with other clinicians caring for the patient.
  - With the patient's consent, all consultants should agree on an approach to treatment and should communicate regularly about her progress.
- Do not neglect drug dependency.
  - If necessary, address drug dependency. The patient should understand why long-term narcotic use has no place in management.

FOLLOW-UP

→ As noted above, patients likely will need to be seen several times. Although multiple appointments are arranged out of necessity, one advantage is that they often give the clinician and patient an opportunity to develop a strong rapport.

→ Do not hesitate to engage in topics other than the pain component. Learning about the whole person usually helps the clinician diagnose the etiology of the pain and understand its effects.

→ Document carefully in the progress notes and on the problem list.

BIBLIOGRAPHY

Balasch, J., Creus, M., Fabreques, F. et al. 1996. Visible and nonvisible endometriosis at laparoscopy in fertile and infertile women and in patients with chronic pelvic pain: a prospective study. *Human Reproduction* 11(2):387–391.

Carlson, K.J., and Eisenstat, S.A. 1995 *Primary care of women*. St. Louis, Mo.: Mosby.

Gelbaya, T.A., El-Halwagy, H.E. 2001. Focus on primary care: chronic pelvic pain in women. *Obstetrics and Gynecology Survey* 56(12):57–64.

Harris, R.D., Holtzmann, S.R., and Poppe, A.M. 2000. Clinical outcome in female patients with pelvic pain and normal pelvic U.S. findings. *Radiology* 216(2):440–443.

Hornstein, M.D., Surrey, E.C., Weisberg, G.W. et al. 1998. Leuprolide acetate depot and hormonal add-back in endometriosis: a 12 month study. *Obstetrics and Gynecology* 91(1):16–24.

Howard, F.M., Perry, C.P., Carter, J.E. et al. 2000. *Pelvic pain diagnosis and management*. Philadelphia: Lippincott Williams & Wilkins.

Mathias, S.C., Kuppermann, M., Liberman, R.F. et al. 1996. Chronic pelvic pain: prevalence, health-related quality of life, and economic correlates. *Obstetrics and Gynecology* 87(3):321–327.

Matorras, R., Rodriquez, F., Pijoan, J.L. et al. 1996. Are there any clinical signs and symptoms that are related to endometriosis in infertile women? *American Journal of Obstetrics and Gynecology* 174(2):620–623.

McGowan, L.A., Clark-Carter, D.D., and Pitts, M.K. 1998. Chronic pelvic pain: a meta-analytic review. *Psychology and Health* 13:937–951.

Moore, J., and Kennedy, S. 2000. Causes of chronic pelvic pain. *Bailliere's Clinical Obstetrics and Gynaecology* 14(3): 389–402.

Olive, D.L. 2000. New approaches to the management of fibroids. *Current Reproductive Endocrinology* 27(3): 669–675.

Peters, A.A., van Dorst, E., Jellis, B. et al. 1991. A randomized clinical trial to compare two different approaches in women with chronic pelvic pain. *Obstetrics and Gynecology* 77(5): 740–744.

Reiter, R.C. 1998. Evidence-based management of chronic pelvic pain. *Clinical Obstetrics and Gynecology* 41(2): 422–435.

Rickert, V.I., and Kozlowski, K.J. 2000. Pelvic pain, a SAFE approach. *Obstetrics and Gynecology Clinics of North America* 27(1):181–193.

Schroeder, B., and Sanfilippo, J.S. 1999. Dysmenorrhea and pelvic pain in adolescents. *Pediatric Clinics of North America* 46(3):555–571.

Scialli, A.R. 1999. Evaluating chronic pelvic pain. A consensus recommendation. *Journal of Reproductive Medicine* 44(11):945–952.

12-M

Perimenopausal and Menopausal Symptoms and Hormone Therapy

Menopause, the cessation of menstruation, occurs at an average age of 51 years (American College of Obstetricians and Gynecologists [ACOG] 2000). Ovulatory frequency begins to decrease at approximately 40 years of age (Speroff et al. 1999). This change marks the beginning of the decreased fertility and reduced estrogen production that characterizes the transition to menopause. Forty million American women have reached the menopausal period and an additional 20 million women will be entering this time within the next 10 years (Finkel et al. 2001). As our current life expectancy is greater than 76 years, most of these women will spend one-third of their lives after menopause.

Menopause has been defined by the World Health Organization (1994) as the permanent cessation of menstruation due to loss of ovarian follicular activity and is clinically defined as 12 months of amenorrhea. *Perimenopause* is defined as the 2–8 years before menopause and the one year after the final menses. *Premenopause* is a poorly characterized period before *perimenopause*, and *postmenopause* is the entire span of life following the last menses. Menopause before 40 years of age is considered premature and is defined as *premature ovarian failure* (North American Menopause Society [NAMS] Consensus Opinion 2000).

Induced menopause is the result of a medical or surgical intervention (e.g., bilateral oophorectomy, postoperative compromise of the ovarian blood supply, or ovarian failure due to chemotherapy). When menopause is induced, the cessation of menstrual function occurs precipitously and symptoms vary depending on the age of the woman (NAMS Consensus Opinion 2000). Induced menopause in a young woman may result in severe somatic and affective changes not observed in an older woman whose body has begun to adapt to the hormonal and physiological changes of menopause. In addition, women who have had a surgically induced menopause may be more at risk for serious health problems (e.g., earlier development of heart disease and accelerated bone loss leading to osteoporosis) than are women who experience natural menopause (Manson et al. 2001).

The perimenopause is a time when the initial endocrinological and physiological alterations leading to menopause are observed. During a woman's forties and even thirties, the oocytes begin to undergo rapid depletion leading ultimately to the end of ovulation (NAMS Consensus Opinion 2000). The reduced ovarian function results in reduced levels of estrogen and progesterone. In response, the pituitary releases greater levels of follicle-stimulating hormone (FSH) in an attempt to stimulate the ovary to increase estrogen production (Speroff et al. 1999). As a result, FSH levels are often elevated during this time, though levels of estradiol and luteinizing hormone may stay normal. Persistently elevated levels of FSH overstimulate a still-functional ovary, leading to a further decline in ovarian activity (Speroff et al. 1999).

The gradual decline of estrogen production results in a progressive loss of estrogen-dependent functions: ovulation, menstruation, and vaginal, vulvar, and urethral tissue integrity. As the levels of circulating estrogen decrease, women may begin to experience perimenopausal and menopausal symptoms. The occurrence of vasomotor instability (hot flashes, night sweats), psychological dysfunction (anxiety, mood changes, and irritability), and vaginal and urinary tract atrophy are common and may have a negative impact on quality of life (Brown et al. 2001). The long-term effects of estrogen deficiency—osteoporosis and an increased risk of cardiovascular disease—are also serious consequences (ACOG 2000, NAMS Consensus Opinion 2000, Speroff et al. 1999).

Menstrual cycle irregularity is considered a hallmark of the perimenopausal transition. Menstrual cycle duration may shorten and the amount of flow may decrease (NAMS Consensus Opinion 2000). Patterns of shorter cycles alternating with longer cycles may occur. Cycles may be missed altogether for several months only to recur and return to regularity for a while (NAMS Consensus Opinion 2000). Sexually active women in the perimenopausal transition are considered at risk for pregnancy until at least one year of amenorrhea or until levels of FSH remain consistently elevated above 30 mIU/mL (NAMS Consensus Opinion 2000).

Symptoms of the perimenopausal and menopausal phases vary from woman to woman. Women may begin to experience an array of physical, emotional, and cognitive symptoms long before they experience alterations in their menstrual cycle. Acute symptoms in the perimenopause include vasomotor symptoms, sleep disturbances, and exacerbation of premenstrual syndrome and premenstrual dysphoric disorder (see the **Premenstrual Syndrome and Premenstrual Dysphoric Disorder** chapter) as well as cycle changes (NAMS Consensus Opinion 2000).

Other physiological systems may demonstrate age-related changes not directly related to estrogen depletion. Obesity, diabetes, thyroid disease, and hypertension are observed during the perimenopausal and menopausal years. These physiological alterations occur in concert with many other psychosocial challenges of midlife: Marital, familial, social, and emotional alterations are numerous in the perimenopausal and menopausal woman (ACOG 2000, NAMS Consensus Opinion 2000).

Entrance into these transitional years can present an opportunity to help women make healthy life choices. Developing a flexible, multidimensional health maintenance program is a goal of the health care provider (Finkel et al. 2001). All perimenopausal and menopausal women will benefit from making healthy lifestyle choices. Exercise (weight-bearing/weight-training and aerobic exercises), a nutritious and balanced diet (especially adequate calcium and vitamin D intake), avoidance of tobacco use, moderate alcohol use, and stress management are several desirable choices (ACOG 2000, NAMS Consensus Opinion 2000).

The use of hormone replacement therapy (HRT) is an option for managing perimenopausal and menopausal symptoms and reducing osteoporosis risk. Approximately 30–40% of women in the United States use HRT (Manson et al. 2001). Bisphosphonates and selective estrogen receptor modulators (SERM) are options for reducing osteoporosis risk. Additional options include complementary and alternative medications, and other types of nontraditional treatments for vasomotor and psychological symptom management.

Hormone Replacement Therapy

HRT refers to a combination of estrogen and progestogen that reduces the symptoms of vasomotor instability and the risk of osteoporosis. Women with an intact uterus need progestogen to reduce their risk of developing endometrial cancer (Woodruff et al. 1994). Estrogen replacement therapy (ERT) is appropriate for women without a uterus for whom progestogen is not required (Finkel et al. 2001).

Although many older observational studies have generally supported the use of HRT, newer data from randomized, well-controlled clinical studies have resulted in reconsideration of the use of HRT for menopausal women (Manson et al. 2001). Concerns regarding the effectiveness of lower doses of HRT recently have been evaluated in response to the desire of patients to reduce the potential risks of HRT and to minimize side effects (Speroff et al. 2001). The Women's Heart, Osteoporosis, Progestin, and Estrogen study evaluated the use of various doses of conjugated equine estrogens (CEE) (0.625 mg, 0.45 mg, 0.3 mg) in combination with varying amounts of medroxyprogesterone

acetate (MPA) (1.5 mg, 2.5 mg). Results indicated that lower-dose combinations of CEE and MPA were well-tolerated and provided many of the same benefits of HRT at higher doses (Speroff et al. 2001). Longer-term management recommendations will be developed further as the results of many prospective, well-designed clinical trials become available (ACOG Practice Bulletin 2001).

Benefits of Hormone Replacement Therapy

Menopausal and Vascular Symptoms

Approximately 80% of women in the United States report perimenopausal or menopausal symptoms such as hot flashes, night sweats, insomnia, mood swings, memory loss, fatigue, emotional lability, or depression (Dennerstein et al. 2000, NAMS Consensus Opinion 2000). Evidence from recent randomized clinical trials has continued to show that HRT is an effective therapy in reducing these symptoms, as noted in the Heart and Estrogen/Progestin Replacement Study (HERS) (Hlatky et al. 2002). Although the precise etiology of hot flashes is not known, estrogen therapy reduces their frequency in a dose-dependent manner (NAMS Consensus Opinion 2000). Although hot flashes have been noted to disrupt daily activities and quality of sleep, few quantitative assessments of the impact of hot flashes on quality of life have been performed (Dennerstein et al. 2000). Hot flashes also have been associated with palpitations and feelings of anxiety. Women using HRT for vascular symptoms also may experience improvement in mental health and depressive symptoms (Hlatky et al. 2002).

Genitourinary Symptoms

The use of vaginal estrogen creams and other topical systems can alleviate atrophic vaginal and urogenital effects and have reduced the risk of recurrent urinary tract infections in some clinical trials. Oral HRT has not demonstrated similar findings (Brown et al. 2001). The use of vaginal estrogen creams and systems may still require the administration of a progestogen to prevent endometrial hyperplasia (Finkel et al. 2001).

Osteoporosis

Estrogen plays an important role in inhibiting demineralization of bone. After menopause, bone demineralization occurs faster than bone resorption, resulting in accelerated bone loss. It is estimated that one-quarter of all women older than 60 years will develop osteoporotic vertebral fractures. Of these osteoporotic women, 15% also will have hip fractures in their lifetimes (Marcus et al. 1996). Osteoporosis is responsible for increased mortality and morbidity among postmenopausal women. It is more common than the aggregate of cervical, endometrial, ovarian, and breast cancer (Simon et al. 2001). (See the **Osteoporosis** chapter in Section 10.)

Estrogen administration in menopause can substantially decrease the rate of bone loss and improve bone density (Finkel et al. 2001, Speroff et al. 1999). Unfortunately, if a woman stops HRT, she begins to lose bone mass at the rapid rate noted in early menopause (Cummings et al. 1998). Although estrogen has been considered an appropriate agent for osteoporosis prevention and treatment, few prospective, well-controlled, randomized clinical trials have been performed to confirm the role of estrogen in treating established osteoporosis. The U.S. Food and Drug Administration (FDA) has removed estrogen from the list of medications for treating osteoporosis until the results of several ongoing trials are available. Alternate medications—bisphosphonates (alendronate and risedronate) and raloxifene (a SERM)—have been found to be effective in preventing and treating osteoporosis (National Osteoporosis Foundation [NOF] 1998).

Risks and Controversies of Hormone Replacement Therapy

Endometrial Cancer

Many observational studies have demonstrated clearly that the long-term use of estrogen, unopposed by concomitant or cyclic administration of a progestogen, increases the risk of endometrial cancer by a factor of 8–10 (Manson et al. 2001). The Post-menopausal Estrogen/Progestin Interventions Trial (1995) demonstrated the development of atypical endometrial hyperplasia in 24% of women who were assigned to unopposed estrogen therapy for three years compared to the development of hyperplasia in only 1% of women in the placebo group. The risk increases with duration of exposure and dosage of estrogen, and may persist for up to 10 years after estrogen in discontinued (Grady et al. 1995).

Breast Cancer

The incidence of breast cancer rises as women age. Factors associated with prolonged exposure to estrogen (nulliparity, late or no child-bearing, early menarche) are strongly associated with an increased risk of breast cancer (Speroff et al. 1999). Observational and prospective studies of women using HRT have provided somewhat contradictory results regarding an increased risk of breast cancer (Bush 2001). In some studies, combined estrogen-progestin regimens have been found to increase breast cancer risk more than estrogen alone does (Schairer et al. 2000). A clinical arm of the Women's Health Initiative, which compared outcomes of prospectively randomized women who were taking daily combined conjugated equine estrogen (0.625 mg) and medroxyprogesterone acetate (2.5 mg), was recently discontinued due to a significant risk of invasive breast cancer in the treatment group (Writing Group for the Women's Health Initiative Investigators 2002). The clinical trial of hysterectomized, randomized women taking daily conjugated equine estrogens continues, but results have not been released (Writing Group for the Women's Health Initiative Investigators 2002).

Cardiovascular Disease and Stroke

Although numerous observational studies in the past have supported the use of HRT in menopausal women for preventing heart disease, data from recent randomized, placebo-controlled, clinical trials have challenged its benefit in this regard (Hulley et al. 1998). In the Heart and Estrogen/Progestin Replacement Study (HERS), the effect of HRT on the risk of cardiovascular events and nonfatal myocardial infarction among the 2,763 women with documented coronary disease was similar to the risk in the placebo group. A disturbing finding in this study was a 50% increase of coronary heart disease events among women with known cardiac disease during the first year of the study, although this finding was ultimately offset by the decreased overall cardiovascular risk (Manson et al. 2001). The WHI has also identified an increased risk for cerebrovascular accidents (CVA) or strokes, although the earlier HERS study did not identify a similar risk. The American Heart Association recently has published recommendations for using HRT in managing heart disease risk (Mosca et al. 2001). In women with established cardiovascular disease (CVD), HRT should not be recommended for secondary prevention. Women who are already taking HRT may continue based on noncoronary benefits, risks, and preferences. Women who develop an acute CVD event or stroke, or who require long-term immobilization, should discontinue HRT. Initiation and continuance of HRT for women without CVD also should be based on established noncoronary benefits and patient preference.

The Women's Health Initiative, sponsored by the National Institutes of Health, has produced results that further define the relationship between HRT and coronary disease. The initiative study was designed to define and clarify the risks and benefits of HRT with regard to heart disease, breast and colorectal cancers, and fractures in postmenopausal women. One of the clinical trials, which examined the use of combined conjugated equine estrogens with medroxyprogesterone acetate (Prempro® 0.625 mg/2.5 mg) in women with a uterus, was stopped early after finding that health risks for coronary heart disease, as well as risks for invasive breast cancer, had surpassed benefits (Writing Group for the Women's Health Initiative Investigators 2002). The trials involving estrogen alone for women with a hysterectomy continue and will further define the relationships between ERT and coronary disease and breast cancer. The results of these trials are not necessarily applicable to lower-dose regimens or to other formulations of estrogens and progestins in oral or transdermal use. Also, the data from this study cannot be directly applied to the use of HRT by symptomatic women in the perimenopause nor to women with early or premature menopause (Writing Group for the Women's Health Initiative Investigators 2002).

The North American Menopause Society has reviewed these findings and has recommended that no HRT regimen be used for the primary or secondary prevention of coronary heart disease. Alternate, clinically proven, and established therapies to prevent or reduce coronary heart disease should be utilized.

Venous Thromboembolism

Numerous observational studies have identified an increased risk of deep venous thromboembolism by a factor of 2–3.5 (Grady et al. 2000). Other recent randomized clinical trials have confirmed this increased risk (Grady et al. 1995, Speroff et al. 1996). Both the Women's Health Initiative and the HERS have found a significant increased risk of venous thromboembolism (Hulley et al. 1998, Writing Group for the Women's Health Initiative Investigators 2002). Risk of stroke may also increase as a consequence of increased venous thrombotic events (Finkel et al. 2001).

Gall Bladder Disease

Many of the older observational studies and more recent clinical trials have demonstrated an increased risk of gallstones and cholecystectomy among women using HRT or ERT. The HERS study also noted a significant increased risk of cholecystectomy among women using HRT (Hulley et al. 1998). Metabolic studies indicate that estrogen causes an increase in biliary cholesterol and cholelithiasis (Hulley et al. 1998, Manson et al. 2001).

Colorectal Cancer

Data from observational studies have suggested that women using HRT may have a decreased risk of colorectal cancer. Utilizing results from the Nurses' Health Study, Grodstein and colleagues (1998) found that current hormone users had a relative risk of 0.64. A recent meta-analysis of data revealed significant inconsistencies among the studies regarding the development of colorectal cancer and the use of HRT (Nanda et al. 1999). The Women' Health Initiative also has found a significant decreased risk for colon cancer (Writing Group for the Women's Health Initiative Investigators 2002).

Ovarian Cancer

One large prospective study of postmenopausal women has shown a significant, though small, increase of ovarian cancer with the long-term use of HRT or ERT (for more than 10 years) (Rodriguez et al. 2001). An earlier large prospective study also found a significant increase among women who used HRT for more than six years (Rodriguez et al. 1995). However, Hartge et al. (1988), in a hospital-based, case-control study, found a significantly reduced risk of ovarian cancer in women using HRT. This study was shorter than the later studies, a flaw that may reduce the applicability of these results.

Results of a recent, retrospective, observational study of women at high risk of developing ovarian cancer also have shown a statistically significant increase in risk of developing ovarian cancer among those who used ERT only, especially after 10 years (Lacey et al. 2002).

Neurological Effects

Studies have examined the relationship between the decline in endogenous estrogen and the development of Alzheimer's disease. Estrogen was purported to increase neurotransmitter synthesis or improve blood flow to the brain; however, results from large, randomized, controlled clinical trials have not supported this view (Finkel et al. 2001). The current information released from the Women's Health Initiative did not include data regarding cognitive function (Writing Group for the Women's Health Initiative Investigators 2002).

Additional Therapies

Androgen

Androgens, produced in the ovary and adrenal glands, are the source of all steroidal estrogens (Davis 2000). With the reduction of functional ovarian follicles in the perimenopause and menopause, the burden of androgen production is borne by the adrenal glands (Naftolin 1994). Specifically androstenedione and testosterone undergo "peripheral conversion" in body fat (and possibly brain and bone tissues) to estrone and estradiol (Watts 2002).

Androgens are considered precursors to estrogen production but also have androgenic effects that increase the sense of well-being, improve libido, and possibly reduce osteoporosis risk. Androgens have been added to some HRT regimens for these effects but do not have FDA approval for this use (Watts 2002).

Complementary and Alternative Therapies

Alternatives to conventional hormone therapy are quite common and often are perceived as more gentle, healthy, and free of side effects (ACOG 2001). The phytoestrogens in many legumes have been promoted as an alternative to HRT in managing vasomotor symptoms. Soy beans, in particular, contain isoflavones that function as weak estrogens. Randomized clinical trials have not yet identified the effectiveness of isoflavones in reducing the risk of cardiovascular disease and osteoporosis (Fugh-Berman 2000). Several other herbal and botanical remedies, dietary supplements, vitamins, and minerals also are marketed for managing menopausal symptoms and, in some cases, reducing osteoporosis risk (ACOG 2001). Because these alternatives are sold as supplements, they have not been evaluated for safety and efficacy by the FDA and long-term data are not available. Quality, dosage, and safety issues are also of concern (ACOG 2001).

DATABASE

SUBJECTIVE

→ Symptomatology of the perimenopausal transition is highly variable, regardless of race, socioeconomic status, ethnicity, or culture. Some women report few or no symptoms and others report extreme distress and discomfort.

→ Symptoms may include:
  - Vasomotor instability:
    - Hot flashes (vary in frequency/intensity; may continue for a few months to years)
    - Night sweats
    - Dizziness
    - Nausea
    - Lightheadedness
    - Palpitations
    - Nervousness
    - Insomnia
    - Sleep disturbance
    - Fatigue (secondary to nocturnal hot flashes)
  - Oligomenorrhagia, polymenorrhea
  - Menorrhagia, metrorrhagia, hypomenorrhea, menometrorrhagia, amenorrhea

- Gastrointestinal symptoms: appetite changes, constipation, bloating
- Genitourinary symptoms: vaginal dryness, pruritis, or discharge; urinary urgency, frequency, dysuria, or stress urinary incontinence
- Affective symptoms: depression, irritability, emotional lability, tension, heightened stress response
- Physical discomfort: headaches, breast tenderness, musculoskeletal aches and pains
- Cognitive changes: decreased concentration, forgetfulness, short-term memory loss
- Sexual changes: decreased libido, reduced arousal, dyspareunia

NOTE: Symptoms may be more severe and persist longer in women who undergo early surgical menopause. Symptom severity declines in 1–5 years. However, vaginal atrophy may persist and may worsen with time.

→ Gynecological history:
- Menstrual cycle changes
- Abnormal bleeding patterns
- Change in sexual desire, orgasmic potential, lubrication; dyspareunia
- Use of contraceptives
- Fibroids, endometriosis
- Cancer of the breast, uterus, ovaries, cervix; abnormal cervical cytology

→ Complete medical/surgical history:
- Major medical illness: cardiovascular, liver, gallbladder disease, cancer, diabetes, hypertension, obesity, arthritis, coagulopathies
- Surgeries
- Mental health
- Medications, including current and previous hormone use
- Habits: smoking, drugs, alcohol, exercise, nutrition

→ Psychosocial history:
- Living situation
- Social support
- Economic stability
- Life event changes
- Coping/stress management skills

→ Family history:
- Cardiovascular disease, hypertension, cerebrovascular accident (CVA)
- Breast, uterine, ovarian cancer
- Hypercholesterolemia, triglyceridemia
- Osteoporosis

→ Osteoporosis risk factors (see also the **Osteoporosis** chapter in Section 10):
- Low bone density
- Age
- Caucasian or Asian race
- History of fracture in adulthood
- Family history of osteoporosis
- Small stature, low weight (<127 lbs.) (NOF 1998)
- Smoking

- History of eating disorder, hyperthyroidism, hyperparathyroidism, gastric/small-bowel resection
- Low lifetime calcium intake
- Long-term use of corticosteroids
- Inactivity

→ Cardiovascular risk factors:
- Recent myocardial infarction, CVA, transient ischemic attack
- Acute thrombosis or emboli, coagulation disorders
- Established hypertension
- Family history of early-onset coronary artery disease, hypercholesterolemia, hyperlipidemia, hypertriglyceridemia

---

OBJECTIVE

→ Physical examination (Schnare 2002):
- Height, weight, vital signs: Compare with previous findings, if available. Yearly evaluation of height may assist in diagnosis of vertebral compression fracture of osteoporosis. (See the **Osteoporosis** chapter in Section 10.)
- Mental/sensory status, affect: Assess for signs of anxiety, depression; cognitive function loss; sensory loss; memory loss.
- General: Assess for increased facial hair, increased/decreased skin pigmentation, changes in body contour (kyphosis), stature, carriage, and gait.
- Head, eyes, ears, nose, throat: Assess for masses, lesions. Perform a funduscopic examination and check visual acuity as indicated.
- Neck: Assess for lymphadenopathy.
- Thyroid: Assess for thyromegaly, masses.
- Heart and lungs: Assess for signs of cardiorespiratory disease.
- Back: Assess for scoliosis and kyphosis.
- Breasts: Assess for masses, skin/nipple changes, axillary and supraclavicular lymphadenopathy, galactorrhea, atrophy of breast tissue.
- Abdomen: Assess for organomegaly, masses, scars, tenderness. Monitor for multiple skin folds (may indicate vertebral compression fractures).
- Extremities: Assess for edema, varicosities, skin lesions, peripheral pulses.
- Complete pelvic examination (a lateral recumbent position may be more comfortable for sexually inactive women, women with osteoarthritis, or women with a history of hip fracture):
  - External genitalia/urethra: Assess for thinning or fusion of labia.
  - Vagina: Assess vault (may be foreshortened); assess for paleness/erythema of vaginal epithelium, atrophy of vaginal mucosa, vaginal dryness, loss of rugae, petechial hemorrhage, lesions, signs of infection. Assess muscle tone and for cystocele, rectocele, uterine descent.
  - Cervix: Assess color, texture, patency of os (may become stenotic). Cervical portio may no longer protrude into vagina and become flush with vault.

- Uterus: Assess size, contour, consistency, mobility, tenderness. (The uterus decreases in size after menopause.)
- Adnexa: Assess for pelvic masses, tenderness. (The ovaries should be nonpalpable in a postmenopausal woman.)
- Rectovaginal: Assess for masses; occult blood analysis as needed.
→ Additional objective findings:
  - Wet mount may reveal:
    - An increased number of basal and parabasal cells/white blood cells. (See the **Atrophic Vaginitis** chapter.)
    - Reduced lactobacilli
    - Concomitant infection: bacterial vaginosis, trichomoniasis, candidiasis. (See the appropriate **Vaginitis** chapters.)
  - Cytological evaluation (Pap smear) may reveal atypia associated with atrophic changes of the cervix.
  - Mammography may reveal "fatty replacement" of glandular breast tissue.

ASSESSMENT

→ R/O menopause (natural or surgically induced)
→ R/O premature ovarian failure
→ R/O perimenopausal symptoms
→ R/O osteoporosis
→ R/O cardiovascular disease
→ R/O mental health problems
→ R/O abnormal uterine bleeding
→ R/O pregnancy
→ R/O urinary tract/vaginal infection

PLAN

DIAGNOSTIC TESTS

→ Self-assessment: Self-evaluation of symptoms will be a useful first step in evaluating the perimenopausal and postmenopausal woman.
  - Prospective charting for 1–2 menstrual cycles (or 1–2 months if the cycle is irregular) may be undertaken by the patient using a symptom checklist or calendar method.
  - The method should include a severity rating scale for women to record their symptom experiences. (See the **Premenstrual Syndrome and Premenstrual Dysphoric Disorder** chapter.)
→ Perimenopausal history: Evaluate the woman's complete medical history and risk factors.
→ Additional diagnostic studies related to age, risk status, symptoms:
  - Cytological evaluation of the cervix (Pap smear):
    - The frequency of Pap smear intervals should be based on history and risk factors (Schnare 2002).
      - Consider a Pap smear interval of 1–3 years for women with a history of normal Pap smears.
      - Women with a history of abnormal Pap smears or human papillomavirus infection will require Pap smears every year.
      - For women without a cervix due to hysterectomy for

benign disease, no Pap smear is required. If the hysterectomy was for cervical cancer or severe dysplasia, Pap smears should be performed yearly.

- Atypical (nondysplastic) changes may be observed in women with cervical or vaginal atrophy. Treat with a vaginal estrogen cream and repeat the Pap smear after treatment.
      - Colposcopy may be required if Pap smear abnormality persists or worsens. (See also the **Abnormal Cervical Cytology** chapter.)

    NOTE: Perform careful sampling, as the squamocolumnar junction recedes into the endocervical canal with age.
  - Microscopic examination of vaginal secretions as indicated to assess for the presence of vaginal infection or atrophy
  - Mammography: The use of mammography in the years between 40–50 is controversial, but every two years has been the most widely accepted interval. However, yearly mammograms should be performed after 50 years of age.
  - Complete blood count or hemoglobin/hematocrit as indicated
  - TSH as indicated. (Subclinical thyroid disease exists in up to 17% of women older than 40 years [Schnare 2002].)
  - Urinalysis as indicated
  - Stool for occult blood as indicated
  - Flexible sigmoidoscopy, as indicated
  - Fasting blood glucose, particularly if there is a family history of diabetes
  - Lipid profile: total cholesterol, triglycerides, HDL, LDL. (See the **Hyperlipidemia** chapter in Section 6 for specifics as indicated.)
  - Liver function tests as indicated
  - FSH, estradiol levels as indicated
  - Dual-energy x-ray absorptiometry (DXA) of the spine and hip (particularly in cases where the woman is considering HRT for osteoporosis prevention but requires more data to assist in decision-making). (See the **Osteoporosis** chapter in Section 10.)
    - The World Health Organization (WHO) has developed bone mineral density (BMD) measurements to standardize the diagnostic criteria for osteoporosis. The T-score refers to the number of standard deviations above or below the average BMD for healthy, 27-year-old white women. A T-score of 0 represents the peak bone mass. The WHO has established that T-scores below –2.5 constitute osteoporosis, that T-scores between –1.0 and –2.5 indicate osteopenia, and that T-scores above –1.0 are within the range of normal values (NIH Consensus Statement 2000).
    - The decision to obtain BMD evaluation should be based on an individual risk assessment.
  - Endometrial biopsy (EMB) as indicated for abnormal bleeding in the perimenopausal or menopausal period, or when on HRT
    - Women in higher-risk categories for endometrial changes include those who are obese or who have

Table 12M.1.   HORMONAL PREPARATIONS

Brand Name	Type of Hormone	Available Dosages (mg)
Oral Estrogens		
Cenestin®	Synthetic conjugated estrogens	0.625, 0.9, 1.25
Estrace®	Micronized estradiol	0.5, 1.0, 2.0
Estratab®	Esterified estrogens	0.3, 0.625, 2.5
Menest®	Esterified estrogens	0.3, 0.625, 1.25, 2.5
Ogen®	Estropipate	0.625, 1.25, 2.5
Ortho-Est®	Estropipate	0.625, 1.25
Premarin®	Conjugated equine estrogens	0.3, 0.625, 0.9, 1.25, 2.5
Transdermal Estrogens (Patches)		
Alora®	Transdermal estradiol	0.05, 0.075, 0.1
Climara®	Transdermal estradiol	0.025, 0.05, 0.06, 0.075, 0.1
Estraderm®	Transdermal estradiol	0.05, 0.1
Esclim®	Transdermal estradiol	0.025, 0.0375, 0.05, 0.075, 0.1
Vivelle®/Vivelle-Dot®	Transdermal estradiol	0.025, 0.0375, 0.05, 0.075, 0.1
Vaginal Estrogens		
Estrace Cream®	Micronized estradiol	1.0/gm
Ogen Vaginal Cream®	Estropipate	1.5/gm
Ortho-Dienestrol®	Dienestrol	0.1%
Premarin Vaginal Cream®	Conjugated equine estrogens	0.625 mg/gm
Estring®	Estradiol	2-mg reservoir
Vagifem®	Estradiol vaginal tablets	25 mcg
Progestogens		
Amen®	Medroxyprogesterone acetate	10
Aygestin®	Norethindrone acetate	5
Cycrin®	Medroxyprogesterone acetate	2.5, 5, 10
Megace®	Megestrol acetate	20, 40, 40 suspended
Micronor®	Norethindrone	0.35
Nor-QD®	Norethindrone	0.35
Ovrette®	d,l-norgestrel	0.075
Progesterones		
Prometrium®	Micronized oral progesterone Progesterone vaginal suppository	100, 200 25, 50
Oral Androgens		
Android®	Methyltestosterone	10
Halotestin®	Fluoxymesterone	2, 5, 10
Testred®	Methyltestosterone	10
Estrogen/Androgen or Progestogen Combinations		
Activella®	Estradiol Norethindrone acetate	1.0 0.05
CombiPatch®	Estradiol Norethindrone acetate	0.05 0.14, 0.25
Estratest tablets®	Esterified estrogens Methyltestosterone	1.25 2.5
Estratest HS tablets®	Esterified estrogens Methyltestosterone	0.625 1.25
FemHRT®	Ethinyl estradiol Norethindrone acetate	0.5 1.0
Prempro®	Conjugated estrogens Medroxyprogesterone acetate	0.45, 0.625 1.5, 2.5, 5
Premphase®	Conjugated estrogens (CE) Conjugated estrogens/medroxyprogesterone acetate (MPA)	0.625 0.625 CE with 5 MPA
Ortho-Prefest®	Estradiol Estradiol/norgestimate (repeated 6-day cycle of estradiol for 3 days, then combination of estradiol/norgestimate for 3 days)	1.0 1.0 estradiol/0.09 norgestimate

Source: *Physicians' Desk Reference* 2002; Rugierro, R., personal communication, April 2002.

diabetes, dysfunctional uterine bleeding, anovulation, infertility, high alcohol intake, hepatic disease, or hypothyroidism (Speroff et al. 1999).

- Abnormal uterine bleeding usually is defined as (NAMS Consensus Opinion 2000, Speroff et al. 1999):
  - Heavier uterine bleeding than the patient normally experiences
  - Prolonged uterine bleeding
  - Menstrual cycles more often than every 21 days
  - Spotting between menstrual cycles
  - Bleeding after sexual intercourse

NOTE: Consult a specialist regarding the need for EMB. (See the **Abnormal Uterine Bleeding** chapter.)

TREATMENT/MANAGEMENT

→ Initial and ongoing counseling regarding the perimenopausal and menopausal periods should be initiated when patients are in the thirties and forties and should continue throughout life.

→ Perimenopausal hormone therapy:
- Medical treatment for anovulatory or dysfunctional uterine bleeding in the perimenopausal period is recommended by the NAMS Consensus Opinion 2000.
  - Progestogen therapy: Administration of a progestogen such as medroxyprogesterone acetate, 10 mg/day p.o. for 10–14 days each month for 3–6 months will provide regular withdrawal bleeding. Further evaluation is need-

Table 12M.2.   HORMONE REPLACEMENT THERAPY: TYPICAL PRESCRIBING REGIMENS

Continuous Estrogen Therapy*

- Oral estrogen: 0.3–1.25 mg conjugated equine estrogen (CEE) (or equivalent) taken daily
      OR
- Transdermal patch changed once or twice weekly

*For women without a uterus

Continuous Combined Hormone Therapy†

- Oral estrogen 0.3–1.25 mg CEE (or equivalent), or transdermal patch changed once or twice weekly, PLUS 2.5–5 mg medroxyprogesterone acetate (MPA) (or equivalent progestin), or micronized oral progesterone 100 mg QD at HS (may induce somnolence)
      OR
- Combination estrogen and progestin transdermal patch, changed twice weekly

†Daily continuous use for women with intact uteri to avoid withdrawal bleeding and minimize progestin side effects. Irregular bleeding may occur in the first 6 months. Will require evaluation if abnormal uterine bleeding persists beyond 6 months.

Continuous Estrogen Therapy with Intermittent Progestin

- Oral estrogen 0.3–1.25 mg CEE (or equivalent) taken daily, or transdermal patch changed once or twice weekly
      PLUS
- Progestin: 5–10 mg MPA (or equivalent) taken on calendar Days 1–12 or 14–25. (Progestin regimens every 3 months are considered in some cases but are not recommended without consultation with a specialist.)
      OR
- Micronized oral progesterone 200 mg taken on calendar Days 1–12 or 14–25 at HS (may induce somnolence)

Cyclical Combined Hormone Therapy

- Oral estrogen: 0.3–1.25 mg CEE (or equivalent) taken on calendar Days 1–25
      PLUS
- Progestin: 5–10 mg MPA (or equivalent) taken on calendar Days 1–12 or 14–25
      OR
- Micronized oral progesterone 200 mg taken on calendar Days 1–12 or 14–25 at HS (may induce somnolence)

Vaginal Estrogens

- Vaginal creams: 1–2 g per vagina daily for 1–2 weeks, then gradually tapering to maintenance dose of 1 g, 2 times per week (manufacturers' recommendations may vary)
- Estrogen ring: estradiol ring inserted into vagina every 90 days
- Estrogen tablets for vaginal application: once daily into vagina for 2 weeks; maintenance dose is 1 tablet twice a week. (Recommendations for endometrial protection are not well-established. Consultation is recommended for women with intact uteri.)

Sources: *Physicians' Desk Reference* 2002; Rugierro, R., personal communication, April 2002; Wong, B.C. 2002. Atrophic vaginitis. *Menopausal Medicine* 10(2):9–12.

ed in cases of continued irregular bleeding or in the absence of withdrawal bleeding (Speroff et al. 1999).

- Combined low-dose contraceptive therapy also will provide regular withdrawal bleeding as well as contraceptive benefits and relief of perimenopausal symptoms (NAMS Consensus Opinion 2000). (See the **Abnormal Uterine Bleeding** chapter.)
- A progesterone-releasing intrauterine device (IUD) may be appropriate for women who do not tolerate progestogen side effects (e.g. depression); however, such devices are not FDA-approved (NAMS Consensus Opinion 2000).

→ Postmenopausal hormonal replacement therapy (see **Table 12M.1, Hormonal Preparations** and **Table 12M.2, Hormone Replacement Therapy: Typical Prescribing Regimens**):

- Indications for HRT include management of moderate to severe vasomotor symptoms, genitourinary atrophy, and prevention of osteoporosis. Contraindications for HRT continue to be refined as results of prospective clinical trials are evaluated.
- Absolute contraindications include (*Physicians' Desk Reference [PDR]* 2002):
  - Known or suspected pregnancy
  - Known or suspected breast cancer
  - Known or suspected estrogen-dependent neoplasia
  - Undiagnosed abnormal genital bleeding
  - Active thrombophlebitis or thromboembolic disorders
- Relative contraindications include (*PDR* 2002):
  - Cardiovascular disease
  - Impaired liver function
  - Gallbladder disease
  - Hyperlipidemia
  - Asthma
  - Migraine headaches
  - Epilepsy
  - Uterine fibroids
  - Diabetes
  - Metabolic bone disease
  - Kidney disease
  - Hypertension
  - Depression
- Side effects may include:
  - Genitourinary system:
    - Abnormal vaginal bleeding, breakthrough bleeding, spotting, and increased uterine fibroid size
    - Breast tenderness and enlargement
  - Gastrointestinal:
    - Nausea and vomiting
    - Cramping and bloating
    - Cholestatic jaundice
    - Increased incidence of gallbladder disease
  - Skin:
    - Chloasma, which may persist after discontinuance
  - Central nervous system:
    - Headache, migraine, dizziness
    - Depression
  - Miscellaneous:
    - Increase or decrease in weight
    - Reduced carbohydrate tolerance
    - Edema
    - Changes in libido

→ Nonhormonal therapy:

- Medications for vasomotor symptoms:
  - One of the selective serotonin reuptake inhibitors (SRRIs), venlafaxine, has demonstrated success in reducing symptoms in lower doses than usually considered therapeutic for depression (Loprinzi et al. 2000).
    - Venlafaxine:
      - ➤ 37.5–75 mg/day p.o. is the usual effective dosage range.
      - ➤ May need to start at 25–37.5 mg/day p.o. and increase as tolerated.
      - ➤ The main side effects are dry mouth, anorexia, and nausea.
      - ➤ Anxiety and sedation have been reported. Dosing at HS is recommended.
      - ➤ Sexual dysfunction has been reported at higher doses, but little data are available for the lower doses used in the perimenopause and menopause (Loprinzi et al. 2000).
    - Clonidine:
      - ➤ An alpha adrenergic blocker (a type of cardiovascular agent)
        - ∗ Clinical trials show some benefit in oral or patch form at 0.1 mg/day p.o., but evidence is not consistent.
        - ∗ Significant side effects include sleep difficulties and dry mouth.
        - ∗ Contraindicated in women with hypotension (*PDR* 2002)
    - Propranolol:
      - ➤ A cardiovascular agent and antihypertensive medication
        - ∗ Usual dosage is 40–80 mg/day p.o.
        - ∗ Results from clinical trials have not been consistent (Shoupe 2002).
    - Complementary and alternative therapies:
      - ➤ ACOG has developed recommendations regarding the use of botanical and alternatives for managing vasomotor symptoms, based on consensus and expert opinion. Options include (adapted from ACOG Practice Bulletin 2001):
        - ∗ Soy and isoflavones may be considered in the short-term management of vasomotor symptoms. For women with estrogen-dependent cancers, use of these botanicals should be carefully evaluated. Over prolonged periods, botanicals may improve lipoprotein profiles and provide some protection against osteoporosis.
        - ∗ Black cohosh may be helpful in the short-term management of vasomotor symptoms.

- Vitamins and minerals for bone health:
  - Elemental calcium: 1,000–1,500 mg/day. (See the **Osteoporosis** chapter in Section 10.)
  - Vitamin D: 400 IU/day. (See the **Osteoporosis** chapter in Section 10.)
→ Health maintenance strategies:
  - Elimination of smoking
  - Decrease in excessive alcohol intake
  - Maintenance of a nutritious, high-quality diet
  - Regular exercise and weight-resistance training

CONSULTATION

→ Consultation with a gynecologist who has expertise in the perimenopause and menopause as indicated, in particular for:
  - Abnormal uterine bleeding
  - Indications for endometrial biopsy
  - Abnormal endometrial pathology
  - Abnormal pelvic ultrasonography
  - Suspicious or abnormal mammogram
→ Consultation with a physician may be indicated for an identified underlying medical condition.
→ Consult with a physician in cases where there is continued bone demineralization despite medical therapy.

PATIENT EDUCATION

→ Educate the patient about the natural course of perimenopause and menopause. Provide anticipatory guidance regarding bleeding patterns, vasomotor symptoms, genitourinary symptoms, and emotional and affective changes.
  - Educate regarding lifestyle changes and ongoing health care maintenance.
  - See **Appendix 12M.1, Selected Resources**.
→ Provide accurate information about medical and nonmedical therapies as well as risk/benefit assessment, side effects, and use.
→ Discuss contraceptive options for the sexually active perimenopausal woman, including barrier methods, hormonal contraception, IUDs, and sterilization.
  - Discuss safer sex practices.

FOLLOW-UP

→ Follow-up will vary in response to the therapeutic regimen desired by the perimenopausal and menopausal woman.
→ For women who choose no hormonal or medical therapy:
  - Follow health and risk-assessment screening guidelines. (See **Women's Health Across the Lifespan: An Overview** in Section 1.)
→ For women who choose hormone or other medical therapy:
  - Assess at three months initially, then every year thereafter. Assess more frequently if necessary.
  - Monitor proper medication use.
  - Monitor for neoplasia (ovarian, uterine, breast, colon, etc.).
  - Follow health and risk-assessment screening guidelines. (See **Women's Health Across the Lifespan: An Overview** in Section 1.)

→ Follow up on abnormal laboratory tests as indicated.
→ Document in progress notes and on problem list.

BIBLIOGRAPHY

American College of Obstetricians and Gynecologists (ACOG). 2000. The menopause years. Available at: http://www.medem.com. Accessed on January 26, 2002.

_____. 2001. Practice bulletin: use of botanicals for management of menopausal symptoms. Available at: http://www.acog.org/from_home/publications/misc/pb028.htm. Accessed on January 26, 2002.

Brown, J.S., Vittinghoff, E., Kanaya, A.M. et al. 2001. Urinary tract infections in postmenopausal women: effect of hormone therapy and risk factors. *Obstetrics and Gynecology* 98(6):1045–1052.

Bush, T.L., Whiteman, M., and Flaws, J. 2001. Hormone replacement therapy and breast cancer: a qualitative review. *Obstetrics and Gynecology* 98(3):498–508.

Cummings, S.R., Black, D.M., Thompson, D.E. et al. 1998. Effect of alendronate on risk of fracture in women with low bone density but without vertebral fractures: results from the Fracture Intervention Trial. *Journal of the American Medical Association* 280:2077–2082.

Davis, S.R. 2000. Androgens. In *Menopause: biology and pathobiology*, eds. R.A. Lobo, J. Kelsey, and R. Marcus. San Diego, Calif.: Academic Press.

Dennerstein, L., Dudley, E.C., Hopper, J.L. et al. 2000. A prospective population-based study of menopausal symptoms. *Obstetrics and Gynecology* 96(3):351–358.

Finkel, M.L., Cohen, M.C., and Mahoney, H. 2001. Treatment options for the menopausal woman. *Nurse Practitioner* 26(2):5–15.

Fugh-Berman, A. 2000. Ipriflavone: mechanism and safety. *Alternative Therapies in Women's Health* 1(5):63–65.

Grady, D., Gebretsadik, T., Kerlikowske, K. et al. 1995. Hormone replacement therapy and endometrial cancer risk: a meta analysis. *Obstetrics and Gynecology* 85(2):304–313.

Grady, D., Wenger, N.K., Herrington, D. et al. 2000. Postmenopausal hormone therapy increases risk of venous thromboembolic disease: the Heart and Estrogen/Progestin Replacement Study. *Annals of Internal Medicine* 132:689–696.

Grodstein, F., Martinez, E., Platz, E.A. et al. 1998. Postmenopausal hormone use and risk of colorectal cancer and adenoma. *Annals of Internal Medicine* 128(9):705–712.

Hartge, P., Hoover, R., McGowan, L. 1988. Menopause and ovarian cancer. *American Journal of Epidemiology* 127:990–998.

Hlatky, M., Boothroyd, D., Vittinghoff, E. et al. 2002. Quality-of-life and depressive symptoms in postmenopausal women after receiving hormone therapy. *Journal of the American Medical Association* 287(5):591–597.

Hulley, S., Grady, D., Bush, T. et al. 1998. Randomized trial of estrogen plus progestin for secondary prevention of coronary heart disease in postmenopausal women. *Journal of the American Medical Association* 280(7):605–651.

Lacey, J.V., Mink, P.J., Lubin, J.H. et al. 2002. Menopausal hormone replacement therapy and risks of ovarian cancer. *Journal of the American Medical Association* 288:334–341.

Loprinzi, C.L., Kugler, J.W., Sloan, J.A. et al. 2000. Venlafaxine in management of hot flashes in survivors of breast cancer: a randomized controlled trial. *Lancet* 356:2059–2063.

Manson, J.E., and Martin, K.A. 2001. Postmenopausal hormone therapy. *New England Journal of Medicine* 345(1):34–40.

Marcus, R., Feldman, D., and Kelsey J., eds. 1996. *Osteoporosis.* San Diego, Calif.: Academic Press.

Mosca, L., Collins, P., Herrington, D.M. et al. 2001. Hormone replacement therapy and cardiovascular disease: a statement for healthcare professionals from the American Heart Association. *Circulation* 104:499–503.

Naftolin, F. 1994. The use of androgens. In *Treatment of the postmenopausal woman,* ed. R.A. Lobo. New York: Raven Press.

Nanda, K., Bastian, L.A., Hasselblad, V. et al. 1999. Hormone replacement therapy and the risk of colorectal cancer: a meta-analysis. *Obstetrics and Gynecology* 93:880–888.

National Institutes of Health (NIH) Consensus Statement Online 2000. Osteoporosis prevention, diagnosis, and therapy. March 27–29, 2001.

National Osteoporosis Foundation (NOF). 1998. *Physician's guide to prevention and treatment of osteoporosis.* Washington, D.C.: National Osteoporosis Foundation.

North American Menopause Society (NAMS). 2002. Amended report from the NAMS Advisory Panel on Postmenopausal Hormone Therapy. Available at: http://www.menopause.org/news.html. Accessed on October 14, 2002.

North American Menopause Society (NAMS) Consensus Opinion. 2000. Clinical challenges of the perimenopause: consensus opinion of the North American Menopause Society. *Menopause* 7:5–13.

Physicians' desk reference. 2002. Hormone replacement therapy prescribing guide. Montvale, N.J.: Medical Economics.

Rodriguez, C., Calle, E.E., Coates, R.J. et al. 1995. Estrogen replacement therapy and fatal ovarian cancer. *American Journal of Epidemiology* 141:828–835.

Rodriguez, C., Patel, A.V., Calle, E.E. et al. 2001. Estrogen replacement therapy and ovarian cancer mortality in a large prospective study of U.S. women. *Journal of the American Medical Association* 285(11):1460–1465.

Schairer, C., Lubin, J., Troisi, R. et al. 2000. Menopausal estrogen and estrogen-progestin replacement therapy and breast cancer risk. *Journal of the American Medical Association* 283(4):485–492.

Schnare, S.M. 2002. Comprehensive assessment of the older woman. *Women's Health Care* 1(1):9–14.

Shoupe, D. 2002. Practical strategies for treating hot flashes. *Women's Health: Gynecology Edition* 2(1):49–55.

Simon, J.A., and Mack, C.J. 2001. Preventing osteoporosis and improving compliance with HRT. *Contemporary Obstetrics/Gynecology for the Nurse Practitioner* (Suppl.):4–9.

Speroff, L., Gallagher, J.C., Rise, V.M. et al. 2001. Menopause management: the impact of low-dose HRT. *Contemporary Obstetrics and Gynecology for Nurse Practitioners* (Suppl.):4–26.

Speroff, L., Glass, R.H., and Kase, N.G. 1999. *Clinical gynecologic endocrinology and infertility,* 6th ed. Baltimore, Md.: Williams & Wilkins.

Speroff, L., Rowan, J., Symons, J. et al. 1996. The comparative effect on bone density, endometrium, and lipids of continuous hormones as replacement therapy (CHART Study). *Journal of the American Medical Association* 276:1397–1403.

Watts, N.B. 2002. Therapies to improve bone mineral density and reduce the risk of fracture. *Journal of Reproductive Medicine* 47(1)(Suppl.):82–92.

Wong, B.C. 2002. Atrophic vaginitis. *Menopausal Medicine* 10(2):9–12.

Woodruff, J.D., Pickar, J.H. 1994. Incidence of endometrial hyperplasia in postmenopausal women taking conjugated estrogens (Premarin®) with medroxyprogesterone acetate or conjugated estrogens alone. *American Journal of Obstetrics and Gynecology* 170(5):1213–1223.

World Health Organization (WHO) Scientific Group on Research on the Menopause in the 1990s. 1994. Technical report series 866. Geneva, Switzerland: WHO

Writing Group for the Women's Health Initiative Investigators. 2002. Risks and benefits of estrogen plus progestin in healthy postmenopausal women. *Journal of the American Medical Association* 288(3):321–368.

APPENDIX 12M.1.

Selected Resources

- North American Menopause Society
  P.O. Box 94527
  Cleveland, Ohio 44101
  (440) 442-7550
  www.menopause.org

- National Women's Health Resource Center
  2440 M Street NW, Suite 201
  Washington, D.C. 20037
  (202) 293-6045
  www.healthywomen.org

- Older Women's League
  666 11th Street NW
  Washington, D.C. 20001
   (202) 783-6686

- American Society for Reproductive Medicine
  1209 Montgomery Highway
  Birmingham, Ala. 35216-2809
  (205) 978-5000
  www.asrm.org

- Female Health Links
  www.femalehealthlinks.com

12-N

Polyps—Cervical and Endometrial

Cervical polyps are the most common neoplastic lesions of the cervix, occurring in about 4% of all gynecological patients. Also referred to as *pseudotumors*, they represent a hyperplastic response of normal epithelial tissue. They present most often in perimenopausal women, postmenopausal women, and multigravidas. Cervical polyps are usually found incidentally on pelvic examination and are predominantly asymptomatic. In some cases, polyps may be a cause of abnormal bleeding or discharge. The etiology of a polyp may be inflammatory, traumatic, pregnancy-related (pseudodecidual), or unknown (Adelson et al. 2000). Malignant change within a polyp is rare. Adenosarcomas may be confused clinically and pathologically with benign cervical polyps (Adelson et al. 2000, Hino et al. 1998).

Endometrial polyps are localized overgrowths of endometrial glands, stroma, and blood vessels projecting beyond the endometrial surface. The etiology is unknown. They may be solitary or multiple and may occur with or without generalized endometrial hyperplasia (Grasel et al. 2000). Polyps of endometrial origin occur most commonly in women 40–60 years old. In general, women with endometrial polyps are asymptomatic; however, abnormal bleeding may be a presenting complaint. The prevalence of endometrial polyps in women with abnormal bleeding has been reported to range from 13–50% (Tjarks et al. 2000). The malignancy potential appears to be low, but 10–34% of cases of endometrial cancer in postmenopausal women have been associated with endometrial polyps. In women on tamoxifen, endometrial polyps occur 2–4 times more often (Adelson et al. 2000).

There appears to be an association between cervical and endometrial polyps (Vilodre et al. 1997). In postmenopause, cervical polyps—especially those that are symptomatic—may be associated with endometrial polyps (57% of cases) or neoplasia (Adelson et al. 2000).

DATABASE

SUBJECTIVE

→ Cervical polyps:
- The woman is usually asymptomatic.
- Symptoms may include intermenstrual or postcoital spotting/bleeding, or bleeding after douching or a pelvic examination.
- Abnormal discharge may also be a presenting complaint.

→ Endometrial polyps:
- Most are asymptomatic.
- Symptoms may include a wide range of abnormal bleeding patterns, with premenstrual and postmenstrual spotting being the most common presentations. Menometrorrhagia also may exist.

OBJECTIVE

→ Cervical polyps:
- Are usually an incidental finding on routine speculum examination.
- May appear as a reddish-purple to cherry-red lesion with a long narrow pedicle or as a gray-white lesion with short broad base. Usually smooth and soft.
- May be single or multiple and a few millimeters to 4 cm in diameter.
- May be friable to touch.
- May not be palpable because of soft consistency.
- If large, may dilate cervix.
- Leukorrhea may be present if the cervix is inflamed.

→ Endometrial polyps:
- May protrude from external cervical os if on long pedicle. Otherwise, they are not usually visible on pelvic examination.
- Most arise from uterine fundus, usually the cornual region.
- Are velvety gray, tan, red, or brown.
- Are a few millimeters to several centimeters in diameter. A single large polyp may fill the entire uterine cavity.
- May have a broad base (sessile) or slender pedicle (pedunculated).
- Ultrasound findings may include nonspecific thickened endometrium, focal echogenic areas (bright edges, sharp and smooth), or endocavitary mass surrounded by fluid (Caspi et al. 2000).

ASSESSMENT

→ Cervical polyp
→ R/O endometrial polyp
→ R/O microglandular endocervical hyperplasia
→ R/O prolapsed myoma, retained products of conception, squamous papilloma, adenofibroma, adenosarcoma, and other cervical/endometrial malignancies

PLAN

DIAGNOSTIC TESTS

→ Cervical polyps are usually diagnosed incidentally during a routine pelvic examination.
→ Diagnosis of endometrial polyps generally is made during evaluation of abnormal uterine bleeding—i.e., via endometrial biopsy, dilatation and curettage (D&C), hysteroscopy, sonohysterography, transvaginal ultrasonography, transvaginal saline hysterography, hysterosalpingography, or hysterectomy. Site-specific practice will dictate the diagnostic modalities.
  ▪ If endometrial polyps are discovered, other endometrial pathology should be ruled out.
→ Hysteroscopy now is considered the gold standard for detecting endometrial polyps. It is a more sensitive diagnostic test than uterine curettage and should be performed if a D&C fails to identify causes of abnormal bleeding or if bleeding recurs after a D&C. In the postmenopausal woman, endometrial biopsy and possibly hysteroscopy with D&C should be considered as part of the work-up for cervical polyps (Adelson et al. 2000, Bakour et al. 2000).
→ All polyps should be sent to pathology after removal. Careful pathological examination is important for avoiding misdiagnosis.
→ Additional lab studies/procedures, as indicated, may include but are not be limited to: Pap smear, STD screen of the cervix, wet mounts, CBC, and colposcopy.

TREATMENT/MANAGEMENT

→ Cervical polyps generally can be removed safely in the office.
  ▪ Grasp the base of the polyp with an appropriate-size ring forceps and avulse it with a twisting motion. After removal, gentle curettage or cautery of the base may be performed to help prevent recurrence.
  ▪ Bleeding may be controlled with direct pressure and/or ferric subsulfate (Monsel's solution). Electrocautery or cryocautery also may be used but is rarely required.
  ▪ Send the specimen to pathology for histological diagnosis.
  ▪ If the polyp does not dislodge easily or if the patient has excessive pain, STOP. Refer to a physician for further management.
→ In all cases of suspected endometrial polyps, a thorough endometrial exploration is warranted (Orvieto 1999).
  ▪ Endometrial polyps are generally removed by curettage or hysteroscopic resection. The latter is regarded as optimal

therapy *except* if the hysteroscopic appearance suggests atypicality or a malignant component, in which case D&C is recommended (Cravello et al. 2000).

CONSULTATION

→ For patients with abnormal bleeding when the diagnosis is uncertain.
→ For prolonged/excessive bleeding immediately after cervical polyp removal.
→ For consideration of endometrial evaluation if cervical polyps are diagnosed in a woman older than 50 years.
→ Referral to a physician is indicated if endometrial polyps are suspected and, in some cases, for removal of cervical polyps.

PATIENT EDUCATION

→ Discuss the (usually) benign nature of the condition and methods for polyp removal. Advise that polyps may recur.
→ Ask the patient to return for reassessment if excessive or abnormal vaginal bleeding continues after polyp removal.

FOLLOW-UP

→ Based on case presentation.
→ Review pathology results with the patient and consult with a physician as indicated. Follow-up of endometrial polyps is generally done by the physician caring for the patient.
→ Stable/benign-appearing cervical polyps may simply be observed during the course of a pregnancy.
→ Document in progress notes and on problem list.

BIBLIOGRAPHY

Adelson, M.D, and Adelson, K.L. 2000. Miscellaneous benign disorders of the upper genital tract. In *Textbook of gynecology*, eds. L.J Copeland and J.F Jarrell. Philadelphia: W.B. Saunders.

Bakour, S.H., Khan, K.S, and Gupta, J.K. 2000. The risk of premalignant and malignant pathology in endometrial polyps. *Acta Obstetricia et Gynecologica Scandinavica* 79: 317–320.

Caspi, B., Appelman, Z., Goldchmit, R. et al. 2000. The bright edge of the endometrial polyp. *Ultrasound in Obstetrics and Gynecology* 15:327–330.

Cravello, L., Stolla, V., Bretelle, F. et al. 2000. Hysteroscopic resection of endometrial polyps: a study of 195 cases. *Obstetrics and Gynecology* 93:131–134.

Grasel, R.P., Outwater, E.K., Siegelman, E.S. et al. 2000. Endometrial polyps: MRI imaging features and distinction from endometrial carcinoma. *Radiology* 214:47–52.

Hino, A., Hirose, T., Seki, K. et al. 1998. Adenosarcoma of the uterine cervix presenting as a cervical polyp. *Pathology International* 48:649–652.

Orvieto, R., Bar-Hava, I., Dicker, D. et al. 1999. Endometrial polyps during menopause: characterization and significance. *Acta Obstetricia et Gynecologica Scandinavica* 78:883–886.

Reslova, T., Tosner, J., Resl, M. et al. 1999. Endometrial

polyps: a clinical study of 245 cases. *Archives of Gynecology and Obstetrics* 262:133–139.

Tjarks, M., and Van Voorhis, B.J. 2000. Treatment of endometrial polyps. *Obstetrics and Gynecology* 96(6):886-889.

Vilodre, L.-C., Bertat, R., Petters, R. et al. 1997. Cervical polyp as a risk factor for hysteroscopically diagnosed endometrial polyps. *Gynecologic and Obstetric Investigation* 44:191–195.

12-O

Premenstrual Syndrome and Premenstrual Dysphoric Disorder

Premenstrual syndrome (PMS) is the cyclic recurrence of distressing physical, affective, and behavioral changes during the luteal phase of the menstrual cycle that may result in the deterioration of interpersonal relationships and personal health (Brown et al. 1986, Ugarriza et al. 1998). While many women experience mood and physical changes during the week prior to menses, very few women experience premenstrual symptoms to such a severe extent as to result in a deterioration of their familial or work relationships. However, approximately 5–10% of menstruating women experience symptoms severe enough to interfere with their work or social lives and thus are categorized as having PMS (American College of Obstetricians and Gynecologists [ACOG] 2000).

Although mild to moderate premenstrual symptoms do not result in functional impairment for most women, severe symptoms can significantly disrupt lifestyle and social functioning for a subset of women with PMS. Vocational functioning does not appear to be impaired to the same extent. Studies have noted that fewer than 1% of women regularly missed work due to their symptoms and only 2% felt that their symptoms impaired their work (Logue et al. 1986).

Premenstrual dysphoric disorder (PMDD) is found in approximately 3–5% of women (American Psychiatric Association [APA] 2000). For these women, the symptoms of depression, irritability, and other mood changes are so difficult to manage that there is a significant impact on familial, social, and work relationships (ACOG 2000). Marital discord, parenting difficulties, poor work or school performance, and social isolation are more often observed in women with severe symptoms.

Although premenstrual symptoms may begin at any time after menarche, the average age of onset is 26 years. Over time, the number and severity of symptoms may increase and then later regress as the woman enters the perimenopausal period. The age of onset, progression, and duration of severe premenstrual symptoms have a significant impact on the extent of morbidity associated with these disorders. The woman with either PMS or PMDD who experiences little or no symptom relief may experience more than 200 symptomatic menstrual cycles or 1,400 to 2,800 days of severe premenstrual symptoms before reaching menopause (Yonkers 1997).

PMS is not observed exclusively in any single culture or society. Cultural variations have been noted in numerous cross-cultural studies. These comparisons show some variance in symptom type and severity but indicate that PMS can be identified in women in many different cultural and socioeconomic circumstances (Janiger et al. 1972).

PMS and the Menstrual Cycle

The duration of the menstrual cycle for the most women is 25–35 days. It is divided into phases determined by the cyclic changes of the gonadotropin hormones (follicle stimulating hormone [FSH] and luteinizing hormone [LH]), the ovaries, and the uterus. The follicular phase of the cycle is characterized by the actions of FSH and estradiol on the ovary and endometrium, respectively, resulting in the development of the ovum and preparation of the endometrium for ovulation. The luteal phase is characterized by the dominance of progesterone and LH in the development of the postovulatory endometrium and corpus luteum (Speroff et al. 1999, Ugarriza et al. 1998). PMS is distinguished by signs and symptoms that are manifested during the luteal phase of the menstrual cycle and regress by the end of the full flow of menses (Severino et al. 1995). In general, the signs and symptoms of PMS and PMDD are only experienced by ovulating women; pregnant women, menopausal women, and premenarchal girls do not experience such symptoms. (See **Table 12O.1, Common Signs and Symptoms of PMS.**)

PMS and PMDD

The American College of Obstetricians and Gynecologists has advocated using either the criteria developed by the National Institutes of Health (Hamilton et al. 1984) or the research criteria utilized by Mortola and co-workers (1989, 1990) to define PMS (ACOG 2000). These criteria require documentation of symptoms associated with PMS. They also require that symptoms occur only during the luteal phase of the menstrual cycle and impair some aspect of life, and that other possible diagnostic entities (e.g., hypothyroidism, major depression) are eliminated. PMS and PMDD share many of the same symptoms, but PMDD encompasses a more severe form of PMS that emphasizes emotional and mood alterations of such severity as to interfere with social and work relationships. The APA (2000) has developed similar criteria for the diagnosis of PMDD as well. (See **Table 120.1** and **Table 120.2, Research Criteria for the Premenstrual Dysphoric Disorder**.)

The defining criteria for PMS developed by the National Institute of Mental Health include (Hamilton et al. 1984):

→ An approximately 30% increase in symptom severity when comparing cycle Days 5–10 to the final six days before menses, as measured or determined by rating scales or questionnaires.

→ Documentation of these changes for at least two consecutive cycles.

The defining criteria for PMS developed by Mortola and co-workers (1989, 1990) are:

→ Cyclic manifestations of at least one of the following six affective symptoms:
  ▪ Depression
  ▪ Angry outbursts
  ▪ Irritability
  ▪ Anxiety
  ▪ Confusion
  ▪ Social withdrawal

→ Cyclic manifestations of at least one of the following four somatic symptoms:
  ▪ Breast tenderness
  ▪ Headache
  ▪ Abdominal bloating

  ▪ Swelling of extremities

→ Symptoms are limited to occurrence during the five days before menses in each of the three prior menstrual cycles, and are relieved within four days of the onset of menses, without recurrence until ovulation.

→ Symptoms are reproducible during two cycles of prospective charting.

→ The patient experiences impairment in social or work performance.

→ Symptoms are present in the absence of pharmacotherapeutics, hormone use, or drug or alcohol abuse.

The criteria developed by the APA (2000) for the diagnosis of PMDD require that prospective daily ratings of symptoms occur only in the luteal phase, that at least five of the eleven symptoms characterizing PMDD be present, and that there be a defined level of impairment. In addition, there should be a predictable, symptom-free period before ovulation. Although a woman with PMDD may present with physical and emotional symptoms, the diagnosis of PMDD emphasizes mood and affect alterations that are severe enough to interfere with her social and family relationships and are present during most menstrual cycles in the span of one year. The intention is to delineate women with PMDD from women who may have other psychiatric illnesses with symptoms similar to premenstrual symptoms. The symptoms of PMDD are often as severe as major depressive disorders but of shorter duration (Korzekwa et al. 1997, APA 2000). (See **Table 120.2**.)

Interference with social and familial functioning is a hallmark of women with severe PMS and PMDD. If the interference in interpersonal relationships and social function that occurs in the luteal phase is not addressed, it may extend into the follicular and ovulatory phases of the cycle (Ugarriza et al. 1998).

Table 120.1.   COMMON SIGNS AND SYMPTOMS OF PMS

Emotional/Affective	Physiological/Somatic
Anger	Acne
Anxiety	Bloating or weight gain
Depression, sadness, or hopelessness	Breast swelling or tenderness
Decreased alertness or concentration	Diarrhea
Decreased self-esteem	Fatigue or lethargy
Decreased interest in usual activities	Food craving or overeating
Decreased libido	Edema
Impulsivity	Gastrointestinal complaints
Irritability, agitation, or listlessness	Muscle and joint pain
Mood lability	Nausea
Sleep disturbances (insomnia, hypersomnia)	Sweating
Social isolation	Weight gain
Tearfulness	
Tension	

Source: Logue, C.M., and Moos, R.H. 1986. Perimenstrual symptoms: prevalence and risk factors *Psychosomatic Medicine* 48:388–414; Severino, S.K., and Moline, M.L. 1995. Premenstrual syndrome: identification and management. *Drugs* 49:71–82; Ugarriza, D.N., Klingner, S., and O'Brien, S. 1998. Premenstrual syndrome: diagnosis and intervention. *Nurse Practitioner* 23(9):40–58.

PMS and PMDD also must be distinguished from *premenstrual exacerbation* of an ongoing psychiatric or physical disorder. *Premenstrual magnification* is another term that describes this process, which is considered to be a separate syndrome from PMS and PMDD. Women with conditions such as major depression, dysthymia, anxiety disorders, personality disorders, bipolar disorder, eating disorders, and substance-abuse disorder may experience symptoms throughout the menstrual cycle, but the symptoms are more severe during the luteal phase (Korzekwa et al. 1997).

PMS Pathophysiology

The underlying mechanisms for menstrually related mood syndromes are poorly understood and to date none of the proposed etiological theories has been completely substantiated. Biomedical theories have included hypotheses about hormone imbalances, aldosterone increase, vitamin deficiencies, hypoglycemia, hyperprolactinemia, and psychogenic factors. Genetics, behavioral and environmental factors, stress, and endogenous opiate withdrawal have also been proposed (ACOG 2000, Rapkin et al. 1997, Rubinow et al. 1995).

The strongest theory involves the interactions of ovarian steroids and neurotransmitters. It has been proposed that normal ovarian cycling initiates PMS and PMDD symptoms, as opposed to a hormone imbalance or an irregularity in the hypothalamic-pituitary-ovarian axis. PMS and PMDD may result primarily from changes in the levels of neurotransmitters (particularly serotonin) that develop in response to alterations in ovarian steroids during the menstrual cycle. Women with PMS and PMDD are possibly predisposed to hormone-induced affective instability. However, there is currently no explanation for the varying degrees of sensitivity to ovarian hormone-induced neurotransmitter alterations among women (Rapkin et al. 1997, Rubinow et al. 1995).

Table 120.2.   RESEARCH CRITERIA FOR THE PREMENSTRUAL DYSPHORIC DISORDER

A. In most menstrual cycles during the past year, 5 (or more) of the following symptoms were present for most of the time during the last week of the luteal phase, began to remit within a few days after the onset of the follicular phase, and were absent in the last week after the menses, with at least one of the symptoms being (1), (2), (3), or (4):

(1)   Markedly depressed mood, feelings of hopelessness, or self-deprecating thoughts

(2)   Marked anxiety, tension, feelings of being "keyed up" or "on edge"

(3)   Markedly affective lability (e.g., feeling suddenly sad or tearful or increased sensitivity to rejection)

(4)   Persistent and marked anger or irritability or increased interpersonal conflicts

(5)   Decreased interest in usual activities (e.g., work, school, friends, hobbies)

(6)   Subjective sense of difficulty concentrating

(7)   Lethargy, easy fatigability, or marked lack of energy

(8)   Marked change in appetite, overeating, or specific food cravings

(9)   Hypersomnia or insomnia

(10) A subjective sense of being overwhelmed or out of control

(11) Other physical symptoms, such as breast tenderness or swelling, headaches, joint or muscle pain, a sense of "bloating," weight gain

NOTE: In menstruating females, the luteal phase corresponds to the period between ovulation and the onset of menses, and the follicular phase begins with menses. In nonmenstruating females, (e.g., those who have had a hysterectomy), the timing of luteal and follicular phases may require measurement of circulating reproductive hormones.

B. The disturbance markedly interferes with work, school, or usual social activities, and with relationships (e.g., avoidance of social activities, and decreased productivity and efficiency at work or school).

C. The disturbance is not merely an exacerbation of the symptoms of another disorder, such as major depressive disorder, panic disorder, dysthymic disorder, or a personality disorder, although it may be superimposed on any of these.

D. Criteria A, B, and C must be confirmed by prospective daily ratings during at least 2 consecutive symptomatic cycles. (The diagnosis may be made provisionally before confirmation.)

Reprinted with permission from the *Diagnostic and statistical manual of mental disorders*, 4th ed., text revision. ©American Psychiatric Association, 2000.

Many of the neuroendocrine transmitters associated with the human stress response have been associated with the initiation or aggravation of PMS. The manifestations of PMS may result from a combination of multiple stressors, a heightened stress response, few social supports, and a vulnerable period of biological reactivity.

DATABASE

SUBJECTIVE

→ Very few risk factors have been identified (Korzekwa et al. 1997, Mortola 1992):
- Age: late 20s–late 30s
- Family history: Women with PMS often have mothers, aunts, and sisters with similar symptoms. Genetic factors play a role, as may learned behaviors.
- Previous psychiatric illness
- Oral contraceptive (OC) use: For a subgroup of women, OCs may exacerbate symptoms.

→ PMS history:
- Age at onset of PMS?
- How long has PMS been experienced?
- Has PMS severity decreased or increased since onset?
- What makes the symptoms worse or better?
- What forms of treatment has the patient tried (e.g., pharmacological, self-help)?
- Has there been work absenteeism or decreased work productivity due to PMS?

→ Menstrual history:
- Menstrual regularity
- Menstrual cycle variation related to any chronic condition

→ Lifestyle and health history:
- Physical activity or exercise: level, type, frequency, and amount
- Stress: current and past stressors and PMS exacerbation, relief factors, stress management methods
- Nutrition: food cravings and symptom responses, vitamins, supplements, and complementary and alternative medicines

→ Symptom assessment:
- Several scales and specially designed symptom calendars are available, but the woman can use any calendar to note symptoms and their severity.
- Daily symptom ratings reduce retrospective bias.
- A calendar is essential in differentiating PMS from PMDD.
- A calendar is also useful in differentiating premenstrual exacerbation of an underlying psychiatric or physical disorder.
- PMS symptom calendar: accurate *daily* rating of symptoms and their severity for 2–3 cycles (Mortola et al. 1990).
  - Women fill in their most distressing symptoms, beginning on the first day of their last menstrual period, using a 5-point rating scale (0 = no symptoms, 1 = minimal severity, 2 = mild severity, 3 = moderate severity, 4 = extreme severity).
  - Compare the follicular phase score from Days 3–9 with the luteal score from the last seven days of the cycle.
  - To confirm PMS or PMDD, the calendar should demonstrate at least a twofold increase in the total severity score during the last week of the cycle compared with the total severity score of the early follicular phase.

OBJECTIVE

→ Physical examination:
- Vital signs as indicated
- Weight
- Assessment of affect, mental health
- Thyroid examination
- Breast examination
- Abdominal examination
- Complete pelvic examination
- Additional physical examination components as indicated by history

ASSESSMENT

→ PMS
→ PMDD
→ R/O underlying chronic illness with menstrual cycle exacerbation:
- Psychiatric disorders
- Seizure disorders
- Endocrine disorders (hyperprolactinemia, hypothyroidism)
- Cancer
- Systemic lupus erythematosus

→ R/O chronic illness (physical/psychological) without cyclical exacerbation:
- Anemia
- Autoimmune disorders
- Hypothyroidism
- Diabetes
- Seizure disorders
- Chronic fatigue syndrome
- Collagen vascular disease

→ R/O menstrual/ovarian dysfunction
→ R/O sexual dysfunction
→ R/O dysmenorrhea
→ R/O endometriosis
→ R/O chronic pelvic pain
→ R/O sexually transmitted diseases (STDs)
→ R/O urinary tract infection/vaginitis
→ R/O mastalgia, nodularity, fibrocystic changes
→ R/O situational stress reaction
→ R/O other psychiatric illness:
- Generalized anxiety
- Major depression
- Dysthymia
- Panic disorder
- Bipolar illness
- Personality disorders
- Phobic disorder
- Substance abuse

PLAN

DIAGNOSTIC TESTS

→ Laboratory tests: Currently, there is no physiological or hormonal test that confirms the diagnosis of PMS. However, some laboratory studies may be useful for ruling out other conditions:

- TSH and thyroxine (free T_4) as indicated to rule out hypothyroidism
- Prolactin levels as indicated for galactorrhea or chronic menstrual irregularity
- CBC to evaluate anemia
- Fasting blood sugar and HbA1C evaluations
- FSH to rule out menopausal status if a woman is reporting regular hot flashes and menstrual irregularity
  NOTE: Measurement of estrogen and progesterone levels is not recommended, as these do not demonstrate any differences between women with or without PMS.
- Wet mounts and STD testing as indicated to rule out vaginitis/STDs
- Urinalysis as indicated to rule out cystitis

→ Anxiety and depression questionnaires, when available, can assist in evaluation and referral. (See the **Anxiety Disorders** and **Depression** chapters in Section 14.)

TREATMENT/MANAGEMENT

→ Develop individualized treatment plans to reflect the priorities of the patient and her expectations for management.

→ A multifactorial approach to PMS treatment often can result in a complete or marked reduction of premenstrual symptoms.

→ If pharmacological treatment is necessary, a complementary nonpharmacological approach also can be used.

→ Identify women with PMS, PMDD, and premenstrual magnification or exacerbation of another physical or psychological disorder.

→ Pharmacological treatments:
- Selective serotonin reuptake inhibitors (SSRIs) (Steiner et al. 1995):
  - Work with relative specificity on the serotonergic system and have been used to manage moderate to severe premenstrual symptoms in women with PMS and PMDD.
  - Good treatment choices for premenstrual affective symptoms with or without somatic symptoms.
  - Effective with mood alteration and depression as well as bloating and breast tenderness.
  - Response to these medications is more rapid than that of patients with depression.
  - Have been shown to be relatively safe during the first trimester and late prenatal exposure (Nulman et al. 1997).
    - Fluoxetine:
      ➤ Treatment efficacy has been demonstrated in several placebo-controlled studies (Steiner et al. 1995).
      ➤ Recommended dosage is 20 mg p.o./day in the morning.
      ➤ Recently marketed in a 14-day cycle format to be taken during the last 2 weeks of the menstrual cycle.
      ➤ Side effects include decreased libido (as with all SSRIs), nervousness, nausea, insomnia, and drowsiness.
      ➤ Neurologic development of children exposed to fluoxetine in utero has not been found to have been impaired (Nulman et al. 1997).
    - Sertraline: also been shown to be effective in a placebo-controlled study (Yonkers 1997).
      ➤ Recommended dosage is 50–150 mg p.o./day.
      ➤ Side effects: decreased libido, nausea, diarrhea, insomnia, and somnolence.
    - Paroxetine:
      ➤ Has shown efficacy in reducing severe emotional and somatic premenstrual symptoms (Eriksson et al. 1995).
      ➤ Recommended dosage is 10–30 mg p.o./day.
      ➤ Common side effects include nausea, somnolence, dizziness, asthenia, insomnia, and sweating.
- Tricyclic antidepressants:
  - Clomipramine:
    - A tricyclic antidepressant with serotonergic and noradrenergic reuptake inhibiting properties that reduce affective and somatic symptoms of severe PMS/PMDD (Eriksson et al. 1990, Pearlstein 1994, Steiner et al. 1995, Sundblad et al. 1993).
    - Recommended dosage is 25–75 mg p.o./day during the last 14 days of the cycle.
    - Side effects: dry mouth, fatigue, vertigo, and nausea.
    - Pregnancy risk category C. Animal studies have shown there is a risk to the fetus (*Physicians' Desk Reference [PDR]* 2002).
- Anxiolytics:
  - Alprazolam:
    - Has demonstrated effectiveness for affective symptoms (irritability, depression, and anxiety) (Steiner et al. 1995).
    - Concerns regarding dependence and tolerance with benzodiazepines may limit its use.
    - Recommended dosage is 0.25–0.5 mg p.o. TID for 6–14 days before menses. (Maximum dose is 4 mg/day.)
    - Consultation with a PMS specialist before prescribing is recommended.
    - Common side effects include headache, dizziness, nausea, and nervousness.
    - Pregnancy risk category D. May cause a risk to a human fetus (*PDR* 2002).
  - Buspirone:
    - A nonbenzodiazepine anxiolytic may prove effective for premenstrual anxiety, irritability, and depression.
    - Recommended dosage is 25–60 mg p.o./day during the 12 days before menses (Sundblad et al. 1993).

- Common side effects include headache, dizziness, nausea, and nervousness.
- Pregnancy risk category B. No animal studies have shown a risk and there have been no controlled human studies (*PDR* 2002).

■ Ovarian suppression: A number of investigators have found that temporarily suppressing ovulation can reduce PMS in some women (Korzekwa et al. 1997). Women with PMDD often experience increased symptoms of depression when taking these agents; therefore, differentiation of this diagnosis is critical (Brown et al. 1994, Freeman et al. 1997).

   • Oral contraceptives:
   - Suppression of ovarian function can bring relief of symptom severity for women who experience marked premenstrual pain (dysmenorrhea, endometriosis, or menstrual migraines).
   - Low-dose OCs are safe, with few side effects.
   - Continuous administration of the OC may be appropriate for patients with pelvic pain or severe dysmenorrhea.
   - An OC has been marketed that is compounded with a new progestin, drospirenone, which has anti-mineralocorticoid properties comparable to 25 mg of spironolactone. This OC may be more effective for women experiencing PMS (*PDR* 2002).
   - Side effects: Common nuisance symptoms include breakthrough bleeding and nausea, which resolve with use.

   • Gonadotropin releasing hormones (GnRHs) (Schmidt et al. 1998):
   - GnRH analogs manipulate the menstrual cycle.
   - Physical and somatic symptoms are improved more than the affective symptoms.
   - Anti-estrogens have negative effects on bone metabolism and lipogenesis.
   - Limited in duration of use (no more than 6 months) and provide only short-term relief.
   - Consultation with a PMS specialist before use is recommended.
   - Avoid pregnancy. Pregnancy risk category X (*PDR* 2002).
   - Synthetic androgens (17-alpha ethinyl testosterone derivative [Danazol®]) and GnRH analogs (nafarelin acetate [Synarel®], leuprolide acetate [Lupron®]) may be considered.
   - Consultation with a specialist before prescribing is recommended.

   • Progesterone:
   - Randomized, controlled, clinical trials of progesterone therapy have failed to demonstrate a significant difference between the effects of progesterone and placebo (ACOG 2000).
   - Several topical creams claiming to be derived from progesterone and to reduce PMS symptoms have

been marketed as over-the-counter cosmetics or supplements.
   - Because these "progesterone" creams are sold as cosmetics or supplements, they need not conform to the usual clinical trials demanded for evidence-based therapeutics.
   - Quality and dosage are of concern.

■ Aldosterone inhibitors: Excessive aldosterone secretion has been proposed as a cause of premenstrual fluid retention and has received clinical attention, but this has never been confirmed (Katz et al. 1972).

   • While most women experience a shift in body fluids during the premenstrual period, few actually increase their total body weight.
   • A few women experience marked discomfort related to fluid retention in their extremities, breasts, and abdomen.
   • Fluid retention may be responsible for premenstrual headaches. Spironolactone is both an aldosterone inhibitor and a potassium-sparing, mild diuretic.
   - Dose is 50 mg p.o. BID starting 2–3 days before the anticipated symptoms until menses.
   - Avoid using in women with impaired renal function.
   - Avoid concurrent use with other diuretics, such as furosemide and ethacrynic acid.

■ Prostaglandin inhibitors:
   • Nonsteroidal anti-inflammatory drugs (NSAIDs) may help reduce premenstrual headache and dysmenorrhea.
   • NSAIDs have specific side effects. A recommended dosage should be followed. (See the **Headache** chapter in Section 9 and the **Dysmenorrhea** chapter.)
   • Dysmenorrhea is not considered a premenstrual symptom, but anxiety regarding anticipated pain may be reduced by using NSAIDs.

■ Complementary and alternative medications:
   • Oil of evening primrose (Hardy 2000):
   - Effectiveness has not been substantiated by randomized, placebo, controlled trials.
   - Women may try it before professional evaluation.
   - Marketed under a number of different brand names.
   - Quality and dosage are of concern.
   - No long-term side effects are known, but reported short-term side effects include skin blemishes, nausea, soft stools or diarrhea, and headache.

   • Chaste tree berry: *Vitex agnus-castus* has been used for many centuries as a phytomedicine.
   - Has both progestin and anti-estrogen properties, and may reduce premenstrual symptoms.
   - Studies are limited. Anecdotally, one woman involved in fertility studies experienced ovarian hyperstimulation (Hardy 2000).
   - Dosage is not well-defined because products are not similarly compounded.
   - May reduce the effectiveness of OCs.
   - Side effects include mild nausea and mild rashes.
   - Avoid using in pregnancy, as chaste tree berry may interfere with prolactin secretion (Hardy 2000).

- Diet and nutritional therapy: While little evidence demonstrates that dietary change alone reduces PMS severity, a healthy diet promotes general good health. Pyridoxine and calcium deficiencies have been identified as potential causative factors in PMS symptoms (Ugarriza et al. 1998).
  - Nutritional supplements:
    - Vitamin B_6 (pyridoxine): Its use in premenstrual symptom management is controversial due to poorly controlled studies with contradictory results and the potential side effect of irreversible peripheral neuropathy. For women who want to try vitamin B_6, these recommendations should be followed:
      - Start with 100 mg/day p.o., midcycle to menses.
      - Dosages >100 mg/day may cause damage, including irreversible peripheral neuropathy (ACOG 2000).
      - Side effects of vitamin B_6 excess include numbness and tingling in the arms and legs, shooting pain, headaches, fatigue, dizziness, and weakness.
    - Calcium: Recent evidence has shown a connection between calcium deficiency and PMS.
      - Daily supplementation with 1,200 mg of calcium carbonate may reduce depression, mood swings, headache, bloating, food cravings, and pain, with minimal side effects (Thys-Jacobs et al. 1998).
- Exercise: Research on exercise and the neuroendocrine system suggests that the benefits of a regular exercise program may directly or indirectly alleviate some of the symptoms of PMS and indirectly mediate symptoms through healthy coping behavior (Prior et al. 1987).
- Stress management: Although little is known about stress management and PMS, extensive evidence exists showing the positive effects of stress reduction strategies.
  - Relaxation has been found to result in a 58% reduction in symptoms after 3 months of daily relaxation (Goodale et al. 1990).
  - Stress management may enhance personal and social competency.

CONSULTATION

→ Consultation with a gynecologist who has expertise in PMS management or with an endocrinologist as indicated.

→ Consultation with or referral to a mental health care provider who has expertise in women's health may be necessary.

→ Consultation with a physician may be indicated if there is an identified, underlying medical problem.

PATIENT EDUCATION

→ Education begins with evaluation and self-monitoring. A prospective symptom calendar will help each woman to identify her premenstrual signs and symptoms and to develop treatment and management modalities that can improve her life.

→ There should be detailed discussion of the various etiologic theories of PMS and PMDD and of the rationales for the various treatments to promote better patient understanding and compliance.

→ Useful Web sites with information regarding PMS are:
- American Academy of Family Physicians, familydoctor.org/healthfacts/141/
- American College of Obstetricians and Gynecologists, medem.com/search

FOLLOW-UP

→ The initial visit should entail development of an individual symptom list, a PMS symptom calendar with its use and importance explained, and basic PMS and PMDD information for the patient. A subsequent visit after 2–3 cycles have been charted will be necessary to clarify the diagnosis and assess the response to any modifications identified at the initial exam.

→ A session should be scheduled after 2–3 months to assess treatment success.

→ Women should be advised to continue monitoring their symptoms using a PMS symptom calendar.

→ Refer the patient to a specialty clinic or health care provider with expertise in PMS as indicated. Use community mental health resources if the patient requires ongoing psychosocial support.

→ Follow up on abnormal laboratory tests. Refer the patient's partner for evaluation/treatment of identified STDs.

→ Treat or refer for treatment/management as indicated if there is any identified, underlying medical condition.

→ Document in progress notes and on problem list.

BIBLIOGRAPHY

American College of Obstetricians and Gynecologists (ACOG). 2000. Premenstrual syndrome: ACOG Practice Bulletin No. 15. *International Journal of Gynecology and Obstetrics* 73 (2000):183–191.

American Psychiatric Association (APA). 2000. *Diagnostic and statistical manual of mental disorders*, 4th ed., pp. 771–774. Washington, D.C.: APA.

Brown, C.S., Ling, F.W., Anderson, R.N. et al. 1994. Efficacy of depot leuprolide in premenstrual syndrome: effect of symptom severity and type in a controlled trial. *Obstetrics and Gynecology* 84:779–786.

Brown, M., and Zimmer, P. 1986. Personal and family impact of premenstrual symptoms. *Journal of Obstetrical, Gynecological, and Neonatal Nursing* 150:363–369.

Eriksson, E., Hedberg, M.A., Andersch, B. et al. 1995. The serotonin reuptake inhibitor paroxetine is superior to the noradrenaline reuptake inhibitor maprotiline in the treatment of premenstrual syndrome. *Neuropharmacology* 12:167–176.

Eriksson, E., Lisjo, P., Sundblad, C. et al. 1990. Effect of clomipramine on premenstrual syndrome. *Acta Psychiatrica Scandinavia* 81:87–88.

Freeman, E.W., Sondheimer, S.J., and Rickels, K. 1997. Gonadotropin-releasing hormone agonist in the treatment of premenstrual symptoms with and without ongoing dysphoria: a controlled study. *Psychopharmacology Bulletin* 33:303–309.

Goodale, I., Domar, A., and Benson, H. 1990. Alleviation of premenstrual syndrome symptoms with the relaxation response. *Obstetrics and Gynecology* 75:649–655.

Hamilton, J.A., Parry, B.L., Alagna, S. et al. 1984. Premenstrual mood changes: a guide to evaluation and treatment. *Psychiatric Annals* 14:426–435.

Hardy, M. 2000. Herbs of special interest to women. *Journal of the American Pharmaceutical Association* 40(2):234–243.

Janiger, O., Riffenburgh, M., and Kersh, M. 1972. A cross-cultural study of premenstrual symptoms. *Psychosomatics* 13:226–235.

Katz, F., and Romfh, P. 1972. Plasma aldosterone and renin activity during the menstrual cycle. *Journal of Clinical Endocrinology and Metabolism* 34:819–821.

Korzekwa, M.I., and Steiner, M. 1997. Premenstrual syndromes. *Clinical Obstetrics and Gynecology* 40:574–576.

Logue, C.M., and Moos, R.H. 1986. Perimenstrual symptoms: prevalence and risk factors *Psychosomatic Medicine* 48: 388–414.

Mortola, J.F. 1992. Issues in the diagnosis and research of premenstrual syndrome. *Clinical Obstetrics and Gynecology* 35:587–598.

Mortola, J.F., Girton, L., and Yen, S.C. 1989. Depressive episodes in premenstrual syndrome. *American Journal of Obstetrics and Gynecology* 161:1682–1687.

Mortola, J.F., Girton, L., Beck, L. et al. 1990. Diagnosis of premenstrual syndrome by a simple, prospective, and reliable instrument: the calendar of premenstrual experiences. *Obstetrics and Gynecology* 76(2):302–307.

Nulman, I., Rovet, J., Stewart, D.E. et al. 1997. Neurodevelopment of children exposed in utero to antidepressant drugs. *New England Journal of Medicine* 336(4):258–262.

Pearlstein, T.B., and Stone, A.B. 1994. Long-term fluoxetine treatment of late luteal phase dysphoric disorder. *Journal of Clinical Psychiatry* 55:332–335.

Physicians' desk reference. 2002. Montvale, N.J.: Medical Economics.

Prior, J., Vigna, Y., Sciarretta D. et al. 1987. Conditioning exercise decreases premenstrual symptoms: a prospective, controlled 6-month trial. *Fertility and Sterility* 47:402–408.

Rapkin, A.J., Morgan, M., Goldman, L. et al. 1997. Progesterone metabolite allopregnanolone in women with premenstrual syndrome. *Obstetrics and Gynecology* 90:709–714.

Rubinow, D.R., and Schmidt, P.J. 1995. The treatment of premenstrual syndrome—forward into the past (editorial). *New England Journal of Medicine* 332:1574–1575.

Schmidt, P.J., Nieman, L.K., Danaceau, M.A. et al. 1998. Differential behavioral effects of gonadal steroids in women with and in those without premenstrual syndrome. *New England Journal of Medicine* 338:209–216.

Severino, S.K., and Moline, M.L. 1995. Premenstrual syndrome: identification and management. *Drugs* 49:71–82.

Speroff, L., Glass, R.H., and Kase, N.G. 1999. *Clinical gynecologic endocrinology and infertility*, 6th ed. Baltimore, Md.: Lippincott Williams & Wilkins.

Steiner, M., Steinberg, S., Stewart, D. et al. for the Canadian Fluoxetine/Premenstrual Dysphoria Collaborative Study Group. 1995. Fluoxetine in the treatment of premenstrual dysphoria. *New England Journal of Medicine* 332:1529–1534.

Sundblad, C., Hedberg, M.A., and Erikson, E. 1993. Clomipramine administered during the luteal phase reduces the symptoms of premenstrual syndrome: a placebo-controlled trial. *Neuropsychopharmacology* 9:133–145.

Thys-Jacobs, S., Starkey, P., Bernstein, D. et al. 1998. Calcium carbonate and the premenstrual syndrome: effects on premenstrual and menstrual symptoms. Premenstrual Syndrome Study Group. *American Journal of Obstetrics and Gynecology* 179:444–452.

Ugarriza, D.N., Klingner, S., and O'Brien, S. 1998. Premenstrual syndrome: diagnosis and intervention. *Nurse Practitioner* 23(9):40–58.

Yonkers, K.A. 1997. Antidepressants in the treatment of premenstrual dysphoric disorder. *Journal of Clinical Psychiatry* 58(Suppl. 14):4–10.

12-P
Sexual Dysfunction

Sexual dysfunction is generally defined as a disturbance that occurs in one of the four phases of the sexual response cycle—desire phase, arousal phase, orgasm phase, or resolution phase (American Psychiatric Association [APA] 2000). Additional categories in this chapter include dyspareunia and vaginismus. In the *Diagnostic and Statistical Manual of Mental Disorders*, the APA has subtyped sexual dysfunctions as *lifelong* (occurring since the onset of sexual functioning) or *acquired* (developing after a period of normal functioning), *generalized* (occurring with all types of stimulations, situations, and partners) or *situational* (limited to certain types of stimulations, situations, and partners), and affecting one or both partners (APA 2000). "In order for a woman to be considered to have a 'sexual disorder,' the symptoms must be persistent and pervasive and her problem must cause *her* personal distress. If it is bothering only her partner, then by definition she does not have sexual dysfunction" (Berman et al. 2001, p. 68).

Desire Phase Disorder

Low desire is now the most common presenting complaint of the patients seen in many sex-therapy specialty clinics (Pridal et al. 2000). The cause of low desire is often difficult to sort out due to the complexity of factors influencing desire. Desire phase dysfunctions *include hypoactive sexual desire* (HSD) and *sexual aversion*. Differential diagnosis of these two dysfunctions is important for treatment planning. Sexual aversion that is the result of trauma, such as childhood sexual abuse or adult rape, requires treatment of the trauma before treatment of the desire disorder.

Hypoactive Sexual Desire

HSD is defined by the APA as a deficiency or absence of sexual fantasies and desire for sexual activity (Criterion A). The disturbance causes marked distress or interpersonal difficulty (Criterion B). The dysfunction is not better accounted for by some other psychiatric syndrome, such as major depression, and is not due exclusively to the direct physiological effects of a substance (including medications) or a general medical condition (Criterion C) (APA 2000). The woman doesn't seek sexual stimulation, doesn't feel distressed about the lack of sexual activity, and may never be aware of any spontaneously occurring "wanting" of sexual expression. If sexual activity happens with her partner, the woman usually does not find it emotionally unpleasant. There may be some resentment toward the partner for pressing sex, but the negative emotions are not centered on sex itself (Pridal 2000). The average age of onset for women is 33 years (Kelly 2001).

When HSD is the primary dysfunction, the capacity to experience arousal and orgasm may remain, but lack of adequate desire makes arousal and orgasm more difficult to achieve. However, HSD may be the result of distress about disturbances in arousability or orgasm (APA 2000).

According to Kaplan (1979), sexual desire originates in the sex center of the brain (hypothalamus), is dependent on hormones (testosterone, luteinizing hormone-releasing hormone [LH-RH]) in both men and woman, and is influenced by emotions (fear, anger). Suppressing sexual appetite can be a learned survival skill that is appropriate in the context of the patient's life, as when a sexual situation is perceived as either emotionally or physically dangerous.

Physical causes commonly include severe stress states, certain drugs and illnesses, weakness, pain, body-image concerns, and low testosterone levels, as in menopause. The symptoms of testosterone deficiency in women include (Rako 1996):
→ Global loss of sexual desire; lack of sexual fantasy and sexual dreams
→ Decreased sensitivity to sexual stimulation in the nipples and clitoris
→ Decreased arousability and capacity for orgasm
→ Diminished vital energy and sense of well-being
→ Loss of muscle tone
And in some women:
→ Thinning and loss of pubic hair
→ Genital atrophy unresponsive to estrogen
→ Dry and brittle scalp hair; dry skin

Psychological factors include major depressive disorder, dysthymia, obsessive-compulsive disorder, and an anxiety disorder (Bartlik et al. 1999). Depression, which is frequently associated with HSD, may precede the loss of desire or become a consequence of such loss. Most antidepressant medications, with the exception of nefazodone, mirtazapine, and buproprion, can inhibit sexual desire, excitement, and orgasm. Patients with HSD tend to have deeper and more intense sexual anxieties, greater amounts of hostility and/or resentment in their relationships, and more tenacious defense mechanisms than do patients with arousal or orgasm phase problems. Sexual therapy focuses on sorting out the physiological, psychological, and relationship factors that contribute to HSD. (See **Table 12P.1, Psychic Factors Associated with Hypoactive Sexual Desire**.) In practice, the two most common psychosocial etiologies are sexual trauma (sexual abuse, assault, incest) and unresolved relationship dynamics.

Table 12P.1. PSYCHIC FACTORS ASSOCIATED WITH HYPOACTIVE SEXUAL DESIRE

Milder Sources of Anxiety

Performance fears (including body image-concerns)

Anticipation of lack of pleasure in the act

Mild residual guilt about sex and pleasure

Simple overconcern about pleasing the partner

Failure to communicate one's own needs

Repeated nonpleasurable, ungratifying sexual experiences

Insensitive or inept partner

Anxious and pressuring partner

Residues of antisexual injunctions from childhood

Midlevel Sources of Anxiety

Unconscious fear of romantic success

Unconscious fear of intimacy

Unresolved grief following miscarriage or stillbirth

Unresolved feelings regarding abortion

Fear of pregnancy

Fear of contracting HIV/AIDS

Relationship problems (intimacy, power struggles, territoriality)

Deeper Sources of Anxiety

Complex intrapsychic conflicts involving early emotional development

Early learning to inhibit sexual feeling in response to destructive, intrusive, or abusive family interaction

Unresolved hostility and resentment in the relationship

Source: Adapted from Kaplan, H.S. 1979. *Disorders of sexual desire*, pp. 78–92. New York: Simon & Schuster.

HSD may be further specified by type:

→ Lifelong HSD—total lack of sexual desire throughout a person's life

→ Acquired HSD—loss of previously present desire (e.g., after childbirth)

→ Situational HSD—lack of desire in particular situations but not in others

→ Generalized HSD—current lack of desire regardless of situational variables

→ Due to psychological factors

→ Due to combined factors

Sexual Aversion Disorder

Sexual aversion is defined by the APA as "aversion to and active avoidance of genital sexual contact with a sexual partner" (Criterion A). The disturbance causes marked distress or interpersonal difficulty (Criterion B). This disorder is the most severe form of sexual inhibition. The diagnosis is made when the disturbance is not part of another psychiatric disorder, such as major depression (Criterion C) (APA 2000). History often includes severely negative parental attitude(s) toward sex; sexual trauma (incest, rape); constant pressuring, coercion, or bargaining for sex; repeated unsuccessful attempts to please a sexual partner; relentless, unsuccessful attempts to overcome a sexual dysfunction; and/or unresolved conflicts in sexual identity or orientation (Crooks et al. 1987).

Some individuals with severe sexual aversion disorder may experience panic attacks and report symptoms of extreme anxiety, feelings of terror, faintness, nausea, palpitations, dizziness, and breathing difficulties in a sexual situation (APA 2000). Often the patient describes sex as an ordeal, disgusting, or repulsive. She may use various strategies to avoid sex, such as going to sleep earlier or later than the partner, traveling, neglecting personal appearance, abusing a substance, or overinvolving herself in work, social, or family activities (APA 2000).

Sexual aversion may be further specified by type:

→ Lifelong—total avoidance throughout a person's life

→ Acquired—loss of previously present desire (e.g., after childbirth)

→ Situational—total avoidance in particular situations but not in others

→ Generalized—global avoidance regardless of situational variables

→ Due to psychological factors

→ Due to combined factors

Arousal Phase Disorder

Sexual Arousal Disorder

According to the APA, a *sexual arousal disorder* is diagnosed when the following conditions are present: "persistent or recurrent inability to attain or maintain, until completion of the sexual activity, an adequate lubrication-swelling response of sexual excitement" (Criterion A). The disturbance causes marked distress or interpersonal difficulty (Criterion B). The dysfunction is not better accounted for by another psychiatric diagnosis and is not due exclusively to substance use or a general medical condition (Criterion C) (APA 2000).

Physiologically, arousal response in women is characterized by increased vasocongestion in the genital area and expansion of the posterior end of the vagina. The woman may notice a feeling of pressure or fullness in her pelvis and/or a twitching in the pubococcygeus muscle (Berman et al. 2001). This is followed by development of lubrication, which is pushed through the semipermeable membrane of the vagina as a result of increased vasocongestion in the sponge-like tissue surrounding the vagina. In addition to lubrication, the cervix and uterus lift out of the way of the vaginal barrel and there is swelling of the outer third of the vagina. Lubrication is the same psychophysiological response as erection in the male and is governed by the same neurophysiological pathways (primarily the parasympathetic part of the autonomic nervous system). The same psychic factors that are associated with inhibited sexual desire can cause anxiety in the arousal stage and block sexual response and lubrication. (See **Table 12P.1**.)

Subtypes should be specified:
→ Lifelong—total lack of arousal throughout life
→ Acquired—loss of previous ability to become aroused
→ Generalized—total lack of arousal regardless of type of stimulation or situation
→ Situational—lack of arousal in some situations but not others
→ Due to combined factors

One physiological cause could be hysterectomy, which can injure the uterovaginal and cervical plexus (Berman et al. 2001). This can decrease lubrication and sensation. The uterus and cervix no longer pull up out of the way, there may be scar tissue along the vaginal barrel, shortening of the vagina, and decreased blood flow to the genitals, which inhibits the vasocongestion that produces lubrication. Loss of the cervix may cause loss of pelvic floor orgasms from deep vaginal penetration.

Uterine embolization for the treatment of uterine fibroids is another surgery that can affect arousal. This relatively new procedure injects small particles of plastic into the uterine artery to block the blood supply to the fibroids (Berman 2001). Newer techniques attempt to spare the vaginal branches of the uterine artery to prevent the loss of uterine contractions and sensations after this procedure.

Nerve and vascular damage from childbirth can affect arousal weeks or months after delivery. Atherosclerosis can reduce blood flow to the arteries supplying the pelvis and genitals. This can lead to fibrosis in the vaginal wall and smooth muscle of the clitoris, and possibly to inhibition of the release of nitric oxide (Berman 2001). Smoking is another source of restriction of blood flow through the pelvic arteries.

Orgasm Phase Disorder

Female orgasmic disorder is defined by the APA as "a persistent or recurrent delay in, or absence of, orgasm following a normal sexual excitement phase" (Criterion A). This diagnosis requires a subjective judgment by the practitioner, based on what would be reasonable given the patient's age, sexual experience, and adequacy of the sexual stimulation she receives. The clinician needs to determine whether the sexual activity is adequate in focus, intensity, and duration. The disturbance must cause marked distress or interpersonal difficulty (Criterion B). The dysfunction is not due to some other psychiatric disorder nor to the direct physiological effects of a substance or a general medical condition (Criterion C) (APA 2000).

Three basic elements are necessary for orgasm to occur: effective stimulation, sufficient relaxation, and absence of learned inhibition of orgasmic response. Not having an orgasm may affect body image, self-esteem, or satisfaction with the relationship.

Whether or not lack of orgasm (anorgasmia) is a problem should be decided by the patient. Some women who are anorgasmic enjoy their sexual experiences anyway. Others view a lack of orgasm as sexual failure and feel frustrated and ashamed. Anorgasmia does not preclude arousal, lubrication, and enjoyment of the sexual experience.

Female orgasmic disorder is broken down into subtypes:
→ Lifelong (primary) or acquired (secondary)
→ Generalized or situational (including coital anorgasmia)
→ Due to psychological factors
→ Due to combined factors

Primary Anorgasmia (Subtype: Lifelong)

The woman has never experienced orgasm by any means, including masturbation or with a partner. It is estimated that approximately 5–20% of women have never had an orgasm (Heinman et al. 1998). These women often lack knowledge of their own sexuality, including their response patterns and anatomy. While orgasmic women usually learn through self-stimulation, few women with primary anorgasmia masturbate. Often they fear loss of control.

Secondary Anorgasmia (Subtype: Acquired)

The woman has had orgasms at one time but no longer does. A physical component may be associated; thus, a general health history is important to rule out conditions such as diabetes or multiple sclerosis. (It is doubtful, however, that anorgasmia would be the first symptom of these conditions.) Physiological causes can include the use of medications, damage to pelvic nerves from surgery, or clitoridectomy (a practice in some cultures in Africa, the Middle East, and Asia) (Berman et al. 2001). Use of antidepressants called selective serotonin reuptake inhibitors, such as fluoxetine, are known to cause anorgasmia. Often, the development of acquired anorgasmia reflects a major change in the woman's life, such as marriage, a new full-time job, a new or deteriorating relationship, or extreme stress.

Additional contributing factors may include concern that family members will overhear the sexual encounter, lack of sufficient arousal time for orgasm to occur, or preoccupation with the fear of losing the ability to achieve orgasm. It is important for the health care provider to inquire about changes that occurred around the time orgasm response stopped.

Situational Anorgasmia

The woman has orgasms only in certain situations (e.g., with masturbation but not with a partner, with coitus only and no other forms of stimulation, or with a certain partner only). It is important to determine the conditions under which the patient is orgasmic and her requirements for orgasm. Women can increase the likelihood of orgasm as they expand their experiences with stimulation and gain more knowledge of their bodies.

Coital Anorgasmia

This woman is often orgasmic with manual or oral stimulation from a partner but not from intercourse alone. The condition is so common that health practitioners must be careful not to consider it a dysfunction unless it is a problem for the patient. According to the Hite Report (1976), only about 30% of women routinely experience orgasm during intercourse without additional simultaneous stimulation of the clitoral area. Another 30% are orgasmic during intercourse with simultaneous clitoral stimulation. In a small study of 2,600 women, 38% had not had an orgasm during intercourse (Ellison 2000).

Dyspareunia

Dyspareunia is defined by the APA as recurrent or persistent genital pain in either a male or female before, during, or after sexual intercourse (Criterion A). Occasional pain during coitus that is not persistent or recurrent or is not causing marked distress is not considered dyspareunia. For females, the pain ranges from mild to severe and can occur in various places in the genitals. The disturbance must cause marked distress or relationship difficulty (Criterion B). The disturbance is not caused exclusively by vaginismus or lack of lubrication, a psychiatric disorder, or the direct physiological effects of a substance or general medical condition (Criterion C) (APA 2000).

Subtypes should be specified:
→ Lifelong or acquired
→ Generalized or situational
→ Due to psychological factors
→ Due to combined factors

The most common cause of occasional discomfort is lack of lubrication due to insufficient arousal. Intercourse with insufficient lubrication irritates the vaginal walls and increases the possibility of vaginal infection. Dyspareunia can result from vaginal infections, vaginal atrophy during menopause, or postoperatively from vaginal or vulvar procedures. Foam, sponges, spermicidal jelly or cream, condoms, condom lubricant, nonoxynol-9, and diaphragms also may cause irritation in sensitive women. If a physical cause of the pain goes untreated, ongoing attempts at penetration can result in vaginismus. Dyspareunia also can be caused by an emotional issue or relationship problem. It is often a combination of physiological and psychological factors (Berman et al. 2001, Binik et al. 2000) and therefore takes effort to sort out.

The primary focus of care should be to legitimize the presenting complaint of pain, evaluate the degree of interference or disruption of sexual response, and evaluate the pain-coping strategies. Women who have had coital pain for a long time present with complaints of arousal disorder or desire disorder, not with the primary complaint of pain (Binik et al. 2000).

Vaginismus

Vaginismus is defined by the APA as "recurrent or persistent involuntary spasm of the perineal muscles surrounding the outer third of the vagina when vaginal penetration with penis, finger, tampon, or speculum is attempted" (Criterion A). The disturbance must cause marked distress or interpersonal difficulty (Criterion B). It is not caused by a psychiatric disorder or the direct physiological effects of a substance or general medical condition (Criterion C) (APA 2000).

Subtypes should be specified:
→ Lifelong or acquired
→ Generalized or situational
→ Due to psychological factors
→ Due to combined factors

Contraction of the vaginal muscles is the physical manifestation of an emotional response to penetration. The muscle contractions may be mild enough to allow for some vaginal penetration, accompanied by the discomfort of not being able to fully relax the pubococcygeus muscle. The contraction of the vaginal opening can also be quite severe, preventing penetration by anything. The patient has psychologically associated pain with penetration, most often connected to some kind of trauma. The trauma can be either in consensual or nonconsensual situations. Traumatic associations may include sexual abuse, a first-time sexual experience, a painful vaginal examination, tampon insertion, chronically painful intercourse, strong religious taboos about sex, repeated attempts at penetration by a partner with erectile difficulties, or pain associated with physical problems, such as pelvic inflammatory disease or endometriosis. The vagina "closes off" in an attempt to avoid further pain, even after the cause has been resolved. An additional factor is fear—of cancer, pregnancy, HIV infection, sexually transmitted diseases, or lesbian orientation. Desire, arousal, lubrication, and orgasm may be unaffected by vaginismus. Inability to have intercourse may cause distress, shame, and feelings of inadequacy. Some women may not desire intercourse but seek treatment only because they desire pregnancy. These women will seek treatment for infertility or unconsummated marriages.

Vaginismus is considered primary if the woman has never been able to tolerate penetration. In secondary vaginismus, a woman has previously enjoyed intercourse but developed spasms after some type of traumatic penetration. Situational or selective vaginismus happens with a specific partner only. Vaginismus is considered rare but is probably under-reported.

Desire Phase Disorders

DATABASE

SUBJECTIVE

Hypoactive Sexual Desire (HSD)

→ The patient usually complains of having no interest in sexual contact or sexual experience.
→ The patient rarely entertains thoughts of having sex, and if those thoughts occur, she rapidly dismisses them.

→ Lubrication and orgasm may occur on a reflexive level; only desire for a sexual encounter is inhibited.

→ Low sexual desire may be associated with (LoPicolo 1980):

- History or current complaints of depression
- Catholicism
- Presence of sexual dysfunction
- Aversion to oral-genital contact
- Aversion (in both males and females) to female genitals
- No history of masturbation or discontinued masturbation
- History of relationship problems assessed by the clinician but denied by the couple

Sexual Aversion

→ The patient may report feelings ranging from disgust to extreme, irrational fear of sexual activity (Schover et al. 1982).

→ The patient may experience intense anxiety, including panic attacks, at the mere thought of having sexual contact.

→ The patient may report physiological symptoms such as sweating, increased heartbeat, nausea, or diarrhea.

→ The patient may describe the sexual experience as an ordeal—disgusting or repulsive.

→ The patient rarely has orgasms and often has no desire to change the condition.

→ History to evaluate desire phase disorders should include:

- Complete medical/surgical history:
  - Surgical removal of adrenals, ovaries, or pituitary
  - Disfiguring surgery
  - Any major pelvic surgery or injury
  - Acquired disability
  - Epilepsy
  - Pituitary tumor
  - Thyroid deficiency
  - Addison's disease
  - Cushing's disease
  - Hepatitis
  - Advanced malignancies
  - Degenerative diseases
  - Pulmonary diseases
  - Chronic fatigue syndrome
  - HIV positivity
  - Low levels of hormones, especially total testosterone <20 ng/dL
- Obstetrical/gynecological/contraceptive history:
  - Suction or forceps delivery, episiotomy
  - Perimenopause, menopause, and postmenopause
- Medication history:
  - Illicit drug use/abuse, use of cigarettes and/or alcohol
  - Antihypertensives (especially beta-blockers, reserpine, and alpha-methyldopa)
  - Sedative-hypnotics
  - Anti-anxiety drugs
  - Antidepressants
  - Narcotics
  - Phenothiazines
  - Amphetamines
  - Antihistamines
  - Adrenal steroids in high doses
  - Neurotoxic industrial agents
  - Chemotherapy
  - Oral contraceptives
- Psychosocial history to assess current life situation for severe stress/depression:
  - Loss of job, death of a family member, first 6–8 months postpartum, strict breast-feeding, relationship difficulties
- Review of systems, especially weight gain, weight loss; vegetative symptoms of depression, such as not eating or sleeping
- Sexual history:
  - Situational or generalized lack of desire, including masturbation
  - Severity of lack of desire
  - The couple's and individual's actual sexual behavior, including types of behaviors (coital, manual, oral-genital) and the frequency of behaviors not currently engaged in
  - The couple's and individual's motivation to change the situation
  - Frequency of and subjective reaction to sexual thoughts, masturbation, sexual fantasies, erotic dreams, erotic books, magazines, films
  - Extramarital sexual behaviors
  - Relationship factors that keep one or both partners from feeling sexual, including the degree of hostility and resentment
  - Past experiences of sexual trauma (incest, molestation, sexual assault, date rape)
  - Associated dyspareunia, lack of orgasm
- See **Appendix 12P.1, General Assessment Questions for Sexual Functioning** for more general questions regarding sexual functioning.
  NOTE: Detailed sexual history-taking may be beyond the scope of practice of the primary care provider unless he or she has received training in human sexuality.

OBJECTIVE

→ Complete pelvic examination if there is a complaint or history of pelvic pain or dyspareunia.

→ Additional physical examination components based on history.

ASSESSMENT

→ Desire phase disorder: lifelong, acquired, situational, or generalized

→ R/O hypoactive sexual desire

→ R/O sexual aversion

→ R/O concomitant sexual dysfunction

→ R/O concomitant medical, psychiatric illness

→ R/O prescription and/or recreational-drug effects

→ Assess contributing stress factors

→ Assess motivation and readiness for referral for therapy

PLAN

DIAGNOSTIC TESTS

NOTE: Desire disorders are difficult to diagnose. The key diagnostic issue is the distinction between HSD as the primary diagnosis versus HSD as secondary to a medical, psychiatric, or other sexual dysfunction.

→ Laboratory tests may include:
- Plasma testosterone levels on at least two different occasions
- Estradiol, prolactin
- Estrogen/testosterone ratio
- Percentage of circulating unbound testosterone (free) and total testosterone
- Fasting blood sugar
- Thyroid function tests
- LH, FSH
- Additional laboratory tests based on history

TREATMENT/MANAGEMENT

→ Judge the extent of the dysfunction, taking into account factors that affect sexual functioning, such as age, sex, occupation, and context of the individual's life.
- Simple behavioral intervention generally is not sufficient to reawaken sexual feelings.
→ Treat identified underlying physiological causes. Desire often will return when feelings of well-being return.
→ A regular exercise program can contribute to relaxation, sense of well-being, body-image improvement, and management of depression, although it usually will be only part of a total plan.
→ Consider testosterone supplementation if total testosterone is <20 ng/dL (Berman et al. 2001, Rako 1996, Reiss 2001). Normal total testosterone range is 20–50 ng/dl. Testosterone supplementation is still in early stages of research. Many practitioners have found compounding pharmacies to be helpful in adjusting dosages. Periodic monitoring of blood levels of testosterone and physical symptoms is necessary to prevent unwanted side effects, such as irritability or hair growth.
- Berman et al. (2001) recommend oral methyltestosterone for increasing libido and topical testosterone cream for increasing vaginal and labial sensation and for building up atrophic tissues.
  - Oral methyltestosterone with estrogen is available in two fixed combinations of the prescription drug Estratest® (2.5 mg methyltestosterone, 1.25 mg estrogen) or Estratest H.S.® (half strength—1.25 mg methyltestosterone, 0.625 mg estrogen). Testosterone cream, obtained from compounding pharmacies, preferably should have a dosage of 2% and a range of 1–3% (Berman et al. 2001). The cream should be applied, in carefully monitored amounts, 3 times a week at HS and 30 minutes before sex if it occurs outside of the 3-times-a-week application schedule.

- Rako (1996) recommends an effective oral dose of methyltestosterone of 0.25–0.8 mg/day. Most women benefit from 0.3–0.6 mg. This is far less methyltestosterone than what is in Estratest®. Rako also recommends topical testosterone compounded to order and used once a day on the labia but only until libido has improved and the capacity for stimulation has been restored. After that, oral supplementation should be adequate.
- Reiss (2001) recommends assessment of the woman's body hair as an indicator of starting dosages: Start with a low dosage if there is little body hair and muscle development or if there is above-average body hair, more muscle development, and a testosterone level >40 ng/dL. Prescribe higher dosages if the woman has more hair and muscle development and a testosterone level <20 ng/dL. Reiss prescribes testosterone in gel, capsules, and sublingual drops provided by compounding pharmacies.
  - The dosage of the prescribed gel is 0.2–0.4% beginning with 1 g (a quarter teaspoon); the lower dose (0.2%) is for women who have average blood levels of total testosterone. According to Reiss (2001), blood levels of total testosterone range between 30–80 ng/dL. A higher dose (0.4%) is used if blood levels are low. The gel is rubbed on the inner arm or thigh, perineum, and/or the inner labia. The quantity can be increased by 50% every 4 weeks.
  - The capsules are available in 0.5–5 mg strength, with a starting dosage of 2.5 mg twice a day with meals.
  - Sublingual drops (1 mg per drop) start with 2 drops a day, taken in the morning (Reiss 2001).

NOTE: Testosterone should be discontinued at the first sign of excess. Symptoms may take a few weeks to clear up; then, testosterone can be restarted at a lower dose.

→ Treatment of a primary sexual dysfunction (e.g., dyspareunia, anorgasmia) often alleviates lack of desire.
→ Progress in treating desire phase dysfunctions is relatively slow and the prognosis much less successful than for arousal and orgasm phase dysfunctions.
- If there has been no sexual interaction for many years in a relationship, the prognosis for therapy is very poor.
→ Refer for sex therapy as indicated. Do not refer during a crisis period.
- Sex therapy is not appropriate when HSD is secondary to depression.
→ If underlying depression is suspected, refer the patient to a psychiatrist for medication and/or psychotherapy.
→ Refer for individual psychotherapy as indicated.
→ Refer for couple therapy as indicated.
→ See "Bibliotherapy" in "Patient Education," below.

CONSULTATION

→ Refer for sex therapy, individual psychotherapy, or couple therapy as indicated.
→ Consult with a psychotherapist as needed to evaluate signs of depression or anxiety.
→ Consult with a pharmacist as needed to clarify the effects of

various drugs on sexual desire. Compounding pharmacies and resources for locating them include (Berman et al. 2001, Reiss 2001):

- The International Academy of Compounding Pharmacists
  P.O. Box 1365
  Sugar Land, Tex. 77487
  (800) 927-4227, FAX: (281) 495-0602
  iacpinfo@iacprx.org
  www.iacprx.org
  The Web site can locate local compounding pharmacies.
- Urgent Care Pharmacy
  227 Winchester Place, Suite 106
  Spartanburg, S.C. 29209
  (800) 692-6982, FAX: (888) 235-9350
  urgentcarepharmacy@msn.com
- Kronos Compounding Pharmacy
  3675 South Rainbow
  Las Vegas, Nev. 89103
  (800) 723-7455, FAX: (800) 238-8239
  www.kronospharmacy.com
- Women's International Pharmacy
  2 Marsh Court
  Madison, Wis. 53718
  (608) 221-7800

  12012 North 111th Avenue
  Youngtown, Ariz. 85363
  (623) 214-7700
  Toll free numbers: (800) 279-5708, FAX: (800) 279-8011
  www.womensinternational.com
→ The primary care provider may be serving as a consultant to the therapist who refers a patient for physical and gynecological examinations.

PATIENT EDUCATION

→ Introduce the idea of alternate ways for the male partner to have an orgasm besides intercourse (e.g., self-masturbation, partner masturbation, rubbing penis on outside of the patient's body).
→ Reassure the patient who has underlying depression or severe stress that sexual desire often returns when depression or stress is alleviated.
→ Discuss the loss of desire as an adaptive response that may provide an opportunity for self-reflection.
→ Loss of desire is common after childbirth, miscarriage, and therapeutic abortion. Desire usually returns after cessation of breast-feeding. Teach the patient to focus on ways to maintain touching while awaiting the return of desire.
→ Bibliotherapy is indicated in cases that appear to stem from mild to midlevel sources of anxiety:
  - Barbach, L. 1975. *For Yourself: The Fulfillment of Female Sexuality*. New York: Doubleday. This is an easy-to-read, self-help book with basic information about taking responsibility for one's own sexuality. It discusses orgasm, the sexual response cycle, sources of sexual confusion, masturbation, and partner exercises.

- Barbach, L. 1982. *For Each Other: Sharing Sexual Intimacy*. New York: Signet. This is an easy-to-read, self-help book that provides excellent information and exercises. Chapters 11–13 focus on normal sexual desire, lack of sexual interest, and reconnecting.
- Berman, J., and Berman, L. 2001. *For Women Only: A Revolutionary Guide to Overcoming Sexual Dysfunction and Reclaiming Your Sex Life*. New York: Henry Holt and Co. This book is an easy-to-understand, self-help update on female sexual anatomy and sexual response changes. It combines psychological and physiological discussions of sexual problems.
- Loulan, J.A. 1984. *Lesbian Sex*. San Francisco: Spinsters/Aunt Lute. This book is about female sexuality in general. It originally was written for lesbians, but it applies to heterosexuals, as well. The book is full of self-help exercises to do alone or with a partner; it discusses desire issues on pages 87–89.
- Haines, S. 1999. *The Survivor's Guide to Sex: How to Have an Empowered Sex Life After Child Sexual Abuse*. San Francisco: Cleis Press. This is an excellent, easy-to-read, self-help book covering many aspects of sexual healing. Chapter 2 covers sexual desire.
- Goodwin, A.J., and Agronin, M.E. 1997. *A Woman's Guide to Overcoming Sexual Fear and Pain*. Oakland, Calif.: New Harbinger Publications. This is another excellent, easy-to-read, self-help guide focusing on psychosocial and physiological education about sexuality.

NOTE: The above listed books could be sold at practice site.

FOLLOW-UP

→ Individualized, based on case presentations and needs of the patient.
→ Document in progress notes and on problem list.

Arousal Phase Disorder

DATABASE

SUBJECTIVE

→ Symptoms may include:
  - Lack of lubrication or lack of subjective feeling of arousal
  - Decreased clitoral or labial sensation, decreased clitoral or labial engorgement, or lack of ballooning out of posterior vagina
  - Pain during intercourse (dyspareunia)
  - Vaginal discomfort/irritation or dysuria following intercourse
→ Several physical conditions may contribute to a lack of lubrication:
  - Lack of effective stimulation
  - Chronic use of antihistamines
  - Chronic yeast infections
  - Acute or chronic bacterial vaginosis or trichomoniasis

- Marijuana use before a sexual experience
- Hysterectomy
- Lack of estrogen resulting from surgical removal of the ovaries, chemotherapy, or menopause
- Adhesions/scarring resulting from vaginal/pelvic surgery
- Endometriosis
- Intact/tight hymen
- Fatigue

→ A complete history—medical, surgical, obstetrical, gynecological, contraceptive, medication, habits, and psychosocial—should be obtained.

- Specific history to assess arousal phase disorders should include the following:
  - Alcohol and/or marijuana use in association with sex
  - The presence of anger or anxiety before, during, or after sex
  - The experience of pleasurable sensations in the vagina or clitoris
  - The experience of painful sensations in the vagina or clitoris
  - Changes in pulse rate and respiration when aroused
  - Swelling or engorgement of genital tissue when aroused
  - The degree of vaginal lubrication or dryness, use of artificial lubricant
  - The degree of difficulty concentrating during sexual activity. What interferes?
  - The amount of focus on upsetting or unpleasant thoughts
  - The amount of focus on what aspects of her partner turn her on or off
  - If the lack of arousal is lifelong, acquired, situational, or generalized
  - The patient's awareness regarding effective stimulation (Is it enough? Would she like more or less of something?) and her ability to communicate her needs to her partner
  - Partner cooperation
  - Mutually consensual sexual encounters
  - Stress level
  - Preoccupation with other aspects of life
  - If coitus is prolonged

→ See the general assessment questions in **Appendix 12P.1**.

OBJECTIVE

→ Complete pelvic examination to assess for evidence of infections, lesions, or other pathology.
→ Bimanual examination to note any tenderness in introitus, vagina, or pelvis.
→ Additional physical examination components based on history.

ASSESSMENT

→ Arousal phase disorder: lifelong, acquired, situational, or generalized

→ R/O vaginal/pelvic pathology
→ R/O psychological factors

PLAN

DIAGNOSTIC TESTS

→ Wet mount of vaginal secretions
→ Endocervical samples for *Neisseria gonorrhoeae* and *Chlamydia trachomatis*
→ Additional laboratory tests as indicated

TREATMENT/MANAGEMENT

→ Discuss and encourage the use of artificial, water-based lubricants, which may be all that is needed to stimulate the patient's own lubrication. Brand names include Probe®, Astroglide®, PrePair Personal Lubricant®, Wet®, Lubrin®, and Replens®.
→ Bibliotherapy is indicated in cases that appear to stem from milder sources of anxiety. See Barbach (1975, 1982) and Berman et al. (2001).
→ Probe for feelings of apathy, anger, fear, boredom.
→ Kaplan (1979) suggests the following behavioral model for sexual tasks:

- Sensate focus I—taking turns pleasuring or caressing the other's body without genital stimulation.
- Sensate focus II—taking turns pleasuring the other's body with gentle, undemanding genital stimulation that does not proceed to orgasm.
- Slow, teasing genital stimulation by the partner. The vulva, clitoris, vaginal entrance, and nipples are caressed. This stimulation is interrupted if the woman feels she is near orgasm and is continued a little later, when arousal has diminished somewhat.
- Coitus is withheld until the woman is well-lubricated.
- Slow, teasing, undemanding intromission in the female superior position under the patient's control for the purpose of focusing on her vaginal sensations.

→ Refer for sex therapy as indicated.
→ Refer for individual psychotherapy as indicated.
→ Refer for couple therapy as indicated.

CONSULTATION

→ Refer for sex therapy, individual psychotherapy, or couple therapy as indicated.
→ The primary care provider might be serving as a consultant to the psychotherapist who refers the patient for physical or gynecological examination.

PATIENT EDUCATION

→ Encourage the patient to take responsibility for her arousal by learning specifically what she needs to do to become aroused and communicating this information to her partner.
→ Refer for bibliotherapy. See Barbach (1975, 1982) and Berman et al. (2001).
→ Reassure the patient that using an artificial lubricant is not an indicator of failure.

→ Explain the similarities and differences between the male and female sexual response cycle.
→ Make available brief, informative, patient-education flyers.

FOLLOW-UP

→ Individualized, based on case presentation and needs of the patient.
→ Document in progress notes and on problem list.

Orgasm Phase Disorder

DATABASE

SUBJECTIVE

→ See the introductory section for subcategories of this disorder and contributing factors.
→ A complete history—medical, surgical, obstetrical, gynecological, contraceptive, medication, habits, and psychosocial—should be obtained.
  ■ A specific history of orgasm phase disorder should include:
    • Evaluation of whether the lack of orgasm is lifelong (primary), acquired (secondary), situational, generalized, or coital.
      – If the patient says she is anorgasmic, ask if she has ever had an orgasm by *any* means.
      – Does she know what an orgasm is?
      – Can she bring herself to orgasm on her own?
      – Does she use her finger, a vibrator, or other means?
      – When she is with her partner, what type of stimulation does she receive and for how long?
      – Does she fear letting go? If so, what gets in the way?
    • Lifelong (primary) anorgasmia:
      – The patient's experiences with masturbation
      – Knowledge of location of clitoris
      – History of masturbation (does she stop stimulation before orgasm?)
      – Outcome of becoming orgasmic
      – Partner pressure for orgasm
      – Responsible party for arousal and orgasm
      – Breath-holding, teeth-gritting during arousal
      – Tightening of stomach and pelvis to produce orgasm
    • Acquired (secondary) anorgasmia:
      – Changes in relationship and health, stress level
      – Medications
      – Stress reduction or relaxation practices
      – Past events that aroused the patient to orgasm
      – The ability to communicate needs to a partner
      – Partner receptivity
      – Preoccupation with losing the ability to achieve orgasm
    • Situational anorgasmia:
      – Under what circumstances the patient is orgasmic and anorgasmic (manual, oral, vibrator, self, partner); orgasm relationship to a certain partner and/or partner technique

• Generalized anorgasmia:
  – Use of antidepressant medication, illnesses involving nerve damage
• Coital anorgasmia:
  – History of orgasm during intercourse, with or without additional clitoral stimulation; partner pressure to have coital orgasms; expectation for simultaneous orgasms with partner
→ See the general assessment questions in **Appendix 12P.1**.

OBJECTIVE

→ Complete pelvic examination to assess for genital neuropathy.
→ Assess for physical signs associated with diabetes or multiple sclerosis.

ASSESSMENT

→ Orgasm phase disorder: lifelong, acquired, situational, generalized, or coital
→ R/O concomitant medical illness such as diabetes or multiple sclerosis
→ R/O prescription and/or recreational-drug effects
→ Assess contributing stress factors

PLAN

DIAGNOSTIC TESTS

→ Pelvic examination to assess for genital neuropathy
→ Appropriate diagnostic tests to assess for diabetes or multiple sclerosis as indicated
→ Additional laboratory tests based on history

TREATMENT/MANAGEMENT

Primary Anorgasmia

→ Give permission for self-exploration.
→ Provide education regarding anatomy, physiology, and sexual norms.
→ Provide education regarding appropriate and effective stimulation.
→ Relaxation of inhibition.
→ Discuss methods to help focus the patient's attention. Suggest using fantasy for distraction from performance anxiety during stimulation.
→ Refer for bibliotherapy. See Barbach (1975, 1982).
→ Recommend using a water-based lubricant for self-exploration and partner stimulation.
→ Recommend taking plenty of private time to explore genitals, noting which parts feel more pleasurable than others when stimulated. Have the patient locate the clitoris and stimulate it in various ways until she finds the way that feels best (Barbach 1975).
→ Recommend reading a romantic or erotic fantasy for stimulation and distraction from performance anxiety.
→ Introduce the idea that arousal is ultimately the patient's responsibility.

→ Teach relaxation and pelvic breathing so the patient can breathe deeply as she approaches orgasm. Remind the patient to relax her jaw muscles.

→ Suggest using a vibrator if the patient requires more intense stimulation.

→ Refer for psychotherapy as indicated to resolve unconscious fears of orgasm.

Secondary Anorgasmia

→ Remind the patient that stress can be a sexual inhibitor; advise that stress reduction is beneficial.

→ Discuss the importance of setting aside a special, unhurried time for sex.

→ Demonstrate deep pelvic breathing and jaw relaxation. Instruct the patient to use slow, deep pelvic breathing to prevent blockage of orgasm.

→ Give permission for self-exploration and leisurely sexual experimentation. Validate sexual feelings.

→ Refer for bibliotherapy. See Barbach (1975, 1982). The patient should note information on risk-taking, communication, blocks to orgasm, orgasm-expanding potential, and orgasm with a partner.

→ Recommend using a water-based lubricant for self-exploration and partner stimulation.

→ Introduce the idea that the patient's arousal is ultimately her own responsibility.

→ Suggest using a vibrator if the patient requires more intense stimulation.

→ Discuss methods to help focus the patient's attention. Suggest using fantasy for distraction from performance anxiety during stimulation.

Situational Anorgasmia

→ Give permission to have any kind of orgasm. Help the patient increase her self-esteem about her sexuality without pressure for orgasm through intercourse.

→ Introduce the idea of communicating with her partner about preferences for stimulation.

→ Discuss methods to help focus the patient's attention. Suggest using fantasy for distraction from performance anxiety during stimulation.

→ Refer for bibliotherapy. See Barbach (1975, 1982).

Coital Anorgasmia

→ Suggest heightened arousal before intercourse.

→ Teach Kegel exercises to enhance vaginal sensations.

→ Suggest combining clitoral stimulation (manual or vibrator) with intercourse.

→ Suggest having intercourse in a position in which the clitoris can be reached by hand or a vibrator, or tilting the female pelvis upward to maximize contact during intercourse.

CONSULTATION

→ Consult with a physician as indicated to assess whether physical illness may be a contributing factor.

→ Consult with a pharmacist as indicated to determine if medication might be implicated.

PATIENT EDUCATION

Primary Anorgasmia

→ Reassure the patient that nothing is "wrong" with her, that she needs to explore herself more.

→ Use pictures or a hand-held mirror to educate the patient about female anatomy. Discuss the need for clitoral stimulation.

→ See "Treatment/Management," above.

Secondary Anorgasmia

→ See "Treatment/Management," above.

Situational Anorgasmia

→ See "Treatment/Management," above.

Coital Anorgasmia

→ See "Treatment/Management," above.

FOLLOW-UP

→ Individualized based on case presentation and needs of the patient.

→ Document in progress notes and on problem list.

Dyspareunia

DATABASE

SUBJECTIVE

→ History to include detailed pain specifics, such as quality, quantity, location, duration, timing of occurrence, and aggravating/relieving factors. Additional questions should focus on the degree of interference with sexuality, relationships, and personal well-being (Binik et al 2000).

→ A complete history—medical, surgical, obstetrical, gynecological, contraceptive, medications, habits, and psychosocial.

■ Question the patient specifically about the use of soap on her genitals (e.g., antibacterial, scented, or other soap that may cause dermatitis); "scrubbing" of genitals; excessive use of douches; genital eczema; and detergent used for washing underwear.

■ Question the patient specifically about previous vaginal or pelvic surgeries or other pelvic trauma, such as rape, childbirth, or accidents.

→ Pain description (Binik et al. 2000):
  • Location:
    – Ask where the pain is exactly. This is more difficult to answer if the pain is not localized or it "travels" around.
    – Ask if the pain is vulvar, vaginal, deep, or some combination of locations.
    – Ask if a gynecological exam could "recreate" a similar pain.

– Ask if self-examination with a hand-held mirror could help localize the pain.
- Quality:
  – Ask if the pain is burning, sharp, dull, aching, shooting, hot, etc.
- Pain elicitors and time course:
  – Ask what activities (not just sexual activities) create the pain and how long it lasts (seconds, hours, or days).
- Intensity:
  – Ask the patient to rate the pain on a scale of 0–10 (no pain versus worst pain).
  – Ask the patient to rate the degree of distress caused by the pain (not distressing versus extremely distressing).
- Meaning:
  – Ask the patient how she explains to herself that she has this pain.
  – Does her theory ascribe a physiological or psychological basis to the cause of dyspareunia?

OBJECTIVE

→ Bimanual examination to note any tenderness in introitus, vagina, or pelvis.
→ Assess for unstretched or rigid hymen.

ASSESSMENT

→ Dyspareunia: lifelong, acquired, situational, or generalized
→ R/O anxiety and depression

PLAN

DIAGNOSTIC TESTS

→ Wet mount of vaginal secretions
→ Endocervical samples for *N. gonorrhoeae* and *C. trachomatis*
→ Additional laboratory tests as indicated by history

TREATMENT/MANAGEMENT

→ Specific to underlying cause(s). See the appropriate chapters.
→ Education regarding anatomy, physiology, and sexual norms and techniques.
→ Kegel exercises
→ Increase noncoital, nonpenetrating stimulation.
→ Increase lubrication (natural or artificial; avoid nonoxynol-9 or anything with fragrance due to irritation).
→ Systematic desensitization of pain
→ Woman controls speed and depth of penetration
→ Change coital positions.
→ Relationship counseling
→ Eliminate soap for washing genitals or recommend a nonsoap such as Aveeno

CONSULTATION

→ The primary care provider may serve as a consultant to the

mental health professional who is referring the patient with dyspareunia for physical and gynecological examination.
→ Consult with a physical therapist for assessment of pelvic floor muscles.
→ Consult with a physician as indicated in difficult cases.

PATIENT EDUCATION

→ Specific to underlying cause(s). See the appropriate chapters.
→ Discuss ways to avoid positions or movements that aggravate the pain.
→ Discuss pain-coping strategies.

FOLLOW-UP

→ Individualized, based on case presentation and needs of the patient.
→ Document in progress notes and problem list.

Vaginismus

DATABASE

SUBJECTIVE

→ The degree of vaginal spasm is on a continuum—partial (penetration is possible but painful) to complete (nothing can penetrate).
→ A complete history—medical, surgical, obstetrical, gynecological, contraceptive, medications, habits, and psychosocial.
- Specific questions regarding:
  - The presence of desire, arousal, lubrication, and orgasm
  - History of pain related to penetration
  - Fear of penetration, "ripping"
  - Partner sensitivity to the patient's pain
  - The patient's ability to communicate needs to her partner
  - Erectile difficulty in partner
  - Use of lubricant
  - Attempts to penetrate virginal hymen
- See "Subjective" under "Dyspareunia."

OBJECTIVE

→ Vaginismus is diagnosed primarily by pelvic examination. A past or present pelvic examination may be connected to the trauma. Discuss this possibility with the patient. Work together to make examination as comfortable as possible.
→ See "Objective" under "Dyspareunia."
→ Assess for involuntary contraction of vaginal muscles upon touching the vulva or digitally entering the vagina.

ASSESSMENT

→ Vaginismus: lifelong, acquired, situational, or generalized
→ R/O anxiety and depression

PLAN

DIAGNOSTIC TESTS

→ See "Dyspareunia."

TREATMENT/MANAGEMENT

→ Treatment can be protracted, especially when vaginismus is associated with trauma.
→ Treatment is threefold:
  ▪ Education and behavioral reconditioning techniques until vaginal spasms disappear
  ▪ Psychodynamic therapy to resolve the phobic elements
  ▪ Couple therapy to gain essential partner cooperation and communication
→ The provider may be able to initiate educational and behavioral reconditioning. However, the patient should be referred to a sex therapist, marriage counselor, social worker, or psychologist with special training in resolving sexual dysfunction.
→ Dispel myths about anatomy, sexual response cycle, and intercourse.
→ Discuss the meaning of intercourse for the patient and her partner.
→ Give the patient permission to say "no" to intercourse verbally rather than decline it physically.
→ Reassure the patient that because the vaginal muscle reaction is a learned response to the fear of pain, it can be unlearned.
→ Clarify for the patient and partner that while the patient can learn to prevent the contractions, she does not consciously will them to occur (Kaplan 1979).
→ Teach Kegel exercises and ask the patient to perform approximately 100/day.
  ▪ She should concentrate on a final squeeze of the muscles of the pelvic floor (pubococcygeus) so she can get maximum relaxation after the squeeze.
  ▪ She should consciously try to relax the muscles of the pelvic floor even further after initially relaxing them.
→ Behavioral reconditioning includes:
  ▪ Teaching relaxation and pelvic breathing
  ▪ Gentle self-insertion of graduated dilators to allow adaptation to vaginal penetration and to associate it with feeling calm and in control
  NOTE: The general principle is to start with very thin objects and work up to an object the size of the partner's penis. Often the patient's or the partner's finger is used instead of an object, starting with the smallest finger. The patient is in total control of the timing, depth, and movement. (The partner can serve as a coach for relaxation breathing if the patient is comfortable with this.) An inexpensive dilator is the plastic outside casing of a syringe, which comes in a variety of sizes. *Use lots of lubricant* (water-based, nonirritating, unscented). The step-by-step insertion process is generally as follows:
    • Perform relaxation and deep pelvic breathing.
    • Lubricate the vagina.
    • Insert the smallest object and remain in a prone position for a while. If anxiety arises, talk about it. Stop at any time. Do not do anything that is painful. The whole point is to become relaxed and comfortable.

• Repeat the above steps with each graduated object. The patient determines readiness.
• The partner inserts his smallest finger. Work up to insertion of a larger finger, possibly two fingers. When the patient is ready, she can signal her partner to begin very slight movement of his finger.
• Insert penis (the most difficult part). When the patient feels ready for penis insertion, she should be in total control. It is helpful if she holds her hand on the partner's penis and directs it inside herself. She should hold the penis inside her with no movement by either partner. When she feels ready for movement, she can move slightly or direct her partner to gently move his penis.

CONSULTATION

→ The primary care provider may serve as a consultant to the mental health professional who is referring the patient with dyspareunia for physical and gynecological examination.
→ Consult with a physician as indicated in difficult cases.

PATIENT EDUCATION

→ See "Treatment/Management, above."

FOLLOW-UP

→ Individualized, based on case presentation and needs of the patient.
→ Document in progress notes and on problem list.

BIBLIOGRAPHY

American Psychiatric Association (APA). 2000. *Diagnostic and statistical manual of mental disorders*, 4th ed., text revision. Washington, D.C.: the Author.

Barbach, L. 1975. *For yourself: the fulfillment of female sexuality*. New York: Doubleday.

_____. 1982. *For each other: sharing sexual intimacy*. New York: Signet.

Bartlik, B., Legere, R., and Anderson, L. 1999. The combined use of sex therapy and testosterone replacement therapy for women. *Psychiatric Annals* 29(1):27–33.

Berman, J., and Berman, L. 2001. *For women only: a revolutionary guide to overcoming sexual dysfunction and reclaiming your sex life*. New York: Henry Holt and Co.

Binik, Y.M., Bergeron, S., and Khalife, S. 2000. Dyspareunia. In *Principles and practice of sex therapy*, 3rd ed., eds. S.R. Leiblum and R.C. Rosen, pp. 154–180. New York: Guilford Press.

Crooks, R., and Bauer, K. 1987. *Our sexuality*, 3rd ed. Menlo Park, Calif.: Benjamin/Cummings.

Ellison, C.R. 2000. *Women's sexualities: Generations of women share intimate secrets of sexual self-acceptance*. Oakland, Calif.: New Harbinger Publications.

Heinman, J.R., and Meston, C.M. 1998. Empirically validated treatment for sexual dysfunction. *Annual Review of Sex Research* 8:148–194.

Hite, S. 1976. *The Hite Report: a nationwide study of female sexuality*. New York: Dell Books.

Kaplan, H.S. 1979. *Disorders of sexual desire*. New York: Simon & Schuster.

Kelly, G.F. 2001. *Sexuality today: the human perspective*, 7th ed. Boston: McGraw-Hill.

Leiblum, S.R., and Rosen, R.C. 2000. *Principles and practice of sex therapy*, 3rd ed. New York: Guilford Press.

LoPicolo, L. 1980. Low sexual desire. In *Principles and practice of sex therapy*, eds. S.R. Leiblum and L.A. Pervin, pp. 27–64. New York: Guilford Press.

Loulan, J.A. 1984. *Lesbian sex*. San Francisco: Spinsters/Aunt Lute.

Pridal, C.G., and Lo Picolo, J. 2000. Multielement treatment for desire disorders: integration of cognitive, behavioral, and systemic therapy. In *Principles and practice of sex therapy*, 3rd ed., eds. S.R. Leiblum and R.C. Rosen, pp. 57–81. New York: Guilford Press.

Rako, S. 1996. *The hormone of desire: the truth about sexuality, menopause, and testosterone*. New York: Harmony Press.

Reiss, U. 2001. *Natural hormone balancing for women*. New York: Pocket Books.

Schover, L., Friedman, J., Weiler, S. et al. 1982. Multiaxial-problem oriented system for sexual dysfunction. *Archives of General Psychiatry* 39:614–619.

APPENDIX 12P.1.

General Assessment Questions for Sexual Functioning

These questions are useful in bringing up the topic of sexual functioning:

General Profile (sexual problem history)

Which sexual problems, if any, have concerned you in the past or are current concerns?

What is the specific problem?

What is the onset, course, duration, and severity?

Get specifics:

When did the problem start? Have you always had it?

Why did you come in about it now?

How frequently do you have sex? What percentage of the time do you have the problem?

Is it different with different partners? If so, have you any idea why?

Are you usually fairly turned on when you have the problem? Or does the problem appear after you get turned on and then turned off? Or does the problem arise because you are just not that turned on?

What do you think contributes to the problem?

When is there no problem?

What other attempts have either or both partners made to solve the problem? How did they work? (Gives the clinician an idea of what didn't work. The clinician should note attempts that have made the problem worse.)

What do you think is the ideal way for you and your partner to function in bed, in your daily living, in other aspects of the relationship?

Follow-up Questions as indicated:

What do you consider a sexual stimulus?

What do you consider a sexual response?

What reinforces your sexual response?

What inhibits your sexual response?

What would be a complete or satisfying sexual experience?

How does using birth control affect your sexual response?

How does using safer sex practices affect your sexual response?

How does your concern about HIV/AIDS affect your sexual response?

Are there symptoms of premenstrual syndrome (in you or your partner) that affect your sexual response?

How does your or your partner's monthly cycle affect your sexual response?

What have been the effects of pregnancy (3 trimesters of pregnancy and postpartum up to 2+ years) on your sexual response?

Is infertility an issue? How does it affect your feelings about yourself as a sexual person? How has it affected the sexual dynamics between you and your partner?

How do you feel emotionally about foreplay (amount, kinds, partner communication)?

How would you describe your ability to let go to arousal?

How has your sexuality been different in different stages of development (teen, young adult, adult, older adult)?

What would increase your willingness to have sexual relations?

How does focusing on your biological clock affect your sexual responses and behaviors?

12-Q

Toxic Shock Syndrome

Toxic shock syndrome (TSS) is an acute illness characterized by multisystem organ failure. In 1978, the first description of TSS appeared in the scientific literature. Is was described as an acute, severe, multisystem disease occurring in seven children and adolescents who presented with a sudden onset of high fever, sore throat, headache, diarrhea, and erythematous rash with subsequent desquamation, liver abnormalities, renal failure, and central nervous system symptoms (e.g., confusion) (Todd et al. 1978). The disease was associated with strains of staphylococci that produced an epidermal toxin.

The unique characteristics of TSS were subsequently noted in seven patients in Wisconsin. Six of the seven patients were menstruating woman. In response to this clustering of cases, a statewide TSS surveillance system began in Wisconsin. Thirty-eight cases were reported between 1975 and mid-1980. Of these cases, 37 occurred in women. Of the 37 women, 35 had symptoms during menses and 97% of the menstruating women reported tampon use during the onset of the illness. In addition, *Staphylococcus aureus* was cultured from vaginal and cervical sites in 74% of the women from whom specimens were collected. Recurrent TSS episodes were noted in 28% of the 35 menstruating women, with all recurrences reportedly during menses (Davis et al. 1980).

In 1980, the Center for Disease Control (CDC) began national TSS surveillance to monitor trends, assess the magnitude, and determine risk factors associated with the disease (CDC 1980). Initial results from this surveillance noted that more than 90% of TSS cases were reported in menstruating women of childbearing age (American Academy of Pediatrics [AAP] 2000, CDC 1990). A mortality rate of 5% also was noted. Continuing investigations discovered several risk factors associated with TSS, including menstruation, tampon use (especially continuous use of tampons for 24 hours during menstruation), young age, *S. aureus* colonization of the genital tract, and a low-level antibody titer to toxic shock syndrome toxin-1 (TSST-1). Subsequent studies further delineated a number of tampon characteristics that were associated with an increased risk of TSS, including super absorbency, the use of carboxymethylcellulose or polyacrylate rayon in tampon fibers, vagina/cervical microabrasions resulting from tampon use, and the capacity of the tampon to bind to magnesium (Berkeley et al. 1987, Hanrahan 1994, Kass 1989, Kass et al. 1987, Lanes et al. 1990).

In 1980, the CDC developed a case definition delineating specific signs and symptoms required for the diagnosis of TSS. (see **Table 12Q.1, CDC Case Definition for Toxic Shock Syndrome.**) A significant decline in reported cases was observed late in 1981 after a particular tampon product (Rely®) was withdrawn from the market. Since that time, the national incidence of TSS has continued to decline. This decline has been attributed to several factors, including changes in the composition of remaining tampon products (i.e., decreased absorbency and removal of polyacrylate material from tampon fibers), education of professionals and the public about TSS, labeling of tampon packages regarding product absorbency and early signs of TSS, and a possible change in the use of catamenial products by women (e.g., more women choosing not to use tampons or not to use tampons continuously) (AAP 2000, Bloch 2001, Hanrahan 1994).

Nonmenstrual TSS (NMTSS) cases also have been documented in men and women. NMTSS currently accounts for more than half of the TSS cases reported annually (AAP 2000). It can occur in any patient with possible foci of *S. aureus* infection (e.g., surgical sites, wounds, and nasal packing) and is not associated with *S. aureus* that produces TSST-1. Although rare, NMTSS in women using diaphragms, cervical caps, and the contraceptive sponge has been documented (AAP 2000, Schwartz et al. 1989). There is an increased mortality rate observed in NMTSS compared to menstruation-associated TSS (AAP 2000, Bloch 2001).

The pathogenesis of TSS reportedly involves the multiplication of *S. aureus* in the foreign body or tissue wound that results in an increased production of TSST-1. TSST-1 is absorbed and causes decreased vasomotor tone and leakage of intravascular fluid. which can lead to rapid hypotension, tissue ischemia, and multisystem organ failure (AAP 2000, Fitzpatrick et al. 2001). Ninety percent of adults have antibodies to TSST-1. It has been proposed that in these individuals, TSST-1 that produces *S. aureus* may be part of the normal nasal and vaginal flora. Colonization by this strain of *S. aureus* would lead to antibody production and afford protection against TSS caused by TSST-1-producing *S. aureus*. Adults who lack these antibodies would remain susceptible to TSST-1-mediated by TSS.

Transmission of TSST-1-producing *S. aureus* between persons or nosocomially is rare. When nosocomial transmission does occur, it is usually after a surgical procedure (AAP 2000, Bloch 2001). The incubation period is approximately 12 hours for nosocomial-related TSS; in contrast, menstrual-related TSS usually occurs 3–4 days after menstruation begins (AAP 2000). The overall mortality rate for TSS remains approximately 5%; however, adults older than 45 years have an increased risk of mortality (AAP 2000).

Since 1987, a toxic shock-like syndrome (TSLS) caused by group A streptococcus has been documented (Gallo et al. 1990) and should be included in the differential diagnosis of patients who are being evaluated for TSS (AAP 2000, Bloch 2001, Fitzpatrick et al. 2001). TSLS can occur in persons of all ages but has an increased incidence in very young children (usually in association with varicella), the elderly (persons 75 years old or older), and persons with diabetes mellitus, chronic pulmonary or cardiac conditions, human immunodeficiency virus infection, or alcohol or injection-drug use (AAP 2000, Chambers 2001). Symptoms similar to TSST-1-producing *S. aureus* TSS are noted in this condition, including shock, renal failure, and adult respiratory distress syndrome (ARDS). However, bacteremia and deep soft-tissue infection, which are uncommon in *S. aureus*-associated TSS, occur in most of these patients (AAP 2000, Stevens 2001) and the symptoms are not related to menses in women.

Most patients present with a history of a viral illness, minor trauma, recent surgery, or varicella infection (AAP 2000, Fitzpatrick et al. 2001, Stevens 2001). In almost half of the patients with TSLS, there is no identified portal of entry for the pathogen (Stevens 2001). Necrotizing fasciitis develops in 50–70% of patients with soft tissue infection. Multisystem organ failure and shock occur as a result of cytokine production stimulated by pyogenic exotoxins A, B, and C (Chambers 2001, Stevens 2001). The mortality rate is 25–50%, with an increased rate observed in adults compared to children (AAP 2000, Fitzpatrick et al. 2001).

DATABASE

SUBJECTIVE

→ Predisposing factors may include:
  - Menses with tampon use (usually within five days of symptom onset)

Table 12Q.1.   CDC CASE DEFINITION FOR TOXIC SHOCK SYNDROME

The following are CDC criteria used for diagnosing toxic shock syndrome:

1. Fever: temperature ≥38.9° C (102° F)

2. Rash: diffuse macular erythroderma

3. Desquamation: 1–2 weeks after the onset of the initial rash, especially involving the palms and soles

4. Hypotension: systolic blood pressure <90 mm Hg for adults or <5th percentile by age for children, or orthostatic syncope

5. Involvement of three or more of the following organs:

   Gastrointestinal system: vomiting or diarrhea at the onset of symptoms

   Musculoskeletal system: severe myalgia or creatine kinase >2 times normal levels

   Mucous membranes: vaginal, oropharyngeal, or conjunctival hyperemia

   Renal system: serum BUN or creatinine ≥2 times normal levels or >5 WBC/HPF on microscopic urinalysis in the absence of a urinary tract infection

   Hepatic system: bilirubin or transaminase levels ≥2 times normal levels

   Hematological system: platelets <100,000/mm^3

   CNS system: disorientation or altered consciousness without focal neurological signs when a fever and neurological signs are absent

6. Negative results for the following tests (if obtained):

   Cultures of blood, throat, cerebrospinal fluid

   Serology for Rocky Mountain spotted fever, leptospirosis, or measles

---

Source: Center for Disease Control (CDC). 1980. Toxic shock syndrome—United States. *Morbidity and Mortality Weekly Report* 29:227–229.

- History of TSS.
- History of recent surgery, wound, or nasal packing
→ The patient may report one or more of the following symptoms (AAP 2000, Bloch 2001, Fitzpatrick et al. 2001):
  - Sudden onset of high fever (≥38.9° C/102° F)
  - Headache
  - Erythema of conjunctiva and/or oropharynx
  - Myalgias/arthralgias
  - Muscle weakness
  - Nausea
  - Vomiting
  - Frequent, profuse diarrhea
  - Chills
  - Lightheadedness
  - Syncopal episode(s)
  - Dermatological manifestations:
    • Early manifestations that may be reported during the first few days of illness include:
      – Transient, generalized, erythematous rash
      – Red palms and soles
      – Petechiae (uncommon)
      – Generalized nonpitting edema
      – And/or vesicles/bullae (uncommon)
    • Late manifestations that may be reported one week or more after initial symptoms include:
      – Generalized, pruritic, erythematous, maculopapular rash (1–2 weeks after the initial symptoms)
      – Scaling of skin, which may be generalized or specific to the fingers, palms, toes, soles (10–21 days after the initial symptoms)
      – Loss of hair and/or nails (1–6 months after the initial symptoms)

OBJECTIVE

→ Physical examination may reveal the following (AAP 2000, Bloch 2001, CDC 1990, Fitzpatrick et al. 2001):
  - Elevated temperature (≥38.9° C/102° F)
  - Hemodynamic signs associated with shock, including decreased blood pressure (systolic <90 mm Hg) and increased pulse and respirations
  - The patient may appear disoriented or confused
  - Erythema of conjunctiva, tongue, pharynx, tympanic membranes, and/or vagina
  - Dermatological findings may vary depending on the stage of illness and may include the following:
    • Early findings noted during the acute phase of the illness:
      – Generalized, erythematous, macular rash
      – Generalized, nonpitting edema
      – Erythema of palms and soles
      – Petechiae (uncommon)
      – Vesicles/bullae (uncommon)
      – Possible evidence of a surgical or traumatic wound (usually not inflamed and often without purulent discharge)

    • Dermatological findings noted after the acute phase of illness include:
      – Generalized, maculopapular rash usually occurring 1–2 weeks after the acute phase
      – Desquamation of fingers, palms, toes, and soles (may be generalized) usually occurring 10–14 days after the acute phase
      – Evidence of hair and nail loss usually occurring 1–6 months after acute illness
→ In ARDS with pleural effusion, an initial pulmonary assessment of patients with dehydration may be within normal limits. However, once the patient is hydrated, pleural effusion may be evident (decreased breath sounds, fremitus, and dullness to chest percussion).
→ Pelvic examination may reveal erythema of vaginal mucosa, vaginal ulceration(s), blood, and/or the presence of a tampon in the vaginal vault.

ASSESSMENT

→ TSS
→ R/O streptococcal TSS
→ R/O ARDS
→ R/O acute renal failure
→ R/O myocardial dysfunction
→ R/O cerebral edema
→ R/O disseminated intravascular coagulation (DIC)
→ R/O gastroenteritis from other causes (e.g., bacterial or viral pathogens)
→ R/O septic shock from other causes (e.g., meningococcus)

PLAN

DIAGNOSTIC TESTS

→ The diagnosis of TSS is based on clinical manifestations that meet the CDC case definition. (See **Table 12Q.1**.)
  - No specific laboratory test is available for confirming a TSS diagnosis. However, the laboratory tests below will provide information about the status of the patient and possibly isolate the pathogen responsible for her symptoms, lending support to a TSS diagnosis (AAP 2000, Fitzpatrick et al. 2001).
  - If TSS is suspected, these tests should be ordered in consultation with a physician:
    • CBC with differential: will reveal >90% mature and immature neutrophils and may demonstrate decreased hematocrit
    • Ferritin level: will be decreased
    • Clotting studies may reveal the following:
      – Platelet count: decreased if DIC is present
      – Prothrombin time: prolonged if DIC is present
      – Partial thromboplastin time: prolonged if DIC is present
      – Fibrin split products: increased if DIC is present
    • Serum chemistry panel will be abnormal when the following results are reported:

– Elevated liver enzymes (alanine aminotransferase, aspartate aminotransferase)
– Increased creatinine phosphokinase
– Decreased protein and albumin
– Decreased calcium
– Decreased phosphorous
– Elevated BUN
– Elevated creatinine

• Cultures:
– Blood cultures are positive in fewer than 5% of cases because TSS is caused by an *S. aureus* toxin (AAP 2000).
– Cultures obtained from vaginal foci are positive for *S. aureus* in 85% of menstruation-related TSS cases and in 40–60% of infected foci-related NMTSS cases (Bloch 2001). However, up to one-third of isolates of *S. aureus* from NMTSS cases do not demonstrate TSST-1; TSST-1-producing organisms can be part of the normal nasal and genital flora in adults. Therefore, the presence or absence of TSST-1 in an *S. aureus* isolate is helpful diagnostically (AAP 2000). Antimicrobial susceptibility testing should be performed on cultures that isolate *S. aureus* to determine if the strain is methicillin-resistant (AAP 2000).

• Serum antibody testing for the presence of TSST-1: A significant increase in titer in patients with a history of clinical manifestations of TSS would support a TSS diagnosis. However, the presence of antibody to TSST-1 can occur in asymptomatic patients and negative or low TSST-1 antibody titers have been reported in patients with nonmenstrual TSS (Chesney 1989, Jacobson et al. 1989).

• Urinalysis: will reveal pyuria with more than 5 leukocytes per high-power field.

• Streptococcal antibodies (e.g., serial antistreptolysin O, antideoxyribonuclease B, etc.): will not demonstrate rising titers in patients with *S. aureus* TSS (a positive result indicates streptococcal infection) (AAP 2000).

• EKG: will demonstrate decreased voltage throughout the pericardium, nonspecific ST-T wave changes, and flattened T waves.

• Hemodynamic monitoring should be performed when the patient is admitted to the hospital. It will reveal:
– Increased pulmonary wedge pressure, central venous pressure, and left ventricular end-diastolic pressure
– Decreased cardiac index

TREATMENT/MANAGEMENT

→ The major cause of morbidity and mortality associated with TSS is hypovolemia and shock. Therefore, the immediate treatment of a suspected TSS patient is establishing a peripheral intravenous line to provide hydration and prevent further hemodynamic collapse (Bloch 2001).

→ Any potentially infected foreign body (e.g., a tampon or nasal packaging) should be identified and removed immediately (AAP 2000, Bloch 2001).

→ Necessary drainage and irrigation of identified infected sites should be managed by the consulting physician.

→ The decision regarding antibiotic therapy should be made by the consulting physician who is admitting the suspected TSS patient to the hospital. Antibiotic therapy should include agents that are effective against *S. aureus* and ß-lactamase-resistant organisms.

→ The need for immediate hospitalization should be explained to the patient and take place with individual(s) accompanying her to the ambulatory setting.
  ■ If the patient's nearest relative or significant other is not accompanying her, that person should be notified as soon as possible because of the morbidity and mortality associated with TSS.

CONSULTATION

→ TSS is a life-threatening disease.
  ■ Delays in diagnosis and interventions are associated with an increased risk of mortality.
  ■ Immediate consultation with a physician is warranted for *all* patients suspected of having TSS. The consulting physician is responsible for the patient's treatment plan.

PATIENT EDUCATION

→ When appropriate, the patient and family should be educated about the immediate treatment of TSS (i.e., the need for stabilization and hospitalization).

→ The consulting physician and the patient should discuss the cause of TSS, as well as diagnostic tests, therapeutic options, possible complications, strategies for preventing future episodes, and follow-up care. Reviewing and/or reiterating these points may be necessary when the patient returns for follow-up care. Women with menstruation-related TSS should be educated about the possibility of a recurrence.

→ Education of all menstruating women and other patients at risk of TSS about the signs and symptoms of TSS and ways to prevent its occurrence (e.g., avoiding the use of high-absorbency tampons, using tampons for a limited period of time [≤18 hours per day] during menses, and using a diaphragm/cervical cap properly) should be included in primary health care visits.

FOLLOW-UP

→ Follow-up of the patient should be per recommendation of the consulting physician.

→ Document in progress notes and problem list.

BIBLIOGRAPHY

American Academy of Pediatrics (AAP). 2000. *2000 red book: report of the Committee on Infectious Diseases*, pp. 576–581. Elk Grove, Ill.: American Academy of Pediatrics.

Berkeley, S.F., Hightower, A.W., Broome, C.V. et al. 1987. The relationship of tampon characteristics to menstrual toxic shock syndrome. *Journal of the American Medical Association* 258(7):917–920.

Bloch, K. 2001. Bacterial infections. Staphylococci. In *Current diagnosis and treatment in infectious diseases*, eds. W.R. Wilson and M.A. Sande, pp. 480–481. New York: Lange Medical Books/McGraw-Hill.

Center for Disease Control (CDC). 1980. Toxic-shock syndrome—United States. *Morbidity and Mortality Weekly Report* 29:227–229.

Centers for Disease Control and Prevention (CDC). 1990. Reduced incidence of menstrual toxic-shock syndrome—United States, 1980–1990. *Morbidity and Mortality Weekly Report* 39(25):421–423.

Chambers, J.F. 2001. Infectious diseases: bacterial and chlamydial. In *2002 current medical diagnosis and treatment*, eds. L.M. Tierney, Jr., S.J. McPhee, M.A. Papadakis et al., pp. 1399–1404. New York: Lange Medical Books/McGraw-Hill.

Chesney, P.J. 1989. Clinical aspects and spectrum of illness of toxic shock syndrome: overview. *Reviews of Infectious Diseases* 11(Suppl. 1):S1–S7.

Davis, J.P., Chesney, P.J., Wand, P.J. et al. 1980. Toxic-shock syndrome: epidemiologic features, recurrence, risk factors, and prevention. *New England Journal of Medicine* 303(25): 1429–1435.

Fitzpatrick, T.B., Johnson, R.A., Wolff, K. et al. 2001. *Color atlas and synopsis of clinical dermatology. Common and serious diseases*, pp. 624–626. New York: McGraw-Hill.

Gallo, U.E., and Fontanarosa, P.B. 1990. Toxic streptococcal syndrome. *Annals of Emergency Medicine* 19(11):1332–1334.

Hanrahan, S.N. 1994. Historical review of menstrual toxic shock syndrome. *Women and Health* 21:141–165.

Jacobson, J.A., Kasworm, E., and Daly, J.A. 1989. Risk of developing toxic shock syndrome associated with toxic shock syndrome toxin 1 following nongenital staphylococcal infection. *Reviews of Infectious Diseases* 11(Suppl. 1): S8–S13.

Kass, E.H. 1989. Magnesium and the pathogenesis of toxic shock syndrome. *Reviews of Infectious Diseases* 11(Suppl. 1):S167–S175.

Kass, E.H., and Parsonnet, J. 1987. On the pathogenesis of toxic shock syndrome. *Reviews of Infectious Diseases* 9 (Suppl. 5):S482–S489.

Lanes, S.F., and Rothman, K.J. 1990. Tampon absorbency, composition, and oxygen content and risk of toxic shock syndrome. *Journal of Clinical Epidemiology* 43(12): 1379–1385.

Schwartz, B., Gaventa, S., Broome, C.V. et al. 1989. Nonmenstrual toxic shock syndrome associated with barrier contraceptives: report of a case-control study. *Reviews of Infectious Diseases* 11(Suppl. 1):S43–S49.

Stevens, D.L. 2001. Streptococcus pyogenes. In *Current diagnosis and treatment in infectious diseases*, eds. W.R. Wilson and M.A. Sande, pp. 507–508. New York: Lange Medical Books/McGraw-Hill.

Todd, J., Fishaut, M., Kapral, F. et al. 1978. Toxic shock syndrome associated with phage-group-I staphylococci. *Lancet* 2:1116–1118.

12-RA Urinary Tract Disorders
Urinary Tract Infection

Urinary tract infection (UTI) refers to the invasion of microbial uropathogens in the lower or upper urinary tract, or both. Infection may be divided into lower urinary tract infection, commonly referred to as *bladder infection* or *cystitis*, and upper urinary tract infection, referred to as *kidney infection* or *pyelonephritis*. Lower urinary tract infection refers to the inflammation of the bladder mucosa caused by the presence of urinary pathogens in the bladder and is often characterized by urinary frequency, dysuria, urgency, suprapubic discomfort, and malodorous urine. Such infections are often recurrent; however, they are usually uncomplicated, easily treated, and no threat to future health (Stamm et al. 2001).

Pyelonephritis is an infection of the pelvis and parenchyma of the kidney and is usually the result of an infection that has ascended from the lower urinary tract. Once in the parenchyma, certain virulent strains of uropathogens may cross the renal epithelial barrier into the bloodstream, resulting in urosepsis (Wult et al. 2001). Clinical manifestations of pyelonephritis may include those of lower tract infections as well as severe flank pain, abdominal pain, fever, chills, malaise, nausea, and vomiting. One-third of patients with symptoms of uncomplicated lower tract infections may also have unrecognized infection of the upper urinary tract (Johnson et al. 1987, Rubin et al. 1992).

Lower urinary tract infections are the most common infection affecting women. Twenty-five to 35% of women will experience a lower urinary tract infection at least once in their lifetime and 25–50% of these women will experience recurrent episodes (Scholes et al. 2000, Stamm et al. 1991). An estimated 6–8 million acute, uncomplicated UTIs occur in women annually in the United States, where an estimated $1 billion is spent annually on the evaluation and treatment of ambulatory cases of lower urinary tract infections (Scholes et al. 2000).

There are three possible routes by which bacteria can invade and spread within the urinary tract: the lymphatic, hematogenous, and ascending pathways. Ascent of bacteria within the urethra is the most common pathway of infection. Intestinal flora are almost invariably the source of pathogens. *Escherichia coli* is the most common uropathogen and accounts for 80–90%

of UTIs (Nicolle 2001, Stamey 1996). *Staphylococcus saprophyticus* is the pathogen responsible for approximately 20% of UTIs in young women (Ishihara et al. 2001, Raz 2001). Other uropathogens include Klebsiella species, *Proteus mirabilis*, *Pseudomonas*, *Staphylococcus aureus*, *Staphylococcus epidermidis*, and Group D enterococcus.

Colonization of the vaginal epithelium, followed by colonization of the urethral epithelium, are the most important events in the pathogenesis of UTIs in women (Schaeffer 2001, Stamey 1996). This dynamic, noninflammatory process is characterized by the attachment of the uropathogen pili onto host cell receptors in the vaginal and periurethral mucosa. The normal bacterial flora of the vaginal intoitus and periurethral mucosa interfere with attachment of uropathogens by competing for receptor sites. Lactobacilli inhibit the attachment of uropathogens to introital and uroepithelial cells (Reid et al. 1987, Thomas et al. 1989).

Immunoglobulins secreted by the cervix inhibit bacterial adherence and colonization of the introital mucosa (Iravani 1990). Vaginal pH also influences colonization. Vaginal fluid is bactericidal at a pH of 4.0; in premenopausal women, estrogen influences the acidic pH of the vagina (Raz 2001). Vaginal pH of 6.5 or greater, often seen in hypoestrogenemic genital mucosa, supports the growth of all Gram-negative bacilli (Iravani 1990, Stamey 1980).

The combination of diaphragm and spermicidal is associated with profound disturbances of normal vaginal flora. There appears to be a marked increase in *E. coli* colonization, an increase in vaginal pH, and a decrease in lactobacilli with diaphragm use (Scholes et al. 2000, Stamm et al. 1989). There is no association between colonization and personal habits (Chow et al. 1986, Scholes et al. 2000).

The role of sexual activity in the pathogenesis of urinary tract infections has long been the subject of investigation. If uropathogens have not colonized the urogenital epithelium, intercourse alone will not cause an infection. Therefore, the importance of intercourse as a precipitant of urinary tract infections is limited to women who are inherently susceptible to urogenital colonization (Fowler 1989). Colonized women experiencing four or more episodes of intercourse per month are at further risk of recurrent UTIs (Scholes et al. 2000).

Ascending colonization of the proximal urethra and inoculation of the urine comprise the subsequent steps in the pathogenesis of urinary tract infections. The lower urinary tract exhibits several defense mechanisms that increase its resistance to bacterial invasion. The flushing action of urination removes uropathogens, and the urine acidity, osmolality, organic acids, and urea content inhibit bacterial growth (Iravani 1990).

The lower urinary tract secretes tissue factors such as oligosaccharides, uromucoids, immunoglobulins (IgA, IgG, and secretory IgA), and bladder mucopolysaccharides that inhibit, prevent, or detach the bacteria on urothelial mucosal cells. These factors appear to be deficient in women susceptible to UTIs (Iravani 1990, Stamey 1996).

Uncomplicated pyelonephritis most commonly occurs secondary to infected urine flowing back through the ureters into the renal pelvis. This occurrence is commonly referred to as *reflux*. Patients at risk for pyelonephritis are those infected with uropathogens with chromosomal virulence factors that enable the uropathogens to infect the upper urinary tract or bloodstream (Schilling et al. 2001, Stamey 1980). Complicated pyelonephritis occurs in the presence of congenital ureterovesical reflux, urinary obstruction, foreign bodies, urinary calculi, neurogenic bladder, and diabetes (Nicolle 2001).

Traditionally, the diagnosis of a lower urinary tract infection was based on a urine culture with $\geq 10^5$ uropathogen colony forming units (CFU) per mL from a clean-catch midstream urine specimen (Stamey 1980). However, only 40–80% of women with symptoms of a lower urinary tract infection demonstrate this quantity of bacteriuria (Fowler 1989, Stamey 1980). The remaining symptomatic patients will have urine cultures that may contain colony counts of 10^2–10^5 CFU/mL or may contain no identifiable pathogen.

Low colony counts are frequently found in infections caused by *E. coli*, *Staphylococcus saprophyticus*, enterococci, Klebsiella species, and *S. aureus* (Thomas et al. 1989). Urine cultures with low colony counts may result from early or subsiding infections, previous use of antibiotics, bacteriostatic agents in the urine, hydration, or diuresis (Stamey 1980, Thomas et al. 1989). It is currently recommended that a urine culture with a uropathogen of 10^2 CFU/mL or greater from symptomatic women be considered sufficient for the diagnosis of a lower urinary tract infection (Fowler 1989, Stamey 1980, Thomas et al. 1989). The recommended microbiological criterion for diagnosis of suspected acute pyelonephritis is $\geq 10^4$ CFU/mL (Rubin et al. 1992).

Antibiotic therapy is usually initiated for the treatment of presumptive or documented urinary tract infections. Antimicrobials used to treat urinary tract infections should have the following characteristics: excellent Gram-negative coverage, high urinary excretion in active form, minimal effect on the bowel and vaginal flora, low potential to develop bacterial resistance, ease of administration, good patient tolerance, and low cost (Iravani 1990). In addition to the preceding characteristics, antibiotics used to treat pyelonephritis must achieve adequate renal tissue levels. Community resistance patterns also should be considered. For example, 15–20% of urinary pathogens from non-nosocomial, uncomplicated urinary tract infections are now resistant to trimethoprim-sulfamethoxazole, 30–40% are resistant to ampicillin, and 20–30% are resistant to cephalothin (Stamm et al. 2001).

Recently there has been extensive investigation of the appropriate length of treatment for urinary tract infections. Conventional duration has been 7–10 days of antimicrobial therapy. However, studies have shown that more than 90% of women with lower urinary tract infections are cured within three days of antibiotic therapy (Bump 1990, Norby 1990, Stamm et al. 2001). The advantages of short-course therapy (1–5 days) include decreased incidence of side effects and adverse reactions, increased patient compliance, less development of bacterial resistance, less effect on the vaginal flora, less effect on bladder mucopolysaccharides, and lower cost. Short-course therapy is recommended for the treatment of nonpregnant women who have acute, uncomplicated lower UTIs. Renal infections will not respond to short-course therapy (Stamm et al. 2001, Talan 2000).

Contraindications to short-course therapy include pyelonephritis, known structural or functional abnormalities, diabetes, immunosuppressive conditions, and use of in-dwelling catheters. Short-course therapy in pregnancy and pediatrics is under investigation. Historically, a minimum of 10–14 days of antibiotic therapy was thought to be required to treat uncomplicated pyelonephritis and complicated urinary tract infections. Currently it is believed that seven days of therapy are sufficient to treat uncomplicated pyelonephritis (Stamm et al. 2001). Sicker patients may require hospitalization for parenteral antibiotics and hydration, anti-emetics, and pain control.

Following the initial episode, recurrent infections are frequent—2–6 per year in 85% of women (Iravani 1990, Stamey 1980). Susceptibility to recurrent infections is lifelong and is related to biological deficiencies that allow bacteria to adhere to vaginal epithelium and uroepithelium. The urogenital epithelium of women susceptible to recurrent urinary tract infections has been shown to have more attachment sites for uropathogens than does urogenital epithelium of women resistant to infections (Fowler 1989, Thomas et al. 1989). The primary risk factor for recurrent UTIs in women is the increased number of urogenital epithelial attachments sites (Schaeffer 2001). Until recently, uropathogenic *E. coli* (UPEC) were presumed to be predominately extracellular. Recent studies indicate that some cases of recurrent UTIs may be secondary to UPEC invasion of and persistence in bladder epithelial cells (Schilling et al. 2001).

Anatomical or functional abnormalities of the urinary tract are found in fewer than 5% of women with recurrent infections (Scholes et al. 2000, Stamey 1980, Stamm et al. 1989).

Depending on the frequency and nature of infections, women with recurrent urinary tract infections require special antibiotic treatment, which may include continual prophylaxis, postcoital prophylaxis, or self-treatment. Future trends in the management of recurrent UTIs in women include the application of a vaginal or oral lactobacillus probiotic to restore the normal lactobacilli-dominant flora (Stamm et al. 2001). The use of carefully selected, avirulent *E. coli* strains to colonize the bladder and prevent colonization by virulent strains is being pursued. In addition, anti-adhesive vaccines are being developed to prevent UTIs in women (Stamm et al. 2001).

DATABASE

SUBJECTIVE

→ Risk factors include:
- History of UTIs
- The patient is sexually active
- Increased frequency of coitus
- New sexual partner
- Child-bearing age
- Postmenopausal
- Use of barrier methods of contraception/spermicides
- Recent urogenital instrumentation
- Diabetes
- Urinary stones or history of stones
- Immunosuppressive conditions
- History of hysterectomy
- History of cystocele repair
- History of urethral dilatations
- Childhood urinary tract infections
- In-dwelling catheter
- Neurogenic bladder
- First-degree female relative with history of UTIs

→ Symptoms may include:

Lower Urinary Tract Infection

- Urinary frequency with small voids
- Dysuria/internal burning with urination
- Poor sensation of emptying
- Suprapubic tenderness
- Gross hematuria
- Urinary urgency
- Stress/urge incontinence
- Nocturia
- Tenesmus
- Malodorous urine
- Cloudy urine

Upper Urinary Tract Infection

- May have any of the above symptoms plus:
  - Fever ≥38.3° C/101° F
  - Severe flank pain
  - Abdominal pain
  - Nausea/vomiting
  - Chills
  - Malaise

OBJECTIVE

Lower Urinary Tract Infection

→ Abdominal examination: Patient may have suprapubic tenderness.

→ Pelvic examination: absence of vulvar erythema, excoriation, or abnormal vaginal discharge (unless there is a concomitant vaginal/cervical infection)
→ Urine microscopy (**NOTE:** Within specific *E. coli* species groups, there is a wide variation in the degree of pyuria):
- 10+ white blood cells (WBCs)/high power field (uncentrifuged urine)
- ± red blood cells (RBCs)
- + bacteria
→ Urine dipstick (**NOTE:** Not proven to be sufficiently sensitive or specific [Stamm et al. 2001]):
- ± WBCs
- ± RBCs
- + nitrites
- + leukocyte esterase
→ Urine culture with a single uropathogen $\geq 10^2$
NOTE: Cultures consistent with mixed uropathic flora may represent a low colony count UTI. "Mixed cultures" may also occur in diluted urine.
→ Temperature <37.8° C/100° F
→ Absence of costovertebral angle (CVA) tenderness

Upper Urinary Tract Infection

→ Abdominal examination: Patient may have suprapubic tenderness, abdominal tenderness.
→ Back examination: Patient may have CVA tenderness.
→ Urine microscopy:
- 10+ WBCs (uncentrifuged urine)
- ± RBCs
- + bacteria
→ Urine dipstick:
- + WBCs
- ± RBCs
- + nitrites
- + leukocyte esterase
→ Urine culture with a urinary pathogen $\geq 10^4$
→ Temperature ≥38.3° C/101° F

ASSESSMENT

Lower or upper urinary tract infection
→ R/O vaginitis, sexually transmitted disease (STD), pelvic inflammatory disease
→ R/O urinary obstruction/urinary stone
→ R/O interstitial cystitis
→ R/O neurogenic bladder
→ R/O musculoskeletal strain
→ R/O congenital anomalies
→ R/O papillary necrosis
→ R/O diverticulosis/diverticulitis
→ R/O surgical abdomen

PLAN

DIAGNOSTIC TESTS

→ Obtain urine culture and sensitivity for:
- First urinary tract infection

- Recurrent urinary tract infection without a culture in the past year
- Previous urine culture with a pathogen other than *E. coli/ S. saprophyticus*
- Resistance pattern on previous sensitivities
- Suspicion of pyelonephritis
- Subjective/objective data equivocal
- Gross hematuria
- Diabetes

→ Vaginal/cervical specimens and vaginal wet mount as indicated to rule out vaginitis/STD.

→ Women experiencing recurrent urinary tract infections may also require additional diagnostic tests based on their history and presentation. These additional tests include:

- Kidney, ureters, bladder (KUB) x-ray to rule out stones:
  - Previous stone or family history of stones
  - A pathogen other than *E. coli/Staphylococcus*
  - Patients younger than 40 years with a positive urine culture and gross hematuria
- Renal ultrasound to assess kidney size and rule out hydronephrosis or renal tumor:
  - Flank discomfort
  - Nonsmoker younger than 40 years with recurrent positive urine culture and gross hematuria
  - History of urinary tract infections/pyelonephritis in childhood/early childhood (>1 cm difference in renal length may indicate current or history of vesicoureteral reflux)
  - Persistent microscopic hematuria (>5 RBCs/HPF)
- Postvoid residual (**NOTE:** >100 cc should be considered abnormal):
  - Patient relates feeling of inability to completely empty bladder
  - Patient relates changes in stream or obstructive symptoms
  - History of bladder repair
  - Large cystocele on examination
  - Use of antihistaminics, decongestants, anticholinergics
  - History of urethral dilatations
  - Wheelchair-confined patients
  - Pessary/diaphragm users with device in place
  - Women with a medical illness such as diabetes, neurological conditions (e.g., multiple sclerosis), and lower-back problems, which can cause peripheral neuropathy
  - Following first episode of pyelonephritis
- Cystogram to rule out vesicoureteral reflux:
  - History of childhood urinary tract infections
  - History of pyelonephritis
  - Large cystocele
- Cystoscopy to rule out bladder tumors/stones, intravesical abnormalities:
  - Gross hematuria (cystoscopy is mandatory for the presence of gross hematuria without positive urine culture)
  - Persistent microscopic hematuria >5 RBCs/HPF
  - Numerous urinary tract infections (more than six per year)
- Intravenous pyelogram (IVP) to rule out renal tumors, stones, or hydronephrosis:

- Anyone with gross hematuria and a negative urine culture
- Smokers with gross hematuria regardless of culture result
- High suspicion of a stone
- Hydronephrosis
- Equivocal renal ultrasound/KUB

TREATMENT/MANAGEMENT

Lower Urinary Tract Infections

→ Medication regimens (Stamm et al. 2001, Talan 2000):

- Trimethoprim and sulfamethoxazole double strength, 1 tablet p.o. BID for 3–5 days
- Trimethoprim 100 mg, 1 tablet p.o. BID for 3–5 days (a good alternative for patients with sulfa allergy)
- Nitrofurantoin 50 mg, 1 tablet p.o. QID for 3–5 days
- Nitrofurantoin monohydrate 100 mg, 1 tablet p.o. BID for 3–5 days
  NOTE: Nitrofurantoin and nitrofurantoin monohydrate are contraindicated in patients with a G6PD deficiency.
- Cephradine 250–500 mg, 1 tablet p.o. QID for 3–5 days
- Cephalexin 250–500 mg, 1 tablet p.o. QID for 3–5 days
- Ciprofloxacin 250–500 mg, 1 tablet p.o. BID for 3–5 days
  NOTE: Caution is advised in using fluoroquinolones routinely in order to preserve their low resistance rates.
- Levofloxacin 250 mg, 1 tablet p.o. QD for 3–5 days
- Ofloxacin 200 mg, 1 tablet p.o. BID for 3–5 days
- Amoxicillin/clavulanate potassium 250–500 mg, 1 tablet p.o. TID for 3–5 days
- Ampicillin 500 mg, 1 tablet p.o. QID for 3–5 days.
  NOTE: This drug is recommended less frequently for the treatment of UTIs due to a high number of resistance patterns.
- Phenazopyridine hydrochloride for bladder discomfort: 100–200 mg, 1 tablet p.o. BID–TID prn.

Pyelonephritis

→ Medication regimens (Stamm et al. 2001, Talan 2000):
  NOTE: A portion of patients with pyelonephritis will require hospitalization for parenteral antibiotics/fluid replacement, pain management, and anti-emetics. The following list of medications may be used to treat pyelonephritis in ambulatory settings; however, these patients will require close follow-up.

- Trimethoprim and sulfamethoxazole, 1 tablet p.o. BID for 7–14 days
- Trimethoprim 100 mg, 1 tablet p.o. BID for 7–14 days
- Ciprofloxacin 500 mg, 1 tablet p.o. BID for 7–14 days
- Levofloxacin 250 mg, 1 tablet p.o. QD for 7–14 days
- Ofloxacin 200 mg, 1 tablet p.o. BID for 7–14 days
- Amoxicillin/clavulanate potassium 500 mg, 1 tablet p.o. QID for 10–14 days
- Garamycin (in cases of severe symptoms) 80–120 mg IM plus any of the above regimens
- Pain and antipyretic medications as indicated

Recurrent Urinary Tract Infections

→ Medication regimens (Stamm et al. 2001, Talan 2000):
- Continual prophylaxis: used in women experiencing more than 4–6 lower urinary tract infections per year or after one episode of pyelonephritis. Duration of prophylaxis ranges from 3–6 months, a minimum of 6 months following pyelonephritis/urosepsis.
  - Nitrofurantoin 50 mg, 1 tablet p.o. at HS
  - Trimethoprim 100 mg, 1 tablet p.o. at HS
  - Cephradine 250 mg, 1 tablet p.o. at HS
  - Cefuroxime 250 mg, 1 tablet p.o. at HS
  - Cephalexin 250 mg, 1 tablet p.o. at HS
  - Trimethoprim and sulfamethoxazole double strength, ½ tablet p.o. at HS
  - Ciprofloxacin 250 mg, ½ tablet every other day at HS

  NOTE: Avoid using fluoroquinolones as prophylactic agents unless sensitivities reflect resistance to other agents.
- Postcoital prophylaxis: used for women in whom infections are directly related to coital activity. Any of the above medications are to be taken within 30 minutes before or after intercourse. Must consider frequency of intercourse: If frequency is greater than 4 times per week, use daily prophylaxis instead.
- Self-treatment: used for women experiencing urinary infections less than 6 times per year. The patient self-treats with any of the above medications for 1–3 days.

→ Other management considerations:
- Vaginal pH: Consider local (urogenital) estrogen therapy in perimenopausal/menopausal women. Use Acigel® for patients with increased vaginal pH in whom topical estrogen therapy is contraindicated. Also screen for and treat bacterial vaginosis.
- Consider an alternative method of birth control in women using diaphragms.

CONSULTATION

→ For presence of urinary stones, hydronephrosis, structural abnormalities
→ For abnormal findings on cystogram, renal ultrasound, KUB, IVP
→ For postvoid residuals >50 cc
→ For cystoscopy
→ For diagnosis of pyelonephritis requiring hospitalization
→ For diagnosis of urosepsis
→ For gross hematuria with negative urine culture
→ For recurrent infections in wheelchair-confined patients
→ As needed for prescription(s).

PATIENT EDUCATION

→ Discuss compliance with prescribed mediation therapy.
→ Advise the patient to avoid alcohol, caffeine, chocolate, hot spicy foods, and citrus while symptomatic.
→ Advise the patient to prevent constipation and diarrhea. (See the **Constipation** and **Diarrhea** chapters in Section 7.)

→ Advise the patient to have vaginal symptoms assessed and treated.
→ Advise the patient to avoid vaginal douching.
→ Advise the patient to urinate 6–8 times a day.
→ Advise the patient to urinate 30–60 minutes after intercourse.
→ Advise the patient to avoid the use of artificial sweeteners, which adversely affect bladder mucopolysaccharides.
→ Discuss factors that may help control recurrent bacterial vaginosis. (See the **Bacterial Vaginosis** chapter.)

FOLLOW-UP

→ Post-treatment cultures usually are not recommended except in cases of pyelonephritis.
→ If this is the first or an occasional lower urinary tract infection, follow-up for ambulatory pyelonephritis should include early phone contact with the patient to assess her response to treatment and after completion of antibiotic therapy to discuss possible referrals, diagnostic tests, and prophylaxis.
→ For patients with recurrent lower urinary tract infections, follow-up visits initially should occur every 2–3 months while on continual prophylaxis, then every 4–6 months depending on the medication regimen and frequency of infections.
→ Explore other contraceptive options if the patient uses a diaphragm.
→ Document in progress notes and on problem list.

BIBLIOGRAPHY

Bump, R.C. 1990. Urinary tract infections in women: current role of single dose therapy. *Journal of Reproductive Medicine* 35:785–791.

Chow, A.W., Percival-Smith, R., and Bartlet, K.H. 1986. Vaginal colonization with *E. coli* in healthy women. *American Journal of Obstetrics and Gynecology* 154:120–126.

Fowler, J.E. 1989. *Urinary tract infections and inflammation,* pp. 13–35, 71–91. Chicago: Yearbook Medical Publishers.

Iravani, A. 1990. Advances in the understanding and treatment of urinary tract infections in young women. *Urology* 37(6): 503–511.

Ishihara, S., Yokoi, S., Ito, M. et al. 2001. Pathologic significance of *Staphylococcus saprophyticus* in complicated urinary tract infections. *Urology* 57(1):17–20.

Johnson, J.R., and Stamm, W.E. 1987. Diagnosis and treatment of acute urinary tract infections. *Infectious Disease Clinics of North America* 1:773–791.

Nicolle, L.E. 2001. Urinary tract pathogens in complicated infection and in elderly. *Journal of Infectious Diseases* 183 (Suppl. 1):S5–S8.

Norby, S.R. 1990. Short-term treatment of uncomplicated lower urinary tract infections in women. *Reviews of Infectious Diseases* 12(3):458–467.

Raz, R. 2001. Hormone replacement therapy or prophylaxis in postmenopausal women with recurrent urinary tract infection. *Journal of Infectious Diseases* 183(Suppl. 1):S74–S76.

Reid, G., and Sobel, J.D. 1987. Bacterial adherence in the

pathogenesis of urinary tract infections: a review. *Reviews of Infectious Disease* 9:470–482.

Rubin, R., Beam, T., and Stamm, W. 1992. An approach to evaluating antibacterial agents in the treatment of urinary tract infections. *Clinical Infectious Diseases* 14:S246–S251.

Schaeffer, A.J. 2001. What do we know about the urinary tract infection-prone individual? *Journal of Infectious Diseases* 183(Suppl. 1):S66–S69.

Schilling, J.D., Mulvey, M.A., and Hultgren S.J. 2001. Structure and function of *Escherichia coli* type 1 pili: new insight into the pathogenesis of urinary tract infection. *Journal of Infectious Diseases* 183(Suppl. 1):S36–S40.

Scholes, D., Hooton, T.M., Roberts, P.L. et al. 2000. Risk factors for recurrent urinary tract infections in young women. *Journal of Infectious Diseases* 183(Suppl. 1):536–540.

Stamey, T.A. 1980. *Pathogenesis and treatment of urinary tract infections.* Baltimore, Md.: Waverly.

_____. 1996. Update on the pathogenesis and management of urinary tract infections in women. *Monographs in Urology* 17(5):67–80.

Stamm, W.E. 2000. Risk factors for recurrent urinary tract infection in young women. *Journal of Infectious Diseases* 182:1177–1182.

Stamm, W.E., Hooton, T.M., Johnson, J.R. et al. 1989. Urinary tract infections: from pathogenesis to treatment. *Journal of Infectious Diseases* 159(3):400–406.

Stamm, W.E., Mckevitt, M., Roberts, P.L. et al. 1991. Natural history of recurrent urinary tract infections in women. *Review of Infectious Diseases* 13:77–89.

Stamm W.E., and Norby S.R. 2001. Urinary tract infections: disease panorama and challenges. *Journal of Infectious Diseases* 183 (Suppl. 10):S1–S4.

Talan, D.A. 2000. Short-course therapy for acute uncomplicated cystitis and pyelonephritis. *Infections in Urology* 13(5A): S14–S18.

Thomas, S., and Bhatia, N.N. 1989. New approaches in the treatment of urinary tract infections. *Urogynecology* 16: 897–909.

Wult, B., Bergsten, G., Samuelsson, M. et al. 2001. The role of P fimbriae for colonization and host response induction in the human urinary tract. *Journal of Infectious Diseases* 183 (Suppl. 1): S43-S46.

Sandra L. Lindholm-Norman, R.N., M.S., N.P.

12-RB Urinary Tract Disorders
Female Urinary Incontinence

Urinary incontinence (UI) is defined by the International Continence Society as a condition in which involuntary loss of urine is a "social or hygienic problem and is objectively demonstrated" (Stilling Burkhart 2000). UI is an underdiagnosed and underreported condition affecting the physical, psychological, social, and economic well-being of women and their families.

A review of epidemiological data on UI reflects a prevalence rate among community-dwelling women older than 60 years of between 17–55%. Among younger and middle-age females, the prevalence ranges from 12–47%, and at least 11.5 million nursing home residents are affected by UI (Burgio et al. 2000, Culligan et al. 2000, Sampselle 2000, Stilling Burkhart 2000). The economic cost of managing UI in the United States has been estimated to be $16–$26 billion annually (Sampselle 2000, Stilling Burkhart 2000).

Significant psychosocial sequelae are associated with incontinence. Depression, embarrassment, fear, guilt, lowered self-esteem, a sense of dependency, social isolation, and sexual abstinence frequently are reported by women with urinary incontinence (Dugan et al. 2000).

An intact bladder, urethra, and neurological system, as well as competent urethral sphincter mechanisms, are necessary for continence. The detrusor, a smooth muscle under voluntary control, is the external layer of the muscular coat of the bladder. Normally, a stable detrusor relaxes and expands in response to increasing bladder volumes without involuntary contractions or sensory symptoms. The urethral sphincter mechanism consists of the following: an intrinsic, urethral, smooth-muscle sphincter that extends from the bladder outlet through the pelvic floor; a distal, intrinsic, urethral, striated sphincter that surrounds the urethra; and an extrinsic, periurethral, striated muscle.

As the bladder fills with urine, the intrinsic urethral sphincter provides the resistance to keep the intraurethral pressure greater than that of the bladder to prevent urine leakage. The extrinsic periurethral muscles strengthen the resistance of the intrinsic mechanisms when bladder or intra-abdominal pressures increase. Continence is maintained as long as the intraurethral pressure is greater than the bladder pressure. During micturition,

a voluntary contraction of the detrusor increases the bladder pressure so it exceeds the intraurethral pressure. Voiding occurs when a voluntary contraction of the detrusor is synchronized with voluntary relaxation of the urethral sphincter mechanisms (Keane et al. 2000, Stilling Burkhart 2000).

The parasympathetic nervous system is responsible for the most detrusor innervation. The detrusor increases its contractile force and frequency in response to cholinergic activity. The bladder base and proximal urethra are innervated by the sympathetic nervous system primarily through alpha receptors that contract the bladder neck and urethra when stimulated. Innervation of the striated urethral sphincter is through the somatic nervous system, although the striated sphincter is thought to receive other innervation, as well (Keane et al. 2000, Stilling Burkhart 2000).

There are six classifications of urinary incontinence that may occur alone or in combination: stress, urge, mixed, overflow, functional, and transient. The most common types are stress, urge, mixed, and transient.

Transient incontinence is often secondary to existing, reversible conditions and is always alleviated by treatment. Transient causes of incontinence are implicated in up to one-third of elderly people (Resnick 1992). The mnemonic DIAPPERS is used to recall the etiologies of transient incontinence: **D**elirium/confusional state, **I**nfection, **A**trophic urethritis/vaginitis, **P**harmaceuticals, **P**sychological, **E**xcessive excretion (e.g. congestive heart failure, hyperglycemia), **R**estricted mobility, and **S**tool impaction (Stilling Burkhart 2000). Medications that may precipitate incontinence include anticholinergics, diuretics, antidepressants, antipsychotics, sedatives/hypnotics, narcotic analgesics, those containing alcohol, calcium channel blockers, and alpha adrenergic blockers/agonists (Cheater et al. 2000).

Stress urinary incontinence (SUI) is an involuntary loss of urine during activities that increase intra-abdominal pressure, such as coughing, laughing, sneezing, walking, and jumping. It is thought to occur as a result of weakened pelvic floor muscles or sphincter pathology. These anatomical changes allow increases in intra-abdominal pressure to exceed the intraurethral pressure, thereby allowing urine leakage (Cheater et al. 2000). Urine leakage is intermittent and usually occurs in small quantities. Stress incontinence is not usually associated with urinary frequency, urgency, dysuria, or nocturia except in the presence of concomitant conditions. Among ambulatory women, SUI is the most common type of incontinence, accounting for 50–70% of cases (Cheater et al. 2000).

Mixed incontinence is a combination of both stress and urge incontinence. Approximately one-third of women with urge incontinence also have stress incontinence. The two types of incontinence may present as separate conditions or they may be causally related. Usually, either the stress or urge component is most problematic.

Overflow incontinence occurs as a result of bladder overdistention. It is usually due to a hypoactive or underactive detrusor muscle secondary to medications, fecal impaction, diabetes, lower-spinal-cord injury, or disruption of the motor innervation of the detrusor (as in multiple sclerosis). Less common in women, overflow incontinence occurs as a result of obstruction such as occurs in severe genital prolapse, surgical overcorrection of a cystocele/urethral hypermobility, or poorly fitted pessary (Culligan et al. 2000, Stilling Burkhart 2000).

Functional incontinence is caused by factors outside the lower urinary tract, such as impaired mobility, reduced cognition and environmental limitations. It is diagnosed by exclusion (Cheater et al. 2000, Culligan et al. 2000, Stilling Burkhart 2000).

For information on *urge incontinence*, refer to the **Overactive Bladder** chapter.

DATABASE

SUBJECTIVE

→ Risk factors include:
- Confusional state
- Use of sedative-hypnotics, diuretics, anticholinergics, alpha-adrenergic agents, calcium channel blockers
- Restricted mobility
- Stool impaction
- Neurological conditions
- Urinary tract infection/inflammation
- Obesity
- Atrophic urethritis/vaginitis
- Pelvic floor relaxation
- Excessive urine production (e.g., diuretics, diabetes)
- Diabetes
- Increased body mass index
- Hysterectomy/pelvic surgery
- Estrogen deficiency
- Obstetrical factors: parity, vaginal delivery, advanced maternal age at first delivery, large infant birth weight
- Genetic predispositions (connective tissue factors)

→ Symptoms may include:

Stress Incontinence
- Patient reports involuntary leakage of urine precipitated

by events that increase intra-abdominal pressure (e.g., cough, laugh, sneeze, exercise).

Urge Incontinence
- See the **Overactive Bladder** chapter.

Mixed Incontinence
- The patient reports symptoms associated with both stress and urge incontinence.

Overflow Incontinence
- The patient reports constant, small-volume urinary loss, frequency, urgency, small voids, poor sensation of emptying.

Transient/Functional Incontinence
- The patient may report mixed symptoms often similar to those of overactive bladder.

OBJECTIVE

→ Pelvic examination:

Stress Incontinence
- May observe the effects of hypoestrogenemia on vulvar and vaginal tissues.
- May observe presence of cystocele, rectocele, or prolapsed uterus or urethra.
- Decreased strength of pubococcygeal muscle.
- Positive Q-tip test: With the patient in a supine position, a lubricated, cotton-tip applicator is placed in the urethra at the urethrovesical junction.
  - The angle formed by the applicator and the floor is measured while the patient is resting and during a Valsalva maneuver.
    - An angle <15° during the Valsalva maneuver indicates good anatomic support.
    - An angle >30° indicates poor anatomical support.
    - An angle of 15–30° is considered inconclusive.
- Positive stress test: Urine leakage is observed when the patient is asked to cough.
  - This maneuver may be performed in the lithotomy or standing position.
- Normal postvoid residual: Postvoid residuals are easily determined by straight catheterization immediately after the patient has voided or by ultrasound.
  - A normal postvoid residual is 0–50 cc of urine.
  - Postvoid residuals >100 cc should be considered abnormal and may be indicative of other, less common types of incontinence, such as overflow or reflux.

Mixed Incontinence
- Objective findings may be any combination of those found with stress and urge incontinence.

Urge Incontinence

- See the **Overactive Bladder** chapter.

ASSESSMENT

→ Stress urinary incontinence
→ Urge incontinence
→ Mixed urinary incontinence
→ R/O transient/functional incontinence
→ R/O neurological conditions
→ R/O overflow incontinence/abnormal postvoid residual

PLAN

DIAGNOSTIC TESTS

→ Initial diagnostic tests for all types of incontinence should include:
  - Urinalysis
  - Urine culture and sensitivities
  - Postvoid residual
→ Other tests may include:
  - 48–72 hour bladder diary
  - Q-tip test
  - Stress test
  - Cystourethroscopy/cystometrics

TREATMENT/MANAGEMENT

(Culligan et al. 2000, Dmochowski et al. 2000)

Stress Incontinence

→ Topical estrogen for women with vulvar or vaginal hypo-estrogenemic states in whom estrogen therapy is not contraindicated
  NOTE: Oral estrogen alone is not effective for treating urinary incontinence.
  - Estrogen supplementation may increase urethral vascularity, tone, and the alpha-adrenergic responsiveness, which may increase bladder outlet resistance.
→ Kegel exercises to strengthen voluntary periurethral and pelvic muscles and pelvic visceral structures
→ Vaginal weights: A set of five graduated, conical weights (lightest is 20 g, heaviest is 70 g) worn intravaginally twice a day for 15 minutes
  - This strengthens pelvic floor muscles, ensures proper performance of Kegel exercises, and provides sensory biofeedback and a measure of patient progress.
→ Advanced pelvic floor rehabilitation (i.e., biofeedback, electrical stimulation, electromagnetic field therapy)
→ Vaginal pessaries: These mechanical devices of various shapes are made of latex rubber. They are worn intravaginally to stabilize the ureterovesical junction and increase urethral closure pressures.
  - Especially helpful in patients with a cystocele who are not candidates for surgery.
  - Devices must be fit properly to not make incontinence worse.
→ Pharmacological therapy: It is based on a high concentra-

tion of alpha-adrenergic receptors in the bladder neck, bladder base, and proximal urethra. Sympathomimetic drugs with alpha-adrenergic agonist activity cause muscle contraction of the bladder neck, bladder base, and proximal urethra, thereby increasing bladder outlet resistance.
  - Pharmacological therapy for stress incontinence results in significant reduction of stress incontinence in 19–60% of patients (Urinary Incontinence Guideline Panel 1992).
  - Therapeutic regimens include:
    • Pseudoephedrine 30–60 mg, 1 tablet p.o. BID
    • Imipramine 5–50 mg p.o. at HS
→ Surgical intervention: Its primary goal is to elevate the bladder neck, restoring normal urethrovesical anatomy.
  - There are currently more than 150 surgical procedures to correct stress incontinence, most of which suspend the bladder neck and urethra with a sling.
    • Approaches may be vaginal or abdominal depending on the type of repair.
  - Traditional repairs commonly used to correct stress incontinence are the Marshall-Marchetti-Krantz, Raz, Burch, Stamey, and Pereyra procedures.
  - Recent surgical advances for sling procedures are cadaveric or autologous fascial grafts and tension-free vaginal tape.
  - Success rates for surgical interventions range from 75–90% for five years, with the highest success occurring in younger patients.
  - Other surgical interventions include periurethral bulking agents, such as silicone, collagen, and polydimethylsiloxane. Less commonly used are artificial and urinary diversion.

Mixed Incontinence

→ Treatment for mixed incontinence depends on which component of incontinence is most problematic for the patient. A combination of the above options may be used. Often, treatment of one component, either stress or urge incontinence, will improve or resolve the second component.

CONSULTATION

→ Some patients presenting with urinary incontinence may need to be referred to or co-managed with a urologist or urogynecologist for additional diagnostic work-up.
  - Specialized diagnostic tests may include cystoscopy, uroflowmetry, cystometrogram, cystogram, and urethral pressure profile.
→ Referral to a urologist is indicated in the following situations:
  - Persistent diagnostic uncertainty that may affect therapy
  - High morbidity associated with nonspecific therapy
  - Failed empiric therapy
  - Suspicion of obstruction
  - Postvoid residuals >50 cc
  - Patients with a known neurological condition
  - Impending surgical intervention

PATIENT EDUCATION

→ Explain the basic anatomy and physiology of the bladder and urethra, normal bladder function, and probable etiology of the patient's incontinence.

→ Explore how the patient's urinary incontinence is affecting her life.

→ Discuss treatment options, their success rates, and potential side effects.

→ Teach the correct method of practicing Kegel exercises through palpation and verbal feedback.

- Kegels should be performed in a series of ten, sustaining the contraction for 3–10 seconds with equal periods of relaxation.
- Instruct the patient to increase the number of Kegels performed daily until she reaches 100.
- Instruct the patient to perform Kegels before coughing, sneezing, bending, etc.
- It is also helpful to explore times when patients can practice Kegels, such as when they are standing in grocery lines, stopped for traffic lights, or watching television commercials.

FOLLOW-UP

→ Follow-up visits are used to evaluate the response to treatment and to reconsider treatment options if necessary.

→ Follow-up should be at 4–12 week intervals depending on the severity of incontinence and type of treatment.

→ Document in progress notes and on problem list.

BIBLIOGRAPHY

Burgio, K.L., Lochler, J.L., and Goode, P.S. 2000. Combined behavioral and drug therapy for urge incontinence in older women. *Journal of the American Geriatric Society* 48(4): 370–374.

Cheater, F.M., and Castleden, C.M. 2000. Epidemiology and classification of urinary incontinence. *Bailliere's Clinical Obstetrics and Gynaecology* 14(2):207–226.

Culligan, P.J., and Heit, M. 2000. Urinary incontinence in women: evaluation and management. *American Family Physician* 62(11)2433–2444.

Dmochowski, R.R., and Appell, R.A. 2000. Advancements in pharmacologic management of the overactive bladder. *Urology* 56(Suppl. 6A):41–49.

Dugan, E., Cohen, S.J., Bland D.R. et al. 2000. The association of depressive symptoms and urinary incontinence in older women. *Journal of the American Geriatric Society* 48(4): 413–416.

Keane, D.P., and O'Sullivan, S. 2000. Urinary incontinence: anatomy, physiology and pathophysiology. *Bailliere's Clinical Obstetrics and Gynaecology* 14(2):227–249.

Resnick, N.M. 1992. Urinary incontinence in older adults. *Hospital Practice* (October 15):139–184.

Sampselle, C.M. 2000. Behavioral intervention for urinary incontinence in women: evidence for practice. *Journal of Midwifery & Women's Health* 45(2):94–103.

Stilling Burkhart, K. 2000. Urinary incontinence in women: assessment and management in the primary care setting. *Nurse Practitioner Forum* 11:192–204.

Urinary Incontinence Guideline Panel. 1992. *Urinary incontinence in adults: clinical practice guideline.* AHCPR Publication No. 92-0038. Rockville, Md.: Agency for Health Care Policy and Research.

Sandra L. Lindholm-Norman, R.N., M.S., N.P.

12-RC   Urinary Tract Disorders
Overactive Bladder

Overactive bladder (OAB) is a complex of symptoms resulting from detrusor muscle instability. As OAB is a highly prevalent disorder that is vastly underreported, controversy exists concerning its prevalence. In the United States, prevalence estimates range from 17–71 million women (Wein et al. 1999).

Symptoms of OAB include urinary frequency (more than eight voids/day), urgency (a sudden, strong desire to urinate), nocturia (a need to void more than two times/night), and urge incontinence (involuntary loss of urine associate with a strong sensation to urinate). These symptoms occur because the detrusor muscle is overactive and contracts inappropriately during the filling phase (Cheater et al. 2000, Keane et al. 2000, Wein et al. 1999). It has been postulated that a common feature in all cases of detrusor instability is a change in the properties of the smooth muscle of the detrusor that predisposes to unstable contractions (Cheater et al. 2000). The International Continence Society definition subdivides OAB into detrusor instability (not due to neurologic disease) and detrusor hyperreflexia (due to neurologic disease) (Wein et al. 1999).

Recent studies indicate that patients with OAB have a significant decrease in quality of life and are more adversely affected than those with stress incontinence. This presumably is due to the differences in symptoms: Compared to stress urinary incontinence, OAB is more difficult to predict; more likely to negatively impact daily activity, sexual practices, sleep patterns, and social and occupational activity; and results in the loss of large volumes of urine (Wein et al. 1999).

The goal of managing OAB is to improve symptoms and thus improve quality of life. Management consists of strategies to facilitate bladder filling and urine storage by decreasing contractility, increasing capacity, and decreasing sensation. The primary modalities of treatment are behavioral, physical (pelvic floor rehabilitation), and pharmacologic.

DATABASE

SUBJECTIVE

→ Risk factors include:
- Dementia/confusional state
- Use of sedative-hypnotics, diuretics, anticholinergic agents, calcium channel blockers
- Restricted mobility
- Stool impaction
- Neurological conditions
- Urinary tract infection/inflammation
- Urogenital estrogen deficiency
- Pelvic floor relaxation
- Excessive urine production (e.g., diuretic use, diabetes)
- Diabetes
- Dietary intake of caffeine, alcohol, or carbonated beverages
- Pelvic surgeries that disrupt innervation of the bladder
- Foreign bodies
- Bladder neoplasia
- Environmental barriers to toileting

→ Among symptoms, the patient may report:
- Involuntary leakage of urine associated with a strong urge to void
- Precipitating events such as the sound of running water, hands in warm water, exposure to cold temperature, anxiety, or coitus
- Urinary frequency and/or nocturia
- Strong urges to void, with small voids

OBJECTIVE

→ Pelvic examination:
- Anatomical support of the vagina and urethra may be good or poor
- The strength of pubococcygeal muscle may be good or poor

- Possible effects of hypoestrogenemia on vulvar, vaginal, and periurethral tissue
- Normal postvoid residual (>100 cc)
  NOTE: A high post-void residual is indicative of overflow incontinence.
→ Neurological examination: Neurological signs (e.g., hyperreflexia, paraesthesias) are usually absent but may be present with detrusor hyperreflexia.
  - Observe general coordination, mobility, and orientation.
  - May examine sacral reflex by stroking skin adjacent to the anus, which normally should result in reflex contraction of the external anal sphincter.
  - May test patellar, ankle, and plantar reflexes.
  - May test the sensory function of sacral dermatomes using a light touch and a pinprick on the perineum and around the thigh and foot.
→ Laboratory:
  - Normal urinalysis
  - Negative urine culture
  - Negative urine cytology

ASSESSMENT

→ Overactive bladder
→ R/O urinary tract infection
→ R/O bladder malignancy
→ R/O stress incontinence
→ R/O mixed incontinence
→ R/O functional incontinence
→ R/O overflow incontinence
→ R/O neurological conditions

PLAN

DIAGNOSTIC TESTS

→ Diagnostic tests may include:
  - 48–72 hour p.o. intake/output diary
  - Specialized diagnostic tests such as cystoscopy, uroflowmetry, cystometrogram, cystogram, and urethral pressure profile
  - Urinalysis, urine culture and sensitivity, and urine cytology if it has not already been obtained.

TREATMENT/MANAGEMENT

(Culligan et al. 2000, Dmochowski et al. 2000, Elliot et al. 2001, Payne 1999, Stilling Burkhart 2000)

→ Dietary modification:
  - Eliminate bladder irritants (i.e., caffeine, alcohol, carbonated beverages); avoid excessive intake of acidic foods, beverages.
  - Maintain fluid intake below 2,000 cc every 24 hours.
  - Stop oral fluids 2–3 hours before bedtime.
→ Habit training:
  - Also known as timed voiding, habit training is the establishment of a routine voiding schedule.

- The patient is asked to void, usually every 2–4 hours, whether or not she feels the need to.
- The goal of this strategy is to keep the patient dry rather than to improve bladder function.
→ Bladder training:
  - Also known as bladder retraining, this strategy consists of a voiding schedule with progressively longer intervals between mandatory voidings using concomitant distraction/relaxation techniques.
  - The goal of bladder training is to restore normal bladder function.
→ Relaxation training:
  - The patient is taught relaxation techniques to use when the sensation of urinary urgency occurs, allowing her to make it to the bathroom to void.
    - Relaxation techniques include slow, deep breathing and imagery.
    - Contracting the pelvic floor muscles (Kegel) in combination with a relaxation technique can enhance detrusor relaxation.
→ Biofeedback:
  - The efficacy of this newer treatment continues to be investigated.
→ Exercises to strengthen pelvic floor muscles include:
  - Kegels (repetitive contractions of pelvic floor muscles)
→ Pharmacological therapy:
  - May be used indefinitely or for short periods until other treatment modalities (e.g., bladder retraining) become effective.
  - Anticholinergics:
    - Are direct, smooth-muscle relaxants
    - Are contraindicated in patients with narrow-angle glaucoma
    - Most common side effects include constipation, dry mouth, and blurred vision
  - Options include:
    - Oxybutynin chloride extended release (Ditropan XL®): 5 mg, 10 mg, or 15 mg, 1 tablet p.o. QD, maximum dose 30 mg QD
    - Oxybutynin chloride (Ditropan®): 5 mg, ½–1 tablet p.o. BID–QID
    - Tolterodine tartrate (Detrol®): 2 mg, 1 tablet p.o. BID
    - Tolterodine tartrate long-acting (Detrol LA®): 4 mg, 1 tablet p.o. QD
  NOTE: Recent studies indicate that the long-acting formulations of oxybutynin chloride and tolterodine tartrate are more effective and have fewer anticholinergic side effects than their original formulations.
    - Flavoxate 100 mg, 1 tablet p.o. BID–TID
    - Propantheline bromide 7.5–30 mg, 1 p.o. BID–QID
      - A smooth-muscle relaxant with ganglionic blocking effects
      - Less used due to a high incidence of side effects, including dry mouth, visual blurring, xerostomia, nausea, constipation, tachycardia, drowsiness, confusion, and urinary retention

- Other therapies:
  - Imipramine 10–100 mg, 1 tablet p.o. at bedtime or BID
    - This is a tricyclic antidepressant with both anti-cholinergic and alpha-agonist properties. It decreases bladder contractions and increases urethral resistance to outflow.
    - Side effects include postural hypotension, fatigue, dry mouth, and dizziness, as well as cardiac conduction disturbances in the elderly.
  - Estrogen (intravaginal) cream, tablets or ring. Local estrogen replacement is often more effective that the oral route in treating OAB; the estradiol ring appears to be the most effective.
→ Electrical stimulation:
  - Pelvic floor electrical stimulation: Though widely used in Europe, acceptance has been slower in the United States.
  - Neuromodulation of the sacral nerve roots: Electrodes are surgically implanted in the sacral foramina. This is a promising new surgical intervention. But because it is costly and invasive, it should be reserved for patients who are unresponsive to more conservative options.
→ Intravesical treatment:
  - Intravesical instillation of capsaicin and resiniferatoxin: These are experimental but promising agents for treating detrusor hyperreflexia.

CONSULTATION

→ Some patients presenting with urinary incontinence may need to be referred to or co-managed with a urologist for additional diagnostic work-up.
→ Referral to a urologist or urogynecologist is indicated in the following situations:
  - Persistent diagnostic uncertainty that may affect therapy
  - High morbidity associated with nonspecific therapy
  - Failed empiric therapy
  - Suspicion of obstruction
  - Patients with a known neurological condition

PATIENT EDUCATION

→ Explain basic anatomy and physiology of the bladder and urethra, normal bladder function, and probable etiology of patient's incontinence.

→ Explore how the patient's urinary incontinence is affecting her life.
→ Discuss treatment options and their potential side effects and success rates.
→ Teach skills necessary to practice behavioral interventions (i.e., dietary modifications, bladder retraining, timed voidings, pelvic floor restrengthening, etc.).

FOLLOW-UP

→ Follow-up visits are used to evaluate the response to treatment and to reconsider treatment options if necessary.
→ Follow-up should be at 4–12 week intervals depending on the severity of incontinence and type of treatment.
→ Document in progress notes and on problem list.

BIBLIOGRAPHY

Cheater, F.M., and Castleden, C.M. 2000. Epidemiology and classification of urinary incontinence. *Bailliere's Clinical Obstetrics and Gynaecology* 14(2):183–205.

Culligan, P.J., and Heit, M. 2000. Urinary incontinence in women: evaluation and management. *American Family Physician* 62(11):2433–2444.

Dmochowski, R.R., and Appell, R.A. 2000. Advancements in the pharmacologic management of the overactive bladder. *Urology* 56(6A):41–49.

Elliott, D.S., Lightner, D.J., and Blute, M.L. 2001. Medical management of the overactive bladder. *Mayo Clinic Proceedings* 76(4):353–355.

Keane, D.P., and O'Sullivan, S. 2000. Urinary incontinence: anatomy, physiology and pathology. *Bailliere's Clinical Obstetrics and Gynaecology* 14(2):207–226.

Payne, C.K. 1999. Advances in nonsurgical treatment of urinary incontinence and overactive bladder. *Campbell's Urology* 1(1):2–20.

Stilling Burkhart, K. 2000. Urinary incontinence in women: assessment and management in the primary care setting. *Nurse Practitioner Forum* 11(4):192–204.

Wein, A.J., and Rovner, E.S. 1999. The overactive bladder: an overview for primary care providers. *International Journal of Infertility* 44(2):56–66.

12-RD Urinary Tract Disorders
Interstitial Cystitis

Interstitial cystitis (IC) is a chronic syndrome of the lower urinary tract characterized by irritative voiding symptoms and pelvic pain in the presence of sterile and cytologically negative urine. The prevalence of IC among women is unknown; however, three published studies estimate that it ranges from 10–30 per 100,000 to 501 per 100,000, with more than 1 million patients in the United States (Jones et al. 1997). IC is underdiagnosed in this country, particularly in its less severe form; it is believed that women with *urethral syndrome*, *urgency-frequency syndrome*, *trigonitis*, misdiagnosed and recurrent *urinary tract infections*, *chronic pelvic pain* of unknown etiology, and men with chronic nonbacterial *prostatitis/prostadynia* may have IC (Lipsky 1999, Parsons et al. 1996). The median age at diagnosis is 42–46 years and the average time from symptom development to diagnosis is 5–7 years. Eighty-five percent of patients diagnosed with IC are women (Parsons et al. 1996). IC has been reported in early childhood (Park 2001).

Interstitial cystitis is associated with a complex of symptoms: urinary frequency with small voids, dysuria, nocturia, urinary urgency, suprapubic/pelvic/perineal pain, dyspareunia, and anterior vaginal wall discomfort (Parsons 2000). The syndrome is characterized by periods of exacerbations and remissions. Worsening of symptoms is frequently reported during stress, the perimenstrual phase, and after sexual intercourse and ingestion of acidic, alcoholic, spicy, caffeinated, and carbonated products (Koziol 1994). Associated conditions include irritable bowel syndrome, allergies, fibromyalgia, migraines, chronic fatigue immune dysfunction syndrome, endometriosis, vulvodynia/vulvar vestibulitis, systemic lupus erythematosus, Sjögren's syndrome, and Hashimoto's thyroiditis (Ratner 2001).

The etiology of IC remains controversial. Most investigators believe there are several subsets of IC with different etiologies, which may explain why patient responses to treatments vary so widely. There are two main etiologic theories for IC. According to the first, IC may be the result of a defect in bladder epithelium cytoprotection and increased bladder mast cells. Defective cytoprotection with increased urothelial permeability may allow mast cell secretagogues and potassium to penetrate the bladder lining and activate sensory nerves and bladder mast cells (Theoharides et al. 2001). According to the second theory, IC may be the result of excessive sympathetic vasomotor activity that produces regional ischemia, tissue necrosis, and pain (Ratliff et al. 2001).

The diagnosis usually can be made upon a complete history, thorough pelvic exam, urinalysis, urine culture, urine cytology, and voiding log. Optional diagnostic tests include cystoscopy/hydrodistention (considered to be the gold standard), potassium sensitivity test, and urodynamics. A bloody effluent, petechial hemorrhages distributed throughout the bladder, and a small bladder capacity also are suggestive. Hunner's ulcers are present in fewer than 10% of patients with IC (Parsons 2000). In the near future, urinary markers may be used in the diagnosis (Erickson 2001).

DATABASE

SUBJECTIVE

→ Risk factors include:
- Female patient

→ Symptoms may include:
- Urinary frequency with small voids
- Urinary urgency
- Nocturia
- Burning sensation during urination
- Suprapubic discomfort, which is often related to bladder filling and is relieved by voiding
- Deep dyspareunia
- Pelvic/perineal/anterior vaginal wall pain
- Exacerbation of symptoms by certain foods, substances, or stress
- Chronicity of symptoms with periods of exacerbations and remissions
- Symptoms unrelieved by antibiotic therapy

OBJECTIVE

→ The patient may present with:
- Negative urinalysis and cultures

- Negative urine cytology
- Suprapubic/pelvic tenderness
- Anterior vaginal wall or perineal discomfort
- Absence of vaginitis or cervicitis, unless there is a concomitant infection

ASSESSMENT

→ Probable interstitial cystitis
→ R/O urinary tract infection
→ R/O vaginal/cervical infection/sexually transmitted disease
→ R/O bladder tumor
→ R/O endometriosis, ovarian/uterine masses
→ R/O iatrogenic etiologies (i.e., allergy medication, chemo-therapeutic agents, radiation)

PLAN

DIAGNOSTIC TESTS

→ Diagnostic tests may include:
- Urinalysis
- Urine culture and sensitivities
- Vaginal wet mount
- Vaginal and cervical cultures
- Voiding diary
- Potassium sensitivity testing
- Bladder hydrodistention and cystoscopy under anesthesia

TREATMENT/MANAGEMENT

→ All patients in whom interstitial cystitis is suspected should be referred to a urologist with experience in treating this condition.
→ Most patients with IC experience relief of their symptoms, although treatment modalities are nonspecific and usually noncurative.
- Symptom relief is often partial and intermittent.
→ Treatment options include (Hanno 1997, Molwin 2000, Parsons 2000):
- Systemic therapy:
  - Antihistamines block H_1 histamine receptor sites. The release of histamine causes bladder pain, hyperemia, and fibrosis.
    - Hydroxyzine hydrochloride 25–50 mg p.o. at HS or diphenhydramine 25–50 mg p.o. at HS
  - Cimetidine (Tagamet®), a histamine H_2 antagonist
  - Anti-inflammatories inhibit mast cell degranulation that releases prostaglandins
  - Anticholinergics and antispasmodics inhibit bladder smooth muscle contraction
    - Oxybutynin chloride extended release (Ditropan XL®) 5–30 mg p.o. QD
  - **NOTE:** Refer to the **Overactive Bladder** chapter for a more complete list of suggested anticholinergics.
  - Heterocyclic antidepressants exert analgesic action by inhibiting serotonin uptake at the presynaptic neurons. The prolonged availability of serotonin at the neuronal synapses increases the pain threshold.

- Tricyclics have some anticholinergic activity and block pain arousal.
- Amitriptyline 10–50 mg p.o. at HS
NOTE: It is recommended that the clinician start with low doses and titrate up slowly.
- Pentosan polysulfate sodium is a relatively new medication and the only oral one that is FDA-approved specifically for treating IC. This medication is believed to act by adhering to the bladder mucosa, thus helping to maintain/enhance the uroepithelial protective lining.
- Heparin is given subcutaneously or intravenously to restore the defective mucus layer of the bladder wall.
- Urine alkalization
  - 2 Tums® p.o. TID buffer acidic urine
- Transcutaneous electrical nerve stimulation (TENS): Application of high-frequency, conventional TENS is based on the gate theory of pain control, in which counterstimulation of the nervous system modifies the perception of pain.
- Gabapentin and carbamazepine are antiseizure medications for treating neuropathic pain.
- Narcotics are prescribed for managing acute pain.
- Selective serotonin reuptake inhibitors treat underlying depression/anxiety. (See the **Depression** and **Anxiety Disorders** chapters in Section 14.)

- Intravesical pharmacotherapy was previously the mainstay of treatment and is the standard against which treatments are measured.
  - Dimethyl sulfoxide (DMSO): Its pharmacological properties include anti-inflammatory, analgesic, muscle relaxant, and collagen dissolution.
  - Heparin restores the defective mucus layer of the bladder wall and has anti-allergic and anti-inflammatory properties.
  - Cocktails: Mixtures of various medications that may include DMSO, heparin, sodium bicarbonate, bipuvicaine, lidocaine, and steroids.

- Surgery:
  - Simple hydrodistention is diagnostic as well as therapeutic. It causes ischemia or mechanical damage to the submucosal nerve plexus and stretch receptors, resulting in less pain and urinary frequency.
  - Most patients with IC respond to nonsurgical treatment.
  - Surgery is the last resort after various forms of conservative treatment have failed.
  - Fewer than 1–2% of patients require any of the following surgical procedures:
    - Transurethral resection of ulcers
    - Laser photoirradiation of ulcers/fissures
    - Bladder denervation
    - Enterocystoplasty, the aim of which is to replace most of the diseased bladder with healthy bowel.
    - Urinary diversion is a last resort. A continent pouch and catheterizable stoma are created from bowel; the entire bladder and urethra may be removed.

CONSULTATION

→ Referral to a urologist is required for all patients with suspected IC who are refractory to conservative therapy.

PATIENT EDUCATION

→ Teach the patient to avoid foods and beverages that appear to incite or aggravate IC symptoms. These include alcohol, caffeine, citrus fruits/juices, hot spicy foods, chocolates, berries, and processed tomato products.
→ Teach the patient to avoid foods and products that contain artificial sweeteners, which affect the bladder epithelium.
→ Teach bladder retraining.
→ Explore the impact of IC on the patient's life.
→ Explore methods of stress reduction.

FOLLOW-UP

→ Patients with IC require easy access to care and close collaboration with their care provider.
→ Frequent assessment of symptoms and evaluation of treatment are important.
→ Follow-up is more frequent during periods of exacerbations and depends on the severity of the patient's symptoms.
→ Document in progress notes and on problem list.

BIBLIOGRAPHY

Erickson, D. 2001. Urine markers of interstitial cystitis. *Urology* 57(Suppl. 6A):15–21.

Hanno, P. 1997. Analysis of long-term Elmiron therapy for interstitial cystitis. *Urology* 49(Suppl. 5A):93–99.

Jones, C.A., and Nyberg, L. 1997. Epidemiology of interstitial cystitis. *Urology* 49(Suppl. 5A):2–9.

Koziol, J.A. 1994. Epidemiology of interstitial cystitis. *Urology Clinics of North America* 21:7–20.

Lipsky, B.A. 1999. Prostatitis and urinary tract infections in men: What's new; what's true? *American Journal of Medicine* 106:327–334.

Molwin, R. 2000. *The interstitial cystitis survival guide*, pp. 92–93. Oakland, Calif.: New Harbinger Publications.

Park, J.M. 2001. Is interstitial cystitis an underdiagnosed problem in children? A diagnostic and therapeutic dilemma. *Urology* 57(Suppl. 6A):30–31.

Parsons, C.L. 2000. Interstitial cystitis: clinical manifestations and diagnostic criteria in over 200 cases. *Neurourological Urodynamics* 9(3):241-250.

Parsons, C.L., and Parsons, J.K. 1996. Interstitial cystitis. In *Female urology,* 2nd ed., ed. S. Raz. Philadelphia: W.B. Saunders.

Ratliff, T.L., Klutke, C.G., and McDougall, E.M. 2001. The etiology of interstitial cystitis. *Urology Clinics of North America* 21:21–30.

Ratner, V. 2001. Current controversies that adversely affect interstitial cystitis patients. *Urology* 57(Suppl. 6A):89–94.

Theoharides, T.C., Kempuraj, D., and Sant, G.R. 2001. Mast cell involvement in interstitial cystitis: a review of human and experimental evidence. *Urology* 57(Suppl. 6A):47–55.

Winifred L. Star, R.N., C., N.P., M.S.
Melanie Deal, R.N., C., N.P., M.S.

12-SA Vaginitis
Atrophic Vaginitis

The *atrophic vagina* is a result of decreasing estrogen levels, which lead to incomplete maturation and gradual loss of the glycogen-rich squamous epithelium. When estrogen levels fall below a certain physiological level, atrophy ensues. Consequently, the protective vaginal microflora are not supported or maintained, lactobacilli disappear, and reduced lactic-acid production leads to an increased pH. The epithelium is thus rendered susceptible to the overgrowth of various opportunistic bacterial organisms (e.g., streptococci, staphylococci, coliforms, diphtheroids), which may induce superficial infection.

Most atrophism is a result of natural menopause. The degree of vaginal atrophy varies widely according to the individual woman and the status of her hormones. Peripheral conversion of androstenedione provides a source of estrogen, and there is some ovarian estrogen secretion for years after menopause. In many cases, women produce sufficient estrogen to maintain a mature vaginal epithelium.

Other conditions associated with relative estrogen deficiency include radiation therapy, chemotherapy, ovariectomy, ovarian failure of any cause, anti-estrogen medications (e.g., medroxyprogesterone, tamoxifen, danazol, leuprolide, and nafarelin), certain immunological disorders, and premenarche, postpartum, or the lactational state (Bachmann et al. 2000). Cigarette smoking increases the risk for symptomatic atrophic vaginitis. Postmenopausal women who engage in sexual intercourse usually experience milder levels of atrophy.

Only 10–40% of postmenopausal women have symptoms of atrophic vaginitis. Possible sequelae of atrophy are a narrowed and contracted introitus, urethral caruncle, and kraurosis vulvae; a friable, nonrugated vagina; and postcoital or postexamination peri-introital and posterior fourchette lacerations (Bachmann et al. 2000, Pandit et al. 1997).

DATABASE

SUBJECTIVE

→ See **Table 12SF.1, Vaginal Infections.**

→ History may include any of the factors presented in the introductory section.
→ Assess for the use of agents that may cause contact irritation: perfumes, powders, deodorants, panty liners, perineal pads, soaps, spermicides, and tight-fitting or synthetic clothing (Bachmann et al. 2000).
→ Symptoms may include:
- Vaginal dryness (a hallmark symptom)
- Pruritus
- Vulvar irritation, burning
- Dyspareunia
- Abnormal vaginal discharge (described in "Objective," below)
- Vaginal spotting/bleeding
- Dysuria, frequency, urgency, hematuria, stress incontinence

→ The patient may be asymptomatic.

OBJECTIVE

→ External genitalia:
- Diminished elasticity of skin
- Sparse, brittle pubic hair
- Lax, wrinkled labia majora
- Thinning and shrinking of labia minora
- Fusing of labia minora with labia majora
- Atrophic clitoris
- Eversion of mucosa of urethral meatus
→ Vagina:
- Narrowed introitus
- Smooth, shiny, flat, thin rugae
- Dry, initially pale walls, later with diffuse erythema
- Discharge may be odorous, thin, watery, thick, purulent, serosanguinous or bloody, gray, yellow, or green
- Ecchymosis, petechial hemorrhages may be present
- Advanced atrophy may result in adhesions or occlusion (kraurosis)

→ Cervix: Small, pale, or erythematous; petechial hemorrhages may be present.
→ Uterus: small or nonpalpable
→ Adnexa, rectovaginal examination: within normal limits (WNL) unless there is coexistent pathology.
  NOTE: A virginal speculum may be required.

ASSESSMENT

→ Atrophic vaginitis
→ R/O concomitant vaginitis/sexually transmitted disease (STD)
→ R/O contact irritation
→ R/O urinary tract infection
→ R/O urethral caruncle/prolapse
→ R/O endometrial hyperplasia
→ R/O uterine cancer
→ R/O squamous intraepithelial lesion/cervical cancer

PLAN

DIAGNOSTIC TESTS

→ Wet-mount microscopy (10x and 40x power)
  ■ Saline:
    • Intermediate/parabasal/basal squamous epithelial cells
    • Increased WBCs
    • Lactobacilli absent
    • Assess for clue cells, trichomonads
  ■ Potassium hydroxide (KOH), 10–20%:
    • WNL unless there is a concomitant infection
    • Assess for amine odor, hyphae, spores
→ pH 5.5–7.0
→ Maturation index: increased intermediate and parabasal cells identified.
→ Gram stain: intermediate/parabasal/basal cells, numerous bacteria identified.
→ Pap smear as indicated; may show atypia.
→ Tests for *Neisseria gonorrhoeae* and *Chlamydia trachomatis*, as indicated.
→ Urinalysis with culture and sensitivities as indicated.
→ Endometrial biopsy as indicated by history and physical examination.
→ Additional labs may include, but are not limited to: CBC, RPR, or VDRL.

TREATMENT/MANAGEMENT

→ Topical estrogen therapy is the mainstay of treatment. It is available in many different delivery systems, including:
  ■ Estrogen vaginal creams
    • Dosage is usually ½–1 applicator for 1–2 weeks (or until relief of symptoms), tapering to ¼–½ applicator 1–3 times a week. (Manufacturers' recommendations may vary. See the *Physicians' Desk Reference* [*PDR*]).
  ■ Estradiol vaginal rings
    • Replace every 90 days.
  ■ Estrogen vaginal tablets
    • One tablet daily for 2 weeks. Maintenance dose is 1 tablet twice weekly (Wong 2002).

NOTE: With the use of estrogen vaginal cream or vaginal tablets in low doses, estrogen absorption is not likely to produce significant systemic effects. However, in a woman with an intact uterus, supplementation with periodic progestin (e.g., 10–13 days a month every 2–3 months), may be necessary to prevent endometrial hyperplasia. Estradiol vaginal rings induce vaginal epithelial maturation without causing endometrial stimulation; thus, their use does not require regular progestin supplementation (*PDR* 2002, Wallis et al. 1998).
  ■ Oral estrogen replacement therapy (ERT) may be used alternatively or in addition to vaginal therapy, especially when systemic estrogen effects are desired.
  NOTE: Supplementation with progestin is necessary when prescribing oral therapy in a nonhysterectomized woman. Standard systemic ERT alone may not eliminate symptoms of atrophic vaginitis in up to 25% of women (Wong 2002).
  ■ See the **Perimenopausal and Menopausal Symptoms and Hormone Therapy** chapter for a complete list of medications and dosages. Regimens vary. Consult with a physician as indicated. (See the *PDR* for further information.)
→ Tapered doses of vaginal estrogen may be used in a postpartum, breast-feeding woman as indicated without adverse effects on breast milk production or the infant (Kaufman et al. 1994).
→ When estrogen therapy is used to treat atrophic vaginitis, *Candida* and trichomonads that were previously unable to survive in a glycogen-poor vagina may be incited to proliferate and a symptomatic infection may ensue. Treat accordingly.
→ When estrogen replacement therapy is contraindicated, vaginal lubrication with Lubrin® or Replens® may be tried. Lubricants for coitus may include Astroglide®, K-Y Jelly®, Surgilube®, and other brands.
→ Treat concomitant, identified vaginitis and STDs as indicated. (See the appropriate chapters.)

CONSULTATION

→ As indicated.
→ As needed for prescription(s).

PATIENT EDUCATION

→ Discuss the etiology and nature of the condition.
→ Advise all patients regarding vulvovaginal hygiene. (See "Patient Education" in the **Candidal Vulvovaginitis** chapter.)
→ Encourage sexual intercourse as tolerated and appropriate. Lubricants may be helpful.
→ Dilation of the vagina may be helpful in alleviating some of the atrophic changes. A well-lubricated finger, dildo, or candle may be used. A warm tub bath may help relaxation during the dilation process. Graduated dilators may also be provided to the patient by the clinic or office.

FOLLOW-UP

→ As necessary for the individual case.

→ If an STD is identified, treat appropriately. (See the related chapters.) Refer the patient's partner for evaluation and therapy. Discuss safer sex practices. (See **Table 13A.2, Safer Sex Practices** in the **Chancroid** chapter in Section 13.)

→ Document in progress notes and on problem list.

Winifred L. Star, R.N., C., N.P., M.S.
Melanie Deal, R.N., C., N.P., M.S.

12-SB Vaginitis
Bacterial Vaginosis

Despite the fact that *bacterial vaginosis* (BV) is the most common cause of abnormal vaginal discharge in women of childbearing age, its pathogenesis and etiology remain unclear (Hillier et al. 1999, Schwebke 1999). BV is defined as a polymicrobial syndrome in which lactobacilli, the normally predominant bacteria in the vagina, are replaced by a mixture of other microbes. This syndrome is attributed to a complex synergism between certain facultative and anaerobic bacteria, and mycoplasmas, most commonly *Gardnerella vaginalis*, *Prevotella* (formerly *Bacteroides* species), *Bacteroides ureolyticus*, *Fusobacterium nucleatum*, *Peptostreptococcus*, *Mycoplasma hominis*, and *Mobiluncus* (Hillier et al. 1999, Pybus et al. 1999). All of these bacteria, except *Mobiluncus*, are present in normal vaginal flora (Hillier et al. 1999). Concentrations of these bacteria are 100 to 1,000 times greater among women with BV while concentrations of normal lactobacilli are decreased (Hillier et al. 1999, Rauh et al. 2000). BV is best described, then, as an "imbalance in the vaginal ecosystem" and not as "...an introduction of [foreign] pathogens..." (Rauh et al. 2000, p. 220).

Although experts agree that BV results from an imbalance in normal vaginal flora, the triggers that create this imbalance remain unidentified (Hay 1998, Hillier et al. 1999, Pybus et al. 1999). Host characteristics of susceptibility are still under investigation. It is thought that lactobacilli serve a protective role in the vagina by creating a physical barrier to other bacteria, by outcompeting other microbes for nutrients, by releasing toxic byproducts (e.g., hydrogen peroxide), and by contributing to the creation of an acidic, and therefore hostile, environment (Barbes et al. 1999, Eschenbach et al. 2000, Hillier et al. 1999, Pybus et al. 1999). BV may arise, then, if local environmental conditions favor growth of the anaerobes and mycoplasmas and/or cause inhibition of lactobacilli. Vaginal pH is postulated to be a critical factor in the vaginal ecosystem (Pybus et al. 1999). Therefore, factors that alter the vaginal pH, such as hormonal fluctuations, menstruation, presence of semen, genetic host factors, and the type of lactobacilli, may result in BV (Eschenbach et al. 2000, Hillier et al. 1999, Priestley et al. 1997, Rauh et al. 2000, Shalev 1996). Additionally, studies show that cyclic fluctuations in vaginal flora occur (Eschenbach et al. 2000, Hillier et al. 1999, Priestley et al. 1997). These fluctuations may leave a woman vulnerable to bacterial overgrowth at particular times in her menstrual cycle. Once the anaerobes and mycoplasmas dominate, they produce a characteristic malodorous, milky vaginal discharge composed of the microbes' by-product amines: putrescine, cadaverine, and trimethylamine (Hillier et al. 1999). However, many women with this condition are asymptomatic.

Bacterial vaginosis makes up 30–50% of all cases of vaginitis (Shalev et al. 1996). Estimated prevalence rates vary greatly among practice settings (Calzolari et al. 2000). The prevalence of BV is approximately 5–15% among women attending gynecology clinics, 15–20% among pregnant women, and 35% among women attending sexually transmitted disease (STD) clinics (Calzolari et al. 2000). Incidence of BV also varies by ethnicity. For African Americans, the risk for BV is more than twice as high as it is for Caucasian and Asian women. Likewise, Hispanic women have a much higher risk for BV (Hillier et al. 1999). The cause for this ethnic disparity is unclear and merits further investigation. The covariation of race and social class in the United States confounds the ability to distinguish racial from socioeconomic factors (Rauh et al. 2000). One study suggested that this ethnic disparity may be attributable to differences in genital hygienic practices. For example, douching is more common in African American populations (Rajamanoharan et al. 1999).

BV is not generally considered an STD and there is no known clinical counterpart in males (Hay 1998, Hillier et al. 1999). Women with BV are typically older (older than 30 years) than those with STDs. An STD can be defined as "a disease that results from the transmission of a microorganism from one person to another during sexual activity and in which we seek to treat or counsel the sex partner to prevent transmission to another person" (Schmid 1999, p. S19). While BV does not fall under this strict definition, some association of this infection with sexual activity remains (Calzolari et al. 2000, Hillier et al. 1999). For example, women with new or multiple sexual partners are at higher risk for BV. There is a high concordance rate in lesbian partnerships (Fethers et al. 2000, Hillier et al. 1999, McCaffrey et al. 1999). *G. vaginalis* may be recovered from the urethra of a male sex partner. Also, there is a much higher rate of BV in sexually experienced women compared to sexually inexperienced women. However, BV also has characteristics that are not associated with sexual activity: It may be found in virgins, and treatment of male partners does not improve cure or recurrence rates (Morris et al. 2001, Schmid 1999).

Many placebo-controlled studies have demonstrated that treatment of the male partner neither improves clinical outcome nor reduces recurrence of BV (Hillier et al. 1999). While men may harbor BV-related organisms in the urethra, there is no benefit to treatment of the male partner (Chambliss 2000, Colli et al. 1997, Hay 1998, Hillier et al. 1999).

Recurrence is a common problem in BV. Up to 30% of women have recurrences of BV in the first month after treatment and up to 70% in three months (Hay 1998, Hillier et al. 1999, Schmid 1999). Possible causes include reinfection by a male partner colonized with BV-associated microorganisms, persistence of BV-associated microbes that were inhibited but not killed, failure to re-establish a normal lactobacillus-dominant vaginal ecosystem, and/or other host factors (Hillier et al. 1999).

BV may cause serious infection in some cases. Sequelae may include pelvic inflammatory disease (PID) and postoperative infections (post-cesarean section wound infection, posthysterectomy vaginal cuff cellulitis, and post-therapeutic abortion endometritis) (Centers for Disease Control and Prevention [CDC] 2002, Soper 1999). Pregnancy-related risks of BV include chorioamnionitis, premature labor and delivery, premature rupture of membranes, and postpartum endometritis (Hillier et al. 1999, Pybus et al. 1999, Rauh et al. 2000). The presence of BV has been shown to increase susceptibility to HIV infection (Al-Harthi et al. 1999, Hillier et al. 1999, Rauh et al. 2000).

DATABASE

SUBJECTIVE

→ See **Table 12SF.1, Vaginal Infections.**
→ Predisposing risk factors may include:
  ▪ Low oxidation-reduction potential of the vagina
  ▪ Elevated vaginal pH
  ▪ Reduction in H_2O_2-producing lactobacilli
  ▪ Age older than 30 years
  ▪ Multiple sexual partners
  ▪ New sexual partner
  ▪ History of an STD
  ▪ Douching
  ▪ Menses
  ▪ Low socioeconomic status
  ▪ Immunological status
  ▪ Hormonal factors
  ▪ Intrauterine device (oral contraceptives and condoms may be protective)
→ Symptoms may include:
  ▪ None in 40–50% of cases
  ▪ Malodorous discharge (the most common symptom, described as "fishy," most evident after sexual intercourse)
  ▪ Increased milky discharge

  ▪ Burning, pruritus, external dysuria in some cases
  ▪ Intermenstrual spotting (rare), pelvic pain (in subclinical endometritis)
→ History should include:
  ▪ Gynecological
  ▪ Sexual, including sexual practices, number and gender of partners, recent change of partner, partner signs and symptoms
  ▪ Contraceptive use
  ▪ Medical
  ▪ Allergies to foods, medications, products, or environmental factors
  ▪ Medications
  ▪ Drug and alcohol habits, exercise, nutrition, stress
  ▪ Review of systems
  ▪ Onset and timing of symptoms, and their relation to menstrual cycle and sexual activity
  ▪ Characteristics of discharge: color, quantity, quality, odor
  ▪ Location of pruritus, if present
  ▪ Aggravating or relieving factors
  ▪ Associated symptoms
  ▪ Other:
    • Use of self-treatment measures and home remedies (which may cause contact irritation)
    • Over-the-counter medication
    • Spermicides
    • Feminine hygiene deodorant products, douches, bath additives, etc.
    • Type of soap, detergent, toilet paper
    • Use of pads or tampons
    • Sexual paraphernalia
    • Type of undergarments and clothing

OBJECTIVE

→ Vital signs as indicated (usually unnecessary in uncomplicated infection)
→ Abdominal examination, including lymph nodes, as indicated
→ Pelvic examination:
  ▪ External genitalia: thin, homogeneous, gray-white discharge pooling at introitus (yellow-green tints may also be seen)
  ▪ Bartholin's, urethral, Skene's glands: assess or palpate for abnormal discharge, masses
  ▪ Vagina: thin, homogeneous, gray-white discharge adherent to walls; bubbles present in 10–15% of cases; erythema absent unless there is a concomitant infection
  ▪ Cervix: thin discharge covering ectocervix; os clear; erythema rare; cervical motion tenderness absent in uncomplicated cases
  ▪ Uterus, adnexa, rectovaginal: tenderness may be present with associated pelvic infection
NOTE: Because BV is not a tissue pathogen, signs of acute inflammation are usually absent.
→ Additional examination components, depending on case presentation, may include skin, oral cavity, lymph nodes, and pubic hair.

ASSESSMENT

→ Bacterial vaginosis
→ R/O physiological leukorrhea
→ R/O other/concomitant vaginal infection
→ R/O STD/PID

PLAN

DIAGNOSTIC TESTS

NOTE: Symptoms alone are unreliable for a diagnosis. Use Amsel's criteria to assess BV: abnormal discharge, amine odor ("whiff test"), increased pH, and the presence of clue cells. Three of the four must be present to make the diagnosis (CDC 2002). Sample carefully from the lateral or posterior fornices of the vagina to avoid cervical mucus (Hillier et al. 1999).

→ Discharge: usually thin, homogenous, gray-white (the weakest sign, due to the subjectivity of the examiner)
→ Wet-mount microscopy (view under 10x and 40x power)
  ■ KOH (10–20%):
    • Amine or "fishy" odor (sniff the slide if odor isn't apparent)
    • Assess for the presence of hyphae (indicative of concomitant yeast vaginitis).
  ■ Saline:
    • Clue cells—epithelial cells stippled with bacteria in at least 20% of sample. Must be distinguished from "false clue cell," an epithelial cell covered with small numbers of normal lactobacilli. Clue cells are highly suggestive of BV, but by themselves they are not pathognomonic (Kaufman et al. 1994).
    • Decreased/absent lactobacilli
    • Usually no or few WBCs, but this varies. If a large number of WBCs are found, think concomitant vaginal infection/STD.
    • Assess for the presence of motile trichomonads (indicative of concomitant *Trichomonas vaginalis* vaginitis).
→ pH: >4.5, usually in the >5.0–6.0 range. Swab from posterior and lateral fornices of the vagina and place sample directly on pH paper or place pH paper on discharge from the speculum after removing it.
  NOTE: Elevated pH also may result from lubricant, tap water, cervical mucus, semen, amniotic fluid, trichomoniasis, or recent douche.
→ A Gram stain may be used to identify the presence of large, Gram-positive rods (lactobacilli); small, Gram-variable cocci and rods (*G. vaginalis* and other anaerobes); and curved rods (*Mobiluncus*). The sample is then scored using Nugent's criteria: 0–3 = normal; 4–6 = intermediate flora; 7–10 = bacterial vaginosis. This method is 86–89% sensitive and 94–96% specific compared to Amsel's criteria (Hillier et al. 1999, Schwebke 1999).
→ Vaginal culture is *not* advised to establish the diagnosis or as a test-of-cure because *G. vaginalis* may be isolated from 40–50% of normal women.

→ Pap smears are unreliable.
→ Newer, commercially available tests may be helpful (CDC 2002):
  ■ DNA probe-based test for increased *G. vaginalis* (Affirm™ VP III)
  ■ Test for elevated pH and trimethylamine (Fem Exam® test card)
  ■ Test for elevated pH and proline aminopeptidase (Pip Activity TestCard™)
→ Testing for *Neisseria gonorrhoeae* and *Chlamydia trachomatis* should be performed in women at risk for STD. In the absence of a cervix, urethral or urine specimens may be substituted.
→ Additional laboratory tests should be individualized and may include but are not limited to: RPR or VDRL, CBC, urinalysis, urine culture and sensitivities, hepatitis B antigen and antibody, serological HIV, and pregnancy test.

TREATMENT/MANAGEMENT

→ In nonpregnant women, treatment is advised for all symptomatic women with a confirmed diagnosis (CDC 2002). It is reasonable to consider treating an asymptomatic woman before surgical abortion, gynecological surgery, or invasive procedures (CDC 2002).
→ Recommended regimens (CDC 2002):
  ■ Metronidazole 500 mg p.o. BID for 7 days
                        OR
  ■ Metronidazole vaginal gel 0.75%, 1 full applicator (5 g) intravaginally once a day for 5 days
                        OR
  ■ Clindamycin cream 2%, 1 full applicator (5 g) intravaginally at bedtime for 7 days
→ Alternative regimens (lower efficacy than recommended regimens) (CDC 2002):
  ■ Metronidazole 2 g p.o. in a single dose
                        OR
  ■ Clindamycin 300 mg p.o. BID for 7 days
                        OR
  ■ Clindamycin ovules 100 g intravaginally once at bedtime for 3 days
    NOTE: Alcohol should not be consumed during treatment with metronidazole and for 24 hours thereafter. Both oral and dermal clindamycin have been associated with pseudomembranous colitis, which is characterized by severe, persistent diarrhea; severe abdominal cramps; and passage of blood or mucus. Symptoms may begin up to several weeks following therapy. The drug should be discontinued if significant diarrhea develops. Clindamycin cream and ovules are oil-based and might weaken latex condoms or a diaphragm. Refer to the product labeling for further information (CDC 2002, *Physician's Desk Reference* 2002, Zambrano 1991).
→ Recurrent infection:
  ■ Switch the drug of choice or use local therapy if oral therapy has failed (CDC 2002, Eschenbach et al. 1992, Mead 1989).

- Some specialists recommend using a longer course of therapy (e.g., 10–14 days rather than 5–7 days) (Mead 2001).
- A maintenance regimen (after an initial longer course of metronidazole gel) consisting of a single application of metronidazole gel twice weekly for 3–6 months also has been recommended by some specialists (Mead 2001).

NOTE: *Candida* infection rates may increase with long-term therapy. If *Candida* cultures are positive in a woman using long-term gel, fluconazole 150 mg p.o. once a week may be used, provided there are no contraindications (Mead 2001).

- A substantial number of women will relapse after long-term gel is discontinued. Consult with a specialist.
- Intravaginal lactobacillus may prevent recurrences (studies are under way) (CDC 2002, Mead 2001).
- Periodic acidification of the vagina with vinegar douches is generally ineffective for treating or preventing recurrences (Eschenbach et al. 1992).

→ Male partner therapy:
- Treatment of the male partner does not seem to influence the response to therapy or the relapse/recurrence rate in the female; thus, routine treatment of male sex partners is not recommended (CDC 2002).
- If the male has acute symptoms of an STD, a history of prostatitis, or epididymitis, refer him for evaluation and therapy.

→ Treatment during pregnancy:
- All symptomatic pregnant women should be tested and treated (CDC 2002). Recommended regimens:
  - Metronidazole 250 mg p.o. TID for 7 days
    OR
  - Clindamycin 300 mg p.o. BID for 7 days
- Some specialists recommend that women at high risk for preterm delivery (i.e., those who have previously delivered a premature infant) be screened and treated.
- Data are inconclusive regarding the benefit of treating asymptomatic women at low risk for preterm delivery.

→ HIV-infected patients should receive the same treatment regimen as individuals who are HIV-negative.

CONSULTATION

→ For refractory cases
→ For treatment during pregnancy, as indicated
→ If the male has acute symptoms of an STD, a history of prostatitis, or epididymitis, refer him for evaluation and therapy
→ In cases of pseudomembranous colitis secondary to clindamycin
→ As needed for prescription(s)

PATIENT EDUCATION

→ Explain that many factors are related to changes in vaginal flora predisposing to BV: menstruation, hygienic habits, contraceptive methods, immunological status, medications, and hormonal factors.
→ Explain that evidence of sexual transmission remains unclear. Explain how intercourse may introduce BV-associated organisms into the vagina and that alkaline semen may promote vaginal microbial overgrowth, as well. However, routine partner treatment is not advised.

→ When BV is diagnosed in an asymptomatic patient, discuss the finding. Upon further questioning, a woman may recognize the symptom complex and opt for treatment.
→ Stress the importance of completing the full course of medication unless severe side effects occur.
→ Review the common side effects of metronidazole: a metallic taste, nausea, occasionally dark urine, vomiting, diarrhea, and headache.
- Advise against alcohol use during and for 24 hours after medication, as a disulfiram-like reaction may occur.

→ Discuss vaginal health and hygiene measures. The patient should understand that a foul odor in the vulvovaginal area is not normal unless infection is present. Reassure her that some vaginal discharge is normal and discuss the characteristic cyclical changes. (See also the **Candidal Vulvovaginitis** chapter.)
→ Advise of the possibility of *Candida* vaginitis secondary to an oral antibiotic and discuss the indications for prophylactic therapy (if there is a history of antibiotic-induced candidiasis).
→ Provide guidelines on safer sex practices. (See **Table 13A.2, Safer Sex Practices** in the **Chancroid** chapter in Section 13, and **Table 12I.1, Recommendations for Individuals to Prevent STD/PID** in the **Pelvic Inflammatory Disease** chapter.) Encourage condom use with new, multiple, and/or nonmonogamous partners.
→ Address routine health maintenance issues as indicated.

FOLLOW-UP

→ Advise the patient to return for further evaluation if signs and symptoms of infection have not cleared after the week of treatment or if infection recurs. Assess compliance with the medication regimen.
→ Pregnant women who are at high risk for preterm delivery should have a follow-up evaluation one month after completion of treatment to ensure the efficacy of medication (CDC 2002).
→ Follow up on all identified concomitant STDs. Refer to specific chapters for treatment and follow-up. Discuss the importance of partner evaluation and treatment if an STD is identified. Continue to encourage safer sex practices.
→ Newly diagnosed, HIV-positive persons should be referred to the appropriate provider or agency for early intervention services.
→ Newly diagnosed, hepatitis B antigen-positive individuals should undergo liver function tests and receive counseling regarding the implications of their positive status and the need for immunoprophylaxis of sex partners and household members. (See the **Hepatitis—Viral** chapter.)
→ Document in progress and on problem list.

Winifred L. Star, R.N., C., N.P., M.S.
Melanie Deal, R.N., C., N.P., M.S.

12-SC Vaginitis
Candidal Vulvovaginitis

Candidiasis is the second most common cause of vaginitis, after bacterial vaginosis, in women of childbearing age (Dun 1999, Sobel 1999). The causative agents of this fungal infection are various strains of the yeast species *Candida. Candida* are dimorphic organisms that display one of two phenotypes at different developmental phases: the blastospore (a bud-like phenotype) and the hyphae (a filamentous form). *Candida albicans* is responsible for 80–90% of the cases of vulvovaginal candidiasis. Non-*albicans* species, such as *Candida glabrata, Candida tropicalis, Candida lusitaniae, Candida parapsilosis,* and *Candida guillermondii,* are less common causes of infection. However, the prevalence of non-*albicans* species has been increasing in recent years (Palacin et al. 2000, Sobel 1999). The increase is troubling because these species are more resistant to the common azole therapy and because they are more difficult to diagnose via microscopic examination. Non-*albicans* species do not exhibit the hyphal phenotype (Dun 1999, Eckert et al. 1998).

Yeast is a ubiquitous organism that is a normal cohabitant of the mucocutaneous and alimentary tract. *Candida* can be found in or on the mouth, throat, skin, scalp, vagina, fingers, nails, bronchi, lungs, and gastrointestinal tract (Dun 1999). Yeast also may grow in the intertriginous areas: vulva, groin, axilla, under the breasts, and the coronal sulcus of the penis (most often in uncircumcised men). *Candida* may colonize the vagina as a harmless commensal or as a pathogen. About 20–25% of healthy, asymptomatic women will have positive vaginal cultures for yeast (Fidel et al. 1996).

Yeast organisms gain access to the vagina mostly from the nearby perianal area. In the colonization phase, which is usually asymptomatic, yeast and resident vaginal flora exist as commensal organisms. Infection may develop when specific changes in the host response or the local environment occur. The triggers for this pathogenesis remain unclear.

An estimated 75% of women experience at least one episode of vulvovaginal candidiasis (VVC) in their lifetime; 40–50% will experience a recurrence (Sobel 1999). Approximately 5% of women who develop candidiasis will suffer from intractable recurrent vulvovaginal candidiasis (RVVC) (Sobel 1999).

By strict definition, yeast vaginitis is not considered a sexually transmitted disease (STD). Yet sexual transmission may occur. Male sexual partners of infected women are four times more likely to have an asymptomatic genital colonization with *Candida* than are male partners of uninfected women (Sobel 1999). However, the role that this transmission plays in the pathogenesis of infection is not known (Sobel 1999). Routine treatment of male partners is not currently recommended.

RVVC, usually defined as four or more clinically proven infections per year, is a perplexing, frustrating problem (CDC 2002, Fidel et al. 1996). It may be caused secondarily by immunosuppressive therapy, uncontrolled diabetes, or hormone replacement therapy. However, for many women, the cause of RVVC is idiopathic. Although most treatment is successful, it does not prevent recurrence. In 50% of idiopathic RVVC cases, recurrent episodes occur in a few days to three months of treatment cessation (Fidel et al. 1996).

The mechanisms of RVVC are ill-defined. RVVC may result from a spectrum of factors originating from the infecting organism (antimycotic resistance, phenotype switching, intestinal reservoir) or from host factors (T-cell dysregulation, reproductive hormones). There is conflicting evidence for many of these proposed mechanisms. Studies investigating the etiology and pathogenesis of RVVC are ongoing. However, most experts agree on a few points. First, RVVC is most likely caused by relapse and not by reinfection. Relapse may occur because most antifungal agents are fungistatic rather than fungicidal. Second, there is a higher prevalence of non-*albicans* species in RVVC than in other vaginal candidal infections. Non-*albicans* species are more resistant to common azole therapies. *C. albicans* accounts for only 62–79% of RVVC-causing species. Finally, there is a growing body of evidence suggesting that local T-cell mediated immunity may play a defining role in causing RVVC (Fidel et al. 1996, Sobel 1999, Spinillo et al. 1997). Azole-resistant strains of *C. albicans* have been isolated but are an uncommon cause of VVC or RVVC (Dun 1999, Sobel 1999).

New evidence has changed an old paradigm of the relationship between vaginal candidiasis and HIV positivity. Early studies suggested that recurrent vaginal candidiasis, like oropharyngeal and esophageal candidiasis (common opportunistic infections in HIV-positive individuals), was a clinical marker for immunocompromise in HIV-positive women (Sobel 1999). More recent studies have demonstrated that although HIV-positive women are more likely to be colonized with *Candida*, they are not more likely than HIV-negative women to develop candidiasis from this colonization. Rates of candidiasis are similar between HIV-positive and HIV-negative women. Vaginal candidiasis is not related to lower median CD4 count in HIV-positive women (Schuman et al. 1998, Sobel 1999). Researchers have noted that HIV-positive women are more often colonized with non-*albicans* species of *Candida* (Schuman et al. 1998, Spinillo et al. 1997).

Therapeutic agents used to treat yeast vaginitis can be classified into four groups: dyes (gential violet) and miscellaneous compounds (such as boric acid); polyenes (amphotericin B, nystatin, candicidin); imidazoles (clotrimazole, miconazole, butoconazole, tioconazole, ketoconazole); and triazoles (terconazole, fluconazole). The last group is the first in a relatively new generation of azoles for which in vitro studies have shown excellent activity against *C. glabrata* and *C. tropicalis* (Rinaldi 1988); however, more data in humans are needed to determine whether these products offer any advantage over the imidazoles.

DATABASE

SUBJECTIVE

→ See **Table 12SF.1, Vaginal Infections.**
→ Predisposing factors include:
- Pregnancy:
  - The highest risk is in the third trimester. Recurrence is more common. A possible mechanism: High estrogen levels increase the glycogen content of the vagina, providing a favorable climate for yeast overgrowth and enhancing vaginal cell affinity for yeast (Sobel 1999).
- Antibiotics:
  - Broad-spectrum agents (e.g., tetracyclines, oral cephalosporins, and ampicillins) reduce the protective lactobacilli of the gut/vagina, allowing resident yeast proliferation.
- Diabetes, uncontrolled:
  - Increased urinary/vaginal glucose provides an enriched medium for yeast growth.
- Immunocompromised conditions and metabolic factors: AIDS, endocrinopathies (diabetes, hypothyroidism, Cushing's syndrome, etc.), anemia, hematological malignancies (lymphoma, leukemia, Hodgkin's disease), autoimmune diseases (lupus, rheumatoid arthritis, temporal arteritis), and zinc immunosuppressive drugs (Summers et al. 1993).
  - These conditions/factors increase susceptibility to fungal infection, probably by altering cell-mediated immunity.
- Oral contraceptives or hormone replacement therapy:
  - Pharmacological doses of hormones may affect the glycogen status of vaginal epithelium, leading to an enriched substrate for yeast growth. High-estrogen pills are implicated more often.

- Other possible precipitating factors (the evidence is anecdotal and limited, as these factors have not been well-studied):
  - Stress, obesity, menses, trauma, poor hygiene, fomites, warm weather, fever, contraceptive sponges, commercial douches, and feminine hygiene deodorant products.
    - These factors may alter the symbiotic relationship between resident flora in the vagina.
  - Irritants such as perfumed soap and toilet paper, chlorinated pools, and topical anesthetics may cause a reactive vulvitis that can be confused with yeast infection.
→ Symptoms may include (Dun 1999, Eckert et al. 1998, Sobel 1999, Sonnex et al. 1999):
- Pruritus (38% of patients):
  - The primary symptom, located in the vulva; may be mild to severe; may be exacerbated in evening hours; usual onset one week before onset of menses; may improve during menstruation.
- Burning:
  - Often accompanies pruritus; may follow intercourse or be secondary to excoriation from scratching (semen itself also may cause postcoital burning).
- Dysuria (external); urinary urgency, frequency (reflexogenic)
- Dyspareunia
- Abnormal vaginal discharge:
  - Not a classic symptom and rarely the presenting complaint. However, most patients have a slight discharge at some stage of infection. It may be thin, creamy, thick/curd-like (occurs more often in pregnancy); usually odorless or may smell sour or "yeast-like."
- Dryness in the vulvovaginal area
- Soreness and swelling of the vulvovaginal area
- Partner complains of transient penile rash, redness, pruritus, or burning following intercourse.
→ History should include:
- Gynecological
- Sexual (including practices and number and gender of partners; partner signs and symptoms)
- Contraceptive use
- Medical
- Allergies (foods, medications, products, environmental factors)
- Medications
- Habits (drugs, alcohol), exercise, nutrition, stress
- Review of systems
- Family history (diabetes, allergies)
- Onset and timing of symptoms and their relation to menstrual cycle/sexual activity
- Location of pruritus: mons, vulva, vagina, perineum, perianal, generalized
- Characteristics of discharge: color, quantity, quality, odor
- Aggravating/relieving factors
- Associated symptoms
- Other: use of self-treatment measures and home remedies; OTC medication; use of spermicides, feminine hygiene

deodorant products, douches, bath additives, etc.; type of soap, detergent, toilet paper; use of pads or tampons, sexual paraphernalia; type of undergarments and clothing.

OBJECTIVE

→ Ideally, an examination is performed when the patient is symptomatic, has not douched for 2–3 days, has not applied intravaginal cream or contraceptive spermicide for several days to one week, and is not menstruating.
→ Vital signs as indicated (usually unnecessary in uncomplicated infection).
→ Abdominal examination, including inguinal lymph nodes, as indicated.
→ A systematic, thorough examination of the vulvovaginal area should be performed, keeping in mind other potential causes of genital infection.
  ▪ Vulva:
    • May see erythema, edema, excoriation, discharge; erythema may extend to perianal area, crural folds, inner thighs, buttocks; satellite pustules may appear at edges of the affected area.
  ▪ Bartholin's, urethral, Skene's glands:
    • Usually WNL; assess for discharge.
  ▪ Vagina:
    • May see thin, creamy, or thick/curd-like white or yellow discharge, erythema; a pseudomembrane may cover the vaginal walls.
  ▪ Cervix:
    • May see adherent thin, creamy, or thick/curd-like white or yellow discharge; erythema.
→ Uterus, adnexa, rectovaginal examination: usually WNL unless there is concomitant pathology.

ASSESSMENT

→ Candidal vulvovaginitis
→ Candidal vulvitis
→ Candidal vaginitis
→ Recurrent Candidal (vulvo)vaginitis
→ R/O physiological leukorrhea
→ R/O other causes of vaginitis: bacterial vaginosis, trichomoniasis, cytolytic vaginitis, atrophic vaginitis, chemical/mechanical causes
→ R/O idiopathic focal vulvovestibulitis
→ R/O foreign body
→ R/O contact (reactive) vulvitis
→ R/O diabetic vulvitis
→ R/O allergic reaction
→ R/O cutaneous candidiasis of the vulva
→ R/O tinea cruris
→ R/O other vulvar dermatoses (e.g., psoriasis, seborrheic dermatitis, eczemoid dermatitis)
→ R/O STD
→ R/O urinary tract infection
→ R/O infection in partner
→ Assess psychosomatic factors

PLAN

DIAGNOSTIC TESTS

→ Wet mount microscopy (10x and 40x power) is the principal diagnostic method.
  ▪ KOH 10–20%:
    • Spores or branching/budding pseudomycelia (hyphae) may be identified.
      – C. glabrata spores are of variable size, spherical-ovoid, in groups or clusters (but may appear singly), and smaller than a red blood cell. C. glabrata does not form pseudohyphae or hyphae and is not easily recognized on microscopy (CDC 2002).
      – C. albicans spores, in contrast, are uniform in size, isolated, and almost always associated with hyphae (Kaufman et al. 1994).
    • Amine odor may be present in cases of bacterial vaginosis/T. vaginalis vaginitis.
    NOTE: Obtain specimens from more than one area. Half of the women who are culture-positive for yeast will have a negative KOH wet mount. Cotton fibers, scratches on the slide, and Leptothrix (nonfungal vaginal commensal) all appear as long, string-like filaments and thus may be confused with hyphae.
  ▪ Saline:
    • Lactobacilli are usually present.
    • WBCs may be increased.
    • Assess for clue cells, motile trichomonads.
    NOTE: If excessive WBCs are identified, consider trichomoniasis or other STD.
→ pH 4.0–4.7 (4.5 is most common)
  NOTE: Collect a specimen from the mid-third of the lateral vaginal wall. Tap water, cervical mucus, or the presence of bacterial vaginosis/trichomoniasis may result in alkaline readings.
→ Gram stain:
  ▪ Spores and budding hyphae may be seen.
→ Cultures for yeast:
  ▪ Should not be used in the absence of symptoms. 10–20% of women are commensally colonized by yeast (CDC 2002).
  ▪ Should be obtained in recurrent/resistant cases to confirm the diagnosis, to identify unusual species, and with suspected candidiasis when the KOH prep is negative (CDC 2002).
  ▪ Nickerson's, Sabouraud's, Mycosel, or blood agar media may be used. Yeast can be grown at room temperature; some non-albicans species may take 10 days to grow.
→ Pap smear:
  ▪ May identify Candida if present in large numbers.
  ▪ Testing for Chlamydia trachomatis and Neisseria gonorrhoeae should be performed for women at risk for these infections.
→ Additional labs as indicated may include but are not limited to: CBC, herpes culture, urinalysis, urine culture and sensitivities, VDRL or RPR, fasting blood glucose, and pregnancy test.

TREATMENT/MANAGEMENT

→ If *Candida* is identified in an asymptomatic woman, it does not require treatment (CDC 2002).

→ In some situations, a presumptive diagnosis of yeast vulvovaginitis may lead to empirical antifungal therapy.

→ Avoid overtreatment of leukorrhea without other symptoms and in the absence of clinical pathology.

→ Acute therapy:
  ■ Recommended regimens (CDC 2002):
    • Intravaginal agents (* = over-the-counter preparation):
      – Butoconazole 2% cream 5 g intravaginally for 3 days*
        OR
      – Butoconazole 2% cream 5 g (butaconazole 1-sustained release), single intravaginal application
        OR
      – Clotrimazole 1% cream 5 g intravaginally for 7–14 days*
        OR
      – Clotrimazole 100 mg vaginal tablet for 7 days
        OR
      – Clotrimazole 100 mg vaginal tablet, 2 tablets for 3 days
        OR
      – Clotrimazole 500 mg vaginal tablet, 1 tablet in a single application
        OR
      – Miconazole 2% cream 5 g intravaginally for 7 days*
        OR
      – Miconazole 100 mg vaginal suppository, 1 suppository for 7 days*
        OR
      – Miconazole 200 mg vaginal suppository, 1 suppository for 3 days*
        OR
      – Nystatin 100,000-unit vaginal tablet, 1 tablet for 14 days
        OR
      – Tioconazole 6.5% ointment 5 g intravaginally in a single application*
        OR
      – Terconazole 0.4% cream 5 g intravaginally for 7 days
        OR
      – Terconazole 0.8% cream 5 g intravaginally for 3 days
        OR
      – Terconazole 80 mg vaginal suppository, 1 suppository for 3 days
    • Oral agent: Fluconazole 150 mg tablet, 1 tablet in a single dose.

  NOTE: Creams and suppositories are oil-based and may weaken latex condoms and diaphragms (CDC 2002). The clinician must decide between 1-, 3-, 7-, or 14-day antifungal therapy based on the patient's history and clinical presentation. Single- and/or 3-day therapies are indicated for patients with infrequent, episodic infection of mild to moderate severity and may not be effective for chronic cases and during pregnancy (CDC 2002, Sobel 1999). Single-dose oral fluconazole has been shown to be comparable in efficacy to topical azole therapy in many studies (Langdon 1994). For the occasional infection unresponsive to a single course of standard therapy, treat with a second course (Sparks 1991). High relapse rates after therapy can be controlled by continuing treatment for at least two weeks or longer (Kaufman et al. 1994). Nystatin is not as effective as the azole drug regimens.

→ Pregnancy:
  ■ Only topical azole therapies, applied for 7 days, are recommended (CDC 2002).

→ HIV-infected women with acute infection may be treated with CDC-recommended regimens. See above.

→ Yeast vulvitis:
  ■ Mild: Apply a vaginal antifungal cream to the vulvar area BID–TID.
  ■ Severe/extensive: Apply vaginal antifungal preparations both vaginally and to the affected vulvar areas.
  ■ See the **Red Lesions of the Vulva** chapter.

→ Pruritus/inflammation control:
  ■ A low- to midpotency corticosteroid cream or ointment applied sparingly BID–TID to the affected area.
    • Options include:
      – Hydrocortisone 1% (nonfluorinated)
      – Nystatin and triamcinolone acetonide
      – Triamcinolone acetonide 0.1%
    NOTE: Avoid using fluorinated steroids for extended periods, as skin atrophy may result. (See **Table 12TB.1, Potency Ranking of Some Commonly Used Topical Corticosteroids** in the **White Lesions of the Vulva** chapter.)

→ Alternative acute therapy:
  ■ A complete list of alternative therapies is beyond the scope of this chapter.
  ■ Gentian violet 1% painted on the vulva and in the vagina 4 times at intervals of approximately 7 days (Droegemueller 2001). Do not use the solution in the presence of vulvar excoriation or ulceration.

→ Partner therapy:
  ■ In the presence of balanitis (erythema, pruritis, or irritation of glans penis) or penile dermatitis, a topical antifungal agent may be beneficial (CDC 2002).

→ Therapy for recurrent yeast:
  ■ The following general principles may be applied to manage recurrent infection (Kaufman et al. 1994, Sobel 1999, Sparks 1991):
    • The diagnosis must be confirmed by culture.
    • Treat with 7–14 days of topical therapy or, alternatively, a 150 mg oral dose of fluconazole repeated 3 days later. A maintenance antifungal regimen may be initiated (see below) (CDC 2002).
    • Identify and attempt to eradicate all predisposing factors, if possible.
    • Make no assumptions regarding the efficacy of previously used therapies.

- When the patient does not respond to antifungal therapy, consider other causes of vulvovaginitis and vulvar disease (e.g., trichomoniasis, bacterial vaginosis, cytolytic vaginitis, atrophic vaginitis, allergic hypersensitivity/contact vulvitis, lichen sclerosus, vestibulitis, essential vulvodynia, lichen planus, etc.).
- Oral corticosteroids, immunosuppressive drugs, and high-dose estrogen hormone should be discontinued if possible.
- Consider culturing the mouth and ejaculate of the partner.
- If the patient is diabetic, advocate good glucose control.
- Enhance the patient's diet with a vitamin/mineral supplement.
- See "Patient Education," below, regarding health maintenance and additional general principles.

■ Recommended maintenance/suppressive therapies, to be continued for 6 months, include (CDC 2002):
- Clotrimazole 500 mg vaginal suppository once weekly
- Ketoconazole 100 mg oral dose once daily
- Fluconazole 100–150 mg oral dose once weekly
- Itraconazole 400 mg oral dose once monthly or 100 mg dose once daily

NOTE: Ketoconazole may be hepatotoxic (hepatotoxicity is estimated to occur in 1:10,000 to 1:15,000 of exposed persons [CDC 2002]). Refer to the *Physicians' Desk Reference* (*PDR*) and consult with a physician before prescribing. Liver function tests should be performed before initiating therapy and every 3–4 months during therapy. Ketoconazole is contraindicated in pregnancy and not for use in uncomplicated, infrequent/acute vaginal yeast infections.

→ Non-*albicans* VVC (CDC 2002):
■ Optimal treatment is unknown.
■ Therapeutic options include:
- Longer-duration therapy (7–14 days) with a non-fluconazole azole drug.
- If there is a recurrence, 600 mg boric acid in a gelatin capsule intravaginally once daily for 14 days.
  - Ongoing regimens suggested by some specialists include boric acid 300–600 mg intravaginally QOD, then twice weekly for up to 6 months (Mead 2001).
- Topical 4% flucytosine—refer to a specialist.
- For continued recurrence, a maintenance regimen of 100,000 units of nystatin via daily vaginal suppositories.

→ Additional considerations:
■ Treat concomitant vaginal infections appropriately. See specific chapters.

CONSULTATION

→ For recurrent infection as indicated.
→ When considering systemic therapy.

PATIENT EDUCATION

→ Discuss the cause, precipitating factors, and possible transmission of infection.

→ In cases where no pathology is identified and the only complaint is leukorrhea, reassure the patient regarding the absence of infection and educate her regarding the normality of cyclical discharge.
→ Advise the patient that self-treatment with OTC products should be reserved for women who have been previously diagnosed with yeast vulvovaginitis and who are experiencing a recurrence of the same symptoms (CDC 2002).
→ Review/discuss vulvovaginal health and hygiene:
■ All-cotton underwear, loose clothing, avoidance of panty hose
■ Proper wiping technique (i.e., front to back)
■ White, unscented toilet paper
■ Avoidance of chemical irritants such as strong bath or laundry soap, feminine hygiene products, bath additives, plastic-covered or scented peripads, scented tampons, talcum powder, commercial douches, and chlorinated swimming pools (Bachmann et al. 2000)
■ Avoidance of mechanical irritants (e.g., tight-fitting clothing, tampons, dildos, vibrators, bicycling)
■ Ideally, use only water to wash vulva (if necessary, Aveeno® or other hypoallergenic soap may be used with a thorough rinse). Pat the area dry or use a hair dryer on a low setting. Avoid over-cleaning (the woman may do this to attempt to eradicate a vaginal infection/STD).
■ Hand-wash undergarments with a mild soap and thoroughly rinse. No fabric softeners. Line drying is preferable.
■ For recurrent infection, "sterilize" underclothing in a microwave oven for five minutes on high while the garment is still wet from laundering or soak it in bleach overnight and rinse thoroughly. Alternately, boiling or washing at temperatures exceeding 70° C may sterilize undergarments (Kaufman et al. 1994). Disposable underwear or panty liners may be used.
→ Stress the importance of completing the full course of prescribed medication. Continue intravaginal medications throughout menses (use with a peripad instead of a tampon).
→ Advise abstinence from sexual intercourse during treatment for infection.
→ Provide guidelines on safer sex practices. (See **Table 13A.2, Safer Sex Practices** in the **Chancroid** chapter in Section 13.)
■ Encourage condom use with new, multiple, or nonmonogamous partners.
■ Advise that oral-genital sex or anal-vaginal sex without interceding wash may precipitate infection and may need to be curtailed. Clean fingers may need to be substituted for oral sex during masturbation by partner.
→ Sex toys, douche tips, diaphragms, cervical caps, etc., may act as fomites and thus should be cleaned properly after use.
→ Discuss risk factors for recurrent infections: diabetes, immunosuppression, and antibiotic or corticosteroid use. Most women will have no predisposing conditions (CDC 2002).
■ When treating with systemic medication, advise the patient regarding potential side effects (refer to the *PDR*). Explain that 30–40% of women will have recurrent infection after maintenance therapy is discontinued (CDC 2002).

→ Suggest that women with recurrent infection avoid tampon use until they are symptom-free for 3–6 months.

→ Advise the use of prophylactic antifungal agents when antibiotics are taken by women with a history of recurrent infection.

→ When gentian violet is used, advise the patient to wear old underwear or use pads or liners because the product stains. Intercourse should be avoided for 3–4 days post-treatment.

→ Advise the patient to keep boric acid capsules, which look like jelly beans, out of the reach of children; they may cause esophageal ulcers if swallowed.

FOLLOW-UP

→ Acute, uncomplicated cases require no follow-up. Advise the patient to return for re-evaluation if symptoms do not abate after therapy.

→ With the advent of OTC antifungal agents (miconazole, clotrimazole), a patient may opt to self-treat "yeast" vaginitis symptoms. If the patient remains symptomatic after OTC therapy, she should be instructed to see a health care provider for a thorough investigation of signs and symptoms, identification of the infectious agent(s) involved, and therapy based on specific clinical findings.

→ A patient treated for recurrent infection should be monitored for compliance with treatment regimens and assessed regularly to monitor the effectiveness of therapy and the occurrence of side effects (CDC 2002).

→ Follow up on STD test results and treat identified, concomitant STDs (see specific chapters). Discuss the importance of partner evaluation and treatment if an STD is identified.

→ Address additional medical concerns as indicated.

→ Document in progress notes and on problem list.

Winifred L. Star, R.N., C., N.P., M.S.
Melanie Deal, R.N., C., N.P., M.S.

12-SD Vaginitis
Cytolytic Vaginitis

Lactobacilli-overgrowth syndrome, also known as *cytolytic vaginitis* or *Döderlein's cytolysis*, is a condition caused by accelerated exfoliation and increased turnover of squamous epithelial cells in the vagina. Stress may be a precipitating factor. The condition also may arise in women who have been treated or overtreated for vaginal discharge with a variety of antibiotics and antifungal agents. The resultant overgrowth of lactobacilli, which then become the predominant microorganism, breaks down the vaginal mucosa through increased acid production and lysis of the epithelial cells' cytoplasm (Hutti et al. 2000, Kaufman et al. 1994). Some researchers question the existence of this type of vaginitis (Hutti et al. 2000).

DATABASE

SUBJECTIVE

→ See **Table 12SF.1, Vaginal Infections.**
→ Symptoms may include:
  ▪ A nonodorous, increased, or profuse discharge of thick, pasty, or "flaky" quality
  ▪ A mild burning sensation of the vulva that is worse after intercourse
  ▪ Dyspareunia
  ▪ Pruritus (usually absent)
→ Symptoms may be more pronounced in the luteal phase.

OBJECTIVE

→ Vulva is usually WNL or with slight edema and erythema.
→ Vagina may demonstrate an increased presence of a nonodorous, thick, white, opaque discharge.
→ Cervix, uterus, adnexa, and rectovaginal exams are WNL unless there is co-existent pathology.

ASSESSMENT

→ Cytolytic vaginitis or Döderlein's cytolysis
→ R/O Candidal vaginitis
→ R/O other causes of vaginitis
→ R/O squamous intraepithelial lesion

PLAN

DIAGNOSTIC TESTS

→ Wet mounts (10x and 40x power):
  ▪ Saline:
    • Increased number of epithelial cells and cellular debris from squamous cell disintegration
    • Large number of rods (lactobacilli) of varying lengths
    • "False clue cell" (stippled appearance of epithelial cells due to adherence of lactobacilli)
    • Few or no white blood cells
  ▪ KOH (10–20%):
    • No hyphae, no amine odor
→ pH: 3.5–4.5
→ Gram stain: many lactobacilli and Gram-positive rods of varying lengths, fragments of cytoplasm, "stripped" nuclei, and a lack of significant pathogenic bacteria or yeast
→ Vaginal cultures: normal flora or lactobacilli; not normally performed

TREATMENT/MANAGEMENT

→ Alkaline douches: 1 tsp baking soda/pint of warm water, douche once or twice weekly as needed. May be repeated as needed during symptomatic periods without resorting to excessive use (Kaufman et al. 1994).
  NOTE: This therapy is designed to reduce the lactobacillus population.
→ Sitz bath: 2–4 tsp of baking soda in 2 inches of bath water. Sit in the tub twice daily for 15 minutes each time. Take sitz bath 2–3 times in the first week of treatment, then 1–2 times weekly as needed to prevent recurrences (Hutti et al. 2000).
→ Avoid overtreatment of a normal vaginal discharge.

CONSULTATION

→ As indicated.

PATIENT EDUCATION

→ Discuss possible mechanisms for the condition.

→ Reassure the patient that without clinical evidence of infection, leukorrhea is usually physiological. Discuss cyclical changes in normal vaginal discharge.

→ Advise the patient not to seek over-the-phone treatment by a provider or self-overtreat vaginal symptoms, which may lead to improper therapy for vaginitis or treatment of normal vaginal discharge.

→ Stress good health maintenance: proper nutrition, rest, exercise, and stress reduction.

FOLLOW-UP

→ Individualized according to the case presentation.

→ Document in progress notes and on problem list.

Winifred L. Star, R.N., C., N.P., M.S.
Melanie Deal, R.N., C., N.P., M.S.

12-SE Vaginitis
Trichomonas vaginalis Vaginitis

Trichomoniasis is the third most common cause of vaginal infection in women of childbearing age after bacterial vaginosis and candidiasis. *Trichomonas vaginalis*, the causative agent in trichomoniasis, is a single-cell, anaerobic pathogenic protozoan that infects the squamous epithelium of the human genitourinary tract (Petrin et al. 1998). This organism possesses five flagella that give the protozoan its characteristic twitching motility (Krieger et al. 1999). Vaginal pH is a critical, growth-limiting factor for this organism. Its optimum pH is 5.5–5.8. Interestingly, most women with trichomoniasis are co-infected with other urogenital organisms of pathogenic potential, such as *Ureaplasma urealyticum* and/or *Mycoplasma hominis*, *Gardnerella vaginalis*, *Neisseria gonorrhoeae*, various species of *Candida*, and *Chlamydia trachomatis* (Krieger et al. 1999). The significance of this co-infection is unknown. Humans are the only natural host for *T. vaginalis*, which is never considered a normal vaginal commensal (Petrin et al. 1998).

More than 170 million people are infected worldwide annually, including 2–3 million women in the United States (Nyirjesy 1999, Patel 1998, Petrin et al. 1998). Prevalence rates vary depending on the population studied, from 5% in family planning patients to 75% in commercial sex workers (duBochet et al. 1998). The prevalence rate in the general population is estimated to be 5–10%. Rates are higher in women with a concomitant sexually transmitted disease (STD) (Krieger et al. 1999).

T. vaginalis is transmitted almost exclusively sexually. In women, the incubation period for trichomoniasis is 4–28 days following exposure (Petrin et al. 1998). Female partners of infected men harbor the organism from 67–100% of the time, and male partners of infected women, 14–60% of the time (Krieger et al. 1999).

Nonsexual transmission, although possible, is extremely rare. The organism, if allowed to dry, dies quickly outside the human body. It may live longer (up to 45 minutes) in wet environments (e.g., toilet seats, wet washcloths or clothing, bath water, douche nozzles) (Krieger et al. 1999, Petrin et al. 1998). The consensus view, however, is that trichomoniasis is acquired by direct genital contact (Krieger et al. 1999).

In women, sites of infection include the vagina (most common) and urethra, bladder, Bartholin's and Skene's glands, and endocervix (less common). In men, the organism lives in the anterior urethra (most common) and external genitalia, epididymis, semen, and prostate gland.

There are three clinical presentations of *T. vaginalis*: acute, with all of the classic signs and symptoms; chronic, the most common type, with abnormal discharge, milder symptoms, and no gross tissue changes; and asymptomatic carrier state, with no symptoms, normal physical findings, and trichomonads identified on wet mount of vaginal discharge (Petrin et al. 1998).

T. vaginalis can cause changes in the squamous epithelium of the cervix—cytological and histological changes that may be confused with koilocytotic atypia associated with human papillomavirus (Krieger et al. 1999). While there may be an association between trichomoniasis and cervical dysplasia or cancer, no causal relationship has been established (Krieger et al. 1999, Viikki et al. 2000).

Refractory cases of trichomoniasis have been reported. They are most commonly caused by re-infection from an untreated partner or by nonadherence to the prescribed treatment regimen (Clinical Effectiveness Group 1999, duBochet et al. 1998). True clinical resistance to treatment is rare. Often this resistance is relative, and prolonged, higher doses of metronidazole may eradicate the trichomonads (duBochet et al. 1998, Freeman et al. 1997, Lewis et al. 1997). High-level resistance occurs in approximately 1:2,000 to 1:3,000 cases (Sobel et al. 1999).

Trichomoniasis has been associated with potentially serious obstetric sequelae, such as premature rupture of membranes, preterm labor and delivery, and low birth weight (Coco et al. 2000, Krieger et al. 1999, Oleszczuk et al. 2000). Perinatal transmission occurs in up to 5% of female babies born to infected mothers. Usually this is a self-limited infection in perinates (Krieger et al. 1999). Gynecologic sequelae specific to *T. vaginalis* infection are minimal—this organism is not viewed as a causative agent for pelvic inflammatory disease (PID) (Westrom et al. 1999). However, trichomoniasis may result in increased HIV transmission (Petrin et al. 1998).

DATABASE

SUBJECTIVE

→ See **Table 12SF.1, Vaginal Infections.**

→ Predisposing/risk factors include:
- Multiple sexual partners
- History of trichomoniasis or other STD
- Infected sexual partners
- Concomitant STD/bacterial vaginosis (BV)
- Menstrual blood/cervical mucorrhea
- Maternal-fetal transmission during birth (infant infection is usually transitory)
- Low socioeconomic status
- Poor personal hygiene

→ Symptoms may include:
- Vaginal discharge: a cardinal symptom, may be profuse and foul-smelling
- Vulvar pruritus
- Vulvar tenderness, soreness, irritation, erythema
- Dysuria, frequency
- Dyspareunia
- Abnormal vaginal spotting or bleeding
- Male partner with a penile discharge (men are usually asymptomatic; 36–50% of cases resolve within two weeks of exposure [Patel 1998])
- Symptom exacerbation during or following menses
- Symptoms may be most acute during pregnancy.
- The patient may be asymptomatic (25–50% of cases [Petrin et al. 1998]).

→ History should include:
- Gynecological
- STD
- Sexual, including sexual practices, number and gender of partners, recent change of partners, partner signs and symptoms, history of STD in partner
- Contraceptive use
- Medical
- Allergies
- Medications
- Habits
- Description of symptoms
- Aggravating or relieving factors
- Associated symptoms
- Self-treatment measures

OBJECTIVE

→ Vital signs as indicated (usually unnecessary in uncomplicated infection)

→ Abdominal examination, including lymph nodes, as indicated

→ Pelvic examination:
- Vulva:
  - Abnormal discharge
  - Erythema of the vestibule, labia minora
  - Edema, usually of the labia minora
  - Abrasions, excoriations of the interlabial sulci, perineum
  - Intertrigo of the labia majora, crural folds, or inner thighs may be present
  - Chronic irritation may produce lichenification and pigment changes of the skin.
- Urethra, Bartholin's, or Skene's glands:
  - An abnormal discharge may be milked from the meatus or duct openings.
- Vagina:
  - Yellow-gray-green, creamy, purulent, thin, watery, or frothy discharge
  - Foul odor
  - Erythema
  - Granular-appearing or -feeling surface
  - Swollen papillae
  - Ecchymosis, petechiae
  - Pseudomembrane formation—small, thin, gray areas that are spottily distributed or an uninterrupted membrane that cannot be wiped off
- Cervix:
  - Punctuate hemorrhages ("strawberry cervix" in 2–3% of cases), abnormal discharge
- Uterus/adnexa, rectovaginal examination:
  - WNL unless there is concomitant infection/pathology

ASSESSMENT

→ *T. vaginalis* vaginitis
→ R/O concomitant BV, Candidal vaginitis
→ R/O concomitant STD/PID
→ R/O urinary tract infection
→ R/O vaginitis emphysematosa
→ R/O vaginal streptococcal infection

PLAN

DIAGNOSTIC TESTS

→ Wet-mount microscopy (10x and 40x power) is the principal diagnostic method; it is the most accessible and cost-effective. Estimated sensitivity is 50–80% (Okuyama et al. 1998, Patel 1998, Wiese et al. 2000).
- Saline:
  NOTE: The slide should be kept warm and viewed promptly after collection.
  - Motile trichomonads (elongated, slightly larger than WBCs); flagella noted; trichomonads may congregate in a mass and appear quiescent.
  - Increased WBCs (usually >10/high power field)
  - Predominance of mature squamous epithelial cells
  - Reduced number of lactobacilli
  - Clue cells may be present with concomitant BV
- KOH (10–20%):
  - Amine or "fishy" odor (related to anaerobes present)
  - Hyphae of *Candida* may be present

→ pH: ≥6.0. Collect a specimen from the lateral vaginal wall or lateral fornix.

→ Pap smear may reveal trichomonads or inflammatory atypia. The estimated sensitivity and specificity is 35–85% and

78–100%, respectively (Wiese et al. 2000). If Pap is used as the sole criterion, there is an error rate of 48% (Petrin et al. 1998, Wiese et al. 2000). A confirmatory culture or wet mount should be performed before treatment.

→ Cultures:
- The most sensitive and specific diagnostic method—may be performed in selected cases where *T. vaginalis* is suspected but the saline wet mount is negative.
- Diamond's media or InPouch TV® has been recommended (Mead 2001).
- Disadvantages: expense, limited availability in some areas, up to a seven-day waiting period for diagnosis.

→ Immunofluorescence tests and enzyme-linked immunosorbent assays are utilized in research protocols but are expensive and not practical or available in everyday clinical practice.

→ Detection methods by polymerase chain reaction (PCR) are being developed for vaginal, seminal, urethral, and Pap-stained specimens.

→ Microscopic urinalysis may show evidence of *T. vaginalis*.

→ Sensitive testing for *N. gonorrhoeae* and *C. trachomatis* should be performed.

→ Additional laboratory tests should be individualized and may include but are not limited to: RPR or VDRL, CBC, urinalysis, urine culture and sensitivities, hepatitis B antigen and antibody, serological HIV, and pregnancy test.

TREATMENT/MANAGEMENT

→ Recommended regimen (Centers for Disease Control and Prevention [CDC] 2002):
- Metronidazole 2 g p.o. in a single dose.

→ Alternate regimen (CDC 2002):
- Metronidazole 500 mg p.o. BID for 7 days

→ Treatment failures:
- If either of the above regimens fails, re-treat with metronidazole 500 mg p.o. BID for 7 days. In cases of repeated failure, treat with a single dose of metronidazole, 2 g p.o. once a day for 3–5 days (CDC 2002).
- Patients with a culture-proven infection who fail to respond to the above therapies and in whom re-infection has been ruled out should be managed in consultation with an STD expert. Included in the evaluation of these patients should be a determination of the susceptibility of *T. vaginalis* to metronidazole.
  • Consultation is available from the CDC, (770) 488-4115, www.cdc.gov/std/ (CDC 2002). **NOTE:** Significant nausea may develop when doses exceed 2 grams/day. Thus, patient motivation must be strong to continue treatment. An antiemetic may be necessary—refer to the *Physicians' Desk Reference*. Patients allergic to metronidazole can be managed by desensitization (CDC 2002). Adverse effects such as seizures and peripheral neuropathy have been reported in patients treated with metronidazole. Consult with a physician before larger-dose therapy.

→ Partner therapy:
- Sex partners of infected women should be treated with metronidazole.

→ Pregnancy:
- See the recommended regimen above.

→ HIV-infected patients should receive the same treatment regimen as HIV-negative individuals.

CONSULTATION

→ As needed for prescription(s).

→ For a resistant infection when considering larger-dose therapy. Consider consulting with an STD expert for culture-documented treatment failures.

PATIENT EDUCATION

→ Discuss the etiology and transmission of infection, lifestyle behaviors that put the patient at risk, and methods to reduce the risk and spread of infection.
- In rare cases, nonsexual transmission may need to be addressed.
- In addition, asymptomatic carriage may occur for long periods of time; thus, the current partner should not necessarily be implicated. However, treatment of both sexual partners is advisable.

→ Provide guidelines on safer sex practices. (See **Table 12I.1, Recommendations for Individuals to Prevent STD/PID** in the **Pelvic Inflammatory Disease** chapter and **Table 13A.2, Safer Sex Practices** in the **Chancroid** chapter in **Section 13.**) Encourage condom use with new, multiple, or nonmonogamous partners.

→ Discuss vaginal health and hygiene as indicated. (See the **Candidal Vulvovaginitis** chapter.)

→ Stress the importance of completing the full course of prescribed medication.

→ Advise sexual abstinence or at least the use of condoms during the course of treatment for infection.

→ Review the common side effects of metronidazole: a metallic taste, nausea, occasional vomiting, diarrhea, and headache.
- Advise against ingestion of alcohol during and for 24 hours after medication usage, as a disulfiram-like reaction may occur.

→ Advise about the possibility of *Candida* vaginitis secondary to an oral antibiotic and discuss the indications for prophylactic therapy.

→ Allow the patient to vent her feelings of surprise, shame, fear, or anger when discussing this infection as an STD.

FOLLOW-UP

→ Advise the patient to return for further evaluation if the signs and symptoms of infection have not cleared after the week of treatment, and if there are signs of recurrent infection.
- Assess compliance with the medication regime.

→ Follow up on cervical testing and treat any identified concomitant STDs (see the appropriate chapters). Discuss the importance of partner evaluation and treatment if an STD is identified.

→ Refer newly diagnosed, HIV-positive persons to the appropriate provider for early intervention services.

→ Offer hepatitis A vaccine to women at risk for sexual transmission of this virus (e.g., users of illegal injection and noninjection drugs). (See the **Hepatitis—Viral** chapter.)

→ Offer hepatitis B vaccine to all women seeking treatment for an STD who have not been previously vaccinated. (See the **Hepatitis—Viral** chapter for further information.)

→ Newly diagnosed, hepatitis B antigen-positive individuals should undergo liver function tests and receive counseling regarding the implications of their positive status and the need for immunoprophylaxis of sex partners and household members. (See the **Hepatitis—Viral** chapter.)

→ Address additional medical concerns as indicated.

→ Continue to encourage safer sex practices.

→ Document in progress notes and on problem list.

Winifred L. Star, R.N., C., N.P., M.S.
Melanie Deal, R.N., C., N.P., M.S.

12-SF Vaginitis
Vaginal Infections

Table 12SF.1. VAGINAL INFECTIONS

Findings	Candidiasis	Trichomoniasis	Bacterial Vaginosis	Atrophic Vaginitis	Cytolytic Vaginitis
Causative Organism	*Candida albicans* *C. glabrata* *C. tropicalis* *C. lusitaniae* *C. parapsilosis* *C. guillermondii*	*Trichomonas vaginalis*	Polymicrobial	Nonspecific atrophic changes caused by ↓ estrogen	↑ Exfoliation and turnover of squamous epithelium
Characteristics of Discharge	Mild to profuse Thin to thick, white, curd-like discharge; adherent to vagina/cervix	Yellow, gray, green odorous discharge Consistency varies; ± bubbles	White to gray/yellow-green Thin, homogeneous, odorous discharge; adherent to walls and at introitus; ± bubbles	Yellow or blood-tinged Thin, scant, watery discharge	Thick white discharge
Vulvovaginal Findings	May see erythema, excoriation, edema	May see erythema and edema; "strawberry patches" of cervix in 2% of cases	Discharge pooling at introitus; ± erythema	Pale, shiny, thin, nonrugated vaginal walls; ± petechial hemorrhage	WNL
Diagnostic Tests	pH: 4.0–4.7 KOH wet mount: hyphae, spores Saline wet mount: ↑ WBCs Gram stain: budding *Candida* Culture: positive for *Candida* species	pH: >6.0 KOH wet mount: amine odor Saline wet mount: Motile trich, ↑ WBCs, ↓ lactobacilli Culture: + trich Pap smear: + trich	pH: 5.0–6.0 KOH wet mount: amine odor Saline wet mount: Clue cells, ↓ lactobacilli, ± WBCs Gram stain: *G. vaginalis*, *Mobiluncus*, other bacterial morphotypes	pH: 5.5–7.0 KOH wet mount: WNL Saline wet mount: ↑ parabasal cells, ↓ lactobacilli, ↑ WBCs Gram stain: parabasal cells, + bacteria	pH: 4.0–4.5 KOH wet mount: WNL Saline wet mount: ↑ epithelial cells, ↑ lactobacilli, "false clue cells," ± WBCs Gram stain: lactobacilli, gram + rods
Treatment Regimens	Antifungal therapy, boric acid	Metronidazole	Metronidazole, clindamycin	Estrogen therapy	Baking-soda douche or sitz baths; avoid overtreating normal leukorrhea

©2003 W. Star

Winifred L. Star, R.N., C., N.P., M.S.
Melanie Deal, R.N., C., N.P., M.S.

12-SG Vaginitis
Bibliography

Al-Harthi, L., Roebuck, K.A., Olinger, G.G. et al. 1999. Bacterial vaginosis-associated microflora isolated from the female genital tract activates HIV-1 expression. *Journal of Acquired Immune Deficiency Syndrome* 21:194–202.

Bachmann, G.A., and Nevadunsky, N.S. 2000. Diagnosis and treatment of atrophic vaginitis. *American Family Physician* 61(10):3090–3096.

Barbes, B., and Boris, S. 1999. Potential role of lactobacilli as prophylactic agents against genital pathogens. *AIDS Patient Care and STDs* 13(12):747–751.

Calzolari, E., Masciangelo, R., Milite, V. et al. 2000. Bacterial vaginosis and contraceptive methods. *International Journal of Gynecology and Obstetrics* 70:341–346.

Centers for Disease Control and Prevention (CDC). 2002. Sexually transmitted disease treatment guidelines 2002. *Morbidity and Mortality Weekly Report* 51(RR–6):42–48.

Chambliss, M.L. 2000. Bacterial vaginosis and treatment of sexual partners. *Archives of Family Medicine* 9:647–648.

Clinical Effectiveness Group 1999. National guideline for the management of *Trichomonas vaginalis*. *Sexually Transmitted Infections* 75(Suppl. 1):S21–S23.

Coco, A.S., and Vandenbosche, M. 2000. Infectious vaginitis: An accurate diagnosis is essential and attainable. *Postgraduate Medicine* 107(4):63–74.

Colli, E., Landoni, M., Parazzini, F. et al. 1997. Treatment of male partners and recurrence of bacterial vaginosis: a randomized trial. *Genitourinary Medicine* 73:267–270.

Droegemueller, W. 2001. Infections of the lower genital tract. In *Comprehensive gynecology*, 4th ed., eds. M.A. Stenchever, W. Droegemueller, A.L. Herbst et al., pp. 641–705. St. Louis, Mo.: Mosby.

duBochet, L., McGregor, J.A., Ismail, M. et al. 1998. A pilot study of metronidazole vaginal gel versus oral metronidazole for the treatment of *Trichomonas vaginalis* vaginitis. *Sexually Transmitted Diseases* 25(3):176–179.

Dun, E. 1999. Antifungal resistance in yeast vaginitis. *Yale Journal of Biology and Medicine* 72:281–285.

Eckert, L.O., Hawes, S.E., Stevens, C.E. et al. 1998. Vulvovaginal candidiasis: clinical manifestations, risk factors, management algorithm. *Obstetrics and Gynecology* 92:757–765.

Eschenbach, D.A., and Mead, P.B. 1992. Vaginitis update. *Contemporary OB/GYN* 37(12):54–70.

Eschenbach, D.A., Thwin, S.S., Patton, D.L. et al. 2000. Influence of the normal menstrual cycle on vaginal tissue, discharge, and microflora. *Clinical Infectious Diseases* 30: 901–907.

Fethers, K., Marks, C., Mindel, A. et al. 2000. Sexually transmitted infections and risk behaviours in women who have sex with women. *Sexually Transmitted Infections* 76:345–349.

Fidel, P.L., and Sobel, J.D. 1996. Immunopathogenesis of recurrent vulvovaginal candidiasis. *Clinical Microbiology Reviews* 9(3):335–348.

Freeman, C.D., Klutman, N.E., and Lamp, K.C. 1997. Metronidazole: a therapeutic review and update. *Drugs* 54(4):679–708.

Hay, P.E. 1998. Recurrent bacterial vaginosis. *Dermatology Clinics* 16(4):769–773.

Hillier, S., and Holmes, K.K. 1999. Bacterial vaginosis. In *Sexually transmitted diseases*, 3rd ed., eds. K.K. Holmes, P.F. Sparling, P.-A. Mårdh et al., pp. 563–586. New York: McGraw-Hill.

Hutti, M.H., and Hoffman, C. 2000. Cytolytic vaginosis: an overlooked cause of cyclic vaginal itching and burning. *Journal of the American Academy of Nurse Practitioners* 12(2):55–57.

Kaufman, R.H., and Faro, S. 1994. *Benign diseases of the vulva and vagina*, 4th ed. St. Louis, Mo.: Mosby-Year Book.

Krieger, J.N., and Alderete, J.F. 1999. *Trichomonas vaginalis* and trichomoniasis. In *Sexually transmitted diseases*, 3rd ed., eds. K.K. Holmes, P.F. Sparling, P. Mårdh et al., pp. 587–604. New York: McGraw-Hill.

Langdon, S. November 1994. *Vaginitis*. Outline presented at the STD intensive for clinicians. San Francisco STD/HIV Prevention Training Center, San Francisco.

Lewis D.A., Habgood, L., White, R. et al. 1997. Managing vaginal trichomoniasis resistant to high-dose metronidazole therapy. *International Journal of STD & AIDS* 8:780–784.

McCaffrey, M., Varney, P., Evans, B. et al. 1999. Bacterial vaginosis in lesbians: evidence for lack of sexual transmission. *International Journal of STD & AIDS* 10:305–308.

Mead, M. (moderator). 2001. What's new in vaginitis diagnosis and treatment. *Contemporary OB/GYN* 46(11):14–42.

Mead, P.B. 1989. Reconsidering bacterial vaginosis. *Contemporary OB/GYN* 34(6):76–89.

Morris, M.C., Rogers, P.A., and Kinghorn, G.R. 2001. Is bacterial vaginosis a sexually transmitted infection? *Sexually Transmitted Infections* 77:63–68.

Nyirjesy, P. 1999. Vaginitis in the adolescent patient. *Pediatric Clinics of North America* 46(4):733–745.

Okuyama, T., Takahashi, R., Mori, M. et al. 1998. Polymerase chain reaction amplification of *Trichomonas vaginalis* DNA from Papanicolaou-stained smears. *Diagnostic Cytopathology* 19(6):437–440.

Oleszczuk, J.J., and Keith, L.G. 2000. Vaginal infection: prophylaxis and perinatal outcome—a review of the literature. *International Journal of Fertility* 45(6):358–367.

Palacin, C., Tarrago, C., and Ortiz, J.A. 2000. Sertaconazole: pharmacology of a gynecological antifungal agent. *International Journal of Gynecology and Obstetrics* 71:S37–S46.

Pandit, L., and Ouslander, J.G. 1997. Postmenopausal vaginal atrophy and atrophic vaginitis. *American Journal of Medical Science* 314(4):228–231.

Patel, K. 1998. Sexually transmitted diseases in adolescents: focus on gonorrhea, chlamydia, and trichomoniasis—issues and treatment guidelines. *Journal of Pediatric Health Care* 12(4):211–217.

Petrin, D., Delgaty, K., Bhatt, R. et al. 1998. Clinical and microbiological aspects of *Trichomonas vaginalis*. *Clinical Microbiology Reviews* 11(2):300–317.

Physician's desk reference. 2002. 56th ed. Montvale, N.J.: Medical Economics.

Priestley, C.J., Jones, B.M., Dhar, J. et al. 1997. What is normal vaginal flora? *Genitourinary Medicine* 73:23–28.

Pybus, V., and Onderdonk, A.B. 1999. Microbial interactions in the vaginal ecosystem, with emphasis on the pathogenesis of bacterial vaginosis. *Microbes and Infection* 1:285–292.

Rajamanoharan, S., Low, N., Jones, S.B. et al. 1999. Bacterial vaginosis, ethnicity, and the use of genital cleaning agents: a case control study. *Sexually Transmitted Diseases* 26(7): 404–409.

Rauh, V.A., Culhane, J.F., and Hogan, V.K. 2000. Bacterial vaginosis: a public health problem for women. *Journal of the American Medical Women's Association* 55(4):220–224.

Rinaldi, M.G. 1988. The microbiology of terconazole: results of in vitro studies. In *Clinical perspectives: terconazole, an advance in vulvovaginal candidiasis therapy,* ed. J.D. Sobel. New York: BMI/McGraw-Hill.

Schmid, G.P. 1999. The epidemiology of bacterial vaginosis. *International Journal of Gynecology and Obstetrics* 67: S17–S20.

Schuman, P., Sobel, J.D., Ohmit, S.E. et al. 1998. Mucosal candidal colonization and candidiasis in women with or at risk for human immunodeficiency virus infection. *Clinical Infectious Diseases* 27:1161–1167.

Schwebke, J.R. 1999. Diagnostic methods for bacterial vaginosis. *International Journal of Gynecology and Obstetrics* 67:S21–S23.

Shalev, E., Battino, S., Weiner, E. et al. 1996. Ingestion of yogurt containing *Lactobacillus acidophilus* compared with pasteurized yogurt as prophylaxis for recurrent candidal vaginitis and bacterial vaginosis. *Archives of Family Medicine* 5:593–596.

Sobel, J.D. 1999. Vulvovaginal candidiasis. In *Sexually transmitted diseases,* 3rd ed., eds. K.K. Holmes, P.F. Sparling, P.-A. Mårdh et al., pp. 629–639. New York: McGraw-Hill.

Sobel, J.D., Nagappan, V., and Nyirjesy, P. 1999. Metronidazole-resistant vaginal trichomoniasis—an emerging problem. *New England Journal of Medicine* 341(4):292–293.

Sonnex, C., and Lefort, W. 1999. Microscopic features of vaginal candidiasis and their relation to symptomatology. *Sexually Transmitted Infections* 75:417–419.

Soper, D.E. 1999. Gynecologic sequelae of bacterial vaginosis. *International Journal of Gynecology and Obstetrics* 67: S25–S28.

Sparks, J.M. 1991. Vaginitis. *Journal of Reproductive Medicine* 36(10):745–752.

Spinillo, A., Capuzzo, E., Gulminetti, R. et al. 1997. Prevalence of and risk factors for fungal vaginitis caused by non-albicans species. *American Journal of Obstetrics and Gynecology* 176:138–141.

Summers, P.R., and Sharp, H.T. 1993. The management of obscure or difficult cases of vulvovaginitis. *Clinical Obstetrics and Gynecology* 36(1):206–214.

Viikki M., Pukkala, E., Nieminen, P. et al. 2000. Gynecological infections as risk determinants of subsequent cervical neoplasia. *Acta Oncologica* 39(1):71–75.

Wallis, L.A., and Barbo, D.M. 1998. Hormone replacement therapy (HRT). In *Textbook of women's health,* ed. L.A. Wallis, pp. 731–746. Philadelphia: Lippincott-Raven.

Westrom, L., and Eschenbach, D. 1999. Pelvic inflammatory disease. In *Sexually transmitted diseases,* 3rd ed., eds. K.K. Holmes, P.F. Sparling, P.-A. Mårdh et al., pp. 783–809. New York: McGraw-Hill.

Wiese, W., Patel, S.R., Patel, S.C. et al. 2000. A meta-analysis of the Papanicolaou smear and wet mount for the diagnosis of vaginal trichomoniasis. *American Journal of Medicine* 108:301–308.

Wong, B.C. 2002. Atrophic vaginitis. *Menopausal Medicine* 10(2):9–12.

Zambrano, D. 1991. Clindamycin in the treatment of obstetric and gynecologic infections: a review. *Clinical Therapeutics* 13(1):50–58.

Winifred L. Star, R.N., C., N.P., M.S.
Claire L. Appelmans, R.N., C., W.H.C.N.P., M.S.

12-TA Vulvar Disease
Red Lesions of the Vulva

The normal flesh color of the skin of the vulva is due in large part to superficial capillary blood flow muted by the epidermal skin cell layers. When skin becomes erythematous, the capillaries are more visible; the degree of redness depends on dilatation and engorgement of the capillary bed and thickness of the overlying epidermis. Local immune inflammatory responses cause vasodilatation, with diffuse erythema usually signaling a benign process.

With carcinomatous lesions, a tumor angiogenesis factor (development of blood vessels) promotes an increase in the number of surface capillaries. This "neovascularization" occurs in all overt squamous cell carcinomas. Thus, localized *red lesions of the vulva* are more suspicious for a neoplastic process. In other cases, redness may be due to fewer cell layers between the surface skin and underlying vasculature, as occurs in *Paget's disease* and *acute reactive vulvitis*.

In summary, red lesions of the vulva result from inflammation, neovascularization of a neoplasm, or thinning of the epidermal surface (Friedrich 1983). This chapter will cover *cutaneous candidiasis*, *contact dermatitis* (*reactive vulvitis*), and *Paget's disease*. (See the **Folliculitis**, **Psoriasis**, and **Fungal Infections** chapters in Section 3, **Dermatological Disorders**.)

Cutaneous Candidiasis

Yeast, or *Candida*, vaginal infections may produce symptoms on the vulvar tissues as a result of local reactions to allergenic/endotoxic substances from vaginal organisms (Kaufman et al. 1994). However, a primary *cutaneous candidiasis* may arise de novo, affecting the keratinized, superficial, epidermal layers of the vulva. *Candida albicans* is the most commonly encountered species, but infection with other *Candida* species or dermatophytes (e.g., those that cause tinea infections) may occur. Common reasons for overgrowth of the organism—normally found in the gut, mouth, and vagina—include vaginal pH changes and antibiotics that deplete the normal lactobacilli of the gastrointestinal (GI) tract, allowing resident yeast to flourish. However, any change in a woman's health status may put her at risk for infection. Pregnancy, broad spectrum antibiotic use, impaired cell-mediated immunity, oral contraceptives with high estrogen

potency, loss of skin integrity such as that associated with chronic incontinence, and diabetes are some predisposing factors (Ridley et al. 1999). Vulvar *Candida* manifestations are especially prevalent in diabetics and may be a presenting symptom of the disease. It has been suggested that dietary factors—e.g., refined carbohydrates supplying simple sugars such as sucrose or lactose, alcohol, and yeast-containing foods—also may play a role (Friedrich 1983, Gomel et al. 1990).

DATABASE

SUBJECTIVE

→ *Candida* vaginitis may co-exist.
→ Symptoms include:
- Intense pruritus
- Burning
- Bleeding of vulvar skin secondary to scratching/excoriation
- Swelling
- Superficial dysuria
- Superficial or frictional dyspareunia
→ History to include:
- Complete gynecological, contraceptive, sexual history
- Vaginitis or sexually transmitted disease (STD) history
- Recent use of antibiotics or other regular medications
- Feminine hygiene products and douching history
- Chronic use of sanitary pads/pantyliners
- Clothing history (e.g., type of panties, tight pants)
- Type of soap, detergent, toilet paper used
- Partner symptomatology
- General medical history and state of health
- Pregnancy
- Stress
- Family history of diabetes

OBJECTIVE

→ Areas most commonly affected are the posterior fourchette and perineum due to likely vaginal co-infection, but may include:

- Labia majora
- Genitocrural folds
- Lower abdominal folds (pannus)
- Inner aspects of thighs
- Mons pubis
→ External genitalia may exhibit:
  - Erythema with indistinct margins or satellite lesions that may be pustular, papulosquamous, or crusting
  - Edema, excoriation, or maceration
  - Fine, gray sheen overlying erythema
  - Fissuring of interlabial sulci or posterior fourchette
  - Intertriginous areas thick and white
→ The vagina may exhibit:
  - A normal or abnormal discharge
  - Vaginal walls within normal limits (WNL) or erythematous
→ Cervix:
  - May be WNL or an adherent white, thick discharge or erythema may be present.
→ Uterus, adnexa, rectovaginal examination WNL unless there is co-existent pathology.

ASSESSMENT

→ Cutaneous candidiasis of the vulva
→ R/O *tinea cruris*
→ R/O concomitant vaginal candidiasis
→ R/O reactive vulvitis
→ R/O Paget's disease
→ R/O other dermatoses (e.g., squamous hyperplasia [lichen simplex chronicus], psoriasis, lichen planus, seborrheic dermatitis, eczemoid dermatitis [Kaufman et al. 1994])
→ R/O diabetes
→ R/O concomitant STD

PLAN

DIAGNOSTIC TESTS

→ Potassium hydroxide (KOH) prep using 10–20% KOH added to scrapings from affected skin surface
  NOTE: Use a scalpel or spatula to obtain scrapings from the affected area of vulvar skin, spread on a clean glass slide, add 1–2 drops of KOH, and cover with coverslip. Heat gently or allow to "fix" at room temperature for 20–30 minutes before examining under a microscope (Hall 2000). The presence of both spores and hyphae indicate candidal infection; hyphae alone suggest dermatophyte infection.
→ KOH and saline wet preps of vaginal discharge to rule out concomitant vaginitis
  NOTE: Use a moist saline cotton swab to obtain a specimen from the vaginal walls. Spread on clean microscope slides. Add a drop of normal saline for saline prep, cover, and evaluate under a microscope. For KOH prep, add a drop of KOH to a separate slide specimen and cover; this will lyse epithelial cells and provide easier visibility of *Candida* spores/hyphae.
→ For further confirmation, obtain cultures for *Candida*. (See the **Candidal Vulvovaginitis** chapter.)

→ FBS to rule out diabetes may be indicated with recurrent or chronic infection.
→ Laboratory tests as indicated to rule out concomitant STD

TREATMENT/MANAGEMENT

→ Vaginal antifungal agents should be used concurrently when treating cutaneous vulvar candidiasis.
→ Antifungal creams such as azoles are the mainstays of treatment for *Candida*. In severe cases, combined therapy with corticosteroids may be considered for relief of inflammation/pruritus. Some examples include:
  - Miconazole nitrate 2%: Apply to the affected area BID for 14 days. Use sparingly in intertriginous areas.
  - Nystatin and triamcinolone acetonide: Apply sparingly to the affected area BID. Discontinue if symptoms persist after 25 days.
    NOTE: Fluorinated topical steroids such as triamcinolone acetonide should be used cautiously due to the potential for adverse side effects. The immunosuppressive effects of high-potency steroids may cause flares or prolongation of fungal infections. Long-term use of topical steroids may lead to atrophy, striae, telangiectasia, or steroid rebound dermatitis (Black et al. 2002).
  - Hydrocortisone cream 1–2.5%: Apply sparingly to the affected area TID–QID (this product does not contain an antifungal—only an anti-inflammatory/antipruritic agent).
→ Oral antifungal medications for *Candida* may be considered for severe cases of vulvovaginal candidiasis. Limited data exist on their use for treating cutaneous candidiasis (Black et al. 2002).
  - Fluconazole: 150 mg tablet p.o. in a single dose. The potential for serious hepatotoxicity and development of antimicrobial resistance should be considered in selecting this therapy. In refractory cases, longer oral therapy may be helpful; the daily dose should be based on the severity of infection and the patient's response to therapy (*Physicians' Desk Reference [PDR]* 2002).
  - Itraconazole: 100 mg tablet p.o. daily for 7 days or 200 mg tablet p.o. QD for 1–7 days.
    NOTE: Oral griseofulvin is not recommended; it may intensify candidal infection (Hall 2000).
→ Alternative therapy may consist of:
  - Intravaginal boric acid: Insert 600 mg in a 0 gel capsule, per vagina at HS, twice weekly for 1 week.
  - Gentian violet 1% aqueous solution: Paint on vulvovaginal area once a week for 2–3 weeks.
    NOTE: Gentian violet stains garments. Do not use in the presence of severe vulvar excoriation/ulceration. The potential for reactive vulvitis or allergic reaction is substantial.
→ For soothing of the vulva, especially with weeping lesions, Burow's solution may be tried: Wet dressings or sitz baths, 15–30 minutes TID as necessary (Hall 2000). (See **Table 12TA.1, Tips for Treating Skin Lesions**.)
→ For severe pruritus, H_1-receptor antagonist oral antihistamines may be considered (caution the patient about possible drowsiness as a side effect):

- Diphenhydramine hydrochloride: 25 mg or 50 mg caplet p.o. TID
- Hydroxyzine hydrochloride: 25 mg p.o. may be prescribed at HS.
- Cetirizine hydrochloride: 5 mg or 10 mg p.o. daily as a single dose, usually at HS

CONSULTATION

→ As indicated for assessment of lesion or therapeutic failure.
→ As needed for prescription(s).
→ Refer the patient to the appropriate health care provider as indicated if diabetes is diagnosed.

PATIENT EDUCATION

→ Discuss the etiology and nature of the infection.
→ Advise the patient that, although relief of symptoms may occur in 2–3 days, topical antifungals should be used for 2 weeks to reduce the possibility of recurrence (*PDR* 2002).
→ Review and discuss vulvovaginal health and hygiene:
  - Use of all-cotton underwear and loose clothing
  - Avoidance of unnecessary pantyliner use
  - Proper wiping technique
  - White unscented toilet paper
  - Avoidance of strong bath or laundry soap
  - Thorough rinsing of underclothes after washing; line drying
  - Avoidance of feminine hygiene deodorant products and excessive douching

- Ideally, wash the vulvar area with water only. May use Aveeno®, Dove®, Basis®, or hypoallergenic soap. Pat dry or use a hair dryer on a low setting. (See the **Candidal Vulvovaginitis** chapter.)
→ Encourage good health maintenance: a well-balanced diet without excessive simple sugars, refined carbohydrates, dairy and yeast products, or alcohol; adequate rest and exercise; and stress reduction.
→ Advise regarding the desirability of sexual abstinence during the course of treatment.
→ Caution regarding the concurrent use of vaginal therapeutics and condoms—mineral oil in creams may weaken latex, leading to condom breakage.

FOLLOW-UP

→ The patient should return as necessary if symptoms do not improve with treatment.
→ Address additional medical concerns as indicated.
→ Refer sexual partner(s) to a health care provider for evaluation and treatment as indicated for recurrent infection.
→ Document in progress notes and on problem list.

Contact Dermatitis (Reactive Vulvitis)

Reactive changes in the skin of the vulva can be due to a wide variety of physical and chemical stimuli. Most cases are secondary to either a nonimmunological local irritant or represent a cell-mediated allergic response to a circulating antigenic substance.

Table 12TA.1.   TIPS FOR TREATING SKIN LESIONS

1. Start with *mild* agents, increase potency as acuteness subsides. DO NOT begin with the most potent variety of topical corticosteroid.
2. Most products should be massaged in gently for 5–10 seconds.
3. For many conditions, instruct the patient to continue treating the skin for 4–10 days after the dermatosis has cleared.
4. Ointment bases should be used more often than cream bases. The greasiness allows the medicine to penetrate the skin better and may alleviate dryness and remove scales.
5. Cream bases are indicated when treating intertriginous and hairy areas.
6. Long-term use of fluorinated steroids should be avoided because of the potential for skin atrophy, striae, and telangiectasia, especially on intertriginous areas, the face, and the anal area. Some commonly prescribed fluorinated topical steroids are betamethasone, fluocinonide, fluocinolone, and triamcinolone.
7. Agents containing neomycin (e.g., Mycolog®) may precipitate allergy. Mycolog II® does not contain neomycin.
8. Strong topical steroids should not be prescribed for use on widespread areas. The potent steroids have a definite systemic effect.
9. Long-term use of local steroids may result in diminished effectiveness (tachyphylaxis).
10. Wet dressings or sitz baths (warm, hot, or cold) may be used to treat any pruritic, oozing, or crusting dermatosis. Burow's solution (aluminum sulfate, calcium acetate, and boric acid) is often the prescribed agent. Wet dressings should be applied with a clean soaked gauze, with additional solution added via bulb syringe so the gauze does not dry out. The dressing should be left in place for 15–20 minutes and may be applied TID. The solution should be made fresh every time. Sitz baths may be substituted for wet dressings; the same general principles apply regarding timing and frequency.
11. Become familiar with all agents prescribed: their indications, use, and possible side effects. Refer to the *PDR*.
12. Generic products are relatively less expensive. Use of a brand name, however, ensures the correct potency and bioavailability of the agent, the delivery system, and ingredients in the base.

Source: Adapted with permission from Hall, J.C. 2000. *Sauer's manual of skin diseases*, 8th ed. Philadelphia: Lippincott Williams and Wilkins.

The clinical presentation of primary irritant versus allergic reaction is often indistinguishable and may mimic other dermatoses; thus, pinpointing the specific etiology is difficult and good history-taking is important. In most vulvovaginal reactions, the offending agent is a primary irritant. Perspiration, friction, heat, and pressure are all factors that aggravate the reaction.

Many factors and substances can cause *reactive vulvitis*, including scratching, rubbing, bicycle or horseback riding, coitus, saliva, seminal fluid, vaginal discharge, sanitary pads/pantyliners, latex condoms, lubricants, spermicides, synthetic fabrics, fabric dyes, detergents, soap, perfumed oils, feminine hygiene deodorant products, bath oils and additives, over-the-counter remedies, bromine compounds in hot tubs and swimming pools, and oleoresin, as in poison oak or ivy.

Sensitization may also occur with repeated use of many topical medications, particularly antibiotics, caustic agents, and cytotoxic agents such as fluorouracil. Plant contact produces classic allergic contact dermatitis (Black et al. 2002, Hall 2000).

DATABASE

SUBJECTIVE

→ A good history is indispensable to diagnosis. Ask about exposure to all of the aforementioned potential irritants as well as systemic medication being taken.
→ Symptoms include:
  ■ Pruritus
  ■ Burning
  ■ Tenderness, pain
  ■ Irritation
  ■ Superficial/external dysuria, with urinary retention in severe cases

OBJECTIVE

→ Intertriginous areas—e.g., interlabial, genitocrural folds, and the groin—are most susceptible to reactions.
→ Diffuse or localized vulvar erythema may occur and may be symmetrical.
→ Edema, exudate, weeping of the area may occur.
→ Excoriation or ulceration may occur.
→ Papulovesicular lesions or bullae may develop.
→ Scaling, thickening, white plaques or lichenification may occur (features of chronic contact dermatitis) as a result of rubbing/scratching.
→ In allergic reactions, redness and wheals at the point of contact are the initial signs; in 24–48 hours, vesicles and bullae form.
→ Vagina, cervix, uterus, adnexa, and rectovaginal examination will be WNL unless there is co-existent pathology.
  NOTE: Lesion distribution may give a clue to the etiology; the pattern/morphology of lesions may reflect the type of irritant. For example:
  ■ Localized introital erythema can be due to coital trauma, vaginal discharge, hygiene products (e.g., deodorant suppositories, douches), or lubricants.

■ Diffuse reaction can be due to fabric irritants, dyes, soap, detergent, perfumed oils, or "saddle burn" (Friedrich 1983).
■ Linear streaks can be due to poison ivy/oak.
■ An elongated oval can be due to pantyliners.

ASSESSMENT

→ Reactive vulvitis (contact dermatitis)
→ R/O *Candida* vulvitis or vulvovaginitis
→ R/O tinea cruris
→ R/O other dermatoses (e.g., squamous cell hyperplasia [lichen simplex], seborrheic dermatitis, psoriasis, lichen planus, bullous diseases)
→ R/O STD (e.g., human papillomavirus or herpes simplex virus)

PLAN

DIAGNOSTIC TESTS

→ Pap smear, STD testing, KOH prep, or wet mounts as indicated to rule out fungal vulvitis or vaginitis.
→ Fungal cultures may be indicated if the diagnosis is uncertain or *Candida glabrata* fungal vaginal infection is suspected.

TREATMENT/MANAGEMENT

→ Elimination and avoidance of the identified precipitating irritant is crucial.
→ Symptomatic measures for relief and treatment of inflammation include:
  ■ Cool baths or wet dressings with Burow's solution 15–30 minutes BID–QID. Works well for an acute oozing, crusting lesion.
  ■ A low-potency topical corticosteroid (e.g., hydrocortisone ointment or cream) 1–2.5%. Apply a small amount to the affected areas BID–TID until the skin is restored to normal. (See **Table 12TA.1, Tips for Treating Skin Lesions.**) **NOTE:** An ointment base is most useful for penetrating the steroid and removing dryness and scales. A cream base is indicated if the lesion affects a hairy or intertriginous area; however, it may be too drying. Occlusive dressings should not be applied to the vulva (Hall 2000).
→ Topical anesthetics should be avoided.
→ For severe pruritus, H_1-receptor antagonist oral antihistamines may be considered (caution the patient about possible drowsiness as a side effect):
  ■ Diphenhydramine hydrochloride: 25 mg or 50 mg caplet p.o. TID
  ■ Hydroxyzine hydrochloride: 25 mg p.o. may be prescribed at HS
  ■ Cetirizine hydrochloride: 5 mg or 10 mg p.o. daily as a single dose, usually at HS
→ Systemic corticosteroids are indicated for severe allergic reactions and are used in tapering doses for about 3 weeks. Consult with a physician.
→ Alternative therapy may include:
  ■ Compresses of warmed or chilled tea bags applied to the vulva or held in place by a sanitary pad.

- Compresses of Aveeno Bath® mixed with water, chilled, and applied as paste.

CONSULTATION

→ As indicated for assessment of the condition or when systemic corticosteroids are indicated.
→ As needed for prescription(s).

PATIENT EDUCATION

→ Emphasize elimination of predisposing substances.
→ Advise the patient to keep her hands off of the affected area except to apply wet dressings and topical steroid. The itch-scratch cycle is detrimental to resolution of dermatitis. Suggest wearing white cotton gloves at bedtime.
→ Be sure the patient understands how to apply wet dressings and topical steroid medication.
→ Advise the patient that contact dermatitis usually resolves within a few days with sitz baths and emollients, and that allergic reactions may take weeks to resolve.
→ Suggest that the patient use a hair dryer on a low setting after baths and wet dressings to dry the vulvar area thoroughly.
→ Advise the patient to limit or avoid certain foods that stimulate pruritus: chocolate, nuts, cheese, coffee, and spicy foods (Hall 2000).

FOLLOW-UP

→ Return visit in 1–4 weeks or as needed for reassessment.
→ Document in progress notes and on problem list.

Paget's Disease

Paget's disease of the vulva is a slowly progressive, intraepithelial neoplasia that is histologically identical to Paget's disease of the breast. The disease affects areas of the body that contain numerous apocrine glands and represents an unusual differentiation of the primitive stem cell of the epidermis. There appear to be two varieties of Paget's disease: intraepithelial extramammary Paget's and pagetoid changes within the skin associated with an underlying adenocarcinoma of the apocrine gland, found in fewer than 20% of cases. Intraepithelial Paget's disease tends to recur locally, without a propensity for invasion.

Paget's disease with underlying apocrine carcinoma can be aggressive, with regional lymph-node metastases. An underlying carcinoma of the breast or GI tract may exist concomitantly. Primary carcinoma of the rectum, urethra, or bladder may also be present, especially when Paget's affects the perineum. The prognosis for Paget's disease is good if it occurs without underlying adenocarcinoma or lymph node metastasis (DiSaia et al. 2002, Morrow et al. 1998, Ridley et al. 1999).

DATABASE

SUBJECTIVE

→ Caucasian women are most commonly affected.
→ Median age at onset is 65 years.
→ The patient may be asymptomatic, but often pruritus and/or soreness of the vulva is present for years before the diagnosis.

→ Symptoms generally include:
  - Itching
  - Soreness or tenderness

OBJECTIVE

→ Clinical features may include:
  - Lesion(s), variable in size, with eczematoid appearance
  - Well-demarcated lesion(s) with irregular, well-defined borders
  - Localization to one labium or entire vulva
  - Red and white areas representing ulceration and hyperkeratosis
  - Erythema with superficial white coating ("cake-icing effect," almost pathognomonic)
  - Velvety red or bright-pink, scaly lesions of variable size; alternately grayish-white, speckled lesions
  - Moist, oozing excoriations or friable ulcers
  - An induration or mass underlying epithelium
  - Extension to the perineum, perianal area, thigh, or vagina
→ Because the disease process is multifocal, not all lesions may be clinically evident. A high recurrence rate may be associated with inadequate excision of contiguous disease (Morrow et al. 1998) or to "silent" areas of involvement at other sites (Friedrich 1983).
→ Perform a breast and rectal examination to rule out other primary lesion(s).
→ The vagina, cervix, uterus, adnexa, and rectum are WNL unless there is co-existent pathology.
→ A good description and diagram of the lesion is helpful.

ASSESSMENT

→ Paget's disease
→ R/O squamous cell carcinoma in situ (vulvar intraepithelial neoplasia [VIN] III)
→ R/O malignant melanoma
→ R/O dermatoses (e.g., squamous cell hyperplasia [lichen simplex chronicus], psoriasis, lichen planus)
→ R/O *Candida* infection
→ R/O acute or chronic reactive vulvitis
→ R/O co-existent carcinoma(s)

PLAN

DIAGNOSTIC TESTS

→ A delay in diagnosis may occur if a lesion is mistaken for dermatitis.
→ Biopsy of the lesion for histopathology is the definitive method of assessment. An adequate margin of normal-appearing tissue must be obtained (DiSaia et al. 2000, Morrow et al. 1998, Ridley et al. 1999).
→ Fine-needle aspiration (FNA) to evaluate subcutaneous masses for adenocarcinoma
→ Certain histochemical staining techniques and monoclonal antibody tests can distinguish Paget's disease from VIN III and malignant melanoma.

→ A work-up to exclude extensive disease may include:
- Barium enema
- Computerized tomographic scan
- Clinical breast examination
- Mammography
- Proctosigmoidoscopy
- Colposcopy of the vulva, vagina, and cervix

→ Pap smear, STD testing, wet mounts, and other diagnostic tests as indicated

TREATMENT/MANAGEMENT

→ Primary therapy includes (DiSaia et al. 2002, Morrow et al. 1998, Ridley et al. 1999):
- Wide local excision of the lesion
- For larger areas, superficial "skinning" vulvectomy with wide margins to a depth inclusive of all adnexal structures

→ Secondarily, more extensive vulvectomy and inguinal lymphadenectomy are performed if invasive carcinoma is identified.

→ Wide local excision, laser therapy, 5-FU, and bleomycin have been used for recurrent disease.

CONSULTATION

→ As necessary for initial evaluation of the lesion.

→ Refer to a physician for biopsy procedure and FNA per site-specific policy.

→ Due to the nature of the disease, the patient should be referred to a gynecologist or gynecological oncologist for management.

PATIENT EDUCATION

→ Explain the etiology of the disease, treatment, and potential sequelae. The physician responsible for care of the patient will detail the particulars.

→ Paget's disease may require disfiguring surgery resulting in alterations in self-image or sexual function. Provide counseling before surgery.

→ Patients need social and psychological support through phases of treatment for this disease. Refer to appropriate support services.

FOLLOW-UP

→ As recurrence is common, patients will require visits every six months indefinitely. Examination includes careful visual inspection, mammography, colorectal evaluation, Pap smear, and colposcopic evaluation.

→ Patients should be instructed to report promptly any recurrent itching, pain, or soreness of the vulva.

→ Biopsies of all suspicious lesions should be undertaken promptly.

→ For recurrent disease, repeated local excisions may be necessary.

→ Document in progress notes and problem on list.

BIBLIOGRAPHY

Black, M.M., McKay, M., Braude, P.R. et al. 2002. *Obstetric and gynecologic dermatology*, 2nd ed. London: Mosby International.

Del Rosso, J.Q., Zellis, S., and Gupta, A.K. 1998. Itraconazole in the treatment of superficial cutaneous and mucosal *Candida* infections. *Journal of the American Osteopathic Association* 98(9):497–501.

DiSaia, P.J., and Creasman, W.T. 2002. *Clinical gynecologic oncology*, 6th ed. St. Louis, Mo.: Mosby.

Drake, L.A., Dorner, W., Goltz, R.W. et al. 1995. Guidelines of care for contact dermatitis. *Journal of the American Academy of Dermatology* 32:109–113.

Fischer, G., Spurrett, B., and Fischer, A. 1995. The chronically symptomatic vulva: aetiology and management. *British Journal of Obstetrics and Gynaecology* 102:773–779.

Friedrich, E.G., Jr. 1983. *Vulvar disease*, 2nd ed. Philadelphia: W.B. Saunders.

Gomel, V., Munro, M.G., and Rowe, T.C. 1990. *Gynecology: a practical approach*. Baltimore, Md.: Williams & Wilkins.

Hall, J.C. 2000. *Sauer's manual of skin diseases*, 8th ed. Philadelphia: Lippincott Williams & Wilkins.

Kaufman, R.H., and Faro, S. 1994. *Benign diseases of the vulva and vagina*, 4th ed. St. Louis, Mo.: Mosby Year Book.

Kovacs, S.O., and Hruza, L.L. 1995. Superficial fungal infections: getting rid of lesions that won't go away. *Postgraduate Medicine* 98(6):61–75.

Lever, W.F. 1990. *Histopathology of the skin*, 7th ed. Philadelphia: J.B. Lippincott.

Marren, P., and Wojnarowska, F. 1996. Dermatitis of the vulva. *Seminars in Dermatology* 15(1):36–41.

Misas, J.E., Cold, C.J., and Hall, F.W. 1991. Vulvar Paget's disease: fluorescein-aided visualization of margins. *Obstetrics and Gynecology* 77(1):156–159.

Morrow, C.P., and Curtin, J.P. 1998. *Synopsis of gynecologic oncology*, 5th ed. Philadelphia: Churchill Livingstone.

Parker, L.P., Parker, J.R., Bodurka-Bevers, D. et al. 2000. Paget's disease of the vulva: pathology, pattern of involvement, and prognosis. *Gynecologic Oncology* 77:183–189.

Physicians' desk reference. 2002. Montvale, N.J.: Medical Economics.

Ridley, C.M., and Neill, S.M., eds. 1999. *The vulva*, 2nd ed. Oxford: Blackwell Science.

Winifred L. Star, R.N., C., N.P., M.S.
Claire L. Appelmans, R.N., C., W.H.C.N.P., M.S.

12-TB *Vulvar Disease*
White Lesions of the Vulva

Factors contributing to the appearance of *white lesions of the vulva* include hyperkeratosis (i.e., overgrowth of the horny, keratinized layer of the epidermis), depigmentation, and relative avascularity. There has been a lack of uniform terminology for and classification of these lesions. However, in 1987 the International Society for the Study of Vulvar Disease (ISSVD) reclassified the most common white vulvar lesions, the vulvar dystrophies, into *non-neoplastic epithelial disorders of skin and mucosa*. Categories include *lichen sclerosus*, *squamous cell hyperplasia* (formerly hyperplastic dystrophy), and *other dermatoses* (Committee on Terminology of the ISSVD 1990).

The etiology of these various disorders is still unclear. Technically, *dystrophy* means defective nutrition or metabolism, but the definition adds little to the understanding of the phenomenon. Factors that may contribute to the pathogenesis of the non-neoplastic disorders include chronic trauma (scratching), contact irritants, chronic fungal infections, allergic responses, nutritional deficiencies (folic acid deficiency, vitamin A deficiency secondary to achlorhydria/poor diet), metabolic disturbances (5 alpha-reductase deficiency), autoimmune disorders, familial disposition, and psychoneuroses. Further research is needed to establish cause-and-effect relationships (Kaufman et al. 1994, Koo et al. 2001).

One controversial issue is these disorders' potential for malignant transformation. It was originally thought that all white lesions of the vulva were premalignant, but this is now known to be incorrect. Most researchers believe there is little threat that non-neoplastic epithelial disorders will progress to invasive carcinoma; however, either of these pathologies may co-exist with premalignant lesions on the same vulva. Recent prospective studies indicate progression from chronic vulvar dystrophy to cancer on the order of 1–5%. Concern for malignant potential is greater when a lesion that contains atypical hyperplasia on initial biopsy (6% incidence) is present or when vulvar pain, itching, and scratching are chronic. A "mixed" lesion—squamous cell hyperplasia superimposed on a background of lichen sclerosus—is at slightly increased risk for atypia and development of invasive cancer (Black et al. 2002, DiSaia et al. 2002).

By definition, cases of atypia are now all placed in the category of vulvar intraepithelial neoplasia (VIN). Women are at greater risk for cancer progression when lesions do not respond to standard therapy and if they continue to have severe itching that causes chronic scratching (Kaufman et al. 1994, Rodke et al. 1988).

This chapter will cover assessment and management of lichen sclerosus and squamous cell hyperplasia. (See also the **Vulvar Intraepithelial Neoplasia** chapter.)

Lichen Sclerosus

Lichen sclerosus accounts for about 70% of non-neoplastic disorders. Former names included lichen sclerosus et atrophicus, atrophic leukoplakia, kraurosis vulvae, senile atrophy, and atrophic vulvitis. However, the epithelium in lichen sclerosus is metabolically active, not atrophic. The cause is unknown, but associated factors include autoimmune disease, heredity, achlorhydria, and decreased testosterone levels. Areas of squamous hyperplasia, often caused by scratching, may coexist with lichen sclerosus. This condition was formerly called *mixed dystrophy* but is now referred to as lichen sclerosus with squamous cell hyperplasia (DiSaia et al. 2002, Kaufman et al. 1994).

DATABASE

SUBJECTIVE

→ May occur at any age; most women are older than 50 years.

→ Affected children may have spontaneous resolution in adolescence, but most have persistent disease into adulthood.

→ Affected women of reproductive age often have remission during pregnancy with postpartum re-exacerbation.

→ The patient may be asymptomatic.

→ Symptoms may include:
  ▪ Pruritus—generally the primary symptom, but it may be sporadic or only mild and may not correlate with the size and severity of lesions
  ▪ Soreness, pain
  ▪ Dyspareunia

- Excoriations, ulcerations, bruising, skin thickening
→ History to include:
  - Vaginal infections
  - Allergies
  - Use of feminine hygiene products
  - History of diabetes, nutritional deficiencies
  - Family history, especially with regard to diabetes, cancer, and skin disorders

OBJECTIVE

→ Clinical features include (Kaufman et al. 1994):
  - Location on vulva is variable and the pattern often is bilaterally symmetrical
  - Initially a low, irregular lesion
  - A "cigarette paper" or "parchment-like" appearance (commonly extends to the anal area in a keyhole configuration)
  - Adhesion of the labia minora to majora
  - Edema or agglutination of the prepuce and frenulum that may bury the clitoris (phimosis)
  - Constriction or stenosis of the vaginal introitus
  - White maculopapules that may progress to well-defined plaques
  - Splitting of skin in midline (between the clitoris and urethra, in the perineum, or especially at the fourchette)
  - Fissures in skin folds
  - Small hematoma/telangiectasia of skin or mucosa
  - Blisters or ulcers in some cases
→ Vagina, cervix, uterus, adnexa, and rectum are within normal limits (WNL) unless there is co-existent pathology.
→ Other affected areas may include the trunk, neck, forearm, axilla, under the breasts, vulva, skin folds adjacent to the thighs, and inner aspects of the buttocks approximating the anus (Kaufman et al. 1994).
→ A diagram and good description of the lesion are helpful for monitoring response to therapy.

ASSESSMENT

→ Lichen sclerosus
→ R/O other dermatoses (e.g., squamous cell hyperplasia [lichen simplex chronicus], psoriasis, lichen planus)
→ R/O vitiligo
→ R/O VIN
→ R/O vulvar cancer
→ R/O *Candida* infection
→ R/O condyloma acuminata

PLAN

DIAGNOSTIC TESTS

→ A delay in diagnosis often results in progressive loss of vulvar architecture before effective therapy is initiated.
→ Multiple punch biopsies from selected areas of the vulva—especially from fissured, indurated, ulcerated, or thickened-appearing areas—are mandatory for diagnosis, as areas of hyperplasia and atypia cannot be determined by visual inspection alone. Biopsy specimens should be obtained from outer, advancing margins of a lesion.
  - If the appearance of all abnormal areas is similar, only one biopsy is necessary.
  - Ulcerations can be biopsied at different sites of the lesion border. But preferably, the entire ulcer should be excised.
  - Toluidine blue staining is highly sensitive for the detection of VIN (Joura et al. 1998).
→ Pap smear, sexually transmitted disease (STD) testing, wet mounts, and other diagnostic tests as indicated.

TREATMENT/MANAGEMENT

→ VIN or malignancy must be ruled out before initiating local therapy.
→ Local measures for relief of pruritus, ulcerations, and excoriations include (Friedrich 1983):
  - Wet dressings: 5% aluminum acetate (Burow's solution [Domeboro®]). Dilute 1:10 to 1:20, saturate gauze, apply/reapply for 20–30 minutes every day or more often as necessary. Alternately may use Domeboro® tablets or powder (follow the directions on the product); keep the solution refrigerated.
  - Sitz baths (versus wet dressings) may be tried with Burow's solution or with natural or artificial sea water (prepackaged powders are available at aquarium supply stores).
→ Treatments of choice for this disorder are Group I topical corticosteroids (Black et al. 2002, Hall 2000):
  - Clobetasol propionate 0.05% ointment: Apply a small amount to the affected areas once daily for 4–6 weeks, then 1–3 times weekly for 3 months. Therapy may be continued at less-frequent intervals or with a less-potent steroid (Black et al. 2002, Hall 2000).
  - Betamethasone dipropionate 0.05% ointment: Apply a small amount to the affected areas once daily for 4–6 weeks, then 1–3 times weekly for 3 months. Therapy may be continued with a less-potent steroid (Black et al. 2002, Hall 2000).
→ Testosterone is no longer recommended for treating this disorder. Though it may relieve pruritus in some individuals, testosterone has not been shown to be any more effective in bringing about histologic or clinical improvement than petrolatum alone and has been associated with clitoromegaly, vulvar pain, and virilization (Bracco et al. 1993, Sideri et al. 1994).
→ Other less commonly used therapies include (Kaufman et al. 1994):
  - Progesterone 10 mL in oil (50 mg/mL) in 40 g petrolatum has been used in conjunction with topical corticosteroids with varying success.
→ Treat any associated vulvovaginal infection as indicated.
→ Wide local excision for lesions with atypia.
→ Vulvectomy is reserved for persistent or extensive disease or progressive atypia (the recurrence rate after vulvectomy is high).

CONSULTATION

→ Refer to a physician as indicated for initial assessment, biopsy, and/or therapy for a refractory condition, depending on the policies of the practice setting.
→ As needed for prescription(s).
→ For wide local excision and more extensive surgery, refer to a physician.

PATIENT EDUCATION

→ Explain that the disease has no definitive etiology.
→ In some cases, lesions will not disappear, but continued topical therapy can slow disease progression and prevent skin tearing.
   - Symptoms may persist despite improvement in skin appearance.
   - Topical corticosteroids can be continued for relief of pruritus.
   - Additional relief measures for pruritus should be outlined. (See "Treatment/Management," above.)
→ Discuss factors that will improve overall health—e.g., proper diet, stress reduction, and exercise.
→ Assess the patient's coping strategies and provide suggestions for support as indicated.
→ Refer for psychosocial support as indicated.

FOLLOW-UP

→ As with many vulvar diseases, ongoing evaluation of the treated areas to monitor for disease recurrence is of utmost importance. Following excision, lichen sclerosus has been known to recur in 50% of cases.
→ Examinations should be performed on a regular basis (i.e., every 3–6 months) initially. After stabilization, patient visits may be semi-annual.
→ Biopsies of all progressive, recurrent, persistent, or suspicious lesions should be performed, especially from ulcerated, granular, or nodular areas.
→ Instruct patients to report any changes in vulvar tissue and encourage them to continue regular visits even if they are symptom-free.
→ Document in progress notes and on problem list.

Squamous Cell Hyperplasia

This condition has been known by a number of different terms. Previously called *leukoplakia*, *hyperplastic dystrophy*, and *neurodermatitis*, most squamous cell hyperplasia actually represents lichen simplex chronicus. It is one of the most common pruritic dermatoses. Lichenification, or thickening of the epidermis (parakeratosis) with subsequent leathery accentuation of normal skin markings, is the result of rubbing or scratching and is perpetuated by the "itch-scratch" cycle (Black et al. 2002, Hall 2000).

Squamous cell hyperplasia is associated with epithelial thickening or overgrowth of the horny layer of the epidermis. Thus, the lesion is most often hyperpigmented but may also be hypopigmented. Other dermatoses (e.g., chronic reactive vulvitis, psoriasis, and eczema) also have these nonspecific features.

This disorder is thought to be triggered initially by a contact dermatitis, insect bite, candidiasis, or other minor irritation the patient often does not remember. Pruritus is often exacerbated by anxiety, stress, or fatigue—hence the term neurodermatitis. Often, the condition may co-exist with other dermatoses such as lichen sclerosus, but these are histologically distinct entities.

Cancerous potential is related to associated cellular atypia of the lesion, known as VIN. The co-existence of lichen sclerosus with squamous cell hyperplasia increases the risk of atypia.

DATABASE

SUBJECTIVE

→ Any age from childhood through adulthood
→ Symptoms include:
   - Intense pruritus that often is worse at night, often provoking scratching during sleep
   - Excoriations, scratch marks
   - Soreness, pain

OBJECTIVE

→ Clinical features include:
   - A hyper- or hypopigmented patch ranging from small to extensive and often bilaterally symmetrical
   - Lichenification (a thickened leathery appearance) often with fissures, excoriation
   - A raised, well-circumscribed lesion
   - Dusky red vulva, or hazy cast, especially if in conjunction with candidal intertrigo
   - White and red patches possibly appearing within the same lesion
   - The areas most frequently involved: labia majora, interlabial grooves, outer labia minora, or clitoral hood
   - A lesion possibly extending to the groin and thighs
→ Squamous cell hyperplasia may coexist with lichen sclerosus, with features of both appearing on same vulva. (See "Objective" in the "Lichen Sclerosus" section.)
→ KOH prep fails to reveal dermatophytes or *Candida*.
→ The vagina, cervix, uterus, adnexa, and rectum are WNL unless there is co-existent pathology.
→ A diagram and good description of the lesion are helpful.

ASSESSMENT

→ Squamous cell hyperplasia (lichen simplex chronicus)
→ R/O lichen sclerosus
→ R/O cutaneous candidiasis
→ R/O other dermatoses (e.g. psoriasis, eczema, contact dermatitis, lichen planus)
→ R/O VIN
→ R/O invasive cancer

PLAN

DIAGNOSTIC TESTS

→ The possibility of malignancy should be considered before initiating local therapy, especially if the co-existence of lichen sclerosus is suspected.

→ Multiple punch biopsies from outer margins of a lesion:
  ■ Multiple specimens may be obtained from opposite edges of the lesion.
  ■ If the appearance of all abnormal areas is similar, only one biopsy is necessary.
  ■ Toluidine blue staining is highly sensitive for detecting VIN (Joura et al. 1998).

→ Pap smear, STD testing, wet mounts, and other diagnostic tests as indicated.

TREATMENT/MANAGEMENT

→ Breaking the "itch-scratch" cycle is key to successful treatment.

→ Topical corticosteroids are the treatment of choice. Treatment may be initiated with a brief course of high- or moderate-potency topical steroid cream to control pruritus, followed by switching to a less potent steroid for longer therapy until the condition is resolved (Black et al. 2002, Zellis et al. 1996). Options include:

■ Clobetasol propionate 0.05%: Apply a small amount to the affected area(s) once daily for 3–4 weeks, then decrease the frequency of use or switch to a lower-potency steroid such as:
  • Triamcinolone acetonide cream/ointment 0.1%—a small amount to the affected areas BID
  • Fluocinolone acetonide cream/ointment 0.025–0.01% —a small amount to the affected areas BID

Table 12TB.1.   POTENCY RANKING OF SOME COMMONLY USED TOPICAL CORTICOSTEROIDS

Group I (Super Potent)

Diprolene® AF cream 0.05% (betamethasone dipropionate, augmented)
Diprolene® ointment 0.05% (betamethasone dipropionate, augmented)
Psorcon® cream/ointment 0.05% (diflorasone diacetate)
Temovate® cream/ointment/gel 0.05% (clobetasol propionate)
Ultravate® cream/ointment 0.05% (halobetasol propionate)

Group II (Potent)

Cyclocort® ointment 0.1% (amcinonide)
Diprosone® ointment 0.05% (betamethasone dipropionate)
Elocon® ointment 0.1% (mometasone furoate)
Florone® ointment 0.05% (diflorasone diacetate)
Halog® cream 0.1% (halcinonide)
Lidex® cream/ointment/gel 0.05% (fluocinonide)
Maxiflor® ointment 0.05% (diflorasone diacetate)
Maxivate® cream/ointment/lotion 0.05% (betamethasone dipropionate)
Topicort® cream/ointment 0.25% (desoximetasone)
Topicort® gel 0.05% (desoximetasone)

Group III (Potent)

Aristocort® cream HP 0.5% (triamcinolone acetonide)
Aristocort® A ointment 0.1% (triamcinolone acetonide)
Cloderm® cream 0.1% (clocortolone pivalate)
Cyclocort® cream/lotion 0.1% (amcinonide)
Dermatop® emollient cream 0.1% (prednicarbate)
Diprosone® cream 0.05% (betamethasone dipropionate)
Florone® cream 0.05% (diflorasone diacetate)
Halog® ointment/solution 0.1% (halcinonide)
Lidex® E cream 0.05% (fluocinonide)
Maxiflor® cream 0.05% (diflorasone diacetate)
Pandel® cream 0.1% (hydrocortisone buteprate)
Valisone® ointment 0.1% (betamethasone valerate)

Group IV (Midstrength)

Cordran® ointment 0.05% (flurandrenolide)
Elocon® cream/lotion 0.1% (mometasone furoate)
Kenalog® cream/ointment 0.1% (triamcinolone acetonide)
Synalar® ointment 0.025% (fluocinolone acetonide)
Topicort® LP cream 0.05% (desoximetasone)
Westcort® ointment 0.2% (hydrocortisone valerate)

Group V (Midstrength)

Cordran® cream 0.05% (flurandrenolide)
Diprosone® lotion 0.05% (betamethasone dipropionate)
Kenalog® lotion 0.1% (triamcinolone acetonide)
Kenalog® ointment 0.025% (triamcinolone acetonide)
Locoid® cream/ointment 0.1% (hydrocortisone butyrate)
Synalar® cream 0.025% (fluocinolone acetonide)
Tridesilon® ointment 0.05% (desonide)
Valisone® cream 0.1% (betamethasone valerate)
Westcort® cream 0.2% (hydrocortisone valerate)

Group VI (Mild)

Aclovate® cream/ointment 0.05% (alclometasone dipropionate)
Aristocort® cream 0.1% (triamcinolone acetonide)
DesOwen® cream/ointment/lotion 0.05% (desonide)
Kenalog® cream/lotion 0.025% (triamcinolone acetonide)
Locoid® solution 0.1% (hydrocortisone butyrate)
Locorten® cream 0.03% (flumethasone pivalate)
Synalar® cream/solution 0.01% (fluocinolone acetonide)
Tridesilon® cream 0.05% (desonide)
Valisone® lotion 0.1% (betamethasone valerate)

Group VII (Mild)

Topicals with hydrocortisone, dexamethasone, flumethasone, prednisolone, and methylprednisolone

NOTE: Trade names appear first; generic names are in parentheses. Potency descends with each group to Group VII. There is no significant difference between agents within Groups II through VII. In Group I, Temovate cream/ointment is most potent.

Source: Adapted with permission from Hall, J.C., 2000. *Sauer's manual of skin diseases*, 8th ed. Philadelphia: Lippincott Williams & Wilkins.

- Hydrocortisone cream/ointment 0.5% or 1%—a small amount applied to the affected areas BID

NOTE: Fluorinated steroids may cause skin atrophy. Once severe pruritus is controlled, a fluorinated steroid should be replaced with a nonfluorinated steroid—e.g., hydrocortisone. Occlusive dressings to the vulva are not recommended. (See **Table 12TB.1, Potency Ranking of Some Commonly Used Topical Corticosteroids**.)

→ Hormonal creams are of no value in this condition.

→ For severe pruritus, H_1-receptor antagonist oral antihistamines may be considered. Prescribe with caution; they may cause drowsiness (*Physicians' Desk Reference* 2002):

- Diphenhydramine hydrochloride: 25–50 mg p.o. at HS or TID
- Cetirizine hydrochloride: 5–10 mg p.o. as a single daily dose at HS
- Hydroxyzine hydrochloride: 25 mg p.o. TID or at HS

→ Severe pruritus unresponsive to topical therapy may require intralesional injections of triamcinolone, 5 or 10 mg/mL diluted 2:1 in saline. Treatment may be repeated every 2 or 3 weeks.

→ Wide local excision for lesions with atypia.

→ Vulvectomy is reserved for persistent or extensive disease or progressive atypia (the recurrence rate after vulvectomy is high).

CONSULTATION

→ For suspected VIN.

→ For intralesional injections; may require physician referral depending on site-specific practices.

→ As needed for prescription(s).

PATIENT EDUCATION

→ See "Patient Education" in the "Lichen Sclerosus" section.

→ Advise avoidance of potential local irritants. Tips include:

- Completely avoid washing vulva with soap. Use only plain water for bathing.
- Wear all-cotton, white underpants.
- Use mild laundry soap to launder underwear. Rinse well and line dry.
- Avoid using feminine hygiene deodorant products on vulva.
- Use white, unscented toilet paper.

FOLLOW-UP

→ Refer to "Follow-up" in the "Lichen Sclerosus" section.

→ Recurrent squamous cell hyperplasia must be treated as a new lesion.

→ Document in progress notes and on problem list.

BIBLIOGRAPHY

Ambros, R.A., Malfetano, J.H., Carlson, J.A. et al. 1997. Non-neoplastic epithelial alterations of the vulva: recognition, assessment, and comparisons of terminologies used among the various subspecialties. *Modern Pathology* 10(5):401–408.

Ball, S.B., and Wojnarowska, F. 1998. Vulvar dermatoses: lichen sclerosus, lichen planus, and vulval dermatitis/lichen simplex chronicus. *Seminars in Cutaneous Medicine and Surgery* 17(3):182–188.

Black, M.M., McKay, M., Braude, P.R. et al. 2002. *Obstetric and gynecologic dermatology*, 2nd ed. London: Mosby International.

Bracco, G.L., Carli, P., and Sonni, L. 1993. Clinical and histologic effects of topical treatments of vulval lichen sclerosus. *Journal of Reproductive Medicine* 38:37–40.

Committee on Terminology of the International Society for the Study of Vulvar Disease. 1990. New nomenclature for vulvar disease. *Journal of Reproductive Medicine* 35:483–484.

DiSaia, P.J., and Creasman, W.T. 2002. *Clinical gynecologic oncology*, 6th ed. St. Louis, Mo.: Mosby.

Fischer, G., Spurrett, B., and Fischer, A. 1995. The chronically symptomatic vulva: aetiology and management. *British Journal of Obstetrics and Gynaecology* 102:773–779.

Friedrich, E.G., Jr. 1983. *Vulvar disease*, 2nd ed. Philadelphia: W.B. Saunders.

Hall, J.C. 2000. *Sauer's manual of skin diseases*, 8th ed. Philadelphia: Lippincott Williams & Wilkins.

Joura, E.A., Zeisler, H., Lösch, A. et al. 1998. Differentiating vulvar intraepithelial neoplasia from non-neoplastic epithelial disorders: the toluidine blue test. *Journal of Reproductive Medicine* 43(8):671–674.

Kaufman, R.H., and Faro, S. 1994. *Benign diseases of the vulva and vagina*, 4th ed. St. Louis, Mo.: Mosby Year Book.

Kaufman, R.H., Friedrich, E.G., Jr., and Gardner, H.L. 1989. *Benign diseases of the vulva and vagina*, 3rd ed. Chicago: Year Book Medical.

Koo, J., and Lebwohl, A. 2001. Psychodermatology: the mind and skin connection. *American Family Physician* 64(11): 1873–1878.

Marren, P., and Wojnarowska, F. 1996. Dermatitis of the vulva. *Seminars in Dermatology* 15(1):36–41.

Physicians' desk reference. 2002. Montvale, N.J.: Medical Economics.

Rodke, G., Friedrich, E.G., and Wilkinson, E.J. 1988. Malignant potential of mixed vulvar dystrophy (lichen sclerosus associated with squamous cell hyperplasia). *Journal of Reproductive Medicine* 33(6):545–550.

Sideri, M., Origoni, L., Spinaci, L. et al. 1994. Topical testosterone in the treatment of vulvar lichen sclerosus. *International Journal of Gynaecology and Obstetrics* 46:53–56.

Sinha, P., Sorinola, O., and Luesley, D.M. 1999. Lichen sclerosus of the vulva: long-term steroid maintenance therapy. *Journal of Reproductive Medicine* 44(7):621–624.

Wilkinson, E.J., Kneale, B., and Lynch, P.J. 1986. Report of the International Society for the Study of Vulvar Disease, Terminology Committee. *Journal of Reproductive Medicine* 31:973.

Zellis, S., and Pincus, S.H. 1996. Treatment of vulvar dermatoses. *Seminars in Dermatology* 15(1):71–76.

Winifred L. Star, R.N., C., N.P., M.S.
Claire L. Appelmans, R.N., C., W.H.C.N.P., M.S.

12-TC Vulvar Disease
Dark Lesions of the Vulva

Any stimulus that increases the number of melanocytes or the production of melanin will result in color changes or hyperpigmentation of vulvar skin. The vulva's skin color is darker than that of the rest of the body due to the large number of melanocytes concentrated there. Ten percent of all vulvar lesions are *dark lesions*. Their features are dissimilar, and benign-appearing lesions may actually be cancerous. Ideally, all dark lesions of the vulva should be biopsied for a histological diagnosis (Friedrich 1983).

Dark lesions of the vulva to be covered in this chapter are *lentigo, nevi, seborrheic keratoses,* and *melanoma.* Vulvar intraepithelial neoplasia (VIN), which also may present as a dark lesion, is detailed in a separate chapter. Information on consultation, patient education, and follow-up for dark lesions is combined at the end of this chapter. Other conditions that may present as dark lesions are squamous cell hyperplasia, *Pediculosis pubis,* and scabies. (See the **White Lesions of the Vulva** chapter or Section 3, **Dermatological Disorders.**)

Lentigo

A lentigo is a uniformly hyperpigmented lesion of the skin where melanocytes produce excess amounts of melanin. Because no cytologic atypia is associated with lentigenes, no malignant potential is associated with this type of lesion. The findings are similar to those for vulvar melanosis, except that the lesions of melanosis are larger and often irregularly shaped, sometimes appearing as a melanoma (Black et al. 2002, Rahman et al. 1996).

DATABASE

SUBJECTIVE

→ Appears in mid-adult life
→ No relationship to sun exposure
→ Patient is generally asymptomatic

OBJECTIVE

→ Clinical features include:

▪ Hyperpigmented macule with sharp margins located anywhere on the vulva
▪ Resembles a freckle
▪ Light brown to black
▪ Usually smaller than 5 mm and never larger than 1 cm
▪ Surrounded by skin that appears normal
→ Atypical cells may exist above the basal layer.
→ The vagina, cervix, uterus, adnexa, and rectum are within normal limits (WNL) unless there is co-existent pathology.
→ A good description and diagram of the lesion is helpful.

ASSESSMENT

→ Lentigo
→ R/O vulvar melanosis
→ R/O junctional nevi
→ R/O melanoma
→ R/O basal cell carcinoma
→ R/O VIN
→ R/O other dermatoses

PLAN

→ Biopsy is diagnostic and curative.
→ No other specific therapy is indicated.
→ Pap smear, sexually transmitted disease (STD) testing, wet mounts, and other diagnostic tests as indicated.

Nevi

Nevi, or moles, are clusters of neural crest cells derived from melanocytes in the epidermis and Schwann cells of the dermal nerves. Three main groups develop—junctional, compound, and intradermal nevi—as maturation from the basal layer of the epithelium occurs. With this transformation over time comes a diminished potential for melanoma transformation (i.e., junctional and compound nevi have greater malignant potential). Although by definition malignant neoplasia is not a feature of nevi, about 30–50% of melanomas arise from pre-existing nevi.

However, *dysplastic* nevi (usually multiple lesions present; not commonly found on the vulva) and *congenital* nevi (present since birth) do carry increased risks for development of malignant melanoma, especially in persons with a family history of melanoma. The dysplastic type usually appears in adolescence and may continue to appear even after 35 years of age; it may be inherited or sporadic (Black et al. 2002, Friedrich 1983, Kaufman et al. 1994). Congenital nevi have a lifetime malignancy potential of 5–20%, especially if the lesion is larger than 2 cm (Consensus Conference 1984).

Vulvar melanosis is often confused with nevi. Melanosis usually presents as pigmented macules with slightly irregular margins. (See "Lentigo," above). Similar vaginal pigmented lesions also may exist (Kaufman et al. 1994).

DATABASE

SUBJECTIVE

→ Not usually recognized until after puberty, when lesions tend to darken.
→ The patient is generally asymptomatic. She may report a raised area of vulvar skin or an irritation.
→ The lesion may be stable for years or enlarge slowly.

OBJECTIVE

→ Five clinical types of nevi have been described (Lever 1990):
  ■ Flat: usually junctional nevi, looks like lentigo
  ■ Slightly elevated: usually compound nevi
  ■ Papillomatous: majority intradermal nevi
  ■ Dome-shaped: usually intradermal nevi
  ■ Pedunculated: intradermal nevi
→ Clinical features of nevi include:
  ■ Oval or cuboidal shape
  ■ Size varies from 1 mm to 2 cm
  ■ Both a macular and papular component
  ■ Depth of color varies from flesh-colored to light tan to dark brown to black
→ Clinical features of dysplastic nevi (Seykora et al. 1996) include:
  ■ Lesion >5 mm
  ■ A macular component is always present. If a papular component also is present, it is usually in the center of an ovoid macule.
  ■ Borders are characteristically regular but ill-defined and fuzzy.
  ■ Usually brown or tan color, often variegated. Pink colors often are present.
  ■ Substantial asymmetry, excessive variegation, focal black or gray areas should raise suspicion of melanoma.
→ The vagina, cervix, uterus, adnexa, and rectum are WNL unless there is co-existent pathology.
→ A good description and diagram of the lesion are important.

ASSESSMENT

→ Nevi
→ R/O lentigo

→ R/O melanoma
→ R/O melanosis
→ R/O VIN
→ R/O basal cell carcinoma
→ R/O seborrheic keratosis
→ R/O accessory breast tissue
→ R/O other dermatoses

PLAN

DIAGNOSTIC TESTS

→ Biopsy to establish histopathological diagnosis
→ Pap smear, STD testing, wet mounts, and other diagnostic tests as indicated

TREATMENT/MANAGEMENT

→ Pigmented nevi should be removed under the following conditions (Kaufman et al. 1994):
  ■ If they are subject to irritation, as on vulva
  ■ If the lesion darkens or acquires an inflamed appearance
  ■ If it grows
  ■ If it becomes multicolored
  ■ If there is associated ulceration, bleeding, or pain
  NOTE: Increased size, bleeding, ulceration, or "satellite lesions" may indicate malignancy. Such lesions should be excised promptly.
→ Excision should include 0.5–1 cm of normal skin and subcutaneous tissue. Removal of an entire lesion allows for more definitive pathologic distinction between a nevus and melanoma (Pariser 1998).
→ Destructive techniques are not advisable, as they make histological evaluation impossible.
→ Benign vulvar melanosis is generally managed conservatively, but a biopsy is necessary to establish an accurate diagnosis.
→ Papular or hairy moles have a low malignant potential, so removal is not urgent unless there is pain or bleeding.
→ Excision of congenital hairy nevi should be deep enough to remove the hair follicle to prevent recurrence.

Seborrheic Keratosis

In the postmenopausal years, seborrheic keratosis is the most common tumor of the skin, though it is relatively unusual on the vulva. The lesion exists exclusively on hair-bearing skin and comprises proliferative basal epidermal cells and melanocytes that grow in an upward, controlled manner. Clinical features vary and there is a variety of histopathological patterns (Toussaint et al. 1999.) Malignant potential is rare but has been reported (Friedrich 1983, Kaufman et al. 1994).

DATABASE

SUBJECTIVE

→ The patient may be asymptomatic or may report a raised lesion.

OBJECTIVE

→ Early lesions appear as hyperpigmented macules and tend to be ovoid or elongated.
→ Fully developed lesions appear as papular, waxy, stuck-on plaques with a flat top.
→ Similar lesions appear elsewhere on the body.
→ Lesions appear singly or in large numbers.
→ Size varies from a few millimeters to several centimeters.
→ Lesions may be flesh-colored or black, but most are dark brown and greasy.
→ Lesions look like they could be picked or shaved off.
→ A lesion may also be macular.
→ Sudden onset of multiple lesions may signal unrelated internal malignancy.
→ The vagina, cervix, uterus, adnexa, and rectum are WNL unless there is co-existent pathology.
→ A good description and diagram of the lesion are helpful.

ASSESSMENT

→ Seborrheic keratosis
→ R/O nevi or lentigines
→ R/O melanoma
→ R/O VIN
→ R/O condyloma acuminata

PLAN

DIAGNOSTIC TESTS

→ Biopsy to establish a histopathological diagnosis if a lesion is removed
→ Pap smear, STD specimens, wet mounts, and other diagnostic tests as indicated

TREATMENT/MANAGEMENT

→ No treatment is necessary unless a lesion is large, disfiguring, or painful.
→ Simple excision may remove the entire lesion and is diagnostic and curative.

→ A lesion may be scraped off with a dermal curet after freezing it with ethyl chloride. Send the specimen to pathology.

Melanoma

Melanoma is a rare malignant degeneration of melanocytic cells, generally of the skin, and makes up 10% of all vulvar cancers. In women, 5% of melanomas arise in the vulva.

High-risk categories for developing melanoma include (DiSaia et al. 2002): a family history of melanoma; poor or no tanning ability; moles that are blue-black, speckled, splotchy, or jagged on the border; a change in size, shape, or color of mole; or a mole larger than a dime.

There are three varieties: lentigo maligna, superficial spreading (the most common), and nodular melanoma. Melanomas may arise de novo or from pre-existing junctional or compound nevi (30% of cases). Prognosis for survival primarily depends on the depth or level of tumor invasion rather than the size of the tumor. Until quite recently, Clark's Staging Classification has been used for staging melanomas. (See **Table 12TC.1, Clark's Staging Classification by Levels**.) A newer staging system has been adopted by the American Joint Committee on Cancer. As both systems are currently in use, they are both included here (DiSaia et al. 2002). (See **Table 12TC.2, New Staging System for Melanoma Adopted by the American Joint Committee on Cancer**.)

Ten-year survival rates for Levels I to II, III, IV, and V tumors are 100%, 83%, 65%, and 23%, respectively. Other factors influencing survival are urethral and vaginal extension, presence or absence of regional lymph nodes, and distant metastases (Barclay 1991, DiSaia et al. 2002, Dunton et al. 1995, Ridley et al. 1999).

DATABASE

SUBJECTIVE

→ Mostly found in women older than 50 years.
→ Affects Caucasians almost exclusively.
→ The patient often is asymptomatic.

Table 12TC.1.   CLARK'S STAGING CLASSIFICATION BY LEVELS

Level	Definition
I	In situ melanoma: all demonstrable tumor is above the basement membrane in the epidermis
II	Melanoma extends through the basement membrane into the papillary dermis
III	The tumor fills the papillary dermis and extends to the reticular dermis but does not invade it
IV	The tumor extends into the reticular dermis
V	The tumor extends into the subcutaneous fat

Source: Reproduced with permission from DiSaia, P.J., and Creasman, W.T. 2002. *Clinical gynecologic oncology*, 6th ed., p. 233. St. Louis, Mo.: Mosby.

→ Symptoms may include:
- A "lump"
- Pruritis
- Bleeding
- Irritation
- Enlargement of a "mole"
- A change in "mole" pigmentation
- A "mole" with irregular borders

→ A lesion may be present for variable duration before discovery.

→ A family history of "moles"

OBJECTIVE

→ The labia majora, labia minora, or clitoris are common sites of involvement.

→ Follows ABCDE mnemonic for melanoma:
- Asymmetrical morphology
- Border irregularity
- Color variegated
- Diameter >6 mm
- Elevation of the lesion above the skin surface

→ The vagina, cervix, uterus, adnexa, and rectum are WNL unless there is co-existent pathology.

→ A good description and diagram of the lesion(s) are important.

Lentigo Maligna

→ Rare on vulva

→ Resembles a flat freckle

→ Has a speckled appearance

→ May be extensive although superficial

Superficial Spreading

→ The most common type affecting vulva

→ Usually elevated

→ May be ulcerated

→ May be 2–3 cm in diameter

→ Fairly good prognosis if detected early

Nodular Melanoma

→ Raised, irregular surface

→ Small diameter but deep involvement

→ Variable degrees of pigmentation

→ Some amelanotic varieties exist

→ Increased frequency of nodal metastasis

→ Poor prognosis

ASSESSMENT

→ Melanoma

→ R/O lentigo

→ R/O nevus or dysplastic nevus

→ R/O vascular skin tumors

→ R/O seborrheic keratosis

→ R/O VIN

→ R/O furuncle

→ R/O basal cell carcinoma

→ R/O other dermatoses

PLAN

DIAGNOSTIC TESTS

→ Biopsy is essential to establish a histopathological diagnosis.

→ Serial photographs may be helpful in lesion follow-up.

→ Pap smear, STD testing, wet mounts, and other diagnostic tests as indicated.

TREATMENT/MANAGEMENT

→ If the presenting lesion is small, a punch biopsy may be performed. Larger lesions require excision of larger areas.

→ Definitive therapy by a physician after the histopathological diagnosis is established. Management remains controversial.

Table 12TC.2.   NEW STAGING SYSTEM FOR MELANOMA ADOPTED BY THE AMERICAN JOINT COMMITTEE ON CANCER

Stage	Criteria
Ia	Localized melanoma ≤0.75 mm or Level II* (T1N0M0)
Ib	Localized melanoma ≥0.76 mm to 1.5 mm or Level III* (T2N0M0)
IIa	Localized melanoma 1.5 mm to 4 mm or Level IV* (T3N0M0)
IIb	Localized melanoma >4 mm or Level V* (T4N0M0)
III	Limited nodal metastases involving only one regional lymph node basin, or less than 5 in-transit metastases, but without nodal metastases (any T, N1M0)
IV	Advanced regional metastases (any T, N2M0) or any patient with distant metastases (any T, any N, M1 or M2)

* When the thickness and level of invasion criteria do not coincide within a T classification, thickness should take precedence.

Source: Reprinted with permission from Ketcham, A.S., and Balch, C.M. 1985. Classification and staging systems. In *Cutaneous melanoma: clinical management and treatment results worldwide*, eds. C.M. Balch and G.W. Milton. Philadelphia: J.B. Lippincott.

Treatment selection varies depending on the consulting gynecological oncologist. Options include:

- Wide local excision: The trend is toward greater use of this therapy for varying depths of tumor invasion.
- Radial vulvectomy with bilateral inguinal and/or pelvic lymphadenectomy may be necessary for deep tumor invasion.
- Pelvic exenteration for urethral or bladder extension.
- Radiation in selected cases.

CONSULTATION *(pertinent to all dark lesions)*

→ For all suspicious lesions.
→ Refer to a physician for biopsy procedure per site-specific policy.
→ Refer to a physician for surgical procedures and treatment regimens that fall outside the scope of the clinician's practice.
→ Refer to a physician (preferably a gynecological oncologist) all patients with melanoma.

PATIENT EDUCATION/FOLLOW-UP *(pertinent to all dark lesions)*

→ Advise the patient to inspect her vulva periodically and report significant changes in skin appearance and increased pain and/or bleeding of vulvar lesion(s). The frequency of self-examination and clinical examinations is individualized according to case presentation.
→ Serial photographs may be helpful in lesion follow-up.
→ Depending on the initial pathology, the decision to biopsy similar, recurring, benign-appearing lesions should be individualized. Consult with a physician. If there is any doubt, biopsy.
→ Patients with malignant melanoma need more aggressive management. Education and psychological support are paramount. The physician responsible for the patient's care will educate her regarding the nature of the disease, necessary treatment, surgical alternatives, potential complications, and required follow-up.
→ Sexual dysfunction is a common complication of radical vulvar surgery. Psychosexual support is extremely important for the patient's successful recovery.
→ Referral for counseling may be necessary if the patient undergoes major surgical intervention or experiences disturbances in self-image that interfere with social/sexual relationships.
→ Document in progress notes and on problem list.

BIBLIOGRAPHY

Ambros, R.A., Malfetano, J.H., Carlson, J.A. et al. 1997. Non-neoplastic epithelial alterations of the vulva: recognition, assessment and comparisons of terminologies used among the various subspecialties. *Modern Pathology* 10(5):401–408.

Apgar, B.S., and Cox, J.T. 1996. Differentiating normal and abnormal findings of the vulva. *American Family Physician* 53(4):1171–1180.

Barclay, D.L., 1991. Premalignant and malignant disorders of the vulva and vagina. In *Current obstetric and gynecologic diagnosis and treatment*, 7th ed., ed. M.L. Pernoll, pp. 923–936. Norwalk, Conn.: Appleton & Lange.

Black, M.M., McKay, M., Braude, P.R. et al. 2002. *Obstetric and gynecologic dermatology*, 2nd ed. London: Mosby International.

Consensus Conference. 1984. Precursors to malignant melanoma. *Journal of the American Medical Association* 251:1864–1866.

DiSaia, P.J., and Creasman, W.T. 2002. *Clinical gynecologic oncology*, 6th ed. St. Louis, Mo.: Mosby.

Dunton, C.J., and Berd, D. 1999. Vulvar melanoma, biologically different from other cutaneous melanomas. *Lancet* 354:2013–2014.

Dunton, C.J., Kautzky, M., and Hanau, C. 1995. Malignant melanoma of the vulva: a review. *Obstetrical and Gynecological Survey* 50(10):739–746.

Friedrich, E.G., Jr. 1983. *Vulvar disease*, 2nd ed. Philadelphia: W.B. Saunders.

Grendys, E.C., and Fiorica, J.V. 2000. Innovations in the management of vulvar carcinoma. *Current Opinion in Obstetrics and Gynecology* 12:15–20.

Happle, R. 1995. What is a nevus? *Dermatology* 191:1–5.

Jaramillo, B.A. 2000. Managing vulvovaginal melanomas. *Contemporary OB/GYN* 45(4):85–100.

Kaufman, R.H., and Faro, S. 1994. *Benign diseases of the vulva and vagina*, 4th ed. St. Louis, Mo.: Mosby Year Book.

Lever, W.F. 1990. *Histopathology of the skin*, 7th ed. Philadelphia: J.B. Lippincott.

Morgan, M.A., and Mikuta, J.J. 1999. Surgical management of vulvar cancer. *Seminars in Surgical Oncology* 17:168–172.

Morrow, C.P., and Curtin, J.P. 1998. *Synopsis of gynecologic oncology*, 5th ed. Philadelphia: Churchill Livingstone.

Pariser, R.J. 1998. Benign neoplasms of the skin. *Medical Clinics of North America* 82(6):1285–1307.

Rahman, S.B., and Bhawan, J. 1996. Lentigo. *International Journal of Dermatology* 35(4):229–239.

Ridley, C.M., and Neill, S.M., eds. 1999. *The vulva*, 2nd ed. Oxford, United Kingdom: Blackwell Science.

Rogers III, R.S., and Gibson, L.E. 1997. Mucosal, genital, and unusual variants of melanoma. *Mayo Clinic Proceedings* 72:362–366.

Seykora, J., and Elder, D. 1996. Dysplastic nevi and other risk markers for melanoma. *Seminars in Oncology* 23(6):682–687.

Toussaint, S., Salcedo, E., and Kamino, H. 1999. Benign epidermal proliferations. *Advances in Dermatology* 14:307–357.

Venes, D., and Thomas, C.L., eds. 2001. *Taber's cyclopedic medical dictionary*, 19th ed. Philadelphia: F.A. Davis.

Winifred L. Star, R.N., C., N.P., M.S.
Claire L. Appelmans, R.N., C., W.H.C.N.P., M.S.

12-TD Vulvar Disease
Small Lesions of the Vulva

Small lesions of the vulva rarely exceed 1 cm in diameter. They may be white, red, dull-blue, or variegated in color. In general, small vulvar lesions have little in common. Etiologies differ and may include viruses, embryological remnants, trauma, duct blockage, or neoplasia. Although some lesions have a classic, textbook appearance, others can be diagnosed only by histopathology. Some growths are more prone to occur only in specific anatomic locations of the vulva (Friedrich 1983).

This chapter will cover several of the more common small lesions of the vulva, including *epidermal cysts* (*sebaceous cysts*), *acrochordons* (*skin tags*), *hidradenitis suppurativa*, *hemangiomas*, *caruncles* (*urethral*), and *Fox-Fordyce disease*. *Condylomata acuminata* is covered in the **Sexually Transmitted Diseases** section. *Molluscum contagiosum* and *furuncles* and *carbuncles* are in the **Dermatological Disorders** section.

Epidermal Cysts

Epidermal cysts are the most common small lesions of the vulva. Often erroneously called "sebaceous cysts," they are lined with keratinizing squamous epithelium and contain cellular debris with a sebaceous appearance and odor. Most of these cysts arise from pilosebaceous ducts that have become occluded (Kaufman et al. 1994). True sebaceous cells, however, are rarely found. Infection, fibrosis, or calcification may develop in an epidermal cyst (Friedrich 1983).

DATABASE

SUBJECTIVE

→ The patient may be aware of a lump, bump, or "knobby" sensation on the vulva. Cyst(s) may slowly enlarge.
→ The patient is seldom symptomatic in other ways, unless secondarily infected.

OBJECTIVE

→ Lesions characteristically:
- Arise on the labia majora
- Are multiple (but may be single), round, yellow, nontender

- Range from 5 mm to 2 cm in diameter; usually <1 cm
- Are solid, firm to palpation; feel like a "BB shot"
- Have caseous, gritty, foul-smelling material inside
→ Possible signs of secondary infection include tenderness or erythema.

ASSESSMENT

→ Epidermal cyst
→ R/O syringoma
→ R/O nodular melanoma
→ R/O hidradenoma
→ R/O accessory breast tissue
→ R/O fibroma
→ R/O lipoma

PLAN

DIAGNOSTIC TESTS

→ Excision for histopathological diagnosis when a larger, isolated epidermal cyst cannot be recognized by inspection alone.

TREATMENT/MANAGEMENT

→ None, unless the cyst is annoying or cosmetically unacceptable to the patient.
→ Can be removed under local anesthesia. Alternately, a 20-gauge needle can be inserted into the cyst and the contents expressed under gentle pressure. This treatment usually offers only temporary relief, as cyst contents tend to reaccumulate.
→ Acutely infected cysts may be treated with warm soaks or packs, and incision and drainage (I & D). Excision may be necessary to prevent recurrence.

CONSULTATION

→ Usually it is not indicated.
→ Refer the patient to a physician for removal under local anesthesia or for I & D in cases of abscess formation.

PATIENT EDUCATION

→ Reassure the patient and explain the benign nature of the condition. Treatment is not usually recommended unless the patient is bothered by the cyst(s).

FOLLOW-UP

→ None specifically, unless a secondary infection occurs.
→ Have the patient return for reassessment after therapy as indicated.
→ Document in progress notes and on problem list.

Acrochordons

These soft, fibroepithelial polyps are fleshy growths that are usually referred to as *skin tags*. The cause is unknown and there is no malignant potential.

DATABASE
SUBJECTIVE

→ Usually asymptomatic.
→ The patient may be aware of a bump or small, fleshy growth on the vulva, adjacent medial aspect of the thigh, or peri-anal area.

OBJECTIVE

→ The structure is usually solitary, flesh-colored (though the tip may be lighter), soft, wrinkled, polypoid. It is usually on a pedicle but occasionally sessile. It resembles an empty sac of skin. Multiple skin tags are usually widely separated.
→ Size ranges from several millimeters to >1 cm. Giant acrochordons may exist.
→ Repeated trauma or irritation may lead to swelling, ecchymosis, or ulceration. Twisting of the stalk may cause infarction (Friedrich 1983, Kaufman et al. 1994).

ASSESSMENT

→ Acrochordon
→ R/O condyloma acuminata
→ R/O accessory breast tissue
→ R/O hidradenoma
→ R/O neurofibroma

PLAN
DIAGNOSTIC TESTS

→ Excisional biopsy may be indicated when the lesion is >1 cm or if there is doubt about the diagnosis (Friedrich 1983).

TREATMENT/MANAGEMENT

→ None indicated, unless the patient is disturbed by the lesion or in cases of chronic irritation.
→ A lesion may be removed by a variety of methods:
  ▪ Under local anesthesia, cut the lesion close to the surface and apply ferric subsulfate (Monsel's solution), silver nitrate, or a single suture to control bleeding as indicated (Kaufman et al. 1994).

▪ Electrocautery, cryosurgery, laser (Friedrich 1983)

CONSULTATION

→ Referral to a physician may be necessary for removal.

PATIENT EDUCATION

→ Reassure and explain the benign nature of the condition. Treatment is not usually advocated unless the patient is bothered by the lesion.

FOLLOW-UP

→ None specifically. Have the patient return for reassessment after therapy as indicated.
→ Document in progress notes and on problem list.

Hidradenitis Suppurativa

Hidradenitis presents as a chronic, suppurative, dermatological condition affecting predominantly the vulva and axillae, and occasionally the breasts, buttocks, or thighs. It is a disorder of keratinic occlusion of follicles resulting in an inflammation of the follicles and extending to adjacent eccrine and apocrine glands. Eventual perifolliculitis leads to abscess formation contributing to the destruction of the pilosebaceous unit and, often, adnexal structures. The role of hormonal influence has been controversial. There appears to be an association with androgens (which appear to enhance keratin production), as the disorder rarely affects prepubertal women (Brown et al. 1998).

This is not a true pyoderma; rather, bacterial infection is secondary. Various staphylococci, streptococci, and Gram-negative rods can be isolated from the sinuses. Several authors have suggested that this disorder may be another cutaneous manifestation of Crohn's disease due to a significant comorbidity of the two disorders, with Crohn's disease typically preceding the onset of hidradenitis (Brown et al. 1998, Ridley et al. 1999, Tsianos et al. 1995). The disorder appears to have a genetic component.

Successful therapy depends on early diagnosis. Prognosis is associated with the extent of disease progression. Early recognition and treatment make a cure almost certain; with extensive disease, prognosis is not as favorable. Spontaneous resolution is rare.

DATABASE
SUBJECTIVE

→ Risk factors for this disorder include:
  ▪ Usually an age of 11–30 years
  ▪ Blacks are affected more often than other races.
  ▪ A pattern of family history suggesting autosomal dominant inheritance
  ▪ Residence in a hot and humid geographic region
→ Onset is gradual with early symptoms of pruritus, erythema, local hyperhidrosis.
→ Often begins with a recurrent, firm, pea-size, anogenital pustule that may rupture spontaneously.
→ Over time, multiple abscesses form with varying degrees of discomfort and resultant scarring.

→ Exacerbation of symptoms often is associated with the menstrual cycle, stress, hot weather.

→ Noticeable malodor and soiling of clothes may cause the patient to avoid social contact, sexual relationships.

→ In severe cases, physical discomfort may preclude sexual intercourse or limit ambulation.

OBJECTIVE

→ Pustular lesions vary in size, are often nodular, or there is surrounding erythema or cellulitis in any of the apocrine-bearing skin of the mons pubis, labia majora, groin, perianal area, axillae, inframammary areas, or areola of breasts.

→ Comedonal plugs, often with communicating sinus tracts

→ Hypertrophic induration, scarring, and eventual fibrosis

→ A foul-smelling, purulent discharge from draining sinuses

→ With perianal disease, there may be fistulae that drain into the anus.

→ Rarely, septicemia may develop.

ASSESSMENT

→ Hidradenitis suppurativa

→ R/O pyodermas (e.g., furuncles, carbuncles)

→ R/O infected epidermoid cysts

→ R/O pyogenic granuloma

→ R/O vulvar carcinoma (e.g., basal cell carcinoma, squamous cell carcinoma)

→ R/O sexually transmitted disease (e.g., granuloma inguinale, lymphogranuloma venereum)

→ R/O Crohn's disease

→ R/O pilonidal cyst

PLAN

DIAGNOSTIC TESTS

→ None is usually necessary. The diagnosis generally can be made on basis of history and clinical presentation.

→ A culture may be obtained for identifying pathogenic bacteria.

→ A work-up for septicemia if the patient is febrile.

TREATMENT/MANAGEMENT

→ Initiate therapy as early as possible in the course of disease to limit progression to fibrosis and scarring.

→ Instruct the patient to clean the area BID or TID with antibacterial soap (e.g., Liquid Lever 2000®, Dial®) to minimize odor by controlling commensal organisms on skin.

→ Broad-spectrum antibiotics are usually the mainstay of nonsurgical interventions; a prolonged course (usually 2–3 months) is necessary for anti-inflammatory action (Ridley et al. 1999):

- Tetracycline: 250 mg p.o. QID or 500 mg p.o. BID
- Minocycline: 100 mg p.o. BID
- Clindamycin 1% solution, lotion: Apply to affected areas BID.
- Metronidazole: 250 mg p.o. TID or 375 mg. p.o. BID

NOTE: There is a potential for blood dyscrasias with long-term use of metronidazole; monitor leukocytes before and during therapy. Advise the patient to avoid alcohol during and for 3 days after use. (See *Physicians' Desk Reference* [*PDR*].)

→ Oral retinoids have been used with equivocal results, as relapse can occur soon after discontinuation (Brown et al. 1998).

- Isotretinoin: 40–80 mg p.o. daily for 15–20 weeks

NOTE: Oral retinoids are Pregnancy Category X and should not be provided to pregnant or lactating women, or to women of reproductive age unless they are using a reliable method of contraception. Advise the patient to avoid vitamin A and alcohol. The package insert contains a sample consent form. (See *PDR*.)

→ Hormonal therapy with high-estrogenic, low-androgenic oral contraceptive pills:

- Ethinyl estradiol 35 μg, cytoproterone acetate 2 mg (Diane 35®): 1 tablet p.o. daily. This is not available in the United States but may be ordered by individuals through Canadian mail order and Internet pharmacies.
- Ethinyl estradiol 35 μg, norethindrone 0.4 mg: 1 tablet p.o. daily
- Ethinyl estradiol 30 μg, drospirenone 3 mg (Yasmin®): 1 tablet p.o. daily

→ I & D of abscesses may be necessary, ideally when the lesion(s) is/are "pointing."

→ Intralesional corticosteroid injection provides symptomatic relief in some cases:

- Triamcinolone 5 or 10 mg/mL diluted 2:1 in saline. Treatment may be repeated every 2 or 3 weeks.

→ Surgery is the definitive treatment (Brown et al. 1998).

- Often this is preceded by medical management due to the extensive nature of such surgery.
- Wide excision provides a cure only for the particular area excised.
- Healing by granulation appears to be as successful as skin grafting.
- "Unroofing" and marsupialization are commonly performed; recurrence is not uncommon with this approach.
- Carbon dioxide laser treatment may be suitable for mild to severe disease; development of contractures is less likely due to the tissue-sparing nature of this treatment.

CONSULTATION

→ Refer to a dermatologist or surgeon as appropriate for evaluation, prescription(s), or surgical management.

→ As needed for I & D of abscess formations.

→ Refer to a mental health provider for counseling related to self-image and social concerns.

PATIENT EDUCATION

→ Advise the patient to avoid irritants such as deodorants and perfumed soaps, as well as constrictive clothing and synthetic fabrics.

→ Recommend avoiding exposure to heat and activities that provoke sweating.

→ Advise obese patients that weight loss often ameliorates sweating and may improve the condition.

→ As this condition is often very disfiguring, offer psychological support and encouragement to pursue necessary treatment.

→ Encourage the patient to maintain social connections.

FOLLOW-UP

→ Tailored to the individual patient and response to therapy.

→ Document in progress notes and on problem list.

Hemangiomas

Unlike true neoplasms, *hemangiomas* are malformations of blood-vessel origin. Three forms affect the adult vulva: the cherry angioma, the angiokeratoma, and the pyogenic granuloma (Friedrich 1983).

DATABASE
SUBJECTIVE

Cherry Angioma

→ Generally asymptomatic but may bleed as a result of surface trauma.

→ Commonly appears in fourth or fifth decade of life.

→ May present as a source of postmenopausal bleeding.

Angiokeratoma

→ Most develop during childbearing years.

→ Associated with or aggravated by pregnancy.

→ Usually asymptomatic unless irritated or ulcerated as a result of trauma.

Pyogenic Granuloma

→ More rare than cherry angioma and angiokeratoma.

→ Usually arises during pregnancy (analogous to gingival granuloma). May regress postpartum but usually lingers and recurs.

→ Most symptomatic of vulvar hemangiomas, commonly with bleeding and chronic purulent exudate.

OBJECTIVE

Cherry Angioma

→ Tiny, compressible papules, usually 2–3 mm; frequently multiple; located mostly on the labia majora.

→ Bright red to dark blue color.

→ Can demonstrate blanching by running a fingernail over the lesion in a linear fashion, which may help differentiate this lesion from others.

Angiokeratoma

→ May be single or multiple; slightly lobulated, irregular, or papular with verrucous surface; located mostly on the labia majora.

→ Dark-bright red, brown, blue, purple, or black color.

→ Size range is 0.2–2.0 cm; usually not as abundant as cherry angioma.

Pyogenic Granuloma

→ Usually a single lesion with a beefy red surface, often with a raised collar of skin surrounding the base; crust may cover the lesion; may be sessile or pedunculated; located mostly on the labia majora.

→ Dull red to reddish brown color, friable if traumatized.

→ May be tender to palpation with underlying induration.

→ Size range is 0.5–2.0 cm; usually the largest of vulvar hemangiomas.

ASSESSMENT

Cherry Angioma

→ Assess as a source of postmenopausal bleeding

Angiokeratoma

→ R/O melanoma, nevi, condyloma

Pyogenic Granuloma

→ R/O basal cell carcinoma, malignant melanoma, hidradenoma

PLAN
DIAGNOSTIC TESTS

→ Excisional biopsy is warranted with angiokeratoma or pyogenic granuloma when the diagnosis is uncertain or with rapid lesion growth or bleeding.

TREATMENT/MANAGEMENT

Cherry Angioma

→ Usually requires no therapy but may be treated with excision, cryosurgery, electrocautery, or laser in cases of repeated bleeding (Friedrich 1983, Kaufman et al. 1994).

Angiokeratoma

→ Can be treated with local excision if trauma causes pain or bleeding or if the nature of the tumor cannot be clinically determined (Kaufman et al. 1994).

Pyogenic Granuloma

→ Should be treated with wide excision. If the patient is pregnant, treatment may be deferred until postpartum (Friedrich 1983, Kaufman et al. 1994).

CONSULTATION

→ As indicated for assessment of a lesion.

→ Referral to a physician may be necessary for biopsy and treatment.

→ Discuss the benign nature of lesions and indications for treatment.

FOLLOW-UP

→ As indicated following therapy, if any.
→ Pyogenic granulomas may recur.
→ Document in progress notes and on problem list.

Caruncle (Urethral)

Although not a disorder of the vulva per se, a *urethral caruncle* is commonly found during pelvic examination. Urethral caruncles develop from ectropia of the posterior urethral wall, incident to postmenopausal shrinkage of vaginal mucosa, with subsequent mucosal changes caused by trauma and environmental conditions. Other causes for caruncle development are chronic irritation and infection of the urethral meatus. The term *caruncle* has been used to describe various urethral lesions, with prolapse of the urethral mucosa the entity most often mistaken for a caruncle. Urethral mucosal prolapse is a "sliding out" of the mucosa through the external meatus and is common during premenarchal or postmenopausal years due to estrogen deficiency (Kaufman et al. 1994).

DATABASE

SUBJECTIVE

→ The patient is usually asymptomatic.
→ The patient may notice a growth or lump.
→ Pain, bleeding, dysuria, or hematuria may be present.
→ In some cases, extreme sensitivity to friction may prohibit coital activity or the wearing of undergarments.
→ Lesion size does not always correspond to degree of discomfort; even small lesions may be extremely tender. In contrast, prolapse of urethral mucosa causes little pain or discomfort.
→ Voiding difficulties may occur if edema is present.

OBJECTIVE

→ Appears as a red, fleshy tumor in the distal portion of urethral mucosa, usually at the posterior meatus; bleeds easily on contact.
→ Usually single and sessile but may be pedunculated.
→ Size ranges from a few millimeters to 1 cm.
→ Carcinoma should be suspected if there is tenderness, induration, swelling, or masses along the entire length of the urethra, together with enlarged inguinal lymph nodes (Kaufman et al. 1994).

ASSESSMENT

→ Urethral caruncle
→ R/O prolapse of the urethral mucosa
→ R/O hemangioma
→ R/O varices
→ R/O condyloma acuminata
→ R/O polyps
→ R/O carcinoma

PLAN

DIAGNOSTIC TESTS

→ Biopsy is rarely indicated but should be performed when carcinoma is suspected. Topical or locally injected anesthesia should be used before sampling. A small sample is sent for histopathological diagnosis.

TREATMENT/MANAGEMENT

→ Topical or oral estrogen may be prescribed. (See the **Perimenopausal and Menopausal Symptoms and Hormone Therapy** chapter for dosage schedules.)
→ Large or pedunculated lesions may be fulgurated or treated with laser (under local anesthesia) or cryotherapy.
→ Surgery may be required for large lesions.

CONSULTATION

→ As indicated for biopsy and/or therapy.

PATIENT EDUCATION

→ Discuss the benign nature of the condition and indications for treatment.
→ Discuss the medication regimen.

FOLLOW-UP

→ As indicated by the treatment plan.
→ Urethral caruncles may recur.
→ Document in progress notes and on problem list.

Fox-Fordyce Disease

This entity, also known as *apocrine miliaria*, is a rare disorder of the apocrine gland duct at its opening into the hair follicle. It is characterized by chronic, excessive keratinization of the follicular epithelium, multiple microcyst formation caused by rupture of the sweat ducts, and leakage of apocrine secretions into the surrounding epidermis. This results in intense pruritus, the hallmark of the disease. Although the etiology is unclear, it is believed to be associated with hormonal factors because of its onset following puberty, exacerbation with menses, and spontaneous resolution with menopause (Black et al. 2002, Kaufman et al. 1994, Miller et al. 1995).

DATABASE

SUBJECTIVE

→ Only occurs in women of reproductive age.
→ May affect the vulva, axilla, or both.
→ Symptoms include intense pruritus; may be exacerbated by the menstrual cycle, anxiety, or activities that stimulate sweating (Patrizi et al. 1998).
→ The condition often improves with pregnancy or estrogen-containing oral contraceptives.

OBJECTIVE

→ The mons pubis is most often affected; axillary involvement helps establish the diagnosis.
→ Closely grouped, discrete, tiny, flesh-colored papules ranging from 1–3 mm in diameter.
→ No surrounding erythema or induration; normal skin overlies and surrounds papules, unless there is secondary lichen simplex chronicus (squamous hyperplasia).
→ Scratch marks or lichenification may be present.

ASSESSMENT

→ Fox-Fordyce disease
→ R/O syringoma
→ R/O pediculosis pubis or scabies
→ R/O lichen simplex chronicus

PLAN

DIAGNOSTIC TESTS

→ Punch biopsy for transverse histologic sectioning

TREATMENT/MANAGEMENT

→ Effective treatment is very difficult. The following have been used with variable success (Stashower et al. 2000):
- Topical clindamycin solution containing clindamycin phosphate, 10 mg/mL in equal volume with isopropyl alcohol, propylene glycol, and water: Apply solution to affected areas BID; taper frequency of use as symptoms improve.
- Estrogen-containing oral contraceptive pills
- Triamcinolone acetonide 0.1% cream: Apply BID or TID for initial relief of pruritus. Other Group IV to V topical steroids also may be used. (See **Table 12TB.1, Potency Ranking of Some Commonly Used Topical Corticosteroids** in the **White Lesions of the Vulva** chapter.)
NOTE: Fluorinated topical steroids, such as triamcinolone acetonide, should be used cautiously due to the potential for adverse side effects. Long-term use of topical steroids may lead to atrophy, striae, telangiectasia, or steroid rebound dermatitis (Black et al. 2002).
- Tretinoin cream 0.025%: Apply at HS every other day.
→ Anti-acne measures may be helpful. (See the **Acne Vulgaris** chapter in Section 3, **Dermatological Disorders**.)

CONSULTATION

→ Refer to a dermatologist if standard interventions are ineffective.

→ As needed for prescription(s).

PATIENT EDUCATION

→ Discuss the nature of the condition and different therapies. The chronic nature of the condition may be frustrating for the patient. Offer support as indicated.

FOLLOW-UP

→ As indicated by the treatment modality and symptom recurrence.
→ Document in progress notes and on problem list.

BIBLIOGRAPHY

Black, M.M., McKay, M., Braude, P.R. et al. 2002. *Obstetric and gynecologic dermatology*, 2nd ed. London: Mosby International.

Brown, T.J., Rosen, T., and Orengo, I.F. 1998. Hidradenitis suppurativa. *Southern Medical Journal* 91(12):1107–1114.

DiSaia, P.J., and Creasman, W.T. 2002. *Clinical gynecologic oncology*, 6th ed. St. Louis, Mo.: Mosby.

Friedrich, E.G., Jr. 1983. *Vulvar disease*, 2nd ed. Philadelphia: W.B. Saunders.

Kaufman, R.H., and Faro, S. 1994. *Benign diseases of the vulva and vagina*, 4th ed. St. Louis, Mo.: Mosby Year Book.

Miller, M.L., Harford, R.R., and Yeager, J.K. 1995. Fox-Fordyce disease treated with topical clindamycin solution. *Archives of Dermatology* 131:1112–1113.

Pariser, R.J. 1998. Benign neoplasms of the skin. *Medical Clinics of North America* 82(6):1285–1307.

Patrizi, A., Orlandi, C., Neri, I. et al. 1998. Fox-Fordyce disease: two cases in patients with Turner syndrome. *Acta Dermato-Venereologica* 79:83–84.

Physicians' desk reference. 2002. Montvale, N.J.: Medical Economics.

Ridley, C.M., and Neill, S.M., eds. 1999. *The vulva*, 2nd ed. Oxford, United Kingdom: Blackwell Science.

Stashower, M.E., Krivda, S.J., and Turiansky, G.W. 2000. Fox-Fordyce disease: diagnosis with transverse histologic sections. *Journal of the American Academy of Dermatology* 42:89–91.

Toussaint, S., Salcedo, E., and Kamino, H. 1999. Benign epidermal proliferations. *Advances in Dermatology* 14:307–357.

Tsianos, E.V., Dalekos, G.N., Tzermias, C. et al. 1995. Hidradenitis suppurativa in Crohn's disease: a further support to this association. *Journal of Clinical Gastroenterology* 20(2):151–153.

Winifred L. Star, R.N., C., N.P., M.S.
Claire L. Appelmans, R.N., C., W.H.C.N.P., M.S.

12-TE Vulvar Disease
Large Lesions of the Vulva

Large lesions of the vulva most often start as small ones and thus may go unnoticed until they reach a significant size. Embarrassment and fear may prolong the delay in presenting to a clinician for care. This chapter covers *Bartholin's cyst/abscess* and *verrucous carcinoma. Squamous cell carcinoma* and *lymphogranuloma venereum* begin as ulcerative conditions and may progress to large vulvar lesions. These entities are detailed in other **Vulvar Disease** chapters and in the **Sexually Transmitted Diseases** section.

Bartholin's Cyst/Abscess

The Bartholin's glands are two mucus-secreting, glandular structures within the posterolateral vulvar vestibule that provide minimal vulvar lubrication. Cysts of the gland arise within the duct system as a result of duct occlusion, resulting in subsequent mucus retention. Most cysts are unilocular and involve the main duct; however, deeper, multilocular cysts also may form.

The cause of most cysts remains unknown, but obstruction is believed to result from various factors: congenital stenosis or atresia of the duct, thickened mucus near the duct opening, mechanical trauma, and, occasionally, improperly placed episiotomies and sutures. Although Bartholin's neoplasms are rare, Bartholin's cyst formation in a woman older than 40 years should arouse suspicion for a neoplasm (Friedrich 1983, Kaufman et al. 1994).

An abscess forms when cystic fluid becomes infected. It was originally thought that abscesses were primarily caused by gonorrheal infection, but further research has shown that a wide spectrum of organisms are involved. Most infections occur secondary to any number of anaerobic, aerobic, or facultative organisms, including *Escherichia coli*, bacteroides, proteus, and peptostreptococcus species. *Chlamydia trachomatis* also has been identified as an involved pathogen, usually recovered from the cervix. Screening for sexually transmitted infections of the abscess and the cervix remains an important part of assessment. There has been one case report in the literature of bartholinitis-associated, toxic shock-like syndrome secondary to streptococcal exotoxin (Cort 1997, Kaufman et al. 1994, Shearin et al. 1989).

DATABASE
SUBJECTIVE

Cyst

→ Patients are mostly asymptomatic.
→ Symptoms may include:
  ■ Minor discomfort during intercourse
  ■ Interference with walking, sitting, or intercourse, in the presence of larger lesions

Abscess

→ Multiple sexual partners increase the risk for a sexually infection.
→ Usually develops rapidly within 2–3 days.
→ May rupture spontaneously within 72 hours.
→ Symptoms may include:
  ■ Varying degrees of pain or tenderness
  ■ Difficulty sitting or walking
  ■ Dyspareunia
  ■ Few systemic symptoms, unless there is extensive inflammation

OBJECTIVE

Cyst

→ May be an incidental finding on routine pelvic examination.
→ Clinical features include:
  ■ Visible round or ovoid mass causing crescent-shaped vestibular entrance (posterior part of labia majora)
  ■ Nontender but tense, palpable swelling; usually unilateral
  ■ No erythema or inflammation evident
  ■ Size usually ranges from 1–4 cm but may reach 8–10 cm

Abscess

→ Clinical features include:
  ■ Very tender, fluctuant mass; usually unilateral
  ■ Edema, erythema of overlying skin

- Labial edema, distortion of labia on the affected side
- Size rarely >5 cm
- Impending rupture evidenced by an area of softening or "pointing"
→ Bilateral abscess formation suggests gonococcal infection.

ASSESSMENT

→ Bartholin's cyst
→ Bartholin's abscess
→ R/O carcinoma of Bartholin's gland
→ R/O sexually transmitted disease (STD)

PLAN

DIAGNOSTIC TESTS

→ Cultures of purulent abscess fluid and cervix for *Neisseria gonorrhoeae* and *C. trachomatis* to rule out an associated STD.
→ Additional tests may include:
- CBC in cases of severe gland infection or inflammation
- VDRL or RPR as indicated

TREATMENT/MANAGEMENT

→ Most small, asymptomatic Bartholin's cysts require no therapy.
→ Treatment is indicated for:
- Rapid cyst enlargement
- Increased pain, pressure, introital obstruction
- Hemorrhage into cyst cavity
- Abscess formation
→ The aim of therapy for both cysts and abscesses is to create

a fistulous tract from the dilated duct to the vestibule (Friedrich 1983). Options include:
- Incision and drainage (I & D) and insertion of a Word catheter (single lumen #10 catheter with a 1-inch stem and inflatable balloon, a sealed stopper on one end) provides definitive treatment for symptomatic cysts and acute abscess formation:
  - Under local anesthesia, a small incision is made into the cyst/abscess. Purulent fluid is allowed to drain out. The balloon tip is inserted into the cyst cavity, filled with 2–4 cc of water, and left in place for 30 days, with the catheter stem up in the vagina.
    – This "fistulization" method allows for patency of incision until epithelialization ensures a permanent ostium. Sitz baths several times a day initially may speed the healing process (Cort 1997, Kaufman et al. 1994). (See **Figure 12TE.1, Word Catheter Ready for Insertion (Top) and After Inflation (Bottom)** and **Figure 12TE.2, Inflatable Bulb-Tipped Catheter Used to Treat Bartholin's Cysts and Abscesses**.)
- Marsupialization for cysts with tendency for recurrent abscess formation. Under local or general anesthesia, a vertical incision is made in the vaginal mucosa over the cyst. The cyst wall is then sutured to the vaginal mucosa medially and skin of the introitus laterally, inferiorly, and superiorly. (See **Figure 12TE.3, Incision and Suturing for Marsupialization**.)
  - A permanent outlet for gland secretions remains.
  - When general anesthesia is necessary, the patient is admitted to outpatient surgery.

Figure 12TE.1.   WORD CATHETER READY FOR INSERTION (TOP) AND AFTER INFLATION (BOTTOM)

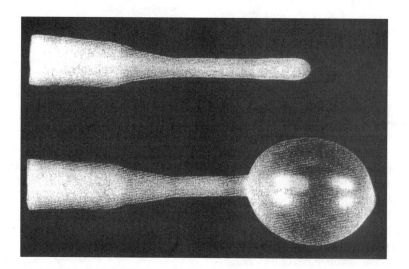

Source: Reprinted with permission from Friedrich, E.G., Jr. 1983. *Vulvar disease*, 2nd ed., p. 71. Philadelphia: W.B. Saunders.

- For persons who have acutely infected cysts, some clinicians elect to treat with antibiotics before performing this procedure (Cort 1997, Kaufman et al. 1994).
→ Broad-spectrum antibiotics may be utilized for early treatment of bartholinitis. Although this approach may provide some initial symptomatic relief and prevent further soft-tissue involvement, it also may delay ripening or pointing of the abscess (Hill et al. 1998).
  - Cephalexin: 500 mg p.o. QID for 7–14 days
  - Amoxicillin 500 mg, clavulanic acid 125 mg: 1 tablet p.o. BID for 7–14 days
→ An acute abscess treated only with sitz baths may spontaneously rupture within 72 hours; however, recurrence is likely.
→ Excision of the gland (bartholinectomy) is not recommended due to increased morbidity (cellulitis, hemorrhage, hematoma, incomplete removal and subsequent recurrence, painful scar-tissue formation) (Cort 1997).
  - This procedure is reserved for patients with huge, multilocular, or recurrent painful cysts.
→ A recently developed procedure called the *window operation* has been advocated as a more effective way to treat Bartholin's cysts and recurrent abscesses. Under local anesthesia, a small piece of skin, including the cyst wall, is excised in an oval shape. Suturing is performed along the excised margin.
  - A new mucocutaneous junction forms within 4 weeks.
  - Postoperative antibiotics are given in cases of acute inflammation (Cho et al. 1990).
→ Other treatment options include:
  - Silver nitrate insertion (Mungan et al. 1995)
  - CO_2 laser

Figure 12TE.2.   INFLATABLE BULB-TIPPED CATHETER USED TO TREAT BARTHOLIN'S CYSTS AND ABSCESSES

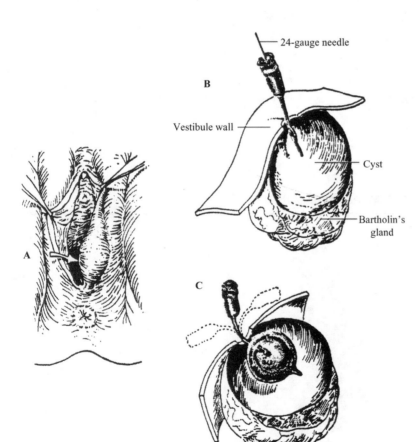

24-gauge needle

Vestibule wall

Cyst

Bartholin's gland

A. An arrow indicates the location for a stab wound in a cyst or abscess.

B. Insertion of the catheter in the stab wound.

C. Inserted catheter initiated with 2–4 mL of water.

Source: Reprinted with permission from Word, B. 1964. New instrument for office treatment of cysts and abscesses of Bartholin's glands. *Journal of the American Medical Association* 190:777–778. © 1964, American Medical Association.

→ Women older than 40 years with primary Bartholin's cyst formation should be referred to a physician for cyst removal to rule out a neoplasm.

CONSULTATION

→ Refer to a physician as indicated for the I & D procedure and placement of a Word catheter.
→ Patients with recurrent symptomatic cysts and recurrent abscess formation should be referred to a gynecologist for marsupialization.
→ Women older than 40 years with primary Bartholin's cyst formation should be referred to a physician for cyst removal to rule out a neoplasm.

PATIENT EDUCATION

→ Reassure patients who have asymptomatic cysts on routine pelvic examination that the condition is benign. Advise them to report increased cyst growth, pain, and/or obstruction interfering with daily activities or sexual intercourse.
→ Discuss the etiology and nature of an acute abscess.
→ Advise regarding STD potential and the need for STD testing and cultures of abscess.
→ Reinforce that, ideally, the Word catheter is to be left in place for 30 days. It is very difficult to replace the catheter once it falls out.
→ Detail symptom-relief measures after I & D or marsupialization. These include sitz baths, OTC analgesics (e.g., acetaminophen 325 mg p.o. every 4 hours prn pain), and rest.
→ After marsupialization, the physician should discuss follow-up measures with the patient.

→ Advise women with multiple sexual partners regarding safer sex practices. (See **Table 13A.2, Safer Sex Practices** in the **Chancroid** chapter in Section 13.)

FOLLOW-UP

→ A follow-up appointment prn and in 4–6 weeks for reassessment and removal of the Word catheter.
→ Document in progress notes and on problem list.

Verrucous Carcinoma

Verrucous carcinoma is a lesion that clinically resembles a giant condyloma, except that verrucous cells display inversion or downward growth into the dermis. This carcinoma is an unusual variant of squamous cell carcinoma. It is slow-growing and locally invasive, and tends to recur locally despite radical excision. The disease does not spread by lymphatic or hematological channels; thus, distant metastases do not occur. Its etiology is unknown. Invasive squamous cell carcinoma and vulvar intraepithelial neoplasia (VIN) may co-exist with verrucous carcinoma (DiSaia et al. 2002, Friedrich 1983, Mehta et al. 2000).

DATABASE

SUBJECTIVE

→ Seen more commonly in older women
→ Symptoms may include:
  ▪ Large, cauliflower-like growth
  ▪ Pruritus, bleeding

Figure 12TE.3.   INCISION AND SUTURING FOR MARSUPIALIZATION

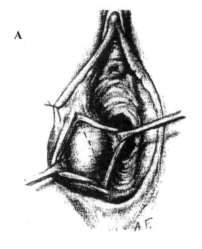 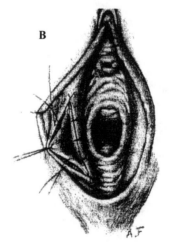

A. Incision for marsupialization.

B. Marsupialization.

Source: Tancer, M.L., Rosenberg, M., and Fernandez, D. 1956. Cysts of the vulvovaginal (Bartholin's) gland. *Obstetrics and Gynecology* 7:609. Reprinted with permission from the American College of Obstetricians and Gynecologists.

OBJECTIVE

→ Clinical features may include:
- A large/gigantic condylomatous lesion
- A dramatic appearance
- May involve extensive areas of the vulva and oral cavity
- May resemble invasive cancer

→ The vagina, cervix, uterus, adnexa, and rectum are within normal limits unless other pathologies co-exist.

ASSESSMENT

→ Verrucous carcinoma
→ R/O condyloma acuminata
→ R/O VIN
→ R/O invasive squamous cell carcinoma
→ R/O granuloma inguinale
→ R/O lymphogranuloma venereum

PLAN

DIAGNOSTIC TESTS

→ Biopsy must be done to establish a histopathological diagnosis.
→ Pap smear, STD testing, wet mounts, VDRL or RPR, and other diagnostic tests as indicated.

TREATMENT/MANAGEMENT

→ Refer to a physician for wide local excision.
→ Radiation is contraindicated, as it may convert a lesion to highly malignant cancer.
→ Acitretin: 25 mg p.o. daily has been used with some success for treating recurrence in patients who are a poor surgical risk. The dose may be decreased to 10 mg daily for maintenance therapy (Mehta et al. 2000).
→ Podophyllin, trichloroacetic acid, bichloroacetic acid are ineffective.

CONSULTATION

→ Usually sought due to the dramatic appearance of a lesion. Refer to a physician, as needed, for biopsy.
→ Refer to a gynecologist or gynecological oncologist for treatment.

PATIENT EDUCATION

→ A physician should discuss the nature of the disease and its management with the patient.
→ Psychological support is needed due to the disfiguring nature of the disease presentation.

FOLLOW-UP

→ Lesion tends to recur locally; additional surgery is warranted.
→ Semi-annual gynecological visits should be maintained.
→ Advise the patient to inspect the vulva carefully on a regular basis.
→ Document in progress notes and on problem list.

BIBLIOGRAPHY

Cho, J.Y., Ahn, M.O., and Cha, K.S. 1990. Window operation: an alternative treatment method for Bartholin's gland cysts and abscesses. *Obstetrics and Gynecology* 76:886–888.

Cort, M.B. 1997. Bartholin's gland cyst and abscess. In *Ob/Gyn Secrets*, eds. H.L. Frederickson and L. Wilkins-Haug. Philadelphia: Hanley & Belfus.

DiSaia, P.J., and Creasman, W.T. 2002. *Clinical gynecologic oncology*, 6th ed. St. Louis, Mo.: Mosby.

Friedrich, E.G., Jr. 1983. *Vulvar disease*, 2nd ed. Philadelphia: W.B. Saunders.

Grendys, E.C., and Fiorica, J.V. 2000. Innovations in the management of vulvar carcinoma. *Current Opinion in Obstetrics and Gynecology* 12:15–20.

Haley, J.C., Mirowski, G.W., and Hood, A.F. 1998. Benign vulvar tumors. *Seminars in Cutaneous Medicine and Surgery* 17(3):196–204.

Hill, D.A., and Lense, J.J. 1998. Office management of Bartholin gland cysts and abscesses. *American Family Physician* 57(7):1611–1616.

Kaufman, R.H., and Faro, S. 1994. *Benign diseases of the vulva and vagina*, 4th ed. St. Louis, Mo.: Mosby Year Book.

Mehta, R.K., Rytina, E., and Sterling, J.C. 2000. Treatment of verrucous carcinoma of vulva with acitretin. *British Journal of Dermatology* 142:1195–1198.

Morgan, M.A., and Mikuta, J.J. 1999. Surgical management of vulvar cancer. *Seminars in Surgical Oncology* 17:168–172.

Morrow, C.P., and Curtin, J.P. 1998. *Synopsis of gynecologic oncology*, 5th ed. Philadelphia: Churchill Livingstone.

Mungan, T., Ugur, M., Yalçin, H. et al. 1995. Treatment of Bartholin's cyst and abscess: excision versus silver nitrate insertion. *European Journal of Obstetrics and Reproductive Biology* 63:61–63.

Shearin, R.S., Boehlke, J., and Karanth, S. 1989. Toxic shock-like syndrome associated with Bartholin's gland abscess: case report. *American Journal of Obstetrics and Gynecology* 160:1073–1074.

Word, B. 1964. New instrument for office treatment of cysts and abscesses of Bartholin's gland. *Journal of the American Medical Association* 190:777–778.

Winifred L. Star, R.N., C., N.P., M.S.
Claire L. Appelmans, R.N., C., W.H.C.N.P., M.S.

12-TF   Vulvar Disease
Ulcerative Lesions of the Vulva

Ulcers form as a result of a defect in skin integrity caused by localized destruction of both the epidermis and dermis. Strictly speaking, when only the epidermis is involved, the lesion should be referred to as an erosion. Most ulcerative lesions of the vulva are the result of an infectious process, with sexually transmitted diseases (STDs) heading the list. Most noninfectious vulvar ulcers are associated with primary dermatologic diseases. However, any open genital lesion is susceptible to bacterial or fungal superinfection that may contribute to ulceration, depending on the patient's health status. Genital ulcers may appear as solitary, multiple, or granulomatous, or as "heaped up" (Black et al. 2002).

Carcinomas of the vulva may present as ulcerative lesions and should be considered in the differential diagnosis of ulcerative lesions, especially when the appearance of the lesion changes little over time (Friedrich 1983).

This chapter will cover *squamous cell carcinoma* and *basal cell carcinoma*. Additional ulcerative lesions affecting the vulva—such as herpes simplex, syphilis, chancroid, lymphogranuloma venereum, and granuloma inguinale—are covered in the **Sexually Transmitted Diseases** section.

Squamous Cell Carcinoma

Malignancies of the vulva account for 3–5% of all genital cancers in women and 1–2% of all female cancers in general. There are various histologies and wide differences in the biological behaviors of these tumors. The largest group is made up of squamous cell carcinomas. Other carcinomas of the vulva include basal cell carcinoma, verrucous carcinoma, and malignant melanoma. (See the **Large Lesions of the Vulva** and **Dark Lesions of the Vulva** chapters.)

Invasive squamous cell carcinoma arises from the squamous epithelium of the skin and mucous membrane of the vulva (between the vaginal introitus and the outer labia majora). The cancer affects mainly women older than 60 years; however, the disease has recently occurred in younger age groups (15% of cases are in women under age 40 years). Environmental factors, smoking, and viral infection—especially with human papillo-mavirus (HPV)—play a role in the etiology of this disease when it occurs in younger women. In many cases, the initial lesion appears to arise from an area of vulvar intraepithelial neoplasia (VIN). Among older women, squamous cell vulvar cancer usually arises from a background of non-neoplastic epithelial disorders. Fifteen to 20% of patients may have an antecedent, concomitant, or subsequent cervical carcinoma that is either in situ or invasive (Ansink 1996, Crum et al. 1997, DiSaia et al. 2002, Jones et al. 1997).

If left untreated, vulvar squamous cell carcinoma has potentially disabling and fatal consequences, but early diagnosis and treatment may mean a cure. Unfortunately, the disease state in most cases is quite advanced at the time of diagnosis. Local extension of the malignancy to the urethra, perineum, vagina, and anorectum is common. In more advanced stages, the pubic bone, skin of the leg, and bladder may become involved. The hallmark of the disease is lymphatic spread that is systematic and predictable, first to the superficial groin nodes and then to the deeper pelvic-wall lymphatics (DiSaia et al. 2002, Jones et al. 1997).

Several different methods have been devised to determine the depth of tumor invasion in superficially invasive disease. Microinvasive squamous cell carcinoma (Stage la) has been defined by the International Society for the Study of Vulvar Disease as a lesion ≤2 cm in diameter with ≤1 mm of stromal invasion (Wilkinson et al. 1986). Because the risk of lymph-node metastasis in these cases is minimal, radical therapy can be avoided (Jones et al. 1997, Van der Velden et al. 1996).

For advanced tumors, staging of vulvar cancer is done utilizing the FIGO (International Federation of Gynecology and Obstetrics) system, which incorporates a TNM (tumor-node-metastasis) classification. Patients are staged based on the size and location of the lesion, the clinical status of inguinal nodes, and the presence or absence of demonstrable metastases (DiSaia et al. 2002, Morrow et al. 1998). (See **Table 12TF.1, International Federation of Gynecology and Obstetrics (FIGO) Staging of Invasive Cancer of the Vulva.**)

The prime factor determining the patient's prognosis is the presence or absence of inguinal-node metastasis. A risk-scoring formula developed by the Gynecology Oncology Group (GOG) also has been utilized to identify patients at low risk for metastases or recurrence, allowing for more conservative therapy. The GOG criteria continue to be evaluated. About 20% of patients with positive groin nodes will have pelvic lymph node metastases; the pelvic nodes are almost never affected without groin node involvement (DiSaia et al. 2002, Morrow et al. 1998).

Survival depends on the extent of disease at the time of diagnosis. The five-year survival rate after complete surgical intervention—radical vulvectomy plus inguinal and pelvic lymphadenectomy—for Stages I and II disease is approximately 90%. In contrast, only 20% of patients with pelvic node metastases will survive five years or more. Recurrences are usually seen within 1–2 years after therapy. Local recurrences are more common than distant ones and are usually near the site of the primary lesion (DiSaia et al. 2002, Morrow et al. 1998).

Surgical treatment of the disease varies and depends on clinical staging. The undesirable effects of radical vulvectomy include sex-organ removal, potential wound-healing complications, and lymphedema. Increasingly, less radical surgical approaches—especially in younger patients—are gaining favor. Psychosexual alterations may be a major component of recovery, and ongoing support is vital for patient acceptance of her changed body image.

DATABASE

SUBJECTIVE

→ Risk factors may include:
- Chronic vulvar irritation or pruritus; chronic rubbing or scratching
- VIN
- HPV infection
- History of non-neoplastic disorder (e.g., lichen sclerosus with squamous cell hyperplasia)
- Obesity, diabetes, hypertension, arteriosclerosis; may reflect increased incidence with aging
- Low socioeconomic status
- Immunodeficiency; may exist in younger subsets of women

Table 12TF.1. **INTERNATIONAL FEDERATION OF GYNECOLOGY AND OBSTETRICS (FIGO) STAGING OF INVASIVE CANCER OF THE VULVA**

Stage 0	Tis			Carcinoma in situ, intraepithelial carcinoma
Stage I	T1	N0	M0	Tumor confined to the vulva and/or perineum—2 cm or less in greatest dimension (no nodal metastasis)
Stage Ia				Lesions 2 cm or less in size confined to the vulva or perineum and with stromal invasion no greater than 1.0 mm* (no nodal metastasis)
Stage Ib				Lesions 2 cm or less in size confined to the vulva or perineum and with stromal invasion greater than 1.0 mm (no nodal metastasis)
Stage II	T2	N0	M0	Tumor confined to the vulva and/or perineum—more than 2 cm in greatest dimension (no nodal metastasis)
Stage III	T3	N0	M0	Tumor of any size with
	T3	N1	M0	(1) Adjacent spread to the lower urethra and/or the vagina, or the anus, and/or
	T1	N1	M0	(2) Unilateral regional lymph node metastasis
	T2	N1	M0	
Stage IVa	T1	N2	M0	Tumor invades any of the following: upper urethra, bladder mucosa, rectal mucosa,
	T2	N2	M0	pelvic bone, and/or bilateral regional node metastasis
	T3	N2	M0	
	T4	Any N	M0	
Stage IVb	Any T	Any N	M1	Any distant metastasis including pelvic lymph nodes

*The depth of invasion is defined as the measurement of the tumor from the epithelial-stromal junction of the adjacent most superficial papilla to the deepest point of invasion.

Source: Adapted with permission from DiSaia, P.J., and Creasman, W.T. 2002. *Clinical gynecologic oncology*, 6th ed., p. 217. St. Louis, Mo.: Mosby.

→ Classically occurs in women 60–70 years old; 15% of cases are in women younger than 40 years; no racial predisposition.

→ No remission or exacerbation.

→ A woman may have had symptoms for 2–16 months before seeking attention. Often the patient has undergone medical treatment for 12 months or longer without biopsy or referral for definitive diagnosis.

→ Up to 20% of cases are asymptomatic.

→ Symptoms may include:

  ▪ Chronic, long-term pruritus
  ▪ Lump, mass (more than 50% of cases), ulcer, warty growth
  ▪ External dysuria
  ▪ Contact bleeding
  ▪ Vague discomfort or pain

→ A complete health history should be taken.

OBJECTIVE

→ Most lesions are on the labia majora, labia minora, or clitoris, but any vulvar site is possible.

→ One-third of tumors are bilateral or midline (increased incidence of nodal spread).

→ Lesions may have *widely* variable presentation:

  ▪ Size varies from <1 cm to very large
  ▪ Usually unifocal, localized, well-demarcated
  ▪ May be multifocal or confluent (less often)
  ▪ White, pink, red, or pigmented
  ▪ Flat, nodular, papular, or exophytic
  ▪ Edges may be sharply rolled with underlying induration
  ▪ Dry or exudative
  ▪ Ulcerated (one-third of cases)
  ▪ Friable, bleeding
  ▪ Painless or tender
  ▪ Possible secondary infection

→ Physical examination should include careful assessment of:

  ▪ The extent of the lesion: Visual inspection should note the proximity to the urethra, vagina, labial-crural folds, and anus.
  ▪ The mobility of the lesion: Palpate well.
  ▪ The skin of the inguinal area, mons pubis, perineum: Palpate for associated lesion, nodules.
  ▪ Inguinal lymph nodes: Inspect and palpate well; note enlargement, fixation, ulceration, suppuration (indicates advanced disease).
  ▪ Integrity of pelvic floor
  ▪ Peripheral pulses
  ▪ The uterus, adnexa, and rectum for abnormalities

→ A good description and diagram of the lesion are important.

ASSESSMENT

→ Squamous cell carcinoma

→ R/O VIN

→ R/O non-neoplastic epithelial disorder

→ R/O syphilis

→ R/O granuloma inguinale

→ R/O lymphogranuloma venereum

→ R/O genital herpes simplex

→ R/O condyloma acuminata

→ R/O tuberculosis of the vulva

→ R/O concomitant vaginal/cervical neoplasia

PLAN

DIAGNOSTIC TESTS

→ Biopsy must be obtained to establish a histopathological diagnosis. Punch biopsy (under local anesthesia) from the center of the lesion may be undertaken if the lesion is small. Lesions ≤1 cm may be totally excised under local anesthesia; consult with or refer to a physician.

→ Pap smear, STD testing, wet mounts, VDRL or RPR, and other diagnostic tests as indicated.

→ Colposcopy of the vagina and cervix should be performed to rule out concomitant neoplasia.

→ Cystoscopy and/or anoscopy should be performed if bladder or rectal involvement is suspected.

→ Preoperative studies vary and depend on the extent of disease and general health of the patient. Additional tests may include CBC, urinalysis, complete biochemical profile, chest x-ray, EKG, proctoscopy, barium enema, intravenous pyelogram, bone scan, and CT scan.

TREATMENT/MANAGEMENT

→ Refer the patient to a gynecological oncologist.

→ Treatment is individualized based on lesion size, location, depth of tumor invasion, lymphatic involvement, health and wishes of the patient, condition of the unaffected vulva, the presence or absence of other gynecological problems, and other sites of genital tract neoplasia (Morrow et al. 1998).

→ Treatment options include (DiSaia et al. 2002):

  ▪ Wide local excision
  ▪ Wide local excision with superficial inguinal lymphadenectomy
  ▪ Simple (unilateral) vulvectomy with unilateral or bilateral inguinal lymphadenectomy
  ▪ Radical vulvectomy with unilateral or bilateral inguinal and pelvic lymphadenectomy
  ▪ Combined radiation and surgery. Radiation alone is not used as primary therapy but may be used for inoperable, locally recurrent disease
  ▪ Pelvic exenteration for advanced disease
  ▪ Chemotherapy (under investigation)

CONSULTATION

→ As necessary for initial assessment.

→ Referral to a physician for initial biopsy procedure may be necessary.

→ Refer to a gynecologist or gynecological oncologist for treatment.

PATIENT EDUCATION

→ The physician responsible for the patient's care should discuss the etiology and nature of the condition with her and outline the details of management. Components include surgical alternatives, potential complications, recovery, and sexuality issues.

→ Despite the potentially overwhelming nature of the disease, successful treatment with acceptable morbidity and long-term survival are possible. Hope is an important message.

→ Psychosocial support is extremely important for the patient's ongoing health and well-being. An advanced practice nurse in oncology may be utilized for patient education and support. Referrals for psychosexual counseling may be necessary for successful recovery and ability to cope.

FOLLOW-UP

→ The patient generally will be followed by the physician responsible for her care. Specific return visits are scheduled according to the individual patient's needs and site-specific clinical practices.

→ Biopsy of any recurring, suspicious-appearing lesions should be undertaken promptly.

→ Document in the progress notes and on problem list.

Basal Cell Carcinoma

Basal cell carcinoma is a locally invasive malignancy that generally does not metastasize. It is commonly found on exposed body surfaces but is rare on the vulva, accounting for only 2–3% of all vulvar cancer. General cure rates are 100%, and if margins are tumor-free, the prognosis is excellent. Regional lymph nodes and lungs have been affected in some cases. Local recurrences are common—they occur in about 20% of cases. A mixed basal-squamous cell carcinoma also may exist; this lesion has a poorer prognosis than pure basal cell carcinoma alone (Benedet et al. 1997, Feakins et al. 1997).

There are multiple theories about the histogenesis of the disorder; a discussion is beyond the scope of this chapter. The tumor's origin is thought to be immature, incompletely differentiated, "pluripotential" cells of the basal epithelium, hair shaft, or glands (Kaufman et al. 1994).

DATABASE

SUBJECTIVE

→ Most often affects Caucasian women in the postmenopausal years; median age is 63 years.

→ The patient may be asymptomatic.

→ Symptoms may include:
- Pruritus, irritation, or burning
- The presence of a nodule or mass
- Chronic ulceration
- Bleeding or discharge if the lesion is large

OBJECTIVE

→ Lesions are usually found on the labia majora; other sites may include the labia minora, clitoris, mons pubis, and posterior fourchette.

→ Clinical presentation may include:

- Pearly, "rolled edge," or "rodent" ulcer (one-third of basal cell carcinomas present as ulcers)
- A polypoid or nodular lesion usually <2 cm in diameter
- Red or brown pigmentation that can present as a freckle-like lesion
- Necrotic debris or crusts may appear at the lesion base.
- Secondary infection may occur with subsequent ipsilateral inguinal adenopathy.

→ The lesion may extend beyond the limits of physical borders. A good description and diagram of the lesion are important.

→ The vagina, cervix, uterus, adnexa, and rectum are WNL unless other pathologies co-exist.

ASSESSMENT

→ Basal cell carcinoma
→ R/O mixed basal-squamous cell carcinoma
→ R/O concomitant squamous cell carcinoma
→ R/O syphilis
→ R/O nevus
→ R/O melanoma
→ R/O genital herpes simplex
→ R/O hidradenitis suppurativa

PLAN

DIAGNOSTIC TESTS

→ Biopsy must be done to establish a histopathological diagnosis. Consult with or refer to a physician.

→ Pap smear, STD testing, wet mounts, VDRL or RPR, and other diagnostic tests as indicated.

TREATMENT/MANAGEMENT

→ Wide and deep local excision, including area of normal-appearing tissue, is the treatment of choice. Multiple sections through the tumor should be excised to rule out concomitant squamous cell carcinoma or melanoma. Refer to a physician.

→ Lymph node dissection is individualized depending on the potential for metastasis.

→ 5-fluorouracil is not recommended, as it may mask invasive basal cell cancer.

CONSULTATION

→ As necessary for initial assessment of a lesion.
→ Refer to a physician for biopsy as necessary.
→ Refer to a gynecologist or gynecological oncologist for treatment.

PATIENT EDUCATION

→ The physician responsible for the patient's care should discuss both the etiology and the nature of the condition with her and detail the particulars of management.

FOLLOW-UP

→ Because recurrence is fairly common, ongoing clinical

observation of the vulvar area should be done at least semi-annually.

→ Advise the patient to inspect her vulvar area regularly.

→ Recurrent tumors may require more aggressive therapy.

→ Document in progress notes and on problem list.

BIBLIOGRAPHY

Ansink, A. 1996. Vulvar squamous cell carcinoma. *Seminars in Dermatology* 15(1):51–59.

Apgar, B.S., and Cox, J.T. 1996. Differentiating normal and abnormal findings of the vulva. *American Family Physician* 53(4):1171–1180.

Barclay, D.L. 1991. Premalignant and malignant disorders of the vulva and vagina. In *Current obstetric and gynecologic diagnosis and treatment*, 7th ed., ed. M.L. Pernoll, pp. 923–936. Norwalk, Conn.: Appleton & Lange.

Benedet, J.L., Miller, D.M., Ehlen, T.G. et al. 1997. Basal cell carcinoma of the vulva: clinical features and treatment results in 28 patients. *Obstetrics and Gynecology* 90(5): 765–768.

Black, M.M., McKay, M., Braude, P.R. et al. 2002. *Obstetric and gynecologic dermatology*, 2nd ed. London: Mosby International.

Crum, C.P., McLachlin, C.M., Tate, J.E. et al. 1997. Pathobiology of vulvar squamous neoplasia. *Current Opinions in Obstetrics and Gynecology* 9:63–69.

DiSaia, P.J., and Creasman, W.T. 2002. *Clinical gynecologic oncology*, 6th ed. St. Louis, Mo.: Mosby.

Feakins, R.M., and Lowe, D.G. 1997. Basal cell carcinoma of the vulva. *International Journal of Gynecological Pathology* 16(4):319–324.

Friedrich, E.G., Jr. 1983. *Vulvar disease*, 2nd ed. Philadelphia: W.B. Saunders.

Grendys, E.C., and Fiorica, J.V. 2000. Innovations in the management of vulvar carcinoma. *Current Opinion in Obstetrics and Gynecology* 12:15–20.

Hall, J.C. 2000. *Sauer's manual of skin diseases*, 8th ed. Philadelphia: Lippincott Williams & Wilkins.

Jones, R.W., Baranyai, J., and Stables, S. 1997. Trends in squamous cell carcinoma of the vulva: the influence of vulvar intraepithelial neoplasia. *Obstetrics and Gynecology* 90(3):448–452.

Kaufman, R.H., and Faro, S. 1994. *Benign diseases of the vulva and vagina*, 4th ed. St. Louis, Mo.: Mosby Year Book.

Morgan, M.A., and Mikuta, J.J. 1999. Surgical management of vulvar cancer. *Seminars in Surgical Oncology* 17:168–172.

Morrow, C.P., and Curtin, J.P. 1998. *Synopsis of gynecologic oncology*, 5th ed. Philadelphia: Churchill Livingstone.

Piura, B., Rabinovich, A., and Dgani, R. 1999. Basal cell carcinoma of the vulva. *Journal of Surgical Oncology* 70: 172–176.

Ridley, C.M., and Neill, S.M., eds. 1999. *The vulva*, 2nd ed. Oxford, United Kingdom: Blackwell Science.

Van der Velden, J., and Hacker, N. 1996. Prognostic factors in squamous cell cancer of the vulva and the implications for treatment. *Current Opinion in Obstetrics and Gynecology* 8:3–7.

Wilkinson, E.J., Kneale, B., and Lynch, P.J. 1986. Report of the International Society for the Study of Vulvar Disease, Terminology Committee. *Journal of Reproductive Medicine* 31:973.

Winifred L. Star, R.N., C., N.P., M.S.
Mary M. Rubin, R.N., C., PH.D., C.R.N.P.

12-TG Vulvar Disease
Vulvar Intraepithelial Neoplasia

Vulvar intraepithelial neoplasia (VIN), a premalignant condition characterized by disorganized epithelial maturation, nuclear enlargement, and nuclear atypia, has been recognized since the early twentieth century. It may include partial involvement of the epithelial layer or extend throughout its full thickness. By definition, VIN is confined to the epithelial layer above the basement membrane of the epidermis with no extension to the underlying dermis (Trimble et al. 1996).

Vulvar intraepithelial disorders have been grouped as follows (Committee on Terminology of the International Society for the Study of Vulvar Disease 1990, Wilkinson et al. 1986):

I. Squamous (may include human papillomavirus [HPV] change)
A. VIN 1 (mild dysplasia)
B. VIN 2 (moderate dysplasia)
C. VIN 3 (severe dysplasia or carcinoma in situ)
II. Other
A. Paget's disease (intraepithelial)
B. Melanoma in situ, level I.

The International Society of Vulvar Disease is considering a change in terminology but has not yet come to a consensus.

In the past, VIN 3 was referred to by various names: *Bowen's disease, Bowenoid papulosis, carcinoma in situ simplex, erythroplasia of Queyrat,* and *squamous cell carcinoma in situ.* To mitigate the confusion with nomenclature and because the biology and histology of all of these entities are indistinguishable, today the more appropriately used terminology is VIN (Wilkinson 1994, Wilkinson et al. 1995).

The etiology of VIN is essentially unknown, but its increasing incidence in younger women, multifocal distribution, and association with other lower genital tract neoplasia suggest a possible viral origin (Basta et al. 1999). Unlike the continuum from pre-invasive to invasive disease in cervical neoplasia, evidence for the same progression has not been clearly established for vulvar neoplasia (Jones et al. 1997).

Neoplasia results from cellular changes precipitated by an oncogenic stimulus, which is then modified by the host reaction.

The chromosomal makeup of the epithelial cell's deoxyribonucleic acid is altered, new cell properties emerge, and uncontrolled replication occurs. The incidence of VIN has dramatically increased over the last 20 years (Iverson et al. 1998). The disease now affects younger women, most of whom are younger than 50 years. VIN is closely associated with the presence of HPV, especially HPV-16 and HPV-18. Careful inspection of the entire lower genital tract is warranted, as carcinoma in situ of the cervix is an associated finding in approximately 20% of patients with VIN; in addition, vaginal and anal neoplasia may co-exist (Singer et al. 2000, Wilkinson et al. 1995).

Although the malignant potential of VIN appears to be low, progression of VIN 3 to cancer does occur (Ghurani et al. 2001). Early invasive disease is seen in 6–10% of patients with VIN, with elderly and immunocompromised women at increased risk (Abercrombie et al. 1998). Progression of VIN to invasive carcinoma may occur over time, but the frequency is unknown; it is estimated to be about 2–4% (Gross et al. 1997). Aggressiveness of the lesions cannot be based on clinical factors such as symptoms, lesion location, and past history. Depending on host defense mechanisms in some patients, there is also a possibility that VIN will not progress to an invasive disease state if left untreated. (See the chapters **White Lesions of the Vulva ["Lichen Sclerosus"], Red Lesions of the Vulva ["Paget's Disease"],** and **Dark Lesions of the Vulva ["Melanoma"]**.)

DATABASE

SUBJECTIVE

→ Potential risk factors may include (Gordon 1993, Singer et al. 2000):
- Intraepithelial neoplasia in other lower genital tract sites
- HPV infection
- Multiple sexual partners
- Smoking
- Immunodeficiency
- Chronic vulvar irritation
- Lighter skin pigmentation

→ Onset is generally in women younger than 50 years. It can occur in teenagers and women in their 20s.
→ 50% of women are asymptomatic.
→ Symptoms may include (Gordon 1993, Wright et al. 1995):
  ■ Pruritus (most common)
  ■ Vulvar pain, irritation, burning, swelling
  ■ Recalcitrant vulvar warts, lumps, nodules, tumor
  ■ Bleeding, discharge, vulvar ulceration
  ■ Vulvar discoloration
  ■ Dyspareunia
  ■ Urinary tract symptoms

OBJECTIVE

→ Lesions, possibly subtle, may first be noted during routine pelvic examination.
→ The distribution of lesions may include:
  ■ Labia minora
  ■ Perineum
  ■ Perianal
  ■ Labia majora
  ■ Clitoris
→ Multifocal distribution is more common in 30–50-year-olds. Malignant transformation is <5% unless the patient is immunodeficient.
→ Unifocal distribution is more common in postmenopausal women, especially those older than 60 years. The incidence of superficial invasion is greater in this age group.
→ VIN I-II lesions (Singer et al. 2000):
  ■ Well-localized and delineated
  ■ Slightly elevated, white, and rough
  ■ Red-brown hue and/or red and white patches (less common)
→ VIN III lesions (Singer et al. 2000):
  ■ Widely variable appearance
  ■ Papular or macular
  ■ Multifocal or unifocal; extensive areas may be involved
  ■ Red, moist, crusted, sharply demarcated
  ■ Small, isolated red or white patch
  ■ Distinct white hyperkeratotic "leukoplakia" patches
  ■ Combination of red and white areas with superficial scaling
  ■ Condyloma-like
  ■ Hyperpigmented, entirely or at lesion margins
→ Lesions that are ulcerated, indurated, granular, raised, and irregular may indicate invasive disease.
→ The vagina, cervix, uterus, adnexa, and rectum are within normal limits unless there is co-existent pathology.
→ A good description, diagram, and/or photograph of the lesion is important.

ASSESSMENT

→ VIN
→ R/O condyloma
→ R/O invasive cancer
→ R/O other dermatological conditions

PLAN

DIAGNOSTIC TESTS

→ Early diagnosis depends on regular, careful examination of the vulva. An index of suspicion for VIN is an important parameter. White, fissured, ulcerated, nodular, or abnormally raised areas should be biopsied.
→ Histological evaluation of biopsy specimens from suspicious lesions will render a definitive diagnosis. Delineation of the extent of disease is critical and invasion must be ruled out (Burghardt et al. 1998).
  ■ The use of toluidine blue may be of some value in determining biopsy sites, especially with a single, extensive lesion or multiple lesions. However, it can often lead to confusion due to the sensitive and nonspecific nature of the nuclear staining. Often, areas of inflammation may result in false positive staining (Stone et al. 1993).
  ■ Multiple biopsy samples with the Keyes punch or a small punch forceps may be necessary.
→ Colposcopy of the vulva after the application of 3–5% acetic acid may be the most useful approach to identify sites for biopsy. Due to the multicentric aspect of disease of the lower genital tract, the clinician should perform colposcopy of the vagina, cervix, and perianal region to rule out concomitant intraepithelial neoplasia (Anderson et al. 1997, Audisio et al. 1999, Giuntoli et al. 1987, Singer et al. 2000).
→ Careful inspection of the anal canal via proctoscopy is indicated when carcinoma in situ involves the perineum.
→ Determination of skin appendage involvement must be made.
NOTE: In most settings, diagnostic evaluation usually is performed by a physician or an advanced practice clinician; however, practices may vary. Biopsy and colposcopic procedures should be performed by a properly trained, experienced practitioner.
→ Pap smear, genital cultures, sexually transmitted disease testing, wet mounts, and other diagnostic tests as indicated.

TREATMENT/MANAGEMENT

→ If VIN is confirmed, refer the patient to a physician for treatment.
→ Treatment should be individualized based on the patient's age and wishes, location and extent of the lesion, and factors that may increase the risk of invasive disease.
→ Preferred treatment options include (Burghardt et al. 1998, Campion et al. 1991, Julian et al. 1996, Singer et al. 2000):
  ■ Wide local excision: used when VIN diagnosis is indefinite or when invasion cannot be ruled out.
  ■ CO_2 laser vaporization: performed under local anesthesia with colposcopic guidance. It is the most popular therapy after invasion has definitely been ruled out. The therapy may be carried out in stages if the lesion is large. General anesthesia may be necessary if large areas are treated at one time.
  ■ Skinning vulvectomy (with or without skin graft): indicated when VIN is extensive. Refer the patient to a gynecological oncologist skilled in this technique.

→ Alternate (but less acceptable) therapies:
- Topical 5-fluorouracil 2–5%: rarely used due to extreme patient discomfort, poor efficacy, low compliance with the treatment regimen, and high recurrence rates.
- Cryotherapy
- Electrotherapy

NOTE: Occult, invasive squamous cell carcinoma must be ruled out before any local medical or mechanical destructive therapy.

CONSULTATION

→ Referral to a physician often will be necessary for lesion evaluation and an extensive biopsy.

→ Referral to a gynecologist or gynecological oncologist will be necessary to administer specific therapies for extensive pre-invasive or invasive disease.

PATIENT EDUCATION

→ Primary health care providers may discuss the etiology and nature of the disease with the patient. There may also be a preliminary discussion of treatment modalities. The physician responsible for treatment and care should detail the particulars of management and necessary follow-up.

→ As HPV infection is associated with this condition, advise safer sex practices to prevent sexually transmitted diseases. (See **Table 13A.2, Safer Sex Guidelines** in the **Chancroid** chapter in Section 13.)

FOLLOW-UP

→ Long-term follow-up is necessary due to the relatively high risk of recurrence.

→ Site-specific guidelines for follow-up may vary. In general, follow-up examinations include careful visual inspection; colposcopy of the vulva, vagina, and cervix; and a Pap smear every 3–6 months for two years (Spitzer 1999).

→ Psychosexual counseling may be indicated for patients who have an HPV-related VIN diagnosis and for those undergoing significant vulvar surgery.

→ Photograph with colposcopic equipment if it is available.

→ Document in progress notes and on problem list.

BIBLIOGRAPHY

Abercrombie, P.D., and Korn, A.P. 1998. Vulvar intraepithelial neoplasia in women with HIV. *AIDS Patient Care STDs* 12(4):251–254.

Anderson, M., Jordan, J., Morse, A. et al. 1997. *A text and atlas of integrated colposcopy*. St. Louis, Mo.: Mosby.

Audisio, T., Zarazaga, J., and Vainer, O. 1999. A classification of vulvoscopic findings for clinical diagnosis. *Journal of Lower Genital Tract Disease* 3(1):7–18.

Basta, A., Adamek, K., and Pitynski, K. 1999. Intraepithelial neoplasia and early stage vulvar cancer clinical and virological observations. *European Journal of Gynecologic Oncology* 20(2):111–114.

Burghardt, E., Pickel, H., and Girardi, F. 1998. *Colposcopy—cervical pathology textbook and atlas*, 3rd ed. New York: Thieme.

Campion, M. J., Ferris, D., diPaola, F. et al. 1991. *Modern colposcopy: a practical approach*. Augusta, Ga.: Educational Systems.

Committee on Terminology of the International Society for the Study of Vulvar Disease. 1990. New nomenclature for vulvar disease. *Journal of Reproductive Medicine* 35:483–484.

Ghurani, G.B., and Penalver, M.A. 2001. An update on vulvar cancer. *American Journal of Obstetrics and Gynecology* 185(2):294–299.

Giuntoli, R., Atkinson, B., Ernst, C. et al. 1987. *Atkinson's correlative atlas of colposcopy, cytology, and histopathology*. Philadelphia: J.B. Lippincott.

Gordon, A.N. 1993. Vulvar neoplasms. In *Textbook of gynecology*, ed. L.J. Copeland, pp. 1096–1116. Philadelphia: W.B. Saunders.

Gross, G., and Barasso, R. 1997. *Human papillomavirus infection: a clinical atlas*. Berlin and Wiesbaden, Germany: Ulstein-Mosby.

Iverson, T., and Tretli, S. 1998. Intraepithelial and invasive squamous neoplasia of the vulva in incidence, recurrence, and survival rate in Norway. *Obstetrics and Gynecology* 91(6):969–972.

Jones, R.W., Baranyai, J., and Stables, S. 1997. Trends in squamous cell cancer of the vulva: the influence of vulvar intraepithelial neoplasia. *Obstetrics and Gynecology* 90(3):448–452.

Julian, T., and Grosen E. 1996. The modern management of multifocal vulvar intraepithelial neoplasia III. *Colposcopist* 27(2):1–3.

Singer, A., and Monaghan, J.M. 2000. *Lower genital tract precancer: colposcopy, pathology, and treatment*, 2nd ed. London: Blackwell Science.

Spitzer, M. 1999. Lower genital tract intraepithelial neoplasia in HIV infected women: guidelines for evaluation and treatment. *Obstetrics and Gynecology Survey* 54(2):131–137.

Stone, K.I., and Wilkinson, E.J. 1993. Benign and pre-invasive lesions of the vulva and vagina. In *Textbook of gynecology*, ed. L.J. Copeland, pp. 871–888. Philadelphia: W.B. Saunders.

Trimble, C.L., Trimble, E.L., and Woodruff, J.D. 1996. Diseases of the vulva. In *Clinical gynecologic pathology*, eds. E. Hernandez and B. Atkinson, pp. 1–90. Philadelphia: W.B. Saunders.

Wilkinson, E.J. 1994. Premalignant and malignant tumors of the vulva. In *Blaustein's pathology of the female genital tract*, 4th ed., ed. R.J. Kurman, pp. 87–129. New York: Springer-Verlag.

Wilkinson, E.J., Kneale, B., and Lynch, P.J. 1986. Report of the International Society for the Study of Vulvar Disease, Terminology Committee. *Journal of Reproductive Medicine* 31:973.

Wilkinson, E.J., and Stone, I.K. 1995. *Atlas of vulvar disease*. New York: Williams & Wilkins.

Wright, C., Lickrish, G., and Shier, M. 1995. *Basic and advanced colposcopy*. Komoka, Canada: Biomedical Communications.

Winifred L. Star, R.N., C., N.P., M.S.
Linda K. Humphrey, R.N., C., N.P., C.N.S., M.S.

12-TH Vulvar Disease

Vulvodynia

The International Society for the Study of Vulvar Disease (ISSVD) defines *vulvodynia* as chronic vulvar discomfort often characterized by burning, stinging, irritation, or rawness of the vulva (ISSVD Committee 1991). The incidence and prevalence are unknown, and many etiologies have been implicated. The characteristics of vulvodynia, established originally in 1977 by Dodson and Friedrich, include persistent symptoms of longstanding duration, lack of demonstrable pathology, sexual inactivity as a result of symptoms, unsuccessful consultation with multiple physicians, "allergy" to common vaginal preparations, reluctance to accept a psychophysiological cause, and emotional lability or dependency (Lynch 1986).

The approach to vulvodynia has changed since the initial parameters were set up, and continued investigation attempts to establish more appropriate definitions of the disorder. McKay (1992) established subsets of vulvodynia, including dermatoses, infection, vestibulitis, iatrogenic factors, and dysesthetic (essential) vulvodynia. *Vulvar dermatoses* include inflammatory dermatoses—irritant dermatitis, lichen planus, and other erosive conditions—and lichen sclerosus. *Infectious causes* include *Candida*, human papillomavirus (HPV), and herpes simplex virus (HSV). Of these, *Candida* is the most significant infectious agent to consider in evaluating a patient who has vulvodynia, as it may cause a cyclical vulvitis, which is defined as episodic vulvodynia with symptom-free periods between recurrences. Immune response factors, allergy, or hypersensitivity to the *Candida* organism, or changes in the vaginal ecosystem, may be responsible for these cyclical recurrences.

HPV was once thought to be the most likely cause of vulvodynia; however, it is now considered significant only in certain cases. Acute, recurring herpes simplex lesions may cause episodic burning. Nonlesional, recurrent infection may produce symptom patterns associated with pudendal neuralgia.

Vulvar vestibulitis is a syndrome of unknown etiology characterized by chronic, nonspecific inflammation of the area around the minor vestibular glands in the superficial stroma of the vestibular tissue. The condition may be acute, but it is generally chronic and persistent, with resultant severe dyspareunia and

vulvodynia, including erythema, edema, and exquisite vestibular tenderness to touch. Discomfort typically is absent without direct pressure. Researchers have attempted to demonstrate many causes: acute or chronic vulvovaginal infectious processes (especially *Candida* and HPV), altered vaginal pH balance (e.g., in association with estrogen-deficient states, bacterial vaginosis, decreased or absent lactobacilli), autoimmune reactions, irritants (e.g., soaps, douches, and sprays), chemical therapeutic agents, topical medications, postinflammatory tissue damage, and hypersensitivity reactions to an undetermined agent. There is little evidence linking vulvar vestibulitis and HPV. Recent data suggest a disorder of the urogenital sinus-derived epithelium as a possible cause of vestibulitis (Bergeron et al. 1997, Goetsch 1999, Morin et al. 2000, Origoni et al. 1999).

All in all, the etiology of this condition remains obscure; however, vestibulitis represents the most significant component in evaluating vulvodynia of multifactorial origin (Davis et al. 1999; ISSVD 1991; Masheb 2000; McKay 1988, 1989a, 1989b, 1992; Metts 1999).

Iatrogenic factors include the side effects of topical steroids (secondary or periorificial dermatitis due to a rebound inflammatory reaction after steroid medication is withdrawn), complications of CO_2 laser therapy, and sequelae of alcohol injections (McKay 1992).

Papillomatosis may be present in women with vulvodynia. Small papillae may be visible within the vulvar vestibule. These papillae are most likely congenital and are considered a normal anatomic variant (Metts 1999). A causal relationship between vulvar papillae and HPV has not been confirmed (Bergeron et al. 1997).

Dysesthetic (essential) vulvodynia refers to a burning-type pain anywhere from the mon pubis to the anus that is sporadic or constant, focal or diffuse, unilateral or bilateral, and unremitting. It typically occurs in perimenopausal and postmenopausal women. Dyspareunia and point tenderness appear to be less frequent than with vulvar vestibulitis syndrome (Metts 1999, Stewart 2001). Its etiology may lie in a neurological problem related to altered cutaneous perception or damaged sensory nerves.

When considering a diagnosis of dysesthetic vulvodynia, one should attempt to differentiate sensory input (pudendal neuralgia) from nerve injury (reflex sympathetic dystrophy). In pudendal neuralgia, sensory input factors may cause pain that radiates out from the vulva to the perineum, groin, or thighs, similar to the pain found in postherpetic neuralgia. Reflex sympathetic dystrophy (RSD) is an umbrella term for superficial, burning-type pain thought to be due to a previous nerve injury, though it is difficult to prove in most cases. The pain of a sympathetic nerve injury tends to spread beyond its original dermatomal pattern (Davis et al. 1999, Goetsch 1999, Metts 1999).

Proposed etiologies for dysesthetic vulvodynia include HSV, orthopedic problems of the back (osteoporosis, back injury, disc herniation, space-occupying lesion), postsurgical or nonsurgical trauma and sports trauma, and, more rarely, neurofibroma and multiple sclerosis (Davis et al. 1999; McKay 1988, 1989a,

Table 12TH.1. DIFFERENTIAL DIAGNOSIS OF VULVODYNIA: PATTERNS OF DISCOMFORT

Symptom Pattern	Dyspareunia	Physical Findings	"Typical Patient"	Diagnosis	Treatment
Cyclical itching and burning, often related to menses; responds to anticandidal agents but recurs; topical drugs may irritate	Irritation after coitus; severe with flares	Variable erythema and edema, minimal vaginal discharge; fissures may occur with intercourse; episodic scaling and pustules	Premenopausal or receiving estrogen replacement, history of frequent *Candida* infection; frequent use of antibiotics for sinus condition, urinary tract infection, or acne; usually better on anticandidal drugs, but recurrence frequent	Cyclical vulvovaginitis seems related to *Candida* infection, but exact mechanism unknown	4–6 months of low-dose systemic ketoconazole or vaginal anticandidal agents
"Irritated" mucosa; poor tolerance of topical medications; corticosteroids may help, then flare symptoms	Often irritated after coitus	Variable erythema; mucosal telangiectasias, sebaceous hyperplasia, or papular eruption over labia majora	History of frequent or chronic use of fluorinated or full-strength topical steroid; often culture-positive *Candida*	Periorificial dermatitis due to topical steroids or irritant reaction; *Candida* infection common	Taper steroids, treat with anticandidal drugs every other day while patient takes steroids; avoid irritating topical agents
"Irritated" mucosa, relieved after treatment for HPV, but recurrent	Discomfort at entry, after coitus, or both	Papillomatous appearance of mucosal surfaces; +/- condyloma; erythema and hyperemia variable	History of HPV infection or koilocytosis in some; others are simply reaction pattern	Vestibular papillomatosis; HPV (condyloma)	Do not treat papillomatosis unless proven related to HPV; recurrent HPV (condyloma) may be treated with BCA/TCA, laser, +/- 5-FU
Pain mainly with intercourse	Specific pain at entry; may prevent intercourse	Point tenderness to cotton-swab palpation of vestibular gland orifices	Usually sexually active until onset of pain; previous inflammatory episodes likely (including following laser surgery)	Vulvar vestibulitis	Multiple therapies tried: sitz baths, low-potency steroids, coital lubricants, topical anesthetics, interferon, surgery, etc.
Constant burning not related to touch or pressure	Not necessarily	Variable or no erythema; often other perineal symptoms	Usually postmenopausal, often not receiving estrogen replacement	Dysesthetic vulvodynia, pudendal neuralgia	Low-dose amitriptyline to control symptoms

NOTE: HPV = human papillomavirus infection; 5-FU = 5-fluorouracil; TCA = trichloroacetic acid

Source: Adapted with permission from McKay, M. 1992. Vulvodynia: diagnostic patterns. *Dermatology Clinics* 10(2):423–433.

1989b, 1992; Metts 1999). (See **Table 12TH.1, Differential Diagnosis of Vulvodynia: Patterns of Discomfort.**)

Vulvodynia is a chronic pain syndrome. It has been suggested that symptoms of vulvodynia result from multiple factors, including those from interpersonal, biological, and psychological realms, and encompass affective, cognitive, and behavioral aspects of mental health (Masheb et al. 2000).

Researchers have proposed that the nerve-related pain experienced by women diagnosed with vulvodynia may be sympathetically maintained (Masheb et al. 2000). Significantly lower pelvic floor muscle performance—as measured by the inability of muscles to relax fully at rest and to contract effectively on command, as well as muscle instability in both of these states—has been observed in symptomatic women. Irritability and destabilization of the pelvic floor muscles may result from localized stimulation of vulvar nerves (Glazer et al. 1998).

Considering vulvodynia as a chronic pain syndrome requires a multidimensional treatment plan that takes into account not only the physical pain, but factors that affect the perception of pain, as well.

The vulvodynia patient often seeks many health care providers in search of a diagnosis and cure. In some cases, she exhibits much frustration and anger toward the medical establishment for its limited success in diagnosis and treatment. Though often told her problem is primarily psychological, "the patient with vulvodynia is no more psychologically unbalanced than one with atopic dermatitis or acne" (McKay 1992, p. 432). These women present a diagnostic challenge and psychological support is paramount in their care.

DATABASE

SUBJECTIVE

→ The woman is typically a Caucasian in her 20s or 30s (except in cases of dysesthetic vulvodynia, which generally affects postmenopausal women). She may have a long-standing history of vulvodynia (months to years) and may have made many visits to providers.

→ Primary psychological disease may be present in a select group of women. Symptoms of depression are common though typically secondary to symptoms.

→ The initial episode of acute pain may be traced to a specific event: vulvovaginitis, an allergic or irritant reaction to a topical agent (e.g., soap, a steroid, podophyllin or bi- or trichloroacetic acid, or 5-fluorouracil).

→ Exposure (known or unknown) to HPV may have occurred within the preceding 3–9 months or longer.

→ The patient may have a history of recurrent candidiasis, herpes genitalis, HPV, allergies, general or gynecological surgery, orthopedic problems, and/or trauma to the genital area.

→ The symptom constellation may include:
- Vulvodynia (burning, stinging, irritation, or rawness). Pain may be intermittent or constant, localized, or bilateral and/or symmetrical; it is almost always in the vulvar vestibule (the posterior fourchette is most commonly involved).
  - Symptoms most common in vestibulitis. They also may

be reported in dermatoses and cyclical infections (*Candida*, HSV).
  - The patient also may report swelling or redness of the posterior fourchette.
- Itching, erythema, edema, "split" skin, irregularity or roughness of the skin surface, fissures, vaginal discharge
  - Symptoms more common in dermatoses and cyclical infection.
- Symptom recurrence at menses or postcoitally.
  - Symptoms mostly associated with *Candida*, HSV.
  - The patient also may report swelling or redness of the posterior fourchette.
- Precipitation of symptoms by sexual intercourse or pressure exerted on the vestibular area (e.g., by tampon insertion, bicycle or horseback riding, or tight clothing).
  - Symptoms most common in vestibulitis.
- A sensation of pins and needles or "crawling"; episodic, superficial burning that radiates from the vulva to the perineum, groin, thighs; deep aching; itch-burn sensation; lancinating or stabbing pain; burning pain on light touch (by clothing, water, pubic-hair motion); dyspareunia with both intromission and deep penetration.
  - Symptoms mostly associated with dysesthetic vulvodynia due to pudendal neuralgia or RSD.
- Erythema and generalized burning when a topical steroid is withdrawn from use on the vulva (rebound inflammatory reaction, periorificial dermatitis)
- Dyspareunia, decreased coital frequency (may be associated with vulvodynia of any cause)
  - Introital dyspareunia is more common in vestibulitis.
  - Dyspareunia occurring with penile penetration and after intercourse is more common with pudendal neuralgia.

→ Aggravating factors may include:
- Sexual activity: Intromission, masturbation
- Recurrent vulvovaginitis
- Physical activities
- Perspiring
- Rubbing of clothing, tampons
- Topical creams, ointments (lubricants, steroids, anesthetics)

→ Relieving factors may include:
- Tub or sitz baths
- Ice packs
- Bed rest

→ History should include:
- A thorough symptom evaluation (onset, duration, course, location, quality and quantity of pain, associated symptoms, aggravating and alleviating factors)
- Menstrual cycle history
- Previous vulvovaginal infections (e.g., candidiasis, trichomoniasis, bacterial vaginosis, condylomata, herpes, other sexually transmitted diseases [STDs])
- Careful search for mechanical and chemical irritants and use of topical or systemic medication
- Contraceptive history

■ Sexual history, including history of sexual abuse/trauma and sexual dysfunction

■ Sexual-partner history and symptomatology

■ Past and present dermatological and orthopedic conditions

■ Surgical history

■ Habits (drugs, alcohol, exercise, nutrition, etc.)

■ Stress level, psychological history

OBJECTIVE

→ A thorough, systematic examination of the genitalia from the labia majora inward must be performed to assess all potential etiologies of vulvodynia. Diagrams are helpful in detailing anatomic distribution of involved area(s).

→ Clinical features may include:

■ Pelvic examination:

• Labia majora: erythema, edema, papules, pustules, architectural skin changes, fissuring, herpetic lesions; satellite pustules may appear at the edges of the vulva; interlabial fissures may occur.

– Diagnostic considerations include inflammatory dermatoses, lichen sclerosus, infectious states (*Candida*, HPV, HSV), periorificial dermatitis, and post-alcohol scarring.

• Labia minora/vestibule: multiple, small, cutaneous papillae and acetowhitening (see "Diagnostic Tests," below). Papillomatosis may be present normally with or without subclinical HPV infection. Herpetic lesions may be present. Interlabial fissures may occur.

– Diagnostic considerations include HPV/papillomatosis, HSV, and lichen sclerosus.

• Vestibule: The following may be present:

➤ Erythematous foci at 5 o'clock and 7 o'clock (at the ducts of Bartholin's glands)

➤ Exquisite pain to light touch with a saline-moistened cotton swab may be present at the base of the hymen or fourchette, parameatal, or subfrenular areas of the vestibule

➤ Erythema at the introitus

➤ Shallow ulcers adjacent to the hymenal ring

➤ Fissuring of the posterior fourchette

➤ Herpetic lesions

– Diagnostic considerations include vestibulitis, *Candida* infection, and HSV.

• Perineum: A thickened surgical scar, palpable nodule, herpetic lesions, or fissures may be present.

– Diagnostic considerations include pudendal neuralgia, HSV, and lichen sclerosus.

• Vagina: Erythema and abnormal discharge may be present.

– Diagnostic considerations include *Candida* infection, HSV, and pudendal neuralgia.

• Cervix, uterus, adnexa, and rectovaginal examinations are usually within normal limits unless there is co-existent pathology.

■ Additional examination components:

• Sensory testing with a cotton swab and sharp pin in the vestibule and labial areas may be utilized to assess pudendal neuralgia, as other physical findings are non-specific. May need to consult with or refer the patient to a neurologist. Any of the following may be found:

– Allodynia: pain elicited by a stimulus that does not normally cause pain (e.g., light touch)

– Hyperalgesia: an exaggerated response to a painful stimulus

– Hyperpathia: an increased reaction to a repetitive stimulus, a delayed reaction, a radiating sensation, or an after-sensation

– Hypoesthesia: decreased sensitivity to stimuli

– Hyperesthesia: increased sensitivity to sensory stimuli such as pain or touch. It may extend from the mons to upper inner thighs and posteriorly across ischial tuberosities (Bergeron et al. 1997, Goetsch 1999, McKay 1992, Pagano 1999).

→ See also "Diagnostic Tests," below.

ASSESSMENT

→ Vulvodynia

→ R/O inflammatory/erosive vulvar dermatoses: irritant dermatitis, lichen planus, lupus erythematosus, bullous dermatoses, aphthosis, Behçet's syndrome

→ R/O infectious states (*Candida*, HSV, HPV)

→ R/O subclinical HPV infection

→ R/O papillomatosis

→ R/O vulvar vestibulitis

→ R/O iatrogenic vulvodynia

→ R/O dysesthetic (essential) vulvodynia

→ R/O concomitant STDs

→ R/O vulvar intraepithelial neoplasia (VIN)

→ R/O a cervical squamous intraepithelial lesion (SIL)

→ R/O urinary tract infection

→ R/O interstitial cystitis

PLAN

DIAGNOSTIC TESTS

→ Diagnostic tests should primarily be directed to documenting infectious disease states.

→ Potassium hydroxide (KOH) and saline wet mounts of vaginal secretions should be performed to assess for *Candida*, *Trichomonas*, or bacterial vaginosis.

→ Scrapings from affected skin may be taken, placed on a glass slide, mixed with KOH, heated, and viewed microscopically for the presence of *Candida*.

→ Vaginal and vulvar cultures for *Candida* may be performed.

→ pH testing of the vagina may be performed

→ Pap smear, genital cultures, blood chemistries, HIV testing, fasting blood sugar, and other diagnostic tests may be performed as indicated.

→ Acetic acid 3–5% may be applied to the vulva for HPV assessment. Several minutes after application, acetowhitening of the affected area may appear, and small, cutaneous

papillae with an associated vascular pattern may be identified on the mucous membrane of the labia minora, vestibule, or posterior fourchette (papillomatosis). These changes can be seen with the naked eye, a hand-held lens, or a colposcope.
NOTE: Acetowhitening is suggestive but not diagnostic of HPV infection. Papillomatosis may be present normally or in a subclinical HPV infection. Acetowhitening also may be due to tissue inflammation, trauma, allergic or contact dermatitis, lichen sclerosus, pantyhose, or constrictive clothing.

→ Colposcopy of the entire vulva, vagina, and cervix may be utilized to assess for HPV and SIL.

→ Tissue biopsy of anogenital areas may be done for histopathological confirmation of HPV. Biopsies of suspicious or questionable areas should be done to rule out VIN and other dermatoses.
  ▪ Biopsy for direct immunofluorescence should be considered in the differential diagnosis of erosive vulvovaginal conditions (e.g., lichen planus, lupus erythematosus, bullous dermatoses, aphthosis, Behçet's syndrome) (McKay 1992).

→ Serum testing for herpes antibodies is of limited value. If negative, herpes infection can be ruled out. Positive tests indicate circulating antibodies, but they do not help determine the date or time of exposure nor help differentiate oral from genital infection.

→ Molecular hybridization techniques (Southern blot, dot blot, polymerized chain reaction) are specific diagnostic techniques utilized to assess the presence of HPV DNA. Recent development of the hybrid capture assay measures HPV load quantitatively, but it also detects nononcogenic as well as oncogenic subtypes of HPV (Apgar et al. 1999).

→ For vulvar vestibulitis, specific criteria for diagnosis include (Friedrich 1987):
  ▪ Severe pain on vestibular touch or attempted vaginal entry
  ▪ Tenderness to pressure localized within the vulvar vestibule
  ▪ Physical findings confined to vestibular erythema of various degrees
  NOTE: Biopsies usually are not beneficial in diagnosing vestibulitis. If they are performed, histological findings may show a nonspecific chronic inflammation of submucosal tissue surrounding the minor vestibular glands.

→ Sensory testing as described under "Objective" can help assess pudendal neuralgia.

→ Orthopedic and additional neurological assessment, x-rays, CT scan, and MRI can be utilized as necessary to evaluate orthopedic and other causes of essential vulvodynia.

TREATMENT/MANAGEMENT

→ Treatment of a *specific* underlying cause, if identified, is key. See specific treatment modalities below.

→ Psychological support to help the patient deal with the chronicity of the condition and to support her coping mechanisms is an important component of care. Refer her to the appropriate resources: social service, psychological or sexual counseling, stress management.

→ Psychiatric evaluation may be indicated in certain cases.

Vulvar Dermatoses

→ Treat underlying dermatological disorders as identified. See specific chapters.

Cyclical *Candida* Infection

→ A positive culture need not be a criterion for treatment.

→ Long-term (4–6 months) maintenance therapy with local or systemic antifungal agents may be employed in patients who have a variable symptom pattern and in those whose symptoms have been relieved in the past by anticandidal measures. (The key to success is consistent, low-dose *Candida* suppression.) Options include:
  ▪ Local therapy:
    • Antifungal cream (azole): one-half applicator every night at HS.
    NOTE: Topical antifungal creams may further irritate some cyclic vulvovaginitis sufferers. Alternately, boric acid 600 mg, compounded with glycerol as a suppository, at HS for 15 days may be used. Occasional vaginal erythema and irritation may occur (Davis et al. 1999).
  ▪ Systemic therapy:
    • Ketoconazole: 100–200 mg/day p.o. for up to 6 months, tapering to 100 mg/day or every other day after the first 2 months. Alternately, 100 mg/day for 5 days before menses. Antifungal cream may be used every other day or every third day at HS in conjunction with systemic therapy (McKay 1989a, Pagano 1999).
    NOTE: Ketoconazole is hepatotoxic. See the *Physicians' Desk Reference* (*PDR*). Consult with a physician before use. Regimens may vary. Liver function should be monitored in cases of prolonged use.
    • Fluconazole: 150 mg orally once weekly for 2 months, then once every other week for 2–4 months (Metts 1999).

→ It is important to rule out chronic illness such as diabetes and HIV infection.

Herpes Simplex Virus Infection

→ Oral antivirals may be offered (CDC 2002):
  ▪ For primary infection:
    • Acyclovir 400 mg p.o. TID for 7–10 days
      OR
    • Acyclovir 200 mg p.o. 5 times/day for 7–10 days
      OR
    • Famciclovir 250 mg p.o. TID for 7–10 days
      OR
    • Valacyclovir 1 gm p.o. BID for 7–10 days
  ▪ For recurrent infection:
    • Acyclovir 400 mg p.o. TID for 5 days
      OR

- Acyclovir 200 mg p.o. 5 times/day for 5 days
  OR
- Acyclovir 800 mg p.o. BID for 5 days
  OR
- Famciclovir 125 mg p.o. BID for 5 days
  OR
- Valacyclovir 500 mg p.o. BID for 5 days
  OR
- Valacyclovir 1 gm p.o. once daily for 5 days
- For frequent infection (chronic suppressive therapy):
  - Acyclovir 400 mg p.o. BID
    OR
  - Famciclovir 250 mg p.o. BID
    OR
  - Valacyclovir 500 mg p.o. once daily
    OR
  - Valacyclovir 1 gm p.o. once daily
→ See the **Genital Herpes Simplex Virus** chapter in Section 13 for further information.

HPV

→ Spontaneous regression is possible; thus, aggressive therapy should be reserved for intractable symptoms (Bergeron et al. 1990, McKay 1992).

→ Well-localized, small lesions respond well to 50–85% bi- or trichloroacetic acid; larger areas might best be treated with laser therapy or cryotherapy. Instead, the patient may self-administer podofilox 0.5% solution or gel, or imiquimod 5% cream (Baker 2001, Reid 1996).

→ Avoid treating asymptomatic papillomatosis.

→ See the **Human Papillomavirus** chapter in Section 13 for details on therapy for condyloma acuminata.

Vestibulitis

→ In cases where a specific etiology cannot be found, many symptomatic women improve with time and/or are able to adjust satisfactorily to discomfort. Specific therapy may not be necessary.

→ There are no firmly established treatment guidelines. Multiple therapies have been tried to alleviate vestibulitis, including:

- Warm sitz baths (for recent onset and mild signs or symptoms)
- Coital lubricants
- Topical lidocaine hydrochloride 2–5%: Apply with a cotton swab prn and/or 10–15 minutes before intercourse (McKay 1992)
- Topical corticosteroids (low potency): A small amount to affected areas BID regularly. They may need to be used for weeks to months (Boardman et al. 1999). (See **Table 12TB.1, Potency Ranking of Some Commonly Used Topical Corticosteroids** in the **White Lesions of the Vulva** chapter.)
- Local or systemic antifungal agents for chronic, recurrent candidiasis. (See "Cyclical *Candida* Infection," above.)

- Treatment of specific vaginal infections (e.g., bacterial vaginosis, atrophic vaginitis) and cervicitis as indicated
- Alpha-interferon (for a subset of patients with biopsy or hybridization evidence of HPV): 1,000,000 U intradermally to vulvar vestibule 3 times/week for 4 weeks. This regime has not received FDA approval for treating vulvar vestibulitis syndrome, but it is approved for treating condylomata (Bergeron et al. 1997, Davis et al. 1999, Metts 1999). Consult with or refer to a physician. (See the **Human Papillomavirus** chapter in Section 13.)
- Biofeedback, relaxation training, and pelvic-floor-muscle physical therapy may be used to strengthen weakened pelvic floor muscles and relax them, resulting in a reduction in pain (Metts 1999). Refer to an experienced therapist/clinician.
- Flash-lamp excited dye laser has been used successfully (Davis et al. 1999). Refer to a physician.
- Surgical resection of the vestibule (perineoplasty) has proved successful in alleviating the condition (Bergeron et al. 1997, McCormack et al. 1999). This is a radical approach and should be reserved for patients with severe levels of dyspareunia. "Severe" is defined as dyspareunia that completely prevents intercourse at times, has lasted at least 6 months, has not responded to a 6-month trial of conservative therapy, or for which no cause can be identified (Goetsch 1999, Metts 1999). Refer to an experienced physician.

→ Avoid overtreatment with antibiotics, topical irritants (potent steroids and other local medications and products), and locally destructive measures.

→ Prevention of repeated inflammation may include concomitant use of topical antifungal agents when systemic antibiotics are prescribed, and avoidance of potent topical steroids or irritating topical medications (McKay 1992).

Iatrogenic Factors

→ Prevention is the key.

→ Avoid the use of potent steroids on vulva for chronic vulvar dermatoses. A popular offender is a combination of betamethasone (a steroid) and clotrimazole (an antifungal) (McKay 1992).

→ Gradual tapering is necessary to withdraw the patient from chronic topical steroid use. Rebound steroid irritant reactions may be treated with hydrocortisone ointment 1% or with bland emollients such as diaper salve and vegetable shortening (Bergeron 1997, McKay 1991).

→ Avoid the use of alcohol injection as a treatment for vulvar pruritus.

→ A low-oxalate diet plus calcium citrate (200 mg calcium plus 950 mg citrate, 2 tablets p.o. TID) have been used to reduce symptoms (Boardman et al. 1999, Masheb 2000, Metts 1999).

NOTE: Foods high in oxalates include rhubarb, spinach, celery, and peanuts.

Dysesthetic (Essential) Vulvodynia

→ Topical lidocaine ointment 5% may be applied prn for local relief (McKay 1992, Stewart 2001).

→ Pudendal neuralgia may be treated with tricyclic antidepressants:

- Amitriptyline 10 mg p.o. BID. If tolerated, the dose is gradually increased every 2–4 weeks until pain relief is achieved (up to 100 mg/day may be required). Once pain relief is achieved, the dose should be maintained for 4–8 weeks, although it may need to be continued for up to 6 months, then gradually decreased until a maintenance level is established. If the patient is symptom-free for 3–6 months, the dose may be decreased gradually until medication is no longer required (Davis et al. 1999, Metts 1999).

  NOTE: Dosage regimens vary in treating vulvodynia. Management by a physician with experience using these drugs is advised. (See the *PDR* for the side effects of antidepressants.)

- Alternate medications may include nortriptyline, desipramine, trazodone, imipramine, or clonazepam. Management by a physician is advised. (See the *PDR*.)

→ Anticonvulsants or antiviral drugs may be used for postherpetic neuralgia and other neuropathic pain conditions (Ben-David et al. 1999, Stewart 2001):

- Phenytoin 300–400 mg/day p.o. in 2 divided doses. Discontinue if there is no relief in 3 weeks. Higher doses may lead to toxicity. Consult with or refer to a physician.

- Carbamazepine 100 mg/day p.o. increased by increments of 100 mg every 2 days up to 600 mg/day, as needed, for pain control. Consult with or refer to a physician. Hematological, dermatological, or hepatic toxicities may occur; close monitoring is necessary.

- Gabapentin 300 mg orally per day, increasing to BID, TID, then QID to a dose of 1,200 mg per day until symptoms are relieved. The dose is maintained for at least 12 weeks, then tapered individually. Do not use in pregnancy (Ben-David et al. 1999).

- Acyclovir may be used if pudendal neuralgia symptoms suggest a herpes infection (Byth 1998).

CONSULTATION

→ See "Objective" and "Treatment/Management," above.

→ For severe, unremitting cases unresponsive to local measures, refer the patient to a gynecologist or dermatologist skilled in assessing and managing patients who have vulvodynia.

→ For cases in which antidepressant or anticonvulsant therapy is being considered, it may be necessary to consult with or refer to a psychiatrist or neurologist.

→ As needed for prescription(s).

PATIENT EDUCATION

→ Discuss proposed etiologies of various subsets of vulvodynia and the possibility of long-term therapy toward resolution. Inform the patient that a continued search for more definitive etiologies and treatment modalities is under way. Explain that vulvodynia is not contagious (as long as communicable disease agents have been ruled out).

→ Discourage the use of potential irritants to the genital area (e.g., soaps, creams, bubble baths, bath oils, feminine deodorant sprays).

→ Encourage the use of unscented, unbleached, white toilet tissue and sanitary products. Encourage the patient to wear 100% cotton underwear and loose clothing, and to avoid wearing pantyhose.

→ Discuss the importance of a healthy immune system and its role in disease prevention.

→ Encourage the patient to keep a diary of all offending substances and, ideally, to eliminate their use. (See the **Candidal Vulvovaginitis** chapter for patient education regarding vulvovaginal health and hygiene measures.)

→ Excessive douching or use of potent topical steroids should be avoided, as these may result in dermatitis.

→ Explain to the patient that tricyclic antidepressants will block the nerve conduction of most of the pain impulses and are used more for this purpose than for their antidepressant effects.

→ In women with known antibiotic-induced cyclical *Candida* infection, prophylactic topical antifungals should be utilized. The patient should ask her health care provider for a prescription as necessary or OTC products should be used at the onset of taking medication.

→ Make sure the patient understands how to properly apply a topical steroid when it is used to treat vestibulitis. (See **Table 12TA.1, Tips for Treating Skin Lesions** in the **Red Lesions of the Vulva** chapter.)

→ Lubricants may be used with intercourse to ease penile entry.

→ Explain that even after surgery, vulvodynia may return.

FOLLOW-UP

→ Support is essential for the patient's psychological health.

→ Psychological or psychosexual counseling may be necessary in refractory cases. Provide appropriate referrals. Communicate with the patient about how she is coping.

→ Arrange a return-visit schedule that best meets the patient's needs. It varies with case presentation.

→ Document in progress notes and on problem list.

→ Resources:

- National Vulvodynia Association
  P.O. Box 4491
  Silver Springs, Md. 20914-4491
  (301) 299-0775, www.nva.org

- Vulvar Pain Foundation
  P.O. Box 177
  Graham, N.C. 27253
  (336) 226-0704
  www.vulvarpainfoundation.org

BIBLIOGRAPHY

Apgar, B.S., and Brotzman, G. 1999. HPV testing in the evaluation of the minimally abnormal Papanicolaou smear. *American Family Physician* 59(10):2794–2801.

Baker, D.A. 2001. Management options for non-HIV viral STDs. *Women's Health in Primary Care* 1(4):237–248.

Barclay, D.L. 1991. Premalignant and malignant disorders of the vulva and vagina. In *Current obstetric and gynecologic diagnosis and treatment*, 7th ed., ed. M.L. Pernoll, pp. 923–936. Norwalk, Conn.: Appleton & Lange.

Ben-David, B., and Friedman, M. 1999. Gabapentin therapy for vulvodynia. *Anesthesia & Analgesia* 89(6):1459–1460.

Bergeron, C., Ferenczy, A., Richart, R.M. et al. 1990. Micropapillomatosis labialis appears unrelated to human papillomavirus. *Obstetrics Oncology* 76(2):281–286.

Bergeron, S., Binik, Y., Khalife, S. et al. 1997. Vulvar vestibulitis syndrome: a critical review. *Clinical Journal of Pain* 13(1):27–42.

Boardman, L., and Peipert, J. 1999. Vulvar vestibulitis: Is it a defined and treatable entity? *Clinical Obstetrics and Gynecology* 42(4):945–956.

Byth, J.L. 1998. Understanding vulvodynia. *Australasian Journal of Dermatology* 39:139–150.

Centers for Disease Control and Prevention (CDC). 2002. Guidelines for treatment of sexually transmitted diseases. *Morbidity and Mortality Weekly Report* 51(RR-6):12–17.

Chafe, W., Richards, A., Morgan, L. et al. 1988. Unrecognized invasive carcinoma in vulvar intraepithelial neoplasia. *Gynecologic Oncology* 31:154–162.

Cho, J.Y., Ahn, M.O., and Cha, K.S. 1990. Window operation: an alternative treatment method for Bartholin's gland cysts and abscesses. *Obstetrics and Gynecology* 76:886–888.

Consensus Conference. 1984. Precursors to malignant melanoma. *Journal of the American Medical Association* 251:1864–1866.

Cornell, R.C., and Stoughton, R.B. 1984. The ranking of topical steroids in psoriasis. *Dermatologic Clinics* 2(3):399.

Cort, M.B. 1991. Bartholin's gland cyst and abscess. In *Ob/Gyn secrets*, eds. H.L. Frederickson and L. Wilkins-Haug. Philadelphia: Hanley & Belfus.

Dalziel, K.L., and Wojnarowska, F. 1991. The treatment of vulvar lichen sclerosus with a very potent topical steroid (clobetasol propionate 0.05%) cream. *British Journal of Dermatology* 124:461–464.

Davis, G.D., and Hutchison, C.V. 1999. Clinical management of vulvodynia. *Clinical Obstetrics and Gynecology* 42(2):221–233.

DePetrillo, A., Krepart, G., Roy, M. et al. 1987. Less radical surgery for vulvar cancer. *Contemporary OB/GYN* 30(1):160–175.

DiSaia, P.J., and Creasman, W.T. 1989. *Clinical gynecologic oncology*, 3rd ed. St. Louis, Mo.: C.V. Mosby.

Friedrich, E.G., Jr. 1983. *Vulvar disease*, 2nd ed. Philadelphia: W.B. Saunders.

_____. 1987. Vulvar vestibulitis syndrome. *Journal of Reproductive Medicine* 32:110–114.

Glazer, H.I., Jantos, M., Hartmann, E.H. et al. 1998. Electromyographic comparisons of the pelvic floor in women with dysesthetic vulvodynia and asymptomatic women. *Journal of Reproductive Medicine* 43(11):959–962.

Goetsch, M.F. 1999. Vulvar vestibulitis. *Contemporary OB/GYN* 44(10):56–63.

Gomel, V., Munro, M.G., and Rowe, T.C. 1990. *Gynecology: a practical approach*. Baltimore, Md.: Williams & Wilkins.

Hammill, H.A. 1989. Unusual causes of vaginitis. *Obstetrics and Gynecology Clinics of North America* 16(2):337–345.

International Society for the Study of Vulvar Disease (ISSVD). 1991. Vulvar vestibulitis and vestibular papillomatosis. Report of the ISSVD committee on vulvodynia. *Journal of Reproductive Medicine* 36(6):413–415.

International Society for the Study of Vulvar Disease, Terminology Committee (ISSVD Committee). 1990. New nomenclature for vulvar disease. *Journal of Reproductive Medicine* 35:483–484.

Jones, H.W., Wentz, A.C., and Burnett, L.S. 1988. *Novak's textbook of gynecology*, 11th ed. Baltimore, Md.: Williams & Wilkins.

Kaufman, R.H., Friedrich, E.G., Jr., and Gardner, H.L. 1989. *Benign diseases of the vulva and vagina*, 3rd ed. Chicago: Year Book Medical.

Kistner, R.W. 1986. *Gynecology: principles and practice*, 4th ed. Chicago: Year Book Medical.

Lerner, A.B. 1972. Pigmented nevi. *Modern Medicine* 17:131.

Lever, W.F. 1990. *Histopathology of the skin*, 7th ed. Philadelphia: J.B. Lippincott.

Lynch, P.J. 1986. Vulvodynia: a syndrome of unexplained vulvar pain, psychologic disability, and sexual dysfunction. *Journal of Reproductive Medicine* 31(9):773–780.

Mann, M.S., Kaufman, R.H., Brown, D., Jr. et al. 1992. Vulvar vestibulitis: significant clinical variables and treatment outcome. *Obstetrics and Gynecology* 79(1):122–125.

Masheb, R.M., Nash, J.M., Brondolo, E. et al. 2000. Vulvodynia: an introduction and critical review of a chronic pain condition. *Pain* 86:3–10.

McCormack, W.M., and Spence, M.R. 1999. Evaluation of the surgical treatment of vulvar vestibulitis. *European Journal of Obstetrics and Gynecology and Reproductive Biology* 86:135–138.

McKay, M. 1988. Subsets of vulvodynia. *Journal of Reproductive Medicine* 33:695–698.

_____. 1989a. Vulvodynia: a multifactorial clinical problem. *Archives of Dermatology* 125:256–262.

_____. 1989b. Vulvodynia and pruritus vulvae. *Seminars in Dermatology* 8(1):40–47.

_____. 1991. Vulvitis and vulvovaginitis: Cutaneous considerations. *American Journal of Obstetrics and Gynecology* 165(4 Part 1):1176–1182.

_____. 1992. Vulvodynia: diagnostic patterns. *Dermatology Clinics* 10(2):423–433.

McKay, M. Frankman, O., Horowitz, B.J. et al. 1991. Vulvar vestibulitis and vestibular papillomatosis. Report of the ISSVD committee on vulvodynia. *Journal of Reproductive Medicine* 36(6):413–415.

Metts, J.F. 1999 Vulvodynia and vulvar vestibulitis: challenges in diagnosis and management. *American Family Physician* 59(6):1547–1556.

Misas, J.E., Cold, C.J., and Hall, F.W. 1991. Vulvar Paget's disease: fluorescein-aided visualization of margins. *Obstetrics and Gynecology* 77(1):156–159.

Morgan, L.S., and Wilkinson, E.J. 1988. Meeting the challenge of superficially invasive carcinoma. *Contemporary OB/GYN* 31(5):181–185.

Morin, C., Bouchard, C., Brisson, J. et al. 2000. Human papillomaviruses and vulvar vestibulitis. *Obstetrics and Gynecology* 95(5):683–687.

Morrow, C.P., and Townsend, D. 1981. *Synopsis of gynecologic oncology*, 2nd ed. New York: John Wiley.

Origoni, M., Rossi, M., Ferrari, D. et al. 1999. Human papillomavirus with co-existing vulvar vestibulitis syndrome and vestibular papillomatosis. *International Journal of Gynecology and Obstetrics* 64:259–263.

Pagano, R. 1999. Vulvar vestibulitis syndrome: an often unrecognized cause of dyspareunia. *Australian and New Zealand Journal of Obstetrics and Gynaecology* 39(1):79–83.

Physicians' desk reference. 2003. Montvale, N.J.: Medical Economics.

Reid, R. 1996. The management of genital condylomas, intraepithelial neoplasia, and vulvodynia. *Obstetrics and Gynecology Clinics of North America* 23(4):917–991.

Reid, R., Greenberg, M.D., Daoud, Y. et al. 1988. Colposcopic findings in women with vulvar pain syndromes. A preliminary report. *Journal of Reproductive Medicine* 33(6): 523–533.

Richart, R., Boronow, R.C., Hacker, N. et al. 1988. Microscopic vulvar Ca: a new concept. *Contemporary OB/GYN* 32(4):117–136.

Rodke, G., Friedrich, E.G., and Wilkinson, E.J. 1988. Malignant potential of mixed vulvar dystrophy (lichen sclerosus associated with squamous cell hyperplasia). *Journal of Reproductive Medicine* 33(6):545–550.

Roy, M. 1988. VIN: latest management approaches. *Contemporary OB/GYN* 31(5):170–179.

Russel, P., and Bannatyne, P. 1989. *Surgical pathology of the ovaries.* Edinburgh, Scotland: Churchill Livingstone.

Sauer, G.C. 2000. *Manual of skin diseases*, 8th ed. Philadelphia: Lippincott Williams & Wilkins.

Sedlis, A., Homesley, H., Marshall, R. et al. 1988. Evaluating risk factors for vulvar cancer. *Contemporary OB/GYN* 32(3):67–74.

Shearin, R.S., Boehlke, J., and Karanth, S. 1989. Toxic shock-like syndrome associated with Bartholin's gland abscess: case report. *American Journal of Obstetrics and Gynecology* 160:1073–1074.

Stewart, D.E., Psych, D., Whelan, C.I. et al. 1990. Psychosocial aspects of chronic, clinically unconfirmed vulvovaginitis. *Obstetrics and Gynecology* 76(5 Part 1):853–856.

Stewart, E.G. 2001. Vulvodynia: diagnosing and managing generalized dysesthesia. *OBG Management* 13(6):48–57.

Thomas, C.L., ed. 1989. *Taber's cyclopedic medical dictionary*, 16th ed. Philadelphia: F.A. Davis.

Wilkinson, E.J. 1987. *Pathology of the vulva and vagina.* New York: Churchill Livingstone.

Wilkinson, E.J., Kneale, B., and Lynch, P.J. 1986. Report of the International Society for the Study of Vulvar Disease, Terminology Committee. *Journal of Reproductive Medicine* 31:973.

Word, B. 1964. New instrument for office treatment of cysts and abscesses of Bartholin's gland. *Journal of the American Medical Association* 190:777–778.

Mary M. Rubin, R.N., C., PH.D., C.R.N.P.

12-U
Vaginal Intraepithelial Neoplasia

Vaginal intraepithelial neoplasia (VAIN), a premalignant condition characterized by disorganized epithelial maturation, nuclear enlargement, and nuclear atypia, has been recognized for several decades. It may include partial involvement of the epithelial layer or extend throughout its full thickness. Consistent with other sites for intraepithelial neoplasia of the lower genital tract, VAIN is confined to the epithelial layer above the basement membrane of the epidermis with no extension to the underlying dermis (Anderson et al. 1996).

Before 1960, VAIN was rarely mentioned in the literature. More recently, there has been an increasing awareness of the disease with the implementation of colposcopic evaluation of the entire lower genital tract following an abnormal Pap smear. About 90% of VAIN lesions are found in the upper one-third of the vagina (Burke et al. 1991). The exact incidence and prevalence of VAIN are unknown, but they are thought to be much less than that of cervical intraepithelial neoplasia (CIN) (Anderson et al. 1996). It is estimated that about 1.5% of patients with CIN (3% of those with a high-grade squamous intraepithelial lesion [HSIL]) have concomitant VAIN or will develop it at some later date (Campion et al. 1991). Although most VAIN goes into remission after treatment, 5% of cases may progress from occult foci to invasion in spite of close follow-up (Sillman et al. 1997). Unfortunately, the progressive potential of low-grade VAIN to high-grade VAIN is not yet established; however, evidence of progression of high-grade VAIN to invasive cancer has been demonstrated (Rome et al. 2000). VAIN lesions are found 71% of the time in patients with cervical or vulvar neoplasia (Dodge et al. 2001, Stone et al. 1993). Squamous vaginal carcinoma is relatively rare but accounts for about 1–3% of all genital tract malignancies (Singer et al. 2000).

Categorization of VAIN lesions is consistent with classification of intraepithelial neoplasia in other lower genital tract sites (Zaino et al. 1994):

1. VAIN 1 = mild dysplasia or human papillomavirus (HPV) changes (low-grade squamous intraepithelial lesion [LSIL])
2. VAIN 2 = moderate dysplasia (HSIL)
3. VAIN 3 = severe dysplasia or carcinoma in situ (HSIL)

DATABASE

SUBJECTIVE

→ Risk factors may include (Abercrombie et al. 1995, Singer et al. 2000, Weiderpass et al. 2001, Zaino et al. 1994):
- Prior treatment for an abnormal Pap smear
- Abnormal Pap smear with a normal cervix and satisfactory colposcopy exam
- Hysterectomy with prior history of CIN
- Diethylstilbestrol (DES) daughters with wide transformation zones
- Multiple sexual partners
- HPV infection
- Smoking
- Immunosuppression

→ Lesions are usually asymptomatic.

→ Symptoms may include:
- Vaginal pain, soreness, burning, swelling
- Vaginal warts, lumps, nodules, presence of a tumor
- Bleeding, discharge

OBJECTIVE

→ Lesions are usually first noted during routine pelvic examination or at the time of colposcopic examination for an abnormal Pap. Features are widely variable and appearance can include (Gross et al. 1997, Singer et al. 2000):
- Focal or multifocal lesions
- Slightly elevated, white, keratinized, rough areas
- Condylomatous-like lesions
- Red patches
- Hyperpigmentation
- Gross vaginal lesion(s) with or without increased vascularity
- Ulcerated, indurated, raised, exophytic, or nodular area(s), which may indicate invasive disease

→ The cervix, uterus, adnexa, vulva, and rectum are within normal limits unless there is co-existent pathology.

→ Vaginal infections, atrophy, adenosis, and trauma often can produce features that mimic high-grade VAIN or vaginal cancer (Singer et al. 2000).

→ A good description, diagram, or photograph of the lesion is important.

ASSESSMENT

→ VAIN
→ R/O condyloma
→ R/O invasive vaginal cancer
→ R/O other vaginal infections, trauma, and pathology

PLAN

DIAGNOSTIC TESTS

→ Early diagnosis depends on regular, careful examination of the vagina visually as well as with palpation. Index of suspicion for VAIN is an important parameter. The multiple factors listed above will help identify women at greatest risk.

→ Colposcopy of the vagina after application of 3–5% acetic acid should be performed to identify the most appropriate sites for biopsy. White, ulcerated, fissured, nodular, abnormally raised areas and those with increased vascularity should be biopsied. Colposcopy of the cervix and vulva also may be performed to rule out concomitant intraepithelial neoplasia (Anderson et al. 1997, Campion et al. 1991, Wilkinson et al. 1995).

NOTE: In most settings, diagnostic evaluation usually is performed by a physician or an advanced practice clinician; however, practices may vary. A properly trained, experienced practitioner should perform biopsy and colposcopic procedures.

→ Histological evaluation of the biopsy specimen from suspicious lesions must be done to render a definitive diagnosis before treatment. Delineation of the extent of disease is critical and invasion must be ruled out. Multiple biopsy samples with a punch biopsy forceps may be necessary. Care must be taken to determine the appropriate depth of the sample, as the vaginal mucosa can be very thin and other pelvic structures are in close proximity (Burghardt et al. 1998).

→ Pap smear, genital cultures, STD testing, wet mounts, and other diagnostic tests as indicated.

TREATMENT/MANAGEMENT

→ If VAIN is confirmed, refer the patient to a physician for treatment.

→ The choice of treatment should be individualized and depends on the age of the patient, the extent and location of the lesion, the presence of the cervix, the availability of equipment, and the surgical expertise of the practitioner.

→ Treatment options include (Cheng et al. 1999, Diakomanolis et al. 1996, Singer et al. 2000):
  ■ Observation: very effective in VAIN I, as many lesions will revert to normal or never progress.
  ■ 5% fluorouracil: successfully used for eradication of multifocal, low-grade lesions, especially HPV but often results in severe excoriation of normal tissue.
  ■ Trichloroacetic acid: successfully used for eradication of focal, low-grade lesions.
  ■ CO_2 laser: effective with extensive lesions for ablative or excisional treatment. It is done under colposcopic guidance with local or general anesthesia.
  ■ Cryosurgery: used for small, well-defined lesions. It can damage surrounding tissue and there is a risk of bowel and bladder damage. Failure rates are fairly high, most often due to incomplete destruction.
  ■ Loop electro-surgical excision: used for small, well-defined lesions. It can damage surrounding tissue and there is a risk of bowel and bladder damage.
  ■ Surgical excision, focal or wide: recommended for posthysterectomy lesions.

NOTE: Follow the triage rules for conservative ablative treatment. The following are mandatory (Campion et al. 1991):
  ■ Expert systematic colposcopy
  ■ Complete visualization of the disease
  ■ Cytologic, colposcopic, and histologic exclusion of invasion or glandular disease
  ■ Representative biopsy of the most abnormal lesions
  ■ Treatment under colposcopic visualization
  ■ Close follow-up

CONSULTATION

→ Referral to a physician usually will be necessary for extensive lesion evaluation, especially in the posthysterectomy patient.

→ Referral to a gynecologist or gynecological oncologist will be necessary to administer specific therapeutic modalities.

PATIENT EDUCATION

→ The primary health care provider may discuss the etiology and nature of the disease with the patient. The physician responsible for care should detail the particulars of treatment and management, and necessary follow-up.

→ As HPV infection is associated with this condition, advise safer sex practices to prevent sexually transmitted diseases. (See **Table 13A.2, Safer Sex Guidelines** in the **Chancroid** chapter in Section 13.)

FOLLOW-UP

→ Long-term follow-up is necessary due to the relatively high risk of recurrence.

→ Site-specific guidelines for follow-up may vary. In general, follow-up examinations include careful visual inspection; colposcopy of the cervix (when present), vagina, and vulva; and Pap smear every 4–6 months for two years.

→ Psychosexual counseling may be indicated.

→ Use of colposcopic photographs is helpful when following the lesion(s) over time.

→ Document in progress notes and on problem list.

BIBLIOGRAPHY

Abercrombie, P.D., and Korn, A.P. 1995. Multifocal lower genital tract neoplasia in women with HIV disease. *Nurse Practitioner* 20(5):68, 74, 76.

Anderson, L.L., and Atkinson, B.F. 1996. In *Clinical gynecologic pathology*, eds. E. Hernandez and B. Atkinson, pp. 129–174. Philadelphia: W.B. Saunders.

Anderson, M., Jordan, J., Morse, A. et al. 1997. *A text and atlas of integrated colposcopy*. St. Louis, Mo.: Mosby.

Burghardt, E., Pickel, H., and Girardi, F. 1998. *Colposcopy—cervical pathology textbook and atlas*, 3rd ed. New York: Thieme.

Burke, L., Antonioli, D.S., and Ducatman, B.S. 1991. *Colposcopy: text and atlas*. Norwalk, Conn.: Appleton & Lange.

Campion, M.J., Ferris, D., diPaola, F. et al. 1991. *Modern colposcopy: a practical approach*. Augusta, Ga.: Educational Systems.

Cheng, D., Ng, T.Y., Ngan, H.Y. et al. 1999. Wide local excision (WLE) for vaginal intraepithelial neoplasia (VAIN). *Acta Obstetrica et Gynecologica Scandinavia* 78(7):648–652.

Diakomanolis, E., Rodokis, A., Sakellaropoulos, K. et al. 1996. Conservative management of vaginal intraepithelial neoplasia (VAIN) by laser CO_2. *European Journal of Gynecologic Oncology* 17(5):389–392.

Dodge, J.A., Eltabbakh, G. H., Mount, S.L. et al. 2001. Clinical features and risk of recurrence among patients with vaginal intraepithelial neoplasia. *Gynecology Oncology* 83(2): 363–369.

Gross, G., and Barrasso, R. 1997. *Human papillomavirus infection: a clinical atlas*. Berlin and Wiesbaden, Germany: Ulstein-Mosby.

Rome, R.M., and England, P.G. 2000. Management of vaginal intraepithelial neoplasia: a series with long-term follow-up. *International Journal of Gynecological Cancer* 10(5): 382–390.

Sillman, F.H., Fruchter, R.G., Chen, Y.S. et al. 1997. Vaginal intraepithelial neoplasia: risk factors for persistence, recurrence, and invasion and its management. *American Journal of Obstetrics and Gynecology* 176(1):93-99.

Singer, A., and Monaghan, J.M. 2000. *Lower genital tract precancer: colposcopy, pathology, and treatment*, 2nd ed. London: Blackwell Science.

Stone, K.I., and Wilkinson, E.J. 1993. Benign and pre-invasive lesions of the vulva and vagina. In *Textbook of gynecology*, ed. L.J. Copeland, pp. 871–888. Philadelphia: W.B. Saunders.

Weiderpass, E., Ye, W., Tammi, R. et al. 2001. Alcoholism and the risk for cancer of the cervix uteri, vagina, and vulva. *Cancer Epidemiology, Biomarkers, and Prevention* 10(8): 899–901.

Wilkinson, E.J., and Stone, I.K. 1995. *Atlas of vulvar disease*. New York: Williams & Wilkins.

Zaino, R.J., Robboy, S.J., Bentley, R. et al. 1994. Diseases of the vagina. In *Blaustein's pathology of the female genital tract*, 4th ed., ed. R.J. Kurman, pp. 131–183. New York: Springer-Verlag.

SECTION 13

Sexually Transmitted Diseases

_____

13-A Chancroid **13-2**
13-B _Chlamydia trachomatis_ **13-9**
13-C Gonorrhea **13-17**
13-D Granuloma Inguinale (Donovanosis) **13-25**
13-E Genital Herpes Simplex Virus **13-29**
13-F Human Papillomavirus **13-37**
13-G Lymphogranuloma Venereum **13-45**
13-H Syphilis **13-50**

Winifred L. Star, R.N., C., N.P., M.S.
Melanie Deal, R.N., C., N.P., M.S.

13-A
Chancroid

Chancroid, or "soft chancre," is a sexually transmitted genital ulcerative disease caused by the Gram-negative bacillus *Haemophilus ducreyi*. It does not cause systemic disease; however, serious sequelae such as extensive destruction or scarring of genital tissue can occur. The disease is most prevalent in the developing countries of Africa, Asia, and Latin America. Chancroid is rare in the United States, but small localized outbreaks have occurred (Ronald et al. 1999).

After a brief rise in incidence in the 1980s, the number of chancroid cases in the United States has again dramatically decreased. In 1995, the number dropped below 1,000 (Ronald et al. 1999). There were only 78 cases reported in the United States in 2000 (Centers for Disease Control and Prevention [CDC] 2001). The global epidemiological picture is different, however. Worldwide incidence of chancroid may now exceed that of syphilis, and in limited areas it is more common than gonorrhea. The World Health Organization estimates the annual incidence is 7 million cases worldwide (Ronald et al. 1999).

In the United States, the incidence of chancroid is higher in persons at lower socioeconomic levels and among military personnel. The primary behavioral factors associated with chancroid are exchange of sex for money or drugs, use of crack cocaine, and use of alcohol (Ronald et al. 1999). Men are affected more than women, by a ratio of 10:1, but the etiology of this disparity is unclear. Women may have lower rates of infection or may have higher rates of asymptomatic lesions. Co-infection with *Treponema pallidum* or herpes simplex virus (HSV) may occur in as many as 10% of patients (CDC 2002, Sweet et al. 2002).

The major means of disease acquisition is sexual. Infection via autoinoculation of fingers or other sites occasionally has been reported. Trauma or abrasion is necessary for the organism to penetrate the epidermis. Transmission by fomites does not play a role (Ronald et al. 1999). Although the incubation period in women has not been well established, it is usually 4–7 days. Prodromal symptoms and systemic illness are not part of the clinical manifestation of chancroid, although mild constitutional symptoms have been reported (Ronald et al. 1999).

Studies in Africa have provided evidence that chancroid is a major risk factor for heterosexual transmission of the human immunodeficiency virus (HIV). The presence of a genital ulcer increases the chance that a sexual partner will become infected. It is thought that a genital ulcer enhances the passage of HIV into vaginal secretions; indeed, chancroid has been established as a cofactor in HIV transmission (CDC 1993, Sweet et al. 2002). A high rate of HIV infection among chancroid patients has been reported in the United States and elsewhere (CDC 2002). There have been some reported treatment failures of chancroid in individuals with HIV (Ronald et al. 1999). Resolution of ulcers in HIV-infected persons may be prolonged (Elkins et al. 2000).

H. ducreyi has demonstrated plasmid-mediated resistance to a variety of antibiotics and a large proportion of isolates are beta-lactamase positive (Jessamine et al. 1990, Ronald et al. 1999). There is no known resistance to macrolides, quinolones, or third-generation cephalosporins (Ronald et al. 1999).

DATABASE

SUBJECTIVE

→ Prostitutes are major carriers.
→ The patient may have a history of travel to areas where chancroid is endemic.
→ Occurs predominantly among lower socioeconomic groups.
→ Most affected individuals are heterosexual.
→ Asymptomatic, subclinical lesions may exist, more commonly in women.
→ Symptoms are less obvious in women.
→ Chancroid is a risk factor for HIV acquisition/transmission.
  ■ Cofactors include other sexually transmitted diseases (STDs).
  ■ Genital herpes may increase susceptibility.
→ Use of systemic/local antibiotics and topical steroids, and an immunodeficient state may modify the clinical presentation of genital ulcers (Ballard 1999).
→ Symptoms may include:
  ■ Vaginal discharge
  ■ External dysuria

- Pain on defecation
- Rectal bleeding
- Dyspareunia
- A "hernia"
- Painful ulcer(s); there is no prodrome. Women are more likely to have a painless ulcer. The patient may be unaware of an ulcer.
- Mild constitutional symptoms

→ Gynecological and medical history:
- Menstrual cycle
- Contraception
- Description of symptoms:
  • Onset
  • Duration
  • Quality/quantity
  • Frequency
  • Course
  • Aggravating/relieving factors
  • Associated symptoms
  • Previous history of same/similar problem
- STD history (including dates/treatment)
- Sensitive questioning regarding recent sexual activity, including date of last exposure, sex practices, sites of exposure, number and gender of partners in past 1–2 months, use of condoms
- Sex partner history (including drug use)
- Acute/chronic illness
- General health
- Medications
- Allergies
- Habits (including use of illegal drugs, both injection and noninjection)
- History of laboratory tests for syphilis, hepatitis B, HIV
- Review of systems (CDC 1991)

OBJECTIVE

→ Examination may be individualized based on case presentation.
→ A thorough STD examination includes (CDC 1991, Graney et al. 1999):
- Vital signs as indicated
- General skin inspection of face, trunk, forearms, palms, and soles for lesions, rashes, discoloration
- Inspection of pharynx and oral cavity for infection, lesions, discoloration
- Abdominal inspection and palpation for masses, tenderness, rebound tenderness
- Inspection of pubic hair for lice, nits
- Inspection of external genitalia for discharge, masses, lesions
- Inspection and palpation of Bartholin's, urethral, and Skene's glands for discharge, masses
- Inspection of vagina for discharge, lesions
- Inspection of cervix for lesions, discharge, eversion, erythema, edema, contact bleeding; assessment for cervical motion tenderness

- Uterine assessment for size, shape, consistency, mobility, tenderness
- Palpation of adnexa for masses, tenderness
- Inspection of perianus and anus for lesions, bleeding, discharge
- Assessment for presence or absence of associated lymphadenopathy. Present in up to 40% of cases. Less common in women (Ronald et al. 1999).
- Rectal examination as indicated

→ Chancroid ulcers most often involve the labia, fourchette, vestibule, clitoris, vaginal introitus, or perineum.
- Peri-urethral and vaginal ulcers also may occur.

→ Extragenital lesions of the breasts, thighs, mouth, and fingers may occur.
→ Characteristics of chancroid lesion:
- Single or multiple lesions may appear.
- Starts as an erythematous papule, becomes pustular, then eroded, then ulcerated over 24–48 hours with an outer zone of erythema. Alternately, papule may persist as a pustule ("dwarf chancroid").
- Deep, ragged with undermined edges
- Sharply demarcated
- Little or no induration (soft chancre)
- Base is a gray or yellow, necrotic, purulent exudate; very friable
- Little surrounding inflammation
- Painful or tender to touch; often painless in women
- May grow to 2–3 cm in diameter; may coalesce and erode through tissue planes resulting in fistulas. More common for women to have multiple ulcers.

→ Progression of disease affects inguinal lymph node area, usually unilaterally, with erythema of overlying skin forming an acute, painful, tender bubo (more than 50% of cases, in 7–10 days; unilateral in two-thirds of cases; less common in females).
→ The bubo may continue to enlarge and spontaneously rupture through the skin (especially if it is >5 cm) with extrusion of thick, creamy, viscous pus. Sinus tracts may form.
→ Inguinal adenopathy may persist for an indeterminate amount of time after the ulcer has healed.
→ Superinfection with *Fusobacterium* or *Bacteroides* species may occur. This may lead to gangrene and severe genital tissue destruction.
→ No signs of systemic infection or spread to distant sites.

ASSESSMENT

→ Chancroid
→ R/O syphilis
→ R/O herpes simplex
→ R/O lymphogranuloma venereum
→ R/O granuloma inguinale
→ R/O folliculitis
→ R/O superinfection, rectovaginal fistula, labial adhesions (complications of chancroid)
→ R/O HIV

→ R/O concomitant STD (e.g., gonorrhea, chlamydia)
→ R/O noninfectious cause of ulcer: trauma, drug eruption, Crohn's/Beçhet's disease
→ R/O metastatic genital cancer (cervical, vulvar, vaginal)

PLAN

DIAGNOSTIC TESTS

→ Distinguish between chancroid and other causes of genital ulcers. (See **Table 13A.1, Clinical Features of Genital Ulcers** and **Figure 13A.1, Sexually Active Patient with Genital Ulcer[s]**.)
→ A culture positive for *H. ducreyi* confirms the diagnosis (sensitivity is ≤80% [CDC 2002]).
→ Using a cotton or calcium alginate swab, obtain a specimen from ulcer base after gently removing necrotic exudate with saline. It is essential to plate out or send the specimen to microbiology immediately, as transport media are not widely available (Lewis 2000).
→ Alternately, aspirate from a bubo may be sent for culture (40–50% sensitive); however, aspirated fluid from the bubo is often sterile. Culture media for chancroid are highly selective (gonococcal agar or Mueller-Hinton agar). Ensure laboratory capabilities.

→ A Gram stain of an ulcer is unreliable, misleading, and not recommended (Lewis 2000).
→ A probable diagnosis of chancroid can be made in the presence of painful genital ulcer(s) plus:
- No evidence of syphilis infection (by dark field examination of ulcer exudate *or* a serological test at least seven days after ulcer onset)
  AND
- The clinical ulcer(s) presentation is typical for chancroid; if present, regional lymphadenopathy also is typical
  AND
- The HSV test results are negative (CDC 2002).
→ A suggestive diagnosis of chancroid includes a combination of painful ulcer(s) with tender inguinal adenopathy. When these signs are combined with suppurative inguinal adenopathy, they are almost pathognomonic for chancroid (CDC 2002).
→ Alternative diagnostic tests for chancroid are not widely available but may include compliment fixation, precipitin, agglutination tests, enzyme-linked immunosorbent assay (ELISA), and direct immunofluorescence (Ballard 1999).
→ Polymerase chain reaction (PCR) testing (>95% sensitivity) is under development but not yet commercially available (Lewis 2000).

Table 13A.1. CLINICAL FEATURES OF GENITAL ULCERS

	Syphilis	Herpes	Chancroid	Lymphogranuloma Venereum	Donovanosis
Incubation Period	9–90 days	2–7 days	1–14 days	3 days–6 weeks	1–4 weeks (up to 6 months)
Primary Lesions	Papule	Vesicle	Pustule	Papule, pustule, or vesicle	Papule
Number of Lesions	Usually one	Multiple, may coalesce	Usually multiple, may coalesce	Usually one	Variable
Diameter	5–15 mm	1–2 mm	Variable	2–10 mm	Variable
Edges	Sharply demarcated, elevated, round, or oval	Erythematous	Undermined, ragged, irregular	Elevated, round, or oval	Elevated, irregular
Depth	Superficial or deep	Superficial	Excavated	Superficial or deep	Elevated
Base	Smooth, nonpurulent, relatively nonvascular	Serous, erythematous, nonvascular	Purulent, bleeds easily	Variable, nonvascular	Red and velvety, bleeds readily
Induration	Firm	None	Soft	Occasionally firm	Firm
Pain	Uncommon	Frequently tender	Usually very tender	Variable	Uncommon
Lymphadenopathy	Firm, nontender, bilateral	Firm, tender, often bilateral with initial episode	Tender, may suppurate, loculated, usually unilateral	Tender, may suppurate, loculated, usually unilateral	None; pseudobuboes

Source: Ballard, R.C. 1999. Genital ulcer adenopathy syndrome. In *Sexually transmitted diseases*, 3rd ed., eds. K.K. Holmes, P.F. Sparling, P.A. Mårdh et al., p. 888. New York: McGraw-Hill. Reproduced with permission from the McGraw-Hill Companies.

→ Diagnostic tests to rule out other causes of genital ulcers and lymphadenopathy include:

- Dark-field or direct immunofluorescence test of serous fluid for *T. pallidum* from genital and nonoral lesion(s) to rule out syphilis. (See the **Syphilis** chapter.)

- RPR (or VDRL) or treponemal tests to rule out syphilis. (See the **Syphilis** chapter.)
- Herpes culture to rule out herpes. (See the **Genital Herpes Simplex Virus** chapter.)
- See "Diagnostic Tests" in the **Lymphogranuloma Venereum** and **Granuloma Inguinale (Donovanosis)** chapters.

Figure 13A.1.   SEXUALLY ACTIVE PATIENT WITH GENITAL ULCER(S)

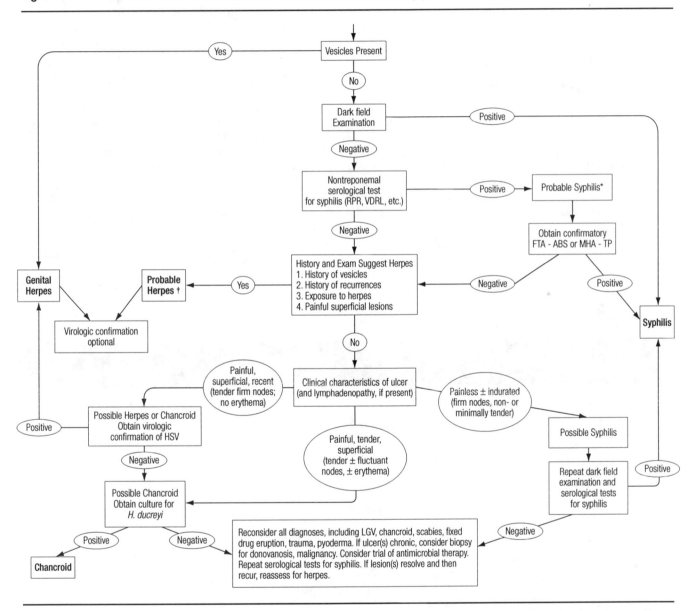

* While awaiting the FTA-ABS results, most clinicians initiate syphilis therapy for patients having dark-field-negative, RPR-positive ulcers that resemble chancres.

† Confirmation of probable herpes is desirable. If the confirmation test for herpes is negative or if the course is atypical, re-evaluate the diagnosis, repeat the serological test for syphilis in 3–4 weeks, consider fixed drug eruption if there is a history of recurrent lesions at the same time, and rule out herpes at the next recurrence.

Source: Reprinted with permission from Piot, P., and Plummer, F.A. 1990. Genital ulcer adenopathy syndrome. In *Sexually transmitted diseases*, 2nd ed., eds. K.K. Holmes, P.-A. Mårdh, P.F. Sparling et al., p. 714. New York: McGraw-Hill. ©The McGraw-Hill Companies.

→ Sensitive testing for *N. gonorrhoeae* and *C. trachomatis*. In the absence of a cervix, a urethral or urine specimen may be obtained.

→ HIV antibody testing should be performed at the time of diagnosis (CDC 2002).

→ Additional tests may include but are not limited to: wet mount, Pap smear, CBC, urinalysis, urine culture and sensitivities, hepatitis B screen, and pregnancy test.

TREATMENT/MANAGEMENT

→ Recommended regimens:
- Azithromycin 1 g p.o. in a single dose
  OR
- Ceftriaxone 250 mg IM in a single dose
  OR
- Ciprofloxacin 500 mg p.o. BID for 3 days
  OR
- Erythromycin base 500 mg p.o. TID for 7 days (CDC 2002).

  NOTE: HIV-infected patients may need longer courses of therapy. The 7-day erythromycin course is suggested by some experts as the preferred regimen when treating HIV-infected patients. Single-dose therapy should only be used in individuals for whom follow-up can be ensured (CDC 2002).

  NOTE: Ciprofloxacin is contraindicated in pregnancy and lactation. The safety and efficacy of azithromycin during pregnancy and lactation have not been established (CDC 2000).

→ Partner therapy:
- All sexual partners exposed within the 10 days preceding a patient's symptom onset should be evaluated and treated with one of the above regimens (CDC 2002).
- Refer to a provider/facility that offers appropriate STD care as indicated.

→ Additional considerations:
- Fluctuant lymph nodes should be aspirated through adjacent healthy skin to prevent rupture. In some cases, repeated aspirations may be necessary. Incision and drainage of buboes may be done in conjunction with antibiotic treatment (Ronald et al. 1999).

  NOTE: Buboes may appear to worsen in the 1–2 days following therapy.
- A broad-spectrum systemic antibiotic is indicated in cases of severe secondary bacterial infection of the ulcer.
- Good hygiene and saline soaks will promote tissue granulation and ulcer re-epithelialization.
- Untreated ulcers will heal in about 5 weeks.

CONSULTATION

→ Because special diagnostic testing is not widely available, consider referral to an STD specialist.

→ As indicated for patient evaluation.

→ For abnormal lab studies as indicated.

Table 13A.2. SAFER SEX PRACTICES

	Safer Sex (Extremely Low or No-Risk Practices)	Probably Safe (Very Low-Risk Practices)	Possibly Unsafe	Unsafe (High Risk)
Behaviors	Abstinence	French (wet) kissing	Cunnilingus	Unprotected vaginal intercourse
	Self-masturbation	Mutual masturbation**	Fellatio	Unprotected receptive anal intercourse
	Monogamous relationship: both partners uninfected and not involved in high-risk activities (e.g., needle-sharing)	Vaginal sex with a male or female condom (put latex or polyurethane condom in place before any penetration)	Anilingus	Unprotected anal penetration
	Hugging,* massaging,* touching,* caressing*	Fellatio with condom***		Multiple sexual partners
	Social (dry) kissing	Cunnilingus with dental dam		Sharing sex toys or douches
	Drug abstinence	Anilingus (rimming) with dental dam		Sharing needles for any purpose
		Contact with urine (water sports; only with intact skin, avoid contact with mouth)		

NOTE: Safer sex practices help prevent HIV infection, chlamydia, gonorrhea, syphilis, trichomoniasis, and chancroid.
*If no breaks or lesions on the skin.
**If no breaks or lesions on the skin. Less effective against HPV transmission.
***Put latex dam or condom in place before contact.

Source: Adapted with permission from Palacio, H. 1999. Safer sex. In *The AIDS knowledge base*, 3rd ed., eds. P.T. Cohen, M.A. Sande, and P.A. Volberding, pp. 903–909. Philadelphia: Lippincott Williams & Wilkins.

→ For patients unresponsive to therapy, refer to a physician.

→ As needed for prescription(s).

PATIENT EDUCATION

→ Discuss the etiology and nature of chancroid, including the mode of transmission, incubation period, symptoms, potential complications, co-association with HIV infection, and importance of partner examination and treatment.

→ Patient-education handouts are a useful adjunct to teaching. Written materials may be obtained from:

- CDC National Prevention Information Network
  P.O. Box 6003, Rockville, Md. 20849-6003
  (800) 458-5231
  www.cdcnpin.org
- American Social Health Association
  P.O. Box 13827, Research Triangle Park, N.C. 27709
  (919) 361-8400
  www.ashastd.org
- Additional resources for patients are:
  - National STD Hotline
    (800) 227-8922 or (800) 342-2437
    En Español: (800) 344-7432
  - For adolescents: www.iwannaknow.org

→ Advise the patient and her partner to finish the full course of medication and return for follow-up. (See "Follow-up," below.)

→ Explain that healing time is related to the size of the ulcer and may require more than two weeks for a large lesion. Scarring may result in extensive cases. Lymphadenopathy resolution is slower than that of ulcers (CDC 2002).

→ Advise abstinence from intercourse until the patient and her partner are treated and cured. They should be instructed to seek care promptly if symptoms recur.

→ Address STD prevention and HIV risk reduction, provide guidelines for safer sex practices, and encourage careful screening of sex partners and committed use of condoms (especially with new, multiple, nonmonogamous partners). (See **Table 13A.2, Safer Sex Practices** and **Table 12I.1, Recommendations for Individuals to Prevent STD/PID** in the **Pelvic Inflammatory Disease** chapter in Section 12.)

→ Allow the patient to vent her feelings of surprise, shame, fear, and anger as indicated. Psychological support may be important for helping the patient gain control over her sexual situation and to prevent future STDs.

FOLLOW-UP

→ Patients should be re-examined 3–7 days after initiation of therapy (CDC 2002). Ulcers usually improve within this time if treatment is successful.

→ Large ulcers may require more than two weeks for complete healing.

→ Fluctuant lymphadenopathy is slower to resolve and may require needle aspiration or incision and drainage.

→ Observe the patient at weekly intervals until the ulcer has completely resolved (CDC 2002).

→ History on follow-up should include:

- Symptom status
- Medication compliance
- Drug reaction and side effects
- Partner therapy
- Sexual exposure
- Use of condoms

→ Treatment failures should arouse suspicion for (CDC 2002):

- HIV infection
- Incorrect diagnosis
- Noncompliance with medication
- Resistance to antibiotic
- Incorrect diagnosis
- Co-existent STD

→ Perform antibiotic susceptibility tests on *H. ducreyi* isolates in patients who are unresponsive to therapy.

→ Syphilis and HIV testing should be repeated in three months if they are initially negative (CDC 2002).

→ HIV-infected patients require close monitoring. Longer courses of therapy may be necessary and healing may be slower. Refer to a physician as indicated.

→ Follow up on all laboratory tests ordered. Treat all concomitant STDs and other identified conditions.

→ Offer the hepatitis A vaccine to women at risk for sexual transmission of this virus (e.g., users of illegal injection and noninjection drugs). (See the **Hepatitis—Viral** chapter in Section 11.)

→ Offer the hepatitis B vaccine to all women seeking treatment for an STD who have not been previously vaccinated. (See the **Hepatitis—Viral** chapter in Section 11 for more information.)

→ HIV-positive results should be conveyed in person by a provider who has received training in the complexities of test disclosure. HIV-positive persons should be referred to the appropriate provider or agency for early intervention services.

→ Newly diagnosed, hepatitis B antigen-positive individuals should have liver function tests and receive counseling regarding the implications of their positive status and the need for immunoprophylaxis of sex partners and household members. (See the **Hepatitis—Viral** chapter in Section 11.)

→ Because chancroid is a state-mandated reportable disease, a morbidity report must be filed with the department of public health.

→ Continue to encourage safer sex practices.

→ Document in progress notes and on problem list.

BIBLIOGRAPHY

Ballard, R.C. 1999. Genital ulcer adenopathy syndrome. In *Sexually transmitted diseases*, 3rd ed., eds. K.K. Holmes, P.F. Sparling, P.-A. Mårdh et al., pp. 887–897. New York: McGraw-Hill.

Centers for Disease Control and Prevention (CDC). 1991. *Sexually transmitted diseases. Clinical practice guidelines.* Atlanta, Ga.: the Author.

_____. 1993. Sexually transmitted diseases treatment guidelines 1993. *Morbidity and Mortality Weekly Report* 42(RR-14):20–22.

_____. 2001. Sexually transmitted disease surveillance 2000. Atlanta, Ga.: the Author.

_____. 2002. Sexually transmitted diseases treatment guidelines 2002. *Morbidity and Mortality Weekly Report* 51(RR-6):11–12.

Elkins, C., Yi, K., Olsen, B. et al. 2000. Development of a serological test for *Haemophilus ducreyi* for seroprevalence studies. *Journal of Clinical Microbiology* 38(4):1520–1526.

Graney, D.O., and Vontver, L.A. 1999. Anatomy and physical examination of the female genital tract. In *Sexually transmitted diseases*, 3rd ed., eds. K.K. Holmes, P.F. Sparling, P. Mårdh et al., pp. 685–697. New York: McGraw-Hill.

Jessamine, P., and Ronald, A.R. 1990. Chancroid and the role of genital ulcer disease in the spread of human retroviruses. *Medical Clinics of North America* 74(6):1417–1431.

Lewis, D.A. 2000. Diagnostic tests for chancroid. *Sexually Transmitted Infections* 76:137–141.

Ronald, A.R., and Albritton, W. 1999. Chancroid and *Haemophilus ducreyi*. In *Sexually transmitted diseases*, 3rd ed., eds. K.K. Holmes, P.F. Sparling, P. Mårdh et al., pp. 515–524. New York: McGraw-Hill.

Sweet, R.L., and Gibbs, R.S. 2002. *Infectious diseases of the female genital tract*, 4th ed. Philadelphia: Lippincott Williams & Wilkins.

Winifred L. Star, R.N., C., N.P., M.S.
Melanie Deal, R.N., C., N.P., M.S.

13-B
Chlamydia trachomatis

Chlamydiae are a group of obligate intracellular microorganisms differentiated from other bacteria by a unique growth cycle. The organisms lack the ability to synthesize high-energy compounds. Thus, in order to survive and grow, they must completely depend on the host cell for energy and nutrients (Schachter 1999).

Two biological forms of the organism exist: the elementary body, which is the infectious, extracellular form, and the reticulate body, which is the replicative, intracellular form (Schachter 1999). A more detailed discussion of the developmental cycle is beyond the scope of this chapter.

There are 15 serotypes of *Chlamydia trachomatis* that are the causative agents for a variety of infections, including trachoma (A, B, B$_a$, C), lymphogranuloma venereum (LGV) (L-1, L-2, L-3), and the genital tract diseases (D-K) urethritis, cervicitis, salpingitis, proctitis, and epididymitis. (Schachter 1999, Sweet et al. 2002). The serotype of *C. trachomatis* that causes genital infections infects only squamocolumnar cells (Schachter 1999).

In industrialized Western countries, *C. trachomatis* is almost exclusively sexually transmitted. Nonsexual transmission may occur if infected genital secretions are inoculated onto mucous membranes, particularly the eye. Infants exposed to chlamydia by passage through the infected cervix at birth may become infected and develop inclusion conjunctivitis and/or newborn pneumonia (Schachter 1999).

Chlamydia is now the number one reportable infectious disease in the United States (Centers for Disease Control and Prevention [CDC] 1996). An estimated 3–4 million cases occur each year in the United States at a cost of $2.2 billion (Cates et al. 1991, Groseclose et al. 1999). The prevalence of chlamydial infection ranges from 2–4% in private practice or primary care settings to 20% in sexually transmitted disease (STD) clinics (Weinstock et al. 1994). The highest incidence of chlamydial infections is among adolescents and young adults (CDC 2001). Approximately 80% of all reported cases are in patients 15–24 years old (CDC 1997). In sexually active female adolescent populations, prevalence ranges vary but are usually greater than 10% (Weinstock et al. 1994).

The incubation period for chlamydia is 6–14 days, but women may harbor the organism for extended periods of time (Golden et al. 2000, Sweet et al. 2002). Studies of transmissibility report varying rates. Rates of infection in women with infected male partners range from 45–50% (Stamm 1999). One study, using a newer diagnostic technology, revealed a transmissibility rate of approximately 70% for both men and women (Quinn et al. 1996). By age 30, an estimated 50% of sexually active women have been exposed to *C. trachomatis* as demonstrated by positive antibody serology (Sweet et al. 2002). Approximately 20–40% of gonorrhea cases are co-infected with chlamydia (CDC 1998).

Chlamydia often is difficult to diagnose due to the high incidence of asymptomatic infections. Seventy percent to 80% of women are asymptomatic (Weinstock et al. 1994). Moreover, most infections do not cause clinical signs. Despite the mild or absent symptoms and clinical signs, chlamydial infections cause more severe tubal inflammation and tubal damage than other organisms do (Weinstock et al. 1994). Thus, chlamydia poses a substantial threat to women's reproductive health.

The clinical manifestations caused by chlamydia, when present, closely parallel those of gonorrhea. Sites of infection in women include the endocervix (most common site), with potential extension to the endometrium, salpinx, and peritoneum; the urethra; the Bartholin's glands; the rectum (5%); and the pharynx (3–6%).

Other, much less common manifestations of chlamydial infection may include perihepatitis or Fitz-Hugh-Curtis (FHC) syndrome, a complication of chlamydia-associated salpingitis; Reiter's syndrome (urethritis, conjunctivitis, arthritis, and characteristic mucotaneous lesions, usually in men); and pneumonia, endocarditis, and meningoencephalitis (all fairly rare) (Stamm 1999). Full discussion of these complications is beyond the scope of this chapter. The reader is referred to a current STD textbook.

C. trachomatis is responsible for 15–55% of nongonococcal urethritis in heterosexual men (CDC 2002). Forty percent to 50% of men with chlamydial infection, however, are asymptomatic (Schachter 1999).

Knowledge of the natural history of chlamydial infections is still unfolding. However, it seems the infection may have the ability to smolder until complications arise. In fact, complications may even develop subclinically. Both *C. trachomatis* and *Neisseria gonorrhoeae* can cause significant tissue damage (e.g., subepithelial inflammation, epithelial ulceration, and scarring), although symptoms are usually less severe and the resultant tissue damage is greater with chlamydia (Stamm et al. 1990, Weinstock et al. 1994).

Sequelae of genital chlamydial infection are significant. They include acute or chronic pelvic inflammatory disease (PID), tubal infertility, and ectopic pregnancy (see related chapters). Moreover, there is an abundant immune response to chlamydial infection. The adverse sequelae may partially result from a delayed hypersensitivity (Schachter 1999). Reinfection is more likely than initial infection to cause adverse health outcomes (Xu et al. 2000). Preventing recurrent infection is vital.

DATABASE

SUBJECTIVE

→ Risk factors include:
- Young age (highest incidence in ages 15–24 years)
- Early age at first intercourse
- New or multiple sexual partners
- Lower socioeconomic status
- Presence of cervical eversion (ectopy)
- Use of oral contraceptives (induces cervical eversion)
- Use of no or nonbarrier contraception
- History of concomitant gonorrhea/other STD
- Sexual partner with nongonococcal urethritis (NGU), gonorrhea, or other STD
- Douching (may precipitate an upper genital tract infection in women with a chlamydia-positive cervix)
- Intrauterine device use (increases risk for chlamydia-associated endometritis)
- See the **Lymphogranuloma Venereum** chapter.

→ Most women don't have symptoms.

→ The patient may present with:
- Endocervicitis:
  - Abnormal vaginal discharge
  - Postcoital or intermenstrual vaginal bleeding or spotting
- Urethral syndrome/urethritis:
  - Dysuria, frequency
  - Usually no suprapubic tenderness or hematuria
  - Onset of symptoms often occurs with a new sexual partner in the past month or with exposure to partner with NGU
  - Symptoms may last longer than in acute cystitis (more than 7–10 days)
  - Less likely to have history of recurrent urinary tract infection (UTI)
- Endometritis/salpingitis:
  - Intermenstrual spotting/bleeding
  - Menorrhagia
  - Dysmenorrhea
  - Dyspareunia
  - Abdominal/pelvic pain
  - Fever, chills, malaise, nausea, vomiting
  - Symptoms usually less severe than those associated with gonorrheal or anaerobic pelvic infection
  - Late symptoms of undiagnosed infection may include chronic pelvic pain, ectopic pregnancy symptoms (see the **Ectopic Pregnancy** chapter in Section 12), and/or unexplained infertility
  - See the **Pelvic Inflammatory Disease** chapter in Section 12.
- Conjunctivitis:
  - Conjunctival irritation, redness
  - See the **Conjunctivitis** chapter in Section 2.
- Pharyngitis:
  - Asymptomatic, not established as a cause of pharyngitis (Weinstock et al. 1994)
- Bartholinitis:
  - Varying degrees of pain/tenderness in Bartholin's gland
  - Difficulty sitting, walking
  - Dyspareunia
  - Few systemic symptoms unless extensive inflammation
  - See the **Vulvar Disease—Large Lesions of the Vulva** chapter in Section 12.
- Proctitis:
  - Usually asymptomatic
  - Clinical manifestations in women haven't been well-studied. Symptoms may include anal irritation, rectal pain, hematochezia, tenesmus, mucous discharge, constipation, painful defecation.
  - See the **Lymphogranuloma Venereum** chapter.
- Perihepatitis (Fitz-Hugh-Curtis syndrome):
  - Severe right upper quadrant (pleuritic) pain (may occur from six days before to 14 days after the onset of lower abdominal pain from salpingitis)
  - Other symptoms may include fever, nausea, vomiting, increased vaginal discharge, menorrhagia, dysmenorrhea, or dyspareunia.
- Reiter's syndrome:
  - Spectrum of urogenital inflammation in men. Remains to be established in women (Rice et al. 1999).
  - Wide range of particular symptoms or nonspecific rheumatic complaints
  - Skin, mouth, nail lesions
  - Conjunctival irritation, redness

→ Gynecological and medical history:
- Menstrual cycle
- Contraception
- Description of symptoms:
  - Onset
  - Duration
  - Quality/quantity
  - Frequency
  - Course

- Aggravating and relieving factors
- Associated symptoms
- Previous history of same or similar symptoms
- STD history (including dates/treatment), activity (including date of last exposure, sex practices, sites of exposure, number and gender of partners in past 1–2 months, use of condoms)
- Sex partner history (including drug use)
- Acute/chronic illness
- General health
- Medications
- Allergies
- Habits (including use of illegal drugs, both injection and noninjection)
- History of laboratory tests for syphilis, hepatitis B, HIV
- Review of systems (CDC 1991)

OBJECTIVE

→ Examination may be individualized based on case presentation. Most women don't have clinical signs.
→ A thorough STD examination includes (CDC 1991, Graney et al. 1999):
- Vital signs as indicated
- General skin inspection of face, trunk, forearms, palms, and soles for lesions, rashes, discoloration
- Inspection of pharynx and oral cavity for infection, lesions, discoloration
- Abdominal inspection and palpation for masses, tenderness, rebound tenderness
- Inspection of pubic hair for lice, nits
- Inspection of external genitalia for discharge, masses
- Inspection and palpation of Bartholin's, urethral, and Skene's glands for discharge, masses
- Inspection of vagina for blood, discharge, lesions
- Inspection of cervix for lesions, discharge, eversion, erythema, edema, contact bleeding; assessment for cervical motion tenderness (CMT)
- Uterine assessment for size, shape, consistency, mobility, tenderness
- Palpation of adnexa for masses, tenderness
- Inspection of perianus and anus for lesions, bleeding, discharge
- Rectal examination as indicated
- Assessment for presence or absence of associated cervical inguinal lymphadenopathy
→ Physical examination components and findings specific to assessment of patients with chlamydial infection may include:
- Temperature: may be elevated in patients with PID, UTI, FHC syndrome, tubo-ovarian abscess (TOA).
- Abdomen: usually within normal limits (WNL) in uncomplicated infections:
  - Possible right upper quadrant tenderness (or liver tenderness) in FHC syndrome

- Generalized tenderness and/or rebound tenderness in endometritis, salpingitis, peritonitis
- Inguinal mass/adenopathy in LGV.
- External genitalia: usually WNL. Erythema, edema, excoriation may be present in concomitant vaginitis.
- Bartholin's, urethral, Skene's glands: usually WNL.
  - Purulent or mucoid exudate (milk the glands, urethra), meatal erythema/swelling may be present in urethritis.
  - Swelling/abscess formation may be present in bartholinitis.
- Vagina: abnormal discharge, blood, pus may be present.
- Cervix: purulent or mucopurulent discharge, edema/erythema of the zone of ectopy, contact bleeding. CMT may be present. (See "Diagnostic Tests," below.)
- Uterus: usually WNL in uncomplicated infections.
  - Tenderness may be present in endometritis.
- Adnexa: usually WNL in uncomplicated infection.
  - Masses/tenderness may be present in salpingitis, FHC syndrome, TOA.
- Rectum: usually WNL in uncomplicated infections.
  - Blood or mucus discharge may be present in proctitis (uncommon in women).
  - Masses/tenderness may be present in salpingitis, FHC syndrome, TOA.
→ Additional assessment of Reiter's syndrome may include:
- Skin:
  - Lesions of keratoderma blennorrhagica occur most commonly on plantar surfaces of the feet. Erythematous macules enlarge and coalesce to form a hyperkeratotic, scaly plaque resembling psoriasis (Colven et al. 1999).
- Mouth:
  - Painless shallow ulcers on palate, tongue, buccal mucosa, lips, tonsillar pillars, or pharynx (Rice et al. 1999).
- Nails:
  - Thickening, brown-yellow discoloration (Rice et al. 1999).
- Extremities:
  - Asymmetrical, polyarticular synovitis-tendonitis often seen initially on tendon insertion sites, the common sites of inflammation (e.g., Achilles tendon, plantar fascia).
  - Arthritis of knees, ankles, and feet, most commonly with knee effusions and fusiform dactylitis ("sausage digits") of fingers, toes; sacroilitis (Rice et al. 1999).
- The HLA-B27 antigen is present in 70–80% of Caucasians and 15–75% of African Americans with Reiter's syndrome. Manifestations of Reiter's syndrome are more severe in these patients (Rice et al. 1999).
→ Anoscopy may be indicated in women with proctitis. Findings include mucopus and erythematous, friable mucosa.
→ A complete and accurate description of any identified lesion or other pertinent physical manifestation should be noted in the "Objective" section of the progress notes.
→ See "Objective" in the **Lymphogranuloma Venereum** chapter.

ASSESSMENT

→ *C. trachomatis* infection
→ Exposure to *C. trachomatis* or other STD
→ Mucopurulent cervicitis
→ R/O chlamydia
→ R/O gonorrhea
→ R/O syphilis
→ R/O other concomitant STD
→ R/O vaginitis
→ R/O urethral syndrome/UTI
→ R/O PID
→ R/O TOA
→ R/O ectopic pregnancy
→ R/O perihepatitis (FHC syndrome). Differential diagnoses include cholecystitis, hepatitis, pleurisy, pneumonia, pyelonephritis, mononucleosis, perforated ulcer, appendicitis, liver/subdiaphragmatic abscess, toxic shock syndrome.
→ R/O Reiter's syndrome
→ R/O LGV

PLAN

DIAGNOSTIC TESTS

→ Mucopurulent cervicitis (MPC) can be caused by *C. trachomatis* (or *N. gonorrhoeae*). However, in most cases, neither organism can be isolated and other nonmicrobiologic determinants (e.g., inflammation in the zone of ectopy) may be involved (CDC 2002).
  - Characteristics include:
    • Yellow or green mucopus on a white, cotton-tip swab of endocervical secretions ("positive swab test")
    • Contact bleeding, erythema, or edema within a zone of cervical eversion (ectopy)
    • >10 polymorphonuclear leukocytes per oil immersion field (x 1,000 magnification) of a Gram stain of endocervical mucus (collected after first gently removing ectocervical vaginal secretions)
→ Selection of the most appropriate laboratory test will depend on availability, laboratory expertise, and *C. trachomatis* prevalence in the population. Experts recommend a test type that is at least 90% sensitive and 97% specific (Region IX Infertility Prevention Project Advisory Committee 1998). Collection and transport requirements vary by test. Refer to the package insert. (See **Table 13B.1, Comparison of Chlamydia Testing Technologies**.)
  - Test options include:
    • Culture: Historically, it has been considered the gold standard for diagnosis of chlamydia. However, this test has been used more restrictively with the advent of the more-sensitive nucleic acid amplification tests. Culture is the only FDA-approved method for pharyngeal and rectal sampling, and it remains a recommended test type for medico-legal cases.
    NOTE: Cultures should be obtained *before* the use of bacteriostatic lubricant. Endocervical cells are necessary for *C. trachomatis* isolation. Ectocervical secretions

should be removed before endocervical sampling. Insert swab 2–3 cm into the endocervical canal (Chernesky 1999). Rayon or cotton-tip swabs on plastic shafts or cytological brushes are preferable. Wood may be toxic to *C. trachomatis*. The specimen should be placed in the proper medium and transported to the laboratory as soon as possible. If a delay is unavoidable, the specimen should be refrigerated (Woods 1996). Depending on clinical presentation, cultures also may be taken from:
  - Urethra:
    ➤ Insert thin swab on flexible-wire shaft 1–2 cm into the urethra and rotate (Chernesky 1999).
  - Eye:
    ➤ With the eyelid everted, swab vigorously over the mucosa.
  - Rectum:
    ➤ Best obtained by direct visualization via anoscopy, but it can be obtained by swabbing 2 cm into the rectum (Chernesky 1999).
  - Bartholin's gland:
    ➤ Strip exudate from gland duct openings.
• Nucleic acid amplification tests (NAATs) are the newest testing modalities. This diagnostic class includes polymerase chain reaction (PCR), ligase chain reaction (LCR), and transcriptase-mediated amplification (TMA) test types. The sensitivities are generally higher than those of all other tests. The advantages of NAATs include use of a single swab for chlamydia and gonorrhea testing, the ability to use urine as a specimen source, and increased sensitivity. The use of these tests on anatomic sites other than the urogenital tract has not been adequately studied. Use culture for anorectal and pharyngeal specimens (Schachter 1999). May be used for medico-legal cases if positive tests are confirmed by a second test (CDC 2002).
  - To collect a urine sample, ensure that the patient has not voided within the past hour. Instruct the patient to void 15–30 cc into a sterile container. Patients should *not* cleanse the genital area. Clearly differentiate this collection method from a "clean catch, midstream" to obtain a urine culture.
• Antigen detection methods. Although these tests are still available, they have lower sensitivities than other commercially available tests:
  - Direct immunofluorescent monoclonal antibody (DFA) tests (MicroTrak®)
  - Enzyme-linked immunosorbent assay (EIA) (Chlamydiazyme®)
• DNA probe:
  - Nonamplified DNA probe (Gen-Probe Pace Assay®)
• Serology:
  - Generally not useful for diagnosing *C. trachomatis* infections (except in LGV and FHC syndrome) due to the high background rate of antichlamydial antibodies in the population.

- The microimmunofluorescence (Micro-IF) assay detects IgG or IgM antibodies.
- Extremely high IgG or IgM levels, IgM antibodies, or fourfold increases in IgG titers are considered diagnostic of recent infection (Sweet et al. 2002).

■ Other diagnostic tests may include:

- Pap smear: may show cellular atypia. If present, sensitive testing for *N. gonorrhoeae* should be considered.
- Cytological detection: a reliable means of diagnosing trachoma and inclusion conjunctivitis (Sweet et al. 2002).

- VDRL or RPR: to rule out syphilis.
- Wet mount: in the presence of an abnormal vaginal discharge.
- Urinalysis: may reveal pyuria (>10 WBCs/HPF spun urine).
- Urine culture: may be negative for common urinary pathogens in acute *C. trachomatis*-associated urethral syndrome.
- Serological HIV testing: should be offered.

Table 13B.1.   COMPARISON OF CHLAMYDIA TESTING TECHNOLOGIES

	Cell Culture	Direct Fluorescent Antibody (DFA)	Enzyme Immunoassay (EIA)	Nucleic Acid Probe	Nucleic Acid Amplification Technology
Name of Test		MicroTrak	Chlamydiazyme	Pace 2	LCR LCx CT Test (Abbott) PCR Amplicor CT Test (Roche) TMA Amplified CT Assay/Aptima (Gen-Probe) SDA /BDProbeTec (Bectin Dickinson)
Collection Site	Endocervical, urethral, urine, rectal, conjunctival, pulmonary	Endocervical, urethral, rectal, conjunctival, nasopharyngeal	Endocervical, urethral, urine, conjunctival	Endocervical, urethral, conjunctival	Male and female urine, endocervical and urethral swabs
Sensitivity	75–85%	70–75%	50–75%	65–75%	90–95%
Specificity	100%	95–99%	95–99%	95–99%	98–99%
Test Advantages	Recommended for medico-legal purposes.	Refrigeration during transport not required.	Refrigeration during transport not required.	One swab for both chlamydia and gonorrhea. Refrigeration during transport not required.	More sensitive. Optional gonorrhea testing on same specimen. Approved for noninvasive urine specimens in addition to genital swabs.
Test Disadvantages	Less sensitive. Longer turnaround time. Technically difficult. Specimen transport, storage times, and temperatures critical. Labor intensive. Quality assurance for specimen adequacy required.	Less sensitive. Technically difficult. Labor intensive.	Poor sensitivity. Quality assurance for specimen adequacy required. Confirmatory testing recommended.	Quality assurance for specimen adequacy required. Confirmatory testing recommended.	Expensive. Contamination possible if specimen not handled properly in the clinic or lab.

Source: Adapted with permission from Bauer, H.M., and Bolan, G. 2000. Diagnosis and treatment of genital chlamydial infections. Oakland, Calif.: California HealthCare Foundation. Based on a template developed in 1998 by the Region IX Infertility Prevention Project Advisory Committee, Region IX Infertility Prevention Project.

- CBC, liver function studies, hepatitis B screen, chest x-ray, ultrasound, pregnancy test: ordered as indicated.
- Laparoscopy: the definitive method for diagnosing salpingitis and perihepatitis.
  - See the **Lymphogranuloma Venereum** chapter and, in Section 12, the **Pelvic Inflammatory Disease** and **Pelvic Masses** chapters.

TREATMENT/MANAGEMENT

→ There has been no reported clinical resistance to *C. trachomatis* (Stamm 1999).
→ Patients with MPC should await results of *C. trachomatis* and *N. gonorrhoea* tests before treatment, unless there is high suspicion of infection or the patient is unlikely to return for follow-up (CDC 2002).
→ The CDC (2002) recommends the following treatment of patients with MPC:
  - Treat appropriately for gonorrhea or chlamydia if tests are positive.
  - Empirically treat for chlamydia and/or gonorrhea in populations with a high prevalence of these diseases and if the patient might be difficult to locate for treatment.
  - Sex partners should be notified, examined, and treated based on the patient's test results. In cases where patients are treated presumptively, partners should receive the same therapy.
→ Recommended treatment regimens for chlamydia (CDC 2002):
  - Azithromycin 1 g p.o. in a single dose
    OR
  - Doxycycline 100 mg p.o. BID for 7 days
    NOTE: Doxycycline is contraindicated in pregnancy (CDC 2002).
→ Alternative regimens (CDC 2002):
  - Erythromycin base 500 mg p.o. QID for 7 days
    OR
  - Erythromycin ethylsuccinate 800 mg p.o. QID for 7 days
    OR
  - Ofloxacin 300 mg p.o. BID for 7 days
    OR
  - Levofloxacin 500 mg p.o. QD for 7 days
    NOTE: Fluoroquinolones are contraindicated in pregnancy (CDC 2002).
→ Partner therapy (CDC 2002):
  - Sex partners should be evaluated, tested, and treated if they had sexual contact with the patient during the 60 days preceding the onset of symptoms in the patient or diagnosis of chlamydia.
  - The most recent sex partner should be evaluated and treated even if the last sexual contact was more than 60 days before symptom onset or diagnosis.
  - Provide referrals to a provider or facility that offers appropriate STD care as necessary.
  - Patients should abstain from sexual intercourse until they and their sex partners have completed treatment, and

abstinence should continue until 7 days after a single-dose regimen or after completion of a 7-day regimen.
  - On January 1, 2001, a new law went into effect in California that allows clinicians to send chlamydia medication home with chlamydia-positive patients for treatment of their sex partners (patient-delivered partner therapy). Refer to the California Chlamydia Coalition's Web site (www.ucsf.edu/castd) for clinical guidelines on this practice.
→ Treatment during pregnancy (CDC 2002):
  - Recommended regimens:
    - Erythromycin base 500 mg p.o. QID for 7 days
      OR
    - Amoxicillin 500 mg p.o. TID for 7 days
  - Alternative regimens:
    - Erythromycin base 250 mg p.o. QID for 14 days
      OR
    - Erythromycin ethylsuccinate 800 mg p.o. QID for 7 days
      OR
    - Erythromycin ethylsuccinate 400 mg p.o. QID for 14 days
      OR
    - Azithromycin 1 g p.o. in a single dose
      NOTE: Erythromycin estolate, doxycycline, and ofloxacin are contraindicated in pregnancy. Although the data are limited, azithromycin is generally considered safe and effective during pregnancy (CDC 2002).
→ Additional considerations:
  - HIV-infected patients with MPC or identified chlamydial infections should receive the same treatment as outlined above (CDC 2002).
  - The mainstay of treatment for Reiter's syndrome is anti-inflammatory medication (e.g., indomethacin or other nonsteroidal agents) (Rice et al. 1999).
    - Consult with a rheumatologist.
    - Underlying chlamydia-associated and/or gonorrhea-associated cervicitis/urethritis should be treated with the recommended drug regimens.
    - See the **Gonorrhea** chapter.
    - Partners of patients with Reiter's syndrome should be referred for treatment.
→ Refer to the **Pelvic Inflammatory Disease** chapter in Section 12 for treatment of FHC syndrome.
→ See these chapters: **Gonorrhea, Syphilis, Lymphogranuloma Venereum,** and others related to sexually transmitted diseases, and, in Section 12, **Pelvic Inflammatory Disease** and **Pelvic Masses**.

CONSULTATION

→ Consultation with a physician is indicated for patients who have PID, TOA, symptoms of ectopic pregnancy, Reiter's syndrome, or complicated LGV.
→ As needed for prescription(s).

PATIENT EDUCATION

→ Discuss the etiology and nature of chlamydial infections, including the mode of transmission, incubation period, symptoms, potential complications, the possibility of co-existent gonorrhea or other STD, and the importance of partner treatment even if the partner is asymptomatic.

- Patient-education handouts are a useful adjunct to teaching. Written materials may be obtained from:
  - CDC National Prevention Information Network
    P.O. Box 6003, Rockville, Md. 20849-6003
    (800) 458-5231, www.cdcnpin.org
  - American Social Health Association
    P.O. Box 13827
    Research Triangle Park, N.C. 27709
    (919) 361-8400, www.ashastd.org
  - Additional resources for patients are:
    - National STD Hotline
      (800) 227-8922 or (800) 342-2437
      En Español: (800) 344-7432
    - For adolescents: www.iwannaknow.org

→ Advise the patient and her partner to finish the full course of medication.

→ Emphasize the importance of partner notification, evaluation, and treatment.

→ Abstinence should be continued until 7 days after a single dose regimen or after completion of a 7-day regimen.

→ The patient and her partner should be instructed to seek care promptly if symptoms recur.

→ Address STD prevention and HIV risk reduction, provide guidelines for safer sex practices, and encourage careful screening of sex partners and committed use of condoms (especially with new, multiple, nonmonogamous partners).

- See Table **13A.2, Safer Sex Practices** in the **Chancroid** chapter and, in Section 12, **Table 12I.1, Recommendations for Individuals to Prevent STD/PID** in the **Pelvic Inflammatory Disease** chapter.

→ Allow the patient to vent her feelings of surprise, shame, fear, and anger as indicated. Psychological support may be important for helping the patient gain control over her sexual situation and prevent future STDs.

FOLLOW-UP

→ Test of cure is not necessary after treatment with doxycycline or azithromycin unless the patient or partner is symptomatic or reinfection is suspected (CDC 2002). Retesting may be considered three weeks after completion of treatment with erythromycin (CDC 2002).
  NOTE: Cultures, if performed less than three weeks after completion of therapy, may yield false-negative results. Nonculture tests performed less than three weeks after completion of therapy may be falsely positive due to continued dead organism excretion (CDC 2002).

→ Rescreening all patients 3–4 months after treatment should be considered (CDC 2002).

→ In pregnancy, repeat testing—preferably by culture—is recommended after completing therapy because recommended regimens may not be highly efficacious and the frequent side effects of erythromycin might discourage patient compliance with this regimen (CDC 2002).

→ When the patient or partner continues to be symptomatic, a return visit is necessary. History on follow-up should include symptom status, medication compliance, drug reaction and side effects, partner therapy, sexual exposure, and use of condoms.

→ Follow up on all laboratory tests ordered. Treat all concomitant STDs and other identified conditions.

→ Negative HIV tests may be repeated in three months. Continue to encourage safer sex.

→ HIV-positive results should be conveyed in person and by a provider who has received training in the complexities of test disclosure. HIV-positive persons should be referred to the appropriate provider or agency for early intervention services.

→ Offer the hepatitis A vaccine to women at risk for sexual transmission of this virus (e.g., users of illegal injection or noninjection drugs). (See the **Hepatitis—Viral** chapter in Section 11.)

→ Offer the hepatitis B vaccine to all women seeking treatment for an STD who have not been previously vaccinated. (See the **Hepatitis—Viral** chapter for further information.)

→ Newly diagnosed, hepatitis B antigen-positive individuals should undergo liver function tests and receive counseling regarding the implications of their positive status and the need for immunoprophylaxis of sex partners and household members. (See the **Hepatitis—Viral** chapter.)

→ Routine *C. trachomatis* screening is recommended for the following categories:
  - Sexually active female adolescents
  - Women 20–25 years old
  - Older women with risk factors (e.g., those with new or multiple sex partners) (CDC 2002)

→ Chlamydia is a mandated reportable disease. A morbidity report must be filed with the department of public health.

→ Patients with FHC syndrome may have chronic upper quadrant pain despite adequate antibiotic therapy; laparoscopic lysis of adhesions may be indicated. Refer to a physician.

→ Document chlamydia diagnosis and complications/sequelae in progress notes and on problem list.

BIBLIOGRAPHY

Cates Jr., W., and Wasserheit, J.N. 1991. Genital chlamydial infections: epidemiology and reproductive sequelae. *American Journal of Obstetrics and Gynecology* 164(6, Part 2): 1771–1781.

Centers for Disease Control and Prevention (CDC). 1991. *Sexually transmitted diseases. Clinical practice guidelines.* Atlanta, Ga.: the Author.

_____. 1996. Ten leading nationally notifiable infectious diseases—United States, 1995. *Morbidity and Mortality Weekly Report* 45(41):883–884.

_____. 1997. *Chlamydia trachomatis* genital infections—United States, 1995. *Morbidity and Mortality Weekly Report* 46(9):193–198.

_____. 1998. Sexually transmitted disease surveillance, 1997. Atlanta, Ga.: the Author.

_____. 2001. Sexually transmitted disease surveillance, 2000. Atlanta, Ga.: the Author.

_____. 2002. Sexually transmitted diseases treatment guidelines 2002. *Morbidity and Mortality Weekly Report* 51(RR–6):32–35.

Chernesky, M.A. 1999. Laboratory services for sexually transmitted diseases: overview and recent developments. In *Sexually transmitted diseases*, 3rd ed., eds. K.K. Holmes, P.F. Sparling, P.-A. Mårdh et al., pp. 1281–1294. New York: McGraw-Hill.

Colven, R., and Spach, R.S. 1999. Generalized cutaneous manifestations of STD and HIV infections. In *Sexually transmitted diseases*, 3rd ed., eds. K.K. Holmes, P.F. Sparling, P.-A. Mårdh et al., pp. 873–892. New York: McGraw-Hill.

Golden, M.R., Schillinger, J.A., Markowitz, L. et al. 2000. Duration of untreated genital infections with *Chlamydia trachomatis*: a review of the literature. *Sexually Transmitted Diseases* 27(6):329–336.

Graney, D.O., and Vontver, L.A. 1999. Anatomy and physical examination of the female genital tract. In *Sexually transmitted diseases*, 3rd ed., eds. K.K. Holmes, P.F. Sparling, P.-A. Mårdh et al., pp. 685–697. New York: McGraw-Hill.

Groseclose, S.L., Zaidi, A.A., DeLisle, S.J. et al. 1999. Estimated incidence and prevalence of genital *Chlamydia trachomatis* infections in the United States, 1996. *Sexually Transmitted Diseases* 26(6):339–344.

Quinn, T.C., Gaydos, C., Shepherd, M. et al. 1996. Epidemiologic and microbiologic correlates of *Chlamydia trachomatis* infection in sexual partnerships. *Journal of the American Medical Association* 276(21):1737–1742.

Region IX Infertility Prevention Project Advisory Committee. Region IX Infertility Prevention Project. 1998 *Clinical guidelines*. San Francisco: the Author.

Rice, P.A., and Handsfield, H.H. 1999. Arthritis associated with sexually transmitted diseases. In *Sexually transmitted diseases*, 3rd ed., eds. K.K. Holmes, P.F. Sparling, P.-A. Mårdh et al., pp. 921–935. New York: McGraw-Hill.

Schachter, J. 1999. Biology of *Chlamydia trachomatis*. In *Sexually transmitted diseases*, 3rd ed., eds. K.K. Holmes, P.F. Sparling, P.-A. Mårdh et al., pp. 391–406. New York: McGraw-Hill.

Stamm, W.E. 1999. *Chlamydia trachomatis* infections of the adult. In *Sexually transmitted diseases*, 3rd ed., eds. K.K. Holmes, P.F. Sparling, P.-A. Mårdh et al., pp. 407–422. New York: McGraw-Hill.

Stamm, W.E., and Holmes, K.K. 1990. *Chlamydia trachomatis* infections of the adult. In *Sexually transmitted diseases*, 2nd ed., eds. K.K. Holmes, P.-A. Mårdh, P.F. Sparling et al., pp. 181–193. New York: McGraw-Hill.

Sweet, R.L., and Gibbs, R.S. 2002. *Infectious diseases of the female genital tract*, 4th ed. Philadelphia: Lippincott Williams & Wilkins.

Weinstock, H., Dean, D., and Bolan, G. 1994. *Chlamydia trachomatis* infections. *Infectious Disease Clinics of North America* 8(4):797–819.

Woods, G.L. 1996. Specimen collection and handling for diagnosis of infectious diseases. In *Clinical diagnosis and management by laboratory methods*, 19th ed., ed. J.B. Henry, pp. 1311–1331. Philadelphia: W.B. Saunders.

Xu, F., Schillinger, J.A., Markowitz, L.E. et al. 2000. Repeat *Chlamydia trachomatis* infection in women: analysis through a surveillance case registry in Washington State, 1993–1998. *American Journal of Epidemiology* 152(12): 1164–1170.

Winifred L. Star, R.N., C., N.P., M.S.
Melanie Deal, R.N., C., N.P., M.S.

13-C

Gonorrhea

Gonorrhea is caused by *Neisseria gonorrhoeae*, a Gram-negative diplococci, and is the second-most common reportable communicable disease in the United States (Centers for Disease Control and Prevention [CDC] 1996). Experts estimate that more than 600,000 cases of gonorrhea occur annually (American Social Health Association 1998, CDC 2002).

Gonococci infect nonsquamous, epithelium-lined mucosal membranes mostly of the urogenital tract and, secondarily, of the rectum, oropharynx, and/or conjunctiva (Hook III et al. 1999). Once inoculated onto the mucosal surface, the gonococci attach to the epithelial cells and enter by phagocytosis (Sparling 1999). Gonococci produce several extracellular products that damage mucosal tissue, but no true extracellular toxin has been identified (Sparling 1999). Most infections remain local; however, gonorrhea can spread via direct tissue extension, the bloodstream, or both.

Although the overall case rate in the United States declined 74% between 1975 and 1997, the rate increased slightly in 1998 and has remained essentially unchanged through 2000 (CDC 2001). In the United States, rates are highest in the South. By age, rates of gonorrhea are highest among both men and women 15–19 years old, followed by those who are 20–24 years old. In men, rates continue to be high among those who are 25–29 years old. Minority populations suffer a disproportionate rate of infection. The covariation of race and social class in the United States confounds the ability to distinguish racial from socioeconomic factors (Rauh et al. 2000). In 1997, African Americans accounted for 77% of reported gonorrhea cases, a rate approximately 30 times higher than that for Caucasians (CDC 2001). The incidence in Hispanics and Native Americans is 2–3 times higher than that in Caucasians (CDC 2001). A portion of this racial disparity may be explained by the fact that reporting of gonorrhea is higher in public clinics, which serve a higher proportion of minority populations (Hook III et al. 1999). Incidence appears to be seasonal, with rates highest in summer and lowest in late winter (Hook III et al. 1999).

Gonorrhea prevalence is sustained by continued transmission via asymptomatically infected individuals and via "core group" transmitters (a subgroup that, because of certain behavioral factors, is more likely to attain and transmit infection) (Hook III et al. 1999).

The mode of transmission is almost exclusively sexual or perinatal. Transmission via fomites or nonsexual means is extremely rare. While many women may be asymptomatic, most have symptoms of infection. Transmission is more efficient from male to female. The estimated risk of transmission from an infected male to an exposed female is about 50–90% (Hook III et al. 1999, Sweet et al. 2002). Co-infection with *Chlamydia trachomatis* occurs in 20–30% of cases (Sweet et al. 2002).

Common sites of gonococcal infection in women are the endocervix (the primary site), urethra, Skene's and Bartholin's glands, and rectum. Colonization of the urethra is present in 70–90% of infected women, although uncommonly in the absence of endocervical disease. In hysterectomized women, however, the urethra is the usual site of infection. Gland infection is rare in the absence of endocervical or urethral infection. Infection of the rectum occurs in 35–50% of women with endocervical gonorrhea and may be the only site of infection in about 5% of cases. Most rectal infections are asymptomatic and result from local spread of infected cervical secretions (Hook III et al. 1999, Sweet et al. 2002).

Pharyngeal infection, caused by orogenital contact and transmission (and occasionally by autoinoculation from anogenital infection), occurs in 10–20% of heterosexual women with gonorrheal infections. It is the sole site of infection in less than 5% of cases. Approximately 90% of these infections are asymptomatic. Infection of the pharynx is transmitted more efficiently by fellatio than cunnilingus (Hook III et al. 1999). Conjunctival infections also may arise. If left untreated, corneal ulceration, perforation, scarring, and eventual blindness may result (Chandler 1999).

The major local complications of infection in women are salpingitis (pelvic inflammatory disease, or PID) and Bartholin's gland abscess. PID occurs in 10–20% of cases. Ascending infection may cause progressive mucosal damage accompanied by a leukocyte response and submucosal abscess formation. Infertility and ectopic pregnancy are serious sequelae of upper genital tract infection (Hook III et al. 1999). Gonorrhea-related PID is more common in the first part of the menstrual cycle. Loss of the mucus plug allows rapid ascent of the organism. The iron in menstrual blood promotes growth of the gonococci, and the type of gonococci that cause tubal infection proliferate at the cervix during menstruation (Bolan et al. 1999, Westrom et al. 1999).

Disseminated gonococcal infection (DGI) is the most common systemic complication. It occurs in 0.5–3% of all patients with untreated gonorrhea (Hook III et al. 1999) and is more common in women than men. Dissemination in women often is associated with menstruation or pregnancy (Hook III et al. 1999, Sweet et al. 2002). More than 80% of DGI patients will have a positive culture for *N. gonorrhoeae* from anogenital or pharyngeal sources or will have a positive contact. DGI is caused by gonococcal bacteremia; the most common clinical manifestations are acute arthritis, teno-synovitis, dermatitis, or a combination of these (Hook III et al. 1999). (See "Objective," below).

Uncommon systemic complications of gonococcal bacteremia include endocarditis, which affects 1–3% of individuals with DGI; and meningitis, with fewer than 25 cases reported (Hook III et al. 1999). Occasionally, perihepatitis may occur (CDC 2002).

Though rare, meningococcal infections may mimic gonococcal infections. Colonization with *Neisseria meningitidis* has been documented in the pharynx, urethra, endocervix, and anus. The inherent pathogenicity of anogenital meningococcal infections is unclear, but case reports have linked meningococcal isolation to urethritis, vaginal discharge, salpingitis, and DGI-like syndromes (Hook III et al. 1999).

In recent years, the growing number of antibiotic-resistant strains has complicated gonorrhea treatment measures. In 2000, approximately 25% of tested gonococcal isolates demonstrated resistance to penicillin, tetracycline, or both (CDC 2001). Resistance can develop slowly over time by an accumulation of chromosomal mutations (chromosomally mediated) or more immediately by acquisition of an antibiotic-resistant plasmid (Hook III et al. 1999). There are chromosomally mediated, resistant strains to penicillin, tetracycline, spectinomycin, and, more recently, to fluoroquinolones. There are plasmid-mediated resistant strains to penicillin and tetracycline.

The CDC maintains surveillance of antimicrobial-resistant gonococcal isolates. Resistance to penicillin and tetracycline has become so common that since 1989 the CDC has recommended primary use of broad-spectrum cephalosporins and fluoroquinolones for treating uncomplicated gonorrhea (Knapp et al. 1997). However, fluoroquinolone resistance is now a growing concern. Rates of fluoroquinolone resistance are high in parts of Asia (10% in Japan and Hong Kong, 62% in the Philippines) and rates are rising in the United States (CDC 2000). In 2000, 1.6% of all isolates tested in the United States demonstrated some form of resistance to this drug class (CDC 2001). Fluoroquinolone resistance is significantly higher in Hawaii (10% of isolates tested) and California (5–7% of isolates tested). Fluoroquinolone use is not advised for infections in these states or for infections acquired in Asia or the Pacific (Bolan 2002; CDC 2000, 2002). No ceftriaxone-resistant strains have been reported (Hook III et al. 1999).

DATABASE

SUBJECTIVE

→ Risk factors include:
- Young age
- Early onset of sexual activity
- Lower socioeconomic status
- Urban residence
- Prostitution
- Illicit drug use
- People who trade sex for drugs
- New or multiple sexual partners
- Exposure to "core group" transmitters. These include people who (Hook III et al. 1999):
  - Have had repeated episodes of gonorrhea
  - Continue to have sex despite symptoms
  - Engage in high-risk behavior (e.g., drugs, prostitution/prostitution patronage)
  - Live in areas of high population density
  - Are of low socioeconomic status
- A partner who has gonorrhea or other sexually transmitted disease (STD)
- History of gonorrhea, PID, or other STD
- Concomitant STD
- No use of contraception
- Use of nonbarrier contraception
- Use of hormonal contraception

→ Symptoms:
- The patient may be asymptomatic or complain of any of the following:
  - Pain and/or swelling of the labia
  - Increased or abnormal vaginal discharge
  - Abnormal vaginal bleeding (e.g., intermenstrual bleeding)
  - Dyspareunia
  - Dysmenorrhea
  - Menstrual irregularity
  - Dysuria
  - Urinary urgency/frequency
  - Lower abdominal/pelvic discomfort, cramping, pain
  - Low-back ache
  - Anal pruritus/discharge
  - Rectal fullness, pressure, pain
  - Mucoid/mucopurulent rectal discharge
  - Tenesmus or painful defecation
  - Constipation or diarrhea
  - Pus or blood in stool
  - Sore throat (most pharyngeal infection is asymptomatic)
  - Nausea, vomiting
  - Fever
  - Malaise
  - Inguinal/cervical adenopathy
  - Skin lesions
  - Joint/tendon pain
  - Migratory polyarthritis
- Symptoms tend to be worse postmenstrually.

- Symptoms also depend on the site of infection.
- Partner(s) may have symptoms of urethral/rectal discharge, dysuria, frequency, redness of urethral meatus, epididymal pain or swelling, lower abdominal pain, rectal pain, tenesmus, and pus or blood in stool.
- See the **Pelvic Inflammatory Disease** and **Pelvic Masses** chapters in Section 12.

→ Gynecological and medical history:
- Menstrual cycle
- Contraception
- Description of symptoms:
  - Onset
  - Duration
  - Quality/quantity
  - Frequency
  - Course
  - Aggravating/relieving factors
  - Associated symptoms
- Previous history of same/similar problem
- STD history (including dates, treatment)
- Sensitive questioning regarding recent sexual activity (including date of last exposure, sex practices, sites of exposure, number and gender of partners, use of condoms)
- Sex-partner history (including travel, drug use)
- Acute or chronic illness
- General health
- Medications
- Allergies
- Habits (including use of illegal drugs, both injection and noninjection; travel history)
- History of laboratory tests for syphilis, hepatitis B, HIV
- Review of systems (CDC 1991)

OBJECTIVE

→ Examination may be individualized based on case presentation.

→ A thorough STD examination includes (CDC 1991, Graney et al. 1999):
- Vital signs as indicated
- General skin inspection of face, trunk, forearms, palms, and soles for lesions, rashes, discoloration
- Inspection of pharynx and oral cavity for infection, lesions, discoloration
- Abdominal inspection and palpation for masses, tenderness, rebound tenderness
- Inspection of pubic hair for lice, nits
- Inspection of external genitalia for discharge, masses, lesions
- Inspection and palpation of Bartholin's, urethral, and Skene's glands for discharge, masses
- Inspection of the vagina for discharge, lesions
- Inspection of the cervix for lesions, discharge, eversion, erythema, edema, contact bleeding; assessment for cervical motion tenderness (CMT)
- Uterine assessment for size, shape, consistency, mobility, tenderness

- Palpation of adnexa for masses, tenderness
- Inspection of perianus and anus for lesions, bleeding, discharge
- Rectal examination as indicated
- Assessment of presence or absence of associated cervical or inguinal lymphadenopathy (CDC 1991)

→ Physical examination components and findings specific to the assessment of patients with gonorrhea may include:
- Temperature: may be elevated in patients with pharyngitis, urethritis, DGI, PID, tubo-ovarian abscess (TOA).
- Throat/neck: pharyngeal injection, cervical lymphadenopathy (may be present with pharyngitis).
- Skin: assess volar aspect of arms, hands, fingers.
  - Cutaneous manifestations of DGI include:
    - A "classic" lesion, a painful necrotic pustule on an erythematous base, approximately 1 mm to 2 cm in diameter. However, such lesions may present as macules, papules, pustules, petechiae, bullae, or ecchymoses. They are usually found on the distal portion of an extremity and usually number less than 30 (Hook III et al. 1999).

    NOTE: A primary cutaneous infection with *N. gonorrhoeae* presents with a localized ulcer of the genitals, perineum, proximal lower extremities, or finger (Hook III et al. 1999).
- Extremity examination: assess small hand joints, wrists, knees, and ankles for tenderness, swelling, erythema, and effusion associated with DGI.
  - Monoarthritis is present in 30–40% of patients with DGI; the rest have multiple joint involvement (Rice et al. 1999). It most commonly involves the wrist, metacarpophalangeal, ankle, and knee joints (Hook III et al. 1999).
- Abdomen: usually within normal limits (WNL) in uncomplicated infections. There may be tenderness and/or rebound tenderness in PID.
- External genitalia: erythema, edema, excoriation may be present.
- Bartholin's, urethral, Skene's glands: purulent or mucoid exudate (milk the glands, urethra); swelling/abscess formation may be present.
- Vagina: abnormal discharge, blood, pus may be present.
- Cervix: purulent or mucopurulent discharge, edema and/or erythema of the zone of ectopy, contact bleeding, and CMT may be present.
  - See details regarding mucopurulent cervicitis (MPC) under "Diagnostic Tests" in the **Chlamydia trachomatis** chapter.
- Uterus: usually WNL in uncomplicated infections; there may be tenderness in acute PID.
- Adnexa: usually WNL in uncomplicated infections; there may be tenderness or masses in PID or TOA.
- Rectum: usually WNL in uncomplicated infection; blood, mucopurulent discharge may be present in rectal infection; there may be tenderness/masses in cul-de-sac area in PID or TOA.

→ Anoscopy, if performed, may reveal erythema, edema, mucopurulent exudate, and friable mucosa usually in the distal 5–10 cm of the rectum.

→ A complete and accurate description of any identified lesion or other pertinent physical finding should be written in the "Objective" section of the progress notes.

→ See the ***Chlamydia trachomatis*** chapter for discussion of objective findings in Fitz-Hugh-Curtis (FHC) and Reiter's syndromes.

→ See the **Pelvic Inflammatory Disease** and **Pelvic Masses** chapters in Section 12, and **Syphilis** and other chapters in this section.

ASSESSMENT

→ Gonorrhea (may be endocervical, urethral, pharyngeal, rectal)

→ Exposure to gonorrhea, other STD

→ R/O gonorrhea

→ R/O *C. trachomatis*

→ R/O MPC

→ R/O syphilis

→ R/O other concomitant STD

→ R/O vaginitis

→ R/O urinary tract infection/urethral syndrome

→ R/O DGI or other arthropathy

→ R/O PID

→ R/O TOA

→ R/O perihepatitis (FHC syndrome)

→ R/O endocarditis/meningitis (rare)

→ R/O *N. meningitidis* infection

PLAN

DIAGNOSTIC TESTS

→ While the choice of a test site depends somewhat on the symptoms and given that the most common site of infection is the cervix, endocervical sampling is recommended. Use a swab with a wire shaft and either a calcium alginate or synthetic fiber tip because swabs with wooden shafts or cotton tips may be toxic to gonorrhea (Emmert et al. 2000, Woods 1996).

→ Cultures historically have been considered the gold standard for diagnosis of gonorrhea; however, this test has been used more restrictively with the advent of the more-sensitive nucleic acid amplification tests. Culture is the only diagnostic method that allows for antimicrobial testing; is the only FDA-approved method for pharyngeal, conjunctival, and rectal specimen sources; and is a recommended test type for medico-legal cases. Culture of an endocervical sample is approximately 80–95% sensitive (Hook III et al. 1999).

■ Endocervical cultures for both *N. gonorrhoeae* and *C. trachomatis* should be obtained *before* using a bacteriostatic lubricant.

NOTE: For gonorrhea testing, it is not necessary to clear cervical mucus. Insert a swab 2–3 cm into the endocervical canal and rotate for 10–30 seconds. In the absence of a cervix, urethral cultures may be obtained. To obtain a specimen, insert a thin swab on a flexible-wire shaft 1–2 cm and rotate (Chernesky 1999).

■ Obtain pharyngeal, rectal, and gland duct cultures as indicated, depending on signs, symptoms, and sites exposed. **NOTE:** Pharyngeal specimens are obtained from the posterior pharynx, tonsils, and tonsillar pillars. Rectal cultures should be obtained by inserting a swab 2–3 cm into the anal canal and pressing laterally to avoid feces. Direct visualization via anoscopy should be used for specimen collection in patients with anorectal symptoms. Gland duct cultures are obtained after stripping exudate from gland duct openings (Chernesky 1999). Specimens for *N. gonorrhoeae* should be stored at room temperature (Woods 1996). Ideally, the specimen should be plated onto a selective medium (i.e., Thayer-Martin). After inoculation, this medium should be placed in a carbon dioxide incubator or candle jar to provide an adequate concentration of carbon dioxide. However, when culture facilities are not readily available, a holding or transport medium should be used (Sweet et al. 2002).

→ A Gram stain of endocervical or urethral secretions may be used as an adjunct to diagnosis in high-prevalence settings.

■ It should not be used for screening asymptomatic women or for diagnosing pharyngeal gonorrhea.

■ Positive stains reveal Gram-negative diplococci within or closely associated with polymorphonuclear leukocytes; the sensitivity of the stain for a cervical sample is 50–70% (Hook III et al. 1999).

→ Nonamplified DNA probe tests are widely utilized. They have sensitivities ranging from 89–97%. The advantage of this method is that it tests for both chlamydia and gonorrhea from a single swab (Hook III et al. 1999).

→ Nucleic acid amplification tests (NAATs) are the newest modalities. This diagnostic class includes polymerase chain reaction (PCR), ligase chain reaction (LCR), and transcriptase-mediated amplification (TMA) tests. The sensitivities, which range from 95–98%, are generally higher than with all other test types. The advantages of NAATs include use of a single swab for both gonorrhea and chlamydia testing, the ability to use urine as specimen source, and increased sensitivity. This technology may be used as a substitute for culture in medico-legal cases. Use confirmatory testing if the results are positive (CDC 2002). These tests have not been adequately studied in anatomic sites other than the urogenital tract. Use culture for anorectal and pharyngeal specimens (Hook III et al. 1999).

■ Instructions for collecting and storing samples vary. Refer to the package insert.

■ To collect a urine sample, ensure that the patient has not voided within the past hour. Instruct the patient to void 15–30 cc into a sterile container. Patients should *not* cleanse the genital area. Clearly differentiate this collection method from a "clean-catch, mid-stream" to obtain a urine culture.

→ Direct-specimen, antigen-detection methods (enzyme-linked immunosorbent assays [Gonozyme®] and fluorescent antibody techniques) are less-sensitive, older tests that should be replaced with newer test types.

→ Serological tests for *N. gonorrhoeae* antibodies are not recommended for screening or diagnosis but may be used as an adjunct.

→ VDRL or RPR to rule out syphilis should be performed.

→ Serological HIV testing should be offered.

→ In cases of suspected DGI:
  ■ Urogenital, oropharyngeal, and rectal specimens should be obtained for culture.
    • Cultures will be positive in more than 80% of patients (Hook III et al. 1999, Mårdh et al. 1990).
  ■ A blood culture may be obtained.
    NOTE: Blood cultures should be collected promptly after suspicion of DGI because the incidence of positive culture decreases quickly after the onset of signs and symptoms (Mårdh et al. 1990). Positive results may be obtained in up to 50% of patients with polyarthritis within two days of symptom onset (Rice et al. 1999).
  ■ Acute and convalescent serum antibody titers may be obtained.
  ■ Synovial fluid may be aspirated from affected joints for culture or Gram stain.
    NOTE: Specimens may be sent directly to the laboratory in a capped syringe or sterile tube for Gram stain and culture, or inoculated directly into a blood culture (Hall et al. 1995). Cultures are often positive in cases where synovial leukocyte counts exceed 40,000 WBC/mm³ (Hook III et al. 1999). A Gram stain is positive in only 10–30% of cases (Dalabetta et al. 1987).
    • *Proven DGI* = positive cultures from joints, blood, skin lesions (fewer than 50% of cases).
    • *Probable DGI* = arthritis/dermatitis syndrome, positive gonococcal cultures from primary mucosal site, negative cultures from blood or other sterile site.
    • *Possible DGI* = arthritis/dermatitis syndrome, positive response to therapy, negative cultures (Hook III et al. 1999).

→ Screening for complement deficiency should be considered in patients with recurrent systemic gonococcal or meningococcal infection (Hook III et al. 1999).

→ Additional tests may include but are not limited to: wet mount, Pap smear, CBC, urinalysis, urine culture and sensitivities, hepatitis B screen, and a pregnancy test.

→ See the ***Chlamydia trachomatis*** chapter and, in Section 12, the **Pelvic Inflammatory Disease** and **Pelvic Masses** chapters.

TREATMENT/MANAGEMENT

→ Patients with MPC should await the results of *C. trachomatis* and *N. gonorrhoea* tests before treatment, unless there is high suspicion of infection or the patient is unlikely to return for follow-up (CDC 2002).

→ The CDC (2002) recommends the following treatment of patients with MPC:
  ■ Treat appropriately for gonorrhea or chlamydia if test results are positive.
  ■ Empirically treat for chlamydia and/or gonorrhea in populations with a high prevalence and if the patient might be difficult to locate for treatment.
  ■ Sex partners should be notified, examined, and treated based on the patient's test results. In cases where patients are treated presumptively, partners should receive the same therapy.

Uncomplicated Anal or Genital Infection

→ Recommended regimens include (CDC 2002):
  ■ Cefixime 400 mg p.o. in a single dose   *[handwritten: Suprax]*
    [handwritten: Cephalosporin]   OR
  ■ Ceftriaxone 125 mg IM in a single dose   *[handwritten: (Rocephin)]*
    [handwritten: Cephalosporin]   OR
  ■ Ciprofloxacin 500 mg p.o. in a single dose
    [handwritten: Quinolone]   OR
  ■ Ofloxacin 400 mg p.o. in a single dose
    [handwritten: Quinolone]   OR
  ■ Levofloxacin 250 mg p.o. in a single dose
    PLUS (if chlamydial infection is not ruled out)
  ■ Azithromycin 1 g p.o. in a single dose
    OR
  ■ Doxycycline 100 mg p.o. BID for 7 days (CDC 2002)
  NOTE: The use of fluoroquinolones to treat gonorrhea is not advised in Hawaii and California. In addition, they should not be used to treat gonococcal infections that may have been acquired in Asia or the Pacific. If fluoroquinolones are indicated (as in the case of significant anaphylaxis-type allergy to penicillin), the clinician should recommend a test-of-cure (Bolan 2002, CDC 2002). Quinolones and doxycycline are contraindicated in pregnancy (CDC 2002).

→ Alternative regimens include (CDC 2002):
  ■ Injectables:
    • Spectinomycin 2 g IM in a single dose (useful when patients are unable to tolerate cephalosporins/quinolones)
      OR
    • Ceftizoxime 500 mg IM in a single dose
      OR
    • Cefotaxime 500 mg IM in a single dose
      OR
    • Cefoxitin 2 g IM in a single dose with probenicid 1 g p.o.
      PLUS (if chlamydial infection is not ruled out)
    • Azithromycin 1 g p.o. in a single dose
      OR
    • Doxycycline 100 mg p.o. BID for 7 days
      NOTE: The above alternative injectable cephalosporins aren't more advantageous than ceftriaxone. Spectinomycin is useful when patients cannot tolerate cephalosporins and quinolones (CDC 2002).

■ Oral quinolones:
  • Gatifloxacin 400 mg p.o. in a single dose
                OR
  • Norfloxacin 800 mg p.o. in a single dose
                OR
  • Lomefloxacin 400 mg p.o. in a single dose
      PLUS (if chlamydial infection is not ruled out)
  • Azithromycin 1 g p.o. in a single dose
                OR
  • Doxycycline 100 mg p.o. BID for 7 days (CDC 2002)
    NOTE: The above alternative quinolones aren't more advantageous than ciprofloxacin, ofloxacin, or levofloxacin. Quinolones and doxycycline are contraindicated in pregnancy (CDC 2002). See "NOTE" above, under the section "Uncomplicated Anal or Genital Infection," regarding use of quinolones in certain geographic areas.

Uncomplicated Pharyngeal Infection

→ Ceftriaxone 125 mg IM in a single dose
                OR
→ Ciprofloxacin 500 mg p.o. in a single dose
      PLUS (if chlamydial infection is not ruled out)
→ Azithromycin 1 g p.o. in a single dose
                OR
→ Doxycycline 100 mg p.o. BID for 7 days (CDC 2002)
  NOTE: Quinolones are contraindicated in pregnancy (CDC 2002). If cephalosporins and quinolones are not tolerated, use spectinomycin. Because spectinomycin is unreliable against pharyngeal infections (52% efficacy), patients who have suspected or known pharyngeal infection should have a pharyngeal culture evaluated 3–5 days after treatment to verify eradication of infection (CDC 2002). See "NOTE" above, under the section "Uncomplicated Anal or Genital Infection," regarding use of quinolones in certain geographic areas.

Adult Gonococcal Conjunctivitis

→ Ceftriaxone 1 g IM in a single dose.
→ Consider lavage of the infected eye once with saline solution (CDC 2002).
→ Ophthalmologic assessment as indicated.
→ Consider co-existent chlamydial infection if the condition does not respond to therapy.

Disseminated Gonococcal Infection

→ Hospitalization is recommended for initial therapy, especially for patients who may not comply with treatment, for those in whom the diagnosis is uncertain, or for those who have purulent synovial effusions or other complications. Details of treatment are beyond the scope of this chapter. Refer to the CDC STD treatment guidelines (CDC 2002).

Treatment in Pregnancy

→ Use a recommended or alternative cephalosporin *plus* erythromycin or amoxicillin for presumed or diagnosed concomitant chlamydial infection (CDC 2002). (See the ***Chlamydia trachomatis*** chapter.)
→ In cases where cephalosporins are not tolerated, use spectinomycin 2 g IM in a single dose (CDC 2002).
→ Quinolones and tetracyclines are contraindicated during pregnancy.

Partner Therapy

→ All sex partners of patients with *N. gonorrhoeae* should be evaluated and treated for *N. gonorrhoeae* and *C. trachomatis* if their last sexual contact was within 60 days before the onset of symptoms or diagnosis of infection in the patient (CDC 2002).
→ The most recent sex partner should be treated if the sexual intercourse was more than 60 days before the onset of symptoms or diagnosis in the patient (CDC 2002). Provide referrals to a provider or facility that offers appropriate STD care as indicated.
→ Patients should not resume sexual intercourse until both patient and partner have been successfully treated (CDC 2002).

Special Considerations

→ Careful inquiry should be made regarding previous hypersensitivity to cephalosporins and penicillins. Cephalosporins should be withheld in those patients with a history of anaphylactic or histamine response to penicillin (*Physicians' Desk Reference [PDR]* 2002).
→ Serious and fatal reactions have been reported in patients receiving ciprofloxacin and theophylline concurrently (*PDR* 2002).
→ For patients sensitive/allergic to cephalosporins, quinolones should be used (except in areas of the world with significant quinolone-resistant *N. gonorrhoeae*. See previous notes.)
  ■ If neither can be tolerated, substitute with spectinomycin (CDC 2002).
→ HIV-infected persons should be treated with the same regimens as those for individuals without HIV (CDC 2002).
→ Observe patients for untoward reactions to IM medication for a period of 30 minutes after administration.
→ See the **Pelvic Inflammatory Disease** and **Pelvic Masses** chapters in Section 12, and ***Chlamydia trachomatis***, **Syphilis**, and other chapters in this section.

CONSULTATION

→ Consultation with a physician is indicated for patients who have PID, DGI, FHC syndrome, endocarditis, or meningitis.
→ Hospitalization is recommended for initial therapy of DGI and the complications thereof, and for patients with endocarditis or meningitis. Hospitalization should be considered for patients with PID. (See the **Pelvic Inflammatory Disease** chapter.)
→ As needed for prescription(s).

PATIENT EDUCATION

→ Discuss the etiology and nature of gonorrhea, including the mode of transmission, incubation period, symptoms, potential complications and the possibility of co-existent chlamydia or other STD, and the importance of evaluation and treatment of sexual partner(s).
  - Patent-education handouts are a helpful adjunct to teaching. Written materials may be obtained from:
    • CDC National Prevention Information Network
      P.O. Box 6003
      Rockville, Md. 20849-6003
      (800) 458-5231, www.cdcnpin.org
    • American Social Health Association
      P.O. Box 13827
      Research Triangle Park, N.C. 27709
      (919) 361-8400, www.ashastd.org
  - Additional resources for patients are:
    • National STD Hotline
      (800) 227-8922 or (800) 342-2437
      En Español: (800) 344-7432
    • For adolescents: www.iwannaknow.org
→ Stress compliance with treatment regimens.
→ Advise abstinence from intercourse until the patient and her partner are treated and cured. They should be instructed to seek care promptly if symptoms recur.
→ Address STD prevention and HIV risk-reduction.
  - Provide guidelines for safer sex practices.
  - Encourage careful screening of sex partners and committed use of condoms/spermicides (especially with new, multiple, nonmonogamous partners).
  - See **Table 13A.2, Safer Sex Practices** in the **Chancroid** chapter, and **Table 12I.1, Recommendations for Individuals to Prevent STD/PID** in the **Pelvic Inflammatory Disease** chapter in Section 12.
→ Allow the patient to vent her feelings of surprise, shame, fear, and anger as indicated. Psychological support may be important in helping the patient gain control over her sexual situation and prevent future STDs.

FOLLOW-UP

→ Test-of-cure is not essential in cases of uncomplicated gonorrhea treated with any of the recommended regimens *except* in fluoroquinolone-treated cases in geographic areas where there is high fluoroquinolone resistance (Bolan 2002, CDC 2002).
  - Ideally, a test-of-cure should be both a culture and a nucleic acid amplification test. If only a nonculture test is used, positive results should be followed up with a culture and susceptibility testing before the patient receives alternative treatment (Bolan 2002).
  - Patients with persistent symptoms after treatment should have a culture done for *N. gonorrhoeae,* with isolates tested for antimicrobial susceptibility (CDC 2002).

→ Recurrence of gonorrhea may be due to reinfection.
  - Advise the patient to return for evaluation if symptoms of infection recur.
  - History on follow-up should include symptom status, medication compliance, drug reaction or side effects, partner therapy, sexual exposure, and use of condoms.
  - All sexual partners of symptomatic patients should be evaluated.
→ Infection with *C. trachomatis* and other organisms should be considered in cases of persistent cervicitis, urethritis, or proctitis (CDC 2002).
→ Follow up on all laboratory tests ordered. Treat all concomitant STDs and other identified conditions.
  - Continue to encourage safer sex.
→ Negative HIV antibody tests may be repeated in three months.
→ HIV-positive results should be conveyed in person by a provider who has received training in the complexities of test disclosure. HIV-positive persons should be referred to the appropriate provider or agency for early intervention services.
→ Offer the hepatitis A vaccine to women at risk for sexual transmission of this virus (e.g., users of illegal injection and noninjection drugs). (See the **Hepatitis—Viral** chapter in Section 11.)
→ Offer the hepatitis B vaccine to all women seeking treatment for an STD who have not been previously vaccinated. (See the **Hepatitis—Viral** chapter for further information.)
→ Newly diagnosed, hepatitis B antigen-positive individuals should have liver function tests and receive counseling regarding the implications of their positive status and the need for immunoprophylaxis of sex partners and household members. (See the **Hepatitis—Viral** chapter.)
→ Routine gonococcal screening of asymptomatic women in high-risk groups should be considered. These include (U.S. Preventive Services Task Force 1996):
  - Women with history of other STD or repeated gonorrhea
  - Prostitutes
  - Women with multiple partners or a sexual partner with multiple sexual contacts
  - Partners of males with gonorrhea or urethritis in the previous three months
  - Adolescents
  - Younger women
  - Drug abusers
→ Because gonorrhea is a state-mandated reportable disease, a morbidity report needs to be filed with the department of public health.
→ See the **Pelvic Inflammatory Disease** and **Pelvic Masses** chapters in Section 12, and *Chlamydia trachomatis,* **Syphilis,** and other chapters in this section.
→ Document gonorrhea diagnosis and complications/sequelae thereof in progress notes and on problem list.

BIBLIOGRAPHY

American Social Health Association. 1998. *Sexually transmitted diseases in America: How many cases and at what cost?* Menlo Park, Calif.: Kaiser Family Foundation.

Bolan, G. 2002. New 2002 STD treatment guidelines. *Medical Board of California Action Report* 82:10–14.

Bolan, G., Ehrhardt, A.A., and Wasserheit, J.N. 1999. Gender perspectives and STDs. In *Sexually transmitted diseases*, 3rd ed., eds. K.K. Holmes, P.F. Sparling, P.-A. Mårdh et al., pp. 117–127. New York: McGraw-Hill.

Centers for Disease Control and Prevention (CDC). 1991. *Sexually transmitted diseases. Clinical practice guidelines.* Atlanta, Ga.: the Author.

_____. 1996. Ten leading nationally notifiable infectious diseases—United States, 1995. *Morbidity and Mortality Weekly Report* 45(41):883–884.

_____. 1998. Sexually transmitted disease surveillance, 1997. Atlanta, Ga.: the Author.

_____. 2000. Sexually transmitted disease surveillance, 1999, supplement. Atlanta, Ga.: the Author.

_____. 2001. Sexually transmitted disease surveillance, 2000. Atlanta, Ga.: the Author.

_____. 2002. Sexually transmitted diseases treatment guidelines 2002. *Morbidity and Mortality Weekly Report* 51(RR–6):36–42.

Chandler, J.W. 1999. Ocular infections associated with sexually transmitted diseases and AIDS. In *Sexually transmitted diseases*, 3rd ed., eds. K.K. Holmes, P.F. Sparling, P.-A. Mårdh et al., pp. 903–911. New York: McGraw-Hill.

Chernesky, M.A. 1999. Laboratory services for sexually transmitted diseases: overview and recent developments. In *Sexually transmitted diseases*, 3rd ed., eds. K.K. Holmes, P.F. Sparling, P.-A. Mårdh et al., pp. 1281–1294. New York: McGraw-Hill.

Dalabetta, G., and Hook III, E.W. 1987. Gonococcal infections. *Infectious Disease Clinics of North America* 1(1):25–55.

Emmert, D.H. and Kirchner, J.T. 2000. Sexually transmitted diseases in women: gonorrhea and syphilis. *Postgraduate Medicine* 107(2):181–197.

Graney, D.O., and Vontver, L.A. 1999. Anatomy and physical examination of the female genital tract. In *Sexually transmitted diseases*, 3rd ed., eds. K.K. Holmes, P.F. Sparling, P.-A. Mårdh et al., pp. 685–697. New York: McGraw-Hill.

Hall, G., and Goodman, N.L. 1995. Microbiology. In *Clinical guide to laboratory tests*, 3rd ed., ed. N.W. Tietz, pp. 899–968. Philadelphia: W.B. Saunders.

Handsfield, H.H. 1991. Recent developments in STDs: I. Bacterial diseases. *Hospital Practice* (July 15):47–56.

Hook III, E.W., and Handsfield, H.H. 1999. Gonococcal infections in the adult. In *Sexually transmitted diseases*, 3rd ed., eds. K.K. Holmes, P.F. Sparling, P.-A. Mårdh et al., pp. 451–466. New York: McGraw-Hill.

Knapp, J.S., Fox, K.K., Trees, D.L. et al. 1997. Fluoroquinolone resistance in *Neisseria gonorrhoeae. Emerging Infectious Diseases* 3(1):142–148.

Mårdh, P.-A., and Danielsson, D. 1990. *Neisseria gonorrhoeae.* In *Sexually transmitted diseases*, 2nd ed., eds. K.K. Holmes, P.-A. Mårdh, P.F. Sparling et al., pp. 903–916. New York: McGraw-Hill.

Physicians' desk reference. 2002. Montvale, N.J.: Medical Economics.

Rauh, V.A., Culhane, J.F., and Hogan, V.K. 2000. Bacterial vaginosis: a public health problem for women. *Journal of the American Medical Women's Association* 55(4):220–224.

Rice, P.A., and Handsfield, H.H. 1999. Arthritis associated with sexually transmitted diseases. In *Sexually transmitted diseases*, 3rd ed., eds. K.K. Holmes, P.F. Sparling, P.-A. Mårdh et al., pp. 921–935. New York: McGraw-Hill.

Sparling, P.F. 1999. Biology of *Neisseria gonorrhoeae.* In *Sexually transmitted diseases*, 3rd ed., eds. K.K. Holmes, P.F. Sparling, P.-A. Mårdh et al., pp. 433–449. New York: McGraw-Hill.

Sweet, R.L., and Gibbs, R.S. 2002. *Infectious diseases of the female genital tract*, 4th ed. Philadelphia: Lippincott Williams & Wilkins.

U.S. Preventive Services Task Force. 1996. Screening for gonorrhea. In *Guide to clinical preventive services*, 2nd ed. Washington. D.C.: U.S. Department of Health and Human Services.

Westrom, L., and Eschenbach, D. 1999. Pelvic inflammatory disease. In *Sexually transmitted diseases*, 3rd ed., eds. K.K. Holmes, P.F. Sparling, P.-A. Mårdh et al., pp. 783–809. New York: McGraw-Hill.

Woods, G.L. 1996. Specimen collection and handling for diagnosis of infectious diseases. In *Clinical diagnosis and management by laboratory methods*, 19th ed., ed. J.B. Henry, pp. 1311–1331. Philadelphia: W.B. Saunders.

Winifred L. Star, R.N., C., N.P., M.S.
Melanie Deal, R.N., C., N.P., M.S.

13-D

Granuloma Inguinale (Donovanosis)

Granuloma inguinale (also called *donovanosis*) is a chronic, progressive bacterial infection found mostly in tropical or sub-tropical countries (O'Farrell 1999). An extremely rare disease in the United States, it is much more common in Papua New Guinea, Northeastern Brazil, French Guyana, the Caribbean, Africa (especially South Africa), aboriginal communities of Australia, and other subtropical and tropical environments. In the United States, there were only three cases reported in 1994 (Centers for Disease Control and Prevention [CDC] 1995). As of 1995, this infection was no longer reportable to the CDC.

The infectious agent in donovanosis is *Calymmatobacterium granulomatis*, a Gram-negative bacterium also called the Donovan body. Although most experts agree that the weight of evidence favors classification of donovanosis as a sexually transmitted disease (STD), some dispute this mode of transmission (Hart 1997, O'Farrell 1999). Primary evidence supporting sexual transmission is as follows: lesions are predominantly genital, the highest prevalence is in age groups most commonly affected by STDs (20–40 years old), and there is frequent occurrence of disease in visitors to endemic areas after sexual exposure. Evidence disputing sexual transmission is as follows: an inconsistent conjugal infection rate (2–50%), infections in children, and occurrence of primary extragenital lesions. However, this "counterevidence" may be explained by the long incubation period of the organism, its low rate of infection, the fact that childhood infection occurs with other STDs, and the great variability of diagnostic skills on the part of health care personnel (Hart 1997). Experts recommend examination of all sexual partners.

Contagion is generally mild and repeated exposure is necessary for most cases of the disease to develop. Nonsexual transmission may occur via autoinoculation of the genital tract from the rectum. Disease occurrence has been identified in the very young and elderly (Sweet et al. 2002). In the Caribbean, a high incidence of squamous carcinoma of the vulva has been reported in premenopausal women with granuloma inguinale (Blanco et al. 1991, Hart 1990, Richens 1991). Disseminated donovanosis has been reported in a neonate born to a mother with a large granulomatous vulvar lesion (O'Farrell 1999).

There are four types of donovanosis: *ulcero-granulomatous* (the most common), *hypertrophic* or *verrucous*, *necrotic*, and *sclerotic* or *cicatricial*. The incubation period generally varies. The average incubation period is 17 days, but a range of 1–360 days has been reported (O'Farrell 1999). The genitals are affected in 90% of cases and the inguinal region in 10%. Disseminated donovanosis is rare, although spread to the liver and bone may occur. Patients often present late in the course of the disease when disfigurement has occurred. Without treatment, scarring and tissue destruction often occur. The most common complication of donovanosis is pseudoelephantiasis, which is more common in women and found in up to 5% of cases (O'Farrell 1999).

In patients with AIDS, donovanosis infection may behave differently and treatment may fail even after extended courses of antibiotics. Also, HIV may slow the healing of ulcers (Jamkhedkar et al. 1998). In South Africa, sexually active individuals infected with granuloma inguinale have highly associated HIV seropositivity (Blanco et al. 1991, Hart 1990)

A host of antibiotics have been used to treat the disease, some potentially toxic and others with variable effectiveness. Donovanosis responds best to lipid-soluble antibiotics such as chloramphenicol, erythromycin, lincomycin, quinolones, and tetracyclines (see "Treatment/Management," below) (Hart 1990, Richens 1991).

DATABASE

SUBJECTIVE

→ Peak ages for granuloma inguinale are 20–40 years old.

→ Affected individuals living in endemic areas may be of lower socioeconomic status and have poor standards of personal genital hygiene (O'Farrell 1999).

→ The patient may have a history of travel to area(s) where granuloma inguinale is endemic.

→ Two percent to 50% of sex partners of patients with the disease are affected (O'Farrell 1999).

→ Co-existent STD (particularly syphilis) is common.

→ The initial lesion may go unnoticed.

→ Symptoms may include:
- Pruritus; may precede or accompany lesion
- Painless lump in genital area
- Ulceration of genital tissues
- Bleeding from ulcerated lesions
- Swelling in inguinal area
- Vaginal discharge or bleeding
- "Cauliflower-like" tumor
- Extragenital lesions (see "Objective," below, for lesion descriptions)

→ Gynecological and medical history:
- Menstrual cycle
- Contraception
- Description of symptoms:
  - Onset
  - Duration
  - Quality/quantity
  - Frequency
  - Course
  - Aggravating/relieving factors
  - Associated symptoms
- Previous history of same/similar problem
- STD history (including dates, treatment)
- Sensitive questioning regarding recent sexual activity, including the date of last exposure, sex practices, sites of exposure, number and gender of partners in the past month, and the use of condoms
- Sex partner history (including travel, drug use)
- Acute/chronic illness
- General health
- Medications
- Allergies
- Habits (including travel outside the United States and use of illegal drugs, both injection and noninjection)
- History of laboratory tests for syphilis, hepatitis B, HIV
- Review of systems (CDC 1991)

OBJECTIVE

→ Examination may be individualized based on case presentation.

→ A thorough STD examination includes (CDC 1991, Graney et al. 1999):
- Vital signs as indicated
- General skin inspection of face, trunk, forearms, and palms and soles for lesions, rashes, discoloration
- Inspection of pharynx and oral cavity for erythema, infection, lesions, discoloration
- Abdominal inspection and palpation for masses, tenderness, rebound tenderness
- Inspection of pubic hair for lice, nits
- Inspection of external genitalia for discharge, masses, lesions
- Inspection and palpation of Bartholin's, urethral, and Skene's glands for discharge, masses
- Inspection of vagina for discharge, lesions

- Inspection of cervix for lesions, discharge, eversion, erythema edema, contact bleeding; assessment for cervical motion tenderness
- Uterine assessment for size, shape, consistency, mobility, tenderness
- Palpation of adnexa for masses, tenderness
- Inspection of perianus and anus for lesions, bleeding, discharge
- Rectal examination as indicated
- Assessment of presence or absence of associated lymphadenopathy

→ Characteristics of granuloma inguinale:
- Lesions generally appear on the labia minora and fourchette, crural folds.
- Lesions of the vagina and cervix also may occur.
  - Vulvar and cervical changes may mimic carcinoma growth.
- Six percent of cases present with extragenital disease. Affected areas may include lip, gums, cheek, palate, pharynx, neck, nose, larynx, chest (O'Farrell 1999).
- The initial lesion is usually a firm, nontender papule or subcutaneous nodule that later ulcerates.
- Four types of donovanosis may occur (O'Farrell 1999):
  - Ulcero-granulomatous (most common)
    - Nontender, fleshy, single or multiple, beefy-red ulcers; bleed easily
  - Hypertrophic or verrucous
    - Ulcer/growth with raised, irregular edge
    - May be dry with a "walnut-like" appearance
  - Necrotic
    - Deep, foul-smelling ulcer causing tissue destruction
  - Sclerotic or cicatricial
    - Extensive formation of fibrous and scar tissue
- Spread to inguinal area produces pseudobubo—a subcutaneous, granulomatous process not involving the lymph nodes.
- Lymphedema of labia and distal tissues may occur in the chronic, active-disease phase; however, lymphatic blockage and fibrosis are rare.
- Secondary infection may produce necrotic debris at ulcer edge (Hart 1990).
- Systemic symptoms are absent except in rare cases of intrapelvic spread, secondary infection, or hematogenous dissemination.
- In some cases, extensive scarring may accompany active disease; depigmented, irregular scars may appear at the border of the healed lesion.

ASSESSMENT

→ Granuloma inguinale (donovanosis)
→ R/O herpes genitalis
→ R/O chancroid
→ R/O lymphogranuloma venereum
→ R/O carcinoma
→ R/O syphilis

→ R/O condyloma lata

→ R/O ulcerated genital warts

→ R/O genital amebiasis

→ R/O concomitant STDs

→ R/O metastatic genital cancer (cervical, vulvar, vaginal)

PLAN

DIAGNOSTIC TESTS

→ Distinguish between donovanosis and other causes of genital ulcers.

- See **Table 13A.1, Clinical Features of Genital Ulcers** and **Figure 13A.1, Sexually Active Patient with Genital Ulcer(s)** in the **Chancroid** chapter.

→ Culture is not recommended for diagnosis due to the fastidious nature of the organism and the lack of adequate culture methods.

→ Tissue smears are the mainstay diagnostic method (O'Farrell 1999).

→ Identification of intracellular Donovan bodies within large mononuclear cells is possible from lesion material stained with Giemsa, Leishman's, or Wright's stain (CDC 2002, Hart 1997).
NOTE: Good technique in obtaining and preparing the slide is important: (1) clean the ulcerated area with saline; (2) with forceps, scalpel blade, punch biopsy instrument, or cotton swab, detach a small piece of tissue from the deep surface of the ulcer (local anesthesia may be necessary); (3) smear it on a glass slide or crush the specimen between two glass slides; (4) air dry, heat fix, then stain. Donovan bodies appear as "safety pin," blue-black organisms (O'Farrell 1999, Richens 1991).

→ Biopsy is recommended for very early, sclerotic, dry, or necrotic lesions and for those with superinfection, and when carcinoma is being ruled out (O'Farrell 1999, Richens 1991). Silver stain is probably the most sensitive (Hart 1997).

→ Pap smears may have identified Donovan bodies.

→ Complement fixation tests have been used in some settings but are not standard approaches to diagnosis.

→ Diagnostic tests to rule out other causes of genital ulcers and lymphadenopathy include:

- Dark-field or direct immunofluorescence test of serous fluid for *Treponema pallidum* from genital and nonoral lesion(s) to rule out syphilis. (See the **Syphilis** chapter.)
- RPR (or VDRL) to rule out syphilis. (See the **Syphilis** chapter.)
- Herpes cultures from genital lesion(s) to rule out herpes. (See the **Genital Herpes Simplex Virus** chapter.)
- See "Diagnostic Tests" in the **Chancroid** and **Lymphogranuloma Venereum** chapters.

→ Perform sensitive testing for *Neisseria gonorrhoeae* and *Chlamydia trachomatis*. In the absence of a cervix, a urethral or urine specimen may be obtained.

→ HIV testing should be offered.

→ Additional tests may include but are not limited to: wet mounts, CBC, urinalysis, urine culture and sensitivities, pregnancy testing, and hepatitis B screen.

TREATMENT/MANAGEMENT

→ Recommended regimens (CDC 2002):

- Doxycycline 100 mg p.o. BID for at least 3 weeks
  OR
- Trimethoprim-sulfamethoxazole 1 double-strength tablet (160 mg/800 mg) p.o. BID for at least 3 weeks

→ Alternative regimens (CDC 2002):

- Ciprofloxacin 750 mg p.o. BID for at least 3 weeks
  OR
- Erythromycin base 500 mg p.o. QID for at least 3 weeks
  OR
- Azithromycin 1 g p.o. once per week for at least 3 weeks
  NOTE: Some specialists recommend adding a parenteral aminoglycoside to the above regimens if improvement is not evident within the first few days of therapy (CDC 2002). (See "Follow-up," below, for further information.)

→ Treatment during pregnancy (CDC 2002):

- Pregnant and lactating women should be treated with the erythromycin regimen and consideration should be given to the addition of a parenteral aminoglycoside (e.g., gentamicin).
- Azithromycin may prove useful for treatment in pregnancy, but data are lacking.
  NOTE: Sulfonamides are relatively contraindicated in pregnancy. Doxycycline and ciprofloxacin are contraindicated in pregnant women (CDC 2002).

→ Examine and treat sex partners who have had sexual contact with the patient within 60 days preceding the onset of the patient's symptoms (CDC 2002).

→ HIV-infected individuals should be treated with the same regimens as those for HIV-negative individuals. Consideration should be given to the addition of a parenteral aminoglycoside (e.g., gentamicin) (CDC 2002).

→ Treatment of sequelae and complications:

- Strictures and fistulae may require surgery.
- Because extragenital lesions may be refractory to antibiotics, surgical curettage plus antibiotic therapy may be necessary.
- Donovanosis may spread to pelvic organs, mimicking pelvic inflammatory disease (PID) or malignancy. Surgical exploration may be indicated for drainage of fluid collections but must be attempted only with antibiotic coverage to prevent dissemination of donovanosis (Richens 1991).

CONSULTATION

→ Given the rarity of this infection in the United States and the necessity of nonstandard diagnostic tests, consider referring the patient to an STD clinic or infectious disease specialist for evaluation.

PATIENT EDUCATION

→ Discuss the etiology and nature of the infection, including the mode of transmission, incubation period, symptoms, diagnostic tests, potential complications, and possible association with increased risk for HIV infection.

- Explain to the patient that an area of depigmentation may occur at the border of the healed lesion (Hart 1990).
- Patent-education handouts are a helpful adjunct to teaching. Written materials may be obtained from:
  - CDC National Prevention Information Network
    P.O. Box 6003
    Rockville, Md. 20849-6003
    (800) 458-5231, www.cdcnpin.org
  - American Social Health Association
    P.O. Box 13827
    Research Triangle Park, N.C. 27709
    (919) 361-8400, www.ashastd.org
- Additional resources for patients are:
  - National STD Hotline
    (800) 227-8922 or (800) 342-2437
    En Español: (800) 344-7432
  - For adolescents: www.iwannaknow.org

→ Advise the patient to finish the full course of medication and return for follow-up (see "Follow-up," below).

→ Discuss the importance of evaluation and treatment of sexual partner(s). Provide referrals to a provider or facility offering appropriate STD care.

→ Advise abstinence from intercourse until the patient and her partner are treated and cured. They should be instructed to seek care promptly if symptoms recur.

→ Address STD prevention and HIV risk-reduction.
- Provide guidelines for safer sex practices.
- Encourage careful screening of sex partners and committed use of condoms (especially with new, multiple, non-monogamous partners).
- See **Table 13A.2, Safer Sex Practices** in the **Chancroid** chapter and **Table 12I.1, Recommendations for Individuals to Prevent STD/PID** in the **Pelvic Inflammatory Disease** chapter in Section 12.

→ Allow the patient to vent her feelings of surprise, shame, fear, and anger as indicated. Psychological support may be important in helping the patient gain control over her sexual situation and prevent future STDs.

FOLLOW-UP

→ Treatment should be continued for three weeks or until all lesions are healed.
- Lesions are generally paler/less visible in a few days and shrink after seven days.
- Total healing may take 3–5 weeks.
- Recurrence rates are higher if antibiotics are discontinued before the primary lesion has healed.
- Patients should be seen during the course of treatment for assessment of response to therapy (weekly or on an individualized basis until lesions are clearly resolving) (CDC 1991). Refer the patient to a specialist if improvement is not evident.

→ History on follow-up should include symptom status, medication compliance, drug reaction and side effects, partner therapy, sexual exposure, and use of condoms (CDC 1991).

→ Syphilis and HIV testing should be repeated in three months if test results are initially negative.

→ Follow up on all laboratory tests ordered. Treat all concomitant STDs and other identified conditions.

→ If ordered, HIV test results should be conveyed in person by a provider who has received training in the complexities of test disclosure. HIV-positive persons should be referred to the appropriate provider or agency for early intervention services.

→ Offer the hepatitis A vaccine to women at risk for sexual transmission of this virus (e.g., users of illegal injection or noninjection drugs). (See the **Hepatitis—Viral** chapter in Section 11.)

→ Offer the hepatitis B vaccine to all women seeking treatment for an STD who have not been previously vaccinated. (See the **Hepatitis—Viral** chapter for further information.)

→ Newly diagnosed, hepatitis B antigen-positive individuals should undergo liver function tests and receive counseling regarding the implications of seropositivity and the need for immunoprophylaxis of sex partners and household members. (See the **Hepatitis—Viral** chapter.)

→ Document in progress notes and on problem list.

BIBLIOGRAPHY

Blanco, J.D., and Gonik, B. 1991. Sexually transmitted diseases. *Current Problems in Obstetrics, Gynecology and Fertility* 14(6):179–233.

Centers for Disease Control and Prevention (CDC). 1991. *Sexually transmitted diseases. Clinical practice guidelines*. Atlanta, Ga.: the Author.

_____. 1995. Summary of notifiable diseases—United States, 1994. *Morbidity and Mortality Weekly Report* 43(53):1–80.

_____. 2002. Sexually transmitted diseases treatment guidelines 2002. *Morbidity and Mortality Weekly Report* 51(RR–6): 17–18.

Graney, D.O., and Vontver, L.A. 1999. Anatomy and physical examination of the female genital tract. In *Sexually transmitted diseases*, 3rd ed., eds. K.K. Holmes, P.F. Sparling, P.-A. Mårdh et al., pp. 685–697. New York: McGraw-Hill.

Hart, G. 1990. Donovanosis. In *Sexually transmitted diseases*, 2nd ed., eds. K.K. Holmes, P.-A. Mårdh, P.F. Sparling et al., pp. 273–277. New York: McGraw-Hill.

_____. 1997. Donovanosis. *Clinical Infectious Diseases* 25:24–32.

Jamkhedkar, P.P., Hira, S.K., Shroff, H.J. et al. 1998. Clinico-epidemiologic features of granuloma inguinale in the era of acquired immune deficiency syndrome. *Sexually Transmitted Diseases* 25(4):196–200.

O'Farrell, N. 1999. Donovanosis. In *Sexually transmitted diseases*, 3rd ed., eds. K.K. Holmes, P.-A. Mårdh, P.F. Sparling et al., pp. 525–532. New York: McGraw-Hill.

Richens, R. 1991. The diagnosis and treatment of donovanosis (granuloma inguinale). *Genitourinary Medicine* 67:441–452.

Sweet, R.L., and Gibbs, R.S. 2002. *Infectious diseases of the female genital tract*, 4th ed. Philadelphia: Lippincott Williams & Wilkins.

Geraldine M. Collins-Bride, R.N., M.S., A.N.P.
Joan R. Murphy, R.N., C., M.S., N.P., C.N.S.

13-E
Genital Herpes Simplex Virus

Genital herpes simplex virus (HSV) is a sexually transmitted disease caused by two types of the herpes virus. *Herpes simplex virus type 2* (HSV-2) causes most genital infections and infections below the waist. *Herpes simplex virus type 1* (HSV-1) is responsible for most oral lesions and infections above the waist, although approximately 15% of primary genital HSV infections are caused by HSV-1 (Fleming et al. 1997).

Both HSV-1 and HSV-2 can infect mucous membranes and/or abraded skin at any site, but the severity and duration of symptoms with an initial infection are not influenced by virus type. Conversely, the virus type and site of infection *do* affect the likelihood of recurrences and their frequency (Mertz et al. 1998).

HSV is the single most common cause of genital ulcers in the United States (Mertz et al. 1998). The infection is transmitted by mucosal contact with HSV-infected secretions. Lesions progress through four stages: vesicular, pustular, ulcerative, and coalescent/crusted (Corey et al. 1983). (See **Figure 13E.1, Clinical Course of Primary Genital Herpes Simplex Virus Infection.**) Humans are the sole known reservoir for HSV, although brief survival of HSV on environmental surfaces has been documented. Fomite and aerosol transmission is unlikely, however. The risk of sexual transmission is estimated to be 10% per year, according to recent studies of monogamous heterosexual couples with discordant HSV serum antibody status (Wald et al. 2001).

It is estimated that 60 million people in the United States (more than 25% of the adult population) have genital HSV infection (Fleming et al. 1997, Handsfield 2001). Based on the National Health and Nutrition Examination Survey (NHANES), a population-based study from 1976–1994, the seroprevalence of HSV infection increased 30% over the last decade. Prevalence rose in all age groups, with the fastest rise (fivefold) among Caucasian teenagers. Seroprevalence was highest among African American women (55%) and African American men (35%), with Caucasian women at 20% and Caucasian men at 15% (Fleming et al. 1997).

Exact incidence rates are difficult to estimate because HSV is not a reportable disease in the United States and most people with HSV are unaware they are infected. In the NHANES study, fewer than 10% of all those who were seropositive for HSV reported a history of genital herpes (Fleming et al. 1997). Reasons cited for lack of recognition of HSV infections include mild disease in most individuals, location of lesions in difficult-to-examine areas, and disparities in health access and health behaviors (Corey 1999). In addition, individuals with prior HSV-1 infections experience clinical symptoms of initial HSV-2 infections that are much less severe and recognizable as herpes than do those individuals without prior HSV-1 infections.

The risk of transmission from an infected male to a female is estimated to be 80–100% (Bryson et al. 1993, Mertz et al. 1992). Women are more likely than men to acquire new HSV-2 infection and to have symptomatic infection (Sweet et al. 2002). Most transmission events are not associated with a recognizable recurrence or prodrome in the source partner. There is an estimated 10% annual transmission rate despite safe sex in monogamous couples, with 70% of HSV transmission occurring during asymptomatic periods (Bryson et al. 1993, Mertz et al. 1992).

The herpes simplex virus is thought to be an important cofactor for human immunodeficiency virus (HIV) acquisition. In HIV-infected individuals, the HIV virus can consistently be detected in genital ulcers caused by HSV-2, which suggests that genital herpes infections likely increase the efficiency of the sexual transmission of HIV (Schacker et al. 1998b). This efficient viral transmission is thought to be due to HSV regulatory proteins that can up regulate the rate of HIV replication (Corey 1999).

Pregnancy does not lead to an increase in the frequency or severity of recurrent herpes outbreaks (Sweet et al. 2002). Although neonatal HSV is associated with severe morbidity and mortality, most pregnant women with a history of recurrent genital herpes can experience a normal pregnancy and vaginal delivery. The highest risk of neonatal HSV occurs with primary maternal infection during or near labor. HSV antibody seroconversion completed by the time of labor confirms no increased risk in neonatal morbidity (American College of Obstetricians and Gynecologists [ACOG] 1999, Brown et al. 1997, Sweet et al. 2002). Given the unreliability of the patient history in identifying HSV-2 seropositive women, some experts now recommend sero-

Figure 13E.1.   CLINICAL COURSE OF PRIMARY GENITAL HERPES SIMPLEX VIRUS INFECTION

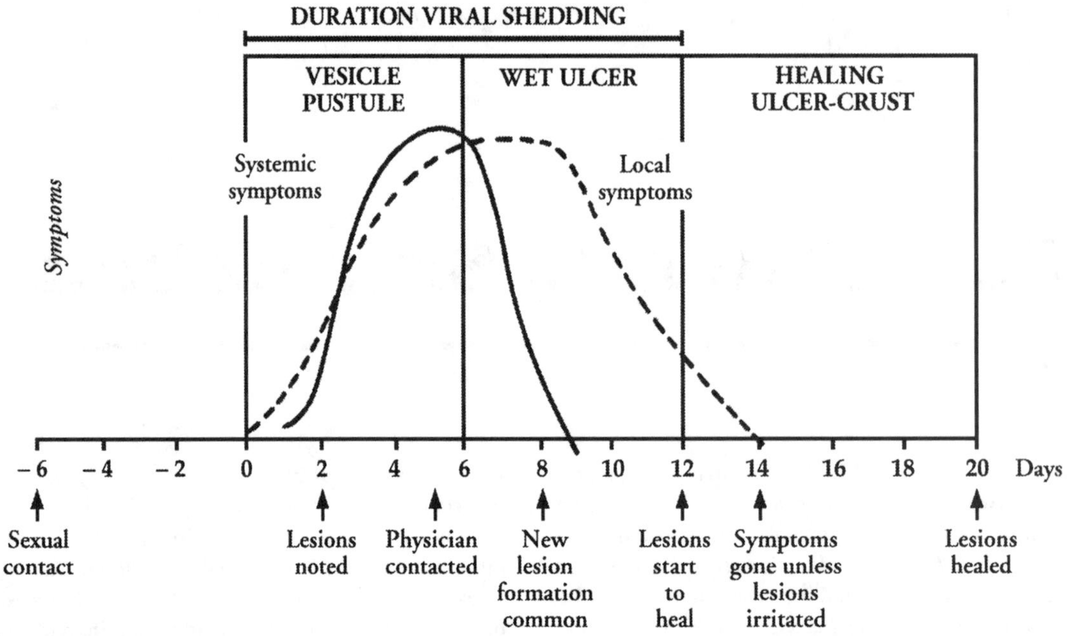

Source: Reprinted with permission from Corey, L., Adams, H., Brown, Z. et al. 1983. Genital herpes simplex virus infections: clinical manifestations, course, and complications. *Annals of Internal Medicine* 98(6):961.

logic screening in pregnancy to identify women at risk for acquiring herpes during pregnancy (Brown et al. 1995). However, there is currently no consensus regarding the exact time during pregnancy that HSV testing would be of greatest benefit.

Clinical Presentations

There are three distinct clinical presentations of HSV infection: primary, nonprimary first episode, and recurrent HSV.

Primary Herpes

Primary herpes is the first clinical episode of HSV in a patient who does not have antibodies to HSV-1 or HSV-2. The incubation period is 1–45 days, with a mean of 5.8 days (Corey et al. 1983). Primary HSV is generally characterized by severe local symptoms with a prolonged duration, commonly with bilateral distribution. Lesions progress from painful and pruritic vesicles to pustules, which often coalesce to form large areas of ulceration. If untreated, new lesions often form by the second week, with healing occurring by the third week after onset (Corey 1999, Corey et al. 1983). (See **Figure 13E.1.**) Systemic symptoms such as fever, malaise, myalgia, and adenopathy often accompany a primary outbreak (ACOG 1999, Corey 1999, Sweet et al. 2002).

Symptoms usually last approximately two weeks, and healing occurs in 1–2 weeks. Therefore, total time of infection from onset of lesions to complete healing is 3–4 weeks. Mean dura-

tion of viral shedding is 11–14 days (Corey 1999, Sweet et al. 2002). Cervical shedding of the virus occurs in 80–86% of women with primary HSV (Sweet et al. 2002). Serum antibody is not present when symptoms appear, then rises in convalescence. (See **Table 13E.1, Traditionally Recognized Characteristics of Clinically Evident True Primary and Recurrent Genital Herpes Infection.**)

Concomitant with primary genital infection, HSV ascends peripheral sensory nerves and enters the spinal root ganglia where it establishes latency. Reactivation is precipitated by multiple factors (Corey 1999). (See "Recurrent Herpes," below.)

Possible complications of primary HSV include aseptic meningitis, HSV keratitis, HSV encephalitis, temporary autonomic nervous system dysfunction, extragenital lesions, erythema multiforme, and herpes pharyngitis. Concomitant yeast infections are extremely common in women (Corey 1999). Primary HSV tends to be more severe in women than in men. Disseminated HSV infection is extremely rare in immunocompetent individuals. Residual scarring from lesions is uncommon (Corey 1999).

Nonprimary First-Episode Herpes

Nonprimary first-episode herpes is the initial clinical outbreak of herpes in a patient who has either HSV-1 or HSV-2 serum antibodies (Corey 1999, Sweet et al. 2002). The infection occurs due to reactivation of the latent virus. The clinical course is less severe, and signs and symptoms are of shorter duration, similar

Table 13E.1. **TRADITIONALLY RECOGNIZED CHARACTERISTICS OF CLINICALLY EVIDENT TRUE PRIMARY AND RECURRENT GENITAL HERPES INFECTION**

Features	True Primary	Recurrent
Incubation period	2–10 days	
Prodrome		1–2 days
Fever	+	
Regional lymphadenopathy	+	
Malaise	+	
Duration of genital symptoms (mean)	Approx. 15 days	Approx. 7 days
Duration of viral shedding (mean)	Approx. 12 days	Approx. 5 days
Number of lesions	Greater	Fewer
Cervical lesions	Common	Uncommon

Source: Reprinted with permission from Sweet, R.L., and Gibbs, R.S. 2002. *Infectious diseases of the female genital tract*, 4th ed., p. 145. Philadelphia: Lippincott Williams & Wilkins.

to recurrent HSV. The only definitive way to determine whether a patient has had a primary or nonprimary outbreak is by serological testing (i.e., in nonprimary first-episode herpes, antibody is present initially and then rises in convalescence). Recent evidence suggests that many "new" herpes infections are actually nonprimary first-episode infections and not primary herpes (Sweet et al. 2002).

Recurrent Herpes

Recurrent HSV is characterized by symptoms, signs, and sites of infection localized to the genital region. Symptoms are usually mild and of shorter duration (the average is 4–5 days) than in primary HSV infection (Corey 1999). Systemic symptoms are usually absent, although recent studies have noted a diverse clinical spectrum in recurrent disease (Corey 1999, Fleming et al. 1997).

Most outbreaks are unilateral and well localized, with a smaller mean number of lesions. Approximately 50% of recurrent HSV outbreaks are preceded by a prodrome. The prodrome occurs several hours to several days before the onset of lesions and is characterized by local symptoms such as paresthesias, itching, pain, and urinary symptoms (Corey 1999, Sweet et al. 2002). Prodromal symptoms generally occur along the distribution of the infected nerve root, signaling an impending herpes outbreak in the region of the skin experiencing symptoms.

The duration of viral shedding is shorter with recurrent HSV (mean duration is 4–5 days). Cervical shedding of HSV with recurrent outbreaks occurs in only about 12% of cases (Sweet et al. 2002). (See **Table 13E.1.**)

Certain "triggers," such as stress, menses, trauma, illness, and sunlight, may reactivate the latent virus and cause recurrent outbreaks (Koelle et al. 2000). There is no scientific evidence that sexual activity affects the onset of recurrences. However, some patients may report that sexual intercourse is a factor in triggering outbreaks.

The average rate of recurrence is approximately 4–5 times per year for the first few years, with a subsequent gradual decrease in frequency (Benedetti et al. 1999). Approximately 50% of patients with primary HSV will have a recurrent outbreak within six months (Corey 1999, Sweet et al. 2002).

Genital HSV-1 infection does not recur as frequently as genital HSV-2 infection. In the first year, the median number of recurrences of HSV-2 is four times greater than that of HSV-1. Recurrence of genital HSV-1 is milder, with a shorter course, than that of HSV-2 (Corey 1999). Medical complications associated with recurrent herpes are minimal; however, the chronic nature of this disease and the unpredictability of recurrences cause considerable psychosocial and psychosexual distress for many patients (Ashley et al. 1999, Conant et al. 1996).

Asymptomatic Infection

Asymptomatic viral shedding of HSV and unrecognized subclinical infections appear to be major factors in HSV transmission (Corey 1999, Handsfield 2001). Asymptomatic HSV is defined as the viral shedding of HSV without clinical signs and symptoms of the disease. Most commonly, this occurs in patients who are antibody seropositive for HSV-1 or HSV-2 and do not have a known history of genital herpes or those who have asymptomatic viral shedding between overt recurrences (Handsfield 2001). Serum antibody is present. Women with a positive history of symptomatic genital HSV have been shown to asymptomatically shed HSV 4–14% of the time, and one-third to two-thirds of women with positive genital cultures do not have clinically evident lesions (Sweet et al. 2002).

The exact rate of asymptomatic viral shedding is unknown. Higher rates occur in women, in HSV-2 infections, and during the first year after initial infection (Corey 1999, Handsfield 2001). Many apparently asymptomatic shedding episodes are associated with mild symptoms that patients can learn to recognize (Handsfield 2001, Koelle et al. 2000, Wald et al. 2000).

DATABASE

SUBJECTIVE

Primary Infection

→ The most common etiology of vulvar ulcers is infection with HSV (Mertz et al. 1998). The severity of symptoms, duration of viral shedding, and duration of lesions are similar in primary HSV-1 and HSV-2 disease (Corey 1999).

→ The patient may have a history of exposure to an infected partner.

→ Symptoms may include:
- Multiple, painful genital lesions (papules, vesicles, pustules, ulcers, fissures)
  - Often bilateral
- Itching, burning, and/or tingling at the site of infection
- Flu-like symptoms—malaise, headache, fever, stiff neck, mild photophobia, myalgias, nausea
  - Systemic symptoms appear early, reach a peak 3–4 days after lesion onset, and gradually recede over the subsequent 3–4 days (Corey 1999).
- Dysuria (both external and internal), urinary retention
- Tender inguinal adenopathy
  - Usually appears during second to third week; often the last symptom to resolve (Corey 1999).
- Sacral paresthesia
- Change in vaginal discharge (amount, color, consistency, odor)
- Dyspareunia/pelvic pain
- Sore throat (in pharyngeal infection; 20% of patients with primary HSV-1 or HSV-2)

→ Symptoms last for approximately 2–4 weeks.

→ See the introductory discussion of "Primary Herpes" and "Nonprimary First-Episode Herpes."

Recurrent Infection

→ Approximately 50% of patients will have a recurrent infection within six months of the primary outbreak (Sweet et al. 2002). Many HSV infections present with atypical symptoms (Handsfield 2001).

→ The patient may be asymptomatic.

→ The patient may present with:
- A history of HSV outbreaks with similar symptoms

→ Symptoms may include:
- Prodromal symptoms: pain, itching, burning, tingling, numbness, and sensitivity (paresthesias) at the site where lesions will develop
  - Symptoms last from 12 hours to two days but may come and go for up to one week.
- Painful, well-localized genital sore(s) (single or small clusters)
- Dysuria (usually external)
- Systemic symptoms (usually absent)

→ Symptoms usually resolve within 7–10 days.

→ See the introductory discussion of "Recurrent Herpes."

OBJECTIVE

→ The patient may present with the following findings:
- Elevated temperature (primary HSV)
- Skin: erythematous plaques consistent with erythema multiforme
- Pharynx: if infected, signs include mild erythema or diffuse ulceration with white exudate. Tender cervical lymph nodes are usually present in association with HSV pharyngitis.
- External genitalia: papules, vesicles, ulcerations, crusted-over lesions, localized erythema/edema
  - Bilateral lesions usually are indicative of primary HSV; unilateral lesions usually are indicative of recurrent HSV.

NOTE: Lidocaine or benzocaine gel (numbing compounds) may be used to facilitate the pelvic examination when painful lesions are present.
- Vagina: leukorrhea, normal or abnormal discharge
- Cervix: may be friable, erythematous; a purulent, bloody, or watery discharge may be present; there may be ulcerative lesions on ectocervix; a necrotic mass may be present; the patient may have cervical motion tenderness.

NOTE: Primary herpes cervicitis occurs in approximately 90% of primary HSV-2 infections, 70% of primary HSV-1 infections, and 70% of nonprimary first-episode HSV-2 infections. Only 15–20% of women with recurrent lesions have concomitant cervical infection (Corey 1999).
- Inguinal and/or generalized lymphadenopathy (primary HSV); inguinal nodes usually are firm, nonfluctuant, and tender.
- Extragenital lesions on fingers (also known as herpetic whitlow), eyes, perianal area, buttocks, thighs, and oropharynx
  - A common complication of primary HSV, uncommon in nonprimary/recurrent HSV

→ Wet mount: no pathogens, unless concomitant infection; may see increased white blood cells.

→ Pap smear may reveal the presence of giant, multinucleated cells (not diagnostic of HSV-2).

→ Results of HSV culture of lesions and/or cervix may be positive (diagnostic of HSV infection or viral shedding).

→ Serological studies reveal a fourfold or greater rise in antibody titer (compare acute and convalescent serum).
- Useful for determination of primary HSV.

→ HSV antibody testing also may be used to document past, asymptomatic, or atypical infection. (See "Diagnostic Tests," below, for further discussion.)

→ See the introductory discussions of "Primary Herpes," "Nonprimary First-Episode Herpes," and "Recurrent Herpes" infections.

ASSESSMENT

→ R/O herpes genitalis
→ R/O extragenital herpes lesions

→ R/O chancroid

→ R/O syphilitic chancre

→ R/O lymphogranuloma venereum

→ R/O fungal infection

→ R/O eczemoid vulvitis (lichen sclerosus/squamous cell hyperplasia)

→ R/O pemphigus/bullous pemphigoid

→ R/O Beçhet's syndrome

→ R/O aphthous ulceration ("canker sore")

→ R/O squamous/basal cell carcinoma

→ R/O trauma

→ R/O Crohn's disease

→ R/O invasive cervical carcinoma

→ R/O HIV

PLAN

DIAGNOSTIC TESTS

→ Herpes culture of genital lesions and/or cervix. Tissue culture remains the most sensitive and specific diagnostic test, distinguishing HSV-1 from HSV-2 (Ashley et al. 1999, Centers for Disease Control and Prevention [CDC] 2002, Sweet et al. 2002).

NOTE: A negative HSV culture *does not prove* that the patient does not have HSV. Cultures are more likely to be positive early in the course of disease (within 72 hours of lesion onset), in the vesicular or pustule lesion stage, and in primary or initial clinical infections (Ashley et al. 1999).

→ Type-specific serologic testing detects the presence of antibodies to HSV antigens. Antibodies develop within the first few weeks of infection and persist indefinitely (CDC 2002). Serologic tests can now distinguish HSV-1 from HSV-2 with glycoprotein tests: gG-2 is specific for HSV-2 and gG-1 or gC-1 is specific for HSV-1 (Ashley et al. 1999). Currently there are several FDA-approved, gG-based, type-specific assays. The sensitivities of these tests vary from 80–98%. False-negative results may occur, especially early in the infection. Specificity rates are greater than 96%. Repeat testing or confirmatory testing may be indicated (CDC 2002). Consider serologic testing to:

■ Detect silent HSV-2 carriers in high-risk patients, such as pregnant women, immunocompromised patients, and those at risk for HIV (Ashley et al. 1999)

■ Distinguish primary from nonprimary first-episode disease

→ Western blot testing and immunoblot can distinguish HSV-1 and HSV-2 but are expensive and time-consuming. They were not developed for commercial use (Ashley et al. 1999).

→ Polymerase chain reaction (PCR), available in some labs, detects HSV DNA in genital lesions and body fluids. Its role is not clearly defined for diagnosis in genital ulcers. It is the test of choice for spinal fluid HSV (CDC 2002).

→ Cytologic testing (Tzanck stain and Pap smear) is unreliable and nonspecific. It is not recommended.

→ RPR or VDRL; dark-field or direct immunofluorescence test of serous fluid for *Treponema pallidum* to rule out syphilis. (See the **Syphilis** chapter.)

→ Consider HIV testing in primary HSV infections, as they are among the most common clinical presentations and manifestations of HIV infections (Corey 1999).

→ Distinguish between herpes and other causes of genital ulcers. (In the **Chancroid** chapter, see **Table 13A.1, Clinical Features of Genital Ulcers** and **Figure 13A.1, Sexually Active Patient with Genital Ulcer[s].**)

→ See "Diagnostic Tests" in the **Chancroid**, **Granuloma Inguinale (Donovanosis)**, and **Lymphogranuloma Venereum** chapters.

TREATMENT/MANAGEMENT

→ There is no known cure for HSV infections.

→ Antiviral chemotherapy is the mainstay of treatment (CDC 2002). Three antiviral medications are now approved for treating HSV: acyclovir, valacyclovir, and famciclovir. The mechanism of action is interference with HSV DNA synthesis.

■ Its major advantage is a high degree of selectivity against HSV-infected cells and a lack of activity against normal cells (Corey 1999).

■ Antivirals neither eradicate latent virus nor affect subsequent risk, frequency, or severity of recurrences after discontinuation of medication (CDC 2002).

First Episodes (Primary and Nonprimary Infection)

→ Recommended regimens (CDC 2002):

■ Acyclovir 400 mg p.o. TID for 7–10 days
OR

■ Acyclovir 200 mg p.o. 5 times/day for 7–10 days
OR

■ Famciclovir 250 mg p.o. TID for 7–10 days
OR

■ Valacyclovir 1 g p.o. BID for 7–10 days

• Treatment may be extended if healing is incomplete after 10 days of therapy (CDC 2002).

• Mean duration of infection is reduced by 3–5 days, viral shedding by 8 days, and time to healing by 7 days (Corey 1999).

• Topical antiviral ointment provides marginal benefit and its use is discouraged.

NOTE: Patients with extremely severe episodes (prostration, central nervous system involvement, urinary retention) may require hospitalization for more aggressive management/intravenous therapy.

Recurrent Infection (Intermittent Therapy)

→ Recommended regimens (CDC 2002):

■ Acyclovir 200 mg p.o. 5 times/day for 5 days
OR

■ Acyclovir 400 mg p.o. TID for 5 days
OR

- Acyclovir 800 mg p.o. BID for 5 days
  OR
- Famciclovir 125 mg p.o. BID for 5 days
  OR
- Valacyclovir 500 mg p.o. BID for 3–5 days
  OR
- Valacyclovir 1 g p.o. QD for 5 days
  - Effective episodic treatment of recurrent herpes requires *initiation of therapy within 1 day of lesion onset* or during the prodrome that precedes some outbreaks (CDC 2002).
  - For episodic treatment, a randomized, controlled trial indicated that a 3-day course of valacyclovir 500 mg twice daily is as effective as a 5-day course. Similar studies have not been done with acyclovir and famciclovir (CDC 2002).

Frequent Infection (chronic suppressive therapy—at least 6 outbreaks/year)

→ Recommended regimens (CDC 2002):
- Acyclovir 400 mg p.o. BID
  OR
- Famciclovir 250 mg p.o. BID
  OR
- Valacyclovir 500 mg p.o. QD
  OR
- Valacyclovir 1 g p.o. QD
  - Valacyclovir 500 mg once a day might be less effective than other valacyclovir or acyclovir dosing regimens in patients who have very frequent recurrences (i.e., 10 or more episodes per year) (CDC 2002).
  - Suppressive therapy reduces the frequency of genital herpes recurrences by 70–80% among patients who have frequent recurrences (i.e., 6 or more recurrences per year) (CDC 2002).
  - Safety and efficacy have been documented among patients receiving daily therapy with acyclovir for as long as 6 years and with valacyclovir or famciclovir for 1 year. Quality of life often is improved in patients with frequent recurrences who receive suppressive compared with episodic treatment (CDC 2002).
  - In the immunocompromised individual, suppressive antiviral therapy is usually recommended due to the increased aggressiveness of HSV and the higher rate of both symptomatic and asymptomatic HSV shedding. Significant reduction in HSV shedding can be seen with suppressive famciclovir therapy (Schacker et al. 1998a).
  - Periodically during suppressive treatment (e.g., once a year), discontinuation of therapy should be discussed with the patient to reassess the need for continued therapy (CDC 2002).
  - Suppressive antiviral therapy reduces but does not eliminate subclinical viral shedding. Therefore, the extent to which suppressive therapy prevents HSV transmission is unknown (CDC 2002, Wald et al. 2000).

- No evidence of clinically significant resistance has been reported with suppressive treatment in immunocompetent individuals (Corey 1999, *Medical Letter on Drugs and Therapeutics* 2002).
- Questions are still unanswered regarding the relevance to humans of in vitro mutagenicity/toxicity studies in animals.
  - In a study by Clive et al. (1991), no mutagenicity was observed in patients receiving acyclovir for recurrent genital herpes.
- Antiviral chemotherapy is generally well-tolerated.
  - The most frequent adverse effects may include nausea, diarrhea, headache, and rash (*Medical Letter on Drugs and Therapeutics* 2002).
  - A thrombotic thrombocytopenic purpura/hemolytic uremic syndrome has been reported in some severely immunocompromised patients on high doses of valacyclovir (*Medical Letter on Drugs and Therapeutics* 2002).

→ Palliative therapy:
- Keep lesions clean and dry.
- May apply cold milk or witch hazel compresses, followed by aloe vera gel or Burow's solution to lesions QID for 30 minutes.
- Warm/cool sitz baths prn followed by a blow dryer on a cool setting
- Pain relief: nonsteroidal anti-inflammatory drugs during prodrome and infection, and topical lidocaine applied to site of lesions

CONSULTATION

→ Consultation with a physician is indicated if the patient has signs/symptoms of severe primary infection requiring possible hospitalization for intravenous acyclovir therapy, details of which are beyond the scope of this chapter.

→ Refer the patient to mental health services for psychological support as necessary.

→ As needed for prescription(s).

PATIENT EDUCATION

→ Discuss the cause and transmission of infection: primary, nonprimary first-episode, and recurrent outbreaks, and latency and asymptomatic shedding.

→ Provide HSV patient-education handouts if available.

→ Allow the patient to express her feelings regarding the diagnosis.

→ Advise abstinence from oral-genital or genital-genital sex with the onset of prodromal symptoms and/or HSV lesions until lesions are completely healed.

→ Emphasize the importance of safer sex practices and the use of condoms. (See **Table 13A.2, Safer Sex Practices** in the **Chancroid** chapter and **Table 12I.1, Recommendations for Individuals to Prevent STD/PID** in the **Pelvic Inflammatory Disease** chapter in Section 12.)

→ Instruct/encourage good perineal hygiene to prevent superimposed infection.

→ Advise frequent hand washing to decrease the risk of autoinoculation.

→ Provide instructions for use of antiviral therapy; discuss intermittent versus chronic suppressive therapy for individuals with recurrences. (See "Treatment/Management," above.)

→ Advise regarding palliative measures. (See "Treatment/Management," above.)

→ Discuss aggravating factors—e.g., illness, stress, fatigue, menses, poor nutrition, irritation/friction, intercourse, and excessive heat/sun. Encourage general health maintenance, appropriate rest, and adequate nutrition.

→ Refer partner(s) for evaluation if any lesions/characteristic symptoms are present.

→ Advise the patient to obtain yearly Pap smears (ACOG 1999).

→ If they become pregnant, women should inform their health care provider of a history of HSV infection in themselves or their sexual partner(s) (ACOG 1999).

→ Refer for psychological support and stress management as indicated.

→ Advise patients to inform prospective partners of the risk of HSV exposure.

  • This is an issue that can be very difficult for patients to cope with; thus, support and guidance are necessary.

→ Provide patients with support group/resource information:

  ▪ American Social Health Association
    P.O. Box 13827
    Research Triangle Park, N.C. 27709
  ▪ National Herpes Help Hotline: (919) 361-8488
    www.ashastd.org
    • Provides a directory of HSV self-help chapters in the United States and Canada, and maintains a list of health care providers/therapists who specialize in treating HSV.
    • Also provides numerous patient brochures, suitable for stocking in the office, about herpes and other STDs.
  ▪ Herpes Help, Glaxo Smith Kline: www.herpeshelp.com
    • Information on herpes by the manufacturer of valacyclovir (Valtrex®) and acyclovir (Zovirax®) with links to other Web sites (Handsfield 2001).

FOLLOW-UP

→ Schedule a follow-up visit after the initial diagnosis to evaluate treatment effectiveness and coping strategies, and to answer any further questions.

→ Annual Pap smears are recommended (ACOG 1999).

→ Re-evaluate suppressive therapy annually.

→ See "Treatment/Management," above.

→ Document in progress notes and on problem list.

BIBLIOGRAPHY

American College of Obstetricians and Gynecologists. 1999. Management of herpes in pregnancy. *ACOG Practice Bulletin No. 8*. Washington D.C.: the Author.

Ashley, R.L., and Wald, A. 1999. Genital herpes: review of the epidemic and potential use of type-specific serology. *Clinical Microbiology Reviews* 12(1):1–8.

Benedetti, J.K., Zeh, J., and Corey, L. 1999. Clinical reactivation of genital herpes simplex virus infection decreases in frequency over time. *Annals of Internal Medicine* 131:14–20.

Brown, Z., Benedetti, J., Watts, D. et al. 1995. A comparison between detailed and simple histories in the diagnosis of genital herpes complicating pregnancy. *American Journal of Obstetrics and Gynecology* 172:1299–1303.

Brown, Z., Seike, S., Zeh, J. et al. 1997. The acquisition of herpes simplex virus during pregnancy. *New England Journal of Medicine* 337:509–515.

Bryson, Y., Dillon, M., Bernstein, D. et al. 1993. Risk of acquisition of genital herpes simplex virus type 2 in sex partners of persons with genital herpes: a prospective couple study. *Journal of Infectious Diseases* 167(4):942–946.

Centers for Disease Control and Prevention (CDC). 2002. Sexually transmitted diseases treatment guidelines. *Morbidity and Mortality Weekly Report* 51(RR–6):12–17.

Chosidow, O., Drouault, Y., Leconte-Veyriac, F. et al. 2001. Famciclovir vs. acyclovir in immunocompetent patients with recurrent genital herpes infections: a parallel-groups, randomized, double-blind clinical trial. *British Journal of Dermatology* 144(4):818–824.

Clive, D., Corey, L., Reichman, R.C. et al. 1991. A double-blind, placebo-controlled cytogenic study of oral acyclovir in patients with recurrent genital herpes. *Journal of Infectious Diseases* 164(4):753–757.

Collins-Bride, G. 1998. Herpes simplex infections. In *Nurse practitioner/physician collaborative practice: clinical guidelines for ambulatory care*, eds. G. Collins-Bride and J. Saxe, pp. 154–157. San Francisco: UCSF Nursing Press.

Conant, M., Berger, T., Coates, T. et al. 1996. Genital herpes: an integrated approach to management. *Journal of the American Academy of Dermatology* 35(4):601–605.

Corey, L. 1999. Genital herpes. In *Sexually transmitted diseases*, 3rd ed., eds. K.K. Holmes, P.-A. Mårdh, P.F. Sparling et al., pp. 391–413. New York: McGraw-Hill.

Corey, L., Adams, H., Brown, Z. et al. 1983. Genital herpes simplex virus infections: clinical manifestations, course, and complications. *Annals of Internal Medicine* 98(6):958–972.

Drugs for non-HIV viral infections. 2002. *Medical Letter on Drugs and Therapeutics* 44(1123):9–16.

Engel, J. 1998. Long-term suppression of genital herpes. *Journal of the American Medical Association* 280:928–929.

Erlich, K., Mills, J., Chatis, P. et al. 1989. Acyclovir-resistant herpes simplex virus in patients with the acquired immunodeficiency syndrome. *New England Journal of Medicine* 320(5):293–296.

Fife, K., Crumpacker, C., and Mertz, G. 1994. Recurrence of resistance patterns of herpes simplex virus following cessation of ≥6 years of chronic suppression with acyclovir. *Journal of Infectious Diseases* 169:1338–1341.

Fleming, D., McQuillon, G., Johnson, R. et al. 1997. Herpes simplex virus type 2 in the United States, 1976 to 1994. *New England Journal of Medicine* 337:1105–1111.

Handsfield, H. 2001. *Genital herpes*. New York: McGraw-Hill.

Koelle, D., and Ward, A. 2000. Herpes simplex virus: the importance of asymptomatic shedding. *Journal of Antimicrobial Chemotherapy* 45:1–8.

Langenberg, A., Corey, L., Ashley, R. et al. 1999. A prospective study of new infections with herpes simplex virus type 1 and type 2. Chiron HSV Vaccine Study Group. *New England Journal of Medicine* 341(19):1432–1438.

Mertz, G., Benedetti, J., Ashley, R. et al. 1992. Risk factors for the sexual transmission of genital herpes. *Annals of Internal Medicine* 116:197–202.

Mertz, K.J., Trees, D., Levine, W.C. et al. 1998. Etiology of genital ulcers and prevalence of human immunodeficiency virus coinfection in 10 U.S. cities. *Journal of Infectious Diseases* 178:1795–1798.

Schacker, T., Hu, H., Koelle, D. et al. 1998a. Famciclovir for the suppression of symptomatic and asymptomatic herpes simplex virus reactivation in HIV-infected persons. *Annals of Internal Medicine* 128(1):21–28.

Schacker, T., Ryncary, A., Goddard, J. et al. 1998b. Frequent recovery of HIV-1 from genital herpes simplex virus lesions in HIV-1 infected men. *Journal of the American Medical Association* 280(1):61–66.

Sensitivity/resistance of herpes simplex virus to zovirax (acyclovir), AVRII-Z. 1993. Research Triangle Park, N.C.: Burroughs Wellcome Co.

Swanson, J., Dibble, S., and Chenity, C. 1995. Clinical features and psychosocial factors in young adults with genital herpes. *Image: The Journal of Nursing Scholarship* 27(1):16–22.

Sweet, R.L., and Gibbs, R.S. 2002. Herpes simplex virus infection. *Infectious diseases of the female genital tract*, 4th ed., pp. 101–118. Philadelphia: Lippincott Williams & Wilkins.

Wald, A., Langenberg, A., Link, K. et al. 2001. Effect of condoms on reducing the transmission of herpes simplex virus type 2 from men to women. *Journal of the American Medical Association* 285:(24):3100–3106.

Wald, A., Zeh, J., Selke, S. et al. 2000. Reactivation of genital herpes simplex virus type 2 infection in asymptomatic seropositive persons. *New England Journal of Medicine* 342:844–850.

Mary M. Rubin, R.N., C., PH.D., C.R.N.P.
Jeanette M. Broering, R.N., M.S., C.P.N.P.
Jennifer L. Tagatz, R.N., C., M.S., F.N.P.

13-F
Human Papillomavirus

Human papillomaviruses are epitheliotropic viruses that infect surface epithelia and mucous membranes and may produce warts or epithelial growths at the site of infection. In addition to causing warts, *human papillomavirus (HPV) infection* is associated with the development of *intraepithelial neoplasia* and *invasive cancer* of the lower genital tract as well as other body sites (Gross et al. 1997a, Singer et al. 2000).

Epidemiological studies indicate that essentially all cervical cancer worldwide has HPV present (Bosch et al. 1995). However, it appears that the presence of HPV infection of the genital tract is essential but not independently sufficient to cause cervical cancer (Walboomers et al. 1999). Cofactors believed to influence the development of lower genital tract intraepithelial neoplasia (*cervical intraepithelial neoplasia* [CIN], *vulvar intraepithelial neoplasia* [VIN], *vaginal intraepithelial neoplasia* [VAIN], *peri-anal intraepithelial neoplasia* [PAIN], and *anal intraepithelial neoplasia* [AIN]) and invasive cancer have been identified. These include smoking, use of oral contraceptives, early onset of sexual activity, multiple partners, infection with other sexually transmitted diseases (STDs), and immunosuppression (Moscicki et al. 2001). Current evidence does not indicate that the presence of visible genital warts (or their treatment) is associated with the development of cervical cancer (Centers for Disease Control and Prevention [CDC] 2002).

Biology

More than 100 subtypes of HPV have been reported and classified based on DNA sequencing, with more being typed and numbered in the order of discovery (Cox et al. 2001, Singer et al. 2000). More than 30 of these subtypes have been associated with lower genital tract disease (Lorincz 1999). Visible genital warts usually are caused by HPV types 6 and 11. Other HPV types in the anogenital region (e.g., types 16, 18, 31, 33, and 35) have been strongly associated with cervical neoplasia (CDC 2002). HPV types 16, 18, 31, 33, and 35 are found occasionally in visible genital warts and have been associated with *external genital squamous intraepithelial neoplasia*. Individuals with visible genital warts can be infected simultaneously with multiple HPV types (CDC 2002). (See **Table 13F.1, Human Papillomavirus [HPV] Types and Common Sites of Infection**.)

Over the last decade, much has been studied about the molecular pathways of HPV oncogenesis. An understanding of cell cycle functions and the make-up of the viral genome and its regulatory mechanisms has begun to enable knowledge-based approaches to triage and management of persons infected with HPV.

Essentially, the episomal (circular) HPV viral genome consists of three regions, each responsible for specific functions. The upstream regulatory region controls viral replication and transcription of some sequences in the early region. The early region (E) consists of seven areas (E1–E7) that encode for oncoproteins important in "early" viral replication. The E6 and E7 areas of high-risk oncogenic HPV types contain tumor promotion properties rarely found in low-risk HPV types, which enable malignant transformation by preventing cell death and immortalizing cancer cells capable of invasion. The late region encodes for structural capsid protein production necessary for the DNA to be infective, as HPV throughout most of its life cycle exists in the host cell without its protein shell. Integration of HPV into the host cellular DNA appears to be the final step in the transformation of normal cells to cancer. Therefore, cancer development, influenced by random events of viral, cofactor, and host interplay, appears to result from the loss of control over normal cell growth and timed cell destruction (apoptosis), occurring with integration and persistence of high-risk HPV into the host cellular DNA (Cox et al. 2001, Lorincz 1999, Singer et al. 2000).

Incidence/Prevalence

It is estimated that approximately 80% of the population has been exposed to HPV. Because there are no mandatory surveillance mechanisms, the exact incidence of this disease is not known. However, prospective data have shown an incidence rate of 14% among sexually active women 20–29 years old (Ho et al. 1998). HPV infection is highly prevalent in young, sexually active populations, with rates up to 20% in some countries. Fre-

Table 13F.1. HUMAN PAPILLOMAVIRUS (HPV) TYPES AND COMMON SITES OF INFECTION

Type of HPV	Usual Epithelial Site	Type of Warts/Lesions
1–4, 7, 10, 26–29, 49, 57, 60, 65, 75–78	Feet, hands, all sites of body	Cutaneous (plantar, common, and flat warts)
5–9, 12, 14–15, 17, 19, 20–25, 36, 47, 50	Face, arms, trunk	Warts, intraepithelial lesions, and invasive cancers, mostly in cutaneous skin of *epidermodysplasia verruciformis* patients
6, 11, 16, 18, 31, 33–35, 39, 40, 42–45, 51–53, 55–59, 61, 62, 64, 66–71, 74	Genital tract and anus, upper respiratory tract, fingers	Benign warts, condyloma, papules, CIN, VIN, VAIN, PIN, PAIN, AIN and anal, genital tract, upper respiratory tract, and subungual cancer
7, 13, 30, 32, 37, 38, 41, 48, 60, 72, 73	Head and neck, all sites of body	Various warty lesions, cysts, keratoacanthomas, melanomas, and squamous cell cancer

Source: Gross, G., and Barrasso, R., eds. 1997. *Human papillomavirus infection: a clinical atlas.* Berlin/Wiesbaden, Germany: Ulstein-Mosby; Lorincz, A.T. 1999. Human papillomavirus. In *Laboratory diagnosis of viral infections*, 3rd ed., eds. E.H. Lennette and T.F. Smith. New York: Marcel Dekker; Singer, A., and Monaghan, J.M. 2000. *Lower genital tract precancer: colposcopy, pathology, and treatment*, 2nd ed. London: Blackwell Science.

quency of HPV infection varies according to the detection method used and the population screened. Statistics suggest that about 1% of the population has clinically gross visible warts and 4% has lesions detected by colposcopy. Another 10% is HPV positive but negative on colposcopic examination, 60% is negative by HPV DNA testing but antibody positive, and only 25% has never been infected (Koutsky 1997).

HPV infection is mostly transient in immunocompetent patients. In some studies, HPV was not detectable in up to 50% of the patients who had been infected within the previous year and who had been tested with the most sensitive DNA assays (Lorincz 1999). However, in a minority of infected individuals, high-risk HPV types persist and place women at risk for cancer many years after exposure (Franco et al. 1999, Ho et al. 1998, Schlect et al. 2001). In addition to persistence of disease, high viral load, especially with high-risk HPV types, influences the development of squamous intraepithelial lesions and, potentially, cancer (Sun et al. 2001).

With the evolution of the AIDS epidemic and extension of life by earlier treatment of women infected with HIV, concern about the incidence of HPV and the development of lower genital tract cancers has risen. Before the availability of antiretroviral drugs, women most likely died before the progression of CIN to cervical cancer (Gross et al. 1997a). Data from the last decade have shown that the incidence of HPV and cervical intraepithelial neoplasia is higher in seropositive women (Jay et al. 2000, Palefsky et al. 1995). In addition to cervical, vaginal, and vulvar intraepithelial neoplasia, anal canal disease and HPV-associated lesions at other body sites have been observed (Del Mistro et al. 2001). Cancer surveillance data support a significantly higher risk of carcinoma in situ and invasive cervical cancers in the HIV-positive population (Gallagher et al. 2001). In 1998, invasive squamous cell cancer of the cervix was added to the list of AIDS-defining diagnoses.

Transmission

Most HPV infection is transmitted by sexual exposure. Although relatively rare, maternal-fetal transmission during labor and delivery may occur in the presence of HPV infection of the birth canal (Cason 1996). In a sexually active person who has been exposed to the virus, the incubation period ranges from three weeks to years. Three months is the average time from viral exposure to the development of clinically apparent warts (Cox et al. 2001).

There is a high correlation between the appearance of clinical warts in the female and the presence of clinical warts in her male sexual partner. Up to 66% of the male partners of women with condyloma have clinically apparent lesions. The infectivity of subclinical HPV-induced disease is not well-documented. However, studies of male partners of women with subclinical HPV disease have shown that 64–70% will have grossly identifiable lesions, 33% will have clinical lesions identified on magnification, and 66% will have subclinical lesions identified by cytology or DNA testing (Cox et al. 2001). No conclusive data exist on the efficiency of female-to-female transmission. Although recurrence and progression rates of the disease are not improved, it is reasonable to consider evaluating any sexual partner of a female patient who presents with clinical condyloma, irrespective of the partner's gender. Evaluating and counseling both partners can be of psychological value to both.

DATABASE

SUBJECTIVE

→ All sexually active women are at risk for exposure to HPV; however, the greatest risk factors include (Kjellberg et al. 2000, Moscicki et al. 2001, Weiderpass et al. 2001):

■ History of multiple sexual partners, especially in the last five years

■ History of contact with a partner who has genital warts

- History of multiple STDs (current or previous)
- Lack of condom use
- Oral contraceptive use
- Age younger than 25 years
- Pregnancy
- Smoking
- Immunosuppression

→ The patient is usually asymptomatic or presents with complaints of painless, warty-appearing growths on her genitals, most commonly occurring at the posterior fourchette, adjacent labia minora, and remainder of the vestibule.
- Growths also may occur on the clitoris, perineum, vagina, cervix, anus, and rectum (Singer et al. 2000).

→ Additional symptoms may include:
- Vulvar pruritus, burning, and/or bleeding
- Vaginal discharge
- Dyspareunia

→ The patient may have a newly diagnosed, abnormal Pap smear or a history of abnormal Pap smear(s).
→ Pregnancy may exacerbate lesion(s).

OBJECTIVE

→ Examination may be individualized based on case presentation.
→ Because HPV often is associated with other STDs, a thorough STD examination should be done.
→ Infection may occur anywhere in the anogenitourinary tract, including the mons pubis, vulva, vagina, urethra, perineum, cervix, peri-anal skin, or rectum, as well as on other body surfaces (CDC 2002, Gross et al. 1997a).
→ Nongenital lesions of the nose, mouth, larynx, or conjunctiva and other body parts also may occur (CDC 2002, Gross et al. 1997a).
→ HPV infection may be categorized utilizing the following method of stratification (Singer et al. 2000):
- Clinical
- Subclinical
- Latent

Clinically Apparent Gross Lesions

→ Lesions have a broad spectrum of clinical appearances (Anderson et al.1997, Burghardt et al. 1998, Gross et al. 1997a, Singer et al. 2000).
→ Lesions in the anogenital area often are visible to the naked eye without any appearance-enhancing techniques.
→ Condyloma acuminata: typically white (leukoplakia) or pink, raised, cauliflower, verrucous lesions.
NOTE: Vulvar vestibular papillae may resemble small condylomata. It continues to be a matter of debate whether HPV plays a role in the etiologic factors of this condition (Fowler 2000).
→ Lesions may appear as slightly raised, discrete, and hyperpigmented brown, white, red, or gray.
→ Vaginal lesions may appear as raised, granular asperites or spikes.

→ Large lesions may become ulcerated and infected.
→ Condyloma may grow markedly during pregnancy.
→ An exophytic lesion can mimic cancer.
→ See also the **Vaginal Intraepithelial Neoplasia** and **Vulvar Intraepithelial Neoplasia** chapters in Section 12.

Subclinical Infection

→ Lesions are detectable only by using enhancing techniques.
→ Acetowhite areas within the anogenital tract are evident after the application of 3–5% acetic acid. They may be seen with the naked eye or with an optical magnifying device such as a colposcope or, in the case of vulvar lesions, with a hand-held magnifying glass (Anderson et al. 1997, Giuntoli et al. 1987, Singer et al. 2000). (See "Diagnostic Tests," below.)
→ Abnormal cervical, vaginal, or anal cytology may be classified under this subgroup.

Latent HPV Disease

→ There are no visible lesions.
→ Detected only by DNA hybridization for HPV. Intraepithelial neoplasia on pathology review is absent.
→ Biologic significance is unclear. Presumably it is noninfectious but may represent a large reservoir for anogenital HPV infections (Singer et al. 2000).
→ Eighty percent of patients may go into sustained clinical remission.
- Those who do not go into remission continue to have active disease with potential neoplastic transformation.

ASSESSMENT

→ HPV: clinical, subclinical, or latent infection
→ Condyloma acuminata (warts)
→ R/O condyloma lata as a manifestation of secondary syphilis
→ R/O a squamous intraepithelial lesion (SIL), also known as a site-specific lesion, such as CIN, VIN, VAIN, PAIN, or AIN
→ R/O verrucous carcinoma or adenocarcinoma
→ R/O concomitant STDs
→ R/O vaginitis

PLAN

DIAGNOSTIC TESTS

→ Inspection with the unaided eye may reveal exophytic condyloma acuminata.
→ Gross visual inspection of the vulva after application of 3–5% acetic acid may reveal discrete, flat, subclinical lesions. However, there is a high false-positive rate of acetowhitening that can lead to overtreatment of normal epithelium when viewed without magnification.
NOTE: Acetowhitening on the vulva also may be due to tissue inflammation, trauma, allergic or contact dermatitis, pantyhose or tight pants, or a variation of normal epithelium.
→ Colposcopy or hand-held magnification of the vulva may enhance the ability to visualize and evaluate lesions throughout the lower genital tract.

→ Biopsies of cervical lesions and vaginal lesions with an atypical appearance should be performed under colposcopic guidance to establish a histopathological diagnosis before treatment is undertaken.

→ Biopsy of vulvar lesions for histopathological diagnosis may be indicated in certain cases (Anderson et al. 1996, CDC 2002):

▪ The diagnosis is uncertain

▪ When a lesion is unresponsive to local therapy or if the disease worsens during therapy

▪ The patient is immunocompromised

▪ Warts are pigmented, indurated, fixed, or ulcerated

→ A Pap smear should be done.

▪ Cervical cytology may identify cellular changes as noted by the presence of koilocytes and other nuclear changes and/or low- or high-grade SIL.

→ Three nucleic acid-based tests are available for detecting and typing HPV: polymerase chain reaction (PCR), the Hybrid Capture system (HC-2), and in situ hybridization (ISH). Only HC-2 is approved by the Food and Drug Administration for clinical use. The other two are limited to special research endeavors (Lorincz 2002).

▪ HC-2 is a highly sensitive, signal amplification-based test that detects and groups low-risk types and high-risk types for clinical reporting.

• There are 13 high-risk or carcinogenic HPV types: 16, 18, 31, 33, 35, 39, 45, 51, 52, 56, 58, 59, and 68.

• There are five low-risk types: 6, 11, 42, 43, and 44.

• Positive test results cannot be used to determine onset of infection or current status of infectivity.

NOTE: Current data do not support the use of type-specific HPV nucleic acid tests in the *routine* diagnosis/management of visible genital warts (CDC 2002).

→ Liquid-based Pap smear sampling now affords the possibility of reflex testing for HPV DNA from the same vial. It is especially useful for future triaging of patients who have equivocal Pap results. (See the **Abnormal Cervical Cytology** chapter in Section 12.)

→ Evaluate for concurrent existence of other STDs, including *Neisseria gonorrhoeae, Chlamydia trachomatis*, and syphilis. Perform vaginal wet smears to rule out *Trichomonas vaginalis* and bacterial vaginosis. (See specific chapters.)

→ Offer HIV testing.

TREATMENT/MANAGEMENT

→ Treat symptomatic warts.

▪ Visible, asymptomatic warts do not require definitive treatment. In untreated patients, visible genital warts may resolve spontaneously, remain unchanged, or proliferate in size and/or number (CDC 2002).

▪ Existing data indicate that currently available therapies may reduce, but probably do not eradicate, infectivity (CDC 2002).

▪ Treatment selection for genital warts should be guided by (CDC 2002):

• Size
• Number
• Anatomic site
  – Warts located on moist surfaces or in intertriginous areas respond better to topical treatment than do warts on drier surfaces.
• Morphology
• Patient preference
• Cost of treatment
• Available resources
• Convenience
• Adverse effects
• Provider experience

▪ In general, evidence does not support the use of one treatment modality over another; many patients require a course of therapy rather than a single treatment (CDC 2002).

→ Treatment regimens are divided into the following categories (see **Table 13F.2, Commonly Used Therapies for Treatment of Genital Warts**):

▪ Patient-applied therapies:

• Podophyllotoxin: Podofilox (Condylox®) 0.5% solution or gel

• Imiquimod (Aldara®) 5% cream

▪ Provider-administered therapies:

• Trichloroacetic acid (TCA) or bichloroacetic acid (BCA) 80–90%

• Podophyllin resin 10–25%

• 5-fluorouracil (5-FU, Efudex®) 3–5%

• Intralesion interferon (Intron A®)

• Surgical removal

• Cryotherapy

• Laser surgery

NOTE: Most patients experience mild to moderate pain/local irritation after treatment.

→ If there is no improvement after three provider-administered treatments or if warts have not completely cleared after six treatments, the treatment modality should be changed (CDC 2002).

→ Thick, keratinized vulvar lesions that do not respond to local therapies should be biopsied to rule out verrucous carcinoma (Singer et al. 2000).

→ Women with exophytic cervical warts must have high-grade squamous intraepithelial lesions excluded before treatment is initiated (CDC 2002). Consult with a physician.

→ Sex-partner examination is not necessary for the management of genital warts; there are no data indicating that re-infection plays a role in recurrences. However, sex partners of patients with warts may benefit from examination to assess the presence of genital warts and other STDs (CDC 2002). Examination of sex partners of women with subclinical HPV infection is not recommended (CDC 2002).

→ Treat concomitant vaginitis or STDs.

→ Obtain Pap smears according to clinical practice guidelines and site-specific protocols. (See the **Abnormal Cervical Cytology** chapter in Section 12.)

- There is no evidence that either the presence of visible genital warts or their treatment is associated with the development of cervical cancer (CDC 2002).
- The presence of genital warts is not an indication for a change in the frequency of Pap smears or for cervical colposcopy (CDC 2002).
- Women with abnormalities on cervical cytology should be evaluated and followed per clinical practice guidelines and site-specific protocols. (See the **Abnormal Cervical Cytology** chapter.)
- Some authors suggest that HIV-infected women at risk for HPV disease be screened every six months by cervical cytology and concurrently by routine colposcopic examination of the vulva, vagina, and cervix. Others advise regular cytologic screening only (Jay et al. 2000).

CONSULTATION

→ Physician consultation is indicated for patients with persistent condyloma that does not respond to therapy after several treatments or for patients with extensive vulvar, vaginal, or cervical disease. Pregnancy may exacerbate HPV and often warrants referral to a physician.
→ Refer to a physician or an experienced advanced practice clinician for colposcopic evaluation and biopsy any patient who has:
- Two consecutive, atypical cervical cytologies
- SIL or CIN on cervical cytology
- Cervical or vaginal lesions visible before application of acetic acid (leukoplakia)

PATIENT EDUCATION

→ Discuss the variable incubation period. Often it is difficult to determine the source-partner of the transmission of the infection.
→ Discuss the issues regarding partner evaluation and treatment. (See "Treatment/Management," above.)
- In ongoing relationships, sex partners usually are infected by the time of the patient's diagnosis, but the partners may be asymptomatic (CDC 2002).
→ The likelihood of transmission to future partners is unknown. Although the use of condoms has not been demonstrated to reduce the risk of reinfection, their use should be emphasized to reduce the risk of other STDs, especially for patients with high-risk behaviors (Davis et al. 2001, Fernandez-Esquer et al. 2000). (See **Table 13A.2, Safer Sex Guidelines** in the **Chancroid** chapter and **Table 12I.1, Recommendations for Individuals to Prevent STD/PID** in the **Pelvic Inflammatory Disease** chapter in Section 12.)
→ Counsel patients who have a history of multiple partners, multiple STDs, and high-risk behaviors, such as unprotected anal receptive intercourse or injection drug use, regarding the risk of HIV infection. (See the **Human Immunodeficiency Virus-1 Infection** chapter in Section 11.)
- Improved efforts are needed to counsel patients, especially adolescents, regarding current knowledge of HPV and HIV (Dell et al. 2000).

→ Discuss the side effects of local ablative therapy.
- Advise patients that recurrence of warts is common in the first few months after treatment. Duration of infectivity after treatment is unknown (CDC 2002).
- Warn patients that persistent hypo/hyperpigmentation is common with ablative therapies. Rarely, treatment can result in chronic pain syndromes (e.g., vulvodynia, hyperesthesia) of the treatment site (CDC 2002).
- Counsel the patient about sexual abstinence during the acute treatment phase, to allow for healing.
→ Reassure the patient that the natural history of genital warts is generally benign and advise her that the HPV types that usually cause external warts are not associated with cancer (CDC 2002).
→ Advise the patient that although visible lesions can be removed, eradication of HPV from the genital tract and long-term effects of the virus are a function of the patient's own healthy immune system. Educate the patient about, and reassure her that, behaviors that promote optimal wellness may enhance the immune system and will help resolve the virus (American Social Health Association 1999). Psychological support is important for the well-being of the patient.
→ Counsel patients regarding the low but real risk of vertical transmission to a neonate during delivery (Cason 1996).
→ Counsel the patient about the need for continued surveillance with Pap smears.
→ The American Social Health Association's HPV Support Program provides support services and publishes a quarterly newsletter, *HPV News*. In addition, the Web site www.ashastd.org provides current information regarding advances in managing the infection and preventing lower-genital-tract cancer. For information about these services, contact the American Social Health Association, P.O. Box 13827, Research Triangle Park, N.C. 27709, (800) 230-6039.

FOLLOW-UP

→ See **Table 13F.2** for the frequency of local therapeutic measures for condyloma.
→ For patients using self-administered therapy, follow-up visits may be useful after several weeks to determine response to treatment (CDC 2002).
→ Offer a three-month follow-up evaluation for patients concerned about recurrences. The patient also may return prn.
→ Follow the recommended time intervals for Pap smears. (See the **Abnormal Cervical Cytology** chapter in Section 12.)
→ Follow up on laboratory tests and treat concomitant STDs. Treat/refer partner(s) as indicated. (See the appropriate chapters.)
→ HIV-positive results should be conveyed in person by a clinician trained in the complexities of test disclosure. HIV-positive persons should be referred to the appropriate provider or agency for early intervention services.
→ Document in progress notes and on problem list.

Table 13F.2.   COMMONLY USED THERAPIES FOR TREATMENT OF GENITAL WARTS

Therapeutic Modality	Clearance Rates	Site-Specific Use	Mechanism of Action	Advantages	Disadvantages/ Additional Information
Podophyllin resin 10–25% solution in tincture of benzoin	38–79%	External genitalia and perianal region. Mucous membrane should be avoided. No use internally on vagina or cervix. Applied directly to wart for up to 4 weeks. Some specialists suggest washing off the preparation 1–4 hours after application.	Local inflammatory response; histologically shows keratinocyte necrosis and abnormal mitoses; causes warts to shrink.	Low cost, relatively convenient	1. Adverse reactions include erythema, pain, burning, swelling, and erosions. 2. Systemic toxicity and fetal demise reported; use in pregnancy prohibited. 3. Stability unreliable. 4. Requires series of clinician visits.
Podophyllotoxin: podofilox (Condylox®) 0.5% solution or gel	68–88%	External genitalia and perianal region. No use internally on vagina or cervix. Patient-applied once in a.m. and p.m. for 3 days in a row followed by 4 days without treatment; repeat cycle up to a total of 4 weeks.	Same as podophyllin	1. Purity, stable shelf life, negligible systemic absorption. 2. Patient-applied, decreasing need for office visits; lower cost. 3. No need to wash off once applied.	1. Same local reactions as podophyllin. 2. Use prohibited in pregnancy.
Trichloroacetic acid (TCA) Bichloroacetic acid (BCA) 80–90% strength	50%	External genitalia and perianal region; internally on vagina or cervix following HPV diagnosis with colposcopically directed biopsy. Applied with wooden tip of Q-tip onto wart and a few mm beyond every 7–12 days up to 6 weeks.	Contact immediately causes superficial destruction of skin lesions and superficial skin necrosis.	1. Low cost, relatively convenient. 2. Approved for use in pregnancy. 3. No need to wash off once applied.	1. Intense transient local pain and tissue necrosis. 2. Requires series of clinician visits.
Imiquimod (Aldara®) 5% cream	72–84%	Apply sparingly to external genitalia and perianal region. No use internally on vagina or cervix. Patient-applied nightly 3 times per week for up to a total of 16 weeks. Wash off in morning.	Cell-mediated immune response resulting in destruction of wart and localized immunity.	1. Low cost, convenient. 2. Patient-applied, decreasing need for office visits.	1. Local adverse reactions include erythema, pain, burning, swelling, and superficial erosions requiring a no-treatment period. 2. Use prohibited in pregnancy due to lack of well-controlled studies.
5-fluorouracil (5-FU, Efudex®) 3–5%	30–50%	Topical application to vulva and off-label use in vagina. Currently rarely used on female or male patients due to severe local reactions and availability of other effective products. Vulva: small amounts to affected areas 2 consecutive days a week for 10 weeks. Vagina: ¼ applicator once a week at bedtime for 10 weeks. Zinc oxide to protect vulva. Hand washing mandatory to prevent irritation of sensitive areas such as eyes.	Interferes with cellular proliferation by disrupting DNA and RNA synthesis.	Most often used as adjuvant therapy following laser or cryotherapy of cervix for treatment of extensive/diffuse vaginal HPV.	1. Complications include acute erosive vulvitis and vaginitis; pain, redness, and discharge are common. 2. Use prohibited in pregnancy.

(continued)

Table 13F.2.   COMMONLY USED THERAPIES FOR TREATMENT OF GENITAL WARTS *(continued)*

Therapeutic Modality	Clearance Rates	Site-Specific Use	Mechanism of Action	Advantages	Disadvantages/ Additional Information
Cryotherapy with liquid nitrogen or cryoprobe	67–88%	Vulva, cervix, perianal, small focal vaginal condyloma. Performed by MD or specially trained NP, PA, or CNM. Use of a cryoprobe in the vagina is not recommended due to the risk of perforation and fistula formation.	Tissue freezing results in membrane rupture and intracellular dehydration, cell death, and localized tissue crushing.	1. Direct application through a variety of devices based on size and location of lesion (cotton swab or cryosurgical probe). 2. Clinically well-tolerated, moderate discomfort. 3. Rarely requires use of local anesthesia; best suited for small lesions.	Postcervical cryotherapy results in heavy, prolonged vaginal discharge for 2–4 weeks. Advise pelvic rest and no tampons, douching, or hot tubs for 2–4 weeks postprocedure.
Surgical methods: electrosurgery, surgical excision via scissors/ blade, curettage	64–72% >3 months clearance rate	Vulvar and perianal condyloma. Performed by MD or specially trained NP, PA, or CNM.	Destruction of lesion by burning or physical removal.	Best suited for small focal lesions.	1. Requires local anesthesia. 2. Mild postoperative pain. 3. Hospitalization may be required for extensive lesions.
Laser therapy (carbon dioxide laser)	72–97%	Cervix, vagina, vulva, anus. Performed by MD.	Direct tissue vaporization. High degree of accuracy in size of area and depth of destruction.	Use when extensive or bulky lesions exist.	1. Complications include short-term pain, swelling, ulceration, infection, or delayed healing. May require hospital stay for pain management for extensive procedures. 2. Most often done in surgical center or operating room, which increases treatment cost. 3. Reservoir of HPV may be contained in adjacent tissue, leading to recurrence of disease at wound site.
Interferon alfa-2b (Intron A®)	36–53%	Genital lesions. Intralesional injection of 1–3 million IU into each lesion 3 times per week for up to 10 weeks.	Antiviral immunopotentiating and antiproliferative activities.	For use with recalcitrant condyloma not responsive to other therapy.	1. Systemic administration results in flu-like symptoms, such as fever, headache, nausea, myalgias, and fatigue. 2. Use in pregnancy contraindicated. 3. Costly 4. Rare use due to variable low efficacy. 5. Not a primary therapy. 6. Necessitates referral to a specialist.

Source: Beutner, K.R. 1997. Therapeutic approaches to genital warts. *American Journal of Medicine* 102(5A):28–37; Centers for Disease Control and Prevention (CDC). 2002. Sexually transmitted diseases treatment guidelines 2002. *Morbidity and Mortality Weekly Report* 51(RR-6):53–57; Cox, T., Buck, H.W., Kinney, W. et al. 2001. Human papillomavirus (HPV) and cervical cancer. *ARHP Clinical Proceedings* March:13–17; Gross, G., Tyring, S.K., von Krogh, G. et al. 1997b. External genitalia: treatment. In *Human papillomavirus infection: a clinical atlas*, eds. G. Gross and R. Barrasso, pp. 365–376. Berlin/ Wiesbaden, Germany: Ulstein-Mosby.

BIBLIOGRAPHY

American Social Health Association. 1999. Healthy choices, healthy lifestyle. *HPV News* 9(4).

Anderson, L.L., and Atkinson, B.F. 1996. Preinvasive lesions of the cervix and vagina. In *Clinical gynecologic pathology*, eds. E. Hernandez and B. Atkinson, pp. 129–174. Philadelphia: W.B. Saunders.

Anderson, M., Jordan, J., Morse, A. et al. 1997. *A text and atlas of integrated colposcopy*. St. Louis, Mo.: Mosby.

Beutner, K.R. 1997. Therapeutic approaches to genital warts. *American Journal of Medicine* 102(5A):28–37.

Bosch, F.X., Manos, M., Munoz, N. et al. 1995. Prevalence of human papillomavirus in cervical cancer: a worldwide perspective. *Journal of the National Cancer Institute* 87: 796–802.

Burghardt, E., Hellmut, P., and Girardi, F. 1998. *Colposcopy, cervical pathology: textbook and atlas*, 3rd ed. New York: Thieme.

Cason, J. 1996. Perinatal acquisition of cervical cancer-associated papillomaviruses. *British Journal of Obstetrics and Gynecology* 103:853–858.

Centers for Disease Control and Prevention (CDC). 2002. Sexually transmitted diseases treatment guidelines 2002. *Morbidity and Mortality Weekly Report* 51(RR-6):53–57.

Cox, T., Buck, H.W., Kinney, W. et al. 2001. Human papillomavirus (HPV) and cervical cancer. *ARHP Clinical Proceedings* March:1–32.

Davis, G., Good, A.E., Rubin, M. et al. 2001. Diagnosis with human papillomavirus—condoms or abstinence? *Journal of Lower Genital Tract Disease* 5(2):99–101.

Dell, D.L., Chen, H., Ahmad, F. et al. 2000. Knowledge about human papillomavirus among adolescents. *Obstetrics and Gynecology* 96(5 Part 1):653–656.

Del Mistro, A., and Chieco Bianchi, L. 2001. HPV-related neoplasias in HIV infected individuals. *European Journal of Cancer* 37(10):1227–1235.

Fernandez-Esquer, M.E., Ross, M.W., and Torres, I. 2000. The importance of psychosocial factors in the prevention of HPV and cervical cancer. *International Journal of STD and AIDS* 11(11):701–713.

Fowler, R.S. 2000. Vulvar vestibulitis: response to hypocontactant vulvar therapy. *Journal of Lower Genital Tract Disease* 4(4):200–203.

Franco, E.L., Villa, L.L., Sobrinho, J.P. et al. 1999. Epidemiology of acquisition and clearance of cervical human papillomavirus infection in women from a high-risk area for cervical cancer. *Journal of Infectious Diseases* 180(5):1415–1423.

Gallagher, B., Zhengyn, W., Schymura, M. et al. 2001. Cancer incidence in New York State acquired immunodeficiency syndrome patients. *American Journal of Epidemiology* 154(6):544–556.

Giuntoli, R., Atkinson, B., Ernst, C. et al. 1987. *Atkinson's correlative atlas of colposcopy, cytology, and histopathology*. Philadelphia: J.B. Lippincott.

Gross, G., and Barrasso, R., eds. 1997a. *Human papillomavirus infection: a clinical atlas*. Berlin/Wiesbaden, Germany: Ulstein-Mosby.

Gross, G., Tyring, S.K., von Krogh, G. et al. 1997b. External genitalia: treatment. In *Human papillomavirus infection: a clinical atlas*, eds. G. Gross and R. Barrasso, pp. 365–376. Berlin/Wiesbaden, Germany: Ulstein-Mosby.

Ho, G.Y., Bierman, R., Beardsley, L. et al. 1998. Natural history of cervicovaginal papillomavirus infection in young women. *New England Journal of Medicine* 338(7):423–428.

Jay, N., and Moscicki, A.B. 2000. Human papillomavirus infections in women with HIV disease: prevalence, risk, and management. *AIDS Reader* 10(11):659–668.

Kjellberg, L., Hallmans, G., Ahren, A. et al. 2000. Smoking, diet, pregnancy, and oral contraceptive use as risk factors for cervical intraepithelial neoplasia in relation to human papillomavirus infection. *British Journal of Cancer* 82(7): 1332–1338.

Koutsky, L. 1997. Epidemiology of genital human papillomavirus infection. *American Journal of Medicine* 102(5A):3–8.

Lorincz, A.T. 1999. Human papillomavirus. In *Laboratory diagnosis of viral infections*, 3rd ed., eds. E.H. Lennette and T.F. Smith. New York: Marcel Dekker.

_____. 2002. HPV testing. In *Integrated textbook and atlas of colposcopy*, eds. B. Apgar, G. Brotzman, and M. Spitzer. Philadelphia: W.B. Saunders.

Moscicki, A.B., Hills, N., Shiboski, S. et al. 2001. Risk for incident human papillomavirus infection and low-grade squamous intraepithelial lesion development in young females. *Journal of the American Medical Association* 285(23): 2995–3002.

Palefsky, J.M., and Holly, E.A. 1995. Molecular virology and epidemiology of human papillomavirus and cervical cancer. *Cancer Epidemiology, Biomarkers, and Prevention* 4(4): 415–428.

Schlect, N.F., Kulaga, S., Robitalle, J. et al. 2001. Persistent human papillomavirus infection as a predictor of cervical intraepithelial neoplasia. *Journal of the American Medical Association* 286(24):3106–3114.

Singer, A., and Monaghan, J.M. 2000. *Lower genital tract precancer: colposcopy, pathology, and treatment*, 2nd ed. London: Blackwell Science.

Sun, C.A., Lai, H.C., Chang, C.C. et al. 2001. The significance of human papillomavirus viral load in prediction of histologic severity and size of squamous intraepithelial lesions of the uterine cervix. *Gynecologic Oncology* 83(1):95–99.

Walboomers, J.M., Jacobs, M.V., Manos, M.M. et al. 1999. Human papillomavirus, a necessary cause of invasive cancer worldwide. *Journal of Pathology* 189:12–19.

Weiderpass, E., Ye, W., Tammi, R. et al. 2001. Alcoholism and the risk for cancer of the cervix uteri, vagina, and vulva. *Cancer Epidemiology, Biomarkers, and Prevention* 10(8): 899–901.

Wilkinson, E.J., and Stone, I.K. 1995. *Atlas of vulvar disease*. New York: Williams & Wilkins.

Winifred L. Star, R.N., C., N.P., M.S.
Melanie Deal, R.N., C., N.P., M.S.

13-G

Lymphogranuloma Venereum

Lymphogranuloma venereum (LGV) is a chronic, systemic, sexually transmitted disease (STD) with variable acute and late manifestations (Perine et al. 1999). LGV is caused by three serotypes of the bacterium *Chlamydia trachomatis*: L1, L2, and L3.

Although LGV is prevalent in the tropical and semi-tropical climates of Africa, India, Southeast Asia, South America, and the Caribbean, it is extremely rare in the United States. There were only 235 cases reported to the Centers for Disease Control and Prevention (CDC) in 1994, which was the last year LGV was a reportable infection in the United States (CDC 1995). In nonendemic areas, most reported cases occur in soldiers, sailors, and travelers who have frequented or lived in high-prevalence areas (Perine et al. 1999).

LGV often has been confused with other ulcerative STDs, such as syphilis, herpes, and chancroid. The pathogenesis of the disease is not yet fully understood and the frequency of infection after exposure is unknown. It is thought that LGV is less contagious than gonorrhea. It cannot penetrate intact skin or mucous membranes and therefore must enter through small abrasions or lacerations in these tissues. Congenital transmission does not occur. Infection, however, may be acquired during passage through an infected birth canal (Perine et al. 1999).

LGV is an aggressive disease, predominantly of lymphatic tissue, with the potential for serious sequelae. Inflammation of infected tissue can lead to abscesses, fistula and sinus tract development, and, if untreated, severe fibrosis and chronic edema. Acute LGV is reported more frequently in men (ratio of 5:1) because women are often asymptomatic in the early stages of the disease. Consequently, because their disease may go undetected, women are more likely than men to suffer late complications.

There are three stages of infection. The primary stage includes a lesion that may take several forms: a papule, an ulcer, a small herpetiform lesion, or nonspecific urethritis. The most common presentation is a small, nonindurated, herpetiform ulcer that appears at the site of infection after an incubation period of 3–12 days or longer. This lesion, present in 3–53% of patients, heals quickly without a scar (Perine et al. 1999).

The most common sites for an acute primary lesion in women are the cervix, the posterior vaginal wall, the fourchette, and the vulva. If located intraurethrally, the ulcer may cause nonspecific urethritis (Perine et al. 1999).

Secondary stage disease is characterized by acute, suppurative, inguinal lymphadenitis with bubo formation (inguinal syndrome) and/or acute hemorrhagic proctitis (anogenitorectal syndrome). In persons exposed via receptive anal intercourse, the most common manifestation of LGV is acute proctitis.

The incubation period for the inguinal syndrome is 10–30 days, but it may be delayed 4–6 months after infection (Perine et al. 1999). Constitutional symptoms including fever, malaise, myalgias, and anorexia are present in the secondary stage. The inflammatory process may persist for several weeks to months. During this time, lymph nodes may abscess, rupture, and form sinus tracts or fistulas. Other systemic manifestations may include hepatitis, meningitis, pneumonitis, and conjunctivitis. The central nervous system may become infected via systemic spread of the organism (Perine et al. 1999).

Most affected individuals recover from LGV after the second stage, but some develop late complications characterized by a chronic inflammatory response with associated genital ulcers, fistulas, rectal strictures, and genital elephantiasis. Antibiotics used during the secondary stage prevent these late complications (Perine et al. 1999, Sweet et al. 2002).

A number of different antimicrobials have been used to treat LGV. Spontaneous remission is possible. Outpatient surgical treatment is limited to aspiration of lymph nodes, and incision and drainage of abscesses. Complications of advanced rectal stricture require more sophisticated surgical procedures and hospitalization. Concomitant STDs are likely in patients with LGV and should be treated accordingly (Perine et al. 1999, Sweet et al. 2002).

DATABASE

SUBJECTIVE

→ LGV is more common in the third decade of life.

→ LGV is seen more frequently in urban areas and among individuals of lower socioeconomic status.

→ The patient may have a history of travel to a country where LGV is endemic.

→ Symptomatic early infection is less common in women. Late complications (ulceration, rectal strictures, hypertrophy of genitals) are more frequent in women.

→ Gynecological and medical history:
  - Menstrual cycle
  - Contraception
  - Description of symptoms:
    • Onset
    • Duration
    • Quality/quantity
    • Frequency
    • Course
    • Aggravating/relieving factors
    • Associated symptoms
  - Previous history of same/similar problem
  - STD history (including dates, treatment)
  - Sensitive questioning regarding recent sexual activity (including date of last exposure), sex practices, sites of exposure, number and gender of partners in past months, and use of condoms
  - Sex partner history (including travel, drug use)
  - Acute/chronic illness
  - General health
  - Medications
  - Allergies
  - Habits (including travel and use of illegal drugs, both injection and noninjection)
  - History of laboratory tests for syphilis, hepatitis B, HIV
  - Review of systems (CDC 1991)

Primary Stage

→ Genital lesions may be asymptomatic. The incubation period ranges from 3–12 days or longer. The lesion heals within a few days with no sequelae.

→ Symptoms include those associated with cervicitis, urethritis, and/or proctitis: abnormal discharge or bleeding, pelvic pain; dysuria, urgency, frequency (urethritis may be mild or asymptomatic); diarrhea, rectal discharge.

→ Relatively few patients present in this stage unless lesions are in the rectum.

→ See "Objective," below.

Secondary Stage

→ Inguinal syndrome:
  - Incubation period is 10–30 days; may be delayed 4–6 months.
  - Symptoms include:

  - Painful swelling of inguinal lymph nodes, usually unilateral, enlarging over 1–2 weeks (the reason most patients seek care)
    – Present in 20–30% of women
  - Constitutional symptoms of fever, malaise, myalgias, arthralgias, headache, anorexia (may precede adenopathy)
  - Lower abdominal pain, back pain (in one-third of cases, due to involvement of deep pelvic/lumbar lymph nodes)
  - Rupture of bubo relieves pain, fever. Relapse of buboes may occur in about 20% of untreated cases.
  - See "Objective," below.

→ Anogenitorectal syndrome:
  - Early symptoms include anal pruritus, mucous rectal discharge.
  - Later symptoms include fever, tenesmus, rectal pain, mucopurulent rectal discharge (a sign of secondary infection), and left lower abdominal pain.
  - See "Objective," below.

→ Other manifestations include:
  - Lesions in mouth, throat
  - Swollen lymph glands in neck area
  - Symptoms of conjunctivitis
  - Skin manifestations
  - See "Objective," below.

Late Stage

→ Symptoms may include:
  - Constipation, passage of "pencil stools" (indicative of rectal stricture), colicky abdominal pain, distention, weight loss
  - Perianal, hemorrhoid-like, tissue growths (a sign of obstruction of lymph/venous drainage of the lower rectum, called *lymphorrhoids* or *perianal condylomas*)
  - "Growths," ulceration at urinary meatus with dysuria, frequency, incontinence (urethrogenitoperineal syndrome)
  - Chronic, painful, genital ulcerations
  - Edema from clitoris to anus, legs
  - See "Objective," below.

OBJECTIVE

→ The examination may be individualized based on case presentation.

→ A thorough STD examination includes (CDC 1991, Graney et al. 1999):
  - Vital signs as indicated
  - General skin inspection of face, trunk, forearms, and palms and soles for lesions, rashes, discoloration
  - Inspection of pharynx and oral cavity for infection, lesions, discoloration
  - Abdominal inspection and palpation for masses, tenderness, rebound tenderness
  - Inspection of pubic hair for lice, nits
  - Inspection of external genitalia for discharge, masses, lesions; inspection and palpation of Bartholin's, urethral, and Skene's glands for discharge, masses

- Inspection of vagina for discharge, lesions
- Inspection of cervix for lesions, discharge, eversion, erythema, edema, contact bleeding; assessment for cervical motion tenderness (CMT)
- Uterine assessment for size, shape, consistency, mobility, tenderness
- Palpation of adnexa for masses, tenderness
- Inspection of perianus and anus for lesions, bleeding, discharge
- Rectal examination as indicated
- Assessment of presence or absence of associated lymphadenopathy

Primary Stage

→ A papular, vesicular, shallow ulcerative, or eroded lesion is most commonly found on the posterior vaginal wall, fourchette, posterior lip of the cervix, vulva, or extragenital area (mouth, fingers, nose). It heals rapidly with no scar.
→ Signs of cervicitis, urethritis (mucopurulent discharge), or salpingitis (lower abdominal tenderness; CMT may be present).

Secondary Stage

→ Inguinal syndrome:
- The patient may present with fever.
- A firm, tender inguinal bubo with overlying erythema (unilateral in two-thirds of cases) enlarges over 1–2 weeks.
  - This occurs in about 20–30% of women.
- In one-third of cases, buboes become fluctuant and rupture; the remainder involute and form a firm mass without suppuration.
- In 20% of cases, femoral lymph nodes are affected and may be separated from inguinal lymph nodes by inguinal ligament (the so-called "groove sign," which is pathognomonic for LGV).
- In 75% of cases, deep iliac lymph nodes are involved. A large pelvic mass is formed that is not likely to suppurate (Perine et al. 1999).
→ Anogenitorectal syndrome (or proctocolitis):
- Rectal mucosa is friable and hyperemic with superficial, irregular ulcerations. A mucopurulent rectal discharge occurs with secondary infection.
- Granulomas and abscesses may form in the bowel wall (a chronic inflammatory process).
- Abdominal examination may reveal left lower quadrant tenderness and palpable, thickened, pelvic colon.

Late Stage

→ The patient may present with:
- Papillary growths, ulceration of urethral meatus
- Recto-vaginal erosion with fistula formation
- Lymphorrhoids in perianal area
- Chronic, progressive lymphangitis; edema; fibrosis of vulva with induration, enlargement, ulceration of genital tissues (esthiomene). Ulcerations are mostly on the labia majora, perineum, crural folds.
- Lymphedema from clitoris to anus, legs (genital elephantiasis)
→ Perirectal abscess formation and anal fissures may occur (may be the only manifestation of chronic anogenital LGV).
→ Rectal stricture may form. Rectal examination may reveal normal consistency to mucosa above stricture but ulcerative and granular below (examination is quite painful). May palpate moveable lymph nodes under the bowel wall.
→ Complete bowel obstruction is rare but may cause perforation and peritonitis, the usual cause of death in LGV.

Other Manifestations

→ Lymphadenitis of the cervical or submaxillary lymph nodes may exist if the primary lesion is in the mouth or pharynx.
→ Follicular conjunctivitis may occur with lymphadenitis of the maxillary and posterior auricular nodes.
→ Other manifestations may include erythema nodosum, erythema multiforme, mediastinal adenitis, pericarditis, hepatitis, pneumonitis, arthritis, aseptic meningitis, and papillary edema.

ASSESSMENT

→ LGV
→ R/O syphilis
→ R/O chancroid
→ R/O herpes genitalis
→ R/O concomitant STDs
→ R/O other possible causes of inguinal lymphadenitis: metastatic cervical, vulvar, or vaginal cancer; Hodgkin's disease; incarcerated hernia; infected lesions of legs, feet; plague; tularemia; tuberculosis
→ R/O salpingitis
→ R/O appendicitis
→ R/O tubo-ovarian abscess
→ R/O incarcerated hernia
→ R/O lymphoma
→ R/O rectal cancer

PLAN

DIAGNOSTIC TESTS

→ Distinguish between LGV and other causes of genital ulcers.
- See **Table 13A.1, Clinical Features of Genital Ulcers** and **Figure 13A.1, Sexually Active Patient with Genital Ulcer(s)** in the **Chancroid** chapter.
→ Definitive diagnosis: isolation of *C. trachomatis* (serotypes L1, L2, or L3) by tissue culture of lymph node aspirate *or* immunofluorescence of *C. trachomatis* inclusion bodies in leukocytes of inguinal lymph node (bubo) aspirate (CDC 1991).
- Material for culture also may be obtained from the ulcer base or rectal lesions.
  NOTE: Material from infected tissue and/or ruptured

buboes poses a health risk to personnel. Universal precautions should be applied.

→ Additional diagnostic tests may include:
- Complement fixation test: titers ≥ 1:64
  NOTE: Titers are usually high initially and do not rise much between acute and six-week convalescent specimens. High or low titers may persist for years. Titers may also represent levels from other chlamydial infections.
- Cytology: elementary and inclusion bodies of *C. trachomatis* may be identified with Giemsa, iodine, and fluorescent antibody-staining methods.
- Polymerase chain reaction (PCR) test
- Radiological procedures: lymphography, barium enema
- Biopsy of rectal tissue to rule out cancer

→ CBC: shows mild leukocytosis with increased monocytes/eosinophils in early disease or more significant polymorphonuclear leukocytosis if superinfection is present.

→ Diagnostic tests to rule out other causes of genital ulcers and lymphadenopathy include:
- Dark-field or direct immunofluorescence test of serous fluid for *Treponema pallidum* from genital and nonoral lesion(s) to rule out syphilis.
  - See the **Syphilis** chapter.
- RPR (or VDRL) or treponemal tests to rule out syphilis.
  - See the **Syphilis** chapter.
- Herpes culture to rule out herpes.
  - See the **Genital Herpes Simplex Virus** chapter.
- See "Diagnostic Tests" in the **Chancroid** and **Granuloma Inguinale Donovanosis** chapters.

→ Sensitive testing for *N. gonorrhoeae* and *C. trachomatis*. In the absence of a cervix, urethral or urine specimen may be obtained.

→ HIV testing should be offered.

→ Additional tests may include but are not limited to: wet mount, Pap smear, urinalysis, urine culture and sensitivities, pregnancy test, and hepatitis B screen.

TREATMENT/MANAGEMENT

→ Recommended regimen (CDC 2002):
- Doxycycline 100 mg p.o. BID for 21 days

→ Alternative regimen (CDC 2002):
- Erythromycin base 500 mg p.o. QID for 21 days
  - Some STD specialists believe that azithromycin 1 g p.o. once weekly for 3 weeks is likely effective.

→ Surgical intervention:
- Antibiotic therapy should precede surgical intervention.
- Surgical treatment of inguinal syndrome should be limited to aspiration of fluctuant lymph nodes and occasional incision and drainage of abscesses (Perine et al. 1999).
- Rectal strictures may require dilation with elastic bougies. Advanced strictures require a variety of surgical procedures.
- Additional indications for surgery include a bowel obstruction, a persistent rectovaginal fistula, and destruction of the anal canal/sphincter or perineum.

NOTE: Ideally, antibiotics should be given for several months before advanced surgery. Patients with chronic or late manifestations of anogenitorectal syndrome (e.g., perirectal abscess, rectovaginal fistula, rectal stricture) should be managed by a physician due to the serious and complex nature of these conditions.

→ Partner therapy:
- All sex partners exposed within the 30 days before the patient's symptom onset should be examined, tested for urethral or cervical chlamydial infection, and treated (CDC 2002). Provide referrals to a provider or facility that offers appropriate STD care.

→ Special considerations:
- Pregnant and lactating women should be treated with erythromycin. Azithromycin may prove useful for treatment in pregnancy, but there are no published data regarding its safety and efficacy (CDC 2002).
- HIV-infected individuals should be treated with the same regimens as those for HIV-negative individuals. Prolonged therapy may be required and symptom resolution may be delayed (CDC 2002).

CONSULTATION

→ Consultation with a physician as indicated for patient evaluation, abnormal laboratory studies, and management.

→ For advanced cases of LGV, referral to a physician is warranted.

→ As needed for prescription(s).

PATIENT EDUCATION

→ Discuss the etiology and nature of LGV, including the mode of transmission, incubation period, symptoms and potential complications, and the importance of partner evaluation and treatment.
- Patent-education handouts are a helpful adjunct to teaching. Written materials may be obtained from:
  - CDC National Prevention Information Network
    P.O. Box 6003
    Rockville, Md. 20849-6003
    (800) 458-5231, www.cdcnpin.org
  - American Social Health Association
    P.O. Box 13827
    Research Triangle Park, N.C. 27709
    (919) 361-8400, www.ashastd.org
- Additional resources for patients are:
  - National STD Hotline
    (800) 227-8922 or (800) 342-2437
    En Español: (800) 344-7432
  - For adolescents: www.iwannaknow.org

→ Advise the patient to finish the full course of medication and return for follow-up (see "Follow-up," below). After antibiotics have been started, the patient's fever and pain should abate and she should feel markedly better within 1–2 days.

→ Advise the patient that buboes are unlikely to suppurate after medication has begun. However, in some cases it may become necessary to needle-aspirate fluctuant buboes to prevent rupture.

- Refer the patient to a physician for this procedure.

→ Chronic or late complications of anogenitorectal syndrome may require surgical management. Procedures should be discussed with the patient by the physician responsible for her care.

→ Advise abstinence from intercourse until the patient and her partner are treated and cured. They should be instructed to seek care promptly if symptoms recur.

→ Address STD prevention and HIV risk-reduction.

- Provide guidelines for safer sex practices.
- Encourage careful screening of sex partners and the committed use of condoms (especially with new, multiple, nonmonogamous partners).
- See Table **13A.2, Safer Sex Practices** in the **Chancroid** chapter and **Table 12I.1, Recommendations for Individuals to Prevent STD/PID** in the **Pelvic Inflammatory Disease** chapter in Section 12.

→ Allow the patient to vent her feelings of surprise, shame, fear, and anger as indicated. Psychological support may be important in helping the patient gain control over her sexual situation and prevent future STDs.

FOLLOW-UP

→ Follow-up visits at one- to two-week intervals should be scheduled for clinical assessment of response to therapy.

→ Advise the patient to return for evaluation if symptoms persist or recur after treatment is completed.

→ History on follow-up should include:

- Symptom status
- Medication compliance
- Drug reaction and side effects
- Partner therapy
- Sexual exposure
- Use of condoms

→ Patients with complicated secondary and/or late-stage disease should be followed by a physician due to the serious and complex nature of the condition. Ongoing medical, surgical, and psychological evaluation and support will be indicated.

→ Serological tests for syphilis should be repeated in three months.

→ HIV antibody tests should be repeated in three months. Continue to encourage safer sex.

→ Follow up on all lab tests ordered. Treat all concomitant STDs and other identified conditions.

→ HIV-positive results should be conveyed in person by a provider who has received training in the complexities of test disclosure. HIV-positive persons should be referred to the appropriate provider or agency for early intervention services.

→ Offer the hepatitis A vaccine to women at risk for sexual transmission of this virus (e.g., users of illegal injection and noninjection drugs). (See the **Hepatitis—Viral** chapter in Section 11.)

→ Offer the hepatitis B vaccine to all women seeking treatment for an STD who have not been previously vaccinated. (See the **Hepatitis—Viral** chapter for further information.)

→ Newly diagnosed, hepatitis B antigen-positive individuals should undergo liver function tests and receive counseling regarding the implications of their positive status and need for immunoprophylaxis of sex partners and household members. (See the **Hepatitis—Viral** chapter.)

→ Document in progress notes and on problem list.

BIBLIOGRAPHY

Centers for Disease Control and Prevention (CDC). 1991. *Sexually transmitted diseases. Clinical practice guidelines.* Atlanta, Ga.: the Author.

_____. 1995. Summary of notifiable diseases, United States, 1994. *Morbidity and Mortality Weekly Report* 43(53):iv, 70.

_____. 2002. Sexually transmitted diseases treatment guidelines 2002. *Morbidity and Mortality Weekly Report* 51(RR–6):18.

Graney, D.O., and Vontver, L.A. 1999. Anatomy and physical examination of the female genital tract. In *Sexually transmitted diseases*, 3rd ed., eds. K.K. Holmes, P.F. Sparling, P.-A. Mårdh et al., pp. 685–697. New York: McGraw-Hill.

Perine, P.L., and Stamm, W.E. 1999. Lymphogranuloma inguinale. In *Sexually transmitted diseases*, 3rd ed., eds. K.K. Holmes, P.F. Sparling, P.-A. Mårdh et al., pp. 423–432. New York: McGraw-Hill.

Sweet, R.L., and Gibbs, R.S. 2002. *Infectious diseases of the female genital tract*, 4th ed. Philadelphia: Lippincott Williams & Wilkins.

Winifred L. Star, R.N., C., N.P., M.S.
Melanie Deal, R.N., C., N.P., M.S.

13-H

Syphilis

Syphilis is a chronic, systemic infection caused by the motile spirochete *Treponema pallidum.* Syphilis rates in the United States have plummeted since the introduction of penicillin in the 1940s. While case rates have continued a downward trend, there was a brief increase in incidence in the 1980s among homosexual men and in the early 1990s among heterosexuals. However, rates again seem to be on the decline (Stamm 1999). In 2000, only 5,979 cases of primary and secondary syphilis were reported to the Centers for Disease Control and Prevention (CDC), which represented the lowest case rate ever recorded (2.5 cases/100,000) (CDC 2001b).

In the United States, syphilis is geographically concentrated in the South and in a small number of urban areas. Approximately 80% of U.S. counties reported no syphilis in 1999 (CDC 2001a). Syphilis is most common among ages 20–39 years and is more common in men than women. As with other sexually transmitted disease (STDs), there is a significant racial disparity in syphilis. However, the underlying cause of this disparity is unclear, as race may be a marker for socioeconomic or other factors. The rate for syphilis among African Americans was more than 21 times that among Caucasians in 1999 (CDC 2000).

The infection spreads mainly through sexual contact but may also occur via nonsexual intimate contact, blood transfusion, or transplacental transmission. *T. pallidum* enters the body through nonevident breaks in the skin or mucous membrane, usually during sexual intercourse (Sparling 1999). The risk of acquisition from an infected partner is about 30% (Sparling 1999).

The first observable reaction occurs in 2–6 weeks (the average is three weeks) and consists of a painless papule or chancre at the site of penetration of the organism, usually the anogenital area (Chapel 1984, Musher 1999). The lesion is usually solitary, but multiple lesions frequently occur. This chancre marks the onset of the primary stage of syphilis. In women, this primary stage often goes unnoticed, delaying diagnosis. Even without treatment, the primary chancre usually disappears in 2–6 weeks (Musher 1999, Sweet et al. 2002).

As local replication occurs, simultaneous dissemination via the lymphatics and bloodstream begins (Musher 1999). In 60–80% of patients, associated regional lymphadenopathy, usually bilateral, appears 7–10 days after chancre development (Chapel 1984, Musher 1999). The secondary or "disseminated" stage of syphilis begins either simultaneously with the primary chancre or, more commonly, 4–10 weeks and up to six months after primary inoculation (Musher 1999, Stamm 1999).

Systemic involvement of all major organ systems occurs in the secondary stage. Flu-like symptoms, a generalized maculopapular skin rash, mucous membrane lesions, and generalized lymphadenopathy may occur. The secondary stage lasts for several weeks or months, with relapse in about 25% of untreated patients (Stamm 1999).

The latent stage, which is without apparent clinical manifestations in most cases, is divided into early latent (shorter than one year duration) and late latent syphilis (longer than one year duration). The lesion-free, asymptomatic, late-latent stage is not considered infectious; however, transplacental infection may still occur. Approximately 30% of untreated individuals develop late or tertiary syphilis (Schwarz et al. 1999, Stamm 1999, Sweet et al. 2002).

Tertiary syphilis may occur from months to many years after the initiation of latency and is characterized by central nervous system (CNS) involvement (although neurosyphilis may occur at any stage), cardiovascular or musculoskeletal system involvement, or gumma formation (CDC 1991, Sparling 1999, Stamm 1999, Sweet et al. 2002). An in-depth discussion of tertiary syphilis is beyond the scope of this chapter. The reader is directed to a current STD textbook.

Co-existence of primary and/or secondary syphilis with AIDS is common (van Voorst Vader 1998). HIV infection affects the clinical course of syphilis. HIV increases the risk for multiple chancres in primary syphilis and a higher frequency of ulcerating secondary syphilis, causes a rapid progression to secondary and tertiary stages of syphilis, and results in more serious sequelae involving the CNS (Stamm 1999, van Voorst Vader 1998, Zenker et al. 1990). Although there may be some delay in seropositivity, the serologic response to syphilis in most HIV-infected patients is either normal or exaggerated (Young 1998).

DATABASE

SUBJECTIVE

→ Risk factors include:

- Age (20–39 years most commonly)
- Low socioeconomic status
- Inner-city dweller
- Resident of the southern United States
- Trading sex for illegal drugs
- Drug abuse (intravenous drug use and crack)
- Prostitution
- Multiple sexual partners
- Concomitant STD
- Prior history of syphilis
- No condom use
- HIV infection (may alter course of syphilis infection)

→ Features include:

Primary Syphilis

- Patient may be asymptomatic
- Anogenital lesion:
  - Usually raised, painless, and indurated with distinct margins, although atypical presentation is not uncommon (Chapel 1978). Locations may include:
    - Vulva
    - Fourchette
    - Vagina
    - Cervix
    - Perineum
    - Anus
- Nongenital lesion:
  - Usually raised, painless, and indurated with distinct margins. Locations may include:
    - Lip(s) (most common nongenital site)
    - Tongue
    - Tonsils
    - Gingiva (rare)
    - Finger
    - Eyelid
    - Breast
    - Nipple
- Inguinal or cervical lymphadenopathy
- Vaginal or urethral discharge
- Rectal pain on defecation, rectal bleeding, mucoid or blood-streaked stool
- No constitutional symptoms

Secondary Syphilis

- Patient may be asymptomatic or exhibit subtle symptomatology.
- Flu-like symptoms (70% of patients):
  - Sore throat, malaise, headache, fever, myalgias, arthralgias, hoarseness, anorexia
  - Weight loss
- Skin rash on trunk, extremities, palms and/or soles (this syphiloderm occurs in 90% of cases):
  - May be pruritic
- Persisting primary chancre (25% of cases)
- Skin and mucous membrane lesions of vulva, perineum, anus, mouth (condyloma lata, "mucous patches")
- Bone pain
- Patchy hair loss
- Neurological complaints:
  - Meningitis symptoms, headache, hearing or vision loss, tingling, weakness, mental changes
- Generalized lymphadenopathy (common)
- Mild hepatitis (10%)
- Nephrotic syndrome (rare)

Latent Syphilis

- The patient is usually asymptomatic.
- Twenty-five percent of untreated patients may relapse to the secondary stage (Musher 1999, Stamm 1999).

Tertiary Syphilis and Neurosyphilis

- Tertiary syphilis is now rare in the United States. It usually occurs in 15–40% of untreated patients (Schwarz et al. 1999).
- A discussion of symptomatology is beyond the scope of this chapter.

→ Gynecological and medical history:

- Menstrual cycle
- Contraception
- Description of symptoms:
  - Onset
  - Duration
  - Quality/quantity
  - Frequency
  - Course
  - Aggravating/relieving factors
  - Associated symptoms
- Previous history of same/similar problem, including VDRL or RPR results, if known
- STD history (including dates, treatment)
- Sensitive questioning regarding recent sexual activity, including:
  - Date of last exposure
  - Sex practices
  - Sites of exposure
  - Number and gender of partners
  - Use of condoms
- Sex partner history
- Acute/chronic illness
- General health
- Medications
- Allergies
- Habits (including use of illegal drugs, both injection and noninjection)
- History of laboratory tests for syphilis, hepatitis B, HIV
- Review of systems (CDC 1991)

OBJECTIVE

→ A thorough STD examination includes (CDC 1991, Graney et al. 1999):

- Vital signs as indicated
- General skin inspection of face, trunk, forearms, and palms and soles for lesions, rashes, discoloration
- Inspection of pharynx and oral cavity for erythema, infection, lesions, discoloration
- Abdominal inspection and palpation for masses, tenderness, rebound tenderness
- Inspection of pubic hair for lice, nits
- Inspection of external genitalia for discharge, masses, lesions
- Inspection/palpation of Bartholin's, urethral, and Skene's glands for discharge, masses
- Inspection of vagina for blood, discharge, lesions
- Inspection of cervix for lesions, discharge, eversion, erythema, edema, contact bleeding; assessment for cervical motion tenderness
- Uterine assessment for size, shape, consistency, mobility, tenderness
- Palpation of adnexa for masses, tenderness
- Inspection of perianus, anus, and rectum for lesions, bleeding, discharge
- Rectal examination as indicated
- Assessment of presence or absence of associated cervical, inguinal lymphadenopathy

→ Physical examination findings specific to patients with syphilis may include:

Primary Syphilis

- External genital chancres (fourchette, vulva, perineum):
  - Single or multiple lesions may occur.
    - Progresses from dull red macule 0.5–1 cm to papule to ulcer (chancre).
    - A classic chancre is round or elongated, covered with grayish exudate, surrounded by indurated margin. Atypical appearance is common (Chapel 1978).
    - May have stippled hemorrhage line or dilated capillaries circling margin.
    - Usually nontender.
- Urethral meatus chancres (1–3% of cases): scant serous/serosanguineous discharge, induration
- Vaginal chancres (fewer than 1% of cases): eroded papules or nodules
- Cervical chancres (5–45% of cases):
  - In most cases, the lesion surrounds external os; remainder are on anterior or posterior lip.
- Nongenital chancres (5% of chancres):
  - May appear on:
    - Lip(s) (most common site)
    - Tongue
    - Tonsils
    - Gingiva (rare)
    - Fingers

- Eyelid
- Breast
- Nipple

- Extragenital lesions may be atypical:
  - Lip: solitary, eroded or ulcerated papule or nodule
  - Tongue: smooth, firm, eroded, or ulcerated plaque
  - Anus: dull, red, indurated, eroded; may also appear as an indurated fissure or hemorrhoid. Anorectal lesions can be palpated on digital examination (Chapel 1984).
- Regional lymphadenopathy:
  - Usually occurs within one week of chancre
  - Nodes nontender, small-to-moderate size, rubbery, nonsuppurative
  - Bilateral inguinal adenopathy with genital/anal chancre
  - Unilateral submental or anterior cervical adenopathy if chancre is in oropharyngeal cavity
  - In some cases, if chancre is on the anus, the lower two-thirds of the vulva, or the cervix, inguinal adenopathy will be absent (Chapel 1984).
- Perform neurological examination as indicated.

Secondary Syphilis

- Fever
- Weight loss
- Skin rash (in about 90% of cases): Appears initially as 0.5–1 cm, faint rose-pink, macular lesions beginning on the trunk and flexor surfaces of upper extremities. Becomes dull red or reddish brown, discrete, scaly papules ranging from 0.5–2 cm in diameter, spreading to the whole body, including palms and soles.
- Split papules: eroded, fissured papules affecting intertriginous areas (especially nasolabial fold, angles of the mouth, behind the ears).
- Condyloma lata: characteristically large, whitish gray, raised, broad papules resembling viral warts, typically on the anus, vulva, or other warm, moist areas.
- Mucosal lesions: "mucous patch"—a raised 7–10 mm, inflammatory papule with oval central erosion and gray membrane.
  - May affect any mucous membrane.
  - Diffuse inflammation may occur on pharynx/tonsils ("syphilitic sore throat").
    NOTE: Cutaneous lesions of secondary syphilis heal in 2–6 weeks without scarring. Relapse of secondary lesions occurs in 25% of cases. Ninety percent of relapses occur within the first year, but relapse may occur up to five years later (Chapel 1984, Sparling 1999, Thin 1990).
- Hair loss (alopecia): patchy loss on scalp, eyelashes, eyebrows. Diffuse thinning also may occur.
- Lymphadenopathy:
  - Inguinal (most common), suboccipital, posterior cervical, axillary, epitrochlear, and femoral. Nodes are discrete, nontender, moderately enlarged, rubbery.

- Other findings: arthritis, bursitis, osteitis, hepatitis, anterior iritis, choroiditis, nephritis/nephrotic syndrome, gastritis, gastric ulcer
- Perform neurological examination as indicated. CNS involvement may include aseptic meningitis, cranial nerve palsies, transverse myelitis, deafness.

Latent Syphilis

- Clinical findings are usually limited to positive nontreponemal and treponemal tests.

Tertiary Syphilis and Neurosyphilis

- Discussion of manifestations is beyond the scope of this chapter.

ASSESSMENT

→ Syphilis—primary, secondary, latent, or tertiary
→ R/O syphilis
→ R/O other types of genital ulcer disease: herpes simplex, granuloma inguinale, lymphogranuloma venereum, chancroid, vulvar cancer
→ R/O other types of orogenital ulceration: Reiter's, Stevens-Johnson's, and Behçet's syndromes, etc.
→ R/O other dermatoses (e.g., fixed drug eruption, psoriasis, pityriasis rosea)
→ R/O concomitant STDs
→ R/O HIV infection
→ R/O mononucleosis
→ R/O Hodgkin's disease
→ R/O lymphoma
→ R/O complications associated with secondary syphilis: arthritis, bursitis, osteitis, hepatitis, nephrotic syndrome, gastritis, gastric ulceration, iritis, choroiditis
→ R/O neurosyphilis

PLAN

DIAGNOSTIC TESTS

→ Index of suspicion is requisite for diagnosis.
→ Serology is the mainstay of laboratory testing for this disease (Young 1998). (See **Table 13H.1, Important Points in the Interpretation of Syphilis Tests**.)
→ Types of tests:

Direct Detection

- Dark-field microscopy: useful in primary and secondary syphilis and provides definitive, immediate diagnosis of *T. pallidum* from lesions (except oral lesions) and tissues. Most specific and sensitive test (Musher 1999).
- DFA-TP (direct fluorescent antibody to *T. pallidum*) can be used for primary and secondary syphilis.
  NOTE: These diagnostic tests are rarely available in mainstream clinical practice.

Indirect Detection/Serological Testing

- Nontreponemal testing: used for screening. Provides indirect evidence of primary or secondary syphilis:
  - VDRL (venereal disease research laboratory)
  - RPR (rapid plasma reagin)
- Treponemal serological tests are used for confirmation of nontreponemal tests (Sweet et al. 2002). Tests include:
  - FTA-ABS (fluorescent treponemal antibody absorption)
  - MHA-TP (microhemagglutination assay for antibody to *T. pallidum*)
  - TP-PA (*T. pallidum* particle agglutination)
  - EIA (enzyme immunoassay methods)
- PCR (polymerase chain reaction) can be used for lesion exudate, CSF, amniotic fluid; available only in research labs.
→ Criteria for diagnosis:
  NOTE: In the vast majority of cases, a diagnosis will be made based on serologic (or presumptive) evidence of disease together with clinical findings and patient history. Direct detection is not widely available.

Primary Syphilis

- Definitive diagnosis is via direct microscopic examination utilizing the following modalities (CDC 2002):
  - Dark-field microscopy of *T. pallidum* from chancre or regional lymph-node aspirate.
    NOTE: Only a trained microscopist should perform this test; therefore, it may not be commonly available. An ideal specimen is serous-rich fluid. Clean the chancre with sterile saline and then abrade the area, squeeze it to produce a serous exudate, then press directly onto a microscope slide and apply cover slip (Sweet et al. 2002). Lymph-node aspirates may also be used: Disinfect the area, inject 0.2 mL of sterile saline into the node, and then aspirate fluid. Immediate, dark-field microscopy by an experienced microscopist to identify *T. pallidum* must be performed after specimen collection (Larsen et al. 1990). If the initial dark-field is negative in a suspect case, repeat the test on two successive days; advise the patient to cleanse the lesion with physiological saline between exams and to avoid topical substances (CDC 1991, Thin 1990).
  - DFA-TP for *T. pallidum*: an alternative when dark-field is not available or for oral lesions.
    NOTE: Lesion material collected on a slide is stained with fluorescein-labeled, anti-*T. pallidum* globulin and examined under a fluorescent microscope (Sweet et al. 2002).
- Presumptive evidence (most commonly obtained) of primary syphilis includes:
  - Typical lesion(s) (chancre)
                    PLUS
  - Reactive nontreponemal test without prior history of syphilis
                    PLUS

Table 13H.1. **IMPORTANT POINTS IN THE INTERPRETATION OF SYPHILIS TESTS**

General Comments on Serology

Serological testing is the mainstay for diagnosing this infection. By the time clinical signs develop, most patients have IgG and IgM antibodies.

Clinicians must fully understand the testing strategy before they order and interpret serological tests for syphilis. They must know whether tests detect or exclude infection, the likely testing patterns for different stages of disease, and the patient's history of infection and treatment status. Additionally, there is no "test of cure" for syphilis.

Nontreponemal Tests (VDRL, RPR)

→ Nonspecific tests that must be confirmed with treponemal testing. Alone, they are insufficient for diagnosing syphilis.

→ Use for screening and to follow treatment response. Use the same test type (and preferably the same laboratory) for sequential testing.

→ Tests are reported as reactive or nonreactive. Quantitative results are reported as a dilution (i.e., 1:4) or as a reciprocal of the dilutions (i.e., 4 dilutions). A fourfold titer change is equivalent to a change of 2 doubling-dilutions (e.g., from 1:16 to 1:4 or from 1:8 to 1:32) (CDC 2002).

→ Rising titers indicate infection, re-infection, or treatment failure.

→ May be nonreactive in the primary stage of syphilis; usually not reactive until at least 7–10 days after the appearance of the chancre (CDC 1991). Test sensitivity at this stage is approximately 70–80% (Young 1998).

→ Initial nonreactive nontreponemal tests should be repeated in 1 week, 1 month, and 3 months in cases where the lesion is suspicious for syphilis and dark-field examination is unavailable (Larsen et al. 1990). In addition, with a suspect lesion, a treponemal test should be performed if the nontreponemal test is nonreactive (Larsen et al. 1990).

→ If the patient with secondary syphilis develops a very high titer, the VDRL or RPR could remain nonreactive due to the prozone phenomenon.* Thus, in all cases where suspicious lesions are present, ask the laboratory to dilute the negative serum and continue the titration.

→ Nonreactive VDRL or RPR may occur in a patient with late symptomatic syphilis, either acquired or congenital. A negative nontreponemal test does not rule out syphilis. False-negative tests may occur in HIV infection due to the prozone phenomenon.*

→ Reactive VDRL or RPR performed on a sample of spinal fluid always represents syphilis unless proved otherwise. CNS involvement (except in cases of tabes dorsalis) also is indicated by elevations of spinal fluid blood cell count and total protein.

→ A sustained, two-dilution rise in titer (e.g., 1:2 to 1:8) performed by the same laboratory is considered minimal evidence of the need for retreatment. The only exception is the adequately treated, congenitally syphilitic patient whose titer may fluctuate without any particular significance.

→ With adequate therapy of primary and secondary syphilis, titers should decline fourfold in 6 months and eightfold in 12 months

(Young 1998). In primary syphilis, nontreponemal tests are usually nonreactive 1 year after treatment, and in secondary syphilis, 2 years after treatment (Thin 1990). For early latent syphilis, a fourfold decline in titer should occur in 12 months and nontreponemal tests should be nonreactive by 2 years after adequate therapy (Young 1998). In late latent syphilis, decreases in titers are variable after treatment is completed (Bolan 1994).

→ VDRL or RPR may remain positive in low titer (serofast state) or in the high-pretreatment titer range for life if the patient receives treatment in the latter part of the infection. In such cases, cure is not based on serological reversal and treatment need not be repeated unless there is other evidence of re-infection. Serofast patients should be re-evaluated for HIV infection (CDC 2002).

→ A reactive VDRL or RPR in the absence of syphilis is called a biological false positive, or BFP (1–2% of cases). A BFP must always be proven to not represent syphilis. BFPs may occur in the following conditions:

■ Infectious mononucleosis
■ Leprosy, malaria
■ Lupus erythematosus and other autoimmune diseases
■ Vaccinia
■ Viral pneumonia and other viral infections
■ Pregnancy
■ Narcotic addiction
■ Acute febrile illness
■ Lyme disease
■ Chronic infections
■ Immunizations

→ Other spirochete infections (e.g., yaws, pinta, bejel) produce positive reactions as well, but these should not be considered false-positive (Meheus at al. 1999).

Treponemal Tests

→ Used for confirmation of nontreponemal tests or clinical suspicion of negative nontreponemal tests and for patients with symptoms of late syphilis (Larsen et al. 1990, Musher 1999, Young 1998).

→ Positive in 90% of primary syphilis cases and always positive in secondary syphilis (Musher 1999).

→ With a suspect lesion, a treponemal test should be performed if the nontreponemal test is nonreactive (Larsen et al. 1990).

→ Correlate poorly with disease activity and should not be used to assess response to treatment.

→ Reactive test indicates past or present infection. In incubating syphilis, however, tests may be negative.

→ One percent false-positive rate in the general population (may be seen in lupus erythematosus, infectious mononucleosis, leprosy).

→ In most cases, once the test is positive it remains so for life; thus, treponemal tests cannot be used to follow response to therapy. Fifteen percent to 25% of cases treated in the early primary stage may revert to nonreactive in 2–3 years (CDC 2002).

*See below, under the section "Secondary Syphilis," for a discussion of the prozone phenomenon.

- Positive treponemal test
                OR
- ≥fourfold titer increase on a quantitative nontreponemal test compared with previous results of the same serologic test for a person with a history of syphilis (CDC 1991, 2002).
- A patient who has clinical evidence of neurologic involvement with syphilis (e.g., cognitive dysfunction, motor or sensory deficits, ophthalmic or auditory symptoms, cranial nerve palsies, and symptoms or signs of meningitis) should have a CSF examination (CDC 2002).

Secondary Syphilis

- A definitive diagnosis includes:
  - Identification of *T. pallidum* from skin/mucous membrane lesions or lymph-node aspirate via dark-field microscopy or DFA-TP
                OR
  - Demonstration of *T. pallidum* on DFA-TP or histological staining of biopsy material from lesions characteristic of secondary syphilis (CDC 1991). **NOTE:** The above testing in the secondary stage of syphilis is difficult to perform and generally is not recommended. Serologic tests give more distinctive results in secondary syphilis (Musher 1999). See below.
- Presumptive evidence includes:
  - Skin/mucous membrane lesions of secondary syphilis, specifically one of the following:
    - Skin lesions, bilaterally symmetrical
    - Condyloma lata
    - Mucous patches on cervix or oropharynx
                PLUS
  - Reactive nontreponemal test (≥1:8) in the absence of a syphilis history
                PLUS
  - A positive treponemal test (if negative, diagnosis of secondary syphilis is most likely excluded)
                OR
  - ≥fourfold titer increase on a nontreponemal test compared with previous results of the same serologic test for a person with a history of syphilis (CDC 1991).
- Additional signs of secondary syphilis that may aid the diagnosis may include:
  - Alopecia
  - Loss of eyelashes, lateral third of eyebrows
  - Iritis
  - Fever and malaise
  - Generalized lymphadenopathy
  - Hepatomegaly and/or splenomegaly (CDC 1991)
- Patients with suspicious findings and/or nontreponemal titers <1:16 should undergo repeat nontreponemal tests and a confirmatory treponemal test (Larsen et al. 1990).
  - Fewer than 2% of patients will have a nonreactive nontreponemal test due to the *prozone phenomenon*. The lab should be asked to dilute the sera and continue

titration if there is a high index of suspicion (Musher 1999, Sweet et al. 2002).
NOTE: The prozone phenomenon occurs when a higher than optimal amount of antibody in the tested sera prevents the flocculation reaction typical of a positive test (Sweet et al. 2002). This phenomenon is more common in HIV-infected individuals (Young 1998).
- Examination of CSF via lumbar puncture usually is not indicated in secondary syphilis but should be considered in patients with signs or symptoms of neurological involvement (e.g., cognitive dysfunction, motor or sensory deficits, ophthalmic or auditory symptoms, cranial nerve palsies, and symptoms or signs of meningitis) (CDC 2002).

Early Latent Syphilis (less than one year):

- Definitive evidence—within the year preceding evaluation, the following criteria are met:
  - Documented seroconversion
  - Unequivocal symptoms of primary or secondary syphilis
                OR
  - Sex partner is documented to have primary, secondary, or early latent syphilis (CDC 2002).
    NOTE: Early latent syphilis cannot be reliably distinguished from late latent syphilis solely on the basis of nontreponemal titers. Nontreponemal titers usually are higher during early latent syphilis (CDC 2002).

Late Latent Syphilis (more than one year):

- Presumptive evidence includes:
  - Absence of signs and symptoms
                PLUS
  - Reactive nontreponemal test and positive treponemal test
                PLUS
  - No history of syphilis or previous tests (CDC 1991, Musher 1999)
- Careful examination of all accessible mucosal surfaces is warranted in all patients who have latent syphilis (CDC 2002).
- A CSF analysis is advised in the following instances (CDC 2002):
  - Neurologic or ophthalmic signs or symptoms
  - Evidence of active tertiary syphilis (e.g., aortitis, gumma, and iritis)
  - Treatment failure
  - HIV infection with late latent syphilis or syphilis of unknown duration
  NOTE: Some specialists recommend performing a CSF examination on all patients who have latent syphilis and a nontreponemal titer ≥1:32 (CDC 2002).
→ Additional considerations:
- Distinguish between syphilis and other causes of genital ulcers. In the **Chancroid** chapter, see **Table 13A.1,**

Clinical Features of Genital Ulcers and **Figure 13A.1, Sexually Active Patient with Genital Ulcer(s)**.

- Use diagnostic tests to rule out other causes of genital ulcers and lymphadenopathy, including appropriate herpes diagnostics. (See the **Genital Herpes Simplex Virus** chapter.)
  - See "Diagnostic Tests" in the **Chancroid, Lymphogranuloma Venereum**, and **Granuloma Inguinale (Donovanosis)** chapters.
- Sensitive testing for *Neisseria gonorrhoeae* and *Chlamydia trachomatis* should be considered to rule out concomitant STDs.
  - In the absence of a cervix, a urethral or urine specimen may be obtained.
- Wet mount of vaginal discharge to rule out concomitant vaginitis, especially trichomoniasis. (See the **Vaginitis** chapters in Section 12.)
- All patients with syphilis should be tested for HIV. If the test is negative, repeat in three months (CDC 2002).
- Additional labs may be ordered as indicated and may include but are not limited to: CBC, urinalysis, urine culture and sensitivities, hepatitis B screen, pregnancy test, CD_4+ cell and lymphocyte counts (if the patient is known to be HIV-positive).
- In an HIV-infected patient, if serological tests are nonreactive or do not seem to fit the clinical picture, alternative diagnostic tests should be employed (e.g., biopsy of lesion, dark-field examination, DFA-TP).

TREATMENT/MANAGEMENT

The treatment and management guidelines outlined below are from the CDC's "Sexually Transmitted Diseases Treatment Guidelines" (CDC 2002).

→ Parenteral penicillin G is the preferred drug in all stages. It is the only therapy with documented efficacy for pregnant women.

Primary and Secondary Syphilis

→ Recommended regimen:
  - Benzathine penicillin G, 2.4 million units IM in a single dose
→ Alternative regimens for nonpregnant, penicillin-allergic patients:
  - Doxycycline 100 mg p.o. BID for 14 days
                    OR
  - Tetracycline 500 mg p.o. QID for 14 days
                    OR
  - Ceftriaxone 1 g daily either IM or IV for 8–10 days (limited data on efficacy; close follow-up essential)
                    OR
  - Azithromycin 2 g p.o. in a single dose (limited data on efficacy; close follow-up essential)
    NOTE: The use of alternative therapies in HIV-infected persons has not been studied.
→ For pregnant, penicillin-allergic patients and in cases where

compliance or follow-up cannot be ensured, penicillin should be given after desensitization. (See CDC 2002, pp. 28–30, and "Additional Considerations," below.)

Latent Syphilis: Early Latent

→ Recommended regimen:
  - Benzathine penicillin G, 2.4 million units IM in a single dose
→ For nonpregnant, penicillin-allergic patients, treatment is the same as for primary and secondary syphilis. See alternative regimens above.
→ Pregnant patients allergic to penicillin should be desensitized and treated with penicillin. (See CDC 2002, pp. 28–30, and "Additional Considerations," below.)
→ All patients with latent syphilis should be evaluated for evidence of tertiary disease. (See "Diagnostic Tests," above.)

Latent Syphilis: Late Latent or Unknown Duration

→ Recommended regimen:
  - Benzathine penicillin G, 7.2 million units total, administered as 3 doses of 2.4 million units IM each at 1-week intervals
→ Alternative regimens for nonpregnant, penicillin-allergic patients include:
  - Doxycycline 100 mg p.o. BID for 28 days
                    OR
  - Tetracycline 500 mg p.o. QID for 28 days
    NOTE: These alternative therapies should be used only in conjunction with close serologic and clinical follow-up. The efficacy of alternative regimens in HIV-infected persons has not been studied.
→ Pregnant patients allergic to penicillin should be desensitized and treated with penicillin. (See CDC 2002, pp. 28–30, and "Additional Considerations," below.)
→ All patients with latent syphilis should be evaluated for evidence of tertiary disease. (See "Diagnostic Tests," above.)

Tertiary Syphilis (gumma and cardiovascular syphilis, *not* neurosyphilis):

→ A CSF examination should be performed before therapy. Complete discussion of management of patients with cardiovascular or gummatous syphilis is beyond the scope of this chapter. The patient should be referred to a physician.

Neurosyphilis

→ A detailed discussion regarding therapy for neurosyphilis is beyond the scope of this chapter. The patient should be referred to a physician.

Syphilis and HIV Infection: Primary and Secondary Syphilis

→ HIV-positive patients with early syphilis may be at increased risk for neurologic complications and may have higher rates of treatment failure. Some specialists recommend CSF examination before treating HIV-infected persons who have early syphilis, with a follow-up CSF examination after treating persons who have initial abnormalities.

→ Recommended regimen:
  ▪ Benzathine penicillin G 2.4 million units IM in a single dose
  ▪ Some experts recommend additional treatments (e.g., benzathine penicillin G administered at 1-week intervals for 3 weeks, as recommended for late syphilis).

→ Penicillin-allergic patients with HIV who have primary or secondary syphilis should be managed and treated according to the recommendations for penicillin-allergic, HIV-negative patients. The use of penicillin alternatives has not been well-studied in HIV-infected individuals.

Syphilis and HIV Infection: Latent Syphilis

→ For early latent syphilis, treatment/management regimens are according to the recommendations for HIV-negative patients with primary and secondary syphilis.

→ CSF examination should be performed in patients with late latent syphilis or syphilis of unknown duration.

→ Recommended regimen for late latent syphilis or syphilis of unknown duration (if CSF examination is within normal limits [WNL]):
  ▪ Benzathine penicillin G, 7.2 million units total administered as 3 doses of 2.4 million units IM each at 1-week intervals

→ Penicillin-allergic patients with HIV whose compliance or follow-up cannot be ensured should be desensitized and treated with penicillin. The use of penicillin alternatives has not been well-studied in HIV-infected individuals.

→ Patients with CSF findings consistent with neurosyphilis should be treated and managed for neurosyphilis. Refer to a physician.

→ Close, careful follow-up of HIV-infected syphilis patients is essential.

Partner Therapy

→ All sex partners of patients with syphilis should be evaluated both clinically and serologically. Provide referrals to a provider or facility that offers appropriate STD care, if necessary.

→ Persons exposed to a patient with primary, secondary, or early latent syphilis within the preceding 90 days should be treated presumptively, even if they are seronegative.

→ Persons exposed more than 90 days before the diagnosis of primary, secondary, or early latent syphilis in a sex partner should be treated presumptively if serological test results are not available immediately and follow-up is uncertain.

→ For partner notification purposes and presumptive treatment of exposed sex partners, patients who have syphilis of unknown duration and nontreponemal titers ≥ 1:32 can be assumed to have early syphilis. However, serological titers should not be used to differentiate early from late latent syphilis for the purpose of determining treatment.

→ Long-term sex partners of patients with late syphilis should be evaluated both clinically and serologically and treated on the basis of the findings.

→ The time periods before treatment that are used to identify at-risk sex partners are:
  ▪ 3 months plus duration of symptoms for primary syphilis
  ▪ 6 months plus duration of symptoms for secondary syphilis
  ▪ 1 year for early latent syphilis

Additional Considerations

→ A CSF examination should be performed of patients with neurological signs or symptoms. (See "Diagnostic Tests," above.)

→ An ocular slit-lamp examination should be performed of patients with signs or symptoms suggesting ophthalmic disease (e.g., uveitis).

→ Syphilis screening during pregnancy should be performed as soon as the patient presents for care. In high-prevalence areas or in high-risk individuals, additional screening is warranted at 28 weeks' gestation and at delivery.

→ Seropositive pregnant women should be considered infected unless it can be documented that prior treatment has been completed and sequential serological antibody titers have declined appropriately.

→ Treatment regimens during pregnancy are the same as for nonpregnant patients, according to the stage of syphilis. (See the previous discussion.)
  ▪ Some experts have recommended that additional therapy (e.g., a second dose of benzathine penicillin 2.4 million units IM) be given 1 week after the initial dose for women who have primary, secondary, or early latent syphilis.
  ▪ Tetracycline and doxycycline are contraindicated during pregnancy.

CONSULTATION

→ Consultation with a physician is indicated for complicated or advanced cases and for treatment failures.

→ If neurosyphilis is suspected, refer the patient to a physician for evaluation and management.

→ As needed for prescription(s).

PATIENT EDUCATION

→ Discuss the etiology and nature of syphilis, including the mode of transmission, incubation period, symptoms, course of disease, potential complications, possible association with HIV infection, and importance of partner evaluation and treatment.
  ▪ Patent-education handouts are a helpful adjunct to teaching. Written materials may be obtained from:
    • CDC National Prevention Information Network
      P.O. Box 6003
      Rockville, Md. 20849-6003
      (800) 458-5231, www.cdcnpin.org

- American Social Health Association
  P.O. Box 13827
  Research Triangle Park, N.C. 27709
  (919) 361-8400, www.ashastd.org
  - Additional resources for patients are:
    - National STD Hotline
      (800) 227-8922 or (800) 342-2437
      En Español: (800) 344-7432
    - For adolescents: www.iwannaknow.org
  NOTE: It is important to discuss the *Jarisch-Herxheimer reaction*. This is a self-limited, acute, febrile reaction that may occur after any therapy for syphilis. It is common among early syphilis patients. Onset may be a few hours after treatment. Symptoms may last for 24 hours and include fever, malaise, headache, musculoskeletal pain, nausea, and tachycardia. The chancre may swell or secondary syphilitic lesions may appear for the first time. Antipyretics may be taken. Women in the second trimester of pregnancy whose treatment precipitates this reaction are at risk for premature labor and/or fetal distress (CDC 2002, Musher 1999).
→ If the patient is on oral medication, advise her to finish the full course. When multiple injections are indicated, advise the patient of the importance of follow-up until therapy is completed.
  - Give instructions for follow-up as indicated for the stage of disease. (See "Follow-up," below.)
→ Advise abstinence from intercourse until the patient and her partner are treated and cured. They should be instructed to seek care promptly if symptoms recur.
→ Address STD prevention and HIV risk reduction.
  - Provide guidelines for safer sex practices.
  - Encourage careful screening of sex partners and the committed use of condoms (especially with new, multiple, nonmonogamous partners).
  - See **Table 13A.2, Safer Sex Practices** in the **Chancroid** chapter and **Table 12I.1, Recommendations for Individuals to Prevent STD/PID** in the **Pelvic Inflammatory Disease** chapter in Section 12.
→ Educate patients to become aware of their VDRL or RPR results.
  - Suggest they keep a diary to facilitate future management.
→ Allow the patient to vent her feelings of surprise, shame, fear, and anger, as indicated. Psychological support may be important in helping the patient gain control over her sexual situation and prevent future STDs.

FOLLOW-UP

→ The importance of follow-up should be stressed. It is especially important for a woman of reproductive age; if inadequately treated, congenital syphilis may occur during an ensuing pregnancy. A pregnant woman at high risk for syphilis should be tested initially, during the third trimester, and at delivery (CDC 2002).
→ History at follow-up examination should include symptom status, medication compliance, drug reaction and side

effects, partner therapy, sexual exposure, and use of condoms.
→ See **Table 13H.1**.

Primary and Secondary Syphilis

→ Clinical and serological examination should be performed at six and 12 months (CDC 2002).
→ Patients with persistent or recurrent signs or symptoms, or a sustained fourfold increase in nontreponemal test titer (compared with the maximum or baseline titer at the time of treatment), should be considered as treatment failures or as re-infected.
  - Evaluate for HIV infection and retreat (see below).
  - A CSF examination should be performed (CDC 2002). Consult with a physician.
→ Persons with probable treatment failure are identified by the failure of nontreponemal test titers to decline fourfold by six months after therapy (CDC 2002). Additional clinical and serological follow-up should be performed.
  - Re-evaluate for HIV infection.
  - A CSF examination is recommended (CDC 2002). Consult with a physician.
  - Retreat if further follow-up cannot be ensured. Retreatment regimen:
    - Benzathine penicillin G, 2.4 million units IM once a week for 3 weeks (unless CSF analysis indicates neurosyphilis) (CDC 2002).

Latent Syphilis

→ Quantitative nontreponemal tests should be repeated at six, 12, and 24 months (CDC 2002).
→ Patients with a normal CSF examination (if performed) should be retreated for latent syphilis if titers increase fourfold, an initially high titer ($\geq 1:32$) fails to decline at least fourfold (two dilutions) within 12–24 months, or signs or symptoms of syphilis develop (CDC 2002). Consult with a physician.

Tertiary Syphilis

→ Limited information is available regarding clinical response and follow-up (CDC 2002).

Neurosyphilis

→ Details about follow-up for neurosyphilis are beyond the scope of this chapter. The patient should be managed by a physician.

Syphilis and HIV Infection: Primary and Secondary Syphilis

→ Re-examination and quantitative nontreponemal tests should be performed at three, six, nine, 12, and 24 months after treatment (CDC 2002).
→ CSF examination after therapy (i.e., at six months) has been suggested by some experts (CDC 2002).

→ If the patient meets criteria for treatment failure, a CSF examination should be performed and retreatment initiated. A CSF examination and retreatment should be strongly considered for those patients who fail to demonstrate a fourfold decrease in nontreponemal titer within 6–12 months after treatment for primary or secondary syphilis (CDC 2002).

■ If a CSF examination is WNL, retreat with benzathine penicillin G, administered as 3 doses of 2.4 million units IM each at weekly intervals (CDC 2002). Consult with a physician.

Syphilis and HIV Infection: Latent Syphilis

→ Re-examination and quantitative nontreponemal tests should be performed at six, 12, 18, and 24 months after treatment (CDC 2002).

→ Repeat a CSF examination and treat accordingly if, at any time, clinical symptoms develop or nontreponemal titers rise fourfold (CDC 2002). Consult with a physician.

→ If nontreponemal titer does not decline fourfold in 12–24 months, repeat a CSF examination and treat accordingly (CDC 2002). Consult with a physician.

Pregnancy

→ Serological titers should be repeated in the third trimester and at delivery. For high-risk women and in high-prevalence areas, serology may be repeated monthly (CDC 2002).

→ Clinical and antibody response should be appropriate for the stage of disease.

→ Advise pregnant women to seek care for decreased fetal movement or contractions associated with the Jarisch-Herxheimer reaction.

Additional Considerations

→ Follow up on all additional laboratory tests ordered. Treat all concomitant STDs and other identified conditions. Continue to encourage safer sex practices.

→ HIV-positive results should be conveyed in person and by a provider who has received training in the complexities of test disclosure. HIV-positive persons should be referred to the appropriate provider or agency for early intervention services.

→ Offer the hepatitis A vaccine to women at risk for sexual transmission of this virus (e.g., users of illegal injection and noninjection drugs). (See the **Hepatitis—Viral** chapter in Section 11.)

→ Offer the hepatitis B vaccine to all women seeking treatment for an STD who have not been previously vaccinated. (See the **Hepatitis—Viral** chapter for further information.)

→ Newly diagnosed, hepatitis B antigen-positive individuals should undergo liver function tests and receive counseling regarding the implications of their positive status and the need for immunoprophylaxis of sex partners and household members. (See the **Hepatitis—Viral** chapter.)

→ A report must be filed with the department of public health, as required by state law.

→ Document in progress notes and on problem list.

BIBLIOGRAPHY

Bolan, G. 1994. Syphilis. Outline presented at the STD intensive for clinicians, Nov. 11–19, STD/HIV Prevention Center, San Francisco.

Centers for Disease Control and Prevention (CDC). 1991. *Sexually transmitted diseases. Clinical practice guidelines.* Atlanta, Ga.: the Author.

_____. 2000. Sexually transmitted disease surveillance, 1999, supplement. Atlanta, Ga.: the Author.

_____. 2001a. Primary and secondary syphilis—United States, 1999. *Morbidity and Mortality Weekly Report* 50(7):113–134.

_____. 2001b. Sexually transmitted disease surveillance, 2000. Atlanta, Ga.: the Author.

_____. 2002. Sexually transmitted diseases treatment guidelines. *Morbidity and Mortality Weekly Report* 51(RR–6):18–25.

Chapel, T.A. 1978. The variability of syphilitic chancres. *Sexually Transmitted Diseases* 5(2):68–70.

_____. 1984. Primary and secondary syphilis. *Cutis* 33(1):4–9.

Graney, D.O., and Vontver, L.A. 1999. Anatomy and physical examination of the female genital tract. In *Sexually transmitted diseases*, 3rd ed., eds. K.K. Holmes, P.F. Sparling, P.-A. Mårdh et al., pp. 685–697. New York: McGraw-Hill.

Larsen, S.A., Hunter, E.F., and Creighton, E.T. 1990. Syphilis. In *Sexually transmitted diseases*, 2nd ed., eds. K.K. Holmes, P.-A. Mårdh, P.F. Sparling et al., pp. 927–934. New York: McGraw-Hill.

Meheus, A.R., and Tikhomirov, E. 1999. Endemic treponematoses. In *Sexually transmitted diseases*, 3rd ed., eds. K.K. Holmes, P.F. Sparling, P.-A. Mårdh et al., pp. 511–515. New York: McGraw-Hill.

Musher, D.M. 1999. Early syphilis. In *Sexually transmitted diseases*, 3rd ed., eds. K.K. Holmes, P.F. Sparling, P.-A. Mårdh et al., pp. 479–486. New York: McGraw-Hill.

Schwartz, M.N., Musher, D.M., and Healy, B.P. 1999. Late syphilis. In *Sexually transmitted diseases*, 3rd ed., eds. K.K. Holmes, P.F. Sparling, P.-A. Mårdh et al., pp. 487–510. New York: McGraw-Hill.

Sparling, P.F. 1999. Natural history of syphilis. In *Sexually transmitted diseases*, 3rd ed., eds. K.K. Holmes, P.F. Sparling, P.-A. Mårdh et al., pp. 463–478. New York: McGraw-Hill.

Stamm, L.V. 1999. Biology of *Treponema pallidum*. In *Sexually transmitted diseases*, 3rd ed., eds. K.K. Holmes, P.F. Sparling, P.-A. Mårdh et al., pp. 467–472. New York: McGraw-Hill.

Sweet, R.L., and Gibbs, R.S. 2002. *Infectious diseases of the female genital tract*, 4th ed. Philadelphia: Lippincott Williams & Wilkins.

Thin, R.N. 1990. Early syphilis in the adult. In *Sexually transmitted diseases*, 2nd ed., eds. K.K. Holmes, P.-A. Mårdh, P.F. Sparling et al., pp. 221–230. New York: McGraw-Hill.

van Voorst Vader, P.C. 1998. Syphilis management and treatment. *Dermatologic Clinics* 16(4):699–711.

Young, H. 1998. Syphilis: serology. *Dermatology Clinics* 16(4):691–698.

Zenker, P.N., and Rolfs, R.T. 1990. Treatment of syphilis, 1989. *Reviews of Infectious Diseases* 12(Suppl. 6):S590–S609.

SECTION 14

Behavioral Disorders

14-A   Alcohol and Other Drug Problems **14-2**
14-B   Anxiety Disorders **14-10**
14-C   Depression. **14-19**
14-D   Domestic Violence **14-30**
14-E   Eating Disorders **14-35**
14-F   Sexual Abuse (Minors and Adult Survivors) **14-46**
14-G   Sexual Assault **14-51**
14-H   Smoking Cessation. **14-64**
14-I   Stress Management **14-69**

14-A
Alcohol and Other Drug Problems

Substance dependence is a chronic and progressive disease characterized by compulsion, loss of control, and continued use in spite of adverse consequences (McLellan et al. 2000, Smith 1990). With early intervention and treatment, the prognosis is positive and recovery is possible.

Substance dependence is also a biopsychosocial problem that has been described as a brain-based disease wherein successful treatment involves "biological, behavioral, and social-context components" (Leshner 1997). It is a family disease that has an impact on each member of the family. Landmark research in the 1980s examined the presence of genetic markers that correlated with the later development of alcoholism (Schuckit 1985). Among women, there are clear links between childhood trauma and substance use and dependence. High rates of violence by intimate partners are reported for women drug users, occurring at 2–3 times the rate for women who do not use drugs (U.S. Department of Health and Human Services [USDHHS] 1997b). The majority of women in treatment for alcohol and other drug problems have experienced rape, incest, or other sexual abuse (Fullilove et al. 1993, Hein et al. 1994).

A recent national survey of women's alcohol and drug use indicated that 50% of nonpregnant women age 26–44 reported use of alcohol in the past month; 17.1% of those women reported a binge pattern of alcohol use (five or more drinks on the same occasion in the past 30 days). Among pregnant women in the same age group, 14% reported alcohol use in the past month, with 3.1% reporting binge use (USDHHS 2002). Among women older than 12 years, 5% had used illicit drugs and 3.5% reported marijuana use. An additional 23% of women reported current tobacco use (USDHHS 2001).

Divorced, separated, or never-married women are more likely than married women to report the use of illicit drugs in the past year (USDHHS 1997a). According to the USDHHS, heavy alcohol use occurs at a higher prevalence among women age 18–25, those with less than a college education, the unemployed, those who had never married or were separated or divorced, those who first used alcohol or drugs at an early age (15 or younger), and those who had had agoraphobia or panic attacks in the previous year (USDHHS 1997a).

Women alcoholics are at greater risk for circulatory disorders, anemia (Hill 1984), and alcoholic cardiomyopathy and myopathy than their male counterparts (Urbano-Marquez et al. 1995). When women and men consume equal amounts of beverage alcohol, the women reach higher peak blood alcohol levels (Jones et al. 1976). All women who use alcohol and drugs are at risk for HIV/AIDS due to the disinhibition of sexual behavior and the potential for unsafe sex. In 1999, 40% of female AIDS cases were due to heterosexual transmission of HIV and 27% were due to injection drug use (Centers for Disease Control and Prevention [CDC] 2001). As of December 2000, 91% of pediatric AIDS cases (<13 years old) were children of mothers who have, or are at risk for, HIV (CDC 2000). Identifying, assessing, and treating pregnant, drug-dependent women who are HIV-positive is critical, as HIV preventive chemoprophylaxis can now be used to significantly reduce the rate of vertical transmission of HIV to the newborn (Connor et al. 1994).

Stressors for women that may contribute to an alcohol or drug problem include family or spousal discord; death of a spouse, child, or family member; poverty; unemployment; role changes; racism; sexism; sexual and/or physical abuse as a child; domestic violence; the stresses of single parenting; homelessness; or being raised in a family affected by alcohol or drug dependency. Women of any ethnic group, socioeconomic class, or age can develop an alcohol or other drug problem (Glick et al. 1990, Mora et al. 1991, Richardson et al. 1990, Wallace 1990).

Currently, the majority of women who are frequent users of drugs or alcohol are polydrug users, using multiple substances on a daily basis or in a binge pattern. Because the use of alcohol and other drugs by women is highly stigmatized, shame, embarrassment, and fear of the criminal justice system are frequent characteristics of addicted women (Allen 1995).

Only recently have substance abuse programs begun to address the specific needs of women. Historically, treatment centers for alcohol and drug problems have utilized male models of treatment and recovery. These types of programs cause women to talk less in co-ed groups (Swacker 1975) and can keep women from feeling comfortable and supported enough to address issues of rape, incest, abuse, or violence. In addition, transportation and child care have been noted historically as barriers to women seeking treatment (Grant 1997).

Women who either abuse or are dependent upon alcohol and/or another drug (see **Table 14A.1, Criteria for Substance Abuse** and **Table 14A.2, Criteria for Substance Dependence**) require assessment and a treatment-oriented intervention. Because women with alcohol and drug problems present fre-

quently to the health care system, health care providers are in an excellent position to act as facilitators and help their patients recover and adopt a clean and sober lifestyle.

Referral for treatment needs to be made to the most appropriate program in the woman's region. Many programs (especially in urban areas) are now tailored to a particular population. Providers should consider the financial status, drug of choice, age, sexual preference, and ethnicity of the woman prior to making a referral. Any referral for substance abuse treatment should include a referral to a 12-Step program such as Alcoholics Anonymous, Narcotics Anonymous, or Cocaine Anonymous.

Table 14A.1. CRITERIA FOR SUBSTANCE ABUSE

A. A maladaptive pattern of substance use leading to clinically significant impairment or distress, as manifested by one or more of the following occurring within a 12-month period:

   1) Recurrent substance use resulting in failure to fulfill major role obligations at work, school, or home (e.g., repeated absences or poor work performance related to substance use; substance-related absences, suspensions, or expulsions from school; neglect of children or household)
   2) Recurrent substance use in situations in which it is physically hazardous (e.g., driving an automobile or operating a machine when impaired by substance use)
   3) Recurrent substance-related legal problems (e.g., arrests for substance-related disorderly conduct)
   4) Continued substance use despite having persistent or recurrent social or interpersonal problems caused or exacerbated by the effects of the substance (e.g., arguments with spouse about consequences of intoxication, physical fights)

B. The symptoms have never met the criteria for *substance dependence* for this class of substance.

Source: Reprinted with permission from American Psychiatric Association. 2000. *Diagnostic and statistical manual of mental disorders*, 4th ed. (text revision). Washington, D.C.: the Author.

Table 14A.2. CRITERIA FOR SUBSTANCE DEPENDENCE

A maladaptive pattern of substance use leading to clinically significant impairment or distress as manifested by three or more of the following occurring at any time in the same 12-month period:

1) Tolerance, as defined by either of the following:
   a) A need for markedly increased amounts of the substance to achieve intoxication or desired effect
   b) Markedly diminished effect with continued use of the same amount of the substance
2) Withdrawal, as manifested by either of the following:
   a) The characteristic withdrawal syndrome for the substance (refer to Criteria A and B of the criteria sets for Withdrawal from the specific substances)
   b) The same (or a closely related) substance is taken to relieve or avoid withdrawal symptoms
3) The substance is often taken in larger amounts or over a longer period than was intended.
4) There is a persistent desire or unsuccessful efforts to reduce or control the substance use.
5) A great deal of time is spent on activities necessary to obtain the substance (e.g., visiting multiple doctors or driving long distances), use the substance (e.g., chain-smoking), or recover from its effects.
6) Important social, occupational, or recreational activities are given up or reduced because of substance use.
7) The substance use is continued despite knowledge of having a persistent or recurrent physical or psychological problem that is likely to have been caused or exacerbated by the substance (e.g., current cocaine use despite recognition of cocaine-induced depression or continued drinking despite recognition that an ulcer was made worse by alcohol consumption).

Source: Reprinted with permission from American Psychiatric Association. 2000. *Diagnostic and statistical manual of mental disorders,* 4th ed. (text revision). Washington, D.C.: the Author.

Most communities now have a 12-Step meeting, many have women's meetings, and some may have meetings that are culturally specific and/or language-appropriate.

Treatment varies based on the individual patient's problem and her ability to participate in an outpatient, inpatient, or residential program (see **Appendix 14A.3, Treatment for Alcohol or Other Drug Problems**). Recovery is, however, a lifelong process and the treatment is only the beginning. Ongoing recovery requires abstinence and participating in recovery activities (see **Appendix 14A.4, Recovery**).

DATABASE

SUBJECTIVE

→ Essentially all women are at risk, although there is a greater risk for those with a family history of alcoholism or other drug dependency.
→ The presence of "past history" suggests the patient should be either in recovery currently or that the active phase of the disease has returned—she currently is using and/or drinking (i.e., has relapsed).

→ There are specific behavioral and historical indicators (see **Table 14A.3, Indicators of Alcohol and/or Drug Use**).
→ Patient states, "My life is out of control, I may need help." Variations of this statement can include other requests for help or denial of the existence of a problem.
→ Denial: "I don't have a problem" or "I used to have a problem, but that's all over now..." (accompanied by subjective and objective evidence of a drug dependency).
→ Minimization: "It's not that bad. You should see how some people drink."
→ Rationalization: "I have so much stress in my life, I have to do something to calm down."
→ Drug and alcohol history to include:
  ■ Psychoactive substances used and year of first use
  ■ Route of administration
  ■ Level of tolerance for each substance
  ■ Past treatment attempts or participation in 12-Step meetings
  ■ Negative consequences of alcohol or drug use (past and present)

Table 14A.3.   INDICATORS OF ALCOHOL AND/OR DRUG USE*

Behavioral	Historical
Mental health problem	Family dissolution
History of childhood abuse/neglect	Alcohol- or drug-abusing partner
Family and personal chaos	Placement of children with caretaker other than biological parent
Inappropriate behavior	Family history of alcohol/drug problems
Mood swings	History of psychiatric treatment
Difficulties with concentration	Child with alcohol or drug-related effects due to in utero exposure
Unpredictable behavior	Many contacts with providers for prescriptions of psychoactive substances
Impulsive actions	Many urgent care/ER visits
Signs of intoxication	
Alcohol on breath	
Slurred speech	
Staggering gait	
Suicidal thoughts, gestures, attempts	
Conflicts with spouse, family	
Domestic violence	
Employment problems	
Missed appointments	
Cited for driving while intoxicated	
Vague history regarding personal or medical problems	

*No one item alone is necessarily indicative of an alcohol or drug problem. These indicators should alert the provider to the need for further evaluation and discussion with the patient.

Source: Adapted with permission from Jessup, M. 1990. The treatment of perinatal addiction: identification, intervention, and advocacy. *Western Journal of Medicine* 152:553–558.

- Codependency issues
- Adult child of alcoholic/addict
- Motivation for abstinence and recovery
- Ability to access treatment (i.e., disability, financial status, intellectual level)
- Complete social history
- Evaluation of mental health
- Evaluation for eating disorder

→ Complete medical history should be obtained.

OBJECTIVE

→ Patient may present with:
- Hair loss
- Dilated or pinpoint pupils, bloodshot or glassy eyes, yellow sclera, toxic amblyopia
- Rhinitis, perforation of nasal septum, epistaxis
- Poor dental hygiene, gum disease, abscesses
- Hypertension, mitral valve disease, anemias, bacteremias, myocarditis
- Tuberculosis, asthma, chronic cough, rales, sinusitis, bronchitis, pulmonary hypertension, nonthrombotic pulmonary hypertension (methamphetamine use), noncardiogenic pulmonary edema, tracheobronchial epithelial disease, other acute pulmonary effects
- Abscesses, cellulitis, septic thrombophlebitis, edema and erythema and/or scars on the hands, palmar erythema, track marks, thrombosed veins, traumatic burns, subdural hemorrhage, bruising, loss of muscle mass
- Gastritis, esophagitis, ulcers, acute and/or chronic hepatitis, hepatomegaly, pancreatitis, chronic constipation or diarrhea, ascites, malabsorption syndrome
- Abnormal vaginal bleeding, decreased vaginal lubrication
- Sexually transmitted diseases, HIV seropositivity
- Overdose, withdrawal symptoms, seizures, tremors, delirium tremens (DTs), blackouts, "grayouts," cognitive and sensory impairment, memory lapses and losses
- Alcoholic myopathy, ataxia
- Malnutrition

ASSESSMENT

→ Alcohol and/or drug dependency
→ Concomitant physical and/or psychiatric illness

PLAN

DIAGNOSTIC TESTS

→ Laboratory tests may include:
- Blood alcohol level
- Toxicology screen
- Glucose tolerance test (GTT)
- Aspartate aminotransferase (AST), alanine aminotransferase (ALT)
- MCH and MCV (elevated with excessive alcohol consumption with or without folic acid or vitamin B_{12} deficiency)
- Uric acid (elevated with excessive alcohol consumption)

- Albumin (decreased)
- Total protein (decreased; may be increased in intravenous drug users without chronic liver disease)
- Serum magnesium and potassium (decreased)

TREATMENT/MANAGEMENT

→ A statement of concern to the patient is important: "I am concerned that you may have an alcohol or drug problem."
→ Patient-specific evidence of alcohol or drug use should be presented to the patient: "These events in your life could be associated with your drug/alcohol use:
- Your history of gastritis, blackouts, marital problems"
- Your arrest for driving under the influence"
- Your mood swings"
- The placement of your child in temporary foster care"
- Your employment difficulties"
→ Patient education: Provide information regarding the potential negative physical, emotional, financial, spiritual, and psychological consequences of continued use of the substance(s).
→ Refer patient for evaluation (and possible treatment).
- Give list of local 12-Step meetings (e.g., Alcoholics Anonymous, Narcotics Anonymous, Cocaine Anonymous).
  - Ideally, the patient should call the local AA or other 12-Step group for a list of meetings (see **Appendices 14A.3** and **14A.4**).

CONSULTATION

→ Consultation with a mental health expert is recommended and required for evaluation of a possible co-existing mental health problem (see **Appendix 14A.1, Co-occurring Disorders**) that may or may not result in prescription of psychotropic or psychoactive medications.
→ Consultation with an expert in the treatment of alcohol and other drug problems is suggested for prescription of mood-altering drugs for a patient in recovery from an alcohol or drug problem (see **Appendix 14A.2, The Use of Mood-Altering Medications by Recovering Persons**).
→ Staff in a substance abuse treatment program may provide consultation to determine appropriate referral—i.e., residential, inpatient, outpatient, methadone maintenance, sober living setting.
→ Consultation and collaboration with other health care personnel providing services or counseling to an addicted person is recommended. Some alcohol- and drug-dependent patients may seek health care providers to obtain prescriptions for psychoactive drugs.

PATIENT EDUCATION

→ Review all previous physical, emotional, financial, spiritual, and psychological effects of the primary drug(s) of abuse to date.
→ State the expected and possible physical effects that may ensue with continued abuse of these drug(s).

→ Ask the patient to describe what she thinks may be the potential negative impact of continued drug abuse on the emotional, financial, spiritual, and psychological realms of her life.

→ Describe the probable impact of continued drug use on the emotional, financial, spiritual, and psychological realms of the patient's life.

→ State that with treatment and application of 12-Step programs, abstinence and recovery are possible.

FOLLOW-UP

→ Ask patient how she is doing in general. Inquire if she contacted, participated in, or completed a course of treatment for an alcohol/drug problem.
  ▪ If yes, support and commend efforts.
  ▪ If no, refer again for treatment and to 12-Step meetings or other self-help support groups.

→ Check on recovery efforts when patient is subsequently seen.

→ Observe for all physical and behavioral signs of resumed alcohol or drug use. Relapse that occurs after a period of sobriety and abstinence usually occurs after an individual has begun to think about returning to alcohol and drug use. Therefore, suggesting that the patient continue to utilize ongoing support services may assist in preventing relapse.

→ If relapse has occurred, repeat steps under "Treatment/ Management."

→ On the rare occasion that a mood-altering drug is indicated, advise patient of issues concerning the use of these drugs by people in recovery from an alcohol or other drug problem (see **Appendix 14A.2**).

→ See **Appendix 14A.4**.

→ Document in progress notes and on problem list, as appropriate, the status of the patient's alcohol or other drug dependency.

BIBLIOGRAPHY

Allen, K. 1995. Barriers to treatment for addicted African-American women. *Journal of the National Medical Association* 87(10):751–756.

Alcoholics Anonymous. 1998. *General Services Branch membership survey.* New York: the Author.

American Psychiatric Association. 2000. Diagnostic and statistical manual of mental disorders, 4th ed. (text revision). Washington, D.C.: the Author.

Centers for Disease Control and Prevention (CDC). 1989. Education about adult domestic violence in U.S. and Canadian medical schools, 1987–1988. *Morbidity and Mortality Weekly Report* 38(20):17–19.

_____. 2000. National Center for HIV, STD, and TB Prevention. *CDC AIDS surveillance report*, p. 21. Atlanta, Ga.: U.S. Department of Health and Human Services, U.S. Public Health Service.

_____. 2001. National Center for HIV, STD, and TB Prevention. HIV/AIDS among U.S. women: minority and young women at continuing risk. Available at: http://www.cdc.gov/ hiv/pubs/facts/women/women.pdf. Accessed on October 3, 2001.

Connor, E.M., Sperling, E.S., Gelber, R.D. et al. 1994. Reduction of maternal-infant transmission of human immunodeficiency virus type 1 zidovudine treatment. *New England Journal of Medicine* 331:1173–1180.

Fullilove, M., Fullilove, R., Smith, M. et al. 1993. Violence, trauma and post-traumatic stress disorder among women drug users. *Journal of Traumatic Stress* 6:533–543.

Glick, R., and Moore, J. 1990. Introduction. In *Drugs in Hispanic communities*, eds. R. Glick and J. Moore. New Brunswick, N.J.: Rutgers University Press.

Grant, B.F. 1997. Barriers to alcoholism treatment: reasons for not seeking treatment in a general population sample. *Journal of Studies in Alcohol* 58:365–371.

Hein, D., and Levin, F.R. 1994. Trauma and trauma-related disorders for women on methadone: prevalence and treatment considerations. *Journal of Psychoactive Drugs* 26(4): 421–428.

Hill, S. 1984. Vulnerability to biomedical consequences of alcoholism and alcohol related problems. In *Alcohol problems in women*, eds. S. Wilsnack and L. Beckman. New York: Guilford Press.

Jessup, M. 1990. The treatment of perinatal addiction: identification, intervention, and advocacy. *Western Journal of Medicine* 152:553–558.

Jones, B.B., and Jones, M.K. 1976. Women and alcohol: intoxication, metabolism, and the menstrual cycle. In *Alcohol problems in women and children*, eds. M. Greenblatt and M. Schuckit. New York: Grune and Stratton.

Kessler, R.C., Crum, R.M., Warner, L.A. et al. 1997. Lifetime occurrence of DSM III-R alcohol abuse and dependence and other psychiatric disorders in the National Co-morbidity Survey. *Archives of General Psychiatry* 54:313–321.

Leshner, A.I. 1997. Addiction is a brain disease and it matters. *Science* 238(3):45–47.

McLellan, A.T., Lewis, D.C., O'Brien, C.P. et al. 2000. Drug dependence, a chronic medical illness. *Journal of the American Medical Association* 284(13):1689–1695.

Meyer, R.E. 1986. How to understand the relationship between psychopathology and addictive disorders: another example of the chicken and the egg. In *Psychopathology and addictive disorders*, ed. R.E. Meyer. New York: Guilford Press.

Mora, J., and Gilbert, M.J. 1991. Issues for Latinas: Mexican American women. In *Alcohol and drugs are women's issues*, ed. P. Roth. Metuchen, N.J.: Women's Action Alliance and Scarecrow Press.

National Institute on Drug Abuse (NIDA). 1999. *Principles of drug addiction treatment.* Publication No. 99-4180. Bethesda, Md.: National Institutes of Health.

Richardson, T.M., and Williams, B.A. 1990. *African-Americans in treatment: dealing with cultural differences.* Center City, Minn.: Hazelden Press.

Ries, R., Russo, D., Wingerson, D.S. et al. 2000. Shorter hospital stays and more rapid improvement among patients with schizophrenia and substance disorders. *Psychiatric Services* 51(2):210–215.

Schuckit, M. 1985. Genetics of alcoholism. University of California-Davis Conference. *Alcoholism: Clinical and Experimental Research* 9(6):475–492.

Smith, D.E. 1990. Introduction. *Western Journal of Medicine* 152:(5):480.

Swacker, M. 1975. The sex of the speaker as a socio-linguistic variable. In *Language and sex: difference and dominance*, eds., B. Thorne and N. Henley. Rowley, Mass.: Newbury House.

United States Department of Health and Human Services. Substance Abuse and Mental Health Administration. Office of Applied Studies. 1997a. *National household survey on drug abuse: main findings 1997*, p. IV, and chapter 4, p. 7. Rockville, Md.: U.S. Department of Health and Human Services.

_____. 1997b. Substance Abuse and Mental Health Administration. *Substance abuse among women in the United States*,

p. 161. Rockville, Md.: U.S. Department of Health and Human Services.

_____. 2001 Substance Abuse and Mental Health Administration. Office of Applied Research and Research Triangle Institute. *National household survey on drug abuse report*, pp. 2–3. Rockville, Md.: U.S. Department of Health and Human Services.

_____. 2002. Substance Abuse and Mental Health Administration. Office of Applied Research and Research Triangle Institute. *National household survey on drug abuse report*, p. 3. Rockville, Md.: U.S. Department of Health and Human Services.

Urbano-Marquez, A., Estruch, R., Fernandez-Sola, J. et al. 1995. The greater risk of alcoholic cardiomyopathy and myopathy in women compared with men. *Journal of the American Medical Association* 274(2):149–154.

Wallace, J. 1990. The new disease model of addiction. *Western Journal of Medicine* 152(5):502–505.

Zweben, J. 1996. Psychiatric problems among alcohol and drug dependent women. *Journal of Psychoactive Drugs* 28(4):347.

APPENDIX 14A.1.

Co-occurring Disorders

Definition and Demographics:

- The co-morbidity of psychiatric illness and alcohol or another drug problem.
- The 1997 National Co-morbidity Study found that 72.4% of women with alcohol abuse disorders had co-occurring mental health problems. Among women with alcohol dependence, 86% of women reported co-occurring disorders in their lifetimes (Kessler et al. 1997).
- Persons with co-occurring disorders can have a poor prognosis in treatment characterized by increased usage rates of higher levels of care (Ries et al. 2000).
- Diagnosis of patients with co-occurring substance abuse and mental health problems is a complex process best conducted in consultation with or by professionals experienced in treating co-occurring disorders. Inexperienced or unknowing health care providers may inappropriately prescribe psychoactive drugs in an attempt to treat what they believe is solely a mental health problem.
- Misperception that an addict/alcoholic may not also have significant mental health problem.
- Patient is unable to seek or tolerate conventional modes of treatment for a substance abuse problem without significant provider input and case management.

Diagnosis and Treatment:

- Long-term evaluation is usually indicated to differentiate between signs of intoxication, alcohol or other drug withdrawal, organic brain damage, developmental disability, or psychiatric symptom re-emergence after detoxification.
- Accurate diagnosis is benefited by a period of sobriety and abstinence from mood-altering chemicals by the patient (Zweben 1996).
- Patients with co-occurring disorders "should have both disorders treated in an integrated way" (National Institute on Drug Abuse [NIDA] 1999) by providers experienced in treating people with co-occurring disorders.

APPENDIX 14A.2.

The Use of Mood-Altering Medications by Recovering Persons

- Generally contraindicated.
- Fractures, dental work, surgical procedures, or psychiatric problems may require prescription of analgesics, anesthetics, or psychoactive medications.
- Prescription of, or advocacy for, prescription of these drugs should be done by those providers with knowledge of substance abuse who are cognizant of the behavioral, medical, and pharmacological issues in the treatment of addicted persons.
- Deprivation of these medications for a bona fide medical indication is inhumane and inappropriate, and could lead to relapse.
- Consultation with a substance abuse treatment specialist prior to prescription is necessary to ensure that medication is essential and to determine safe and effective nonpharmacological alternatives that may be tried prior to the use of medication.
- A minimum number of doses should be prescribed. Prescriptions that can be refilled automatically are not recommended.
- Patient should notify people in her support system (family, friends, 12-Step sponsor) that she will be taking the drug and should create an agreement regarding prevention of relapse and actions she will take if relapse does occur. This should constitute a plan shared by the patient, her support system members, and her prescribing health care provider.
- If medications for a psychiatric illness are prescribed, careful follow-up and dual management by a mental health expert knowledgeable in substance abuse treatment are strongly recommended.

APPENDIX 14A.3.

Treatment for Alcohol or Other Drug Problems

- Assistance to achieve abstinence, introduction to the 12-Step programs, and education about alcoholism and other drug dependencies.
- Process may include an initial treatment for physiological detoxification depending on the patient's physical condition, chronicity of use, and number and types of drugs of choice.
- Detoxification is the first step in the treatment continuum. Detoxification can occur in either an outpatient or inpatient setting and depends on the frequency, amount, and types of drugs used—may not be indicated for all patients.
- Treatment provides tools to maintain sobriety and an introduction to a clean and sober support system.
- Programs focus on education about alcohol and other drug dependency, relapse prevention, and identification of psychological issues that might require long-term attention. Some programs provide intervention and assistance to the family as a whole as well as other social services, such as housing and employment assistance.
- Gender-specific programs include women-oriented outreach strategies, health care information and services, child and family services, vocational rehabilitation, skills training to enhance self-esteem, trauma recovery services, legal assistance, and processes to address sexuality and intimacy.
- Modalities for treatment include outpatient, day treatment, residential, sober living homes, methadone maintenance, in-hospital programs, and therapeutic communities (long-term). Programs vary in length of stay, extent of services, and mode of payment.

APPENDIX 14A.4.

Recovery

- Recovery is a life-long process initiated by treatment or participation in 12-Step program(s).
- Abstinence from all mood-altering drugs is required for a true recovery.
- Recovery requires adherence to a daily program of activities that foster, support, and educate the patient about the recovery process.
- Recovery occurs in the physical, emotional, psychological, and spiritual realms.
- Recovery is characterized by a reduction of chaos, resumption of self-esteem, healing of the physical and emotional wounds, and a willingness, openness, and honesty about the emotional work to be done.
- Staying in treatment for an adequate amount of time is an important determinant of treatment effectiveness and recovery. Research has shown that the "threshold of significant improvement is reached at about three months in treatment. After this threshold is reached, additional treatment can produce further progress toward recovery" (NIDA 1999).
- Recovery may include the licit use of medications for treatment of a mental health disorder. These medications are most appropriately prescribed by a health care provider knowledgeable about alcoholism and other drug dependencies.

14-B

Anxiety Disorders

Anxiety can be an appropriate response to a real and threatening situation. It can be framed as a positive phenomenon that helps "mobilize and direct all available energy toward problem solving abilities and achievement" (Hodiamont 1991). A surge in heart rate, blood pressure, sweating, breathing, and metabolism, and tensing of muscles are the physiologic hallmark changes mediated by the sympathetic nervous system responding to acute stress. This response is called the fight-or-flight response. Anxiety can also represent a mental health disorder; it is the dominant feature in *panic disorder*, *phobic disorders*, and *generalized anxiety disorder*.

Anxiety disorders are the most common psychiatric disorders, surpassing even the depressive and substance abuse disorders. The lifetime prevalence of anxiety disorders varies substantially by disorder and in different populations. In the United States, the lifetime prevalence of panic disorder is 16–35 per 1,000; for all phobias, it is 14 per 1,000 (for agoraphobia, 53–56 per 1,000; for social phobia, 27–133 per 1,000); and for generalized anxiety, it is 25–51 per 1,000 (Eaton 1995). Anxiety disorders are about twice as common in females as in males. Onset is most frequent in adolescence or early adulthood, although recent studies indicate that anxiety may be a significant mental health problem in older adults and the elderly (Stanley et al. 2000). When evaluating anxiety, it is important to identify whether the anxiety is a normal response or a pathological one. If it is a pathological condition, anxiety can be categorized as a specific disorder. Anxiety may also be precipitated by a general medical condition or substance use. It can also be a symptom of, or be present with, other psychiatric disorders.

→ Medical conditions causing anxiety may include:
  - Hyperthyroidism
  - Hyperparathyroidism
  - Hypoglycemia
  - Pheochromocytoma
  - Mitral valve prolapse
  - Vestibular dysfunctions
  - Cardiac arrhythmias
  - Chest pain

  - Complex partial seizures
  - Alcoholism
  - Generalized seizure disorders
→ Drugs known to cause anxiety states include:
  - Stimulant intoxication:
    • Medications:
      – Bronchodilators
      – β-agonists
      – Thyroid preparations
    • Central nervous system stimulants:
      – Caffeine
      – Cocaine
      – Amphetamines
      – Cannabis
  - Central nervous system depressant withdrawal:
    • Alcohol
    • Anti-anxiety agents
    • Sedative hypnotics
    • Barbiturates
    • Opioids

Anxiety presenting with other psychiatric disorders (e.g., major depression, adjustment disorder with anxious mood, eating disorders, and psychotic disorders) is usually related to the psychiatric illness (Andrews 2000). Anxiety is most common when a depressive disorder is present. Sixteen to 42% of patients with anxiety disorders may also meet the criteria for major depression or dysthymia (Ninan et al. 2001).

This chapter addresses the most common specific anxiety disorders in women as they are defined in the *Diagnostic and Statistical Manual of Mental Disorders* (American Psychiatric Association [APA] 2000).

Panic disorder is characterized by a series of recurrent and unexpected episodes of severe anxiety and fear (panic attacks), followed by at least one month of one or more of the following: persistent fear of having another attack, worry about its possible consequences or implications, or a significant behavioral change related to the attacks. During the panic episode, an intense fear or discomfort develops suddenly in the absence of a real danger and peaks within 10 minutes. This fear is accompanied by at least four characteristic associated somatic or cognitive symptoms of anxiety (see "Database," below). It is usually accompanied by a sense of imminent danger, impending doom, and the urge to escape. The definition of panic disorder includes at least two attacks.

Individuals with panic disorders also commonly suffer from what is referred to as "limited-symptom attacks," where the attacks meet all the other criteria but present with fewer than four somatic or cognitive symptoms. The criterion of panic attacks should not be considered when the attacks are a direct physiological effect of a substance, or are better accounted for by other mental health disorders or a general medical condition. Panic disorder is diagnosed with or without agoraphobia, depending on whether the criterion is met (see following discussion of agoraphobia). When panic disorder is not treated or treatment is inadequate, the following complications are common: depression, alcohol abuse, and increased risk of suicide (Sheikh et al. 1999).

Patients suffering from panic disorders will frequently visit primary health care providers (Katon 1986). They respond well when the disorder is recognized and managed appropriately, helping to avert phobic avoidance (e.g., avoidance of common situations or places due to intense anxiety and fear) (Bennett et al. 1998).

The anxiety that is characteristic of a panic attack can be differentiated from generalized anxiety by its discrete, almost paroxysmal nature. Typically it is also more severe.

Agoraphobia is characterized by marked fear of being in public places (e.g., elevators, crowds, lines, bridges); traveling in a car or other means of closed transportation (i.e., bus, train, airplane); or fear of situations from which escape may be difficult or embarrassing, or in which help may not be available if a panic attack occurs. As a result of this fear, the person increasingly restricts activities outside her home, must have a companion if she is away from home, or endures agoraphobia despite intense anxiety. Agoraphobia is usually considered a complication of panic disorders. In most cases, panic attacks precede agoraphobia. When the avoidance is limited to one or few situations, the diagnosis considered should be "specific phobia"; if the avoidance is limited to social situations, the diagnosis considered should be social phobia.

Specific phobia is characterized by a persistent (and recognized as excessive) fear of specific objects (most commonly animals, such as dogs, mice) or situations (e.g., closed spaces [*claustrophobia*], heights [*acrophobia*], or air travel). The level of anxiety or fear varies as a function of the degree of proximity to the phobic stimulus and the degree to which escape from the phobic stimulus is limited.

Social phobia is characterized by significant anxiety symptoms provoked by fear of and avoidance of social interactions and public situations, or endurance of these with intense anxiety or distress. Some common situations that provoke social phobia are drinking, eating, or writing in front of others; speaking on the telephone; dealing with authority; or talking to strangers. Social phobias that affect more women than men include public speaking or performing, and using public restrooms (Weinstock 1999). Patients are afraid of doing something humiliating or embarrassing or they are concerned that others will notice their anxiety symptoms. They also recognize that their fear is unreasonable. Significant functional/social/occupational disability is common in these patients and is associated with financial difficulties. Because of the fear of social situations, patients may not seek care until significant comorbid conditions are present (Liebowitz 1999). Suicidal ideation and attempts occur at higher than expected rates (Brunello et al. 2000).

Generalized anxiety disorder is characterized by excessive anxiety and worry, which is difficult to control, during a number of events or activities occurring over a period of at least six months. The anxiety and worry are associated with the presence, most days, of at least three of the following symptoms: restlessness or feeling keyed up or on edge, being easily fatigued, difficulty concentrating or mind going blank, irritability, muscle tension, and sleep disturbance. This anxiety fluctuates but is present more days than not.

The course of this disorder is generally intermittent with exacerbations and remissions throughout many years. Significant distress or social, functional, and occupational impairment can be caused by the anxiety, worry, or physical symptoms. The anxiety and worry are not confined to features of panic attacks, phobias, or other mental health disorders; they are not due to the physiological effects of a substance (a drug of abuse, a medication) or a general medical condition; and they do not occur exclusively during a mood disorder, psychotic disorder, or pervasive developmental disorder.

DATABASE
SUBJECTIVE

→ Panic disorder:
- Average age of onset is late 20s.
- More common in females
- Patient reports at least four of the following symptoms that occur during at least one of the attacks:
  - Dyspnea or smothering sensation
  - Dizziness, unsteady feelings, or faintness
  - Palpitations or tachycardia
  - Trembling or shaking
  - Sweating
  - Choking
  - Nausea or abdominal distress
  - Depersonalization or derealization
  - Paresthesias (especially perioral and in fingers and/or toes)
  - Hot flashes or chills
  - Chest pain or discomfort
  - Fear of dying
  - Fear of going crazy or doing something uncontrollable
- Patient may complain of nervousness and apprehension between panic attacks, usually focused on the fear of having another attack
- Possible predisposing factors include:
  - Separation anxiety disorder in childhood

- Sudden loss of social supports
- Disruption of important interpersonal relationships
  - Medical history may include:
    - Mitral valve prolapse or thyroid disease may be more prevalent. Other conditions that may be present are asthma, chronic obstructive pulmonary disease, or irritable bowel syndrome (APA 2000).
    - Depression
  - Personal/health history may include:
    - Substance abuse, particularly alcohol or anxiolytics
    - Limited impairment in social or occupational functioning
  - Family history may include panic attacks.
→ Agoraphobia:
  - Average age of onset is 20s or 30s.
  - More common in women and married people
  - Characteristics include:
    - Fear of being in places or situations from which escape might be difficult—closed spaces (e.g., elevators, tunnels), crowds (e.g., churches, theaters, malls), transportation vehicles or facilities (e.g., planes, trains, highways)
    - Fear of being in places or situations in which help might not be available in case a panic attack develops
    - Fear resulting in restriction of activities outside the home, needing a companion for activities outside the home, or enduring agoraphobic situations despite intense anxiety
  - Agoraphobia is usually associated with panic attacks.
  - Personal/health history may include:
    - Moderate to severe social or occupational impairment
    - Early traumatic separation from parents
→ Specific phobia:
  - Age of onset varies.
    - Animal phobias (fear is cued by animals or insects) and natural environment phobias (fear is cued by objects in the natural environment, such as storms) usually begin in childhood.
    - Blood/injury phobias (i.e., witnessing blood or tissue injuries) begin in adolescence.
    - Situational phobias (fear is cued by a specific situation, such as public transportation or enclosed places) has a bimodal age-at-onset with one age in childhood and another peak in the mid-20s (APA 2000).
  - More common in females. Animal, natural environment, and situational types are predominantly present in females. Blood-injection-injury types are also more common in females although to a lesser degree (APA 2000).
  - Phobic stimulus is unrelated to obsessive-compulsive disorder or to post-traumatic stress disorder (PTSD), separation anxiety disorder, social phobia, panic disorder with agoraphobia, or agoraphobia without a history of panic disorder.
    - Phobic stimulus interferes with daily life activities.
  - Characteristics may include:
    - Marked, persistent, excessive, or unreasonable fear of a circumscribed stimulus (other than fear of having a panic attack), or humiliation or embarrassment in certain social situations (social phobia)
    - Anxiety response during exposure to stimuli
    - Avoidance or endurance with extreme anxiety regarding the object or situation
    - Recognizing fear as being excessive or unreasonable
  - Symptoms may include:
    - Feeling panicky
    - Sweating
    - Tachycardia
    - Dyspnea
    - Vasovagal fainting if blood injury-related phobias
  - Personal/health history may include:
    - Social or occupational impairment if the phobic object cannot be avoided
    - Panic disorder with agoraphobia
    - Family history may include same type of anxiety disorders or phobia (i.e., fear of blood and injury, fear of animals)
→ Social phobia:
  - Age of onset is childhood or early adulthood
  - Slightly higher in females
  - Fear and anxiety only occur in social or public situations or in anticipation of such situations
  - Fear of avoidance is not related to the direct physiologic effects of a medication, substance abuse, general medical condition, or other mental disorder (panic disorder with or without agoraphobia, schizoid personality disorder, separation anxiety disorder, body dysmorphic disorder, or pervasive developmental disorder). Social phobics do not have uncued spontaneous panic attacks.
  - Characteristics may include:
    - Marked or persistent fear of scrutiny by others, or when the person is exposed to unfamiliar people in certain social situations. The patient fears that she may act in a way (or show anxiety symptoms) that will be embarrassing or humiliating.
    - Exposure to the feared situation almost always provokes anxiety.
    - Avoidance or endurance with extreme anxiety of the social situation that interferes with the person's normal routine, occupational functioning, and relationships. The patient experiences serious dysfunction or impairment.
    - The patient recognizes this fear as excessive or unreasonable.
  - Symptoms may include:
    - Trembling hands
    - Sweating
    - Blushing or flushing
    - Dry mouth
    - Stuttering or cracking of the voice
    - "Butterflies in the stomach"
    - Somatic manifestations are common: chest pain, palpitations, shortness of breath, dizziness, fatigue, insomnia, or gastrointestinal complaints

- Personal/health history may include:
  - Difficulty maintaining employment, attaining educational goals, or developing relationships
  - Comorbidity with specific phobia, agoraphobia, alcohol abuse, major depression, dysthymia, obsessive-compulsive disorder, schizoid or schizoaffective disorder, bipolar disorder, panic disorder, or somatization disorder (Zamorski et al. 2000). Onset of social phobia may precede depressive disorder or alcoholism. Social phobics often self-medicate with alcohol.
→ Generalized anxiety disorder:
  - Age of onset is most commonly in the 20s and 30s.
  - More common in women
  - Characteristics may include:
    - Fluctuating unrealistic or excessive anxiety or worry about at least two life circumstances for a period of at least six months
    - Anxiety that is not the result of a panic disorder, social phobia, obsessive-compulsive behavior or anorexia nervosa
  - Reports at least six of the following symptoms:
    - Motor tension:
      - Trembling, shaking, or feeling shaky
      - Muscle tension, aches, or soreness
      - Restlessness
      - Easy fatigability
    - Autonomic hyperactivity:
      - Dyspnea or smothering sensation
      - Palpitations, tachycardia
      - Sweating or cold, clammy hands
      - Dry mouth
      - Dizziness or lightheadedness
      - Nausea, diarrhea, or other abdominal distress
      - Hot flashes or chills
      - Frequent urination
      - Trouble swallowing or "lump in throat"
    - Hypervigilance:
      - Feeling keyed up or on edge
      - Exaggerated startle response
      - Difficulty concentrating or mind going blank
      - Trouble falling asleep or staying asleep
      - Irritability
  - Medical history may include:
    - Major depressive episode (considered a predisposing factor)
    - Peptic ulcer
    - Migraine
    - Ulcerative colitis
  - Personal/health history may include mild to moderate social and occupational impairment, or alcohol-abuse disorder in women (Howell et al. 2001).

OBJECTIVE

→ During an acute anxiety attack, the patient may present with:

- Elevated blood pressure
- Tachycardia
- Tachypnea
- Restlessness
- Trembling
- Screaming
- Erythema or pallor
- Sweating
- Cold and clammy hands
→ Other physical findings within normal limits
→ Common finding in panic disorders is a midsystolic apical and/or late systolic murmur on auscultation (an indication of mitral valve prolapse) (see the **Mitral Valve Prolapse** chapter in Section 6).

ASSESSMENT

→ Panic disorder
→ Panic disorder with agoraphobia
→ Agoraphobia:
  - Mild
  - Moderate
  - Severe
→ Specific phobia
→ Social phobia
→ Generalized phobia
→ R/O anxiety disorder due to a general medical condition
→ R/O medication or substance-induced anxiety disorder
→ R/O other underlying mental health disorders
→ R/O somatoform disorders (hypochondriasis and somatization disorder)

PLAN

DIAGNOSTIC TESTS

→ No specific diagnostic tests used in clinical practice
→ Additional diagnostic tests as indicated by database to rule out organic causes of anxiety
→ Echocardiogram if signs of mitral valve prolapse (see the **Mitral Valve Prolapse** chapter in Section 6).

TREATMENT/MANAGEMENT

→ Assess suicide risk in all confirmed cases of anxiety (see the **Depression** chapter).
→ If anxiety is present during the visit:
  - Remain with the patient during the period of anxiety.
  - Approach the patient in a calm, matter-of-fact manner.
  - Place her in a safe, nonstimulating environment.
  - Encourage the patient to express her feelings, describe her symptoms, and relate behaviors that relieve this condition.
→ Anxiety disorders—psychological therapy:
  - All patients with anxiety disorders can benefit from psychological therapy. Of these, cognitive behavioral therapy, psychotherapy, and cognitive therapy have been used extensively. These therapies are time-consuming and require a skilled practitioner. They have been found to be

effective particularly as an adjunct to pharmacotherapy (APA 2000).

- Cognitive behavioral therapy:
  - Relaxation—attempting to break the vicious cycle of anxiety:
    - ➤ Can be used in groups
    - ➤ May be aided by relaxation tape recordings
    - ➤ Encourage daily practice of the technique at home.
    - ➤ Through sessions, encourage the patient to talk about difficulties in achieving relaxation.
  - Guidelines to relaxation techniques include:
    - ➤ Have the patient sit in a quiet room, with dim lights, and in a comfortable chair.
    - ➤ Ask the patient to focus initially on her breathing.
    - ➤ Direct the patient to move slowly through tension and relaxation for each major muscle group.
    - ➤ Direct the patient to maintain tension for 10 seconds and release it instantaneously on cue; at least 2 repetitions of the tension-relaxation cycle.
    - ➤ Give instructions very slowly, allowing the patient to enjoy the feelings of relaxation.
    - ➤ This technique should be taught in a progressive manner, encouraging the patient to practice the relaxation technique independently.
  - Problem-solving techniques suggested by Andrews (2000) include:
    - ➤ Identify the problem.
    - ➤ Write the problem in simple, concrete terms.
    - ➤ Use a specific problem rather than a broad, vague one.
    - ➤ Consider as many solutions as possible, whether they are reasonable or not.
    - ➤ List the solutions without dismissing any out of hand.
    - ➤ Debate the pros and cons of each.
    - ➤ Choose the most practical solution.
    - ➤ Plan the implementation carefully.
    - ➤ Review and evaluate progress.
  - Exposure treatment—used mostly for phobic anxiety states:
    - ➤ Persuade the patient to repeatedly confront the feared object or situation.
    - ➤ The exposure trials progress for longer periods of time.
    - ➤ The length of the exposure is determined by the level of anxiety and the presence of other medical complications (e.g., asthma, heart disease).
    - ➤ The therapist may not be present for the phobic situation.
    - ➤ The patient is to keep a diary monitored by the therapist.
    - ➤ Significant improvement is usually seen within 4–20 sessions and is often maintained for up to 2–4 years.
    - ➤ Therapy is discontinued if the patient fails to habituate within 2 weeks.
  - Systemic desensitization:
    - ➤ The patient draws up a hierarchy of feared stimuli or situations that provoke anxiety, initially only in her imagination, while in a pleasant, relaxed state.
    - ➤ The feared stimuli or situation is then extended into real-life situations.
  - Social skills training and assertiveness training are provided. More effective and satisfying behaviors are substituted through rehearsal with other patients and then practiced in real-life situations. Guidelines include (Edwards 1991):
    - ➤ Instructing patient in these behaviors
    - ➤ Coaching
    - ➤ Modeling
    - ➤ Role reversal
- Psychotherapy:
  - Supportive therapy—counseling to accept responsibility for behavior and actions and, if possible, to work out solutions (Edwards 1991):
    - ➤ Simple, brief technique with limited objectives
    - ➤ Can be given to couples, families, and groups
  - Guidelines for supportive therapy include:
    - ➤ Show concern.
    - ➤ Listen sympathetically.
    - ➤ Allow the patient to release/verbalize emotions or unconscious fears if necessary.
    - ➤ Give reassurance.
    - ➤ Give suggestions and advice about ongoing problems.
    - ➤ Provide encouragement.
    - ➤ Discuss methods of coping with stress.
- Cognitive therapy:
  - Combines exposure with cognitive behavior, restructuring, and distraction techniques (Edwards 1991):
    - ➤ Identify illogical thoughts (e.g., of failure, disease, or death) and objectively discuss the evidence for and against these beliefs.
    - ➤ The patient recognizes the irrationality and damaging effects of her ideas.
    - ➤ Encourage the patient to substitute healthier ideas with the help of positive self-commentaries.
    - ➤ In panic disorder, attempt to substitute normal, rational explanations for abnormal, catastrophic interpretations.

→ Panic disorder and agoraphobia—psycho-pharmacotherapy:
- ■ Psychotherapy, particularly behavioral therapy and cognitive behavioral therapy (CBT), can augment the efficacy of pharmacotherapy. Combining one of those psychotherapy modalities with pharmacotherapy has shown greater and more durable success than pharmacotherapy alone (Bennett et al. 1998, Johnson et al. 1995). Initiating CBT is helpful when patients are being withdrawn from benzodiazepine therapy; on the other hand, adding benzodiazepines early in CBT may also prove helpful in managing panic disorder (Bennett et al. 1998).
- ■ Consultation with a mental health care provider is

indicated (particularly in cases in which short-term psychological treatment has failed).

- Pharmacotherapy categories include tricyclic antidepressants (TCAs), selective serotonin reuptake inhibitors (SSRIs), benzodiazepines, and monoamine oxidase inhibitors (MAOIs) (Bennett et al. 1998). Efficacy is similar with all medications. The selection should be based on the patient's preference and the risk/benefit profile of each treatment option.

  • TCAs:
    - Imipramine hydrochloride is most frequently recommended. To avoid common side effects, start the dose at 10 mg p.o. per day and increase 10 mg every 2–4 days. If the medicine is tolerated, the dose can be increased 25 mg every few days up to 150 mg/day. The maximum dose for outpatients is 200 mg/day in divided doses or a single dose given at HS. For elderly patients, the dose should be halved.
    - Other TCAs recommended are clomipramine, nortriptyline, or desipramine. See the *Physicians' Desk Reference (PDR)* for dosing.
    - Maintenance therapy is recommended with half the dose required for an acute attack. Remission up to a year may be attained with a maintenance dose. To prevent relapse, the medication should be tapered after maintenance for 18 months. TCA, if discontinued abruptly, can cause cholinergic rebound (stomach upset, nausea, vomiting, and abdominal cramping).
    - Resolution of panic symptoms may take 4–6 weeks.
    - TCA treatment is effective for mild depressive symptoms often associated with panic disorders. (See also the **Depression** chapter for a more thorough review of antidepressant therapy.)
    - QD dosing is allowed because of TCAs' long half-life; generic preparations are available at a low cost for most patients.
    - Adverse anticholinergic effects are common in patients on TCAs, especially dry mouth and orthostatic hypotension. Up to 17% of patients find these effects intolerable (see the **Depression** chapter for a review of TCA side effects).
    - One of these cholinergic effects is hyperstimulation reaction. It is characterized by intensified anxiety symptoms, agitation, tachycardia, and insomnia, and may be experienced by 20–30% of patients. These symptoms may last up to 3 weeks. Beginning with a low dose (see above) and gradually increasing the dose are helpful in minimizing this effect. Adding benzodiazepines can also decrease this reaction (see below).
    - β-adrenergic blocking agents are recommended to decrease tachycardia, but when used alone they are not effective therapies for panic disorders.
    - TCAs should be used with extreme caution if the patient has a history of manic or hypomanic symptoms (may precipitate mania in bipolar patients).
    - TCAs can precipitate hypertensive crises. It is speculated that cardiovascular disregulation in panic disorder may increase this risk (Schatzber et al. 1991).
    - Weight gain in patients with panic disorder on TCAs is controversial.
    - TCAs may cause sexual impairment.
    - TCAs are dangerous if overdosed. Prescribe with caution for patients with suicidal ideation. Limit the prescription to a 1-week supply at a time.

  • SSRIs:
    - Fluvoxamine, fluoxetine, and paroxetine have shown to be effective in panic disorder (Bennett et al. 1998). The author recommends initiating with daily oral doses of 25 mg of fluvoxamine, 5–10 mg fluoxetine, or 10 mg of paroxetine as appropriate. Fluoxetine should be started gradually with doses of 2–5 mg/day (using elixir) and increasing the dose by 2 mg every 2–3 days. Most patients respond to doses of 20 mg/day or less.
    - Increased anxiety can be observed if the initial dose is too high. Patients may complain of jitteriness, restlessness, agitation, and insomnia. To avoid these unwanted effects, the initial dose of SSRIs should be low and kept low for several days (APA 2000).
    - SSRIs are relatively safe in overdose, are generally well-tolerated, and do not have anticholinergic or postural hypotension side effects.
    - Therapeutic response may take 4–12 weeks.
    - Sexual dysfunction can be an unwanted side effect.
    - Abrupt withdrawal of SSRIs should be avoided, as this may cause dizziness, headaches, nausea, irritability, and lack of coordination.
    - As with TCAs, SSRIs may precipitate mania in patients with bipolar disorder.

  • Benzodiazepines (BZDs):
    - Alprazolam 2 mg/day, in multiple daily doses (at least TID to QID—to a maximum of 10 mg p.o. per day) is recommended to provide acute relief and as an adjunctive therapy to antidepressant (especially until the antidepressant exerts its full effect). The usual recommended starting dose is 0.25–0.5 mg p.o. QID, increasing as needed or tolerated every 3–4 days. Maintenance dose is 2–6 mg per day.
    - Other BZDs also recommended: lorazepam, diazepam, clonazepam. See *PDR* for dosing. Not as effective as alprazolam for low-grade depression that often accompanies panic disorder.
    - The major benefit of BZDs is rapid symptom relief, as quickly as 1–2 hours after the initial dose. Short half-life of alprazolam may increase interdose recurrence of symptoms and encourage frequent redosing. Clonazepam, a more potent BZD, has a long half-life, which minimizes this risk and can be administered BID–TID.
    - Patients who self-medicate at 2–3 times the therapeutic dose can experience physical dependence in

2–3 weeks. Dependence at therapeutic dosing can occur if taken for more than 6 months.

– Gradual tapering of dose should be initiated after 4–16 weeks. Adding an antidepressant prior to tapering BZDs may prevent recurrence of panic disorder symptoms (Woods et al. 1992).

– Long-term use of BZDs has the potential risk for dependency; prescribing them for patients with personal or family history of substance abuse should be undertaken with caution.

– Transient ataxia and drowsiness are the most common side effects with alprazolam and clonazepam. Usually these side effects subside with dose reduction or continued administration.

– Other adverse effects: slurred speech and amnesia if the dose is too high or mixed with sedatives or alcohol.

– Use of BZDs for long-term treatment is reserved for the few patients with panic disorder who may not respond to first-line therapy with an SSRI or TCA.

• Monoamine oxidase inhibitors (MAOIs):
– Because of the potentially lethal side effects, these medications are considered second- or third-line agents and should be used only in consultation with a psychiatric clinician.

→ Specific phobia:
■ Behavioral therapy (graduated exposure in vivo) is the treatment of choice. BZDs may be used if the patient is unable to engage in psychological treatment and until anxiety levels are somewhat reduced (Argyropoulos et al. 2000).

→ Social anxiety disorder—psycho-pharmacotherapy:
■ CBT and pharmacotherapy are both effective and complementary. The incidence of relapse is lower with CBT than with pharmacotherapy (Liebowitz 1999).
■ Consultation with a mental health care provider is indicated (particularly in cases in which short-term psychological treatment has failed).
■ Patients with comorbid alcohol abuse have poor treatment outcomes.
■ SSRIs: Paroxetine, fluoxetine, and sertraline are emerging as first-line agents for treatment. See panic disorder treatment for review of these medications.
■ BZDs and other anxiolytics: Studies of alprazolam and clonazepam have proven that these agents are effective, but the relapse rates may be high. Long-term use and monotherapy with BZDs are controversial due to the risk of dependence. In general, BZDs should be avoided in patients with a history of alcohol or drug abuse. Buspirone, a nonbenzodiazepine anxiolytic, is sometimes used but has no proven benefit (Brunello et al. 2000).
■ MAOIs: reserved for treatment of refractory patients and should only be prescribed by clinicians familiar with their use.
■ β-blockers: Nonselective adrenergics (i.e., propranolol, nadolol) have been used for patients with performance

anxiety, particularly to control tremor. Typical dose range is 10–80 mg p.o. 1 hour before an anxiety-provoking activity.
■ An electrocardiogram should be performed prior to prescribing β-blockers to rule out the presence of atrioventricular block.
■ Use of β-blockers is contraindicated for asthma and for high-performance athletes.

→ Generalized anxiety disorder (GAD)—psycho-pharmacotherapy:
■ CBT and behavioral therapy are effective psychological treatments.
■ Consultation with a mental health care provider is indicated (particularly in cases in which short-term psychological treatment has failed).
■ Pharmacotherapy:
• BZDs:
– Effective in treatment of GAD. Recommended on a short-term basis (up to 4 weeks) and as an adjunct to psychotherapy.
– Decrease psychic and somatic symptoms of anxiety
– Quick onset of action and relative safety with overdose
– For chronic anxiety, consider long-acting BZDs (e.g., diazepam, chlordiazepoxide, clorazepate, prazepam, halazepam, clonazepam). See *PDR* for doses and side effects.
– When anxiety is limited to a particular situation or to brief, stressful periods, consider short-acting BZDs (e.g., lorazepam, alprazolam, axazepam).
– Patients who self-medicate at 2–3 times the therapeutic dose can experience physical dependence in 2–3 weeks. Dependence at therapeutic dose can occur if taken for more than 6 months. To avoid withdrawal symptoms, gradual tapering of the dose should be initiated after 4–16 weeks and adjunctive therapy may be required (i.e., sedating antidepressants, β-blockers, carbamazepine).
• Buspirone:
– First non-BZD introduced to the market with no risk of dependence and no anticonvulsant, muscle-relaxant, or sedative properties.
– As effective as diazepam at equipotent doses (i.e., 10–60 mg/day). Initiate at 5 mg p.o. TID, may increase dose every 3 days. Maintenance dose is 20–30 mg/day in divided doses (TID).
– Side effects include: dizziness, nausea, gastrointestinal upset, headache, or insomnia.
– Dysphoria may develop at higher doses (i.e., >30 mg/day).
– Advantages of buspirone over BZDs include: non-sedating, minimal impairment of cognitive and psychomotor skills, low abuse and dependence potential, no withdrawal effects after discontinuation, and does not interact with alcohol.
– Disadvantages compared to BZDs include: slow

onset of action, lower satisfaction in patients with chronic anxiety if previous use of BZDs.

- Antidepressants:
  - Nonsedating TCAs and SSRIs are now recommended as first-line therapy for GAD. Patients with comorbid depression seem to respond well to TCAs or SSRIs. Doses must be minimal initially to avoid unwanted side effects (Ballenger et al. 2001).
- β-adrenergic blockers:
  - Still in use despite no proof of efficacy, probably due to fewer side effects and no abuse potential
  - Useful in ameliorating somatic symptoms (e.g., tremor, tachycardia, palpitations)
- Antihistamines:
  - Play a minor role in management of anxiety. Because they have no addictive potential, are used in patients with history of drug abuse and alcoholism.
  - Hydroxyzine provides sedation at the expense of an anticholinergic effect.
- Barbiturate and nonbarbiturate sedatives:
  - Rarely used due to low margin of safety, potential for addiction, development of tolerance, lethality in overdose, and potential for drug interactions.
- Antipsychotics:
  - Limited to anxiety associated with psychotic disorders.

CONSULTATION

→ See "Treatment/Management."
→ Consultation with or referral to a mental health care provider as indicated.
→ If the patient fails to respond to short-term psychological treatment, refer to a mental health professional.
→ Patients receiving MAOIs are usually managed by a mental health professional.

PATIENT EDUCATION

→ Educate the patient regarding the role the autonomic nervous system plays in initiating symptoms.
→ Teach the patient and her family that anxiety disorders are distinct conditions that have a biologic contribution and can be appropriately treated like other illnesses.
→ Teach the patient relaxation techniques. The patient may obtain a tape recording of these techniques. Explain that relaxation will break the vicious cycle of anxiety.
→ Teach the patient hyperventilation control. Approaching her in a calm manner and coaching her through hyperventilation control may decrease the level of arousal. Lampe (1996) suggests the following steps for hyperventilation control:
1) Take a medium-size breath in and hold for 6 seconds.
2) Just before exhaling, think "relax."
3) Exhale.
4) Breathe through the nose: in for 3 seconds and out for 3 seconds.

5) Breathe in a smooth and light fashion.
6) Repeat Step 4 for the next minute.
7) Repeat the entire sequence (Steps 1–6).
→ Engage the family in managing patients with anxiety disorders.
→ Encourage the patient to read the following book:
- Bourne, E.J. 1995. *The Anxiety and Phobia Workbook: A Step-by-step Program for Curing Yourself From Extreme Anxiety, Panic Attacks, and Phobias.* 2nd edition. New York: Fine Communications.
- Assist the patient in recognizing anxious feelings and their precipitating events.
- Discuss appropriate techniques to alleviate anxiety behavior and deal with feelings (see "Treatment/Management").
→ Refer patient to support groups, provide educational materials, and Web resources:
- Anxiety Disorders Association of America
  11900 Parklawn Drive, Suite 100
  Rockville, Md. 20852
  www.adaa.org
- Toastmaster International
  P.O. Box 9052
  Mission Viejo, Calif. 92690
  (949) 858-8255
  www.toastmasters.org

FOLLOW-UP

→ Make sure that the patient has access to care on a 24-hour basis for crisis management, if the need arises.
→ The health care provider should be aware of community resources for mental health care referral.
→ Follow up with the patient at weekly intervals to monitor psychological management.
→ Patients with anxiety disorders may need long-term maintenance therapy. Maintenance treatment should be extended for as long as 6–12 months after full recovery (Argyropoulos et al. 2000). Patient may have a trial off medication if no symptoms for 6–12 months (Zamorski et al. 2000).
→ Document in progress notes and on problem list.

BIBLIOGRAPHY

American Psychiatric Association (APA). 2000. *Diagnostic and statistical manual of mental disorders*, 4th ed. (text revision). Washington, D.C.: the Author.

Andrews, G. 2000. Anxiety disorders: recognition and management. *Australian Family Physician* 29(4):337–341.

Argyropoulos, S.V., Sandford, J.J., and Nutt, D.J. 2000. The psychobiology of anxiolytic drugs, Part 2: pharmacological treatment of anxiety. *Pharmacology and Therapeutics* 88: 231–227.

Ballenger, J.C., Davidson, J.R., Lecrubier, Y. et al. 2001. Consensus statement on generalized anxiety disorder from the International Consensus Group on Depression Anxiety. *Journal of Clinical Psychiatry* 62 (Suppl. 1):53–58.

Bennett, J.A., Moioffer, M., Stanton, S.P. et al. 1998. A risk-benefit assessment of pharmacological treatments for panic disorder. *Drug and Safety* 18(6):419–430.

Brunello, N., de Boer, J.A., Judd, L.L. et al. 2000. Social phobia: diagnosis and epidemiology, neurobiology and pharmacology, comorbidity and treatment. *Journal of Affective Disorders* 60(1):61–74.

Eaton, W.W. 1995. Progress in the epidemiology of anxiety disorder. *Epidemiologic Reviews* 17(1):32–38.

Edwards, J.G. 1991. Clinical anxiety and its treatment. *Neuropeptides* 19(Suppl.):1–10.

Hodiamont, Q. 1991. How normal are anxiety and fear? *International Journal of Social Psychiatry* 37(1):43–50.

Howell, H.B., Brawman-Mintzer, O., Monnier, J. et al. 2001. Generalized anxiety disorder in women. *Psychiatry Clinics of North America* 24(1):165–178.

Johnson, M.R., Lydiard, R.B., and Ballenger, J.C. 1995. Panic disorder: pathophysiology and drug treatment. *Drugs* 49: 328–344.

Katon, W. 1986. Panic disorder: epidemiology, diagnosis, and treatment in primary care. *Journal of Clinical Psychiatry* 43:21–27.

Lampe, L.A. 1996. A management approach to anxiety. *Australian Family Physician* 25(10)1561–1567.

Liebowitz, M.R. 1999. Update on the diagnosis and treatment of social anxiety disorder. *Journal of Clinical Psychiatry* 60 (Suppl. 18):22–26.

Ninan, P.T., and Berger J. 2001. Symptomatic and syndromal anxiety and depression. *Depression Anxiety* 14(2):79–85.

Schatzber, A.F., and Ballenger, J.C. 1991. Decision for the clinician in the treatment of panic disorder: when to treat, which treatment to use, and how long to treat. *Journal of Clinical Psychiatry* 52 (Suppl. 2):26–31.

Sheikh, J.I., and Swales, P.J. 1999. Treatment of panic disorder in older adults: a pilot study comparison of alprazolam, imipramine, and placebo. *International Journal of Psychiatry in Medicine* 29(1):107–117.

Stanley, M.A., and Beck, J.G. 2000. Anxiety disorders. *Clinical Psychology Review* 20(6):731–754.

Weinstock, L.S., 1999. Gender differences in the presentation and management of social anxiety disorder. *Journal of Clinical Psychiatry* 60 (Suppl. 9):9–13.

Woods, S.W., Nagy, L.M., Koleszar, A.S. et al. 1992. Controlled trial of alprazolam supplementation during imipramine treatment of panic disorder. *Journal of Clinical Psychiatry* 12: 32–38.

Zamorski, M.A., and Ward, R.K. 2000. Social anxiety disorder: common, disabling, and treatable. *Journal of the American Board of Family Practice* 13:251–260.

14-C

Depression

Depression is a mental health problem commonly encountered in primary care practice (Webb et al. 2000b). Epidemiological studies show a range of 5–10% of male adults and 10–25% of female adults have at least one depressive illness in their lifetimes (American Psychiatric Association [APA] 2000, Weissman et al. 1995). The prevalence of depression may be as high as 20–30% among patients with a general medical illness, especially illnesses associated with chronic pain. There is no consistent relationship between the prevalence of depressive disorders and race, education, income, or social status.

Current theories concerning the etiology of depression are multifactorial, involving the interaction of biochemical (imbalance of central neurotransmitters and hormonal changes), genetic-hereditary, and environmental factors. (Webb et al. 2000a).

Differences in cognitive styles, biologic factors (brain structure and function), and higher incidence of psychosocial and economic stress in women have been postulated as the reasons for the higher prevalence of depression in women (Webb et al. 2000b).

The assessment of depression is a complex process, as patients present frequently with somatic complaints (such as fatigue, dizziness, abdominal distress, or back pain) rather than dysphoria. This leads to under-recognized depression in the ambulatory care setting (Tylee 1999). Clinicians should consider the diagnosis of depression in patients who present with unexplained physical conditions, pain, anxiety, and/or substance abuse (Webb et al. 2000b). An additional concern with the assessment of depression in the primary care setting is the issue of suicide. More than 60% of suicides are attributed to a major depressive disorder (Agency for Health Care Policy and Research [AHCPR] 1993). Up to 15% of individuals with severe major depressive disorder die by suicide (APA 2000).

Types of Depression

Depression is categorized as a mental disorder by the American Psychiatric Association in the *Diagnostic and Statistical Manual of Mental Health Disorders (DSM-IV TR)* (APA 2000).

According to this classification, depression can occur as part of:
1. A mood disorder—unipolar category (e.g., major depression, dysthymia, or depressive disorders not otherwise specified [patient does not meet the criteria for any specific mood disorder or adjustment disorder with depressed mood])
2. A mood disorder—bipolar category (depression as part of a manic, mixed, or hypomanic episode)
3. A predominant symptom in an adjustment disorder (adjustment disorder with depressed mood)
4. A nonmood psychotic disorder (e.g. schizoaffective disorder)
5. A mood disorder due to a general medical condition
6. A substance-induced mood disorder

This chapter addresses depression as a mood disorder—unipolar category, and as a predominant symptom in adjustment disorder.

Major Depression

A *major depressive episode* is characterized by the DSM-IV TR (APA 2000) as a condition in which the essential feature is either *depressed mood* (feeling sad or empty) or *anhedonia* (loss of interest or pleasure) in all, or almost all, activities. It also includes the presence of at least four associated symptoms, most of them of the neurovegetative type, for a period of at least two weeks (see "Database," below).

The above symptoms should not be accounted for by a medical condition, substance abuse, medication, psychotic disorder, or bereavement. Symptoms must also result in significant impairment of functioning (e.g., social, occupational).

A major depressive disorder is characterized by one or more major depressive episodes and can be classified as either *mild*—few if any symptoms in excess of those required to make the diagnosis and mild impairment in occupational and social functioning; *moderate*—symptoms and impairment between mild and severe; and *severe*—several symptoms in excess required to make the diagnosis and marked interference with occupational or social functioning. It can also be classified as in *partial remission*—only some symptoms or signs remain from major depression previously diagnosed; or in *full remission*—symptoms or signs of the disorder are no longer present, although it is still clinically relevant to note the disorder. *Seasonal affective disorder* is characterized as a "specifier" or subtype of major depressive episodes, referring to its seasonal pattern. It is characterized by the temporal relationship between the onset of a major depressive episode and a particular time of the year (most often fall onset type, called "winter depression") with full remission also at a particular time of the year (in this case, spring or summer). Depression in this specifier can be part of unipolar (most frequently) or bipolar mood disorder (Saeed et al. 1998).

The onset of a major depressive episode may develop over weeks to months. Its duration may be six months or longer, with an eventual complete remission of symptoms in the majority of the cases. However, in 5–10% percent of patients, some symptoms persist for two years or longer. These cases are specified as chronic.

Suicide is the major complication of major depression. A patient with this disorder is 30 times more likely to commit suicide than a nondepressed person (Lowenstein 1985). Evaluation of suicide risk is crucial in all patients with depression and particularly those with comorbid depression and anxiety (Webb et al. 2000b) or comorbidity with alcohol or drug abuse (Gliatto et al. 1999). The most common method of suicide in women is overdosing (Moscicki 1997).

When assessing the patient for major depression, it is also important to rule out a mood disturbance due to a physiological consequence of a specific general medical condition, a substance-induced mood disorder, or other psychiatric disorders that can masquerade as depression. The following etiologies related to a general medical condition or substance-induced condition should be considered:

→ Drug-induced: antihypertensive agents such as reserpine, methyldopa, or clonidine; nonspecific beta-blockers; corticosteroids; cholinergic drugs; benzodiazepines; or barbiturates

→ Drug abuse: alcohol, sedative hypnotics (e.g., barbiturates, narcotics), cocaine or other psycho-stimulant (e.g., amphetamines, nicotine) withdrawal

→ Toxic metabolic disorders: hyperthyroidism (especially in elderly patients), hypothyroidism, Cushing's syndrome, Addison's disease, diabetes mellitus, hypercalcemia, hyponatremia, or renal disease

→ Neurological disorders: stroke, subdural hematoma, chronic headache, multiple sclerosis, brain tumors, Parkinson's and Huntington's diseases, syphilis, dementia, Alzheimer's disease, or uncontrolled pellagra (very rare)

→ Gastrointestinal disease: irritable bowel syndrome, inflammatory bowel disease, cirrhosis, hepatic encephalopathy, or pancreatic carcinoma

→ Pulmonary disease: sleep apnea or reactive airway disease

→ Rheumatologic: systemic lupus erythematosus, chronic fatigue syndrome, fibromyalgia, rheumatoid arthritis, or other autoimmune diseases

→ Other: anemia, recent surgery (including but not limited to mastectomy, hysterectomy), viral infections (especially mononucleosis and influenza), cancer, chronic pain, heart disease, human immunodeficiency virus (HIV) infection, or recent physical trauma (e.g., motor vehicle accident)

Depression may coexist with a number of other psychiatric disorders, such as anxiety (generalized anxiety, social phobia, or panic disorder), substance abuse, eating disorders, or personality disorders (APA 2000, Webb et al. 2000b). The comorbidity of anxiety and depression, in most cases, does not constitute a dual diagnosis but a symptom of depression. In such cases, the effective treatment is antidepressants; antianxiety medications can worsen the depression (APA 2000, Webb et al. 2000b).

Dysthymia

Dysthymia, also known as *depressive neurosis*, is a chronic disturbance of mood involving depressed mood most days for at least two years. In addition to depressed mood, two of the following symptoms must also be present: poor appetite or overeating, insomnia or hyperinsomnia, low energy or fatigue, low self-esteem, poor concentration or difficulty making decisions, and feelings of hopelessness. To fit the diagnosis of dysthymia, the person may be symptom-free for no longer than two months and only if the initial two-year period of the disorder is free of major depressive episode. Major depressive episodes may be superimposed on the dysthymic disorder after the two initial years of dysthymia. As with major depression, symptoms in dysthymia should not be accounted for by a medical condition, substance abuse, or psychotic disorder, and the symptoms must cause clinically significant distress or impair functioning (e.g., social, occupational, or other important functions).

The differential diagnoses of dysthymia and major depression may be difficult, as both disorders share similar symptoms and differ only in duration and severity—dysthymia being less severe but chronic. Dysthymia usually begins without a clear onset and usually has a superimposed major depressive episode, which increases the possibility that the patient will seek treatment. Dysthymia may precede a major depressive episode (early onset) or follow a major depressive episode (late onset) (Barzega et al. 2001).

Adjustment Disorder With Depressed Mood

Adjustment disorder with depressed mood is characterized by the DSM-IV TR (APA 2000) as a maladaptive reaction in which the predominant manifestations are symptoms of depressed mood, tearfulness, and feelings of hopelessness. Symptoms occur as a response to a single or multiple, recurrent, or continuous psychosocial stressor such as divorce, work difficulties, or chronic illness. Some stressors may accompany specific developmental events such as getting married or becoming a parent. This disorder begins within three months of onset of the stressor and lasts no longer than six months. It is usually self-limited and resolves when the stress ceases or a new level of adaptation is achieved. However, if stressors are chronic or have enduring consequences, symptoms may persist for a prolonged period (i.e., longer than six months). Adjustment disorder with depressed mood can occur at any age and the intensity of the stressor does not necessarily reflect the severity of the reaction.

This disturbance is not a result of uncomplicated bereavement nor does it meet the criteria for any specific mental disorder. Individuals from disadvantaged life circumstances experience a high rate of stressors and may be at increased risk for this disorder. In individuals who have a medical condition, the presence of an adjustment disorder may complicate the course of illness (e.g., decreased compliance with the recommended medical regimen or increased length of hospital stay).

DATABASE

SUBJECTIVE

→ Major depression
- Precipitating factors include:
  - Substance abuse
  - Chronic physical illness
  - Psychosocial stressor
  - Childbirth
- Medical health history may reveal:
  - Recent surgery (especially within the last year)
  - Diabetes (diabetes doubles risk of depression) (Lustman 2001)
  - Major depression or dysthymia
  - Coexisting psychiatric disorders (e.g., anxiety disorders, eating disorders, personality disorders)
- Personal/health/social history may reveal:
  - History of childhood adversity (e.g., abuse, neglect)
  - Difficult social situation, social isolation (lack of family, friends, or other social supports), domestic violence
  - Stress related to unemployment, poverty, adolescence
  - Recent loss or unresolved grief
  - Marital conflicts or dysfunctional family patterns
  - Variable social and occupational impairment
    - May be so severe that the individual is not functional even in the routine of daily living (e.g., feeding or clothing herself)
- Family history may be positive for:
  - Depression
  - Bipolar disorder
  - Suicide
  - Substance abuse
  - Anxiety disorder
- Age of onset is usually mid-20s, but may begin at any age.
- Symptoms develop suddenly or over weeks or months.
- Symptoms may have a seasonal pattern.
- The patient reports at least one of the following symptoms most of the day and nearly every day for at least two weeks:
  - Depressed mood—i.e., feeling of sadness, being "blue" or gloomy
  - Anhedonia—i.e., markedly diminished interest or pleasure; loss of interest in friends, family, and work
- Reports at least four of the following associated symptoms during a two-week period, nearly every day, representing a change from previous functioning:
  - Appetite and weight disturbance—in women, most commonly increased appetite and weight gain

- Sleep disturbances—in women, most commonly increased sleep
- Psychomotor agitation or retardation—being unable to remain still (agitation), or slow speech with more pauses than normal and slow body movements (retardation). These may also be observed by others.
- Fatigue and loss of energy
- Feelings of worthlessness and/or excessive guilt that may be delusional (may also be observed by others)
- Decreased cognitive functioning—difficulty concentrating and thinking, with memory loss (may be observed by others)
- Suicidal ideation or attempts—may believe that she or others may be better off dead. May make indirect statements such as, "I've had enough," "I'm a burden," or "It's not worth it" (Gliatto et al. 1999).
- May also complain of:
  - Feeling of helplessness, hopelessness, and inadequacy
  - Hopelessness appears to be necessary for the development of suicidal ideation (Moscicki 1997).
  - Heaviness in head or chest pains
  - Headache, backache, constipation
- Common associated features may include:
  - Guilt (common in women)
  - Tearfulness
  - Anxiety (common in women)
  - Anger or irritability
  - Brooding or obsessive rumination
  - Excessive concern with physical health
  - Panic attacks
  - Phobias
  - Sexual dysfunction, including decreased libido (Phillips et al. 2000)
- Some women mask their sadness or despair, affecting a cheerful manner or even a kind of hectic gaiety. More commonly, however, the affect is flat. Women with depression more frequently experience guilt, anxiety, increased appetite and sleep, weight gain, and comorbid eating disorders (Bhatia et al. 1999).

→ Dysthymia
- Medical history may reveal superimposed major depressive episode (more common in women).
- Personal/health/social history may include:
  - Mild to moderate social and occupational functioning impairment
  - Psychoactive substance dependence or abuse (degree of severity increased by the chronicity of the disorder)
- Family history may include major depression or dysthymia in first-degree relative(s) (APA 2000).
- Onset: childhood through early adulthood (for this reason, dysthymia has often been referred to as *depressive personality).* Early onset is more common in women.
- The patient reports at least two of the following symptoms during periods of depressed mood (associated features are similar to those of major depression):

- Eating disturbances
- Sleeping disturbances
- Low level of energy or fatigue
- Low self-esteem
- Feeling of hopelessness
- Cognitive difficulties
- Poor concentration or difficulty making decisions
  - Most commonly encountered symptoms in dysthymic disorder may be feelings of:
    - Inadequacy
    - Generalized loss of interest or pleasure
    - Social withdrawal
    - Guilt or brooding about the past
    - Subjective irritability or excessive anger
    - Decreased activity, effectiveness, or productivity
  - In individuals with dysthymic disorder, social, emotional, and cognitive symptoms are common. Vegetative symptoms are less common than in persons with a major depressive episode (Barzega et al. 2001).
- → Adjustment disorder with depressed mood
  - Medical health history may reveal chronic illness.
  - Personal/health/social history may reveal:
    - Social impairment, decreased occupational or school performance, excessive substance abuse
  - Age of onset is variable.
  - Symptoms begin within three months of onset of an identifiable psychosocial stressor(s) and last no longer than six months.
  - May report symptoms of:
    - Depressed mood
    - Tearfulness
    - Feelings of hopelessness
  - Symptoms are greater than a normal or expected reaction to the stressor.

OBJECTIVE

- → General appearance may include:
  - Lack of care in grooming
  - Slumped posture
  - Sad facial expression
  - Smiling in the presence of denial or repression (masked depression)
- → Mental status may include:
  - Psychomotor retardation or agitation
  - Long periods of hesitation before answering, or slow speech
  - Affect that is sad, irritable, anxious, angry, tearful, or despondent
  - Thought that is clear and coherent or tangential, circumstantial, or nonsensical
  - Ideas of worthlessness, helplessness, hopelessness, guilt, suicidal thoughts, homicide. With severe depression, delusions and hallucinations may be present.
  - Mood that is persistently elevated, expansive, or irritable, with history of depression

NOTE: In such a case, bipolar disorder must be considered. Without a history of depressive symptoms, persistent elevated mood suggests univocal mania.

ASSESSMENT

- → Major depression
  - Mild, moderate, or severe
  - Single episode or recurrent
  - Seasonal pattern (winter or summer depression)
  - Chronic
  - In partial or full remission
  - R/O uncomplicated bereavement
  - R/O mood disorder due to a general medical condition
  - R/O substance-induced mood disorder
  - R/O bipolar disorder, depressed phase
  - R/O schizophrenia
  - R/O primary degenerative dementia of the Alzheimer's type and multi-infarct dementia (more common in the elderly)
- → Dysthymia
  - R/O major depression
  - R/O major depression in partial remission
- → Adjustment disorder with depressed mood
- → Depressive disorder not otherwise specified
  - R/O uncomplicated bereavement

PLAN

DIAGNOSTIC TESTS

- → There are no useful chemical tests to confirm a diagnosis of depression.
- → Additional diagnostic tests as indicated to rule out organic causes of depression (e.g., thyroid secreting hormone [TSH], complete blood count [CBC], chemistry panel).
- → The Beck Depression Inventory (BDI) (either long form or short form) may be used for suspicion of depression (Dreyfus 1987).
  - The BDI is useful for monitoring treatment response and changes in affective status over time; less useful for initial diagnosis.
- → The Patient Health Questionnaire (PHQ-9) is a self-administered questionnaire that can be used before, during, or after the office visit to detect and quantify the severity of depression and the effectiveness of treatment (Spitzer et al. 1999). This screening tool is available from the Web site of the MacArthur Foundation Initiative on Depression and Primary Care (www.depression-primarycare.org).
- → A baseline EKG should be obtained for all patients over 40 years old when initiating tricyclic antidepressant medication.
- → Blood pressure measurements (lying and standing) and pulse should be obtained when the patient starts tricyclic antidepressant medication.

TREATMENT/MANAGEMENT

- → Treatment of depression depends on the type of depression, severity of symptoms, personal and social impairments related to the depression, and availability of treatment resources (Whooley et al. 2000).

→ Psychotherapy, pharmacotherapy, and electroconvulsive therapy (ECT) have all demonstrated beneficial effect over placebo (Sobin et al. 1996, Thase et al. 1997). The latter is administered only by a specialist for severe cases of depression and will not be addressed in this chapter.

→ Major depression
- With mild and moderate depression, psychotherapy and pharmacotherapy are equally effective (Geddes et al. 2001). Psychotherapeutic modalities include cognitive, cognitive behavioral, interpersonal psychotherapy, problem solving, and nondirective counseling. Other therapies shown to be of benefit include: group therapy, self-help group, diet and exercise programs, and instruction in coping skills (Geddes et al. 2001, Smith 1986, Ward et al. 2000).
- Behavioral therapy is particularly appropriate with underlying psychosocial and abuse issues, family dysfunction, and life transitions.
- Pharmacotherapy is effective in the management of neurovegetative symptoms. Psychotherapy may enhance social functioning.
- Pharmacotherapy is effective for severe depression. The addition of psychotherapy (interpersonal or cognitive) may prove beneficial (Geddes et al. 2001).
- If moderate or severe depression, medical consultation is indicated.
- Light-box therapy, monoamine oxidase inhibitors (MAOIs), or psychotherapy are recommended for fall-winter onset seasonal depression; antidepressants (see below) are recommended for summer depression (Saeed et al. 1998).

→ Dysthymia disorders
- Consultation with a mental health care provider is indicated.
- Education, supportive counseling, antidepressant therapy, psychotherapy, and family therapy are recommended.
- Two selective serotonin reuptake inhibitors (SSRIs) (fluoxetine, sertraline) have been found effective in managing adults with dysthymia (AHRQ 1999).

→ Adjustment disorder with depressed mood
- This condition may be co-managed with a mental health care provider.
- Treatment includes supportive psychotherapy and education, particularly the latter, if the disorder is precipitated by a medical illness (Perry et al. 1992).
- If moderate sleep and eating disturbances are present, tricyclic and SSRI antidepressants may be effective.

→ Pharmacological guidelines: See **Table 14C.1, Antidepressant Medications: Dosages and Side Effects**.
- Antidepressant medications can be divided into "older" antidepressants, which include first-generation and second-generation tricyclics (TCA), heterocyclics, and MAOIs.
- SSRIs are second-generation antidepressants that are now used as a first-line therapy.
- Other newer agents have surfaced. These include: serotonin noradrenaline reuptake inhibitors (SNRIs), norepinephrine reuptake inhibitors (NRIs), reversible inhibitors of monoamine oxidase (RIMAs), 5-HT$_2$ receptor antagonists (5-HT$_2$), 5-HT$_{1A}$ receptor agonists (5-HT$_{1A}$), gabamimetics (Gaba), dopamine reuptake inhibitors (DopRIs) and antagonists (DopAnts), and herbal remedies such as hypericum (St. John's wort).

- Selection of antidepressant therapy should be made based on side effects (beneficial and adverse), cost, patient preferences, and the provider's familiarity with the pharmacology of medications. Antidepressant side effects can ameliorate specific symptoms (e.g., sedation in a patient with insomnia). In addition, the following factors should be considered in selecting a particular antidepressant (Webb et al. 2000b):
  - Prior response to the medication
  - History of first-degree relatives responding to a medication
  - Noxious effect on concurrent medical conditions
  - Interactions with other medications
- An empirical trial of medication is often required to discover which agent will work for an individual patient (Rush et al. 1997).
- The efficacy of older antidepressants and SSRIs for the treatment of depression has been well established (AHCPR 1993, AHRQ 1999). They are equally effective and considered the first line of treatment. Currently, the most common antidepressants used are SSRIs. Although they are more expensive, they have fewer side effects and are better tolerated than tricyclics over time. Discontinuation rates for SSRIs, second-generation tricyclics, and heterocyclics are lower compared to those for first-generation tricyclics (Hotopf et al. 1997). Newer antidepressants are also effective in treating major depression, and the efficacy and total dropout rates are similar to those for older agents (AHRQ 1999)
  - First-generation tricyclics (tertiary): amineptine, amitriptyline, clomipramine, dothiepin, doxepin, imipramine, trimipramine
  - Second-generation tricyclics (secondary): desipramine, lofepramine, nortriptyline, protriptyline
- In general, secondary tricyclics have fewer side effects than the tertiary ones (AHCRP 1993).
  - First-generation heterocyclic antidepressants: amoxapine, bupropion, bupropion sustained release, maprotiline, trazodone.
  - SSRIs: citalopram, fluoxetine, fluvoxamine, paroxetine, sertraline
- Newer antidepressants approved by the Food and Drug Administration include:
  - Mirtazapine, nefazodone, venlafaxine, and venlafaxine, extended release.
  - These antidepressants act on both the serotonergic and noradrenergic systems but lack the anticholinergic and cardiovascular side effects of older agents (Schatzberg 2000).

Table 14C.1. ANTIDEPRESSANT MEDICATION: DOSAGES AND SIDE EFFECTS

Common Antidepressants Generic name	Starting Dose (mg/day)	Therapeutic Dose Range (mg/day)	Side Effects					
			Orthostatic hypotension	Anticholinergic effects*	Sedation/ drowsiness	Insomnia/ agitation	Sexual dysfunction	GI distress
First-Generation Tricyclics (Tertiary)								
Amitriptyline	25–50	75–300	++++	++++	++++	o/+	+	o
Clomipramine	25	75–300	++	+++	+++	o/+	++	o
Doxepin	25–50	75–300	++/+++	+++	+++/++++	o/+	+	o
Imipramine	25–50	75–300	++++	+++	+++	o/+	+	+
Trimipramine	25–50	75–300	++	+	++++			o
Second-Generation Tricyclics (Secondary)								
Desipramine	25–50	75–300	++/+++	+/++	+/++	+	+	o
Nortriptyline	25	75–150	++	+/++	+/++	+	+	o
Protriptyline	10	20–60	++	++	+			o
First-Generation Heterocyclic Antidepressants								
Amoxapine	50	100–400	++	++	++	++		o
Bupropion	150	300–450	o	o/+	o	++/+++	o/+	+
Maprotiline	50	100–225	o	++	++++	o		o
Trazodone	50	75–300	+	o	++++	o		+
Selective Serotonin Reuptake Inhibitors (SSRIs)								
Citalopram	20	20–40	o	+	o/+	+	+++	++
Fluoxetine	20	20–60	o	o/+	o/+	++++	++++	+++
Fluvoxamine	50	50–300	o	o/+	++	++	+++	+++
Paroxetine	20	20–60	o	+	++	++	+++	+++
Sertraline	50	50–200	o	o/+	o/+	+++	++++	++++
Newer FDA-Approved Antidepressants								
Mirtazapine	15	15–45	o/+	++	++++	o/+	o/+	o/+
Nefazodone	50	150–300	+	+	+++	o	+	++
Venlafaxine	37.5	75–225	o	+	o	++	+++	++++

o = absent or rare   + = very low   ++ = low   +++ = moderate   ++++ = high
*Dry mouth, blurred vision, urinary hesitancy, constipation.

Source: Compiled from Agency for Health Care Policy and Research (AHCPR), 1993. Depression in primary care: detection, diagnosis and treatment. Clinical Practice Guideline No. 5. Publication No. 93-0550. Rockville, Md.: U.S. Department of Health and Human Services, U.S. Public Health Service; American Psychiatric Association (APA). 2000. *Diagnostic and statistical manual of mental disorders*, 4th ed. (text revision). Washington, D.C.: the Author; *Nurse practitioner's drug handbook*. 2000. 3rd ed., ed. C. Laufenberg. Springhouse, Pa.: Springhouse; University of California–San Francisco Hospital Pharmacy and Drug Information Analysis Services. 1997. UCSF treatment guidelines: major depression. *Pharmacy and Therapeutics Forum* 45(1):1–3.

- Major side effects for antidepressants include (AHCPR 1993, Whooley et al. 2000):
- Cardiotoxicity/cardiac arrhythmia
  - Patients with known or suspected cardiac disease must have a consultation with a cardiologist before initiating tricyclics or heterocyclic medication.
  - SSRIs do not appear to exert cardiotoxic effects (Roose et al. 1999).
  - Newer FDA antidepressants (e.g., SSRIs) lack the anticholinergic and cardiovascular side effects of older agents (Schatzberg 2000).
  - Dose-dependent blood-pressure elevations may be observed in a minority of patients taking venlafaxine.
  - Monitor blood pressure closely after a dose increase of venlafaxine (Webb et al. 2000b).
- Orthostatic hypotension
  - More common with TCAs, particularly amitriptyline and imipramine
  - Elderly patients and patients with cardiovascular disease are more vulnerable.
- Anticholinergic effects
  - Central (i.e., poor concentration, memory loss, confusion, and temperature fluctuation) or peripheral (i.e., dry mouth, constipation, tachycardia, urinary hesitancy or retention, increase or decrease in sweating, nasal stuffiness, and blurred vision).
  - First-generation TCAs have the highest frequency (40%) followed by second-generation TCAs.
  - To manage these side effects, consider reducing the dose or changing to a less anticholinergic antidepressant.
  - If antidepressants are discontinued abruptly, dose is reduced drastically, or a change to a less anticholinergic drug is made, rebound cholinergic effects may ensue (i.e., dizziness, nausea, diarrhea, malaise, anxiety, insomnia, and restlessness).
- Memory loss or lack of concentration
  - Can be either an anticholinergic effect or a result of depression
- Constipation
  - Consider stool softener (see the **Constipation** chapter in Section 7).
- Sedation/drowsiness
  - May be troublesome for patients with somnolence and/or psychomotor retardation; may be beneficial in anxious, agitated, or insomniac patients. If sedation is unwanted, consider lowering the dose, administer total dose at bedtime, or change to a less-sedating antidepressant.
- Insomnia/agitation
  - To counteract this side effect, provide medication in the morning.
- Seizures
  - All antidepressants may cause seizures in up to 4% of patients. Bupropion is most likely to induce seizures

(administration should not exceed 450 mg/day in divided doses).
- Weight gain
  - High with mirtazapine due to increased appetite
  - TCAs (particularly amitriptyline) usually cause weight gain (AHCPR 1993, Osser 2002)
  - Minimal with SSRIs
  - Not associated with nefazodone, venlafaxine
- Weight loss
  - Minimal with SSRIs and bupropion
- Sexual dysfunction
  - Common with most SSRIs and venlafaxine. Sertraline and paroxetine induce sexual dysfunction in 30–70% of patients (Kennedy et al 2000).
  - Decreasing antidepressant dose, adding bupropion (150 mg in the morning) or changing antidepressant medication to bupropion or nefazodone may improve libido (Phillips et al. 2000).
  - Drug holidays (i.e., skip Friday dose and resume Sunday at noon) may help 50% of patients but may reduce efficacy or lead to serotonin withdrawal symptoms (see below) (Osser 2002).
  - Sildefanil (Viagra®) may be beneficial (should be considered only under psychiatric consultation).
- Gastrointestinal upset
  - Symptoms of nausea and, rarely, diarrhea or vomiting. Most common with SSRIs and venlafaxine.
  - Try lowering the dose or taking medication with meals; change medication if symptoms do not improve (Osser 2002).
- Headaches
  - SSRIs, compared to first-generation tricyclics, cause significantly higher rates of headache (Osser 2002). Headaches may improve after few weeks of treatment.
- To minimize side effects of tricyclic/heterocyclic antidepressants, begin with a low dose and slowly titrate upward every 3–4 days until a therapeutic dose without intolerable side effects is reached.
- Dose first- and second-generation antidepressants, nefazodone, and mirtazapine once daily at HS to increase compliance and tolerability.
- Dose SSRIs (e.g., citalopram, fluoxetine, sertraline) once daily early in the daytime to minimize insomnia.
  - Some SSRIs may produce somnolence; in such cases, change dosing to every HS (e.g., fluvoxamine, paroxetine).
  - Trazodone, venlafaxine, and bupropion require multiple doses for maximum effectiveness. Bupropion also requires multiple doses to minimize the risk of seizures.
- Blood plasma concentrations of some tricyclic antidepressants are recommended to monitor therapeutic doses and toxic levels.
  - Plasma-concentration monitoring of imipramine, amitriptyline, desipramine, and nortriptyline are useful in patients:

– Who do not respond to therapy

– Who do not comply with therapy

– Who have intolerable side effects

– Who are elderly

– Who are taking other medications that may interact (consult pharmacist or the *Physicians' Desk Reference [PDR]*)

• Obtain plasma levels 8–12 hours after the patient has taken the medication within 5–10 days of initiating antidepressant to assess steady state of therapeutic levels.

• Other agents (e.g., alcohol, tobacco) may alter plasma levels of some drugs (consult pharmacist or *PDR*).

■ SSRI use may be associated with undesirable behavioral changes (insomnia, irritability/agitation, nervousness/anxiety, restlessness/akathisia, increased energy, silliness/euphoria, and disinhibition).

• If such changes occur, the patient should be advised to skip a day or two of medication and then resume the medication at a lower dose.

• Frequent follow-up necessary. If these symptoms continue at a lower dose, consultation with or referral to a physician is recommended (Walkup et al. 1999).

• Nine uncommon (<1%) but serious adverse effects have been associated with the SSRIs: bradycardia, bleeding, granulocytopenia, seizures, hyponatremia, hepatotoxicity, serotonin syndrome, extrapyramidal effects, and mania in unipolar depression (AHRQ 1999).

■ Risk of dependency increases with prolonged use of alprazolam, a mild antidepressant and an excellent antianxiety drug.

■ Antidepressant drugs may interact with other medications; interactions may result in increased side effects and/or reduced antidepressant drug levels, depending on the interacting agent.

■ For patients who have recovered from major depression (with normal mood), continued treatment with an antidepressant for at least 6 months decreases the risk of relapse by 70% (AHRQ 1999).

■ Discontinue antidepressant gradually over several weeks to avoid cholinergic rebound effects. Dizziness, nausea, tremor, anxiety, and dysphoria may ensue if SSRIs with a short half-life are stopped abruptly. Discontinuation syndrome is most common with paroxetine, which has a very short half-life, and is less common with fluoxetine, which has a very long half-life.

■ First depressive episode may be adequately treated with medication for 6–12 months, while chronic depression may require several years or lifelong therapy.

■ Elderly patients require special attention, including lower doses of antidepressant. Initial dose should be lowered to one-half or one-third of the adult dose, although effective doses may be similar to adult doses (Whooley et al. 2000).

■ Consultation is indicated when first-line antidepressants are not effective following an adequate trial. Drug trial failure should be considered when a patient has no response after 4 weeks on a full dose with documented therapeutic blood levels. The presence of a general medical condition, a chronic social stressor, and/or substance abuse can contribute to treatment failure.

■ If the patient evidences any potential suicide risk or has a history of suicide attempts, it is recommended that no more than 1 week's supply or a total of 1 g of a heterocyclic antidepressant be prescribed at a time (Hyman et al. 1987).

■ SSRIs, if combined with benzodiazepines, narcotics, alcohol, or diphenhydramine, are a potential risk factor for suicide, especially in women (Stewart 2001).

■ Antidepressants should be avoided in patients with history of manic depressive disorder. These drugs can induce a manic episode.

■ Other psychoactive drugs:

• MAOIs, lithium, carbamazepine, and other antiepileptic agents should be used only in consultation with a psychiatric clinician.

• These medications may be indicated for those who do not respond well to first-line antidepressants.

■ Herbal medicines:

• Hypericum perforatum is a flowering plant with the common name St. John's wort. It has been found to be therapeutically as effective as imipramine (a TCA) in treating patients with mild to moderate depression (Woelk 2000). St. John's wort is expensive and not covered by insurance.

– Average dose of hypericum extract is 350 mg TID.

– Active ingredient has not been standardized; therapeutic level may have to be found by trial and error.

– Anecdotal severe side effects (liver failure, seizures, and death) have been reported to the FDA Web site um.csfan.fda.gov. The FDA has not concluded that these side effects are associated with St. John's wort (Boehnlein et al. 2002).

– Systemic photosensitivity has been reported. On sunny days, advise patients to take 1 pill early in the morning and another at night. Some patients have complained of dry mouth, dizziness, constipation, GI symptoms, nausea, gastrointestinal upset, and confusion (*The Medical Letter* 1997).

– Hypericum can interact with other medications. It should not be used with other antidepressants. Use with SSRIs can cause serotonin syndrome.

– S-adenosylmethionine (SAMe). Advertised as a nutritional supplement. There is some evidence of efficacy (Morelli et al. 2000). It poses the same issues as St. John's wort regarding cost and effective dose. Combining SAMe with antidepressants can lead to serotonin syndrome.

– Recommended dose is 400–1,200 mg/day in 4 divided doses (Morelli et al. 2000).

NOTE: Clinicians should consult additional literature regarding herbal remedies.

■ Light therapy for the treatment of winter depression is delivered with a 10,000-lux light box (best if fluorescent light) in 10–15 minute sessions once a day, gradually increasing to 30–40 minutes once a day. If symptoms worsen, therapy may be increased to BID, with a maximum of 90 minutes a day. During the session, the patient should keep her eyes open but not stare at the light. Therapy can be administered at any time of the day. Positive response may take from 2–4 days up to several weeks. If there is no response by 6 weeks, clinical management should be reevaluated (Saeed et al. 1998).

→ Evaluation of suicide risk
- Assess suicide risk in confirmed cases of depression.
- Assessing risk of suicide requires attention to:
  • Thoughts (ideas, wishes, motives)
  • Intent (degree of probability that patient intends to act on the thoughts)
  • Plans (formulation of a clear, detailed plan)
- Ask the patient in a straightforward manner if she has any suicide thoughts, intent, or plan. Inquiring about suicide will not give the patient the idea or incentive to commit suicide (Gliatto et al. 1999).
- The following questions have been suggested (Buckwater et al. 1990):
  • Have you thought life is not worth living?
  • Have you considered harming yourself?
  • Do you have a plan for harming yourself?
  • Have you ever acted on a plan?
  • Have you ever attempted suicide?
- If possible, ask the patient's family and friends if she has left any clue suggesting suicide (i.e., a written note, a spoken threat, or a previous attempt at self-destruction).
- If the patient is at high risk for suicide, never leave her alone. Obtain immediate psychiatric consultation (Lowenstein 1985).

CONSULTATION

→ See "Treatment/Management."
→ Women who have severe depression accompanied by active suicidal thoughts or plans, or who are refractory to usual treatments should be managed in conjunction with a psychiatrist (Bhatia et al.1999).
→ Primary care clinicians can improve depression outcomes when patients are co-managed with a psychiatrist or psychologist. This is especially important when patients are still persistently depressed eight or more weeks after treatment is initiated (Katon 2002).

PATIENT EDUCATION

→ Educate the patient and her family regarding symptoms of depression and recurrence. Because mental illness is commonly stigmatized, both the patient and her family should be counseled and the importance of complying with prescribed treatment stressed. Monitoring symptoms on a daily or weekly basis helps the practitioner identify gradual improvement or catch early signs of decompensation.
→ Support and validate the patient's feelings of sadness and remind her that depression can be treated.

→ Educate the patient about the side effects of the medication prescribed:
- For anticholinergic drugs, advise techniques that decrease incidence of dry mouth and constipation.
  • Use of sugarless gum, ice chips, and drinking adequate amount of fluids.
- Encourage proper daily dental cleaning to prevent tooth decay, mouth ulcers, and gum disease.
- Encourage the patient to increase intake of fluids, prune juice, and high-fiber foods to prevent constipation.
- Instruct the patient to get up slowly from sitting or lying positions to prevent falls (if the medication has a high orthostatic effect).
- Advise the patient that the full effect of antidepressant medication will not be evident for 10 days to 3 weeks (at adequate therapeutic levels). It may take 4–6 weeks to observe the full therapeutic benefit.
- Advise the patient that sleep, appetite, and energy levels generally improve within a week.
- Instruct the patient to report side effects rather than stop medication on her own.
- Instruct the patient to call if suicidal thoughts are present or her depressive symptoms worsen.
- Advise the patient to consult a health care provider before using over-the-counter medications.
- Advise the patient to consult a health care provider before discontinuing or changing medication.

→ Review patient compliance with medication. Engage the patient in decision-making; stress that medications may take 2–4 weeks to take effect, longer for full effect; the need to continue with medication even when feeling better; explain the risk of stopping the medication too soon. Noncompliance may be due to cost, adverse side effects, ambivalence regarding the disease, and time lag in effectiveness (Mejo 1990).

→ Engage family members in the management of depressive patients:
- To supervise/monitor medication regimen
- To keep follow-up appointments
- To uncover, explore, and modify stressful situations and provide a reassuring, supportive environment
- To decrease social isolation that results from and exacerbates depression
- To encourage the spouse/partner to express feelings of warmth and compassion in regard to the spouse's depressive illness. This has been proven to increase the speed of recovery (McLeod et al. 1992).
- To minimize suicide risk

→ Providing educational materials about medication treatment and engaging patients earlier after initiating treatment may decrease relapse rates (Mundt et al. 2001). Distribution of pamphlets, books, and videotapes can dispel misinformation about therapy and help patients become active partners in their care (Katon 2002).
→ Teach the patient relaxation techniques if indicated.
→ Encourage the patient to participate in a regular exercise

program (demonstrated to have an antidepressant effect, combats weight gain, and improves sleep).

→ Educate the patient about proper nutrition.

→ Encourage the patient to eliminate drug and alcohol use, and seek social support (church, support/advocacy groups).

→ Encourage the patient to engage in a spiritual practice if appropriate.

→ Encourage the patient to avoid situations in which interpersonal conflicts may arise. Less rapid recovery from depressive illness has been found to be significant when there is a conflicted relationship with friends (McLeod et al. 1992).

FOLLOW-UP

→ Ensure that the patient and her family have access to care on a 24-hour basis for crisis management, should the need arise.

→ The patient should be followed at regular intervals to monitor medications and reinforce psychotherapeutic work. For mild to moderate illness, a visit every 10–14 days (or phone follow-up) is recommended during the first 6–8 weeks of treatment.

→ To prevent relapses, the treatment should continue for 4–9 months after the patient's mood has returned to normal (AHRQ 1999). Once-weekly dosing of fluoxetine (90 mg enteric coated capsule) has been found to be as effective as a 20 mg daily dose of fluoxetine for patients who require long-term treatment of depression, and it may be effective in reducing relapse (Schmidt et al. 2000). Patients should be off of the daily dose for seven days before initiating the once-weekly regimen. Not all patients tolerate the once-weekly dose and should revert to the daily dose.

→ Monitor for early signs of recurrence.

→ Maintenance therapy may be needed if there is a high risk of recurrence (history of two or more dysthymia episodes).

→ Document in progress notes and on problem list.

BIBLIOGRAPHY

Agency for Health Care Policy and Research (AHCPR). 1993. Depression in primary care: detection, diagnosis and treatment. Clinical Practice Guideline No. 5. Publication No. 93-0550. Rockville, Md.: U.S. Department of Health and Human Services, U.S. Public Health Service.

Agency for Healthcare Research and Quality (AHRQ). 1999. Treatment of depression: newer pharmacotherapies. U.S. Department of Health and Human Services, U.S. Public Health Service. Rockville, Md. Available at: http://hstat.nlm. nih.gov/hq/Hquest/screen/DirectAccess/db/5. Accessed on October 30, 2002.

American Psychiatric Association (APA). 2000. *Diagnostic and statistical manual of mental disorders*, 4th ed. (text revision). Washington, D.C.: the Author.

Barbui, C., and Hotopf, M. 2001. Amitriptyline versus the rest: still the leading antidepressant after 40 years of randomized controlled trials. *British Journal of Psychiatry* 178:129–144.

Barzega, G., Maina, G., Venturello, S. et al. 2001. Dysthymic disorder: clinical characteristics in relation to age at onset. *Journal of Affective Disorders* 66:39–46.

Bhatia, S.C., and Bhatia, S. 1999 Depression in women: diagnostic and treatment considerations. *American Family Physician* 60:225–240.

Boehnlein, B., and Oakley, L.D. 2002. Implications of self-administered St. John's wort for depression symptom management. *Journal of the American Academy of Nurse Practitioners* 14(10):443–448.

Brasfield, K. 1991. Practical psychopharmacologic considerations in depression. *Nursing Clinics of North America* 16(3): 651–663.

Buckwater, K.C., and Babich, K.S. 1990. Psychologic and physiologic aspects of depression. *Nursing Clinics of North America* 25(4):945–954.

Dreyfus, J.K. 1987. The prevalence of depression in women in the ambulatory care setting. *Nurse Practitioner Journal* 12(4):34–50.

———. 1998. The treatment of depression in an ambulatory care setting. *Nurse Practitioner Journal* 13(7)14–33.

Geddes, J., and Butler, R. 2001. Depressive disorders. *Clinical Evidence* 6:726–742.

Gliatto, M.F., and Rai, A.K. 1999. Evaluation and treatment of patients with suicidal ideation. *American Family Physician* 59:1500–1503.

Hotopf, M., Hardy, R., and Lewis, G. 1997. Discontinuation rates of SSRIs and tricyclic antidepressants: a meta-analysis and investigation of heterogeneity. *British Journal of Psychiatry* 170:120–127.

Hyman, S.E., and Jenike, M.A. 1987. Approach to the patient with depression in primary care medicine. In *Primary care medicine,* 2nd ed., eds. A.H. Goroll, L.A. May, and A.G. Mulley. Philadelphia: J.B. Lippincott.

Katon, W.J. 2002. *Caring for the depressed patient in medical settings.* Paper presented at the 155th annual meeting of the American Psychiatric Association. Philadelphia, Pa., May 18–23, 2002.

Kennedy, S.H., Eisfeld, B.S., Dickens, S.E. et al. 2000. Antidepressant-induced sexual dysfunction during treatment with moclobemide, paroxetine, sertraline, and venlafaxine. *Journal of Clinical Psychiatry* 61:276–281.

Lowenstein, S.R. 1985. Suicidal behavior recognition and intervention. *Hospital Practice* 20:52–71.

Lustman, P.J. 2001. Diabetes doubles risk of depression. *Diabetes Care* 24:1069–1078.

McLeod, J.D., Kessler, R.C., and Landis, K.R. 1992. Speed of recovery from major depressive episodes in a community sample of married men and women. *Journal of Abnormal Psychology* 101(2):277–286.

The medical letter. 1997. St. John's wort. *Medical Letter on Drugs and Therapeutics* 39:107–108.

Mejo, S. 1990. The use of antidepressant medicine: a guide for the primary care nurse practitioner. *Journal of the American Academy of Nurse Practitioners* 2(4):153–159.

Morelli, V., and Zoorob, R.J. 2000. Alternative therapies: Part I. Depression, diabetes, obesity. *American Family Physician* 62:1051–1060.

Moscicki, E.K. 1997. Identification of suicide risk factors using epidemiologic studies. *Psychiatric Clinics of North America* 20:499–517.

Mundt, J.C., Clarke, G.N., Burrough, D. et al. 2001. Effectiveness of antidepressant pharmacotherapy: the impact of medication compliance and patient education. *Depression and Anxiety* 13:1–10.

Nurse practitioner's drug handbook. 2000. 3rd ed., ed. C. Laufenberg. Springhouse, Pa.: Springhouse.

Osser, D.N. 2002. *Algorithm for the pharmacotherapy of depression.* Available at: http://www.mhc.com/Algorithms/Depression/frame1.htm. Accessed on January 7, 2003.

Perry, M.V., Anderson, L.A. 1992. Assessment and treatment strategies for depressive disorders commonly encountered in primary care settings. *Nurse Practitioner Journal* 17(6): 25–36.

Phillips, R.L., and Slaughter, J.R. 2000. Depression and sexual desire. *American Family Physician* 62:782–786.

Roose, S.P., and Spatz, E. 1999. Treatment of depression in patients with heart disease. *Journal of Clinical Psychiatry* 60(Suppl. 20):34–37.

Rush, A.J., and Thase, M.E. 1997. Strategies and tactics in the treatment of chronic depression. *Journal of Clinical Psychiatry* 58(Suppl. 13):14–22.

Saeed, S.A., and Bruce, T.J. 1998. Seasonal affective disorders. *American Family Physician* 57(6):1340–1346.

Schatzberg, A.F. 2000. New indications for antidepressants. *Journal of Clinical Psychiatry* 6(Suppl. 11):9–17.

Schmidt, M.E., Fava, M., Robinson, J.M. et al. 2000. The efficacy and safety of a new enteric-coated formulation of fluoxetine given once weekly during the continuation treatment of major depressive disorder. *Journal of Clinical Psychiatry* 61(11):851–857

Smith, L.S. 1986. In *Psychologic concerns in contemporary women's health: a nursing advocacy approach,* ed. J. Griffith-Kennedy. Menlo Park, Calif.: Addison-Wesley.

Sobin, C., Prudic, J., Devanand, D.P. et al. 1996. Who responds to electroconvulsive therapy? A comparison of effective and ineffective forms of treatment. *British Journal of Psychiatry* 169(3):322–328.

Spitzer, R.L., Kroenke, K., and Williams, J.B. 1999. Validation and utility of a self-report version of PRIME-MD: the PHQ primary care study. *Journal of the American Medical Association* 282:1737–1744.

Stewart, D.E. 2001. Women and selective serotonin receptor inhibitor antidepressants in the real world. *Medscape Women's Health* 6(3):1.

Thase, M.E., Greenhouse, J.B., Frank, E. et al. 1997. Treatment of major depression with psychotherapy or psychotherapy-pharmacotherapy combinations. *Archives of General Psychiatry* 54(11):1009–1015.

Tylee, A. 1999. Depression in the community: physician and patient care perspective. *Journal of Clinical Psychiatry* 60(Suppl. 7):12–16.

University of California-San Francisco Hospital Pharmacy and Drug Information Analysis Services. 1997. UCSF treatment guidelines: major depression. *Pharmacy and Therapeutics Forum* 45(1):1–3.

Walkup, J.T., and Labellarte, M.J. 1999. The ABCs of SSRI side effects. *AACAP News* November–December: 217–221. Available at: http://aafp.org/afpmonographs.xml. Accessed on February 10, 2003.

Ward, E., King, M., Lloyd, M. et al. 2000. Randomised controlled trial of non-directive counselling, cognitive-behaviour therapy, and usual general practitioner care for patients with depression. I: Clinical effectiveness. *British Medical Journal* 321:1383–1392.

Webb, M.R., Dietrich, A., Katon, W. et al. 2000a. Depression in women: diagnostic and treatment considerations. *American Family Physician* 60:225–240.

_____. 2000b. Diagnosis and management of depression. *American Family Physician.* Monograph No. 2. Available at: http://aafp.org/afpmonographs.xml. Accessed on February 10, 2003.

Weissman, M.M., and Olfson, M. 1995. Depression in women: implications for health care research. *Science* 269:799–801.

Whooley, M.A., and Simon, G.E. 2000. Managing depression in outpatients. *New England Journal of Medicine* 346(26): 1942–1950.

Woelk, H. 2000. Comparison of St John's wort and imipramine for treating depression: randomised controlled trial. *British Medical Journal* 321:536–539.

Maureen T. Shannon, C.N.M., F.N.P., M.S.
Julie Richards, R.N., C., W.H.N.P., F.N.P., M.S., M.S.N.

14-D
Domestic Violence

Domestic violence is a syndrome that involves physical, psychological, emotional, financial, and/or sexual abuse toward a person by a family member or intimate partner (Shannon et al. 2000). This problem affects individuals from all ethnic and socioeconomic backgrounds, and often reflects a pattern of family dysfunction and violence. In the United States, approximately 85% of domestic violence incidences that are reported occur to women as the result of a male intimate partner's actions (Centers for Disease Control and Prevention [CDC] 2000a). However, there is evidence of intimate partner violence by women toward men, with 13% of men experiencing psychological or emotional abuse, without physical assault, by women partners (Archer 2000, CDC 2000a, Hamberger et al. 1994). This chapter will focus on domestic violence that involves harm toward a woman by a male partner.

Domestic violence is one of the most pervasive public health problems worldwide. Reports from various countries indicate that 10–50% of women have been victims of physical assault by an intimate male partner (Garcia-Moreno 2000, Heise et al. 1999). In the United States it is estimated that 1–1.5 million women experience physical or sexual assault by an intimate partner each year (CDC 2000a, 2000b). Various population-based surveys in the United States report that 18% to as many as 30% of women have been victims of physical abuse by an intimate partner at some time in their lives (CDC 2000c, Coker et al. 2000, Federal Bureau of Investigation 1998). In addition to physical assault, many women experience sexual and psychological harm by their partners (Coker et al. 2000).

There is a substantial societal cost for increased legal, police, prison, medical, and counseling expenditures incurred as a result of domestic violence. It is believed that battering accounts for 998,000 days of hospitalization, 28,700 emergency room visits, and 39,900 physician visits, with total medical costs approaching $44 million annually (Warshaw 1989).

Currently, no single comprehensive theory of this problem exists to adequately explain its cause. Studies evaluating the effects of alcohol and substance abuse, physiologic variations (e.g., increased testosterone levels in male abusers), social learn-ing, social stratification and powerlessness, pregnancy, cultural support, and patriarchal societies have provided some evidence of a relationship between these factors and the increased rates of domestic violence in various populations (Archer 2000, Bash et al. 1994, Coker et al. 2000, McFarlane et al. 1996, Soler et al. 2000). In addition, theorists have proposed that there are two types of violent relationships. One involves partners who experience psychological conflicts arising from the relationship itself that eventually lead to abuse. The second, which is observed in the majority of domestic violence cases, involves a person with a violence-prone personality (Moss 1991). For this latter group, Walker (1984) describes a cycle of violence consisting of three stages:

→ The tension-building phase in which conflicts and verbal abuse increase

→ The acute battering episode, and

→ The honeymoon phase in which there are expressions of remorse and often promises that harm toward the partner will not happen again.

Research shows that for 75% of abused women battering episodes do not become less frequent or severe, but increase instead (McLear et al. 1989).

The health consequences for women who experience domestic violence are profound and can include low self-esteem, depression, increased drug or alcohol abuse, multiple injuries, sexually transmitted diseases, permanent physical or psychological damage (e.g., post-traumatic stress disorder [PTSD]), pregnancy complications, and death by suicide or homicide (CDC 2001, Kernic et al. 2000, Parker et al. 1994, Parsons et al. 1999). Battering is the single most common injury to women—surpassing rape, muggings, and motor vehicle accidents combined (Randall 1990). Approximately 30% of female homicide victims are killed by their male partners (CDC 2001). Women are not the only ones affected. Children living in homes where domestic violence takes place experience emotional problems such as increased anxiety and anger, as well as an increased incidence of juvenile crime (Hull et al. 1998). In addition, they are at an increased risk of physical abuse, injuries, and death (McKay

1994). Research indicates that violence against a child is 15 times more likely in families with a history of domestic violence, especially if their mothers are being physically abused (McKay 1994, Stacey et al. 1983, Stark et al. 1988). This may be due to a direct physical assault by the abuser or a result of the child trying to protect the intended victim of violence (Hull et al. 1998).

There have been many explanations proposed as to why women who experience domestic violence choose to stay in abusive relationships. Walker (1984) described the concept of *learned helplessness* in which the victim becomes depressed and hopeless after her attempts to end the violence fail (Walker 1984). Researchers now understand battered women in the broader context of victims' reactions to catastrophe, violent crime, and prolonged captivity that can result in psychological problems including PTSD (Moss 1991, Packer 1990). Reasons for staying with an abusive partner include lack of family support, depression, lack of financial independence, the high social approval accorded marriage, lack of assisted community resources, religious beliefs, financial considerations, and concern for her own safety as well as the safety of her children and other relatives (Moss 1991).

In many instances, leaving the relationship does not end the abuse. In one study of 218 battered women, one-third were not living with their attacker at the time of the assault (Berrios et al. 1991). Furthermore, the risk of homicide tends to increase when the woman threatens to leave an abusive partner (Campbell 1986).

Studies indicate that screening for domestic violence by health care providers is not being regularly performed at most clinical sites, despite the American Medical Association's recommendation that it be a routine part of health care for women (American Medical Association 1992, CDC 1998, Parkinson et al. 2001). Explanations for the lack of screening include misinformation, the structure of the prevailing medical model, lack of training, and lack of effective interventions when domestic violence is identified (Waalen et al. 2000). Clinician education is especially important, as misinformation can be decreased with appropriate instruction. Recently, a systems model approach to the education of health care providers, patients, and community agencies was reported to significantly improve awareness of domestic violence in a managed care setting (McCaw et al. 2001). Simple screening tools can be used in various clinical settings to improve identification of women experiencing or at risk for domestic violence (see **Table 14D.1, Abuse Assessment Screen**) (McFarlane et al. 1996).

To meet the needs of women who are at risk for domestic violence, health care providers must assess all women for this problem and recognize it for what it is—a potentially *life-threatening condition* no less dangerous than cancer, cardiovascular disease, or any other major health problem.

DATABASE

SUBJECTIVE

→ All women are at risk for domestic violence regardless of age, race, or socioeconomic status.

→ Patient may describe episodes of physical, sexual, psychological, or verbal abuse directed at herself or others.

→ Patient may present with injuries that are inconsistent with the history described.

→ Patient may have a history of frequent visits to health care providers where she presents with multiple injuries or vague somatic complaints, including headaches, gastrointestinal (GI) complaints, fatigue, sleeplessness, sexual dysfunction, pelvic pain, chest pain, palpitations, allergic skin reactions, musculoskeletal aches, and anxiety.

→ Patient may report history of:

- Missed appointments or presenting for treatment days after an injury
- Alcohol or substance use in patient or her partner
- Eating disorders, depression, panic attacks, suicidal ideation, or suicide attempt(s)
- Pre-term labor or low-birth-weight infant(s) in previous pregnancies

→ Patient may be accompanied by a male partner who is overprotective and does not want the patient to be left alone with the health care provider.

OBJECTIVE

→ Patient may appear restless, angry, defensive, tearful, evasive, withdrawn, or anxious. She may also exhibit an inappropriate affect or avoid eye contact.

→ Patient may present with:

- Patchy alopecia
- Cigarette burns; human bites; multiple injuries in various stages of healing; wounds to the face, head, neck, breasts, or abdomen; wounds from a knife or firearm
- Foreign object(s) in ear, nose, vagina, or rectum
- Conditions associated with stress, including hypertension, obesity, weight loss, and GI ulcers
- Signs or symptoms consistent with sexual assault (see the **Sexual Assault** chapter)
- Multiple contusions, especially to the neck, face, arms, or trunk
- Signs or symptoms indicative of PTSD:
  - Nightmares
  - Exaggerated startle responses
  - Guilt
  - Fearfulness
  - An inability to concentrate

ASSESSMENT

→ Domestic violence
→ R/O physical assault
→ R/O sexual assault
→ R/O potential for death by suicide or homicide
→ R/O substance or alcohol abuse
→ R/O sexually transmitted disease(s) as indicated
→ R/O coexisting psychological disorder in patient
→ R/O coexisting child abuse
→ If violent behavior is atypical for the male partner, rule out

Table 14D.1.   ABUSE ASSESSMENT SCREEN

ABUSE ASSESSMENT SCREEN
(Circle YES or NO for each question)

1. Have you ever been emotionally or physically abused by your partner or someone important to you?
   YES   NO

2. **WITHIN THE LAST YEAR**, have you been hit, slapped, kicked, or otherwise physically hurt by someone?
   YES   NO

   If YES, by whom (*circle all that apply*)

   Husband   Ex-husband   Boyfriend   Stranger   Other   Multiple

   Total number of times _____

3. **SINCE YOU'VE BEEN PREGNANT**, have you been hit, slapped, kicked, or otherwise physically hurt by someone?   YES   NO

   If YES, by whom (*circle all that apply*)

   Husband   Ex-husband   Boyfriend   Stranger   Other   Multiple

   Total number of times _____

   MARK THE AREA OF INJURY ON THE BODY MAP

   SCORE EACH INCIDENT according to the following scale:

   1 = Threats of abuse, including use of a weapon
   2 = Slapping, pushing; no injuries and/or lasting pain
   3 = Punching, kicking bruises, cuts, and/or continuing pain
   4 = Beaten up, severe contusions, burns, broken bones
   5 = Head, internal, and/or permanent injury
   6 = Use of weapon, wound from weapon

   (If any of the descriptions for the higher number apply, use the higher number)

4. **WITHIN THE LAST YEAR**, has anyone forced you to have sexual activities?   YES   NO

   If YES by whom (*circle all that apply*)

   Husband   Ex-husband   Boyfriend   Stranger   Other   Multiple

   Total number of times _____

5. Are you afraid of your partner or anyone you listed above?   YES   NO

6. Name of person completing form

Source: Reprinted with permission from McFarlane, J., Parker, B., and Soeken, K. 1996. Physical abuse, smoking and substance use during pregnancy: prevalence, interrelationships, and effects on birth weight. *Journal of Obstetric, Gynecologic, and Neonatal Nursing* 25(4):314.

organic origin in the abuser (e.g., brain metastasis, subdural hematoma, drug reaction)

PLAN

DIAGNOSTIC TESTS

→ No specific diagnostic tests are required.

→ Necessary tests will depend upon the nature of any injury.

→ X-rays may reveal presence of multiple new and/or healed fractures.

TREATMENT/MANAGEMENT

→ Screen *all* women for domestic violence regardless of age, race, sexual orientation, and socioeconomic or marital status.

→ Assess the patient's safety as well as that of her children or other family/household members who may be at risk for injury or death.

→ Inquire specifically about threats of homicide or suicidal intent.

→ Assess living arrangements and support system (family, friends, community).

→ Refer the patient and her family to community resources, including legal services, shelters, law enforcement agencies, and counseling services.

→ Specific legal guidelines exist regarding the reporting of domestic violence, child abuse, and suicidal or homicidal intent.

→ Notify police only at the request of the patient or when the law requires it.

→ Use caution when prescribing sedatives, tranquilizers, or antidepressants. They could be used by the patient in a suicide attempt.

→ Assist the patient in developing an escape plan (see "Patient Education").

→ Guard patient confidentiality and never give out information pertaining to the patient's whereabouts, health care, or appointment times.

→ Utilize empowerment strategies to build self-esteem in female patients of all ages (see "Patient Education").

→ Assist males—especially children and adolescents—in identifying alternative ways to express anger and to improve communication with females.

CONSULTATION

→ Physician consultation is required in cases involving serious injuries/medical conditions.

→ Social service referral should be made in cases involving child abuse or to identify additional legal, law enforcement, housing, financial, and counseling services.

→ Referral to psychological/psychiatric services should be made in suspected cases of psychological disorders or substance abuse.

→ Assistance should be sought with emergency mental health and/or law enforcement services in instances of suicidal or homicidal intent.

PATIENT EDUCATION

→ Encourage all female patients to pursue education, employment, and other means of self-actualization to empower themselves and build self-esteem.

→ Teach women to control their fertility through available methods of contraception and abortion services.

- This can have an empowering effect as well as help them avoid an unwanted pregnancy, which could lead to more episodes of abuse.

→ Inform teens and young women that violence and abuse are not a normal part of intimate relationships.

- Help them avoid potential abusers—men who seem very jealous, overprotective, or controlling; have a history of substance or alcohol abuse; or exhibit violent behavior toward animals, objects, or other people.

→ Let the patient know she is free to discuss this issue with you and encourage her to do so.

- Explore the health consequences of battering for her, her children, and other family/household members. Teach the patient that children who are abused may be more likely to abuse or be abused as adults.

→ Educate the patient about the cycle of violence and explain that without intervention, violent episodes will likely increase in both frequency and severity.

→ Provide the patient with referral information for legal, law enforcement, shelter, financial, and counseling services.

- The National Hotline on Domestic Violence provides information for staff and victims: (800) 799-SAFE (telecommunications device for the deaf [800] 873-6363).
- The National Coalition against Domestic Violence provides a network of shelters and counseling programs: P.O. Box 34103, Washington, D.C. 20043-4103, (202) 638-6388.

→ Assist the patient with the development of an escape plan.

→ Caution the patient about documents that the abuser may see inadvertently (e.g., referrals, health education materials, work/school excuses, or discharge materials).

FOLLOW-UP

→ See "Consultation."

→ Continue to monitor at future visits. Consider these patients to be high-risk and follow them with more frequent visits and telephone contact.

→ Be aware that changes in life situation (e.g., unemployment, pregnancy, leaving the abusive relationship) may increase the chances of the patient being abused.

→ On rare occasions, the health care provider may be required to testify if the patient decides to pursue legal action against her batterer.

→ Document findings in progress notes and on problem list in a clear, precise, and comprehensive fashion using diagrams, measurements, and photographs (if the patient consents).

- Because this information might be used for legal purposes, adhere to state and local requirements, including those regarding documentation, consent, and specimen collection.

BIBLIOGRAPHY

American Medical Association. 1992. Diagnostic and treatment guidelines on domestic violence. *Archives of Family Medicine* 1:39–47.

Archer, J. 2000. Sex differences in aggression between heterosexual partners: a meta-analytic review. *Psychological Bulletin* 126(5):651–680.

Bash, K.L., and Jones, F. 1994. Domestic violence in America. *North Carolina Medical Journal* 55(9):400–403.

Berrios, D.D., and Grady, D. 1991. Domestic violence risk factors and outcomes. *Western Journal of Medicine* 155:133–135.

Campbell, J. 1986. Nursing assessment for risk of homicide with battered women. *Annals of Nursing Science* 8:36–51.

Centers for Disease Control and Prevention (CDC). 1998. Rural health-care providers' attitudes, practices and training experience regarding intimate partner violence—West Virginia, March 1997. *Morbidity and Mortality Weekly Report* 47(32):670–673.

———. 2000a. Intimate partner violence among men and women—South Carolina, 1998. *Morbidity and Mortality Weekly Report* 49(30):691–694.

———. 2000b. Use of medical care, police assistance, and restraining orders by women reporting intimate partner violence—Massachusetts, 1996–1997. *Morbidity and Mortality Weekly Report* 49(30):485–488.

———. 2000c. Prevalence of intimate partner violence and injuries—Washington, 1998. *Morbidity and Mortality Weekly Report* 49(30):589–592.

———. 2001. Surveillance for homicide among intimate partners—United States, 1981–1998. *Morbidity and Mortality Weekly Report* 50(SS-3):1–15.

Coker, A.L., Smith P.H., McKeown, R.E. et al. 2000. Frequency and correlates of intimate partner violence by type: physical, sexual, and psychological battering. *American Journal of Public Health* 90(4):553–559.

Federal Bureau of Investigation (FBI). 1998. *FBI uniform crime reports.* Washington, D.C.: Department of Justice.

Garcia-Moreno, C. 2000. Violence against women. International perspectives. *American Journal of Preventive Medicine* 19(4):330–333.

Hall, D., and Lynch M.A. 1998. Violence begins at home. *British Medical Journal* 316:1551–1560.

Hamberger, L.K., and Potente, T. 1994. Counseling heterosexual women arrested for domestic violence: implications for theory and practice. *Violence and Victims* 9(2):125–137.

Heise, L.L., Ellsberg, M., and Gottemoeller, M. 1999. Ending violence against women. *1999 Johns Hopkins University School of Public Health, Population Information Program* (Population Reports Series L. 1999, No. 11). Baltimore, Md.: Johns Hopkins University.

Kernic, M.A., Wolf, M.E., and Holt, V.L. 2000. Rates and relative risk of hospital admission among women in violent intimate partner relationships. *American Journal of Public Health* 90(9):1416–1420.

McCaw, B., Berman, W.H., Syme, S.L. et al. 2001. Beyond screening for domestic violence: a systems model approach in a managed care setting. *American Journal of Preventive Medicine* 21(3):170–176.

McFarlane, J., Parker, B., and Soeken, K. 1996. Physical abuse, smoking, and substance use during pregnancy: prevalence, interrelationships, and effects on birth weight. *Journal of Obstetric, Gynecologic, and Neonatal Nursing* 25(4):313–320.

McKay, M.M. 1994. The link between domestic violence and child abuse: assessment and treatment considerations. *Child Welfare* 73(1):29–39.

McLear, S.V., Anwar, R., Herman, S. et al. 1989. Education is not enough: a systems failure in protecting battered women. *Annals of Emergency Surgery* 18(6):651–653.

Moss, V. 1991. Battered women and the myth of masochism. *Journal of Psychosocial Nursing* 29(7):19–23.

Packer, I.K. 1990. Domestic violence: the role of the mental health expert. *Medicine and Law* 9(6):1274–1276.

Parker, B., McFarlane, B., and Soeken, K. 1994. Abuse during pregnancy: effects on maternal complications and birth weight in adult and teenage women. *Obstetrics & Gynecology* 84(3):323–328.

Parkinson, G.W., Adams, R.C., and Emerling, F.G. 2001. Maternal domestic violence screening in an office-based pediatric practice. *Pediatrics* 108(3):E43.

Parsons, L.H., and Harper, M.A. 1999. Violent maternal deaths in North Carolina. *Obstetrics & Gynecology* 94(6):990–993.

Randall, T. 1990. Domestic violence intervention calls for more than treating injuries. *Journal of the American Medical Association* 264(8):939–940.

Shannon, M.T., and Sammons, L.N. 2000. Battered woman/perinatal violence, eds. W.L. Star, M.T. Shannon, L.L. Lommel et al. In *Ambulatory obstetrics,* 3rd ed., pp. 329–337. San Francisco, Calif.: University of California.

Soler, H., Vinayak, P., and Quadagno, D. 2000. Biosocial aspects of domestic violence. *Psychoneuroendocrinology* 25:721–739.

Stacey, W., and Shupe, A. 1983. *The family secret.* Boston: Beacon Press.

Stark, E., and Flitcraft, A. 1988. Women and children at risk: a feminist perspective on child abuse. *International Journal of Health Services* 18(1):97–118.

Waalen, J., Goodwin, M.M., Spitz, A.M. et al. 2000. Screening for intimate partner violence by health care providers. Barriers and interventions. *American Journal of Preventive Medicine* 19(4):230–237.

Walker, L. 1984. *The battered woman syndrome.* New York: Springer.

Warshaw, C. 1989. Limitations of the medical model in the care of battered women. *Gender and Society* 3(4):506–517.

14-E

Eating Disorders

Anorexia nervosa (AN) and *bulimia nervosa* (BN) are characterized by severe disturbances in eating behavior (American Psychiatric Association [APA] 2000). The age of onset of these eating disorders is typically in adolescence or early adult life, with the ratio of females to males 10:1. The etiology of eating disorders is still poorly understood, but genetic, biological, psychological, and cultural factors appear to play a role (Walsh et al. 1998).

Anorexia nervosa and bulimia nervosa seem to be related, occurring concurrently in an estimated 50% of cases. When they occur concurrently, treatment is more difficult and the prognosis is poorer. The prevalence of these conditions has increased considerably over the last 30 years. For anorexia nervosa, the prevalence is approximately 0.5% of females in late adolescence and early adulthood (APA 2000). For bulimia nervosa, the prevalence ranges from 1–3% of college-age women (APA 2000).

Anorexia nervosa is characterized by self-imposed starvation. The anorexic person becomes obsessed with food, weight, counting calories, and vigorous exercise. Bulimia nervosa is characterized by binge eating (eating large amounts of food) followed by some form of purging as a means of controlling weight. The most common means of purging is self-induced vomiting, which frequently happens immediately or soon after a binge. During the binge, patients commonly drink excessive fluids to "float the food" and facilitate regurgitation. Other forms of purging include diuretics, laxative use, and enemas.

The *Diagnostic and Statistical Manual of Mental Disorders (DSM-IV TR)* (APA 2000) specifies two types for each of these disorders. Anorexia nervosa is either the binge eating/purging type or the restricting type. The former is characterized by binge-eating or purging behaviors regularly in the current episode. In restricting type anorexia nervosa, the patient is not regularly engaging in these behaviors during the current episode. Bulimia nervosa is either the purging or nonpurging type, depending on whether the patient is regularly engaging in purging behaviors during the current episode. All criteria outlined in the *DSM-IV TR* for each of these disorders must be present to make the diagnosis. (See **Table 14E.1, Diagnostic Crite-**

ria for Anorexia Nervosa and **Table 14E.2, Diagnostic Criteria for Bulimia Nervosa**.)

Depression is strongly associated with both anorexia and bulimia. Feelings of worthlessness and helplessness are present in the anorexic as a result of her obsession with perfection (Garner et al. 1985). Major depression is more likely to be present in the bulimia patient, and the more severe the bulimia, the higher the likelihood of severe depression. It has been postulated that depression may be a symptom of eating disorders rather than a frequent comorbid condition, as increased or decreased appetite is a symptom characteristic of depressive disorders (Troop et al. 2001). Low self-esteem is characteristic of both disorders. Shame and guilt in relation to eating are experienced in higher levels in anorexics and bulimics than in the normal population, and anxiety levels tend to increase with purgative behavior (Frank 1991).

Anorexic patients have strong self-control, which is manifested as they deprive themselves of food and drink to avoid gaining weight. Conversely, bulimics lack control and discipline. Yet both conditions result from a negative body image and dissatisfaction with body size. For a more thorough discussion of the characteristics of these disorders, see the "Database" section of this chapter.

Other eating disorder diagnoses should be considered when a patient presents with signs and symptoms of AN or BN. The *eating disorder not otherwise specified* (EDNOS) category is also provided in the *DSM-IV TR* (APA 2000) for those patients who have the psychopathology of an eating disorder but do not fully meet the strict criteria of anorexia or bulimia nervosa. A large percentage of patients with eating disorders (25–60%) fall into this category (Andersen et al. 2001, APA 2000). It includes: 1) When the patient meets all criteria for AN, but either has regular menses or her current weight is normal despite significant weight loss; 2) when the patient meets all criteria for BN but the binge eating and compensatory mechanisms are present less than twice a week and for a duration of less than three months; 3) when inappropriate behaviors are displayed regularly by a woman with normal weight after eating small amounts of food or when large amounts of food are chewed and spit out but not swallowed;

and 4) when there are recurring episodes of binge eating without regular use of the inappropriate compensatory behaviors of BN.

The *Diagnostic and Statistical Manual for Primary Care (DSM-PC)* published by the American Academy of Pediatrics also has a classification for those patients who do not meet the *DSM-IV TR* criteria for anorexia or bulimia nervosa (APA 2000, Wolraich et al. 1996). This classification is based on two specific complexes of eating disorders: 1) dieting/body image behavior and 2) purging/binge behavior. It also addresses two levels of pathology for these two behavior patterns: *variations*, which constitute minor deviations from normal but are still a concern to the clinician or the parent, and *problems*, which constitute a serious manifestation and early evidence of an eating disorder. For a complete review of this classification, the reader is referred to an excellent article by Kreipe et al. (1999).

This chapter addresses anorexia and bulimia nervosa as defined in the *DSM-IV TR* (APA 2000). The usual onset of AN is between 14–18 years; it rarely occurs in women over age 40. The course is highly variable. Some women recover fully after one episode, some fluctuate between weight gain and relapse, and others experience unrelenting weight loss, which results in debilitating illness or death (APA 2000). The median time for partial recovery is 60 months and for full recovery, 80 months. Full recovery before 70 months is rare (Vitiello et al. 2000). Women with AN, restricting type, may develop binge eating. If this symptom is persistent and accompanied by weight gain, the diagnosis should change to BN. The mortality rate from AN is approximately 5% per decade of follow-up (Sullivan 1995), the highest of any psychiatric illness. Death usually results from the complications of starvation, electrolyte imbalance, or suicide. The course of BN is usually intermittent over a period of years.

Table 14E.1. DIAGNOSTIC CRITERIA FOR ANOREXIA NERVOSA

A. Refusal to maintain body weight at or above a minimally normal weight for age and height (e.g., weight loss leading to maintenance of body weight less than 85% of that expected or failure to make expected weight gain during period of growth, leading to body weight less than 85% of that expected).

B. Intense fear of gaining weight or becoming fat, even though underweight.

C. Disturbance in the way in which one's body weight or shape is experienced, undue influence of body weight or shape on self-evaluation, or denial of the seriousness of the current low body weight.

D. In postmenarcheal females, amenorrhea—i.e., the absence of at least three consecutive menstrual cycles. (A woman is considered to have amenorrhea if her periods occur only following hormone [e.g., estrogen] administration.)

Specify type:

Restricting type: During the current episode of anorexia nervosa, the person has not regularly engaged in binge-eating or purging behavior (i.e., self-induced vomiting or the misuse of laxatives, diuretics, or enemas).

Binge-eating/purging type: During the current episode of anorexia nervosa, the person has regularly engaged in binge-eating or purging behavior (i.e., self-induced vomiting or the misuse of laxatives, diuretics, or enemas).

Source: Reprinted with permission from American Psychiatric Association. 2000. *Diagnostic and statistical manual of mental disorders,* 4th ed. (text revision). Washington, D.C.: the Author.

Table 14E.2. DIAGNOSTIC CRITERIA FOR BULIMIA NERVOSA

A. Recurrent episodes of binge eating. An episode of binge eating is characterized by both of the following:
1. Eating, in a discrete period of time (e.g., within any two-hour period), an amount of food that is definitely larger than most people would eat during a similar period of time and under similar circumstances, and
2. A sense of lack of control over eating during the episode (e.g., a feeling that one cannot stop eating or control what or how much one is eating).

B. Recurrent inappropriate compensatory behavior in order to prevent weight gain, such as self-induced vomiting; misuse of laxatives, diuretics, enemas, or other medications; fasting; or excessive exercise.

C. The binge eating and inappropriate compensatory behaviors both occur, on average, at least twice a week for three months.

D. Self-evaluation is unduly influenced by body shape and weight.

E. The disturbance does not occur exclusively during episodes of anorexia nervosa.

Specify type:

Purging type: During the current episode of bulimia nervosa, the person has regularly engaged in self-induced vomiting or the misuse of laxatives, diuretics, or enemas.

Nonpurging type: During the current episode of bulimia nervosa, the person has used other inappropriate compensatory behaviors, such as fasting or excessive exercise, but has not regularly engaged in self-induced vomiting or the misuse of laxatives, diuretics, or enemas.

Source: Reprinted with permission from American Psychiatric Association. 2000. *Diagnostic and statistical manual of mental disorders,* 4th ed. (text revision). Washington, D.C.: the Author.

While anorexics may need hospitalization to prevent death from starvation, bulimics are seldom incapacitated by their disease. Instead, they have a high relapse rate. A five-year follow-up study on bulimics indicates that 10–25% of patients continue to meet the criteria for BN, more than 50% continue to have an eating disorder of clinical significance, 40% continue to meet the criteria for major depressive disorder, and self-esteem remains low (Fairburn et al. 2000).

Individuals with anorexia nervosa or bulimia nervosa are usually very secretive. Patients rarely volunteer information about their eating patterns (Ressler 1998). Families and friends may be unaware of their disease for years. Symptoms are often subclinical until the disease is advanced, which places the patients at risk for significant morbidity and mortality before the diagnosis is made. Anorexics usually are detected earlier than bulimics due to the anorexic's obvious physical condition. Diagnosing bulimia may be more difficult because bulimics may appear physically healthy with a normal (or close to normal) weight.

Medical/health, personal, social, and family health histories can provide important clues in diagnosing eating disorders:

→ A routine thorough history (and physical examination) starting early in adolescence may help discover the disease at an earlier stage.

→ Bulimia nervosa has been shown to be related to a history of sexual abuse. This association may complicate the treatment, particularly if there are also concurrent psychiatric comorbid conditions, such as substance abuse, borderline personality disorder, or post-traumatic stress disorder (Wonderlich et al. 1997).

→ Eating disorders as well as attitudes toward shape and weight seem to run in families.

→ A careful dietary history should be obtained for all women that includes eating patterns, attempts at weight loss (dieting may set off an eating disorder), and the presence of any method of purging. Equally helpful is a history of the patient's previous weights and her perceived ideal body weight (Patton et al. 1999).

DATABASE
SUBJECTIVE

Anorexia Nervosa

→ Age of onset is early to late adolescence.

→ More common in women from educated and prosperous homes

→ Amenorrhea (absence of three consecutive cycles) or delayed menarche

→ An anorexic is often someone who:
- Has an intense fear of being fat or gaining weight, even though she is underweight
- Denies or refuses to acknowledge underweight as a problem
- Is frantically preoccupied with food and eating and has an intense fear of becoming fat, even though she is underweight

- Restricts her food intake even though her appetite is not decreased
- Tends to have obsessive-compulsive behavior, manifested in some cases by over-involvement in exercise
- Has a negative attitude toward herself and a distorted body image, viewing herself as larger than she is
- Uses eating or refusing to eat as a way of achieving a sense of control and a "solution" to feelings of powerlessness, ineffectiveness, and incompetence
- May fear loss of control over her eating. In this case, the anorexic patient may binge and purge like a bulimic, suffering from a combination of anorexia and bulimia symptoms. Fifty percent of anorexic patients may exhibit bulimic behavior; the main differentiating factor is the severe weight loss in anorexia (Garner et al. 1985).
- Anorectic individuals of the binge eating type are more likely to have an increased amount of mood liability, abuse alcohol or other drugs, be sexually active, have greater frequency of suicide attempts, and have borderline personality disorder (APA 2000).
- Is described by others as a perfectionist, as a successful individual

→ Medical/health history may reveal:
- Depression: occurs in approximately 50% of anorexics. May be secondary to the physiological sequelae of semi-starvation.
- Comorbidity with an obsessive-compulsive or personality disorder
- Fractures as a result of low estrogen levels, calcium depletion, and increased cortisol secretion, which leads to decreased bone density and, in chronic cases, to osteoporosis (Walsh et al. 1998)
- Excessive dieting, fasting, and/or exercise for weight loss
- Patient requests advice regarding diet for weight loss or prescription for diuretics or laxatives
- Mildly overweight patient prior to onset of anorexia

→ Personal/social history may reveal:
- Poor family communication skills
- Nonexistent family meals or meals that are no longer an enjoyable experience
- Dieting as an important part of the family ritual
- High achievement expected in family. Patient may feel uncomfortable receiving the support/affection that is necessary to reach the high expectations.
- Sexual molestation in early years by a family member or neighbor.
- Decreased interest in sex (more common in restricting type)
- A recent stressful situation

→ Family history may be positive for:
- Anorexia nervosa in sisters and/or mother
- A higher frequency of depression and bipolar disorder in first-degree biological relatives
- Maternal obesity

→ Patient may complain of:
- Feeling of fullness

- Constipation, sometimes accompanied by abdominal pain
- Insomnia and early awakening
- Feeling cold even on hot days
- Symptoms associated with severe weight loss:
  - Dry skin and hair
  - Cold hands and feet
  - General weakness
  - Nausea
  - Loss of appetite (late in illness, rare)
  - Abnormal body hair (lanugo)

Bulimia Nervosa

→ Age of onset is adolescence or early adult life.

→ A bulimic is often an individual who:
- Binge eats, with episodes occurring on average of at least twice a week for at least three months
- Is preoccupied with food and dieting, and has an excessive desire to lose weight. Fears being overweight. This fear manifests itself in a restrictive eating pattern, excessive exercise routines, or purging behavior (self-induced vomiting, misuse of laxatives, diuretics, and rarely enemas or ipecac use).
- Has a distorted body image—believes she is overweight, even though she is normal or slightly below or above her expected weight
- Believes that specific parts of her body are too large (e.g., buttocks, thighs) (Herzog et al. 1991)
- Has low self-esteem, high anxiety levels, and communication problems
- Lacks control and discipline, blaming symptoms on others
- Has compulsive behaviors, which may lead to stealing in order to obtain high-calorie foods and laxatives

→ Medical/health history may reveal:
- Weekly weight fluctuations of up to 20 pounds (Yates et al. 1984)
- Depressive mood, most often major depression or dysthymia
- Coexisting personality disorder, most commonly borderline, antisocial, histrionic, or narcissistic (Ames-Frankel et al. 1992)
- History of anorexia nervosa (up to one-third of patients)
- Overweight in the past
- Excessive exercise (though not as driven as anorexics)
- Excessive use of laxatives, diuretics, or enemas
- Alcohol and drug abuse (particularly amphetamines). Alcohol consumption happens significantly less during binge eating episodes but may precipitate food binging (Wolfe et al. 2000).
- In severe cases, history of convulsions (due to electrolyte imbalance, hypoglycemia, or alcohol binges), esophagitis, pharyngitis, poor dentition, or unusual enamel damage (due to repeated vomiting)

→ Personal/social history may reveal:
- Eating binges that start during, or immediately following, a diet

- Problematic family interactions, parents over-involved or emotionally detached
- Family member(s) extremely concerned about their own weight and/or dieting
- Divorced parents
- Stressful or traumatic situation within six months of disorder onset (e.g., going to college, being criticized for being fat)
- Childhood sexual abuse (more strongly associated with BN than with AN restricting type)
- Sexual promiscuity, lying, stealing, self-mutilation, or other manifestations of a personality disorder (Kreipe et al. 2000)

→ Family history may be positive for:
- Anorexia nervosa or bulimia nervosa in a first-degree relative
- Obesity in parents
- Major depression in a first-degree biological relative
- Alcoholism in first-degree relatives (this is controversial) (Wolfe et al. 2000)

→ Patient may complain of symptoms that are secondary to binge eating, fasting, vomiting, ipecac use, or laxative or diuretic use (Herzog et al. 1991, McGilley et al. 1998):
- Fatigue, nervousness, insomnia (all also related to emotional distress)
- Sensitivity to cold
- Frequent or severe headaches
- Sore throat
- Abdominal pain and distention
- Constipation
- Nausea
- Sensitive teeth
- Menstrual irregularities

→ Less common complaints (seen with increasing severity of disturbance):
- Facial skin dry and scaly, hair thin/fine (lanugo)
- Heartburn
- Racing, irregular heartbeat
- Chest pain
- Salivary gland enlargement
- Edema in hands or feet
- Cramping of muscles in the feet and legs (due to electrolyte imbalance)
- Muscle weakness (due to hyponatremia and electrolyte imbalance)
- Excessive gastric pain and blood in vomitus (should be considered a medical emergency)

→ Obtaining a dietary history and history of eating patterns is essential and will assist in meal planning.

OBJECTIVE

Anorexia Nervosa

→ General appearance: the patient may be wearing layers of clothing to hide her physical appearance and to keep warm.

→ Body weight is 15% below normal or body mass index (calculated as weight in kg/height in m²) is equal to or below 17.5.
→ Delayed puberty and/or menarche
→ The following physical findings may be present as a result of prolonged state of starvation and being underweight:
  ▪ Bradycardia: 44–60 beats per minute
  ▪ Hypotension: 74/40–90/50 (Some blood pressure measurements need to be obtained with a pediatric cuff.)
  ▪ Hypothermia: rectal body temperatures as low as 35.0°–35.6° C
  ▪ Decreased respiratory rate
  ▪ Muscular weakness and/or atrophy
→ Cardiovascular system (Kalager et al. 1978):
  ▪ Heart murmurs
  ▪ Mitral valve prolapse, which can reverse with weight gain (Walsh et al. 2000)
  ▪ Cardiac arrhythmia
  ▪ Decreased peripheral circulation
  ▪ Acrocyanosis
  ▪ EKG abnormalities
  ▪ Raynaud's phenomenon
→ Skin/hair/dental problems:
  ▪ Pale, dry, flaky facial skin
  ▪ Lanugo (fine body hair) around vermillion border of lips, lower border of mandible, and extremities
  ▪ Yellowish or bronze skin color (due to elevated beta-carotene)
  ▪ Alopecia
  ▪ Skin lesions
  ▪ Dental problems if purging type (See bulimia for dental problems related to vomiting.)
→ Mental status:
  ▪ Fixed delusion about body size and shape
  ▪ Thought: dichotomous thinking (all or nothing, black or white)
  ▪ Low sense of self-worth
  ▪ Difficulty thinking clearly
→ Laboratory findings (may be present as a result of starvation and electrolyte imbalance):
  ▪ Mild anemia (normochromic normocytic anemia) (APA 2000). Can have also megaloblastic anemia secondary to vitamin B_{12} or folate deficiency and/or microcytic anemia secondary to iron deficiency (if still menstruating or having gastrointestinal bleeding).
  ▪ Leukopenia
  ▪ Elevated beta-carotene levels
  ▪ Mild elevation of liver function test
  ▪ Mild hypoglycemia
  ▪ Elevated blood urea nitrogen (BUN) level if dehydration, or low if poor protein intake
  ▪ Hypercholesterolemia, often excessively elevated in starvation states
  ▪ Hypercortisolemia, hypomagnesemia, hypozincemia, hypophosphatemia, and hyperamylasemia are occasionally present.

▪ Induced vomiting may lead to metabolic alkalosis (elevated serum bicarbonate), hypochloremia, and hypokalemia, or mixed alkalosis and acidosis if starvation is also present.
▪ Decreased glomerular filtration rate
▪ Decreased concentrating capacity of kidneys
▪ Urinary calculi
▪ Acute renal failure (rare)
▪ Serum thyroxine (T4) levels are usually in the low-normal range; serum triiodothyronine (T3) levels are decreased ("sick euthyroid syndrome").
▪ Low serum estrogen levels

Bulimia Nervosa

→ Most often, bulimics appear healthy or have few physical findings.
→ Body weight is normal or slightly above normal.
→ Physical findings are a product of medical complications that occur from excessive vomiting, binging, restrictive cycles, or abuse of laxatives, diuretics, or emetics. These include:
  ▪ Dental enamel erosion
  ▪ Buccal erosion
  ▪ Increased number of cavities
  ▪ Loss of teeth
  ▪ Abrasion or callus on index or middle finger (near or at first knuckle) of dominant hand (Russell's sign); may be absent but its presence strongly suggests BN.
  ▪ Palatal petechiae (in severe cases)
  ▪ Facial ecchymosis and blood vessel hemorrhages in and around the eyes (in severe cases)
  ▪ Sore, erythematous tongue
  ▪ Epigastric tenderness
  ▪ Dry skin, hair loss, acrocyanosis, and decreased capillary refill
  ▪ Bilateral, nontender parotid or submandibular gland enlargement
  ▪ Cardiac arrhythmias
  ▪ Hypotension or orthostatic hypotension (if hypovolemia from vomiting or laxative use)
  ▪ Hypertension if excessive weight gain
  ▪ Peripheral edema (due to rebound fluid retention)
  ▪ Mental status: dichotomous thinking (all or nothing, black or white), low self-esteem. Obsessive compulsive symptoms as in AN. Displays impulsiveness and novelty-seeking tendencies (Vitiello et al. 2000).
→ Rare complications of bulimia are cardiomyopathy due to ipecac abuse, cardiac arrest, and esophageal tears, and gastric rupture due to induced vomiting.
→ Most laboratory findings are within normal limits unless bulimia nervosa is advanced. Purging type behavior is much more likely to be associated with abnormal lab results, chiefly electrolyte disturbances.
→ Advanced cases may include:
  ▪ Electrolyte imbalance, which may be evidenced by:
    • Metabolic alkalosis (vomiting)/acidosis (diarrhea)
    • Hypokalemia

- Hypochloremia
- Hyponatremia
- Hypocalcemia
- Hypomagnesemia (if large amounts of watery diarrhea)
- Metabolic alkalosis is not seen until the patient is vomiting at least three times a day; it corrects quickly after the cessation of vomiting (Kreipe et al. 1999).
- Elevated cholesterol levels
- Anemia (as a result of malnutrition or hemoconcentration)
- Increased BUN (indicates volume depletion)
- Urine positive for ketone and protein (indicates deficiency in carbohydrate metabolism related to starvation)
- Urine-specific gravity may be elevated if the patient is dehydrated or lowered if the patient is over-hydrated with water to temporarily increase her weight.
- EKG may show flat or inverted T-waves, U-waves, or ST-segment depression.
- Stool for occult blood may be positive if esophageal ulcers, tears, or gastric rupture have occurred (a rare but severe complication).

ASSESSMENT

→ Anorexia nervosa
- Binge-eating/purging type
  - R/O bulimia nervosa
- Restrictive type
  - R/O physical disorders (e.g., occult malignancy, malabsorption syndromes, hyperthyroidism, diabetes mellitus, brain tumors, acquired immunodeficiency syndrome [AIDS])
  - R/O depressive disorder
  - R/O schizophrenia
  - R/O social phobia, obsessive-compulsive disorder, or body dysmorphic disorder
→ Bulimia nervosa
- Purging type
  - R/O anorexia nervosa, restrictive type (purging may be undisclosed)
- Nonpurging type
  - R/O anorexia nervosa, binge-eating/purging type (if binge eating occurs with full criteria for anorexia nervosa)
  - R/O personality disorder (binge eating present but not full criteria for bulimia nervosa)
  - R/O depressive disorder (commonly major depression)
  - R/O schizophrenia
→ Eating disorder not otherwise specified (abnormal eating behavior that does not fully meet the criteria for any specific eating disorder)

PLAN

DIAGNOSTIC TESTS

→ The SCOFF questionnaire (see **Table 14E.3, SCOFF Questionnaire**) has been tested in clinical settings to identify women with eating disorders. It has a sensitivity of 100% and a specificity of 87.5% for both disorders separately and

Table 14E.3. SCOFF QUESTIONNAIRE

Do you make yourself **S**ick because you feel uncomfortably full?
Do you worry that you have lost **C**ontrol over how much you eat?
Have you recently lost more than **O**ne stone (14 pounds/6.3 kg) in a three-month period?
Do you believe yourself to be **F**at when others say you are too thin?
Would you say that **F**ood dominates your life?

NOTE: Score one point for every "yes." A score of 2 or more is a likely indication of anorexia nervosa or bulimia.

Source: Reprinted with permission from Morgan, J.F., Reid, F., and Lacey J.H. 1999. The SCOFF questionnaire: assessment of a new screening tool for eating disorders. *British Medical Journal* 319:1467.

combined. The initial letter of the core concept of each of the five questions provides the acronym SCOFF. If this instrument is validated in the general population, it may provide an effective, acceptable, and simple screening tool for use in diagnosing eating disorders (Morgan et al. 1999).

Anorexia Nervosa

→ No specific diagnostic tests are indicated in clinical practice.
→ Additional diagnostic tests as indicated under "Objective" to rule out complications.
- Routine screening tests (to establish a baseline, not to establish diagnosis) may include:
  - CBC with differential
  - BUN
  - Creatinine
  - TSH
  - Urinalysis
  - Serum electrolytes
    - If vomiting, serum electrolytes should be monitored closely (particularly potassium and carbon dioxide).
- Consider the following tests if the patient is severely malnourished or has persistent symptoms related to cardiac dysfunction:
  - EKG
  - Blood chemistry studies:
    - Calcium level
    - Magnesium level
    - Phosphorus level
    - Liver function tests
  - Urine dipstick for ketones
  - Bone densitometry to assess severity of bone loss, especially if the patient has been underweight for more than six months
  - Estradiol levels
  - FSH/LH and prolactin may be indicated to evaluate amenorrhea (see the **Amenorrhea—Secondary** chapter in Section 12).

Bulimia Nervosa

→ Urine dipstick for ketones, protein, and specific gravity

→ A urine sodium to urine chloride ratio >1.16 is a useful predictor of BN. This may be helpful in early identification and monitoring, particularly for patients vomiting more than seven times per week (Crow et al. 2001).

→ Measure magnesium levels in those who abuse laxatives (Kreipe et al. 2000).

→ Additional diagnostic tests as indicated under "Objective" to rule out complications

- Routine screening tests (to establish a baseline, not to establish diagnosis) may include:
  - CBC with differential
  - Blood chemistry studies
  - BUN
  - Creatinine
  - TSH
  - Lipid profile
  - Urine chemistry and microscopic testing
  - If vomiting, electrolytes should be monitored (particularly potassium and carbon dioxide).
  - EKG baseline may be indicated if patient has persistent symptoms that may affect cardiac function.

TREATMENT/MANAGEMENT

→ The most important role for the nurse practitioner (NP)/primary care provider (PCP) in the management of eating disorders is prevention and early diagnosis. In addition, the NP/PCP can serve as the case manager of a multidisciplinary team.

→ Because dieting may set up an eating disorder, particularly in young girls, weight loss should not be the only intervention in overweight individuals. Rather, the approach should emphasize wellness, establishing sustainable patterns of enjoyable exercise, good nutrition, positive interpersonal relationships, and an ability to manage stress effectively (Patton et al. 1999, Ressler 1998).

- A dietary history and corroboration with family or friends regarding intake may be helpful, especially for high-risk adolescents (e.g., engaging in activities that require a lean figure such as dancing, modeling, or acting).

→ Initiating treatment for the anorexic or bulimic patient may be very difficult because of *denial*, a key feature of these eating disorders.

- If denial is present and the clinician highly suspects an eating disorder, directing questions to the patient that address the diagnostic criteria of the *DSM-IV TR* can help identify patients who have the disorder (APA 2000).

- Many anorexics and bulimics, as well as their families, do not recognize the severity of the disorder. Discussing the signs, symptoms, and laboratory findings can provide the patient with her first awareness of this condition and motivate her and her family to obtain treatment (Powers 1990).

- Anorexia and bulimia patients may respond with anger, shame, and tears as a result of "being discovered."

→ Medical consultation is indicated, and management by a multidisciplinary team experienced in these types of disorders (including physician/nurse practitioner, nutritionist, psychiatrist, social worker, psychologist, or other professionals experienced in eating disorder management) is recommended in confirmed cases.

→ Setting an ideal weight should be an important goal in managing eating disorder patients. Ideal body weight based on expected height may provide a better standard than body mass index measurements in young girls if there is growth failure (Steiner et al. 1998).

→ Patients can benefit from psychological treatment modalities such as individual, group, family, or marital psychotherapy (Becker et al. 1999). Most of the psychological treatment modalities have a psychodynamic and/or cognitive/behavioral orientation, described in depth in Garner et al. (1985). For simple but handy suggestions about the behavioral/cognitive approach to the management of bulimia nervosa—which can also be applied to the anorexic patient—the reader is referred to an excellent article by Yanovsky (1991).

→ Evaluate depression and suicide risk in all eating disorder patients (see the **Depression** chapter).

→ Referral to dental care as indicated for evaluation and treatment of patients who purge with vomiting.

→ Discontinuation of diuretics or laxatives may temporarily lead to fluid retention and weight gain. A moderate restriction of sodium intake on a short-term basis may help if the patient is distressed by the weight gain (Yanovsky 1991).

→ Potassium supplementation is required if hypokalemia is present. For values ≥2.8 mEq, give 20–80 mEq of potassium chloride p.o. every day: QD–TID dosing until normal serum levels are achieved. Patients with potassium levels <2.8 mEq should be considered for parenteral treatment and hospitalization (Herzog et al. 1985). For mild cases, increasing the intake of foods rich in potassium may normalize the potassium level.

Anorexia Nervosa

→ The goals of treatment for AN include normalizing body weight, correcting the emotional preoccupation with weight loss, and preventing relapse (Walsh et al. 1998).

→ Other goals include treating physical complications and associated psychiatric disorders, enhancing the patient's motivation to cooperate with treatment, providing education about healthy nutrition and eating habits, and enlisting family support (APA 2000).

- The minimum goal for weight gain should be 90% of ideal weight for height according to standard tables. A preferred goal is to achieve sufficient weight gain to restore menstruation and ovulation, or normal sexual development if the individual is premenarcheal (APA 2000).

- Restoration of body weight can be accomplished in specialized eating disorder units, with or without patient cooperation. Psychological problems are harder to treat and relapses are common.

■ Specific strategies for gaining weight include admission to an inpatient hospital or day-treatment program, a prescribed 2,000–4,000 calorie diet provided in a controlled environment, and close supervision of meals and exercise.

■ Patients may experience resurgence of anxiety and depression as weight is gained. Therefore, it is important to reassess for signs and symptoms of mood disturbance as normal weight is restored (APA 2000).

→ Psychological treatment modalities should be initiated after urgent medical issues are resolved (APA 2000, Becker et al. 1999).

■ Cognitive behavior psychotherapy, interpersonal therapy, psychodynamic psychotherapy, or family therapy is recommended for the treatment of AN. They all play an important role in ameliorating symptoms and preventing relapse.

■ Family therapy is particularly helpful if there is a family history of eating disorders and if the illness is of early onset and short duration.

→ Medication is now considered in the treatment of anorexia, but it should not be the sole or primary treatment. Antidepressants are ineffective in promoting food intake and weight gain, but they may prevent relapse after weight goals are achieved (Kaye et al. 1997). They may also be helpful in weight maintenance (Kaye et al. 1991). Antidepressants are also commonly considered for patients with anorexia whose depressive, obsessive, or compulsive symptoms persist in spite of, or in the absence of, weight gain.

■ Selective serotonin reuptake inhibitors (SSRIs) are the safest antidepressants. Fluoxetine is most commonly prescribed at doses of 40 mg p.o. QD.

■ Estrogen replacement without weight gain does not appear to reverse osteoporosis and is not generally indicated (Becker et al. 1999).

■ Daily supplementation with a multivitamin that contains at least 400 IU of vitamin D and 1,000–1,500 mg of calcium is recommended.

Bulimia Nervosa

→ The goals of treatment for BN include reducing binge eating and purging, as well as establishing educational counseling and psychosocial interventions.

→ Care should be coordinated by a single provider who is familiar with the entire treatment plan. This helps foster the development of a strong therapeutic relationship.

→ The most common treatment modality is cognitive behavioral therapy with adjunctive antidepressant medication. The combination of psychotherapy and pharmacotherapy is superior to psychotherapy alone (Bacaltchuk et al. 2002).

■ Although cognitive behavioral therapy is the treatment of choice for BN, it is not uniformly effective. Binge eating and purging resolve in approximately 50% of patients who receive this therapy. The remaining patients show partial improvement and a small number do not benefit at all (Wilson 1996).

■ Interpersonal therapy alone is sometimes helpful (Becker et al. 1999).

■ Cognitive behavioral and interpersonal therapies are helpful in the treatment of the comorbid mental disorders that often are present with bulimia: mood, anxiety, personality, interpersonal, and trauma- or abuse-related disorders (APA 2000).

■ Group psychotherapy, particularly if dietary counseling and management are included as part of the program, can be effective (APA 2000).

■ Family therapy is beneficial for adolescents who still live with their parents or if family and/or marital dysfunction are present.

→ Antidepressant medications are an effective component in the initial treatment of BN, particularly when the patient has significant symptoms of depressive, anxiety, obsessive, or impulse disorders. Drug therapy is less effective alone than when combined with intensive psychological treatment (Wilson 1996). The only medication approved by the Food and Drug Administration for BN is fluoxetine hydrochloride (Prozac®). This medication is not contraindicated even if the patient has the potential to commit suicide.

■ Effective doses of fluoxetine hydrochloride for bulimic symptoms are 60–80 mg/day (higher than those used for depression). Titration downward may be needed if the side effects are intolerable (McGilley et al. 1998).

■ The major side effect of fluoxetine is nausea, which subsides after a few days. Anxiety and insomnia occur in 10–15% of patients and may require reducing or discontinuing the medication (Yanovsky 1991).

■ Tricyclic antidepressants and monoamine oxidase inhibitors (MAOIs) are effective for treating depression in bulimics. However, because these drugs tend to have more significant side effects than the SSRIs, they are not usually utilized as a first-line treatment.

■ If antidepressant medication is used, it should be continued for a minimum of 6 months; usually a year of treatment is advisable (APA 2000).

■ When symptoms do not respond to medication, consider whether the patient may be taking the medication shortly before vomiting.

→ Monitor for severe constipation in patients who stop abusing laxatives. In severe cases of constipation—to prevent fecal impaction—osmotic laxatives such as lactulose can be used (Yanovsky 1991). Stimulant laxatives should be avoided, if possible.

CONSULTATION

→ See "Treatment/Management."

→ A list of psychotherapists specially recommended for treating AN and BN can be obtained from:
National Eating Disorders Association
165 W. 46th St., Suite 1108
New York, N.Y. 10036
(212) 575-6200 or (800) 931-2237

For support group information, call (800) 931-2237
www.nationaleatingdisorders.org

PATIENT EDUCATION

→ Clinicians should address the patient's emotions and behaviors associated with their eating disorder in a nonjudgmental and supportive manner. However, clinicians must also be willing to confront the patient when necessary.

→ Educate the patient about the medical consequences and psychological effects of weight reduction and eating disorders. Stress the importance of follow-up treatment if relapses occur.

→ Correct inaccurate beliefs about laxative use for weight control—i.e., how laxatives exert their effect in the large intestine, after most of the calories consumed have already been absorbed in the small intestine.

→ Advise the patient to reduce the risk of constipation by consuming a balanced diet with enhanced dietary fiber and fluid intake, by maintaining a regular exercise program, and by using bulk laxatives if needed (see the **Constipation** chapter in Section 7).

→ Women with eating disorders need to be re-educated and reconditioned regarding their eating attitudes.

- Encourage the patient to follow structured meal planning as an effective way to ensure balanced meals. By planning menus and eating meals at regular times, she will know what and when she will be eating, and thus may be less likely to fast and/or binge. Many patients will resist attempts at meal planning, believing they will become overweight quickly (Mitchell 1991). Be firm, direct, and persistent.

- Stress the importance of eating several times a day at regular intervals to avoid the vicious cycle of fasting/hunger that can lead to binge eating and vomiting in bulimic patients and prolonged fasting in anorexics.

- Allow the patient to initially exclude high-risk binge foods from the diet. It is important that the patient learn that food can be eaten in reasonable amounts.

- Educate the patient about proper nutrition. Advise the patient that a balanced diet (1,800–2,400 calories daily, eaten several times during the day) will not cause weight gain (Marshall 1991).

- Discuss modification of eating habits. Encourage the patient always to sit down to eat, always eat with others, and plan to do something pleasurable after the meal such as taking a walk, taking a bubble bath, or calling a friend.

- Encourage the patient to keep a food diary to increase her understanding of what she eats and to help her recognize which feelings bring on the urge to eat or fast.

- Assist the patient in recognizing the situations, people, thoughts, or feelings that may trigger an urge response (i.e., purge, binge, restrict). Discuss coping mechanisms that will help her avoid this response.

- Encourage the patient to avoid trigger situations until there is some progress in recovery.

→ Teach the patient that discussing these issues with the treatment team members will foster self-monitoring of eating patterns and help her uncover exactly which behaviors/situations precipitate maladaptive eating habits.

→ Establish a contract with the patient (and her family) regarding a target body weight. Also establish a food contract that includes the type, amount, and timing of food intake.

→ Teach the patient an appropriate exercise program, with a focus on physical fitness rather than calorie expenditure. Lead her to understand the compulsiveness of her past behavior and encourage her to exercise in a healthy and enjoyable fashion.

→ Engage family members in the treatment plan.

→ Patients with eating disorders may benefit from educational resources and support groups. These organizations may also provide consultation and a listing of eating disorder professionals. However, providers should be prepared to discuss information gathered online by the patient and her family by verifying its reliability and by clarifying possible misunderstandings or misinformation. Providers should also be aware of the complex dynamics that interacting with Web sites, listservs, and chat rooms can generate and be prepared to address these, if necessary.

→ Resources include:

Academy for Eating Disorders
6728 Old McLean Village Drive
McLean, Va. 22101
(703) 556-9222
www.aedweb.org

Anorexia Nervosa and Related Eating Disorders
    Affiliated with Eating Disorders Awareness and
    Prevention Inc.
www.anred.com

Eating Disorders Awareness and Prevention Inc.
693 Stewart St., Suite 803
Seattle, Wash. 98101
(206) 382-3587
Fax: (206) 289-8501
Toll-free information and referral hotline (800) 931-2237
www.nationaleatingdisorders.org

National Association of Anorexia Nervosa and
    Associated Disorders
P.O. Box 7
Highland Park, Ill. 60035
Hotline: (847) 831-3438
Fax: (847) 433-4632
www.anad.org

FOLLOW-UP

→ Prolonged outpatient treatment and sometimes hospitalization may be required for managing patients with eating disorders. The following are criteria for hospitalization (Kreipe et al. 2000, Powers 1990):

- Temperature below 36° C
- Pulse <45 beats/minute or orthostatic differential >30 beats per minute
- Complications of fluids or electrolyte imbalance
- Rapid weight loss (>10% in two months) or excessive weight loss that cannot be curtailed as an outpatient (>15% overall)
- True loss of appetite
- Inability to "break the cycle" of disordered eating as an outpatient
- Inability to initiate effective outpatient psychotherapy
- Patient is ill longer than a year
- Suicidal ideation is present
- Patient is living in a destructive family environment
- Incest has occurred and has not been discussed openly

→ Weekly outpatient appointments with the multidisciplinary treatment team are usually required on a long-term basis. Relapse is common after all forms of treatment.

→ Much of the follow-up care will be given by the eating disorder therapist. The primary care provider, along with the multidisciplinary team, must co-manage the patient's nutritional status and be alert for medical complications.

- The patient should be seen frequently and weighed every visit to gauge how far she is from her healthy body weight. A weight gain of 0.5–1 pound per week in an outpatient program is realistic.

→ Patients who engage in self-induced vomiting should be referred for a complete dental examination.

→ Ongoing psychological support of the patient and her family is essential.

→ Document in progress notes and on problem list.

BIBLIOGRAPHY

American Psychiatric Association (APA). 2000. *Diagnostic and statistical manual of mental disorders*, 4th ed. (text revision). Washington, D.C.: the Author.

Ames-Frankel, J., Devlin M.J., Walsh B.T. et al. 1992. Personality disorder diagnoses in patients with bulimia nervosa: clinical correlates and changes with treatment. *Journal of Clinical Psychiatry* 53:90–96.

Andersen, A.E., Bowers, W.A., and Watson, T. 2001. A slimming program for eating disorders not otherwise specified: reconceptualizing a confusing, residual diagnostic category. *Psychiatric Clinics of North America* 24(2):271–281.

Bacaltchuk, J., Hay, P., and Trefiglio, R. 2002. Antidepressants versus psychological treatments and their combination for bulimia nervosa (Cochrane Review). In *The Cochrane Library*. Oxford: Update Software.

Becker, A.E., Grinspan, S.K., Klibanski, A. et al. 1999. Eating disorders. *New England Journal of Medicine* 340(14): 1092–1098.

Crow, S.J., Rosenberg, M.E., Mitchell, J.E. et al. 2001. Urine electrolytes as markers of bulimia nervosa. *International Journal of Eating Disorders* 30:279–287.

Fairburn, C.G., Cooper, Z., Doll, H.A. et al. 2000. The natural course of bulimia nervosa and binge eating disorder in young women. *Archives of General Psychiatry* 57:659–665.

Frank, E. 1991. Shame and guilt in eating disorders. *American Journal of Orthopsychiatry* 6(12):303–306.

Garner, D.M., and Garfinkel, P.E. 1985. *Handbook of psychotherapy for anorexia nervosa and bulimia nervosa.* New York: Guilford Press.

Herzog, D.B., and Copeland, P.M. 1985. Eating disorders. *New England Journal of Medicine* 313(5):295–310.

Herzog, D.B., Keller, M.B., Lavori, P.W. et al. 1991. Bulimia nervosa in adolescence. *Developmental and Behavioral Pediatrics* 12(3):191–195.

Kalager, R., Bruback, O., and Bassoe, H.H. 1978. Cardiac performance in patients with anorexia nervosa. *Cardiology* 63(10):1–4.

Kaye, W.H., Weltzin, T.E., Hsu, G. et al. 1997. Relapse prevention with fluoxetine in anorexia nervosa: double blind placebo-controlled study. In *150th Meeting of the American Psychiatric Association, San Diego, Calif., May 17–22.* Research abstract book. Washington, D.C.: American Psychiatric Association.

Kaye, W.H, Weltzin T.E., Hsu L.K. et al. 1991. An open trial of fluoxetine in patients with anorexia nervosa. *Journal of Clinical Psychiatry* 52:464–471.

Kreipe, R.E., and Dukarm, C.P. 1999. Eating disorders in adolescents and older children. *Pediatrics in Review* 20(12): 410–420.

Kreipe, R.E., and Mou, S.M. 2000. Eating disorders in adolescents and young adults. *Obstetrics and Gynecology Clinics of North America* 27(1):101–214.

Marshall, L. 1991. Eating disorders. In *Psychiatric mental health nursing*, eds. F. Gary and C.K. Kavanagh. Philadelphia: J.B. Lippincott.

McGilley, B.M., and Pryor, T.L. 1998. Assessment and treatment of bulimia nervosa. *American Family Physician* 57 (11):243–250.

Mitchell, J.E. 1991. Bulimia nervosa. *Boletin de la Asociacion Medica de Puerto Rico* 83(1):22–24.

Morgan, J.F., Reid F., and Lacey J.H. 1999. The SCOFF questionnaire: assessment of a new screening tool for eating disorders. *British Medical Journal* 319:1467.

Patton, G.C., Selzer R., Coffey C. et al. 1999. Onset of adolescent eating disorders: population based cohort study over three years. *British Medical Journal* 318:765–768.

Powers, P. 1990. Anorexia nervosa: evaluation and treatment. *Neuropsychiatry Comprehensive Therapy* 16(2):24–34.

Ressler, A. 1998. "A body to die for": eating disorders and body-image distortion in women. *International Journal of Fertility* 43(3):133–138.

Steiner, H., and Lock, J. 1998. Anorexia nervosa and bulimia nervosa in children and adolescents: a review of the past 10 years. *Journal of the American Academy of Child and Adolescent Psychiatry* 37(4):352–359.

Sullivan, P.F. 1995. Mortality in anorexia nervosa. *American Journal of Psychiatry* 152:1073–1074.

Troop, N.A., Serpell, L., and Treasure, J.L. 2001. Specificity in the relationship between eating disorder symptoms in remitted and nonremitted women. *International Journal of Eating Disorder* 30:306–311.

Vitiello, B., and Lederhendler, I. 2000. Research on eating disorders: current status and future prospects. *Biology Psychiatry* 47:777–786.

Walsh, B.T., and Delvin, J.D. 1998. Eating disorders: progress and problems. *Science* 280:1387–1390.

Walsh, M.E., Wheat, M.E., and Freund, K. 2000. Detection, evaluation, and treatment of eating disorders: the role of the primary care physician. *Journal of General Internal Medicine* 15:577–590.

Wilson, G.T. 1996. Treatment of bulimia nervosa: when CBT fails. *Behavioral Research Therapy* 34:197–212.

Wolfe, W.L., and Maisto, S.A. 2000. The relationship between eating disorders and substance use: moving beyond co-prevalence research. *Clinical Psychology Review* 20(5):617–631.

Wolraich, M.L., Felice, M.E., and Drotar, D., eds. 1996. *The classification of child and adolescent mental diagnosis in primary care: diagnostic and statistical manual for primary care providers (DSM-PC), child and adolescent version.* Elk Grove Village, Ill.: American Academy of Pediatrics.

Wonderlich, S.A., Brewerton, T.D., Jocis, Z. et al. 1997. Relationship of childhood sexual abuse and eating disorders. *Journal of the American Academy of Child and Adolescent Psychiatry* 36(8):1107–1115.

Yanovsky, S.Z. 1991. Bulimia nervosa: the role of the family physician. *Association of Family Physicians* 44(4):1231–1238.

Yates, A.J., and Sambrailo, F. 1984. Bulimia nervosa: a description and therapeutic study. *Behavioral Research Therapy* 22:503–577.

14-F
Sexual Abuse (Minors and Adult Survivors)

Sexual abuse occurs in a variety of forms, including child sexual abuse (CSA)—i.e., incest, molestation, child pornography, rape (including situations involving a stranger, a date, a marital relationship, care provider/patient sexual relationships, and sexual harassment) (Gise et al. 1988). The focus of this chapter is CSA in minors (under the age of 18) and adult survivors of child abuse. Domestic violence, sexual assault, and sexual dysfunction are discussed in other chapters (see the **Domestic Violence** and **Sexual Assault** chapters and the **Sexual Dysfunction** chapter in Section 12).

Definitions of CSA in the literature vary. The National Center on Child Abuse and Neglect (NCCAN) (1978) defines CSA as an act perpetrated upon a child by a significantly older person with the intent to stimulate the child sexually and to satisfy the aggressor's sexual impulses. This includes sexual abuse committed by another minor when that person is either significantly older than the victim or is in a position of power or control over that child.

Although numerous definitions appear in the literature, Bachmann et al. (1988) cite four major components that are consistently included: 1) the nature and purpose of the sexual activity, 2) the age and relationship of the perpetrator to the child, 3) the child's understanding of the activity, and 4) the type of coercion used.

Sexual abuse can be *assaultive* (producing injury and resulting in severe emotional trauma) or *nonassaultive* (causing little if any physical injury and undetermined amounts of emotional stress) (Kessler et al. 1991). There may only be one occurrence in an individual's life or the abuse may be chronic and long-term. The abuse can be *incestuous* (intrafamilial) or it can be *perpetrated by strangers*.

There is a broad spectrum of sexually abusive behaviors, including provocative nudity and disrobing; genital exposure; observation of the child undressing, bathing, excreting, or urinating (especially in older children capable of performing these functions without assistance); kissing in a lingering or intimate way; fondling; masturbation with the child observing; fellatio; cunnilingus; digital penetration of the anus and/or vagina; penile

penetration of the anus and/or vagina; and "dry intercourse," which is genital contact without penetration (Sgroi et al. 1985). Infants and adolescents are also victims, although the tendency is for victimization to decrease as the child becomes older, starts to question the appropriateness of the behaviors, and is in a position to reject the approaches.

Reported incidences of CSA vary, depending on the populations studied and the setting. For example, one of the highest rates of reported child sexual abuse (66%) was found among a population of pregnant adolescents in a state of Washington study (Boyer et al. 1992), and a 52% incest incidence was found among patients in an urban psychiatric emergency facility (Briere et al. 1989). Russell (1983) conducted a retrospective study of 930 randomly selected women living in San Francisco and found that 38% of these women reported having had at least one CSA experience.

Child sexual abuse is an international problem. For example, 32% of women at the University of Costa Rica (Krugman et al. 1992) and 12% of women in a study in Great Britain report having been sexually abused (Baker et al. 1985).

Sexual abuse occurs regardless of socioeconomic class, occupational stratum, urban or rural residency, education, religion, or ethnic background (Bachmann et al. 1988). Sexual abuse may occur in families across multiple generations and is often associated with dysfunctional family interactions. This can make it difficult to separate the effects of sexual abuse from those of other emotional and/or physical abuse within the family.

Although any child can be at risk for CSA, victims may have the following profile: oldest female in a large family (four or more children) where substance abuse co-exists and that female is thrust into the parenting role. The father/stepfather may be violent, especially toward family members who are not sexually abused. The mother is usually unaware of or disassociated from the abusive relationship and may lack essential mother/child interpersonal skills. The abuse may be kept secret, with only the abuser and victim aware of the abuse in many cases (Gilgun 1984).

Survivors of CSA report difficulties with their own parenting skills and attitudes toward their children. Social isolation, disorganization, fear of disintegration, lack of trust, family unhappiness, and frequent conflict characterize the families of incestuous relationships (Bachmann et al. 1988; Berth-Jones et al. 1990; Cole et al. 1989, 1992; Finkelhor et al. 1990).

Long-term sequelae of CSA can include physical complaints. For example, Paddison et al. (1990) found a relationship between CSA and premenstrual syndrome (PMS). Of PMS sufferers, 33% of women in a high socioeconomic group reported child sexual abuse by a friend, and 52% of women in a low socioeconomic group reported child sexual abuse by a relative. Ninety-five percent of 42 women interviewed in a randomized clinical trial of nonpharmacological treatments for severe PMS reported at least one attempted or completed sexual abuse event (Golding et al. 2000).

Wurtele et al. (1990) reported a 28% incidence of sexual abuse prior to age 14 in women who were experiencing chronic pain (back/neck, myofascial, carpal tunnel syndrome, chronic tension headaches). The authors hypothesized an abuse/muscle tension/chronic pain linkage where musculoskeletal pain syndromes relate to chronic and excessive contraction of the involved muscle groups.

Associations have also been made between chronic pelvic pain and CSA (Harrop-Griffiths et al. 1988, Reiter et al. 1991). Reiter et al. (1991) found a correlation between sexual abuse and somatization in women with chronic pelvic pain. They caution against the use of hysterectomy in this population until thorough medical and psychological evaluations are completed.

Some evidence suggests that early adverse life events such as CSA may predispose individuals to mood and anxiety disorders, possibly by inducing persistent changes in the anterior pituitary gland and the adrenal cortex (Heim et al. 2001). According to this hypothesis, subsequent stress exposures trigger maladaptive neurological and physiological chemical responses, which then result in symptoms of depression and anxiety.

The reported psychological sequelae of CSA include depression, anxiety, low self-esteem, anger, guilt, self-blame, dissociation, obsessive-compulsive symptoms, panic disorders, phobias, and paranoid ideation (Beitchman et al. 1992, Brown et al. 1990, Cahill et al. 1991, Hall et al. 1994, Johnson et al. 2001, Kreidler et al. 1992, Pribor et al. 1992). There is evidence that incestuous experiences with fathers/stepfathers and the use of violence are more traumatic than nonincestuous experiences and may be associated with higher risk of psychiatric sequelae (Beitchman et al. 1992).

Sexual dysfunction among CSA victims is commonly noted and includes desire dysfunction, arousal problems, adverse feeling states, and anorgasmia (Brown et al. 1990, Gise et al. 1988, Mackey et al. 1991). Revictimization and promiscuity have also been reported (Bachmann et al. 1988, Beitchman et al. 1992) and may predispose CSA survivors to sexually transmitted diseases (STDs), including human papillomavirus (HPV), herpes simplex virus (HSV), and human immunodeficiency virus (HIV) (Petrak et al. 2000, Zierler et al. 1991). There is also a strong positive correlation between CSA and substance abuse/addiction (Adams 1998). Scott (1992) studied the impact of CSA on mental health in the Los Angeles community and determined that a history of CSA significantly increased an individual's odds of developing one or more of eight psychiatric disorders in adulthood, including substance abuse/dependence.

Adults who were sexually abused as children may seek therapy in the face of a seemingly unrelated crisis. There has been evidence of increased use of medical and psychiatric services among survivors of CSA (Rosenberg et al. 2000). If the trauma of sexual abuse is to be resolved successfully, therapy is recommended. However, the quality of the individual's support system may be a more important influence than therapy in the person's adjustment to the trauma of sexual abuse (Feinauer 1989).

Victims of CSA present to the clinical setting in a variety of situations. A child victim may enter care immediately after the occurrence for evaluation of injuries or a grown adult woman may present herself several years later with complaints of physical, psychological, emotional, and/or social conditions where CSA is the underlying problem. It is essential that the primary health care provider be sensitive to these issues. Self-esteem and healthy family functioning in adulthood have been associated with having a helpful provider (Palmer et al. 2001).

Continued prevention efforts aimed at eliminating CSA from the community hold extensive potential for improving everyone's quality of life (Scott 1992). Economic benefits would also accrue by eliminating the financial strain of providing care for individuals experiencing the sequelae of CSA.

State laws vary regarding the reporting of child abuse to child protective services (CPS). Victims of CSA who are minors must be removed from the unsafe environment. In the case of suspected child abuse, California law requires reporting to CPS agencies. Health care providers should be familiar with reporting laws in their own states.

The primary objective of the physical examination in the case of current abuse is to address the medical needs of the victim. The secondary purpose is to collect samples that can be used later as evidence. Most police agencies, hospitals, and large health care institutions have prepackaged rape or sexual abuse evidence kits, and guidelines are available to assist care providers in performing a complete and comprehensive examination (Indest 1989, Kessler et al. 1991, Muram 1992). The following sections cover minor children and adult survivors separately.

Minor Child—Under 18 Years Old

DATABASE

SUBJECTIVE

→ Risk factors for CSA include:
  ■ Substance abuse in the home
  ■ Coexisting physical/emotional abuse
  ■ Family mental illness
  ■ Family violence
  ■ Family history of CSA
  NOTE: It is possible that an adolescent will present to a health care setting by herself.
→ An adult may report suspicion of CSA.
→ Use of sexually explicit descriptions by younger children may suggest CSA.
  ■ Most prepubescent children will not be capable of

describing sexual behaviors unless they themselves have been exposed.
→ Child may be able to show sexual behaviors (e.g., fellatio, intercourse, fondling) using anatomically correct dolls.
→ Child may demonstrate hypersexual behavior, including compulsive masturbation, promiscuity, or prostitution.
→ Child may have nightmares/night terrors, phobic reactions, truancy, withdrawal/depression, clinging behaviors, poor school performance, running away episodes, suicidal ideation, poor peer relationships, and other emotional disturbances.
→ Child may report a history of:
- Gastrointestinal (GI) complaints (e.g., anorexia, vomiting, abdominal pain, rectal pain)
- Genitourinary (GU) complaints (e.g., pelvic pain; urinary symptoms; vaginal itching, discharge, and/or pain; unexplained pregnancies)
- Vague somatic complaints (e.g., headaches and muscle aches)
→ Patient may report prior trauma, hospitalizations, or contact with public health and/or social services (e.g., CPS).
→ Subjective data should be collected using direct quotes from the victim and from any adult person involved with bringing the abuse to the attention of the health care provider.

OBJECTIVE

→ See the **Sexual Assault** chapter.
→ The patient may present with:
- Poor hygiene
- Extreme anxiety during pelvic examination
- Vaginitis and STDs—past or current (see the **Vaginitis** chapters in Section 12, and **Sexually Transmitted Diseases**, Section 13)
- Unexplained pregnancy
→ It is also possible that there is no physical evidence of CSA.

ASSESSMENT

→ R/O CSA
→ R/O coexisting forms of child abuse
→ R/O consensual sexual activity between minors
→ R/O substance abuse
→ R/O illness/injury (e.g., STDs, pregnancy, tissue trauma, psychiatric disorders, neurological disorders)
→ R/O potential for death by suicide or homicide
→ R/O presence of long-term sequelae

PLAN

→ See the **Sexual Assault** chapter (the plan may vary depending on the age of the victim).
→ Consultation involves referral to CPS for *any* suspected sexual abuse and/or physical abuse of a child under 18 years old as required by law.
- The patient should be advised that a report is being made.
- In California, health care providers who fail to report suspected abuse are guilty of a misdemeanor punishable by up to six months in jail and/or up to a $1,000 fine. He or

she may also be found civilly liable for damages, especially if the child-victim or another child is further victimized because of the failure to report (California Penal Code 11166). This penal code is part of the Child Abuse and Neglect Reporting Act in California.
- It is not necessary to report a minor when there is consensual sexual activity, unless the patient and partner are of discrepant age (e.g., ages 12 and 16 or older). Review of local legal guidelines is advised.

Adult Survivor of CSA

DATABASE

SUBJECTIVE

→ All women are at risk for CSA regardless of age, race, socioeconomic status, or sexual preference.
→ The patient may report a history of:
- CSA
- Familial and/or personal substance/alcohol abuse
- Family violence/physical abuse
- Abusive relationships with male partners
- Psychological disorder (e.g., depression, suicide attempts, phobic reactions, borderline personality, eating disorders, panic attacks)
- Contact with law enforcement and/or social service agencies (e.g., foster care placement, detention in juvenile hall)
- Prostitution and/or multiple sexual partners
- Multiple visits to health care provider, presenting with vague somatic complaints, including chronic musculoskeletal problems, headaches, sexual dysfunction, severe PMS, chronic pelvic pain, GU and GI complaints, sleep disorders, and/or psychiatric complaints
→ The patient may report early age of first intercourse.

OBJECTIVE

→ There may be no physical evidence of past CSA.
→ The patient may evidence conditions associated with stress, including alopecia, hypertension, obesity, ulcers, or migraine headaches.
→ The patient may appear restless, angry, defensive, anxious, and evasive and may demonstrate inappropriate affect and/or avoidance of eye contact.
→ The patient may present with poor hygiene.
→ During the examination, the patient may demonstrate a hesitation or refusal to undress and/or extreme anxiety reaction or overly compliant behavior during the examination.
→ Unusual scars may be present, including old cigarette burns, lacerations, pelvic trauma (especially in nulliparous women), and tracks from injection drug abuse.
→ There may be evidence of STDs (e.g., HSV, HPV, HIV).

ASSESSMENT

→ R/O CSA
→ R/O psychological disorder
→ R/O substance and/or alcohol abuse

→ R/O current domestic violence

→ R/O existing medical conditions, illnesses, and/or injuries (e.g., pelvic disease, ulcers, musculoskeletal disorders, STDs)

→ R/O potential for death by suicide or homicide

→ R/O presence of long-term sequelae (e.g., sexual dysfunction, panic disorders, promiscuity)

PLAN

DIAGNOSTIC TESTS

→ Determining which tests are necessary will depend on the nature of the complaint, condition, or injury (e.g., cervical cultures and/or serological examinations to rule out STDs or ultrasound to rule out pelvic pathology).

TREATMENT/MANAGEMENT

→ Clinician should explore her/his own feelings regarding CSA to determine if she/he can approach these women in a holistic, sensitive, supportive, and nonjudgmental fashion.

→ Screen *all* women for history of CSA, regardless of age, race, socioeconomic status, marital status, or sexual preference.

→ Assess the patient's living arrangements and support systems.

→ Provide service to address the patient's chief complaint or concern.

NOTE: Usually the patient will not present to the clinic with the complaint of CSA. The history is elicited after she presents with another need (e.g., STD evaluation, pregnancy, pelvic pain, contraception, annual examination).

→ Integrate the history of CSA into the treatment plan for all medical, social, and psychological services.

→ Determine the level of psychosocial support assistance the patient and her family needs.

→ Communicate history of CSA to the patient's other care providers, but only with her consent.

→ Referral for psychological counseling/therapy is recommended for the patient and her family as indicated.

→ Referral to support groups for incest survivors is recommended.

→ Referral to 12-Step programs is recommended for alcohol abuse, substance abuse, codependency, or adult children of alcoholics (depending on history).

→ Referral to other community agencies is recommended depending on patient needs (e.g., parenting classes, family support services, legal support services, social services).

→ Encourage stress management strategies for patients who are feeling the effects of past CSA in their lives (e.g., use of an informed support network [intimate partners, friends], rest, exercise, recreation, adequate nutrition, meditation, and/or contact with a therapist).

CONSULTATION

→ Consult with a physician as indicated regarding medical conditions.

→ Consult with social service agents to provide assistance with legal, financial, and/or housing issues.

→ Consult with psychological/psychiatric services in suspected cases of psychological disorders and/or substance abuse.

PATIENT EDUCATION

→ Educate the patient about CSA—i.e., incidence, possible sequelae, multigenerational factors, and risks to her in future relationships, especially with her own children.

→ Assure the patient that she is not alone. Many women share this problem and respond to it in a variety of ways.

→ Encourage the patient to find means of self-actualization to empower herself and build self-esteem (e.g., through education, employment, community outreach, fertility control, and assertiveness training).

→ In some situations, it may be necessary to educate the patient about what constitutes abuse and validate her experience that what occurred was an abusive event.

→ Inform the patient of the availability of supportive services in the community to discuss CSA. Encourage her to utilize these services.

→ Explain the rationale for all examination procedures and treatments.

■ Advise the patient that if she is experiencing too much discomfort, the examination will be stopped immediately and a reassessment made to evaluate why she is experiencing pain.

→ Counsel the patient regarding high-risk behaviors that could jeopardize her health (e.g., STDs including HIV infection, unwanted pregnancy, abusive relationships).

FOLLOW-UP

→ Continue to monitor at future visits.

→ Be aware that life events/changes may predispose the patient to crisis (e.g., new relationships, pregnancy, death of the abuser).

→ Document appropriately in progress notes and on problem list. The sensitive nature of the subject requires discretion concerning what is written in the medical record.

BIBLIOGRAPHY

Adams, S. 1998. *The social environment of pregnant women and new mothers who use crack cocaine.* Unpublished doctoral dissertation. University of California-San Francisco.

Bachmann, G.A., Moeller, T.P., and Benett, J. 1988. Childhood sexual abuse and the consequences in adult women. *Obstetrics and Gynecology* 71(4):631–642.

Baker, A.W., and Duncan, S.P. 1985. Child sexual abuse: a study of prevalence in Great Britain. *Child Abuse and Neglect* 9:457–467.

Beitchman, J.H., Zucker, K.J., Hood, J.E. et al. 1992. A review of the long-term effects of child sexual abuse. *Child Abuse and Neglect* 16:101–118.

Berth-Jones, J., and Graham-Brown, R.A.C. 1990. Childhood sexual abuse: a dermatological perspective. *Clinical and Experimental Dermatology* 15:321–330.

Boyer, D., and Fine, D. 1992. Sexual abuse as a factor in adolescent pregnancy and child maltreatment. *Family Planning Perspectives* 24(1):4–19.

Briere, J., and Zaidi, L.Y. 1989. Sexual abuse histories and sequelae in female psychiatric emergency room patients. *American Journal of Psychiatry* 146:1602–1606.

Brown, B.E., and Garrison, C.J. 1990. Patterns of symptomatology of adult women incest survivors. *Western Journal of Nursing Research* 12(5):587–600.

Cahill, C., Llewelyn S.P., and Pearson, C. 1991. Long-term effects of sexual abuse which occurred in childhood: a review. *British Journal of Clinical Psychology* 30:117–130.

California Penal Code 1116. Child Abuse and Neglect Reporting Act in California. Available at: http://leginfo.ca.gov/calaw.html. Accessed on February 20, 2003.

Cole, P.M., Woolger, C., Power, T.G. et al. 1989. Incest survivors: the relation of their perceptions of their parents and their own parenting attitudes. *Child Abuse and Neglect* 13:409–416.

_____. 1992. Parenting difficulties among adult survivors of father-daughter incest. *Child Abuse and Neglect* 16:239–249.

Feinauer, L.L. 1989. Relationship of treatment to adjustment in women sexually abused as children. *American Journal of Family Therapy* 17(4):326–334.

Finkelhor, D., Hotaling, G., Lewis, I.A. et al. 1990. Sexual abuse in a national survey of adult men and women: prevalence, characteristics, and risk factors. *Child Abuse and Neglect* 14:19–28.

Gilgun, J.F. 1984. Does the mother know? Alternatives to blaming mothers for child sexual abuse. *Response* Fall Issue:2–4.

Gise, L.H., and Paddison, P. 1988. Rape, sexual abuse, and its victims. *Psychiatric Clinics of North America* 11(4):629–648.

Golding, J.M., Taylor, D.L., Menard, L. et al. 2000. Prevalence of sexual abuse history in a sample of women seeking treatment for premenstrual syndrome. *Journal of Psychosomatic Obstetrics and Gynecology* 21(2):69–80.

Hall, L.A., Sachs, B., Rayens, M.K. et al. 1994. Childhood physical and sexual abuse: their relationship with depressive symptoms in adulthood. *Image: The Journal of Nursing Scholarship* 25(4):317–323.

Harrop-Griffiths, J., Katon, W., Walker, E. et al. 1988. The association between chronic pelvic pain, psychiatric diagnoses, and childhood sexual abuse. *Obstetrics & Gynecology* 71:589–594.

Heim, C., Newport D.J., Bonsall, R. et al. 2001. Altered pituitary-adrenal axis responses to provocative challenge tests in adult survivors of childhood abuse. *American Journal of Psychiatry* 158(4):575–581.

Indest, G.F. 1989. Medico-legal issues in detecting and proving the sexual abuse of children. *Medical Science Law* 29(1):33–46.

Johnson, D.M., Pike, J.L., and Chard, K.M. 2001. Factors predicting PTSD, depression, and dissociative severity in female treatment-seeking childhood sexual abuse survivors. *Child Abuse and Neglect* 25(1):179–198.

Kessler, D.B., and Hyden, P. 1991. Physical, sexual, and emotional abuse of children. *Clinical Symposia* 43(1):2–32.

Kreidler, M.C., and Hassan, M. 1992. Use of an interactional model with survivors of incest. *Issues in Mental Health Nursing* 13:149–158.

Krugman, S., Mata, L., and Krugaman, R. 1992. Sexual abuse and corporal punishment during childhood: a pilot retrospective survey of university students in Costa Rica. *Pediatrics* 90(1):157–161.

Mackey, T.F., Hacker, S.S., Weissfeld, L.A. et al. 1991. Comparative effects of sexual assault on sexual functioning of child sexual abuse survivors and others. *Issues in Mental Health Nursing* 12:89–112.

Muram, D. 1992. Child sexual abuse. *Obstetrics and Gynecology Clinics of North America* 19(1):193–207.

National Center on Child Abuse and Neglect. 1978. *Child sexual abuse: incest, assault and exploitation. Special report.* Publication No. (OHDS) 79-30166. Washington, D.C.: U.S. Department of Health, Education and Welfare.

Paddison, P.L., Gise, L.H., Lebovits, A. et al. 1990. Sexual abuse and premenstrual syndrome: comparison between a lower and higher socioeconomic group. *Psychosomatics* 31(3):256–272.

Palmer, S.E., Brown, R.A., Rae-Grant, N.I. et al. 2001. Survivors of childhood abuse: their reported experiences with professional help. *Social Work* 46(2):136–145.

Petrak, J., Byrne, A., and Baker, M. 2000. The association between abuse in childhood and STD/HIV risk behaviors in female genitourinary clinic attendees. *Sexually Transmitted Infections* 76(6):457–461.

Pribor, E.F., and Dinwiddie, S.H. 1992. Psychiatric correlates of incest in childhood. *American Journal of Psychiatry* 149(1):52–56.

Reiter, R.C., Shakerin, L.R., Gambone, J.C. et al. 1991. Correlation between sexual abuse and somatization in women with somatic and nonsomatic chronic pelvic pain. *American Journal of Obstetrics and Gynecology* 165:104–109.

Rosenberg, H.J., Rosenberg, S.D., Wolford, G.L. II et al. 2000. The relationship between trauma, PTSD, and medical utilization in three high-risk medical populations. *International Journal of Psychiatry Medicine* 30(3):247–259.

Russell, D. 1983. The incidence and prevalence of intra-familial sexual abuse of female children. *Child Abuse and Neglect* 7:133–145.

Scott, K.D. 1992. Childhood sexual abuse: impact on a community's mental health status. *Child Abuse and Neglect* 16:285–295.

Sgroi, S.M., Blick, L.C., and Porter, F.S. 1985. *A conceptual framework for child sexual abuse.* Education Programs Associates course on Adolescent Sexual Abuse, Reporting and Counseling, Berkeley, Calif., December 8, 1992.

Wurtele, S.K., Kaplan, G.M., and Keairnes, M. 1990. Child sexual abuse among chronic pain patients. *Clinical Journal of Pain* 6(2):110–113.

Zierler, S., Feingold, L., Laufer, D. et al. 1991. Adult survivors of childhood sexual abuse and subsequent risk of HIV infection. *American Journal of Public Health* 81(5):572–575.

Jane A. Newhard-Parks, R.N., M.S.N., F.N.P.
Julie Richards, R.N., C., W.H.N.P., F.N.P., M.S., M.S.N.

14-G
Sexual Assault

Sexual assault is defined as any sexual act performed by a person on another person without his or her consent (Moscarello 1991). It is often defined as any form of nonconsenting sexual activity, which encompasses all unwanted sexual acts from fondling to forcible penetration. Most sexual assault definitions have three components: 1) use of coercion, physical force, intimidation, threats, or deception; 2) sexual contact; and 3) nonconsent of the victim (Reynolds et al. 2000). The term *rape* is usually more narrowly defined as sexual intercourse without consent. Statutory rape occurs when a person is defined by statute as being incapable of consenting because she/he is under a specific age. For the purposes of this chapter, the terms sexual assault and rape will be used interchangeably. Sexually assaulted children, sexually assaulted males, and incest survivors have special needs that are not addressed in this chapter.

Sexual assault is one of the fastest-growing violent crimes in the United States (Hampton 1995). The actual prevalence of rape is unknown, but Reynolds et al. (2000) reports that prevalence estimates range from 1.6 per 1,000 U.S. female residents age 12 and older to seven per 1,000 of U.S. women age 18 and older. This is probably a gross underestimate of actual numbers, however, as reported assaults are estimated to represent only 10–30% of the total (Glaser et al. 1991). The National Institute of Justice reports that in the United States, 1 million women become new victims of rape each year (Rose 1999). In the study *Rape in America*, researchers concluded that 12.1 million adult women have been victims of at least one forcible rape during their life. Sixty-one percent of those attacks occurred before the victim was 18 years old (Schafran 1996).

The majority of rapes are committed by men who are not strangers to their victims but are friends, acquaintances, dates, spouses, long-term partners, or relatives (e.g., fathers, uncles, brothers, or cousins) (Schwartz 1991). Marital rape may occur in 10–14% of all marriages, but these numbers are difficult to estimate because 21 states have marital exclusion laws (Schwartz 1991).

The etiology of rape is complex and involves many sociocultural factors, including acceptance of interpersonal violence, adversarial perception of heterosexual relations, acceptance of rape myths, and sex role stereotyping. Schafran (1996) states that health care professionals should receive training about risk factors, indicators, prevalence, and sequelae of violence. There should also be training and education eradicating the rape myths—such as who commits rape and why, and how victims react. McConkey et al. (2001) state that because sexual assault survivors often seek treatment in primary care settings, clinicians should be prepared to evaluate and care for these patients in a nonjudgmental manner.

The evidence as to whether or not certain women are more vulnerable to rape is inconclusive. However, studies have shown that women who were sexually abused as children may be at higher risk for rape as adults. In addition, there is research that connects violence portrayed in the media with violent behavior in society (Schwartz 1991). The American College of Obstetrics and Gynecology (ACOG) recommends that clinicians discuss preventive strategies with patients to decrease the likelihood of a repeat assault (Rose 1999).

About 40% of sexual assault victims sustain physical injuries. One percent of these require hospitalization and 0.1% are fatal (ACOG 1992, Hampton 1995). Although most of the physical injuries sustained during sexual assault are minor and resolve fairly soon, the psychological damage is much more likely to last for months or years after the assault. The psychological sequelae can be long-term and profound. Petter et al. (1998) found that 100% of surveyed survivors reported that the experience continued to have an effect on their lives five years later. Sexual assault is a tragedy with many long-term and profound consequences. Victims who perceive that health care professionals are concerned, kind, and organized in their care are more likely to return for follow-up treatment, procedures, and counseling (Petter et al. 1998).

Burgess et al. (1974) described the response of women to assault as the *rape trauma syndrome*, a constellation of physical and psychological symptoms. The syndrome consists of two phases: *acute* and *delayed,* also referred to as *organizational.*

The *acute* phase may last for hours or days and is characterized by an alteration in coping mechanisms. The woman may appear to be in control of her behavior or completely out of control. She may exhibit disorganization, shock, and disbelief. She may also express fear and anger and have episodes of crying. Other signs and symptoms include anorexia, nausea and vomiting, abdominal pain, pelvic pain, muscle aches, headaches, sleep disturbances such as insomnia and nightmares, vaginal itching and discharge, rectal pain, and emotional problems, including anxiety, sexual dysfunction, depression, and mood swings.

The delayed or organizational phase can last for months or years. The woman may experience flashbacks, phobias, nightmares, suicidal ideation, and gynecological and menstrual complaints. She may also engage in substance use.

Today, the responses of sexual assault survivors to their ordeals often are described in the broader context of *post-traumatic stress disorder* (PTSD) (Ruch et al. 1991). This disorder was added to the *Diagnostic and Statistical Manual of Mental Disorders* in 1980 as an anxiety disorder after it was determined that victims of many types of psychological trauma (e.g., terrorism, war, torture, violent crimes, and natural disasters) exhibit similar symptoms.

To meet the diagnostic criteria for PTSD, a person must have experienced an event outside the range of normal experience and have symptoms that last longer than one month in each of the following areas: 1) persistent re-experiencing of the trauma, 2) avoidance of stimuli associated with the trauma or a numbing of general responsiveness, and 3) persistent symptoms of increased arousal and anxiety (Bownes et al. 1991).

Although after experiencing an assault most women initially meet these criteria, their symptoms usually subside by the fourth month after the rape. However, a proportion of survivors remain symptomatic for years (Bownes et al. 1991). In one study, Rothbaum et al. (1990) found that 94% of rape victims met the criteria for PTSD shortly after the assault, 47% still suffered from PTSD three months after the assault, and 16.5% had persistent symptoms of PTSD 17 years after the attack.

Women who have a history of depression, suicide attempts, substance abuse, sexual abuse, or sexual assault may have a more severe response to a sexual assault (Moscarello 1991). The nature of the assault, the patient's locus of control, coping ability, life stress, personality variables, social networks, and developmental stages also help to determine the intensity of the response (Ruch et al. 1991).

When caring for assault survivors, health care providers must address their medical, legal, and emotional needs. Because the physical injuries sustained are usually minor, many emergency rooms and sexual assault centers are now using specially trained nurses, referred to as sexual assault nurse examiners (SANEs), to care for these patients.

SANE programs were developed in response to a lack of experienced health care providers trained to meet the special needs of assault survivors in a sensitive and standardized fashion. This multidisciplinary approach is intended to provide more comprehensive and compassionate care to the sexual assault survivor (Hatmaker 1997). SANEs receive specialized training regarding the physical and emotional sequelae of rape, crisis intervention counseling, law enforcement procedures, forensics, evidence collection, colposcopy, and the criminal justice system (Emergency Nurses Association 1991). They examine victims, collect evidence, provide counseling and follow-up care, and testify in court. For a listing of SANE programs, see Lenehan (1991).

DATABASE

NOTE: If the assault has occurred within the last 72 hours, it is strongly recommended (and, in some communities, required) that the patient be referred to a designated sexual assault nurse/physician examiner for the completion of an evidentiary examination using a rape kit. The examination may be completed even if the survivor is unsure regarding prosecution. The following regarding the examination is provided for informational purposes only.

SUBJECTIVE

→ The survivor should be interviewed and examined as soon as possible after the incident in a private, quiet, comfortable environment. She may wish to have a family member, partner, friend, rape crisis counselor, or advocate from a sexual assault organization present.

- Patient may describe episode(s) of sexual assault.
- Patient may report history of:
  - Gastrointestinal complaints (e.g., anorexia, nausea, vomiting, abdominal, or rectal pain)
  - Genitourinary complaints (e.g., vaginal itching, discharge, pelvic pain, menstrual complaints)
  - Vague somatic complaints (e.g., headaches, muscle aches, and fatigue)
  - Sleep disturbances (e.g., insomnia, nightmares)
  - Emotional disturbances (e.g., anxiety, depression, suicidal ideation, mood swings, flashbacks, phobias, sexual dysfunction, substance abuse, diminished interest in usual activities)
  - Patient may report feeling detached from others.
  - Patient may be unable to recall important aspects of the trauma.

→ Obtain a *complete* health history from the survivor.

OBJECTIVE

→ Use of an evidence collection protocol is recommended (see **Appendix 14G.1, Sexual Assault Examination and Forensic Report Form**).

- Obtain the patient's consent for examination and evidence collection.
  - Ideally, all evidence should be collected before the patient bathes, urinates, defecates, douches, washes out her mouth, or cleans her fingernails.
- If the assault occurred within 72 hours prior to the examination, an evidence collection kit should be used.
- The patient should undress standing on paper to catch any fibers or debris that may fall from her body or clothing.

- All clothing is kept in separate paper bags, instead of plastic, to discourage bacterial growth.
- Any wet stains should be allowed to air dry before bagging.
- A complete physical examination should be performed in all cases of sexual assault, regardless of the length of time that has elapsed since the assault. Note the following:
  - Mood/affect: patient may appear fearful, angry, disorganized, seem to be in complete control, or have a restricted range of affect.
  - Presence of slurred/incoherent speech or uneven gait
  - Bruises, abrasions, bite marks, laceration, fractures, restraint or strangulation marks, stab and/or gunshot wounds
    ➤ The most common sites of trauma include the genitals, mouth, throat, wrists, arms, breasts, and thighs (Beebe 1991).
  - Presence of foreign objects in vagina, urethra, rectum, ear, nose, or mouth
  - Lacerations, ecchymosis, and edema in the area of the posterior fourchette (the greatest point of stress associated with forced stretching during penile penetration)
    ➤ These mounting injuries may be enhanced for visualization with the application of toluidine blue or the use of colposcopy (Slaughter et al.1992).

ASSESSMENT

→ Sexual assault
→ R/O serious trauma
→ R/O concurrent domestic violence
→ R/O potential for death by suicide or homicide
→ R/O coexisting child abuse
→ R/O substance abuse
→ R/O sexually transmitted diseases (STDs), including HIV and hepatitis B virus
→ R/O pregnancy
→ R/O presence of long-term sequelae (e.g., PTSD)

PLAN

DIAGNOSTIC TESTS

→ It is essential that the chain of evidence not be broken. All specimens should be labeled, dated, sealed, and locked up until the appropriate law enforcement official takes possession of them.
→ Appropriate tests (e.g., x-rays) should be ordered to rule out physical trauma.
→ If bite marks are present, a forensic odontologist should make a cast and document the findings.
→ The victim's head and pubic hair should be combed while she stands over paper.
  - Obtaining pubic hairs is controversial, but some jurisdictions request that they be collected.
→ The oral cavity may be swabbed to recover seminal fluid/sperm. Oral washings may also be done depending upon the lab facilities available.

- The patient may wash out her mouth with clear water after the samples are taken. She then is instructed not to eat, drink, or smoke for 30 minutes, at which time a saliva sample is taken.
→ Blood and saliva samples are taken to determine the ABO secretor status of the victim.
  - ABO factors are found in everyone's blood, but they are also found in other body secretions—semen, saliva, and vaginal secretions—in about 75–80% of the population. The remaining 20–25% are nonsecretors.
→ A Wood's light is used to check the perineum and thighs for blood or semen.
  - The dried secretions are then collected with saline-moistened cotton swabs.
→ Any semen present is collected from the vagina, cervix, or rectum.
  - Because sperm contain DNA, they can be used to identify the assailant.
  - Motile sperm can be detected in the vagina for up to eight hours, from cervical mucus for 2–3 days and from the rectum for an undetermined length of time.
  - Nonmotile sperm can be detected in the vagina for up to 24 hours, from the cervix for up to 17 days, and from the rectum for 24 hours (ACOG 1992).
→ If no sperm are present (i.e., the perpetrator had no ejaculation or had undergone a vasectomy), seminal plasma components (prostatic antigen p30 and acid phosphatase) may be found in the vagina, rectum, mouth, skin, or clothing for up to several hours and can be used to identify semen and the ABO blood type of secretors.
→ Collection of vaginal secretions for DNA fingerprinting is recommended.
→ Collection of saliva to check for major blood group antigens is recommended.
→ Collection of fingernail scrapings to look for the skin and blood of the attacker is recommended.
→ Obtain specimens for blood tests, wet mounts, cultures, and DNA test for the diagnosis and treatment of existing infections (e.g., candidiasis, gonorrhea, chlamydia, syphilis, herpes, HIV, trichomoniasis, hepatitis B, and bacterial vaginosis).
NOTE: HIV testing should be done at the time of the initial examination. If this test is negative, advise the woman to have repeat testing at six weeks, three months, and six months after the initial test. (See "Follow-up," below.)
→ Obtain specimen for pregnancy test if indicated.
→ Toxicology blood/urine screens are *not* routinely performed.

TREATMENT/MANAGEMENT

→ See "Subjective," "Objective," and "Diagnostic Tests."
→ Offer mouthwash, soap, and a clean set of clothes to the patient. She might want to shower after the examination.
→ Many specialists recommend routine, prophylactic antibiotics after a sexual assault.
  - The following regimen is effective against gonorrhea,

chlamydia, trichomoniasis, bacterial vaginosis, and incubating syphilis (Centers for Disease Control and Prevention [CDC] 2002):

- Ceftriaxone 125 mg IM in a single dose, PLUS
- Metronidazole 2 g p.o. in a single dose, PLUS
- Azithromycin 1 g p.o. in a single dose
        OR
- Doxycycline 100 mg p.o. BID for 7 days

  NOTE: Warn the patient not to use alcoholic beverages for 24–48 hours after taking metronidazole.

→ Though the risk of pregnancy is only 2–4%, an emergency contraceptive such as Plan B® or Preven® should be offered. To be effective, the first pill should be taken within the first 72 hours after the assault. Plan B® consists of 2 levonorgestrel 0.75 mg pills. One is taken STAT and the second exactly 12 hours later. If neither is available, the "morning-after" regimen for pregnancy prevention should be offered as follows:

- A total of 200 mcg of ethinyl estradiol plus 2.0 mg norgestrel or 1.0 mg levonorgestrel. Regimens include:
  - Ovral® 2 tablets STAT, then 2 tablets 12 hours later
  - Lo/Ovral®, Nordette®, Levlen®, Triphasil®, or Tri-Levlen® (yellow pills only) 4 tablets STAT, then 4 tablets 12 hours later (Hatcher et al. 1998)
- The following may be used for nausea from the morning-after pill (Hatcher et al. 1998). This is not necessary for Plan B®.
  - Nonprescription drugs:
    - Dimenhydrinate 50 mg tablets, 1–2 tablets p.o. every 4–6 hours
    - Cyclizine hydrochloride 50 mg tablets, 1 tablet p.o. every 4–6 hours
  - Prescription drugs (warn patient not to drink alcoholic beverages or use dangerous equipment):
    - Trimethobenzamide hydrochloride 250 mg tablets, 1 tablet every 8 hours, or 200 mg rectal suppositories, 1 suppository every 8 hours
    - Promethazine hydrochloride 25 mg tablets, 1 tablet every 12 hours, or 25 mg rectal suppositories, 1 suppository every 12 hours

→ Offer tetanus prophylaxis if indicated.

→ Offer hepatitis B prophylaxis (CDC 2002):

- Postexposure hepatitis B vaccination, without hepatitis B immune globulin, should adequately protect against hepatitis B virus infection. If the patient has not been previously vaccinated, the initial dose should be administered at the time of the sexual assault examination, with follow-up doses 1–2 months and 4–6 months after the first dose. See the *Physicians' Desk Reference (PDR)* for drug dosage information.

→ Consider postexposure prevention for HIV prophylaxis (Fong 2001). Consultation with an HIV specialist is recommended.

→ Provide crisis intervention counseling.

→ Provide an informational brochure about sexual assault, if available.

- Copies may be obtained from:
  Texas Department of Health, Bureau of Emergency Management Sexual Assault Prevention and Crisis Services Program
  1100 West 49th St.
  Austin, Tex. 78765-3199
  (512) 834-6700
  www.oag.state.tx.us/newspubs/publications.shtml

→ Another national resource is:
  Rape, Abuse and Incest National Network (RAINN) (800) 656-HOPE or 4673 (24-hour line)

→ If domestic violence is suspected, see the **Domestic Violence** chapter.

CONSULTATION

→ Consultation with a physician is required if serious injuries are evidenced or suspected.

- General guidelines include but are not limited to:
  - History of loss of consciousness
  - Lack of orientation
  - Chest or abdominal pain
  - Head/neck/back injury
  - Limited range of motion of extremities
  - History of foreign object insertion
  - Perineal laceration

→ Consultation with psychological/psychiatric services with special training in sexual assault is necessary if suicidal ideation, substance abuse, or other emotional disturbances are present.

→ Consultation with appropriate law enforcement officials is required regarding the collection, storage, and transportation of evidence. Consultation is also indicated if the assault was part of the broader problem of domestic violence with homicidal intent and/or concurrent child abuse.

→ As needed for prescription(s).

PATIENT EDUCATION

→ Explain the rationale for examination procedures, cultures, and prophylactic medications.

→ Explain side effects of all medications. Refer to the *PDR*.

→ Explain that the examination and evidence collection can be done regardless of whether the woman decides to report the rape to the police.

→ Reassure the patient that women respond to assault in a variety of ways and that her feelings are normal.

→ Provide the patient with the telephone number of a victim assistance program, if available.

→ Explain that in some jurisdictions, a rape survivor can request that her assailant be tested for HIV.

→ Provide the patient with telephone numbers for law enforcement, psychological and medical services, and the HIV hotline.

→ Educate regarding the signs and symptoms of STDs and the importance of follow-up as indicated.

→ Health promotion/maintenance and prevention for all women:

- Because *all* women are at risk for assault, all women should be screened for sexual violence.
- Utilize strategies in your practice that empower women—e.g., allowing women to have control over their health care, talking to the patient while she is still fully clothed, teaching women about their bodies.
- Inform patients that violence is not a normal part of relationships.
- Provide patients with alternative methods of conflict resolution.
- Discourage rigid sex-role stereotyping.
- Teach teens the warning signals regarding date rape and tactics for resisting peer pressure.
- Encourage assertiveness, leadership skill building, and self-defense in female patients.

FOLLOW-UP

→ The patient's emotional status should be re-evaluated 24–48 hours after the initial assessment and, if indicated, long-term counseling offered. Follow-up contacts should be carried out in a very discreet manner.

→ Unless prophylactic treatment was provided, an examination and testing for STDs should be repeated within 1–2 weeks of the assault (CDC 2002). Review signs and symptoms of STDs and advise further follow-up as indicated.

→ Order/perform a pregnancy test as indicated.

→ Serologic tests for syphilis and HIV should be repeated six, 12, and 24 weeks after the assault if the initial tests were negative (these infections are likely in the assailant) (CDC 2002).

→ The sexual assault nurse examiner may be required to testify on behalf of the patient if the case goes to trial.

→ Document in progress notes and on problem list.
- Events should be recorded accurately and injuries documented with drawings or photographs.

BIBLIOGRAPHY

American College of Obstetricians and Gynecologists (ACOG). 1992. *Sexual assault*. Technical Bulletin No. 172. Washington, D.C.: the Author.

Attorney General's Office of Texas. Sexual Assault Prevention and Crisis Services Program. 1998. *Sexual assault prevention division's handbook*, pp. 86–99. Available at: http://www.oag.state.tx.us/newspubs/publications.shtml. Accessed on October 1, 2002.

Bamberger, J.D., Waldo, C.R., Gerberding, J.L. et al. 1999. Postexposure prophylaxis for human immunodeficiency virus (HIV) infection following sexual assault. *American Journal of Medicine* 106:323–326.

Beebe, D.K. 1991. Emergency management of the adult female rape victim. *American Family Physician* 43(6):2041–2046.

Bownes, I.T., O'Gorman, E.C., and Sayers, A. 1991. Assault characteristics and post-traumatic stress disorder in rape victims. *Acta Psychiatrica Scandinavica* 83(1):27–30.

Burgess, A., and Holmstron, L. 1974. Rape trauma syndrome. *American Journal of Psychiatry* 131:981–986.

Centers for Disease Control and Prevention (CDC). 2002. Sexually transmitted disease treatment guidelines—2002. *Morbidity and Mortality Weekly Report* 51(No. RR-6):69–71.

Emergency Nurses Association. 1991. Emergency Nurses Association sexual assault nurse examiners' resource list. *Journal of Emergency Nursing* 17(4):31A–35A, 95.

Fong, C. 2001. Post-exposure prophylaxis for HIV infection after sexual assault: When is it indicated? *Emergency Medical Journal* 18(4):242–245.

Glaser, J.B., Schacter, J., Benes, S. et al. 1991. Sexually transmitted diseases in postpubertal female rape victims. *Journal of Infectious Diseases* 164(4):726–730.

Hampton, H.L. 1995. Care of the woman who has been raped. *New England Journal of Medicine* 332:234–237.

Hatcher, R.A., Trussel, J., Stewart, F. et al. 1998. *Contraceptive technology*, 17th ed. New York: Ardent Media.

Hatmaker, D. 1997. A SANE approach to sexual assault. *American Journal of Nursing* 97(8):80.

Lenehan, G. 1991. Sexual assault nurse examiners: a SANE way to care for rape victims. *Journal of Emergency Nursing* February 17(1):1–2.

McConkey, T.E., Sole, M.L., and Holcomb, L. 2001. Assessing the female sexual assault survivor. *Nurse Practitioner* 26 (7 Part 1):28–39.

Moscarello, R. 1991. Post-traumatic stress disorder after sexual assault: its psychodynamics and treatment. *Journal of the American Academy of Psychoanalysis* 19(2):235–253.

Nwokolo, N.C., and Hawkins, D.A. 2001. Postexposure prophylaxis for HIV infection. *AIDS Reader* 11(8):402–412.

Petter, L.M., and Whitehill, D.L. 1998. Management of female sexual abuse. *American Family Physician* 58(4):920–929.

Reynolds, M.W., Peipert, J.F., and Collins, B. 2000. Epidemiologic issues of sexually transmitted diseases is sexual assault victims. *Obstetrical and Gynecological Survey* 55(1):51–57.

Rose, V.L. 1999. ACOG releases a statement on identification and treatment of adolescent victims of sexual assault. *American Family Physician* 59(6):1688.

Rothbaum, B., Foa, E., Murdock, T. et al. 1990. Post-traumatic stress disorder in rape victims. Unpublished manuscript.

Ruch, L.D., Amedeo, S.R., Leon, J.J. et al. 1991. Repeated sexual victimization and trauma change during the acute phase of the sexual assault trauma syndrome. *Women and Health* 17(2):1–19.

Schafran, L.H. 1996. Topics for our times: Rape is a major public health issue. *American Journal of Public Health* 86(1):15–16.

Schwartz, I.L. 1991. Sexual violence against women: prevalence, consequences, societal factors and prevention. *American Journal of Preventive Medicine* 7(6):363–373.

Slaughter, L., and Brown, C.R. 1992. Colposcopy to establish physical findings in rape victims. *American Journal of Obstetrics and Gynecology* 166(1):83–86.

APPENDIX 14G.1.

Sexual Assault Examination and Forensic Report Form

SEXUAL ASSAULT FORENSIC EXAMINATION

Please print legibly. To be filled out with medical information gathered from the patient. Please inform the patient that, should the case go to court, it may be necessary to gather additional evidence at a later time. Please fill in all spaces with information or N/A.

Name: _____ DOB: _____ Sex: _____ Race: _____

Address: _____ Phone: _____

Patient Brought in By: _____ Agency or Relationship of Escort: _____

Hospital Number: _____ Law Enforcement Case Number: _____

Exam Date: _____ Beginning Time of Exam: _____

VITAL SIGNS: Time _____ Temp _____ Pulse _____ Resp _____ B/P _____

Known Allergies: _____

Current Medications: _____

HISTORY OF ASSAULT: (Patient's description of pertinent details of the assault, if known by patient, such as: orifice penetrated, digital penetration or use of foreign object, oral contact by assailant, oral contact by patient) _____

_____

_____

_____

_____

Date of Assault: _____ Time of Assault: _____ Number of Assailants: _____

Prior to evidence collection, patient has:

___ Douched   ___ Wiped/Washed   ___ Bathed   ___ Showered   ___ Urinated   ___ Defecated

___ Vomited   ___ Had Food or Drink   ___ Brushed Teeth or Used Mouthwash   ___ Changed Clothes

___ Smoked   ___ Other   ___ None of the Above

At time of assault, was:

Contraceptive foam or spermicide present?   ___ Yes   ___ No   ___ Unknown

Lubricant used by assailant   ___ Yes   ___ No   ___ Unknown

What kind?

Condom used by assailant?   ___ Yes   ___ No   ___ Unknown

Tampon present during assault?   ___ Yes   ___ No   ___ Unknown

Patient menstruating?   ___ Yes   ___ No   ___ Unknown

Assailant injured during assault?   ___ Yes   ___ No   ___ Unknown

If known, where? _____

Was there penetration?   ___ Oral   ___ Female Sexual Organ   ___ Anus   ___ Unknown

Did ejaculation occur?   ___ Oral   ___ Female Sexual Organ   ___ Anus   ___ Unknown

                            ___ Other (specify) _____

At time of **exam**, was tampon present?   ___ Yes   ___ No

Menstruation at time of exam?   ___ Yes   ___ No

When was the patient's most recent sexual contact up to one week prior to the assault? _____

Race of that individual? _____

If the response is less than 48 hours, inform the patient of the possibility that bodily fluid samples may be requested from that individual at a later time.

_____

Signature of Examiner

Office of the Attorney General, Sexual Assault Prevention & Crisis Services, 1998

SEXUAL ASSAULT FORENSIC EXAMINATION

Page 2

Patient's Name _____

Significant Past Medical History:

Last normal menstrual period: _____ Vaginal tampons used in the past? _____

G _____ P _____ AB _____

Contraceptives used: _____

Genital surgical procedures: _____

General Appearance: (behavior, affect) _____

Body Surface Injuries: (include all details of trauma: i.e., abrasions, birthmarks)

❏ No body surface injuries noted.

_____

_____

_____

_____

Body Surface Diagrams: Document injuries and observations on the attached body diagrams.

Genital Examination: **Tanner Stage**   ❏ 1   ❏ 2   ❏ 3   ❏ 4   ❏ 5

Labia Majora _____

Labia Minora _____

Hymen _____

Vagina _____

Cervix _____

Perineum _____

Anus _____

Penis _____

Scrotum _____

Check For Sperm: ____ Not Done   ____ Positive   ____ Negative   Motile: ____ Yes   ____ No

Genital Diagrams: Document injuries and observations on the attached genital diagrams.

Document all diagnostic tests and treatment on medical record.

Ending Time of Exam: _____

Impressions From Exam: _____

_____

_____

_____

_____

_____

_____

_____
Signature of Examiner

Office of the Attorney General, Sexual Assault Prevention & Crisis Services, 1998

SEXUAL ASSAULT FORENSIC EXAMINATION   *Page 3*

Patient's Name _____

EVIDENCE ITEMS INCLUDED IN KIT

____ Oral Swabs (4)	____ External Penile Swabs (2)	____ Fingernail Scrapings
____ Oral Smear (1)	____ External Penile Smear (1)	____ Head Hair Combings & Comb
____ Vaginal Swabs (4)	____ Saliva Swabs (2)	____ Head Hair Pulled Standards
____ Vaginal Smear (1)	____ Yellow Blood Tube	____ Foreign Matter
____ Dried Body Fluids	____ Purple Blood Tube	
____ Pubic Hair Combings & Comb	____ Red Blood Tube	
____ Pubic Hair Pulled Standard	____ Tampon, diaper, sanitary pad, sponge	
____ Anal Swabs (4)	____ Panties (if they fit in box)	
____ Anal Smear (1)	____ Other	

EVIDENCE ITEMS *NOT* INCLUDED IN KIT

____ # of paper bags   ____ Photographs   ____ X-rays   ____ Other _____ (specify)

(Available)

(Please list clothing or miscellaneous items)

Article	Description (tears or stains)
_____	_____
_____	_____
_____	_____
_____	_____

PATIENT FOLLOW-UP CARE/LEGAL CHECKLIST:

Gyn/Medical/STD follow-up appointment recommended	____ yes	____ no
Sexual assault counseling referral given	____ yes	____ no
Written and verbal information given to patient	____ yes	____ no
Medical facility received permission to contact patient ____ by telephone	____ by mail	____ permission not obtained
Authorization for Release of Evidence to Law Enforcement Agency completed	____ yes	____ no
Law enforcement/Children's Protective Services notified if child abuse suspected	____ yes	____ no

_____   _____
Signature of Examiner   Printed Name of Examiner

Office of the Attorney General, Sexual Assault Prevention & Crisis Services, 1998

SEXUAL ASSAULT FORENSIC EXAMINATION   *Page 4*

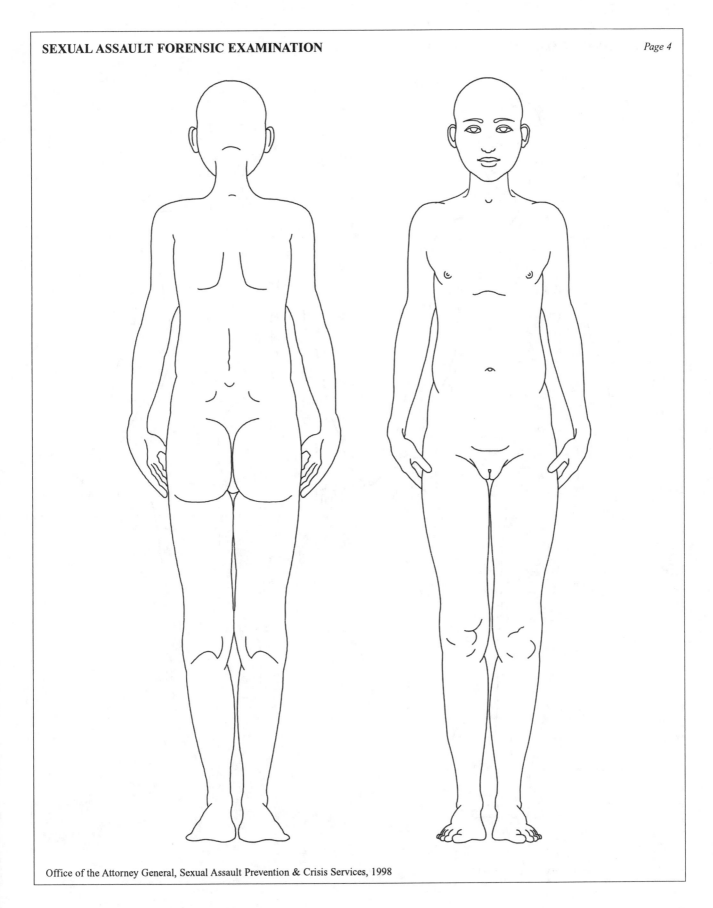

Office of the Attorney General, Sexual Assault Prevention & Crisis Services, 1998

SEXUAL ASSAULT FORENSIC EXAMINATION

Page 5

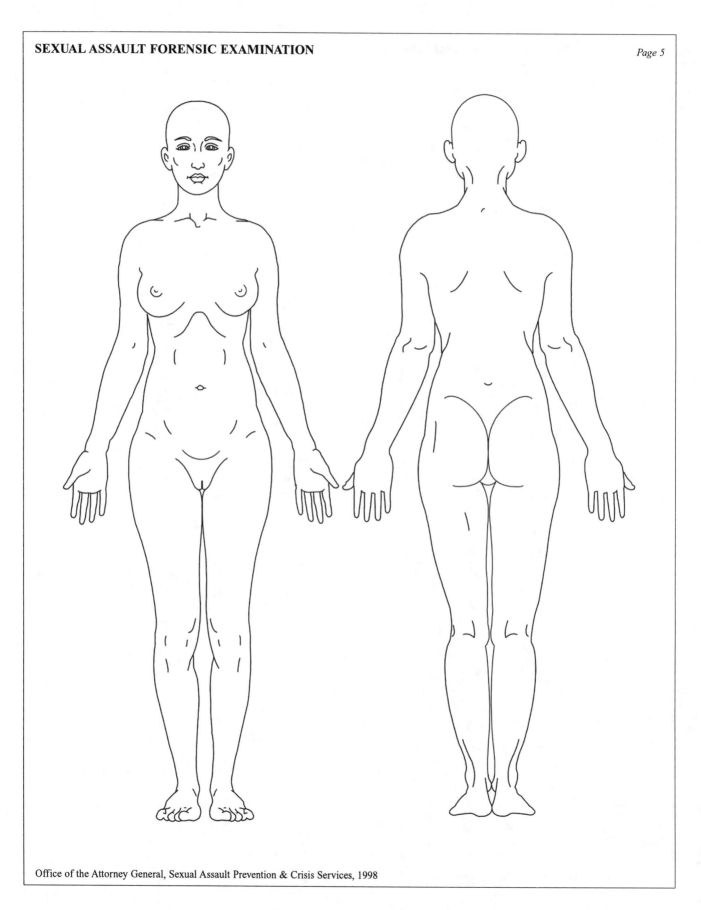

Office of the Attorney General, Sexual Assault Prevention & Crisis Services, 1998

SEXUAL ASSAULT FORENSIC EXAMINATION   *Page 6*

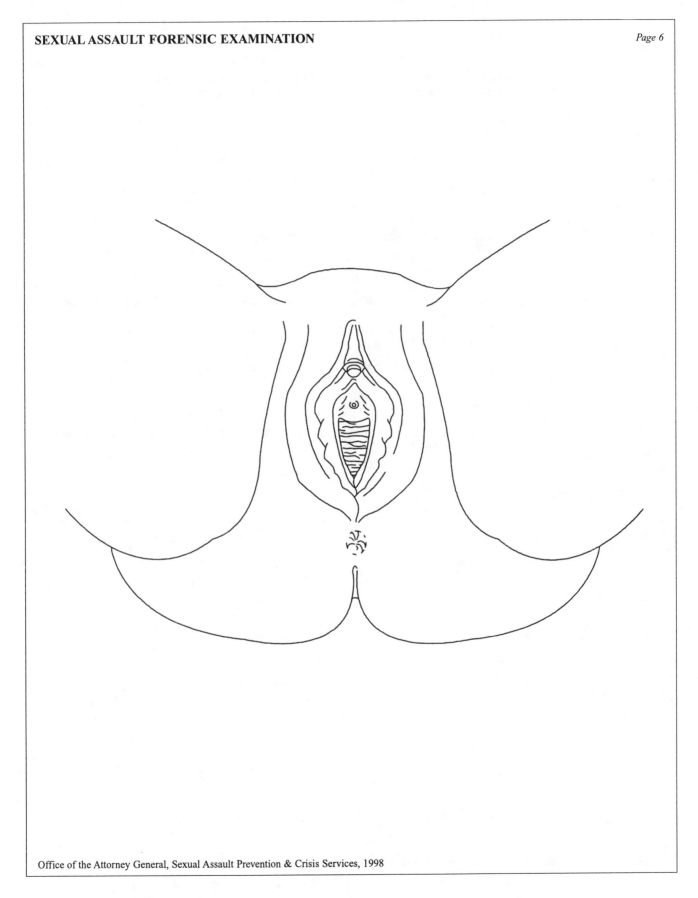

Office of the Attorney General, Sexual Assault Prevention & Crisis Services, 1998

**REQUEST FOR MEDICAL FORENSIC EXAMINATION, TREATMENT,
COLLECTION OF EVIDENCE, AND RELEASE OF MEDICAL RECORDS**

I hereby authorize _____ , a representative of _____
(Name of Examiner)   (Name of Hospital)

to perform a medical forensic examination, treatment, and the collection of evidence. I further permit the photographic

documentation and release of copies of the complete report to the law enforcement agency.

I release _____ and its representatives from legal responsibility or
(Name of Hospital)

liability for the release of this information.

_____   _____
Signature of Patient (parent or guardian)   Signature of Witness

Note: If the parent or guardian is not available for signature, child may be examined for sexual abuse under Texas
Family Code.

Office of the Attorney General, Sexual Assault Prevention & Crisis Services, 1998

RECEIPT OF INFORMATION

I have received the following items (check those that apply):

_____ One sealed evidence kit

_____ # of sealed clothing bag(s)

_____ X-rays or copies of x-rays

_____ Photographs

_____ Other: _____

Name of person releasing articles:

_____

Signature   Printed Name   Date   Time

Received by:

_____

Signature   Printed Name   Date   Time

_____

ID Badge #   Agency

Office of the Attorney General, Sexual Assault Prevention & Crisis Services, 1998

Kellie Sheehan, R.N., C., M.S.N., F.N.P.

14-H
Smoking Cessation

Despite the overall decline of cigarette smoking from 1965 to 1995, tobacco use remains the single most preventable cause of death and disability in the United States (McGinnis et al. 1993). One in five deaths is attributable to smoking. In the United States, smoking causes more deaths each year than the combined deaths from World War I, the Korean War, and the Vietnam War (Jemal et al. 2001).

In the United States, there are an estimated 400,000 deaths per year attributable to smoking. Or put another way, more than 1,000 people die each day from tobacco-related illnesses—the equivalent of the number of passengers in three jumbo jets crashing, without survivors, every day. Yet the public perceives greater health risks from nuclear power plants, acquired immune deficiency syndrome (AIDS), handgun injuries, and suicide than from smoking (Houston 1992). In reality, smoking causes more deaths per year than AIDS, motor vehicle accidents, alcohol, homicide, drugs, and suicide combined (Centers for Disease Control and Prevention [CDC] 2000a).

Eighty-seven percent of lung cancer cases are attributable to smoking. Cancers of the larynx, pharynx, esophagus, bladder, kidney, pancreas, and cervix are attributable, at least in part, to smoking (Wingo et al. 1999). Eighty-five percent of all cases of chronic obstructive pulmonary disease (COPD) are caused by smoking. COPD is the second leading cause of worker disability in the United States (Frank et al. 1993). In terms of health care costs and lost worker productivity, smoking costs an estimated $200 billion a year (Rose 1991). Smoking also increases the risk for cardiac disease and peptic ulcer disease, exacerbates allergies and asthma, and causes premature wrinkling of the skin and periodontal disease (Kahn 1993).

There are special concerns regarding reproduction and fertility for women who smoke. Infertility is more common in smokers as a result of irregular menses and amenorrhea associated with the hormonal changes related to nicotine. Nicotine interferes with the normal release of gonadotropins, which can result in menstrual irregularities as well as hirsutism, early menopause, and accelerated osteoporosis.

It is known that ectopic pregnancy risk is increased by smoking, though exactly why is under investigation. Miscarriage is almost twice as high in smokers as in nonsmokers. There is also increased risk for premature birth, polyhydramnios, placenta previa, and premature rupture of membranes. These complications are thought to be caused by the compensatory hypertrophy of the placenta as it competes for oxygen with the carbon monoxide produced by cigarette smoking (Fredriccson et al. 1992).

Smoking reduces birth weight and, when compared to alcohol, caffeine, and socioeconomic variables, is still the most important factor influencing birth weight. With cigarette consumption of greater than 10 per day, there is increased risk of sudden infant death syndrome. Finally, cleft palate malformation has been identified in some studies as occurring more frequently in children of mothers who smoke (Fredriccson et al. 1992).

History of Tobacco

American settlers adopted the ritual of smoking from Native Americans in the 1800s. In 1884, the cigarette-rolling machine was invented, allowing the mass production of cigarettes. By World War I, tobacco was considered as indispensable as food and was included in ration packets distributed to Americans on the home front (Houston 1992). During World War II, President Franklin D. Roosevelt declared tobacco an essential crop, giving draft deferments to tobacco growers. The American military forces consumed 75% of American tobacco products. The journals of the American Medical Association even accepted cigarette advertisements during this time (Houston 1992).

In 1941, the insightful work of two physicians, Oschner and DeBakey, called attention to the similarity of the curves of increased sales of cigarettes and the increased prevalence of lung cancer (Wynder et al. 1950). Nine years later, Wynder et al. (1950) published the results of a well-designed study linking cigarette smoking with bronchogenic carcinoma.

In 1964, the U.S. Surgeon General issued the first public report linking smoking with negative health consequences.

Despite more than 60,000 documents proving the relationship between smoking and lung cancer, 30% of all other cancers, cardiovascular disease, and COPD, the tobacco industry denied this evidence for years. Spending an estimated $3.5 billion a year on advertising and promotion of its products, the tobacco industry is a powerful political lobby. There is still no regulatory body controlling the tobacco industry's advertising or cigarette production (Houston 1992).

Smoking Cessation

Though more Americans have quit smoking than currently smoke, 46 million Americans still smoke (CDC 2001). The fastest growing group of new smokers is adolescents, with girls outpacing boys. Most current smokers started to smoke as preteens or adolescents.

Seventy percent of smokers see a health care provider at least once a year (Houston 1992). These visits are often a consequence of smoking-related illness, providing an opportunity for intervention and teaching. Most surveys document that 70–90% of smokers want to quit and that more than half will make at least one serious attempt (Houston 1992, Solberg et al. 1990).

Interventions of only two minutes duration, long enough to deliver a smoking cessation message and give out printed self-help materials, have been shown to increase one-year cessation rates (CDC 2000b). Results improve with nicotine replacement and/or bupropion, with success rates at one year varying 16–35% (Jorenby et al. 1999). It is important to recognize that though these numbers may seem small, when dealing with large numbers of smokers, 16–35% can make a huge difference. For example, if just 20% of the 32 million smokers who go to a health care provider this year received a smoking cessation message with pharmacological aids and follow-up, as many as 6.4 million smokers might quit.

Cessation is difficult because nicotine is addictive; nicotine is a psychoactive drug with effects that reinforce smoking behavior despite known health risks. Studies have shown nicotine to be more addictive than heroin or cocaine (Koop 1988). Nicotine replacement therapies are thought to be useful by reducing the withdrawal symptoms associated with abstinence (Benowitz 1993, Lee et al. 1993, Robbins 1993). Even though many smokers initially quit through use of these therapies, after one year the relapse rate is 70% (Jorenby et al. 1999).

Bupropion has been used for depression for many years with an interesting side effect noted by patients; it seems they did not want to smoke as much. In 1996, a second pharmaceutical company studied this phenomenon and found that bupropion did help smokers quit. In May 1997, bupropion was approved by the Food and Drug Administration as an aid for smoking cessation (Dale et al. 2001). Bupropion's exact mechanism of action is unknown, but it is hypothesized that the drug binds to the same receptors in the brain as nicotine, thus reducing the desire to smoke (Ascher et al. 1995).

Jorenby et al. (1999) compared nicotine replacement with the relatively new bupropion for smoking cessation. They found that bupropion alone had higher success rates after one year

(30%) than nicotine patches (16.4%) and higher than placebo (15.6%). There was a slight increased success rate with bupropion and nicotine replacement combined (35.3%) compared with bupropion alone, but this difference was not statistically significant.

Cessation is also difficult due to the variables affecting smoking behavior. There are four categories of forces that drive smoking behavior—the patient, the patient's support network, the value or cultural beliefs of the patient, and the treatment modality chosen (Still 1993). Lennox (1992) reviewed the literature to identify these factors and determine which ones are important for successful cessation. When the uniqueness of the patient's smoking behavior are recognized, intervention strategies can be individualized and are thus more likely to succeed.

Nursing has long been a leader in patient education, and many studies identify nurses as valuable, cost-effective resources for office-based smoking cessation programs (Hollis et al. 1993). Helping patients quit smoking may be the single most important intervention to improve their health.

DATABASE

SUBJECTIVE

→ Obtain a smoking history. Ask, "Do you smoke?" "For how long?" "How much do you smoke?" "Are you interested in quitting?" "Have you ever quit before?" "What made you start again?"
→ If patient has quit, ascertain prior smoking history as above.
  ■ Recent cessation (within the year) increases risk for relapse.
  ■ Offer praise and congratulations for quitting.
  ■ If quitting is recent, offer printed self-help materials and referrals to Nicotine Anonymous, American Lung Association, or American Cancer Society.
  ■ Medical history to include:
    • Illnesses specific to the cardiorespiratory system—e.g., bronchitis, sinusitis, pneumonia, allergies, asthma, COPD, coronary artery disease, myocardial infarction, peripheral vascular disease, Raynaud's disease, hypertension, hypercholesterolemia, blood clots
    • Cancer—e.g., lung, head and neck, mouth, larynx, esophagus, bladder, kidney, pancreas, brain, cervix, breast
    • Gynecological history—infertility, abnormal Pap smears, low-birth-weight babies, complications of pregnancy
    • Gastritis or peptic ulcer disease
→ Family history may reveal cancer, coronary artery disease, peptic ulcer disease, asthma, or COPD.
→ Psychosocial history may include history of depression, substance abuse, or other mental health diagnosis. These conditions can make cessation more difficult. In addition:
  ■ Identify social supports and living situations in terms of other smokers.
  ■ Assess coexistent stressors to determine whether the timing is right to introduce a major lifestyle change.

- Identify any need for possible referrals.
→ Review of systems to include:
  - Respiratory complaints of shortness of breath, productive or nonproductive cough, postnasal drip, wheezing, decreased exercise tolerance, frequent colds, and allergy symptoms
  - Cardiovascular symptoms such as chest pain, leg pain when walking short distances, excessively cold hands or feet, with color change
  - Gastrointestinal symptoms such as abdominal burning or pain, acid indigestion, heartburn, constipation, diarrhea; frequent use of antacids; food intolerance
  - Cosmetic changes noted—e.g., early skin wrinkling, teeth or finger staining

OBJECTIVE

→ General appearance may include:
  - Appears older than stated age
  - Increased facial lines
  - Yellowish stains on fingers, teeth
  - Clothes and hair smelling of tobacco
→ Vital signs may include increase in blood pressure or heart rate if there are cardiorespiratory symptoms.
→ Head, eyes, ears, nose, throat:
  - Assess for presence of periodontal disease:
    - Include bimanual oral examination
    - Assess for oral lesions that may be malignant or premalignant
→ Chest:
  - Generally few findings unless illness present
  - Assess the following:
    - Respirations
    - Quality of cough if observed
    - Anterior-posterior diameter
    - Presence of adventitious sounds
    - Office spirometry/peak expiratory flow rate
→ Extremities:
  - Note color, temperature, and pulses.
  - Note hair distribution—i.e., it is decreased in lower legs and feet with peripheral vascular disease.

ASSESSMENT

→ Identify smoking history, relapse history, motivation to quit.
→ Rule out concomitant physical illness.

PLAN

DIAGNOSTIC TESTS

→ Pulmonary function tests are generally normal unless respiratory illness is present; therefore, not recommended.
→ Cholesterol level—if elevated, this may be useful as a motivator to quit.
→ Additional laboratory tests as indicated by history and physical examination.

TREATMENT/MANAGEMENT

→ Advise patient to stop smoking.
  - If evidence of concomitant illness or signs of abnormality appear on physical examination, use this as an indication of the harmful effects of tobacco and the need to quit.
  - Educate the patient regarding the negative effects of smoking and the benefits of quitting.
→ Help patient pick a quit date.
→ Arrange support, follow-up, and resources.
→ Consider consultation if there is a history of major depression, bipolar disorder, seizure disorder, or AIDS, and if the smoker desires bupropion (Jorenby et al. 1999).
→ Consider consultation if the patient has severe cardiovascular disease or is pregnant and desires nicotine replacement (Benowitz 1993, Hughes 1993).

Pharmacological Adjuncts

→ Bupropion
  - Start about 1–2 weeks before patient's quit date.
  - Start with 150 mg, 1 pill/day for 3 days.
  - Increase to BID. Many patients like to try discontinuing the medication 4–6 months after they have successfully quit. The patient may remain on medication for up to 1 year, though this is individually determined by the patient and health care provider.
→ Nicotine replacement
  - Nicotine patch is a transdermal system absorbed through the skin over 16–24 hours depending on the brand.
    - Patient should start use on her quit date.
    - Instructions for use include:
      - Apply every morning on a dry area of upper arm, stomach, or buttock.
        ➤ Rotate sites, re-using the same site no more frequently than every 7 days.
      - Change every day. The different brands are generally similar in dosage. Taper over 2 months—e.g., 21 mg/day for 4 weeks, 14 mg/day for 2 weeks, and, finally, 7 mg/day for 2 weeks.
    - 21 mg patch is equivalent to trough concentrations (i.e., lowest level of blood nicotine) in smokers averaging 1–2 packs per day.
    - Generally well-tolerated, though 50% of users experience some local skin irritation.
    - Encourage the patient to enroll in a smoking cessation class.
  - Nicotine gum
    - Delivers nicotine through transbuccal absorption.
    - Patient should start use on her quit date if she is not using the nicotine patch, or after successfully tapering with the patch, for "just in case" protection. Instructions for use include:
      - Use only 2 mg gum or one-half of 4 mg gum.
      - Wait 10–15 minutes after drinking any beverage before using gum, as there is decreased absorption in an acidic environment.

- Chew slowly, until there is a tingle or peppery taste, then "park" the gum between the cheek and the gums.
  - Repeat the chewing once the taste disappears, after about 1 minute.
  - The gum lasts 20–30 minutes.
- If using only the nicotine gum, use on a regular schedule. Most people need 10–16 pieces per day.
  - Do not use more than 20 pieces per day.
- Once the patient has quit for 3 months, she should begin to taper use.
  - Taper gradually over 2–3 months.
  - Taper 1–2 pieces per week.
- Encourage the patient to enroll in a smoking cessation class.

CONSULTATION

→ For patients with depression or a history of depression, antidepressant agents may be required. Referral for counseling is recommended.

→ For pregnant patients or those who have cerebrovascular or cardiovascular disease or seizure disorder, consultation with a physician is advised prior to the use of pharmacological adjuncts for smoking cessation.

→ As needed for prescription(s).

PATIENT EDUCATION

→ Inform the patient that quitting smoking is the single most important thing she can do for her health.

→ Encourage the patient to think of quitting smoking as "learning a foreign language." Both efforts require practice. If a relapse occurs, encourage the patient not to give up and to try again.

→ Smoking cessation may take a while to master.
  - On average, it takes three attempts before a smoker quits for good.
  - Encourage the smoker not to feel as if she has a character defect because she did not succeed in the past. Encourage her to try again.

→ Have the smoker write on a 3" x 5" file card the three most important reasons she has for quitting. Have her keep this card in the same place she keeps her cigarettes. Once she has quit, have her pull out the card and read it whenever she has the urge to smoke.

→ Have the patient practice quitting a little every day, at different times of the day.
  - For example, on Monday, advise the patient not to smoke from 6:00 a.m. until 9:00 a.m.; on Tuesday, not to smoke from 9:00 a.m. until 12 noon; on Wednesday, not to smoke from noon until 3:00 p.m.; and so on.
  - Once the week is completed, the smoker will learn which cigarettes were most important and why, and she will then know which cigarettes might prove harder not to have.

→ Have the patient keep a smoking diary.
  - Identifying what triggers smoking is key to determining alternate behaviors to smoking.

→ Give the patient permission to reward nonsmoking behaviors. Rewarded behavior is repeated.

→ Encourage the patient to join a class on quitting smoking.

→ Ask the patient to read as much as possible about the health effects of smoking, the benefits of quitting, and the tobacco industry.

→ Encourage plenty of rest, fresh air, and exercise.

→ Recommend attention to good nutrition.
  - Smokers need an extra amount of folate, betacarotene, and vitamins B_6, E, and C (Baron 1993).

→ Ask the patient to reach out to nonsmokers, to find a "buddy" in her quit-smoking campaign. People with more social support have higher success rates (Lennox 1992).

→ Tell the patient to expect a small weight gain; 7–10 pounds is normal.
  - Being overweight generally is healthier than smoking.
  - Tell the patient to increase the level and frequency of exercise.

→ Advise the patient to be wary of relapse. Advise her to avoid high-risk situations initially, and to learn and practice positive imagery, meditation, or self-hypnosis techniques.

→ Tell the patient to expect to succeed, to be confident.

→ Once the patient has quit for six months, encourage community involvement—e.g., to volunteer on "former smoker" panels, teach a quit smoking class, be a buddy for other "newly quit" smokers.

FOLLOW-UP

→ It is helpful to have a scheduled stop-smoking visit, establish a quit date, and give the patient homework.

→ Establish a "quit day" appointment if possible.
  - Make this a celebratory visit, sign a contract, review strategies for urge control, and offer referral sources.

→ Meet with the patient once every two weeks for one month, every month for three months, then at six months and one year. If the patient chooses a cessation program, then follow up by telephone on or near quit day to offer ongoing encouragement. Offer a support visit at three months.

→ Ask at every visit about the patient's efforts. Do not get discouraged if she has relapsed. Praise her initial effort and explore what caused the relapse.

→ The American Cancer Society and the American Lung Association also offer resources and support groups.

→ Document smoking history and cessation strategies on progress notes. Identify smoking status on problem list as appropriate.

BIBLIOGRAPHY

Ascher, J.A., Cole, J.O., Colin, J.N. et al. 1995. Bupropion: a review of its mechanisms of antidepressant activity. *Journal of Clinical Psychiatry* 56:395–401.

Baron, R. 1993. New developments in clinical nutrition. UCSF Department of Medicine. Primary Care Medicine Update. Continuing Medical Education.

Benowitz, N.L. 1993. Nicotine replacement therapy: What has

been accomplished? Can we do better? *Drugs* 2:157–170.

Centers for Disease Control and Prevention (CDC). 2000a. Tobacco information and prevention service. *Comparative causes of annual deaths in the United States.* Available at: http://www.cdc.gov/health/tobacco.htm or http://www.cdc.gov/tobacco/data.htm. Accessed on October 8, 2002.

_____. 2000b. Receipt of advice to quit smoking in Medicare managed care—United States, 1998. *Morbidity and Mortality Weekly Report* 49(35):797–801.

_____. 2001. State-specific prevalence of cigarette smoking among adults and cigarette smoking in 99 metropolitan areas—United States, 2000. *Morbidity and Mortality Weekly Report* 50:1–3.

Cummings, S.R., Coates, T.J., Richard, R.J. et al. 1989a. Training physicians in counseling about smoking cessation: a randomized trial of the "Quit for Life" program. *Annals of Internal Medicine* 110:640–647.

Cummings, S.R., Rubin, S.M., and Oster, G. 1989b. The cost-effectiveness of counseling smokers to quit. *Journal of the American Medical Association* 261:75–79.

Dale, L.C., Gover, E.D., and Sachs, D.P. 2001. Nicotine-free pill effective in smoking cessation for all categories of smokers. *Chest* 119:1357–1364.

Fagerstrom, K.O. 1978. Measuring degree of physical dependence on tobacco smoking with reference to individuation of treatment. *Addictive Behavior* 3:235–241.

Frank, S.H., and Jaen, C.R. 1993. Office evaluation and treatment of the dependent smoker. *Primary Care* 20:251–268.

Fredriccson, B., and Gilljam, H. 1992. Smoking and reproduction: short and long-term effects and benefits of smoking cessation. *Acta Obstetrica Gynecologica Scandinavia* 71:580–592.

Hollis, J.F., Lichenstein, E., Vogt, T.M. et al. 1993. Nurse-assisted counseling for smokers in primary care. *American College of Physicians* 118:521–525.

Houston, T.P. 1992. Smoking cessation in office practice. *Primary Care* 19:493–507.

Hughes, J.R. 1993. Risk/benefit assessment of nicotine preparations in smoking cessation. *Drug Safety* 8:49–56.

Jemal, A., Chu, K.C., and Tarone, R.E. 2001. Recent trends in lung cancer mortality in the United States. *Journal of the National Cancer Institute* 93:277–283.

Jorenby, D.E., Leischow, S.J., Nides, M.A. et al. 1999. A controlled trial of sustained-release bupropion, a nicotine patch, or both for smoking cessation. *New England Journal of Medicine* 340:685–691.

Kahn, H. 1993. *Nicotine addiction and smoking cessation.* Unpublished manuscript.

_____. 1988. *The health consequences of smoking: nicotine addiction.* A report of the Surgeon General (1988). Available at: http://www.cdc.gov/tobacco/sgr. Accessed on October 8, 2002.

Koop, C.E. 1988. *Smoking: everything you and your family need to know.* Ambrose Video.

Lee, E.W., and D'Alonzo, G.E. 1993. Cigarette smoking, nicotine addiction and its pharmacological treatment. *Archives of Internal Medicine* 153:34–48.

Lennox, A.S. 1992. Determinants of outcome in smoking cessation. *British Journal of General Practice* 42:247–252.

McGinnis, J.M., and Foege, W.H. 1993. Actual causes of death in the United States. *Journal of the American Medical Association* 270:2207–2212.

Robbins, A.S. 1993. Pharmacological approaches to smoking cessation. *American Journal of Preventative Medicine* 9:31–33.

Rose, M.A. 1991. Intervention strategies for smoking cessation: the role of oncology nursing. *Cancer Nursing* 14:225–231.

Solberg, L.I., Maxwell, P.L., Kottke, T.E. et al. 1990. A systematic primary care office-based smoking cessation program. *Journal of Family Practice* 30:647–654.

Still, J.M. 1993. Smoking-cessation therapy: current medical management. *Ob/Gyn Nursing and Patient Counseling* 5:5–9.

Taylor, C.B., Houston-Miller, N., Killen, J.D. et al. 1990. Smoking cessation after acute myocardial infarction: effects of a nurse managed intervention. *Annals of Internal Medicine* 113:118–123.

Wingo, P.A., Reis, L.A., Giovino, G.A. et al. 1999. Annual report to the nation on the status of cancer, 1973–1996, with a special section on lung cancer and tobacco smoking. *Journal of the National Cancer Institute* 91:675–690.

Wynder, E.L., and Graham, E.A. 1950. Tobacco smoking as a possible etiologic factor in bronchiogenic carcinoma. *Journal of the American Medical Association* 143:329–336.

Zahnd, E.G., Coates, T.J., Richard, R.J. et al. 1990. Counseling medical patients about cigarette smoking: a comparison of the impact of training on nurse practitioners and physicians. *Nurse Practitioner* 15:10–18.

Catherine M. Kelber, R.N., M.S., A.N.P., B.C.

14-I

Stress Management

Stress, an unavoidable fact of life for most humans, can have both beneficial and negative effects. Despite extensive research, there remains no consensus definition of stress. Selye (1974) coined the term in the 1930s and described a physiological response pattern that occurs when an individual perceives a threat. This response is mediated by adrenaline and other hormones and includes increased blood pressure, heart rate, muscle tension, and blood clotting. The stress continuum ranges from positive, motivating, creative stress to negative, disabling *distress* or *stress overload*. Prolonged distress can cause organ damage that may lead to disease.

Events that are stress-producing have been well documented in the literature and range from daily hassles, annoyances, and irritants (Monroe 1983) to major life changes such as marriage, divorce, changing jobs or residence, death of a spouse, and illness or injury (Holmes et al. 1967).

Lazarus et al. (1984) devised a transactional model suggesting that an individual's perception of what is stressful and his or her perceived ability to cope with that stressor is key in eliciting the stress response. Stress and coping are affected by environmental, experiential, cognitive, and personality differences. An individual's perceptions and beliefs about the consequences of the actual event also determine the level of stress (Ellis 1975).

Culture and ethnicity are important determinants of perceived stressors, coping patterns, and choice of management strategies. Minority women frequently list finances and maintaining cultural values as stressors (Majumbar et al. 1998, Smyth et al. 1996).

There are countless reactions to stress, including anxiety, depression, somatic symptoms, denial, withdrawal, and substance abuse. Feelings of fear, rage, guilt, shame, and helplessness are common. Symptoms of acute stress can present as restlessness, irritability, fatigue, tension, increased startle reaction, sleep disturbances, and an inability to concentrate (Schroeder et al. 1991).

Chronic stress conditions should be suspected if patients present often with multiple somatic complaints with no apparent underlying cause. Chronic stress also may suggest underlying chronic anxiety or depressive mood disorders. Identified stress-related diseases include hypertension, heart disease, asthma, rheumatoid arthritis, irritable bowel disease, ulcers, headaches, chronic pain, eczema, and recurrent, nonspecific vaginal infections (Manderino et al. 1992).

In the United States, it is estimated that stress-related complaints account for 75% of visits to a medical provider (Charlesworth et al. 1984). Women present more often than men with somatic complaints, anxiety, and depression. The stress experienced by women is thought to be related to increased societal demands, particularly since the 1970s. More and more women are juggling careers, family responsibilities, and personal fulfillment as well as other stressors, including pregnancy, childbirth, menopause, single parenthood, financial insecurity, and physical and sexual assault (Manderino et al.1992). Women may impart different value and meaning to work and family roles than men, which may increase role stress (Simon 1995).

Stress management is a skill that can be learned. There is, however, no simple overall treatment strategy for stress. An approach consisting of multiple modalities is usually necessary. Attention to sources of stress, stress awareness, cognitive appraisal, coping ability, and patient preferences is imperative when designing an optimal management program. Pender (2001) suggests a multidimensional model for intervention that consists of the following:

→ Minimizing the frequency of stress-inducing situations (changing what can be changed in the environment)
→ Psychological preparation to increase resistance to stress (changing attitudes)
→ Counter-conditioning to avoid physiological arousal resulting from stress (altering physiological responses)

Complementary approaches such as acupuncture, bodywork, and aromatherapy have gained increasing acceptance over the last decade in the United States, and scientific evaluation of these modalities is increasingly available. Providers need to become familiar with the literature in order to make prudent recommendations about these modalities (Singleton 1999).

DATABASE

SUBJECTIVE

→ Obtain a description of current somatic symptom complex from the patient.
- Patients may sometimes present stating they are "stressed" but more commonly seek care for a particular symptom or constellation of symptoms.

→ Patient may present with a history of the same symptom or multiple visits for somatic complaints.

→ Assess current and former coping style.
- Helpful questions include, "When you feel this way, what things do you do to make yourself feel better?" or "Have you noticed any changes in your behavior during this period?"

→ Assess current coping level.
- Is coping adequate or is the patient in crisis? Is the patient at risk for harm to herself or others? Could the patient benefit from additional coping strategies?

→ The patient may present with a history and/or family history of psychiatric disorders:
- Anxiety, depression, psychoses, addictive behaviors, phobias, or suicide attempts

→ Obtain obstetrical/gynecological history.
- Current pregnancy, recent delivery or termination, severe premenstrual syndrome, or recent menopause

→ Assess current employment and job satisfaction.
- Schedule, responsibilities, recent changes, or promotions

→ Obtain a psychological history.

- Current/recent/past relationship status and satisfaction, recent major life change(s), social support, parenting responsibilities, history of violence or abuse

→ Obtain medication history.
- Cold preparations, antihypertensives, bronchodilators, steroids, antidepressants, anti-anxiety agents, herbs and nutritional supplements (may mimic or mask stress-related symptoms)

→ Discuss the patient's habits.
- Current or increased use of alcohol, drugs, or cigarettes; nutritional status and any change in eating behavior or appetite; sleep pattern or disruption; caffeine use; usual or current exercise program

→ Conduct an appropriate review of systems for chief complaint and/or history of weight loss or gain, change in sexual desire, suicidal ideation, mood changes (symptoms of anxiety, panic, or depression), inability to perform normal daily activities, fatigue, heat or cold intolerance, polyuria, polydipsia, and polyphagia.

OBJECTIVE

→ Attention should be paid to those systems that:
- Are related to the presenting complaint
- Are subject to target-organ damage from prolonged stress or may cause stress-related symptoms:
  - Blood pressure, pulse
  - General appearance:
    - Sometimes key in diagnosing mood disorders

Figure 14I.1.   BREATHING EXERCISE

1. Sit or lie in a comfortable position.
2. Take 3 deep, slow breaths, inhaling through the nose, exhaling through the mouth.
3. Continue slow breathing and with each inhalation imagine a wave of relaxation flowing through the body.
4. With each exhalation, imagine stress and tension released.
5. Continue the breathing exercise for 5–10 minutes.

Practice at least once daily. May be used prior to anticipated stressful events as needed.

© 2002 Catherine Kelber

Figure 14I.2.   RELAXATION EXERCISE

Sit or lie in a comfortable position. Begin by taking 3 deep cleansing breaths and continue breathing, feeling your body relax. Place your attention on your scalp and forehead, and imagine it relaxing. Relax your face muscles, your mouth, and jaw. Envision a warm, healing, golden light as you inhale. Imagine the light relaxing your neck, shoulders, arms, and fingertips. Relax your chest and abdomen. With continued breathing, breathe in healing energy; breathe out all that you do not need. Imagine the golden light moving down your spine relaxing all your back muscles, your hips, pelvis, and buttocks. Relax your thighs, lower legs, and feet. You are feeling very relaxed and calm and breathing slowly. Pay attention to how your body feels and enjoy it for a few minutes......... When ready, take a few deep breaths, shake your limbs, open your eyes, and become accustomed to your surroundings, bringing with you the sense of relaxation and calm that you need for the day.

Most effective when practiced daily.

©2002 Catherine Kelber

- Rapid, pressured speech may indicate mania or a bipolar disorder
- Exophthalmus may indicate thyroid disease
• Thyroid examination:
  - Evidence of goiter or nodule
• Heart examination
• Neurologic examination, including mental status

ASSESSMENT

→ Stress syndrome, acute or chronic
→ R/O disorders that may need referral for psychiatric, behavioral, or medication therapy
→ R/O other common underlying causes for fatigue, depression, anxiety (e.g., endocrine disorders [thyroid disease, diabetes], anemia, dementia, collagen vascular diseases)

PLAN

DIAGNOSTIC TESTS

→ Thyroid function tests (TFTs), fasting blood sugar (FBS), and/or CBC if appropriate

TREATMENT/MANAGEMENT

→ Refer to psychiatrist if appropriate.
→ Consider short-term treatment with a benzodiazepine (BZD) for acute situational anxiety that interferes with daily functioning.
  ■ Patients should be started on the lowest recommended doses and titrated carefully upward depending on relief of their symptoms.
  ■ Because BZDs have the potential for addiction and withdrawal symptoms, patients should be informed that this medication is only for short-term use and should not be used for chronic, everyday stress.
→ Manage any underlying suspected medication or disease etiologies.
→ Advise adequate nutrition.
  ■ Discontinue caffeine, limit alcohol use
  ■ See Section 16, **General Nutrition Guidelines**.
→ Advise adequate sleep and rest.
→ Prescribe an exercise regimen (including aerobic activity) at least 4–5 days a week.
  ■ Regular exercise has been shown to decrease anxiety, increase productivity, improve body image, and increase psychological well-being (Pender 2001).
→ Refer for "assertiveness" or "time management" training as indicated.
→ Offer assistance with cognitive restructuring techniques.
  ■ These techniques are intended to help the patient identify and change negative thought patterns that trigger and perpetuate self-defeating and stress-producing thoughts (Pender 2001).
→ Advise use of daily scheduled relaxation techniques.
  ■ Progressive relaxation, breathing exercises, biofeedback, meditation, self-hypnosis, yoga, and guided imagery can control physiological responses to stress. (See **Figure**

14I.1, Breathing Exercise and **Figure 14I.2, Relaxation Exercise**.) The use of taped exercises and music enhances the relaxation response in some patients. The choice of technique should depend on the patient's preference.
→ Consider massage therapy for release of muscular tension.
→ Acupuncture, aromatherapy, and craniosacral therapy may provide some benefit and increase a sense of well-being for some patients (Singleton 1999).
→ Help the patient maintain a sense of humor.
  ■ Laughter evokes an endorphin release and decreases anxiety.
    • Suggest viewing comedy on television or video, or reading lighthearted books.

CONSULTATION

→ Physician consultation if required for prescribing controlled drugs.
→ Referral to psychiatrist or psychologist as indicated.

PATIENT EDUCATION

→ Help the patient understand the concept of stress:
  ■ What is stress, and what causes it?
  ■ What are the patient's sources of stress?
  ■ What is the relationship between stress and the patient's somatic symptoms?
  ■ What are the effects of prolonged stress?
  ■ What strategies are available to avoid, prevent, and counteract the effects of stress?

FOLLOW-UP

→ Patients usually need several visits to monitor progress.
  ■ It is unlikely that patients with limited self-awareness will be able to make the connection between symptoms and stress in the first few visits.
  ■ Usually a safe, trusting relationship needs to be established before patients are willing to make major behavioral changes.
  ■ Stress management is a long-term process and requires ongoing support and reinforcement from the provider.
→ Document in progress notes and on problem list.

BIBLIOGRAPHY

Charlesworth, C.A., and Nathan, R.G. 1982. *Stress management—a comprehensive guide to wellness*. Houston: Biobehavioral Press.

_____. 1984. *Stress management: a comprehensive guide to wellness*. New York: Ballantine Books.

Ellis, A.A. 1975. *A new guide to rational living*. North Hollywood, Calif.: Wilshire Books.

Holmes, T.H., and Rahe, R.H. 1967. The social readjustment scale. *Journal of Psychosomatic Research* 11: 213–218.

Lazarus, R.S., and Folkman, S. 1984. *Stress, appraisal and coping*. New York: Springer.

Majumdar, B., and Ladak, S. 1998. Management of family and workplace stress experienced by women of colour from various cultural backgrounds. *Canadian Journal of Public Health* 89(1):48–52.

Manderino, M.A., and Brown, M.C. 1992. A practical, step-by-step approach to stress management for women. *Nurse Practitioner* 17(7):18–28.

Monroe, S. 1983. Major and minor life events as predictors of psychological distress. *Journal of Behavioral Medicine* 6: 189–205.

Pender, N. 2001. *Health promotion in nursing practice.* Los Altos, Calif.: Appleton & Lange.

Schroeder, S.A., Krupp, M.A., Tierney, L.M. et al. 1991. *Current medical diagnosis and treatment.* San Mateo, Calif.: Appleton & Lange.

Selye, H. 1974. *Stress without distress.* New York: Dutton.

Simon, R.W. 1995. Gender, multiple roles, role meaning, and mental health. *Journal of Health and Social Behavior* 36(2): 182–194.

Singleton, J.K. 1999. *Primary care.* Philadelphia: Lippincott.

Smyth, K., and Yarandi, H.N. 1996. Factor analysis of the ways of coping questionnaire for African American women. *Nursing Research* 45(1):25–29.

SECTION 15

Occupational Health

15

Occupational Health

The field of occupational health is focused on recognizing and preventing work-related injury and illness. The primary care provider should include occupational etiology within the differential diagnosis when evaluating and treating patients' symptoms, and consider the physical- and mental-health work demands on them when making decisions about job accommodation or return to work.

Accurately recognizing work-related disorders can be challenging for primary care providers. It is often difficult to obtain and interpret an occupational exposure history. In addition, occupational illnesses can mimic other chronic diseases that have long latency periods. Nevertheless, it is important to identify work site exposures so primary prevention measures can be instituted at the work site to protect the health of current and future workers.

The following are important in managing work-related injury and illness:

→ Recognizing and diagnosing an occupational injury or illness
  ▪ For example, diagnosing occupational dermatitis and asthma resulting from latex glove use
→ Appropriately reporting the illness or injury according to state and federal laws
  ▪ For example, state law requires filing a report of work-related injury within a specified timeframe; many states require mandatory reporting of an elevated blood lead level.
→ Treating an occupational injury or illness, including making recommendations regarding return to work and correcting the workplace hazard
  ▪ For example, prescribing physical therapy and non-steroidal anti-inflammatory agents for an acute back strain, with work restrictions of "no lifting more than 20 pounds" during the recovery phase. Work site recommendations include dividing up the 50-pound loads and raising the work table to keep the load within the lifting zone.
→ Determining if someone is temporarily or permanently disabled from a particular job—based on a work-related

injury/illness—including communicating with a workers' compensation insurance carrier
  ▪ For example, clinically evaluating a keypunch operator for recurrent wrist tendonitis who has had several failed attempts to return to work, even though the number and force of keystrokes have been decreased. Vocational rehabilitation may be indicated for this worker if this benefit is provided in the state's particular workers' compensation benefit package.
→ Rendering a placement decision, in compliance with the Americans with Disabilities Act, regarding an individual's ability—physically and mentally—to do a particular job
  ▪ For example, whether an individual with previous or current illegal substance use qualifies for a driver's license to drive a public bus
→ Making recommendations to employers for reasonable accommodation for any necessary work restrictions based on an individual's health status
  ▪ For example, a woman on chemotherapy for breast cancer may be physically able to work only four hours per day during her treatment.

Women currently make up 46% of the 137 million workers in the United States, with 75% working full-time. In 1999, 3.7 million women held multiple jobs. Three-quarters of women of reproductive age (ages 16–44) are in the workforce (U.S. Department of Health and Human Services [USDHHS] 2001). Many women of color and women with limited language skills work in low-wage, high-hazard jobs, often without access to health care. Musculoskeletal disorders, job stress, and workplace violence are just a few of the work-related conditions impacting women workers. Of note, of the 9 million working women who report back pain, approximately 30% attribute their back pain to their work. Of working African American women with back pain, however, more than 50% attribute their pain to their work (USDHHS 1998).

Of special significance to women's health is the potential impact of occupational and environmental reproductive factors. Both maternal and paternal occupational exposures during the preconception period can negatively impact the ability to conceive and impact the health of the fetus. Maternal exposures during the interpartum and postpartum periods can also impact the health of the infant. The primary care provider should:

→ Complete a preconception occupational and environmental health (OEH) history for both women and men planning a pregnancy. The goal is to identify OEH risk factors and make recommendations to prevent adverse reproductive outcomes.

- For example, a woman painter may be exposed to lead-based paint during burning and scraping operations. She needs to have airborne lead levels measured and may need to be fitted for a respirator.

→ Identify any work restrictions necessary during pregnancy, including making recommendations for reasonable accommodation.

- For example, a pregnant utility worker may be precluded from climbing ladders after 20 weeks gestation. The accommodation could be office work for the remaining 20 weeks of her pregnancy.

→ Evaluate every adverse reproductive outcome for possible OEH risk factors.

- For example, a dental hygienist who has a spontaneous abortion should be evaluated for potential radiation and nitrous oxide exposure at work.

→ Counsel working women on the dual demands of career and child rearing.

- For example, coaching a new mother on breast-feeding techniques she can use upon her return to work or advising her to consider part-time work, if possible.

→ Recognize that women have legal protection against pregnancy discrimination and that the Occupational Safety and Health Act of 1970 entitles all men and women to a safe and healthy workplace. See **Table 15.1, Resources for Pregnancy and Work**.

The Occupational Safety and Health Administration (OSHA) establishes regulatory standards to ensure a safe and healthy workplace. For example, the hazard communication standard requires labeling of hazardous materials and employee training on hazardous substances, and the blood-borne pathogen standard requires training and access to hepatitis B vaccination for those employees reasonably expected to be in contact with blood-borne pathogens in the course of their employment. Further information is on the OSHA Web site: www.osha.gov.

The interface between work and health is important for clinical decision-making in primary care. If there is an injury or an adverse reproductive outcome due to an occupational exposure, there is an opportunity to effect change at the root cause of the problem and prevent similar work-related injury and illness for others.

Table 15.1.   RESOURCES FOR PREGNANCY AND WORK

- American College of Obstetrics and Gynecology and National Institute of Occupational Safety and Health, U.S. Department of Health, Education and Welfare. 1978. *Guidelines on pregnancy and work*. Publication No. 78-118. Washington, D.C.: U.S. Government Printing Office.

- American Medical Association Council on Scientific Affairs. 1984. Effects of physical forces on the reproductive cycle. *Journal of the American Medical Association* 251(2):247–250.

- _____. 1984. Effects of pregnancy on work performance. *Journal of the American Medical Association* 251(15): 1995–1997.

- _____. 1985. Effects of toxic chemicals on the reproductive system. *Journal of the American Medical Association* 253(23): 3431–3437.

- Brown J.W. 1992. United Auto Workers v. Johnson Controls: gender discrimination in the fetotoxic workplace. *Rutgers Law Review* 44(2):479–529.

- Burgel, B.J. 1993. Pregnancy and work restrictions: implications for the occupational health nurse. *American Association of Occupational Health Nurses CE Update*, Volume 5, Lesson 5. Skillman, N.J.: Continuing Professional Education Center.

- Cannon, R.B., Schmidt, J.V., Cambardella, B. et al. 2000. High-risk pregnancy in the workplace. *American Association of Occupational Health Nursing Journal* 48(9):435–446.

- Dodgson, J.E., and Duckett, L. 1997. Breastfeeding in the workplace. *American Association of Occupational Health Nursing Journal* 45(6):290–298.

- Mozurkewich, E.L., Luke, B., Avni, M. et al. 2000. Working conditions and adverse pregnancy outcome: a meta-analysis. *Obstetrics & Gynecology* 95(4):623–635.

- Rayburn, S.K., Yorker, B.A. 1991. Maternal rights in the workplace. *American Association of Occupational Health Nursing Journal* 39(11):534–536.

- Office of Technology Assessment, U.S. Congress. 1985. *Reproductive health hazards in the workplace: summary* (OTA-BA-267). Washington, D.C.: U.S. Government Printing Office.

- U.S. Department of Health and Human Services. 1993. *Case studies in environmental medicine: reproductive and developmental hazards*. Atlanta, Ga.: Agency for Toxic Substances and Disease Registry.

DATABASE

SUBJECTIVE

→ OEH history is critical for accurately diagnosing and managing work-related conditions.

→ For a *basic* OEH history, ask four questions, based on the mnemonic WHACS (Blue et al. 2000):
- W: What do you do?
- H: How do you do it?
- A: Are you concerned about any of your exposures on or off the job?
- C: Co-workers or others exposed?
- S: Satisfied with your job?

→ For a *diagnostic* OEH history, ask:
- Do the symptoms seem to be caused or aggravated by specific activities in the workplace or at home/in the neighborhood?
- Is there a temporal relationship between the symptoms and specific work or home activities? Do these symptoms abate when you are on vacation or away from the environment in question?
- Is there any change(s) in work process that coincide(s) with symptom onset?
- Is there a pattern of similar symptoms in co-workers or neighbors?
- Do you use any protective equipment at work/home? Assess training and maintenance of the equipment.

→ For a *screening* OEH history, see **Figure 15.1, Taking An Exposure History**.

OBJECTIVE

→ Perform a complete physical examination.

→ For exposure, document the route of exposure (i.e., inhalation, skin, ingestion) and amount of dose.

→ Document whether the toxicology of the exposure matches the symptoms/target organ damage.

→ Document applicable OSHA standards, including permissible exposure levels.

→ Document baseline/past medical surveillance data—environmental monitoring data (e.g., noise levels) and/or biological monitoring data (e.g., audiometry results).

→ Document applicable material safety data sheet information (describes toxicology and health hazards for specific hazardous substances, as required by the OSHA hazard communication standard).

→ Document job analysis data if making a placement or return-to-work decision, having obtained from the employer a job analysis that details the physical requirements of the job—e.g., the number of hours/shift, the number of repetitions with dominant arm/pinch grasp, the amount of weight to be lifted, the percent of time in overhead reaching, and if the job requires working in various temperatures or rotating shifts.

ASSESSMENT

→ Occupational exposure:

- Assess exposure relative to OSHA standard.
  NOTE: Biological effects may occur *below* legally established permissible exposure levels.
- R/O nonoccupational exposure.
- R/O contributing nonoccupational exposure (e.g., smoking).

→ Occupational injury or illness:
- R/O nonoccupational injury or illness.
- R/O pre-existing health care condition exacerbated by occupational exposure.

PLAN

DIAGNOSTIC TESTS

→ Commonly ordered tests in occupational health include:
- Spirometry or full pulmonary function tests
  - Evaluate reactive airway disease with histamine/methacholine challenge testing and determine work relationship with serial peak flow measurements at work.
- Liver function tests for hepatotoxins
- Kidney function tests for nephrotoxins
- Neurobehavioral testing for mentation/behavior changes
- Nerve conduction/electromyelogram for paresthesias/motor changes
- Skin patch testing with work site allergens for dermatitis evaluation
- Audiometry for hearing loss
- X-ray/magnetic resonance imaging for musculoskeletal complaints
- Serum heavy metal testing for specific exposure (e.g., lead or cadmium)
- Complete blood count for any exposure affecting the hematopoietic system
- Urinalysis (spot or 24-hour collection) for specific exposures (e.g., arsenic or cadmium)

→ Work site evaluations are a critical tool for both accurate diagnosis and creative management of work-related conditions. These may be obtained in several ways:
- An industrial hygienist (IH) conducts environmental monitoring in the work site to evaluate the extent and scope of the exposure (e.g., collecting wipe samples for lead dust, air monitoring for a methylene chloride level, and/or use of smoke tubes to check adequacy of ventilation). The IH may be employed by the employer, the workers' compensation carrier, or OSHA, or be a consultant.
- Gaining access to the work site by the provider or a consultant to complete a "walkthrough hazard evaluation survey" is often a challenge and should be done with the support of the patient and, if available, a union representative.
- If access to the work site is not possible, a videotape of the work process that shows work tasks and routes of exposure is helpful in designing realistic return-to-work and job modification recommendations.
- A collaborative relationship with the employer facilitates implementation of control measures at the work site.

Figure 15.1.   TAKING AN EXPOSURE HISTORY

Part 1. Exposure Survey

Date: _____   Name: _____

Please circle the appropriate answer.   Birthdate: _____   Sex: M   F

1. Are you currently exposed to any of the following?	metals	no	yes
	dust or fibers	no	yes
	chemicals	no	yes
	fumes	no	yes
	radiation	no	yes
	biologic agents	no	yes
	loud noise, vibration, extreme heat or cold	no	yes
2. Have you been exposed to any of the above in the past?		no	yes
3. Do any household members have contact with metals, dust, fibers, chemicals, fumes, radiation, or biologic agents?		no	yes

If you answered *yes* to any of the items above, describe your exposure in detail—how you were exposed, to what you were exposed. If you need more space, please use a separate piece of paper.

4. Do you know the names of the metals, dusts, fibers, chemicals, fumes, and/or radiation that you are/were exposed to?	no	yes	⇒	If *yes*, list them below.
5. Do you get the material on your skin or clothing?	no	yes		
6. Are your work clothes laundered at home?	no	yes		
7. Do you shower at work?	no	yes		
8. Can you smell the chemical or material you are working with?	no	yes		
9. Do you use protective equipment, such as gloves, mask, respirator, or hearing protectors?	no	yes	⇒	If *yes*, list the protective equipment used.
10. Have you been advised to use protective equipment?	no	yes		
11. Have you been instructed in the use of protective equipment?	no	yes		
12. Do you wash your hands with solvents?	no	yes		
13. Do you smoke at the workplace? no yes At home?	no	yes		
14. Do you eat at the workplace?	no	yes		
15. Do you know of any co-workers experiencing similar or unusual symptoms?	no	yes		

16. Are family members experiencing similar or unusual symptoms?	no	yes
17. Has there been a change in the health or behavior of family pets?	no	yes
18. Do your symptoms seem to be aggravated by a specific activity?	no	yes
19. Do your symptoms get either worse or better at work?	no	yes
at home?	no	yes
on weekends?	no	yes
on vacation?	no	yes
20. Has anything about your job changed in recent months (such as duties, procedures, overtime)?	no	yes
21. Do you use any traditional or alternative medicines?	no	yes

If you answered *yes* to any of the questions, please explain.

(continued)

Figure 15.1.   TAKING AN EXPOSURE HISTORY *(continued)*

Part 2. Work History   Name: _____

A. Occupational Profile   Birthdate: _____ Sex: **M   F**

The following questions refer to your current or most recent job:

Job title: _____   Describe this job:_____

Type of industry: _____   _____

Name of employer: _____   _____

Date job began: _____   _____

Are you still working in this job?   yes   no   _____

If no, when did this job end?_____   _____

Fill in the table below listing all jobs you have worked including short-term, seasonal, part-time employment, and military service. Begin with your most recent job. Use additional paper if necessary.

Dates of Employment	Job Title and Description of Work	Exposures*	Protective Equipment

*List the chemicals, dust, fibers, fumes, radiation, biologic agents (i.e., molds, viruses), and physical agents (i.e., extreme heat, cold, vibration, noise) that you were exposed to at this job.

Have you ever worked at a job or hobby in which you came in contact with any of the following by breathing, touching, or ingesting (swallowing)? If *yes*, please circle.

Acids	Cadmium	Ethylene dibromide	Methylene chloride	Radiation	Trichloroethylene
Alcohols (industrial)	Carbon tetrachloride	Ethylene dichloride	Nickel	Rock dust	Trinitrotoluene
Alkalies	Chlorinated naphthalenes	Fiberglass	PBBs	Silica powder	Vinyl chloride
Ammonia	Chloroform	Halothane	PCBs	Solvents	Welding fumes
Arsenic	Chloroprene	Isocyanates	Perchloroethylene	Styrene	X-rays
Asbestos	Chromates	Ketones	Pesticides	Talc	Other (specify)
Benzene	Coal dust	Lead	Phenol	Toluene	
Beryllium	Dichlorobenzene	Mercury	Phosgene	TDI or MDI	

(continued)

Figure 15.1.   TAKING AN EXPOSURE HISTORY *(continued)*

B. Occupational Exposure Inventory   *Please circle the appropriate answer.*

1. Have you ever been off work for more than one day because of an illness related to work?	no	yes
2. Have you ever been advised to change jobs or work assignments because of any health problems or injuries?	no	yes
3. Has your work routine changed recently?	no	yes

Part 3. Environmental History   *Please circle the appropriate answer.*

1. Do you live next to or near an industrial plant, commercial business, dump site, or nonresidential property?   no   yes

2. Which of the following do you have in your home? Please circle all that apply.

   Air conditioner   Air purifier   Central heating (gas or oil?)   Gas stove   Electric stove
   Fireplace   Wood stove   Humidifier

3. Have you recently acquired new furniture or carpet, refinished furniture, or remodeled your home?   no   yes

4. Have you weatherized your home recently?   no   yes

5. Are pesticides or herbicides (bug or weed killers; flea and tick sprays, collars, powders, or shampoos)
   used in your home or garden, or on pets?   no   yes

6. Do you (or any household member) have a hobby or craft?   no   yes

7. Do you work on your car?   no   yes

8. Have you ever changed your residence because of a health problem?   no   yes

9. Does your drinking water come from a private well, city water supply, or grocery store?

10. Approximately what year was your home built? _____

If you answered *yes* to any of the questions, please explain.

Source: U.S. Department of Health and Human Services. March 2000 (revised). *Case studies in environmental medicine: taking an exposure history.* Atlanta, Ga.: Agency for Toxic Substances and Disease Registry.

TREATMENT/MANAGEMENT

→ Occupational health exposures are managed through a hierarchy of controls, which includes substitution, engineering controls, administrative controls, and personal protective equipment.
- Substitution: substitute a less hazardous substance for the offending agent (e.g., fiberglass substituted for asbestos).
- Engineering controls: focus on the work process by "engineering the problem out" (e.g., ventilation systems to remove lead fumes).
- Administrative controls: focus on reducing the dose to any one person (e.g., job rotation of a specific work task in 4-hour intervals).
- Personal protective equipment: while customarily viewed as temporary until engineering controls can be implemented, this may be the only viable option to control an exposure (e.g., gloves, respirators, earplugs).

→ Temporary modified duty or transitional work is often used until there is recovery and/or a change in the work process.
- This is a critical component of a treatment plan and maintains the injured employee within the social support of the work group.
- It also helps to maintain the employee's income level and prolong her benefits.

→ A work-hardening approach is very valuable, especially with musculoskeletal work injuries; it often includes physical/occupational therapy.

→ Mental health considerations: depression often accompanies injury/illness when there is a loss of full function and fear of losing income, especially if recovery is delayed. Often, timely referral to on-site employee assistance programs is beneficial (Burgel et al. 1986).

→ Reporting requirements:
- "Doctor's First Report of Injury" (or other state-required form). Often there are additional forms the injured employee/employer may have to complete before a workers' compensation claim is initiated.
- "Mandatory Reporting of Occupational Diseases by Clinicians" (CDC 1990). Each state has a listing of the infectious/occupational diseases that must be reported to the local health department.
- There may be additional state-specific requirements. For example, in California, if there is suspected or actual pesticide exposure, the provider must report it to the local health officer within 24 hours.

CONSULTATION

→ Consultation with an occupational health medical/nursing expert, if available

→ Referral to an occupational medicine consultant for toxic exposures when the expected rate of recovery is delayed and for medical/legal evaluations

→ Consultation with patient's employer. Depending on the size and type of industry, some of these resources (e.g., occupational health nurse, industrial hygienist) will be available at the specific industry. The primary care provider can call (with employee permission) to discuss work abilities/work restrictions and/or need for work site evaluation (e.g., ergonomic assessment, environmental sampling).

Table 15.2.   SELECTED OCCUPATIONAL AND ENVIRONMENTAL HEALTH AND SAFETY RESOURCES

- For information and copies of OSHA standards, specific to workplace exposures, with permissible exposure levels and free technical information, contact:
  Occupational Safety and Health Administration
  U.S. Department of Labor
  200 Constitution Ave. N.W.
  Washington, D.C. 20210
  (or check state government listings for nearest regional offices)
  www.osha.gov

- For information on environmental regulations and community right-to-know laws, contact:
  Environmental Protection Agency
  Public Information Center, PM-211B
  401 M St. S.W.
  Washington, D.C. 20460
  (or check state government listings for nearest regional offices)
  www.epa.gov

- Agency for Toxic Substances and Disease Registry
  ATSDR-Chamblee
  1600 Clifton Road N.E.
  Atlanta, Ga. 30333
  www.atsdr.cdc.gov
  www.atsdr.cdc.gov/HEC/CSEM/status.html (for environmental case studies)

- For information about occupational health research, occupational health, and safety professional education, and for free technical information, contact:
  National Institute for Occupational Safety and Health
  1600 Clifton Road N.E.
  Atlanta, Ga. 30333
  www.cdc.gov/niosh/homepage.html

- California Teratogen Registry
  (800) 532-3749

→ Consultation with workers' compensation insurance carriers, especially for case management nursing services for a disabled employee or to request environmental sampling data.

→ Consultation with federal or state OSHA programs. Anonymous complaints about an imminent danger or a hazardous working condition can be made to OSHA by an employee or by the health care provider. Free OSHA consultation for employers may be a component of the specific state OSHA program.

→ Consultation with local health departments, which often have occupational health consultants, poison control centers, or toxicology information lines for health providers. For example, in California there is a teratogen hotline for patients and providers.

→ See **Table 15.2, Selected Occupational and Environmental Health and Safety Resources**.

PATIENT EDUCATION

→ Explain the relationship between exposure and symptoms, and ways to prevent future exposure.

→ Explain the meaning of the workers' compensation system and how best to maximize benefits. The employee needs to inform her work supervisor when a claim is initiated.

→ Clarify the expected rates of recovery and the need to continue modified duty/transitional work, if prescribed.

→ Acknowledge loss, anger, and fear, and refer the patient for counseling if delayed recovery is anticipated.

→ Educate the patient regarding limits of confidentiality in the workers' compensation system.

→ Educate the patient about her legal rights to be informed regarding potential hazards at the work site, specifically as outlined in the OSHA Standards on Hazard Communication (29 CFR 1220.1992) and Access to Employee Exposure and Medical Records (29 CFR 1200.1992).

→ Advocate a self-care approach and empower patients, teaching them to use resources available at their work site

(e.g., the on-site occupational health nurse and/or the union health and safety committee).

FOLLOW-UP

→ Close follow-up, at least weekly, for re-evaluation whenever time off from work is prescribed.

→ Evaluate progression of modified duty assignments during recovery and advance as tolerated until maximum recovery.

→ There is often a requirement that the treating provider for the work-related injury or illness file periodic status reports with the workers' compensation insurance carrier (e.g., every 30–45 days).

→ Document in progress notes and on problem list.

BIBLIOGRAPHY

Blue, A.V., Chessman, A.W., Gilbert, G.E. et al. 2000. Medical students' abilities to take an occupational history: use of the WHACS mnemonic. *Journal of Occupational and Environmental Medicine* 42(11):1050–1053.

Burgel, B.J., and Gliniecki, C.M. 1986. Disability behavior: delayed recovery in employees with work compensable injuries. *American Association of Occupational Health Nurses Journal* 34(1):26–30.

Centers for Disease Control and Prevention. 1990. Mandatory reporting of infectious diseases by clinicians, and mandatory reporting of occupational diseases by clinicians. *Morbidity and Mortality Weekly Report* 39(RR-9):1–28.

U.S. Department of Health and Human Services. March 2000 (revised). *Case studies in environmental medicine: taking an exposure history*. Atlanta, Ga.: Agency for Toxic Substances and Disease Registry.

_____. 1998. *Women: work and health*. Cincinnati, Ohio: National Institute for Occupational Safety and Health and the National Center for Health Statistics.

_____. 2001. *CDC women's safety and health issues at work*. (DHHS [NIOSH] Publication No. 2001-123) Cincinnati, Ohio: National Institute for Occupational Safety and Health.

SECTION 16

General Nutrition Guidelines

Scott Brown, R.D., C.D.E.
Rozane Moon Gee, R.D., M.S., C.D.E.

16

General Nutrition Guidelines

To lead healthier lives, Americans must focus on wellness and preventive medicine. The best way to stay healthy includes a program of regular exercise, adequate rest, and proper nutrition.

Food is what is eaten; *nutrition* is how the food is utilized in the body. Food is the sustenance of life, giving energy for everyday living, affecting weight and height and, to a great extent, strength. The nutrients in food are needed to nourish the body with protein, carbohydrates, fats, vitamins, minerals, and water.

Knowledge of the nutritive content of foods, best sources of the various nutrients, and how to combine them into a healthful, balanced diet is important for women's health care providers. This section provides basic information on the nutritive value of food and guidelines for establishing a healthy diet. The role of the clinician in health promotion and maintenance is discussed.

Variety of Foods

A person needs more than 40 different nutrients (including vitamins and minerals) for good health. These nutrients should come from a variety of foods, not from a few highly fortified foods or supplements. Any food that supplies calories and nutrients can be part of a nutritious diet, but it is the content of the total daily or weekly diet that matters.

No single food can supply all necessary nutrients in the necessary amounts. For example, milk supplies calcium but little iron; meat supplies iron but little calcium. A person must eat a variety of foods, including foods from each of the five major food groups to have a nutritious diet.

The **Food Guide Pyramid, Figure 16.1,** is a general guide from which to choose a healthful diet. It calls for eating a variety of foods to get needed nutrients and the right amount of calories to maintain normal, healthy weight. It starts with 6–11 servings of bread, cereal, rice, and pasta; 3–5 servings of vegetables; 2–4 servings of fruit; 2–3 servings from the milk group; and 2–3 servings from the meat/poultry group. Fats, oils, and sweets, the foods in the small tip of the pyramid, should be eaten in moderation.

Major Nutrients

Of the major categories of nutrients, only three—protein, carbohydrates, and fat—supply energy (measured in calories) to the body. A healthy diet usually consists of 12–15% from protein, 50–65% from carbohydrates, and less than 30% from fats.

Figure 16.1.   THE FOOD GUIDE PYRAMID, A GUIDE TO DAILY FOOD CHOICES

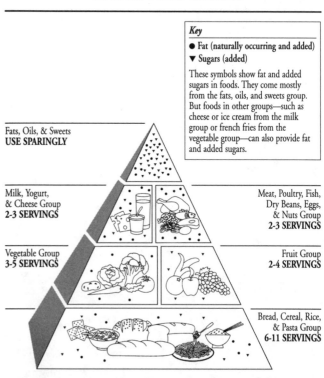

Source: Reprinted from U.S. Department of Agriculture Human Nutrition Information Service. 1992. *The food guide pyramid.* Hyattsville, Md: the Author.

Protein

Every cell in the body contains protein. Protein helps build muscle tissue and is part of the hemoglobin molecule and the antibody system. Protein is also part of bone, cartilage, skin, blood, and lymph. After water and possibly fat, it is the most plentiful substance in the body. Enzymes, which control the processes that keep the body working, are made of protein.

Protein that is eaten is not directly assimilated. Instead, dietary protein must first be broken down into its component parts in the digestive tract and then absorbed into the bloodstream. The building blocks of protein are called *amino acids.* How the amino acids are arranged determines the properties of the resulting protein. The body is able to produce most amino acids, with the exception of eight or nine that must be provided by foods. Indispensable to humans, these are called the *essential amino acids.*

Most Americans get more than enough protein in their diets. Lean meats, poultry, fish, milk, cheese, and eggs provide ample quantities. Bread and cereal, soybeans, chickpeas, and dried beans are also good sources. It is not necessary to load up on meat, poultry, or eggs to get adequate protein. Combining cereal or vegetable foods can also provide adequate amounts. (See "Reduced Meat/Vegetarian Diet," below.)

The amount of protein each person requires is determined by physical size and age. Based on the recommended dietary allowance (National Academy of Sciences 1989), a 120-pound woman between 25–50 years old could satisfy her recommended requirement of 50 grams of protein by eating 3 ounces of tuna, 2 slices of bread, 2 cups of skim milk, and ¾ cup of broccoli. **Tables 16.1, Protein in "Protein" Foods** and **Table 16.2, Protein in Other Foods** illustrate a variety of ways to fulfill the protein requirement and demonstrate how little of the concentrated sources of protein must be eaten to meet the body's needs.

Carbohydrates

Carbohydrates are the major source of energy in the diet. There are two basic types—the *sugars,* or *simple carbohydrates,* and the *starches,* called *complex carbohydrates.*

All carbohydrates are made up of one or more molecules of sugar. The sugars may be single molecules such as *glucose, fructose,* and *galactose,* or double molecules such as *sucrose* (combination of glucose and fructose), *maltose* (combination of two glucose molecules), and *lactose* (combination of glucose and galactose). The starches are branched chains of dozens of molecules of glucose.

All carbohydrates are readily broken down by digestive enzymes into their component sugars and absorbed into the bloodstream. The liver converts the fructose and galactose into glucose, which is the body's main energy source.

The chief sources of carbohydrates are grains, vegetables, fruits, and sugars. The majority of carbohydrates—both complex and simple—are present in foods like corn, wheat, rice, milk, fruits, and vegetables, and in cookies, cakes, and pies.

Grains are the major carbohydrate source for people throughout the world and can also supply a major portion of dietary protein. They are the least expensive, most easily obtainable, and most readily digested form of energy. Since many foods that are high in carbohydrates—bread, cereals, potatoes, and other root vegetables—are relatively inexpensive, the proportion

Table 16.1. PROTEIN IN "PROTEIN" FOODS

Food	Serving Size	Protein (g)
Beef, chuck roast	3 ounces cooked	24.0
Beef, lean ground	¼ pound cooked	23.4
Cheese, cheddar	1 ounce	7.1
Cheese, cottage	½ cup	15.0
Chicken	1 drumstick	12.2
Eggs	2 medium	11.4
Flounder	3 ounces	25.5
Ham, boiled	3 slices (3 ounces)	16.2
Liver, chicken	1 liver	6.6
Milk, skim	1 cup	8.8
Peanut butter	2 tablespoons	8.0
Scallops	3 ounces	16.0
Shrimp	3 ounces	11.6
Tuna, canned	3 ounces drained	24.4
Turkey	3 ounces	26.8
Yogurt	1 cup	8.3

Table 16.2. PROTEIN IN OTHER FOODS

Food	Serving Size	Protein (g)
Banana	1 medium	1.3
Barley	¼ cup raw	4.1
Bean curd (tofu)	1 piece	9.4
Beans, kidney	½ cup cooked	7.2
Bran flakes (40%)	1 cup	3.6
Bread, whole wheat	1 slice	2.6
Broccoli	½ cup	2.4
Bulgur	1 cup cooked	8.4
Lentils	½ cup cooked	7.8
Macaroni	1 cup cooked	6.5
Noodles, egg	1 cup cooked	6.6
Oatmeal	1 cup cooked in water	4.8
Pancakes	3"–4" cakes	5.7
Potato	7 ounces baked	4.0
Potato, sweet	5 ounces baked	2.4
Rice, brown	1 cup cooked	4.9
Rice, white	1 cup cooked	4.1
Soup, tomato	1 cup with milk	6.5
Walnuts	10 large	7.3

of carbohydrates in the diet is greater than that of other nutrients, especially protein, for people at the lower economic levels.

Carbohydrate sources such as fruits and vegetables have a prominent place in a healthy diet. Despite concerns over pesticide residues, which demand strict regulation, the health benefits of eating fresh produce vastly outweigh any risk posed by pesticides. A diet rich in fruits and vegetables, especially the cruciferous vegetables like broccoli and cauliflower, may reduce the risk of certain cancers and is a good source of antioxidant vitamins.

Carbohydrates are necessary to consume for proper nutrition. As the rate of obesity continues, many Americans are exploring high-protein, low-carbohydrate diets. People lose weight while following this type of diet, but there is not evidence that weight loss is maintained over the long term. A low-carbohydrate diet is one is which less than 100 g of carbohydrates are consumed or certain foods are strictly limited. Such foods include fruits, whole grains, milk, or other carbohydrates. Articles from organizations such as the American Dietetic Association, the American Diabetic Association, and the American Heart Association all caution against the use of exploring high-protein, low-carbohydrate diets as a method for achieving a healthy weight. Because it is not yet known how to maintain weight loss over the long term, a woman's health care provider should advise patients to eat healthfully and be physically active. (See "Maintain a Healthy Weight," below.)

Fats

Fats add flavor to food and provide the greatest amount of energy to our body. Within the body, fats carry vitamins A, D, E, and K and are an essential part of the cell structure that makes up body tissue. The fat in our body also serves as cushioning to protect our vital organs.

The American Heart Association recommends that our total daily fat intake be limited to 30% of the diet. (See **Table 16.3**,

Formula to Determine Grams of Fat to Stay Within 30% Limit.) Foods richest in fat include butter, oils, cream, most cheeses, nuts, bacon, and fried foods. There is evidence that high-fat diets may increase the risk of cancer of the colon, breast, and endometrium. Diets low in fat may reduce these risks while assisting in weight control and reducing the incidence of heart disease.

Fats and Cholesterol

There are four main fats in foods: *saturated*, *polyunsaturated*, *monounsaturated*, and *cholesterol*. The first three are fatty acids; cholesterol is a fat-like substance. Of the fatty acids, only saturated fat raises blood cholesterol. Cholesterol obtained from food also can raise blood cholesterol. (See **Table 16.4, Cholesterol and Fat Content of Selected Foods**.)

Saturated Fats

Saturated fatty acids are the main dietary culprits in raising blood cholesterol. They come from both animal and plant products. Saturated fats are usually solid at room temperature and are found largely in meat fat, whole milk products, butter, lard, cocoa butter, coconut oil, palm oil, and palm kernel oil.

During food processing, trans-fatty acid may be formed when manufacturers partially hydrogenate (partially saturate) liquid oils. The *trans-fats* that are formed do appear to raise blood cholesterol levels.

In the case of margarine, the process of hydrogenation allows an oil to be partially hardened and molded into tub or stick form. Hydrogenation increases the time it takes before oils become rancid, so they stay fresh longer. Most of the oils found

Table 16.3. FORMULA TO DETERMINE GRAMS OF FAT TO STAY WITHIN 30% LIMIT

To determine grams of total fat allowed in the daily diet, first multiply the total number of calories by 30%, then divide by 9 (there are 9 calories per gram of fat).

Example: 1,800 calories x .30 = 540 calories from fat

$$\frac{540 \text{ fat calories}}{9} = 60 \text{ g fat (goal of total fat per day)}$$

This chart lists grams of fat recommended per day at several different caloric levels:

Calories	Total Fat to Stay Within 30%
1,200	40 g
1,500	50 g
2,000	67 g
2,500	83 g

Table 16.4. CHOLESTEROL AND FAT CONTENT OF SELECTED FOODS

Food	Cholesterol (mg)	Saturated Fat (g)
Milk, whole (1 cup)	33	5.1
Milk, nonfat (1 cup)	4	0.3
Cheese, cheddar (1 ounce)	30	6.0
Cheese, mozzarella, part skim (1 ounce)	16	2.9
Egg, 1 whole	213	1.7
Egg, white	0	0.0
Butter (1 teaspoon)	11	2.5
Tub margarine-safflower oil (1 teaspoon)	0	0.4
Liver, beef (4 ounces)	545	3.0
Bacon, 4–5 slices	24	5.0
Flounder, sole, clams (4 ounces)	76	0.3
Shrimp (4 ounces)	220	0.3
McDonald's Egg McMuffin	226	4.0
Burger King Whopper w/ cheese	113	17.0
Beans, fruit (not avocado), vegetables	0	0–1.0

in fried fast foods, cookies, pies, doughnuts, and margarine are hydrogenated. Until trans-fats are listed on food labels, here are some easy tips to help avoid them:
→ Eat less fat. Avoid deep-fried foods. Choose lower-fat crackers, cookies, and other processed foods.
→ Use canola or olive oils instead of butter, margarine, or shortening.
→ Look for foods that are labeled "saturated-fat-free." They are also low in trans-fat.

Saturated fat intake should not exceed one-third of the total fat intake (between 7–10%). The remainder of fat intake should come from polyunsaturated or monounsaturated fats.

Polyunsaturated Fats
There are two types of polyunsaturates. One type is *omega-6 fatty acids* found in vegetable oils such as safflower, sunflower seed, soybean, and corn oil. The other type, *omega-3 polyunsaturates*, is found mostly in fish oils. Polyunsaturated fatty acids should be limited to no more than 10% of total calories.

Some studies have shown this kind of fatty acid to be beneficial in reducing risks of heart disease, but these studies are as yet inconclusive. It is, however, beneficial to include fish in the diet regularly. Fish is very low in saturated fat and a better choice than red meat.

Monounsaturated Fats
High amounts of monounsaturates are found in olive, canola, and peanut oils, high-monounsaturated forms of sunflower seed and safflower oils, avocados, and most nuts. Recent research suggest that these may be effective in lowering cholesterol levels when used in place of saturated fatty acids in the diet.

Cholesterol
Cholesterol is a soft, fat-like substance found in all body cells. It is used to form certain hormones, cell membranes, and other important tissues. Because it cannot dissolve in the blood, cholesterol has to be transported to and from the cells by special carriers called *lipoproteins. Low-density lipoprotein* (LDL) is the major cholesterol carrier in the blood. Excess circulating LDL can form plaque on the inner walls of the coronary and cerebral arteries. The LDL-cholesterol level is used as a predictor of heart attack risk. (See the **Hyperlipidemia** chapter in Section 6.)

Approximately one-third to one-fourth of blood cholesterol is carried by another kind of lipoprotein—*high-density lipoprotein* (HDL)—produced mostly in the liver. HDL tends to carry cholesterol away from the arteries and back to the liver, where it is metabolized. It is known as "good" cholesterol because a high level seems to guard against heart attack.

The average American consumes about 400 mg of cholesterol a day. Although some dietary cholesterol is eliminated through the liver, the American Heart Association recommends a daily intake of cholesterol of below 300 mg.

All dietary cholesterol comes from animal products. Egg yolks and organ meats contain the most cholesterol, but some is also found in all meats, fish, poultry, and animal fats. It is rela-

tively easy to reduce blood cholesterol by eating more low-fat (particularly, low in saturated fats), low-cholesterol foods.
→ Low-fat, low-cholesterol diet
  ■ Fats and oils
    • Fats and oils used sparingly in cooking
    • Small amounts of salad dressing and spreads, such as butter, margarine, and mayonnaise, fat-free or reduced-fat dressings and spreads
    • Liquid vegetable oils (lower in saturated fat)
    • Cooking methods requiring little or no fat (boiling, broiling, baking, roasting, poaching, steaming, or microwaving)
  ■ Meat, poultry, fish, dry beans, and eggs
    • Lean cuts of beef (sirloin, round), poultry, fish; not more than 6 ounces (cooked) per day
    • Fresh fish and shellfish, canned fish packed in water
    • Meat and poultry without visible fat/skin
    • Soups and stews without hardened fat
    • Main dishes featuring pasta, rice, beans and/or vegetables. (These foods can be mixed with small amounts of lean meat, fish, or poultry to create a low-fat meal.)
    • Egg yolks (maximum four per week) and organ meats in moderation
  ■ Milk and milk products
    • Skim or 1% extra-light milk and nonfat or low-fat yogurt and cheeses
  ■ Snacks
    • Fresh or frozen fruits and vegetables
    • Air-popped popcorn, low-salt pretzels
    • Less pastry and deep-fried foods

Reduced Meat/Vegetarian Diet

Meats such as beef, pork, veal, and lamb provide protein and many vitamins and minerals the body needs to maintain good health. At the same time, some cuts of meat are high in total fat, saturated fatty acids, and cholesterol. The recommendation is to limit consumption to a total of 6 ounces of lean meat, seafood, or poultry daily. In addition, fish can be substituted for meat, and meatless (vegetarian) meals can be eaten at least twice a week.

The vegetarian diet consists mainly of plant foods—fruits, vegetables, legumes, grains, seeds, and nuts. Eggs and dairy products can be included as well. Plant sources of protein alone can provide adequate amounts of the essential and non-essential amino acids.

Although most vegetarian diets meet or exceed the recommended dietary allowances for protein, they often provide less protein than nonvegetarian diets. This lower protein may be associated with better calcium retention and improved kidney function in individuals with a history of kidney damage. Furthermore, lower protein intakes may result in a lower fat intake with its inherent advantages, because foods high in protein are also frequently high in fat.

A basic principle for preparing meatless meals is the mixing of grains with legumes or low-fat dairy products (see **Table 16.5, Daily Food Guide for Vegetarians**). This provides ample protein from foods that are naturally lower in fat and cholesterol. It is not necessary to add fat or sodium when preparing these foods. The use of cooking oils and spreads, creams, and cheese-based sauces should be limited. Also, use a variety of fruits and vegetables, including a good food source of vitamin C.

Grain products include brown or white rice, barley, pasta, kasha, whole-grain bread, rolls, crackers, and cereals. Legumes include lentils, all beans, chickpeas, tofu, and other soy products. Low-fat dairy products include skim or 1% milk, low-fat or nonfat yogurt, and cheese with 5 g of fat or less per ounce.

Fiber

In the group of polysaccharides (10 or more glucose units), there is *fiber*, the portion of plant foods that human bodies cannot digest. There are two types of fiber: *insoluble* and *soluble*.

Insoluble Fiber

Insoluble fiber, usually referred to as *roughage*, includes the woody or structural parts of plants, such as fruit and vegetable skins and the outer coating (bran) of wheat kernels. Insoluble fiber such as whole-grain cereals, breads, and crackers, and brown and wild rice may help accelerate intestinal transit, slow starch hydrolysis, delay glucose absorption, and guard against colon cancer and other diseases.

Soluble Fiber

Soluble fiber is a substance that dissolves and thickens in water to form gels. Beans, oatmeal, barley, broccoli, raw carrots, and citrus fruits all contain soluble fiber. Oat bran is an especially rich source. There is evidence that soluble fiber may be helpful in improving glucose tolerance and in reducing blood cholesterol levels.

Normal gastrointestinal (GI) tract function is facilitated by both insoluble and soluble fiber. Fiber absorbs water and combats constipation by softening and enlarging the stool. Foods high in fiber also help with weight control, as they tend to be lower in calories, are more filling, and take longer to chew. (See **Table 16.6, High-Fiber Favorites** and **Table 16.7, Sample Menu with Fiber Content in Each Meal**.)

→ Increase fiber in the diet.
- Increase fiber intake gradually—too much, too quickly can cause gas, cramps, and/or diarrhea.
- Obtain fiber from a variety of sources—fruits, vegetables, and grains ensure a variety of nutrients.

Table 16.5.   DAILY FOOD GUIDE FOR VEGETARIANS

Food Group	Suggested Daily Servings	Serving Sizes
Breads, cereals, rice, and pasta	6 or more	1 slice bread ½ bun, bagel, or English muffin ½ cup cooked cereal, rice, or pasta 1 ounce dry cereal
Vegetables	4 or more	½ cup cooked or 1 cup raw
Legumes and other meat substitutes	2–3	½ cup cooked beans 4 ounces tofu or tempeh 8 ounces soy milk 2 tablespoons nuts or seeds (tend to be high in fat, so use sparingly if you are following a low-fat diet)
Fruits	3 or more	1 piece fresh fruit ¼ cup fruit juice ½ cup canned or cooked fruit
Dairy products	Optional—up to 3 servings daily	1 cup low-fat or skim milk 1 cup low-fat or nonfat yogurt 1½ ounces low-fat cheese
Eggs	Optional—limit to 3–4 yolks per week	1 egg or 2 egg whites
Fats, sweets, and alcohol	Go easy on these foods and beverages	Oil, margarine, and mayonnaise Cakes, cookies, pies, pastries, and candies Beer, wine, and distilled spirits

Source: Havala, S., and Dwyer, J. 1993. Position of the American Dietetic Association: vegetarian diets. *Journal of the American Dietetic Association* 93(11):1318. © The American Dietetic Association. Reprinted by permission from the *Journal of the American Dietetic Association*.

Table 16.6.   HIGH-FIBER FAVORITES

Food	Portion Size	Fiber (g)
Apple	large	4.7
Banana	medium	1.8
Orange	medium	3.1
Strawberries	½ cup	2.0
Carrots	½ cup	2.3
Corn	½ cup	3.1
Sweet potato	medium	3.4
Beans, cooked		
pinto	¾ cup	14.2
navy	¾ cup	9.0
kidney	¾ cup	13.8
Bulgur (cracked wheat)	1 cup	8.1
Bran flakes	¾ cup	5.0
Oatmeal	⅔ cup	2.7
Air-popped popcorn	3 cups	3.9
Whole wheat bread	1 slice	2.0
Quaker rice cakes	2 cakes	0.6

Table 16.7.   SAMPLE MENU WITH FIBER CONTENT IN EACH MEAL

Meal	Fiber (g)
Breakfast:	
1 cup shredded wheat with milk	3.0
½ cup strawberries	2.0
1 slice whole wheat bread w/ 1 teaspoon margarine	1.0
Snack:	
3 Triscuits crackers	2.0
Water	
Lunch:	
½ cup split pea soup	5.2
Tuna salad sandwich on whole grain bread w/ lettuce	4.0
1 cup fruit salad (pear, cantaloupe, peach)	4.0
Snack:	
1 large apple, unpeeled	4.7
Dinner:	
½ grapefruit	0.7
Stir-fried chicken and broccoli	2.0
1 cup brown rice	3.3
½ cup vanilla yogurt	
Snack:	
3 cups popcorn, air-popped	3.9
Total	**35.8 g**

- Include plenty of water. Fiber, especially soluble, absorbs large amounts of water. A high-fiber diet can actually cause constipation if not accompanied by liberal amounts of liquids (6–8 glasses a day).
- Include fiber foods in every meal. Breakfast offers an especially good opportunity for incorporating bran, whole-grain cereals, and breads, along with fresh fruits.
- Substitute rather than add. Whole grain breads and flours should be used in place of the more refined varieties. Eat fruits and vegetables with skins intact and bran-containing cereals instead of low-fiber breakfast foods.
- Limit fats. Heavy sauces for high-fiber starch dishes (cheese sauce on broccoli, creamy dressing on salads) should be avoided. Advertisements for "high-fiber" cereals can be misleading because of the undesirable saturated fat content in some of these products.
- It is recommended that healthy adults eat 25–40 g of dietary fiber a day. Most Americans eat far less.

Water

Water is a very important nutrient and is necessary for all the digestive processes. Nutrients dissolve in water to allow them to pass through the intestinal wall and into the bloodstream for use throughout the body. Water carries out waste and helps to regulate body temperature. At least 6–8 glasses of fluids daily are recommended. Coffee and tea, fruit juices and milk, soup, and fruits and vegetables are all sources.

Vitamins and Minerals—RDAs and DRIs

Until recently, the best American standards for micronutrients were the recommended dietary allowances (RDAs). These are a set of guidelines that define the daily amounts of essential nutrients considered to be adequate to meet the known nutritional needs of most healthy persons. The levels are not strict recommendations; instead, they are calculated to be well greater than the requirements of most individuals so that nearly every person's needs will be met without adverse health effects.

As technology advances, so does our ability to measure the micronutrient needs of the human body. In 1993, a new set of guidelines was proposed, creating the dietary reference intakes (DRIs). This umbrella term encompasses four types of nutrient recommendations for healthy individuals: adequate intake (AI), estimated average requirement (EAR), RDA, and tolerable upper intake level (UL). Over the next several years, the Food and Nutrition Board (FNB) of the Institute of Medicine, National Academy of Sciences will be developing updated guidelines to include in the new DRIs. New guidelines for calcium and other B vitamins have already been developed. Until all other micronutrients are reviewed by the FNB, health care practitioners will need to use both the DRIs and existing RDA guidelines and stay abreast of new DRIs as reports are published. (See **Table 16.8, Dietary Reference Intakes [DRIs] and Recommended Dietary Allowances [RDAs].**)

A diet consisting of foods selected from lean meats, low-fat dairy products, whole grains and cereals, legumes, and fresh

Table 16.8. DIETARY REFERENCE INTAKES (DRIs) AND RECOMMENDED DIETARY ALLOWANCES (RDAs)

The nutrient and energy standards known as the recommended dietary allowances (RDAs) are currently being revised. The new recommendations are called dietary reference intakes (DRIs) and include two sets of values that serve as goals for nutrient intake—RDAs and adequate intakes (AIs). The left side of this table presents the new RDA and AI for the 14 nutrients revised to date; the right side presents the 1989 RDA for the remaining nutrients and energy, which will serve until new values can be established.

1997–1998 DRIs

Age (years)[a]	RDAs								AIs					
	Thiamin (mg)	Riboflavin (mg)	Niacin (mg NE)	Vitamin B6 (mg)	Folate (μg DFE)	Vitamin B12 (μg)	Phosphorus (mg)	Magnesium (mg)	Vitamin D (μg)	Pantothenic acid (mg)	Biotin (μg)	Choline (mg)	Calcium (mg)	Fluoride (mg)
Infants														
0.0–0.5	0.2	0.3	2[b]	0.1	65	0.4	100	30	5	1.7	5	125	210	0.01
0.5–1.0	0.3	0.4	4	0.3	80	0.5	275	75	5	1.8	6	150	270	0.5
Children														
1–3	0.5	0.5	6	0.6	150	0.9	460	80	5	2.0	8	200	500	0.7
4–8	0.6	0.6	8	0.6	200	1.2	500	130	5	3.0	12	250	800	1.1
Males														
9–13	0.9	0.9	12	1.0	300	1.8	1,250	240	5	4.0	20	375	1,300	2.0
14–18	1.2	1.3	16	1.3	400	2.4	1,250	410	5	5.0	25	550	1,300	3.2
19–30	1.2	1.3	16	1.3	400	2.4	700	400	5	5.0	30	550	1,000	3.8
31–50	1.2	1.3	16	1.3	400	2.4	700	420	5	5.0	30	550	1,000	3.8
51–70	1.2	1.3	16	1.7	400	2.4	700	420	10	5.0	30	550	1,200	3.8
>70	1.2	1.3	16	1.7	400	2.4	700	420	15	5.0	30	550	1,200	3.8
Females														
9–13	0.9	0.9	12	1.0	300	1.8	1,250	240	5	4.0	20	375	1,300	2.0
14–18	1.0	1.0	14	1.2	400	2.4	1,250	360	5	5.0	25	400	1,300	2.9
19–30	1.1	1.1	14	1.3	400	2.4	700	310	5	5.0	30	425	1,000	3.1
31–50	1.1	1.1	14	1.3	400	2.4	700	320	5	5.0	30	425	1,000	3.1
51–70	1.1	1.1	14	1.5	400	2.4	700	320	10	5.0	30	425	1,200	3.1
>70	1.1	1.1	14	1.5	400	2.4	700	320	15	5.0	30	425	1,200	3.1
Pregnancy	1.4	1.4	18	1.9	600	2.6	*	+40	*	6.0	30	450	*	*
Lactation	1.5	1.6	17	2.0	500	2.8	*	*	*	7.0	35	550	*	*

1989 RDAs

Age (years)	Energy (kcal)	Protein (g)	Vitamin A (μg RE)	Vitamin E (mg α-TE)	Vitamin K (μg)	Vitamin C (mg)	Iron (mg)	Zinc (mg)	Iodine (μg)	Selenium (μg)
Infants										
0.0–0.5	650	13	375	3	5	30	6	5	40	10
0.5–1.0	850	14	375	4	10	35	10	5	50	15
Children										
1–3	1,300	16	400	6	15	40	10	10	70	20
4–6	1,800	24	500	7	20	45	10	10	90	20
7–10	2,000	28	700	7	30	45	10	10	120	30
Males										
11–14	2,500	45	1,000	10	45	50	12	15	150	40
15–18	3,000	59	1,000	10	65	60	12	15	150	50
19–24	2,900	58	1,000	10	70	60	10	15	150	70
25–50	2,900	63	1,000	10	80	60	10	15	150	70
51+	2,300	63	1,000	10	80	60	10	15	150	70
Females										
11–14	2,200	46	800	8	45	50	15	12	150	45
15–18	2,200	44	800	8	55	60	15	12	150	50
19–24	2,200	46	800	8	60	60	15	12	150	55
25–50	2,200	50	800	8	65	60	15	12	150	55
51+	1,900	50	800	8	65	60	10	12	150	55
Pregnancy	+300	60	800	10	65	70	30	15	175	65
Lactation										
1st 6 mo.	+500	65	1,300	12	65	95	15	19	200	75
2nd 6 mo.	+500	62	1,200	11	65	90	15	16	200	75

*Values for these nutrients do not change with pregnancy or lactation. Use the value listed for women of comparable age.

[a]For all nutrients, an AI was established instead of an RDA as the goal for infants; for the B vitamins and choline, the age groupings are 0–5 months and 6–11 months.

[b]The AI for niacin for this age group only is stated as milligrams of preformed niacin instead of niacin equivalents.

Source: Adapted with permission from the National Academy of Sciences. Table of 1989 Recommended Dietary Allowances and 1997–1998 Dietary Reference Intakes (1998). Food and Nutrition Board, National Academy of Sciences. Available at: http://www.nal.usda.gov/fnic/etext/000105.html.

fruits and vegetables will provide ample amounts of vitamins and minerals. A varied diet will provide safe and balanced levels of all essential nutrients. However, if a person's lifestyle prohibits eating wisely most of the time, or if less than 1,200 calories per day are consumed, supplementing the diet with a vitamin/mineral pill that supplies no more than 100% of the RDA (or AI) for each nutrient may be a healthy recommendation.

Self-dosing with vitamins in amounts many times greater than the RDA is usually worthless and may be hazardous. Megadoses of certain vitamins can have drug-like effects quite apart from their usual role as vitamins, and can pose risks just as serious to health as deficiencies of those vitamins (e.g., fat-soluble vitamins are stored in the body and can build up toxic levels if too high a volume is consumed). One out of four Americans takes a daily vitamin/mineral supplement, so it is important that health care practitioners ask patients about the supplements they are taking.

Calcium

Calcium is a mineral important for bone health. However, many women consume inadequate amounts, which increases their risk of osteoporosis later in life. The most critical time to increase calcium consumption is during the years of bone formation and growth, from 11–24 years of age. From ages 9–18, the recommended intake of calcium is 1,300 mg/day, the amount of calcium found in more than four cups of milk. When the critical period of bone formation is over, the recommended intake drops to 1,000 mg/day.

Postmenopausal women who consume less than 1,200 mg of calcium daily and find it difficult to eat enough calories to reach this calcium level may be candidates for calcium supplementation. To attain maximum calcium absorption from the GI tract, some experts believe that calcium supplements should be taken with meals, as lactose and glucose enhance calcium absorption. Others believe calcium supplements should be taken alone, as the phytates and oxalates in food interfere with calcium absorption.

A study by Davis (1989) found that taking a calcium supplement (or milk) with a light meal increased calcium absorption by 10–30% above levels ingested between meals. **Table 16.9, Lower-Fat Calcium Sources** lists some relatively easy to find lower-fat calcium sources that occur naturally in food.

Iron

One major function of iron is the formation of red blood cells. Inadequate iron can lead to iron-deficiency (microcytic) anemia. Many women do not get enough iron-rich food to meet the RDA for iron. Women are likely to ingest fewer calories either because they are dieting or because they have smaller frames that require less food. Iron losses in blood during menstruation and pregnancy can also increase a woman's iron requirements.

Iron-rich foods should be included regularly in the diet. Some excellent sources include lean, fat-trimmed cuts of meat (up to 6 ounces daily), enriched or fortified whole grain products (e.g., hot and cold cereal, bread, crackers, pasta), and dried apricots, prunes, lentils, and beans.

Antioxidant Nutrients
(Vitamins C, E, and Beta-Carotene)

Antioxidants are a group of compounds that help protect the body from damage by unstable molecules known as *free radicals*. Free radicals damage healthy cells and are thought to contribute to cancer, heart disease, immune diseases, cataracts, and aging. The body produces free radicals as byproducts of oxidation, the process by which the body burns fuel. Free radicals can also enter the body from outside (e.g., in cigarette smoke, exhaust fumes, and environmental toxins.)

Our bodies have a fixed level of antioxidants to protect against free radical damage. Additional antioxidant intake depends on the diet. Fruits and vegetables are particularly good sources. These and other sources are listed in **Table 16.10, Antioxidant Food Sources**.

Table 16.9. LOWER-FAT CALCIUM SOURCES

Food	Serving Size	Calcium (mg)
Milk—1%, skim	1 cup	302
Swiss cheese	1 ounce	272
Provolone cheese	1 ounce	214
Part-skim mozzarella cheese	1 ounce	183
Low-fat yogurt (fruit)	1 cup	314
Low-fat yogurt (plain)	1 cup	415
Broccoli (cooked)	1 cup	178
Collard greens (cooked)	1 cup	304
Kale, cooked	1 cup	180
Salmon, canned w/ bone	3 ounces	203
Sardines, canned w/ bone	3 ounces	372

Table 16.10. ANTIOXIDANT FOOD SOURCES

Fruits (2–4 servings daily)
Apricots, cantaloupe, grapefruit, oranges, strawberries, watermelon, peaches

Vegetables (3–5 servings)
Broccoli, carrots, kale, red cabbage, spinach, yams

Whole grains/cereals (6–11 servings)
Whole wheat, rye, pumpernickel, corn or oat bread, muffins or crackers; oatmeal, barley, grits, buckwheat, brown rice, whole-grain cereals

Fish and seafood (up to 6 ounces/day)
Cod, halibut, salmon, lobster, scallops, shrimp, tuna, swordfish

Table 16.11. BODY MASS INDEX

Weight		Height, inches (cm)																							
lb	kg	55.9 (142)	56.7 (144)	57.5 (146)	58.3 (148)	59.1 (150)	59.8 (152)	60.6 (154)	61.4 (156)	62.2 (158)	63.0 (160)	63.8 (162)	64.6 (164)	65.4 (166)	66.1 (168)	66.9 (170)	67.7 (172)	68.5 (174)	69.3 (176)	70.1 (178)	70.9 (180)	71.7 (182)	72.4 (184)	73.2 (186)	74.0 (188)
220	100	49.6	48.2	46.9	45.7	44.4	43.3	42.2	41.1	40.1	39.1	38.1	37.2	36.3	35.4	34.6	33.8	33.0	32.3	31.6	30.9	30.2	29.5	28.9	28.3
218	99	49.1	47.7	46.4	45.2	44.0	42.8	41.7	40.7	39.7	38.7	37.7	36.8	35.9	35.1	34.3	33.5	32.7	32.0	31.2	30.6	29.9	29.2	28.6	28.0
216	98	48.6	47.3	46.0	44.7	43.6	42.4	41.3	40.3	39.3	38.3	37.3	36.4	35.6	34.7	33.9	33.1	32.4	31.6	30.9	30.2	29.6	28.9	28.3	27.7
213	97	48.1	46.8	45.5	44.3	43.1	42.0	40.9	39.9	38.9	37.9	37.0	36.1	35.2	34.4	33.6	32.8	32.0	31.3	30.6	29.9	29.3	28.7	28.0	27.4
211	96	47.6	46.3	45.0	43.8	42.7	41.6	40.5	39.4	38.5	37.5	36.6	35.7	34.8	34.0	33.2	32.4	31.7	31.0	30.3	29.6	29.0	28.4	27.7	27.2
209	95	47.1	45.8	44.6	43.4	42.2	41.1	40.1	39.0	38.1	37.1	36.2	35.3	34.5	33.7	32.9	32.1	31.4	30.7	30.0	29.3	28.7	28.1	27.5	26.9
207	94	46.6	45.3	44.1	42.9	41.8	40.7	39.6	38.6	37.7	36.7	35.8	34.9	34.1	33.3	32.5	31.8	31.0	30.3	29.7	29.0	28.4	27.8	27.2	26.6
205	93	46.1	44.8	43.6	42.5	41.3	40.3	39.2	38.2	37.3	36.3	35.4	34.6	33.7	33.0	32.2	31.4	30.7	30.0	29.4	28.7	28.1	27.5	26.9	26.3
202	92	45.6	44.4	43.2	42.0	40.9	39.8	38.8	37.8	36.9	35.9	35.1	34.2	33.4	32.6	31.8	31.1	30.4	29.7	29.0	28.4	27.8	27.2	26.6	26.0
200	91	45.1	43.9	42.7	41.5	40.4	39.4	38.4	37.4	36.5	35.5	34.7	33.8	33.0	32.2	31.5	30.8	30.1	29.4	28.7	28.1	27.5	26.9	26.3	25.7
198	90	44.6	43.4	42.2	41.1	40.0	39.0	37.9	37.0	36.1	35.2	34.3	33.5	32.7	31.9	31.1	30.4	29.7	29.1	28.4	27.8	27.2	26.6	26.0	25.5
196	89	44.1	42.9	41.8	40.6	39.6	38.5	37.5	36.6	35.7	34.8	33.9	33.1	32.3	31.5	30.8	30.1	29.4	28.7	28.1	27.5	26.9	26.3	25.7	25.2
194	88	43.6	42.4	41.3	40.2	39.1	38.1	37.1	36.2	35.3	34.4	33.5	32.7	31.9	31.2	30.4	29.7	29.1	28.4	27.8	27.2	26.6	26.0	25.4	24.9
191	87	43.1	42.0	40.8	39.7	38.7	37.7	36.7	35.7	34.9	34.0	33.2	32.3	31.6	30.8	30.1	29.4	28.7	28.1	27.5	26.9	26.3	25.7	25.1	24.6
189	86	42.7	41.5	40.3	39.3	38.2	37.2	36.3	35.3	34.4	33.6	32.8	32.0	31.2	30.5	29.8	29.1	28.4	27.8	27.1	26.5	26.0	25.4	24.9	24.3
187	85	42.2	41.0	39.9	38.8	37.8	36.8	35.8	34.9	34.0	33.2	32.4	31.6	30.8	30.1	29.4	28.7	28.1	27.4	26.8	26.2	25.7	25.1	24.6	24.0
185	84	41.7	40.5	39.4	38.3	37.3	36.4	35.4	34.5	33.6	32.8	32.0	31.2	30.5	29.8	29.1	28.4	27.7	27.1	26.5	25.9	25.4	24.8	24.3	23.8
183	83	41.2	40.0	38.9	37.9	36.9	35.9	35.0	34.1	33.2	32.4	31.6	30.9	30.1	29.4	28.7	28.1	27.4	26.8	26.2	25.6	25.1	24.5	24.0	23.5
180	82	40.7	39.5	38.5	37.4	36.4	35.5	34.6	33.7	32.8	32.0	31.2	30.5	29.8	29.1	28.4	27.7	27.1	26.5	25.9	25.3	24.8	24.2	23.7	23.2
178	81	40.2	39.1	38.0	37.0	36.0	35.1	34.2	33.3	32.4	31.6	30.9	30.1	29.4	28.7	28.0	27.4	26.8	26.1	25.6	25.0	24.5	23.9	23.4	22.9
176	80	39.7	38.6	37.5	36.5	35.6	34.6	33.7	32.9	32.0	31.3	30.5	29.7	29.0	28.3	27.7	27.0	26.4	25.8	25.2	24.7	24.2	23.6	23.1	22.6
174	79	39.2	38.1	37.1	36.1	35.1	34.2	33.3	32.5	31.6	30.9	30.1	29.4	28.7	28.0	27.3	26.7	26.1	25.5	24.9	24.4	23.8	23.3	22.8	22.4
172	78	38.7	37.6	36.6	35.6	34.7	33.8	32.9	32.1	31.2	30.5	29.7	29.0	28.3	27.6	27.0	26.4	25.8	25.2	24.6	24.1	23.5	23.0	22.5	22.1
169	77	38.2	37.1	36.1	35.2	34.2	33.3	32.5	31.6	30.8	30.1	29.3	28.6	27.9	27.3	26.6	26.0	25.4	24.9	24.3	23.8	23.2	22.7	22.3	21.8
167	76	37.7	36.7	35.7	34.7	33.8	32.9	32.0	31.2	30.4	29.7	29.0	28.3	27.6	26.9	26.3	25.7	25.1	24.5	24.0	23.5	22.9	22.4	22.0	21.5
165	75	37.2	36.2	35.2	34.2	33.3	32.5	31.6	30.8	30.0	29.3	28.6	27.9	27.2	26.6	26.0	25.4	24.8	24.2	23.7	23.1	22.6	22.2	21.7	21.2
163	74	36.7	35.7	34.7	33.8	32.9	32.0	31.2	30.4	29.6	28.9	28.2	27.5	26.9	26.2	25.6	25.0	24.4	23.9	23.4	22.8	22.3	21.9	21.4	20.9
161	73	36.2	35.2	34.2	33.3	32.4	31.6	30.8	30.0	29.2	28.5	27.8	27.1	26.5	25.9	25.3	24.7	24.1	23.6	23.0	22.5	22.0	21.6	21.1	20.7
158	72	35.7	34.7	33.8	32.9	32.0	31.2	30.4	29.6	28.8	28.1	27.4	26.8	26.1	25.5	24.9	24.3	23.8	23.2	22.7	22.2	21.7	21.3	20.8	20.4
156	71	35.2	34.2	33.3	32.4	31.6	30.7	29.9	29.2	28.4	27.7	27.1	26.4	25.8	25.2	24.6	24.0	23.5	22.9	22.4	21.9	21.4	21.0	20.5	20.1
154	70	34.7	33.8	32.8	32.0	31.4	30.3	29.5	28.8	28.0	27.3	26.7	26.0	25.4	24.8	24.2	23.7	23.1	22.6	22.1	21.6	21.1	20.7	20.2	19.8
152	69	34.2	33.3	32.4	31.5	30.7	29.9	29.1	28.4	27.6	27.0	26.3	25.7	25.0	24.4	23.9	23.3	22.8	22.3	21.8	21.3	20.8	20.4	19.9	19.5
150	68	33.7	32.8	31.9	31.0	30.2	29.4	28.7	27.9	27.2	26.6	25.9	25.3	24.7	24.1	23.5	23.0	22.5	22.0	21.5	21.0	20.5	20.1	19.7	19.2
147	67	33.2	32.3	31.4	30.6	29.8	29.0	28.3	27.5	26.8	26.2	25.5	24.9	24.3	23.7	23.2	22.6	22.1	21.6	21.1	20.7	20.2	19.8	19.4	19.0
145	66	32.7	31.8	31.0	30.1	29.3	28.6	27.8	27.1	26.4	25.8	25.1	24.5	24.0	23.4	22.8	22.3	21.8	21.3	20.8	20.4	19.9	19.5	19.1	18.7
143	65	32.2	31.3	30.5	29.7	28.9	28.1	27.4	26.7	26.0	25.4	24.8	24.2	23.6	23.0	22.5	22.0	21.5	21.0	20.5	20.1	19.6	19.2	18.8	18.4
141	64	31.7	30.9	30.0	29.2	28.4	27.7	27.0	26.3	25.6	25.0	24.4	23.8	23.2	22.7	22.1	21.6	21.1	20.7	20.2	19.8	19.3	18.9	18.5	18.1
139	63	31.2	30.4	29.6	28.8	28.0	27.3	26.6	25.9	25.2	24.6	24.0	23.4	22.9	22.3	21.8	21.3	20.8	20.3	19.9	19.4	19.0	18.6	18.2	17.8
136	62	30.7	29.9	29.1	28.3	27.6	26.8	26.1	25.5	24.8	24.2	23.6	23.1	22.5	22.0	21.5	21.0	20.5	20.0	19.6	19.1	18.7	18.3	17.9	17.5
134	61	30.3	29.4	28.6	27.8	27.1	26.4	25.7	25.1	24.4	23.8	23.2	22.7	22.1	21.6	21.1	20.6	20.1	19.7	19.3	18.8	18.4	18.0	17.6	17.3
132	60	29.8	28.9	28.1	27.4	26.7	26.0	25.3	24.7	24.0	23.4	22.9	22.3	21.8	21.3	20.8	20.3	19.8	19.4	18.9	18.5	18.1	17.7	17.3	17.0
130	59	29.3	28.5	27.7	26.9	26.2	25.5	24.9	24.2	23.6	23.0	22.5	21.9	21.4	20.9	20.4	19.9	19.5	19.0	18.6	18.2	17.8	17.4	17.1	16.7
128	58	28.8	28.0	27.2	26.5	25.8	25.1	24.5	23.8	23.2	22.7	22.1	21.6	21.0	20.5	20.1	19.6	19.2	18.7	18.3	17.9	17.5	17.1	16.8	16.4
125	57	28.3	27.5	26.7	26.0	25.3	24.7	24.0	23.4	22.8	22.3	21.7	21.2	20.7	20.2	19.7	19.3	18.8	18.4	18.0	17.6	17.2	16.8	16.5	16.1
123	56	27.8	27.0	26.3	25.6	24.9	24.2	23.6	23.0	22.4	21.9	21.3	20.8	20.83	19.8	19.4	18.9	18.5	18.1	17.7	17.3	16.9	16.5	16.2	15.8
121	55	27.3	26.5	25.8	25.1	24.4	23.8	23.2	22.6	22.0	21.5	21.0	20.4	20.0	19.5	19.0	18.6	18.2	17.8	17.4	17.0	16.6	16.2	15.9	15.6
119	54	26.8	26.0	25.3	24.7	24.0	23.4	22.8	22.2	21.6	21.1	20.6	20.1	19.6	19.1	18.7	18.3	17.8	17.4	17.0	16.7	16.3	15.9	15.6	15.3
117	53	26.3	25.6	24.9	24.2	23.6	22.9	22.3	21.8	21.2	20.7	20.2	19.7	19.2	18.8	18.3	17.9	17.5	17.1	16.7	16.4	16.0	15.7	15.3	15.0
114	52	25.8	25.1	24.4	23.7	23.1	22.5	21.9	21.4	20.8	20.3	19.8	19.3	18.9	18.4	18.0	17.6	17.2	16.8	16.4	16.0	15.7	15.4	15.0	14.7
112	51	25.3	24.6	23.9	23.3	22.7	22.1	21.5	21.0	20.4	19.9	19.4	19.0	18.5	18.1	17.6	17.2	16.8	16.5	16.1	15.7	15.4	15.1	14.7	14.4
110	50	24.8	24.1	23.5	22.8	22.2	21.6	21.1	20.5	20.0	19.5	19.1	18.6	18.1	17.7	17.3	16.9	16.5	16.1	15.8	15.4	15.1	14.8	14.5	14.1
108	49	24.3	23.6	23.0	22.4	21.8	21.2	20.7	20.1	19.6	19.1	18.7	18.2	17.8	17.4	17.0	16.6	16.2	15.8	15.5	15.1	14.8	14.5	14.2	13.9
106	48	23.8	23.1	22.5	21.9	21.3	20.8	20.2	19.7	19.2	18.8	18.3	17.8	17.4	17.0	16.6	16.2	15.9	15.5	15.1	14.8	14.5	14.2	13.9	13.6
103	47	23.3	22.7	22.0	21.5	20.9	20.3	19.8	19.3	18.8	18.4	17.9	17.5	17.1	16.7	16.3	15.9	15.5	15.2	14.8	14.5	14.2	13.9	13.6	13.3
101	46	22.8	22.2	21.6	21.0	20.4	19.9	19.4	18.9	18.4	18.0	17.5	17.1	16.7	16.3	15.9	15.5	15.2	14.9	14.5	14.2	13.9	13.6	13.3	13.0
99	45	22.3	21.7	21.1	20.5	20.0	19.5	19.0	18.5	18.0	17.6	17.1	16.7	16.3	15.9	15.6	15.2	14.9	14.5	14.2	13.9	13.6	13.3	13.0	12.7
97	44	21.8	21.2	20.6	20.1	19.6	19.0	18.6	18.1	17.6	17.2	16.8	16.4	16.0	15.6	15.2	14.9	14.5	14.2	13.9	13.6	13.3	13.0	12.7	12.4
95	43	21.3	20.7	20.2	19.6	19.1	18.6	18.1	17.7	17.2	16.8	16.4	16.0	15.6	15.2	14.9	14.5	14.2	13.9	13.6	13.3	13.0	12.7	12.4	12.2
92	42	20.8	20.3	19.7	19.2	18.7	18.2	17.7	17.3	16.8	16.4	16.0	15.6	15.2	14.9	14.5	14.2	13.9	13.6	13.3	13.0	12.7	12.4	12.1	11.9
90	41	20.3	19.8	19.2	18.7	18.2	17.7	17.3	16.8	16.4	16.0	15.6	15.2	14.9	14.5	14.2	13.9	13.5	13.2	12.9	12.7	12.4	12.1	11.9	11.6
88	40	19.8	19.3	18.8	18.3	17.8	17.3	16.9	16.4	16.0	15.6	15.2	14.9	14.5	14.2	13.8	13.5	13.2	12.9	12.6	12.3	12.1	11.8	11.6	11.3

NOTE: BMI (metric) = (kg/m^2) x 100; BMI (English) = (lb/in.^{2}) x 100. BMI (metric) x 0.142 = BMI (English); BMI (English) x 7 = BMI (metric).
*BMI 18.5–24.9 = normal; BMI <18.5 = underweight; BMI 25.0–29.9 = overweight; BMI ≥ 30.0 = obesity.

Source: Reprinted with permission from Institute of Medicine. 1990. *Nutrition during pregnancy: Part 1: weight gain, Part 2: nutrient supplements*. Washington, D.C.: National Academy Press. *National Institutes of Health (NIH). National Heart, Lung, and Blood Institute. 1998. *Clinical guidelines on the identification, evaluation, and treatment of overweight and obesity in adults*. NIH Publication No. 98-4083.

Table 16.12. CALORIES USED PER MINUTE OF EXERCISE

Activity	115–150 lbs.	150–195 lbs.
Aerobic dancing	6–7	8–9
Basketball	9–11	11–15
Bicycling	5–6	7–8
Golf	3–4	4–5
Jogging (5 mph)	9–10	12–13
Jogging (7 mph)	10–11	13–14
Rowing machine	5–6	7–8
Skiing (downhill)	8–9	10–12
Skiing (cross-country)	11–12	13–16
Swimming	5–6	7–10
Tennis (doubles)	5–7	7–8
Walking (2 mph)	2–3	3–4
Walking (4 mph)	4–5	6–7

Diet, Weight, and Exercise

Maintain a Healthy Weight

Being underweight or overweight increases the chances of developing health problems. Determining if the weight is healthy depends on the amount of fat, the location of the body fat, and whether there are concomitant weight-related medical problems.

Being overweight is very common in the United States and is linked to heart disease, diabetes, and other illnesses. Being too thin is a less common problem. It occurs with anorexia nervosa and is linked with osteoporosis in women and greater risk of early death in both women and men.

Body mass index (BMI) is used to determine whether weight for height is in a healthy range (see **Table 16.11, Body Mass Index**). The BMI is calculated as weight (in kg) divided by height (in m^2). It can be used to determine if a woman is at health risk because she is underweight (BMI < 18.5), overweight (BMI 25.0–29.9), or obese (BMI ≥ 30.0). The healthy BMI range is 18.5–24.9 (National Institutes of Health [NIH] 1998).

A patient should consider losing weight if she falls above a healthy BMI. Substantial weight loss is difficult, however, and may pose health risks of its own. Before a patient attempts to lose weight, it should be determined how great a risk the weight poses and how much weight needs to be lost to lower that risk. Obese individuals with diabetes and high blood pressure are especially likely to improve their health when extra pounds are shed.

Heredity and metabolism play key roles in keeping some people overweight despite their best efforts to reduce. For such people, striving to attain a recommended weight may be futile and even damaging. Nonetheless, a patient can do well by following healthy eating guidelines and exercising regularly.

Exercise

Healthful eating and exercise improve the odds of losing weight and help maintain health at whatever weight is attained. Inactivity may play an even greater role in weight gain than a high-calorie diet. Exercise can help shed pounds and maintain a healthier weight, as well as improve overall fitness and quality of life.

Aerobic exercise is a good choice because it burns fat from all over the body. It works the larger muscles and uses plenty of oxygen to fuel them. Walking, running, bicycling, and swimming are all aerobic. Thirty minutes or more a day of moderate-intensity activity, like walking, is a good recommendation. A 30-minute walk or three 10-minute walks can produce more or less comparable results. Vigorous or high-intensity aerobic exercise for a certain amount of time may strengthen the heart, but regular, moderate activity can also substantially reduce the risk of disease.

The key is to get up and move. The total energy spent in physical activity is the most important factor. (See **Table 16.12, Calories Used Per Minute of Exercise**.) One can spend 300 calories by running three miles in half an hour or one can spend it in six 10-minute brisk walks throughout the day. The benefits may not be exactly the same, but they are comparable.

Exercise increases the level of HDL, the "good" cholesterol carrier (see "Cholesterol," above). It also lowers blood pressure (significantly lowering both systolic and diastolic blood pressure by an average of 10 points), increases insulin sensitivity in the muscles, and lowers the risk of blood clots.

There is consistent, strong epidemiological evidence that exercise is associated with a lower rate of colon cancer, perhaps increasing the speed with which food travels through the intestinal tract, thus lessening the time the colon is exposed to any potential carcinogens in food. In addition, exercise may stimulate the natural immunity along the mucosal lining of the intestines. For the skeletal system, a moderate, weight-bearing exercise like walking or dancing, rather than swimming, may improve bone mineral density.

Total Energy Requirement

The *basal metabolic rate* (BMR) is the minimum amount of energy needed by the body at rest in the fasting state. This includes cellular metabolism, circulation, and maintenance of body temperature.

Because it is technically difficult to measure an individual's BMR, it is calculated using one of many formulas. Frequently, the calculated BMR is referred to as the basal energy expenditure, or BEE. To be most accurate, these formulas should take into account age, sex, and body surface area.

The following *Harris and Benedict Formula* (Krause et al. 2000) gives the standard BEE for women plus a physical activity factor:

655 + 9.56(W) + 1.85(H) - 4.68(A) = BMR
BMR x physical activity = total calories (kcal) required per day
W = weight in kg   H = height in cm   A = age in years

Physical activity—if:

Sedentary BMR x 1.3 (or 30% additional kcal above BMR)
Moderate BMR x 1.5 (or 50% additional kcal above BMR)
Active BMR x 2.0 (or 100% additional kcal above BMR)

Example: 35-year-old, 5'5" (165 cm), 140-pound (64-kg) moderately active woman

655 + (9.56 x 64 kg) + (1.85 x 165 cm) - (4.68 x 35) = BMR = 1,408
1,408 x 1.5 = *2,112 kcal required per day*

The energy or kcal calculated is the amount required to maintain weight. To lose one pound of weight a week, the average person needs to reduce caloric intake by 3,500 kcal or increase energy expenditure (calories used) by that much.

The Best Nutrition Advice

By adhering to the nutritional guidelines that follow, patients can maintain better health and reduce their chances of developing certain diseases such as heart disease, high blood pressure, and certain cancers.

→ Aim for fitness:
  ▪ Aim for a healthy weight.
  ▪ Be physically active each day.
→ Build a health base:
  ▪ Let the pyramid guide your choices.
  ▪ Choose a variety of grains daily, especially whole grains.
  ▪ Choose a variety of fruits and vegetables daily.
  ▪ Handle and store foods in a safe manner.
→ Choose sensibly:
  ▪ Choose a diet that is low in saturated fat and cholesterol and moderate in total fat.
  ▪ Choose beverages and foods with less sugar.
  ▪ Choose and prepare foods with less salt.
  ▪ If you drink alcoholic beverages, do so in moderation.

Role of the Clinician

Clinicians who care for women should include nutritional services counseling to prevent certain chronic disease. Basic, appropriate nutritional advice should consider the dietary intake of calories, fat (especially saturated fat), cholesterol, fiber, and supplemental vitamins and minerals if indicated, and be culturally appropriate for the individual.

When the clinician, through basic nutritional care, detects serious nutritional problems or complex medical conditions that complicate the care, referral to a registered dietitian or other nutrition professional is required. Special nutritional care usually includes detailed assessments, complex diet modifications, dietary counseling, and close follow-up. Additional reinforcement and follow-up must be provided by the primary care practitioner for successful nutritional interventions to occur and for the new patterns that are set up to be maintained (Abrams et al. 1993).

Basic Nutritional Care For All Women

→ Assess for:
  ▪ Healthy weight
  ▪ Exercise habits
  ▪ Dietary practices
  ▪ Hemoglobin or hematocrit
→ Based on family history, risk factors, and age, consider screening for total cholesterol and, if necessary, a more extensive fasting lipoprotein panel. (See the **Hyperlipidemia** chapter in Section 6.)
→ Assess for nutritional risk factors, making recommendations for dietary change or supplementation. Refer to a dietitian, social services, or substance abuse cessation program if necessary. Nutritional risk factors include:
  ▪ Obesity, eating disorders, food allergies, anemia, extreme underweight, unusual or restrictive dietary patterns
  ▪ Metabolic or chronic diseases
  ▪ Substance abuse (cigarettes, alcohol, or drugs)
  ▪ Adolescence
  ▪ Limited income, education, motivation, or knowledge about food and nutrition
  ▪ Homelessness
→ Emphasize food rather than supplements as the main source of nutrients. Encourage the woman to eat a daily minimum of five servings of fruits and vegetables; six servings of grains; a minimum of two low-fat, calcium-rich dairy products; and moderate amounts of protein-rich foods such as legumes, fish, poultry, and lean meats. Individualize recommendations to reflect the woman's food preferences, lifestyle, cultural context, and economic situation.
→ Recommend vitamin/mineral supplement(s) when it is difficult or impossible for a woman to get adequate dietary intake or when nutritional risk factors (e.g., eating disorders) exist.
→ Document nutritional assessments and interventions in the progress notes and on the problem list.

BIBLIOGRAPHY

Abrams, B., and Berman, C. 1993. Women, nutrition and health. *Current Problems in Obstetrics, Gynecology and Fertility* 16(1):39–41.

American Dietetic Association. 1992. *Eating well—the vegetarian way.* Chicago: the Author.

_____. 1993. Vegetarian diets. *Journal of the American Dietetic Association* 93(11):1317–1318.

_____. 1993. Health implications of dietary fiber. *Journal of the American Dietetic Association* 93:1446–1447.

American Heart Association. 1993. *Cholesterol and your heart.* Dallas, Tex.: the Author.

_____. 1993. *Eat heart smart.* San Francisco: the Author.

_____. 2001. *High protein diets.* Available at: http://www.americanheart.org. Accessed on October 26, 2002.

Brody, J. 1981. *Jane Brody's nutrition book,* pp. 49–50. New York: W.W. Norton.

California Department of Health Services. 1990. *Nutrition during pregnancy and the post-partum period: A manual for health care professionals.* Sacramento, Calif.: Maternal and Child Health Branch, WIC Supplemental Food Branch.

Center for Science in the Public Interest. 1993. The great trans wreck. *Nutrition Action Health Letter* 20(9):10.

_____. 1993. These feet were made for walking. *Nutrition Action Health Letter* 20(10):11.

Davis, R. 1989. Calcium absorption. *American Journal of Clinical Nutrition* 49:372.

Franz, M. 2001. The answer to weight loss is easy—doing it is hard! *Clinical Diabetes* 19(3):105–109.

Havala, S., and Dwyer, J. 1994. Position of the American Dietetic Association: vegetarian diets. *Journal of the American Dietetic Association* 93(11):1318.

Hurley, J. 1990. Rough it up. *Nutrition Action Health Letter* 17(2):8–9.

Institute of Medicine. 1990. *Nutrition during pregnancy: Part 1: weight gain, Part 2: nutrient supplements.* Washington, D.C.: National Academy Press.

Krause, M.V., and Mahan, L.K. 2000. *Food, nutrition, and diet therapy,* 10th ed., p. 871. Philadelphia: W.B. Saunders.

Liebman, B. 1989. Cutting cholesterol. *Nutrition Action Health Letter* 16(7):5.

_____. 1990. CSPI's Fat Savings Plan. *Nutrition Action Health Letter* 17(7).

Metropolitan Life Insurance Co. 1983. *1983 Metropolitan height/weight tables.* New York: the Author.

Morgan, B. 1987. *Nutrition prescription.* New York: Ballantine Books.

National Academy of Sciences. 1998. Table of 1989 Recommended Dietary Allowances and 1997–1998 Dietary Reference Intakes. Food and Nutrition Board, National Academy of Sciences. Available at: http://www.nal.usda.gov/fnic/etext/000105.html.

National Academy of Sciences, National Research Council. 1989. *Recommended dietary allowances,* 10th ed. Washington, D.C.: National Academy Press.

National Institutes of Health (NIH). National Heart, Lung, and Blood Institute. 1998. *Clinical guidelines on the identification, evaluation, and treatment of overweight and obesity in adults.* NIH Publication No. 98-4083.

Owen, A. 1989. *Fiber in your diet.* New York: Healthteam Interactive Communications.

Pennington, J. 1989. *Bowes & Church's food values of portions commonly used,* 15th ed. Philadelphia: J.B. Lippincott.

Shils, M., and Young, V. 1988. *Modern nutrition in health and disease,* 7th ed. Philadelphia: Lea & Febiger.

Spence, W.R. 1990. *Cholesterol—keeping your heart healthy.* Waco, Tex.: Health Edco.

Stein, Karen. 2000. High-protein, low-carbohydrate diets: Do they work? *Journal of the American Dietetic Association* 2000(7):760–761.

U.S. Department of Agriculture. 2000. *Dietary guidelines for Americans, 1980 to 2000.* Available at: http://www.usda.gov/cnpp/Pubs/DG2000/Dgover.PDF. Accessed on October 26, 2003.

_____. Human Nutrition Information Service. 1992. *The food guide pyramid.* Hyattsville, Md.: the Author.

Index

Women's Primary Health Care
Protocols for Practice

Index of Tables, Figures, and Appendices

SECTION 1. WOMEN'S PRIMARY HEALTH CARE—INTRODUCTION
Chapter 1-C Women's Health Across the Life Span: An Overview
Table 1C.1.   Tanner Staging or Sexual Maturity Rating (SMR) of Females **1-10**
Table 1C.2.   Characteristics of Female Adolescent Psychosocial Development **1-11**
Table 1C.3.   Leading Causes of Death for Women by Age Group **1-12**
Table 1C.4.   Health Assessment for Women 13 to 19 Years of Age **1-14**
Table 1C.5.   Risk Assessment, Prevention Measures, and Counseling for Women 13 to 19 Years of Age **1-15**
Table 1C.6.   Health Assessment for Women 20 to 39 Years of Age **1-16**
Table 1C.7.   Risk Assessment, Prevention Measures, and Counseling for Women 20 to 39 Years of Age **1-17**
Table 1C.8.   Health Assessment for Women 40 to 64 Years of Age **1-19**
Table 1C.9.   Risk Assessment, Prevention Measures, and Counseling for Women 40 to 64 Years of Age **1-20**
Table 1C.10.   Health Assessment for Women 65 Years of Age and Older **1-22**
Table 1C.11.   Risk Assessment, Prevention Measures, and Counseling for Women 65 Years of Age and Older **1-23**

SECTION 4. BREAST DISORDERS
Chapter 4-A Breast Cancer Screening
Table 4A.1.   Characteristics of BRCA1 and BRCA2 Mutations **4-3**
Table 4A.2.   Benign Breast Disease and Relative Risk for Subsequent Invasive Breast Cancer **4-3**
Chapter 4-H Galactorrhea
Table 4H.1.   Causes of Chronic Hyperprolactinemia in the Nonpregnant Female **4-21**

SECTION 5. RESPIRATORY/OTORHINOLARYNGOLOGICAL DISORDERS
Chapter 5-A Asthma
Table 5A.1.   Stepwise Approach to Asthma Classification Clinical Features **5-3**
Table 5A.2.   Medications for the Treatment of Asthma **5-5**
Table 5A.3.   Daily Dosages for Inhaled Steroids **5-6**
Table 5A.4.   Types of Medication Used in Asthma **5-6**
Figure 5A.1.   Steps for Using Your Inhaler **5-9**
Chapter 5-D Chronic Obstructive Pulmonary Disease
Table 5D.1.   Patterns of Disease in Advanced COPD **5-18**
Table 5D.2.   Pulmonary Function Tests (PFTs)—Definitions and Results in Obstructive and Restrictive
               Pulmonary Disease **5-19**
Chapter 5-F Influenza
Table 5F.1.   Anti-influenza Medications **5-27**
Chapter 5-J Pneumonia
Table 5J.1.   PORT Criteria and Scoring **5-38**

SECTION 6. CARDIOVASCULAR DISORDERS

Chapter 6-B Deep Vein Thrombosis

Table 6B.1.   Clinical Model for Predicting Pretest Probability for DVT 6-11

Table 6B.2.   Length of Anticoagulation Therapy for DVT 6-13

Figure 6B.1.   Diagnostic Algorithm for Evaluation of Proximal DVT Using Ultrasonography and Venography Based on Pretest Probability 6-12

Chapter 6-C Heart Failure

Table 6C.1.   Drugs Commonly Used for Treatment of Chronic Heart Failure 6-19

Chapter 6-D Hyperlipidemia

Table 6D.1.   Lipid Classification 6-22

Table 6D.2.   Risk Factors for CHD in Women with Hyperlipidemia 6-24

Table 6D.3.   Estimate of 10-Year Risk for Women (Framingham Point Scores) 6-25

Table 6D.4.   CHD Risk Equivalents 6-25

Table 6D.5.   Dietary Recommendations for Hyperlipidemia 6-26

Table 6D.6.   Drug Therapy for Hyperlipidemia 6-27

Chapter 6-E Hypertension

Table 6E.1.   Pharmacologic Therapy for Hypertension (Selected Agents) 6-34

Table 6E.2.   Considerations for Individualizing Antihypertensive Drug Therapy 6-35

Chapter 6-F Mitral Valve Prolapse

Table 6F.1.   Cardiac Conditions for Which Endocarditis Prophylaxis Is Recommended 6-38

Table 6F.2.   Cardiac Conditions for Which Endocarditis Prophylaxis Is Not Recommended 6-38

Table 6F.3.   Procedures for Which Endocarditis Prophylaxis Is Recommended 6-39

Table 6F.4.   Procedures for Which Endocarditis Prophylaxis Is Not Recommended 6-40

SECTION 7. GASTROINTESTINAL DISORDERS

Chapter 7-A Abdominal Pain

Table 7A.1.   Common Anatomical Pain Sites for Specific Disease 7-3

Table 7A.2.   Abdominal Palpation 7-4

Chapter 7-D Constipation

Table 7D.1.   Rome II Criteria for Functional Constipation 7-18

Table 7D.2.   Diseases Associated with Chronic Constipation 7-19

Table 7D.3.   Drugs Associated with Constipation 7-20

Table 7D.4.   Summary of Medications Commonly Used for Constipation 7-21

Chapter 7-E Diarrhea

Table 7E.1.   Differential Diagnosis of Diarrhea 7-25

Chapter 7-G Gastroesophageal Reflux

Table 7G.1.   Composition of Selected Commonly Used Antacids and Antirefluxants 7-36

Table 7G.2.   Medications Used in the Treatment of Gastroesophageal Reflux Disease 7-37

Chapter 7-L Irritable Bowel Syndrome

Table 7L.1.   Rome II Diagnostic Criteria for Irritable Bowel Syndrome 7-61

SECTION 8. MUSCULOSKELETAL DISORDERS

Chapter 8-B Fibromyalgia

Figure 8B.1.   Tender Points in Fibromyalgia Syndrome 8-4

Chapter 8-N Anti-Inflammatory and Analgesic Medication

Table 8N.1.   Anti-inflammatory and Analgesic Medication 8-74

SECTION 9. NEUROLOGICAL DISORDERS

Chapter 9-A Bell's Palsy

Table 9A.1.   Selected Causes of Facial Paralysis 9-4

Table 9A.2.   Bell's Palsy Versus Ramsay Hunt Syndrome 9-4

Table 9A.3.   Polyneuritis Manifestations of Bell's Palsy 9-5

Table 9A.4.   Red Flags in Bell's Palsy 9-5

Table 9A.5.   Cranial Nerve Testing 9-6

Figure 9A.1.   Distribution of the Facial Nerve 9-3

Chapter 9-B Dizziness

Table 9B.1.   Initial Evaluation Tests for Vertigo, Presyncope, Disequilibrium, and Lightheadedness 9-10
Table 9B.2.   Vestibular Suppressants 9-12
Table 9B.3.   Canalith Repositioning Maneuvers 9-14

Chapter 9-C Face Pain

Table 9C.1.   Selected Causes of Face Pain 9-17
Table 9C.2.   Features of Trigeminal Neuralgia 9-18
Figure 9C.1.   Borders of Territory of Sensory Nerves to the Head 9-17
Figure 9C.2.   Characteristic Trigger Zones of Trigeminal Neuralgia 9-18

Chapter 9-D Headache

Table 9D.1.   Headache Classifications 9-24
Table 9D.2.   Pharmacological Therapies for Migraine Headache 9-31
Table 9D.3.   Hormonal Therapies for Migraine Headache 9-34
Table 9D.4.   Pharmacological Therapies for Cluster Headache 9-34
Table 9D.5.   Pharmacological Therapies for Tension-Type Headache 9-35

Chapter 9-E Seizures

Table 9E.1.   Commonly Used Antiepileptic Drugs 9-40

SECTION 10. HEMATATOLOGICAL/ENDROCRINE/IMMUNOLOGICAL DISORDERS

Chapter 10-A Anemia

Table 10A.1.   Classification of Common Anemias by Morphology 10-2
Table 10A.2.   Classification of Common Anemias by Pathogenesis 10-3
Table 10A.3.   Laboratory Findings in Microcytic Anemia 10-4
Table 10A.4.   Laboratory Findings in Normocytic Anemia 10-5
Table 10A.5.   Laboratory Findings in Macrocytic Anemia 10-6
Appendix 10A.1. Patient Education Handout: Dietary Iron 10-12
Appendix 10A.2. Patient Education Handout: Dietary Folate 10-13

Chapter 10-B Chronic Fatigue Syndrome

Table 10B.1.   CDC Working Case Definition of Chronic Fatigue Syndrome or Idiopathic Chronic Fatigue 10-15

Chapter 10-D Systemic Lupus Erythematosus

Table 10D.1.   Diagnostic Criteria for Systemic Lupus Erythematosus 10-26
Table 10D.2.   Manifestations of Systemic Lupus Erythematosus 10-27
Table 10D.3.   Laboratory Tests for Systemic Lupus Erythematosus 10-28
Table 10D.4.   Drugs that Can Cause Lupus-Like Syndrome 10-29
Table 10D.5.   Screening Questionnaire for Systemic Lupus Erythematosus 10-30

Chapter 10-E Thyroid Disorders

Table 10E.1.   Common Thyroid Tests 10-36
Table 10E.2.   Suggested Approach for the Assessment of Thyroid Dysfunction 10-37

Chapter 10-F Type 1 Diabetes Mellitus

Table 10F.1.   Criteria for Diagnosis of Diabetes Mellitus 10-40
Table 10F.2.   Glycemic Control for People with Diabetes 10-41
Table 10F.3.   Time Course of Action of Human Insulin Preparations 10-42
Table 10F.4.   Sample Plan for Premeal Short-Acting (Regular) Insulin Dosing 10-46
Figure 10F.1.   Idealized Insulin Effects of Several Insulin Regimens 10-42
Appendix 10F.1. Resources for Patients with Diabetes 10-50

Chapter 10-G Type 2 Diabetes Mellitus

Table 10G.1.   Categories of Glucose Tolerance 10-51
Table 10G.2.   Criteria for Testing for Diabetes in Asymptomatic, Undiagnosed Individuals 10-52
Table 10G.3.   Comparison of Oral Agents for Type 2 Diabetes 10-53

SECTION 11. INFECTIOUS DISEASES

Chapter 11-A Diarrhea—Infectious

Table 11A.1.   Infec' \s Diarrhea, Selected Organisms 11-3

Figure 11A.1.   Evaluation of Acute Diarrhea 11-5

Chapter 11-B Hepatitis—Viral
Table 11B.1.   Serologic and Molecular Tests for Hepatitis B 11-13

Chapter 11-C Human Immunodeficiency Virus-1 Infection
Table 11C.1.   1993 Revised Classification System for HIV Infection and Expanded Surveillance Case
                Definition for AIDS Among Adults and Adolescents 11-21
Table 11C.2.   Indications for Plasma HIV RNA Testing 11-26
Table 11C.3.   Recommendations for the Use of Drug Resistance Assays 11-28
Table 11C.4.   Prophylaxis to Prevent First Episode of Opportunistic Disease in Adults and Adolescents
                Infected with Human Immunodeficiency Virus 11-29
Table 11C.5.   Indications for the Initiation of Antiretroviral Therapy in Chronically HIV-1 Infected Patients 11-32
Table 11C.6.   Recommended Antiretroviral Agents for Initial Treatment of Established HIV Infection 11-33
Table 11C.7.   Characteristics of Antiretroviral Medications by Class 11-34

Chapter 11-D Lyme Disease
Table 11D.1.   Lyme Disease Surveillance Case Definition (Revised) 11-43

Chapter 11-I Tuberculosis
Table 11I.1.   First-Line Antituberculosis Medications 11-65
Table 11I.2.   Regimen Options for Treatment of Latent Tuberculosis Infection in HIV-Negative Adults 11-66
Table 11I.3.   Regimen Options for Treatment of Latent Tuberculosis Infection in HIV-Infected Adults 11-67

Chapter 11-J Varicella Zoster Virus
Table 11J.1.   Types of Exposure to Varicella or Zoster for Which VZIG Is Indicated for Susceptible Persons 11-72
Table 11J.2.   Candidates for VZIG, Provided Significant Exposure Has Occurred 11-72

SECTION 12. GENITOURINARY DISORDERS

Chapter 12-A Abnormal Uterine Bleeding
Table 12A.1.   Classification of Abnormal Uterine Bleeding 12-4

Chapter 12-B Abnormal Cervical Cytology
Table 12B.1.   The 2001 Bethesda System (Abridged) 12-14
Table 12B.2.   Obtaining a Cytological Sample 12-16
Figure 12B.1.   Management of Women with Atypical Squamous Cells of Undetermined Significance (ASC-US) 12-15
Figure 12B.2.   Management of Women with Atypical Squamous Cells of Undetermined Significance (ASC-US)
                in Special Circumstances 12-16
Figure 12B.3.   Management of Women with Atypical Squamous Cells: Cannot Exclude High-Grade SIL (ASC-H) ... 12-17
Figure 12B.4.   Management of Women with Low-Grade Squamous Intraepithelial Lesions (LSIL) 12-18
Figure 12B.5.   Management of Women with Low-Grade Squamous Intraepithelial Lesions in Special
                Circumstances (Adolescents) 12-19
Figure 12B.6.   Management of Women with Low-Grade Squamous Intraepithelial Lesions in Special
                Circumstances (Postmenopausal Women) 12-20
Figure 12B.7.   Management of Women with High-Grade Squamous Intraepithelial Lesions (HSIL) 12-21
Figure 12B.8.   Management of Women with Atypical Glandular Cells (AGC) 12-22

Chapter 12-C Amenorrhea—Secondary
Figure 12C.1.   Algorithm for Secondary Amenorrhea 12-28

Chapter 12-G Hirsutism
Figure 12G.1.   Hirsutism Scoring 12-56

Chapter 12-H Infertility
Table 12H.1.   Normal Semen Analysis 12-63
Appendix 12H.1. Indications for Intrauterine Insemination 12-74
Appendix 12H.2. Collection of Sample for Semen Analysis 12-74
Appendix 12H.3. Timing of Intrauterine Insemination 12-75
Appendix 12H.4. Assisted Reproductive Technology 12-75

Chapter 12-I Pelvic Inflammatory Disease
Table 12I.1.   Recommendations for Individuals to Prevent STD/PID 12-85

Chapter 12-J Pelvic Masses
Table 12J.1.   Pelvic Masses—Differential Diagnoses 12-88

Chapter 12-K Pelvic Pain—Acute

Table 12K.1.   Causes of Acute Pelvic Pain 12-96
Table 12K.2.   Evaluation of Acute Pelvic Pain 12-98
Table 12K.3.   Physical Examination Features in the Woman with Acute Pelvic Pain 12-98

Chapter 12-L Pelvic Pain—Chronic

Table 12L.1.   Causes of Chronic Pelvic Pain 12-101
Table 12L.2.   Obtaining a Complete History of Chronic Pelvic Pain 12-102
Table 12L.3.   Physical Examination Features in the Woman with Chronic Pelvic Pain 12-103
Table 12L.4.   Laboratory Studies Used in the Evaluation of Chronic Pelvic Pain 12-104
Figure 12L.1.   Pain Questionnaire 12-105
Figure 12L.2.   Pain Map 12-106

Chapter 12-M Perimenopausal and Menopausal Symptoms and Hormone Therapy

Table 12M.1.   Hormonal Preparations 12-115
Table 12M.2.   Hormone Replacement Therapy: Typical Prescribing Regimens 12-116
Appendix 12M.1. Selected Resources 12-120

Chapter 12-O Premenstrual Syndrome and Premenstrual Dysphoric Disorder

Table 12O.1.   Common Signs and Symptoms of PMS 12-125
Table 12O.2.   Research Criteria for the Premenstrual Dysphoric Disorder 12-126

Chapter 12-P Sexual Dysfunction

Table 12P.1.   Psychic Factors Associated with Hypoactive Sexual Desire 12-133
Appendix 12P.1. General Assessment Questions for Sexual Functioning 12-145

Chapter 12-Q Toxic Shock Syndrome

Table 12Q.1.   CDC Case Definition for Toxic Shock Syndrome 12-147

Chapter 12-SF Vaginal Infections

Table 12SF.1.   Vaginal Infections 12-186

Chapter 12-TA Red Lesions of the Vulva

Table 12TA.1.   Tips for Treating Skin Lesions 12-191

Chapter 12-TB White Lesions of the Vulva

Table 12TB.1.   Potency Ranking of Some Commonly Used Topical Corticosteroids 12-198

Chapter 12-TC Dark Lesions of the Vulva

Table 12TC.1.   Clark's Staging Classification by Levels 12-202
Table 12TC.2.   New Staging System for Melanoma Adopted by the American Joint Committee on Cancer 12-203

Chapter 12-TE Large Lesions of the Vulva

Figure 12TE.1.   Word Catheter Ready for Insertion (Top) and After Inflation (Bottom) 12-212
Figure 12TE.2.   Inflatable Bulb-Tipped Catheter Used to Treat Bartholin's Cysts and Abscesses 12-213
Figure 12TE.3.   Incision and Suturing for Marsupialization 12-214

Chapter 12-TF Ulcerative Lesions of the Vulva

Table 12TF.1.   International Federation of Gynecology and Obstetrics (FIGO) Staging of Invasive Cancer of
                 the Vulva 12-217

Chapter 12-TH Vulvodynia

Table 12TH.1.   Differential Diagnosis of Vulvodynia: Patterns of Discomfort 12-225

SECTION 13. SEXUALLY TRANSMITTED DISEASES

Chapter 13-A Chancroid

Table 13A.1.   Clinical Features of Genital Ulcers 13-4
Table 13A.2.   Safer Sex Practices 13-6
Figure 13A.1.   Sexually Active Patient with Genital Ulcer(s) 13-5

Chapter 13-B *Chlamydia trachomatis*

Table 13B.1.   Comparison of Chlamydia Testing Technologies 13-13

Chapter 13-E Genital Herpes Simplex Virus

Table 13E.1.   Traditionally Recognized Characteristics of Clinically Evident True Primary and Recurrent
                 Genital Herpes Infection 13-31
Figure 13E.1.   Clinical Course of Primary Genital Herpes Simplex Virus Infection 13-30

Chapter 13-F Human Papillomavirus
Table 13F.1.   Human Papillomavirus (HPV) Types and Common Sites of Infection **13**-38
Table 13F.2.   Commonly Used Therapies for Treatment of Genital Warts **13**-42

Chapter 13-H Syphilis
Table 13H.1.   Important Points in the Interpretation of Syphilis Tests **13**-54

SECTION 14. BEHAVIORAL DISORDERS
Chapter 14-A Alcohol and Other Drug Problems
Table 14A.1.   Criteria for Substance Abuse **14**-3
Table 14A.2.   Criteria for Substance Dependence **14**-3
Table 14A.3.   Indicators of Alcohol and/or Drug Use **14**-4
Appendix 14A.1. Co-occurring Disorders **14**-8
Appendix 14A.2. The Use of Mood-Altering Medications by Recovering Persons **14**-8
Appendix 14A.3. Treatment for Alcohol or Other Drug Problems **14**-9
Appendix 14A.4. Recovery **14**-9

Chapter 14-C Depression
Table 14C.1.   Antidepressant Medication: Dosages and Side Effects **14**-24

Chapter 14-D Domestic Violence
Table 14D.1.   Abuse Assessment Screen **14**-32

Chapter 14-E Eating Disorders
Table 14E.1.   Diagnostic Criteria for Anorexia Nervosa **14**-36
Table 14E.2.   Diagnostic Criteria for Bulimia Nervosa **14**-36
Table 14E.3.   SCOFF Questionnaire **14**-40

Chapter 14-G Sexual Assault
Appendix 14G.1. Sexual Assault Examination and Forensic Report Form **14**-56

Chapter 14-I Stress Management
Figure 14I.1.   Breathing Exercise **14**-70
Figure 14I.2.   Relaxation Exercise **14**-70

SECTION 15. OCCUPATIONAL HEALTH
Table 15.1.   Resources for Pregnancy and Work **15**-3
Table 15.2.   Selected Occupational and Environmental Health and Safety Resources **15**-8
Figure 15.1.   Taking an Exposure History **15**-5

SECTION 16. GENERAL NUTRITION GUIDELINES
Table 16.1.   Protein in "Protein" Foods **16**-3
Table 16.2.   Protein in Other Foods **16**-3
Table 16.3.   Formula to Determine Grams of Fat to Stay Within 30% Limit **16**-4
Table 16.4.   Cholesterol and Fat Content of Selected Foods **16**-4
Table 16.5.   Daily Food Guide for Vegetarians **16**-6
Table 16.6.   High-Fiber Favorites **16**-7
Table 16.7.   Sample Menu with Fiber Content in Each Meal **16**-7
Table 16.8.   Dietary Reference Intakes (DRIs) and Recommended Dietary Allowances (RDAs) **16**-8
Table 16.9.   Lower-Fat Calcium Sources **16**-9
Table 16.10.   Antioxidant Food Sources **16**-9
Table 16.11.   Body Mass Index **16**-10
Table 16.12.   Calories Used Per Minute of Exercise **16**-11
Figure 16.1.   The Food Guide Pyramid, a Guide to Daily Food Choices **16**-2

Index

Page numbers followed by *t* denote tables; those followed by *f* denote figures

A

Abacavir, **11**-34*t*

Abdominal aortic aneurysm, **7**-5, **7**-8

Abdominal pain, **7**-2–10, **7**-62

Abduction stress test, **8**-32

Abnormal cervical cytology, **12**-13–22

Abnormal uterine bleeding, **12**-3–10, **12**-4*t*

Abscess, Bartholin's, **12**-211–214

Absence seizures, **9**-37

Abuse

elder, **1**-24

screening for, **14**-32*t*

sexual, **14**-46–50

Acanthamoeba, **2**-19

Acarbose, **10**-53*t*

Acebutolol, **6**-34*t*

Acetaminophen, **8**-75*t*, **9**-31*t*

Acetylsalicylic acid, **6**-5, **8**-76*t*

Acne rosacea, **3**-2–4

Acne vulgaris, **3**-5–7

Acoustic neuroma, **9**-10

Acrochordons, **12**-206

Acupuncture, **8**-68

Acute angle-closure glaucoma, **2**-14–16

Acute arterial insufficiency, **7**-5, **7**-7

Acute bronchitis, **5**-15–16

Acute cholecystitis, **7**-14–17

Acute diarrhea, **7**-23, **7**-26, **11**-5*f*

Acute knee pain, **8**-39–43

Acute pancreatitis, **7**-5, **7**-7

Acute pelvic pain, **12**-96–99

Acute sinusitis, **5**-48–50

Acyclovir, **11**-74, **12**-228, **12**-230, **13**-33–34

Adenomyosis, **12**-87–94

Adhesions, **12**-100

Adjustment disorder with depressed mood, **14**-20–23

Adolescents

confidentiality issues, **1**-12–13

counseling of, **1**-15*t*

demographics, **1**-10

health assessments, **1**-14*t*

health care issues for, **1**-10–13

leading causes of death in, **1**-12*t*

preventive health care for, **1**-13, **1**-15*t*

psychosocial development of, **1**-11*t*, **1**-13

risk assessments, **1**-15*t*

sexual activity among, **1**-10–11

sexual maturity rating, **1**-10*t*, **1**-13

ß₂-adrenergic agonists, for asthma, **5**-5–6

Advanced practice nurses

protocols for, **1**-5

reimbursement for, **1**-6

Aeromonas, **11**-3*t*

Agoraphobia, **14**-11–12, **14**-14–16

Albuterol

asthma treated with, **5**-6–7

bronchitis treated with, **5**-16

Alcohol use/abuse

diagnostic tests for, **14**-5

evaluation of, **14**-4–5

hypertension risks, **6**-29, **6**-33

indicators of, **14**-4*t*

in lesbians, **1**-27–28

patient education regarding, **14**-5–6

during pregnancy, **14**-2

psychiatric illness comorbidity with, **14**-8

recovery from, **14**-9

stressors associated with, **14**-2

treatment for, **14**-3–5, **14**-9

Aldosterone inhibitors, **12**-129

Alendronate, **10**-22

Allergic rhinitis, **5**-43–47

Allergy, 2-6–8

Alprazolam, **12**-128, **14**-15

Amantadine, **5**-27

Amebic keratitis, **2**-19–20

Amenorrhea
  definition of, **12**-5
  hypothalamic, **12**-25, **12**-34
  postpill, **12**-26, **12**-34
  secondary, **12**-24–34

Amiloride, **6**-34*t*

Amino acids, **16**-3

Aminosalicylates, **7**-55

Amitriptyline, **9**-21, **9**-33*t*, **9**-35*t*, **14**-24*t*

Amlodipine, **6**-34*t*

Amoxapine, **14**-24*t*

Amoxicillin
  Bartholin's cyst/abscess treated with, **12**-213
  bronchiectasis treated with, **5**-13
  chlamydia treated with, **13**-14
  chronic obstructive pulmonary disease treated with, **5**-21
  group A beta-hemolytic streptococcus treated with, **5**-35
  sinusitis treated with, **5**-49

Amoxicillin-clavulanate
  diverticulitis treated with, **7**-31
  sinusitis treated with, **5**-49, **5**-52

Amoxicillin-clavulanic acid
  bronchiectasis treated with, **5**-13
  chronic obstructive pulmonary disease treated with, **5**-21
  otitis media treated with, **5**-32
  pneumonia treated with, **5**-41

Amprenavir, **11**-36*t*

Anal fissures, **7**-43–47

Analgesics, **8**-74*t*–75*t*

Androgens, **12**-53–60, **12**-65, **12**-112, **12**-115*t*

Anemia
  of chronic disease, **10**-5, **10**-10
  classification of, **10**-2*t*–3*t*
  definition of, **10**-2
  diagnostic tests for, **10**-8–9
  hemolytic, **10**-5–6, **10**-10
  iron-deficiency, **10**-2–3, **10**-4*t*, **10**-9–11
  macrocytic, **10**-6–7
  megaloblastic, **10**-9
  microcytic, **10**-2–5, **10**-4*t*, **10**-8–9
  normocytic, **10**-5–6, **10**-9
  thalassemia, **10**-3–5, **10**-4*t*, **10**-10
  treatment of, **10**-9–11
  vitamin B$_{12}$ deficiency, **10**-10–11

Angina pectoris
  assessment of, **6**-4
  definition of, **6**-2
  diagnostic tests for, **6**-4–5
  facial pain caused by, **9**-19
  gender differences, **6**-2–3
  pathophysiology of, **6**-2
  patient education regarding, **6**-6
  prevalence of, **6**-2
  Prinzmetal's, **6**-2
    signs and symptoms of, **6**-3–4
    stable, **6**-2
    treatment of, **6**-5
    unstable, **6**-2

Angiokeratoma, **12**-208–209

Angioneurotic edema, **7**-6

Angiotensin-converting enzyme inhibitors, **6**-19*t*

Anhedonia, **14**-19

Ankle fracture, **8**-48–51

Ankle pain, **8**-48–51

Ankle sprain, **8**-48–51

Ankylosing spondylitis (AS), **8**-59

Anorexia nervosa
  depression associated with, **14**-35
  diagnostic criteria, **14**-36*t*
  diagnostic tests for, **14**-40
  epidemiology of, **14**-35
  evaluation of, **14**-37–38
  follow-up for, **14**-43–44
  mortality rate, **14**-36
  patient education regarding, **14**-43
  physical examination findings, **14**-38–39
  treatment of, **14**-41–42

Anorgasmia, **12**-134–135, **12**-140–141

Antacids, **7**-36*t*

Anterior blepharitis, **2**-2–3

Anterior cruciate ligament (ACL) tear, **8**-39–40

Anterior drawer test, **8**-41, **8**-49

Anterior uveitis, **2**-22–23

Anticardiolipin antibodies, **10**-28*t*

Anticoagulants, **6**-12–14

Antidepressants
  chronic pelvic pain treated with, **12**-107
  depression treated with, **14**-24*t*
  fibromyalgia treated with, **8**-5
  migraine headache treated with, **9**-33*t*

Antidiarrheal agents, **7**-26, **11**-6

Antiepileptic drugs, **9**-39, **9**-40*t*–41*t*

Antifibrinolytic agents, **12**-9–10

Antifungal drugs, **12**-190

Antihistamines, **5**-45

Antihypertensive therapy, **6**-33, **6**-34*t*–35*t*

Antimicrobial therapy, **11**-6

Antinuclear antibody, **10**-28*t*

Antioxidants, **16**-9

Antiphospholipid antibodies, **6**-8

Antirefluxants, **7**-36*t*

Antiretroviral therapy, **11**-32, **11**-32*t*–37*t*

Antisperm antibodies, **12**-62, **12**-65, **12**-69

Antithrombin III deficiency, **6**-8

Antituberculosis medications, **11**-65*t*–66*t*

Anxiety disorders
  agoraphobia, **14**-11–12, **14**-14–16
  causes of, **14**-10
  description of, **9**-11, **14**-10
  generalized anxiety disorder, **14**-11, **14**-13, **14**-16–17
  panic disorder, **14**-10–12, **14**-14–16
  patient education regarding, **14**-17

prevalence of, **14**-10
social phobia, **14**-11–13, **14**-16
specific phobia, **14**-11–12, **14**-16
treatment of, **14**-13–17
Apocrine miliaria. *See* Fox-Fordyce disease
Apoptosis, **6**-15
Appendicitis, **7**-11–13, **12**-98*t*
Apprehension sign, **8**-20
Arteritis, **9**-19, **9**-30
Arthritis
    osteoarthritis. *See* Osteoarthritis
    rheumatoid, **8**-12–14
Arylpropionic acids, **12**-39
Asherman's syndrome, **12**-24, **12**-30, **12**-63, **12**-69–70
Aspergillus, **5**-48
Aspergillus fumigatus, **5**-37
Aspirin, **9**-31*t*, **9**-35*t*
Assault, sexual. *See* Sexual assault
Assisted reproductive technology, **12**-75
Asthma
    clinical features of, **5**-3*t*
    consultations for, **5**-10
    cough variant, **5**-2, **5**-8
    definition of, **5**-2
    diagnostic tests for, **5**-4
    epidemiology of, **5**-2
    follow-up for, **5**-10
    mild intermittent, **5**-8
    mild persistent, **5**-8
    patient education regarding, **5**-10
    prevalence of, **5**-2
    signs and symptoms of, **5**-3
    spirometry evaluations, **5**-4
    treatment of
        corticosteroids, **5**-6–7
        environmental control, **5**-4
        leukotriene modifiers, **5**-7
        metered-dose inhaler, **5**-9–10
        methylxanthines, **5**-7
        pharmacological, **5**-5–7
        strategies for, **5**-4
Atenolol, **6**-34*t*, **9**-32*t*
Athlete's foot. *See* Tinea pedis
Atopic dermatitis, **3**-8–10
Atorvastatin, **6**-27*t*
Atrophic vaginitis, **12**-167–169, **12**-187*t*
Atypical glandular cells (AGC), **12**-14, **12**-22*f*
Atypical squamous cells, cannot exclude high-grade squamous
    intraepithelial lesion (ASC-H), **12**-13, **12**-17*f*
Atypical squamous cells of undetermined significance
    (ASC-US), **12**-14, **12**-15*f*–16*f*
Auspitz's sign, **3**-45
Avascular necrosis, **8**-36
Azathioprine, **7**-55–56
Azithromycin
    bronchitis treated with, **5**-16
    chancroid treated with, **13**-6
    chlamydia treated with, **13**-14

gonorrhea treated with, **13**-21
granuloma inguinale treated with, **13**-27
group A beta-hemolytic streptococcus treated with, **5**-35
pneumonia treated with, **5**-41
sinusitis treated with, **5**-49
syphilis treated with, **13**-56

B

Bacillus cereus, **7**-25*t*, **11**-3*t*
Bacterial conjunctivitis, **2**-6–8
Bacterial folliculitis, **3**-21–22
Bacterial keratitis, **2**-19–20
Bacterial paronychia, **3**-38
Bacterial pneumonia, **5**-38–39
Bacterial vaginosis (BV), **12**-170–173, **12**-186*t*
Bacteroides fragilis, **5**-51
Bacteroides ureolyticus, **12**-170
Ballance's sign, **7**-4*t*
Barrett's esophagitis, **7**-33
Bartholinitis, **13**-10
Bartholin's cyst, **12**-211–214
Basal body temperature (BBT), **12**-67, **12**-79
Basal cell carcinoma, **12**-219–220
Basal metabolic rate (BMR), **16**-11–12
Basilar joints, osteoarthritis of, **8**-31–32
Bassler's sign, **7**-4*t*
Beclomethasone
    asthma treated with, **5**-6–7
    chronic obstructive pulmonary disease treated with, **5**-21
Beevor's sign, **7**-4*t*
Behavioral disorders
    alcohol abuse. *See* Alcohol use
    anxiety disorders. *See* Anxiety disorders
    depression. *See* Depression
    domestic violence, **14**-30–34
    eating disorders. *See* Anorexia nervosa, Bulimia nervosa
    sexual abuse, **14**-46–50
    sexual assault. *See* Sexual assault
    smoking. *See* Smoking
    stress, **14**-69–72
Bell's palsy, **9**-2–8, **11**-47
Benazepril, **6**-34*t*
Benign paroxysmal positional vertigo (BPPV), **9**-9
Benzathine penicillin G, **13**-56
Benzodiazepines, **14**-15–16
Beta blockers
    angina pectoris treated with, **6**-5
    anxiety disorders treated with, **14**-16
    heart failure treated with, **6**-19*t*, **6**-19–20
    hypertension treated with, **6**-34*t*
    migraine headache treated with, **9**-32*t*
Betamethasone dipropionate, **12**-196
Bethanechol, **7**-37*t*
Biguanides, **10**-53*t*
Bile acid resins, **6**-27*t*
Bilirubin, **11**-12

Biofeedback, **8**-6

Biopsy
breast cancer evaluations, **4**-4–5
endometrial, **12**-114, **12**-116
fine-needle aspiration, **4**-4, **4**-16

Bismuth subsalicylate, **7**-26, **7**-69

Bisoprolol, **6**-19*t*, **6**-34*t*

Bisphosphonates, **10**-22

Bitolterol
asthma treated with, **5**-6
bronchitis treated with, **5**-16

Blackhead, **3**-5

Bleeding
anovulatory, **12**-8–9
gastrointestinal, **7**-39–42
nasal. *See* Epistaxis
postmenopausal, **12**-5, **12**-10
uterine, **12**-3–10

Blue bloater, **5**-18

Blumberg's sign, **7**-4*t*

Body mass index (BMI), **16**-10*t*, **16**-11

Body weight, **16**-11

Bone mineral density, **10**-19, **12**-32

Borrelia burgdorferi, **11**-42

Brainstem disorders, **9**-11

Branhamella catarrhalis, **5**-48, **5**-51

BRCA1, **4**-2–3

BRCA2, **4**-2–3

Breast cancer
biopsy evaluations, **4**-4–5
diagnostic testing for, **4**-4–5
hormone replacement therapy and, **4**-3, **12**-111
incidence of, **1**-8–9
race-based incidence of, **1**-9
risk factors, **4**-2–6
screening for, **4**-2–6
symptoms of, **4**-3–4

Breast disorders
breast cancer. *See* Breast cancer
cysts, **4**-16–17
duct ectasia, **4**-10–11
fat necrosis, **4**-12–13
fibroadenoma, **4**-14–15
galactocele, **4**-18–19
galactorrhea, **4**-20–22
intraductal papilloma, **4**-23–24
mastitis
nonpuerperal, **4**-25–26
periductal, **4**-10–11
nipple discharge, **4**-27–28
Paget's disease, **4**-29–30
periductal mastitis, **4**-10–11
superficial phlebitis, **4**-31–32

Breast Imaging Reporting and Data System (BIRADS), **4**-4

Breast nodularity, **4**-6–9

Breast pain
cyclical, **4**-6
noncyclical, **4**-6, **4**-9

treatment of, **4**-7–9

Breast self-examination, **4**-5

Breathing exercises, for stress management, **14**-70*t*

Bromocriptine, **4**-7, **12**-31, **12**-70

Bronchiectasis, **5**-12–14

Bronchitis
acute, **5**-15–16
chronic
definition of, **5**-17
description of, **5**-17
diagnostic tests, **5**-20
physical examination findings, **5**-19
signs and symptoms of, **5**-17–18
treatment of, **5**-20–22

Bronchodilators, **5**-21

Bronchoscopy, **5**-13

Budesonide
asthma treated with, **5**-6–7
Crohn's disease treated with, **7**-55

Bulimia nervosa
depression associated with, **14**-35
diagnostic criteria, **14**-36*t*
diagnostic tests for, **14**-41
epidemiology of, **14**-35
evaluation of, **14**-38
follow-up for, **14**-37, **14**-43–44
patient education regarding, **14**-43
physical examination findings, **14**-39–40
treatment of, **14**-41–42

Bullous impetigo, **3**-34

Bumetanide, **6**-19*t*, **6**-34*t*

Bupropion, **14**-24*t*, **14**-65–66

Burns
chemical, **2**-11–12
first-degree, **3**-11–13
minor, **3**-11
ocular, **2**-11–12
radiation, **2**-11–12
second-degree, **3**-11–13
thermal, **2**-11–12
third-degree, **3**-11–13

Bursitis, **8**-15–17, **8**-54

Buspirone, **9**-33*t*, **12**-128–129, **14**-16–17

Butalbital, **9**-31*t*

Butoconazole, **12**-177

C

Cabergoline, **12**-31, **12**-70

Calcaneal stress fracture, **8**-53–54

Calcitonin, **10**-22

Calcium, **16**-9, **16**-9*t*

Calcium channel blockers
angina pectoris treated with, **6**-5
hypertension treated with, **6**-34
migraine headache treated with, **9**-32*t*–33*t*

Calmette-Guerin bacillus, **11**-62

Caloric testing, **9**-10*t*
Calymmatobacterium granulomatis, **13**-25
Campylobacter, 7-25*t*, **11**-2, **11**-3*t*, **11**-6
Canalith repositioning maneuvers, **9**-14*t*
Cancer. *See also* Carcinoma
   breast. *See* Breast cancer
   colorectal, **12**-112
   endometrial, **12**-111
   in lesbians, **1**-28
   ovarian, **12**-89, **12**-112
Candida albicans, **2**-10, **5**-48, **12**-174, **12**-189, **12**-224
Candida glabrata, **12**-174
Candida guillermondii, **12**-174
Candida lusitaniae, **12**-174
Candida parapsilosis, **12**-174
Candida paronychia, **3**-38
Candida tropicalis, **12**-174
Candidiasis
   cutaneous, **3**-30–31, **12**-189–191
   oral, **11**-32
   vulvovaginitis, **12**-174–179, **12**-186*t*
Capsaicin, **8**-10
Captopril, **6**-19*t*, **6**-34*t*
Carbamazepine, **9**-21, **9**-40*t*, **12**-230
Carbohydrates, **16**-3–4
Carbuncles, **3**-32–33
Carcinoma. *See also* Cancer
   basal cell, **12**-219–220
   squamous cell, **12**-216–220
   verrucous, **12**-214–215
Cardiac catheterization, **6**-5, **6**-18
Cardiac syncope, **9**-11
Cardiovascular disease, **12**-111
Cardiovascular disorders
   angina pectoris, **6**-2–7
   deep vein thrombosis. *See* Deep vein thrombosis
   heart failure. *See* Heart failure
   hyperlipidemia. *See* Hyperlipidemia
   hypertension. *See* Hypertension
   mitral valve prolapse, **6**-37–41
   palpitations, **6**-42–45
Carnett's sign, **7**-4*t*
Carotidynia, **9**-19, **9**-21
Carpal tunnel syndrome (CTS), **8**-27–30
Carteolol, **6**-34*t*
Caruncle, **12**-209
Carvedilol, **6**-19*t*
Cataracts, **2**-4–5
Cauda equina syndrome, **8**-58, **8**-60, **8**-62, **8**-65
Cavernous sinus thrombosis, **3**-21
CD4+ T lymphocytes, **11**-21
Cefaclor, **5**-32, **5**-52
Cefixime, **5**-49, **13**-21
Cefotaxime, **13**-21
Cefoxitin, **12**-84, **13**-21
Cefpodoxime, **5**-32
Ceftriaxone, **12**-84, **13**-6, **13**-21, **13**-56, **14**-54
Cefuroxime axetil, **5**-35

Celecoxib, **8**-10, **8**-74*t*
Cellulitis, **3**-14–15
Cephalexin, **12**-154
   bacterial folliculitis treated with, **3**-22
   Bartholin's cyst/abscess treated with, **12**-213
   cellulitis treated with, **3**-15
   sinusitis treated with, **5**-49
Cephradine, **12**-154
Cerivastatin, **6**-27*t*
Cervical cytology, abnormal, **12**-13–22
Cervical polyps, **12**-121–123
Cetirizine, **5**-46
Chalazion, **2**-17–18
Chancroid, **13**-2–8
Chandelier sign, **7**-4*t*
Charcot's sign, **7**-4*t*
Chaussier's sign, **7**-4*t*
Chemical burns of eye, **2**-11–12
Cherry angioma, **12**-208–209
Chest pain. *See* Angina
Chest wall pain, **4**-6–9
Chest x-rays
   deep vein thrombosis evaluations, **6**-11
   heart failure evaluations, **6**-18
   pneumonia evaluations, **5**-40
Chickenpox, **11**-69–73
Child sexual abuse (CSA), **14**-46–50
Chlamydia
   diagnostic tests for, **13**-12–14, **13**-13*t*
   epidemiology of, **13**-9
   evaluation of, **13**-10–11
   manifestations of, **13**-9
   physical examination findings, **13**-11–12
   treatment of, **13**-14–15
Chlamydia pneumoniae, **5**-37
Chlamydia trachomatis, **12**-63–64, **12**-96, **12**-182, **12**-211, **13**-9–16
Chlamydial conjunctivitis, **2**-6–8
Chlorpromazine, **9**-32*t*
Chlorpropamide, **10**-53*t*
Chlorthalidone, **6**-34*t*
Cholecystitis, **7**-14–17
Cholesterol, **16**-4*t*, **16**-5
Cholestyramine, **6**-27*t*, **7**-54–55
Choline magnesium trisalicylate, **8**-76*t*
Chondroitin, **8**-10–11
Chronic bronchitis
   definition of, **5**-17
   diagnostic tests, **5**-20
   physical examination findings, **5**-19
   signs and symptoms of, **5**-17–18
   treatment of, **5**-20–22
Chronic cholecystitis, **7**-14–17
Chronic diarrhea, **7**-23, **7**-26
Chronic fatigue syndrome, **10**-14–17
Chronic illness, **1**-3
Chronic knee pain, **8**-43–47
Chronic mesenteric insufficiency, **7**-5, **7**-8

Chronic obstructive pulmonary disease (COPD)
  blue bloater, **5**-18
  chronic bronchitis. *See* Chronic bronchitis
  definition of, **5**-17
  emphysema. *See* Emphysema
  epidemiology of, **5**-17
  pink puffer, **5**-18
  pulmonary function tests, **5**-19
  smoking and, **5**-17
Chronic open-angle glaucoma, **2**-14–16
Chronic pancreatitis, **7**-5, **7**-7
Chronic pelvic pain, **12**-100–108
Chronic sinusitis, **5**-51–52
Cigarette smoking, **1**-9
Cimetidine, **7**-37*t*, **7**-68–69, **8**-9
Ciprofloxacin
  bacterial folliculitis treated with, **3**-22
  chancroid treated with, **13**-6
  diarrhea treated with, **11**-6
  diverticulitis treated with, **7**-31
  gonorrhea treated with, **13**-21
  granuloma inguinale treated with, **13**-27
  infectious diarrhea treated with, **11**-6
  sinusitis treated with, **5**-49
  traveler's diarrhea treated with, **7**-27
  urinary tract infection treated with, **12**-154
Cisapride, **7**-37*t*
Citalopram, **14**-24*t*
Clarithromycin
  bronchitis treated with, **5**-16
  group A beta-hemolytic streptococcus treated with, **5**-35
  Helicobacter pylori treated with, **7**-68
  sinusitis treated with, **5**-49
Claybrook's sign, **7**-4*t*
Clindamycin, **3**-15, **12**-173, **12**-207
Clinical breast examination (CBE), **4**-5, **4**-11
Clobetasol propionate, **12**-196, **12**-198
Clomiphene citrate, **12**-69, **12**-76–80
Clomipramine, **12**-128, **14**-24*t*
Clonazepam, **9**-41*t*
Clostridium difficile, **7**-25*t*, **11**-6
Clostridium perfringens, **11**-3*t*
Clotrimazole, **11**-32, **12**-177
Cluster headache, **9**-28–29, **9**-34*t*
Cocaine, **9**-34*t*
Coccidioides immitis, **5**-37
Coccygodynia, **8**-59, **8**-61, **8**-63
Codeine, **8**-74*t*, **9**-31*t*
Cognitive behavioral therapy (CBT), **14**-14
Colestipol, **6**-27*t*
Colonoscopy
  Crohn's disease evaluations, **7**-54
  gastrointestinal bleeding evaluations, **7**-41
  ulcerative colitis evaluations, **7**-53–54
Colorectal cancer, **12**-112
Colposcopy, **12**-17
Comedone, **3**-5
Common cold. *See* Viral rhinitis

Community-acquired pneumonia (CAP), **5**-37
Complementary and alternative therapies, **12**-112, **12**-129–130, **14**-26
Confidentiality, **1**-12
Congenital adrenal hyperplasia (CAH), **12**-54
Conjunctivitis, **2**-6–9, **13**-22
Constipation, **7**-18–22
Contact allergy conjunctivitis, **2**-7–8
Contact dermatitis, **3**-16–18, **12**-191–193
Contrast venogram, **6**-11
Core needle biopsy, **4**-4
Corneal abrasion, **2**-11–13
Corneal ulcers, **2**-19
Coronary heart disease (CHD)
  definition of, **6**-2
  gender differences, **6**-3
  hyperlipidemia and, **6**-22–23
  hypertriglyceridemia and, **6**-23
  risk factors, **6**-3, **6**-24*t*
Corticosteroids
  asthma treated with, **5**-6–7
  chronic obstructive pulmonary disease treated with, **5**-21
  contact dermatitis treated with, **3**-17, **12**-192
  Crohn's disease treated with, **7**-55, **7**-57
  fibromyalgia treated with, **8**-5
  lichen sclerosis treated with, **12**-196
  low back pain treated with, **8**-66
  potency ranking of, **12**-198*t*
  rheumatoid arthritis treated with, **8**-13
Cough variant asthma, **5**-2, **5**-8
Counseling
  adolescents, **1**-15*t*
  middle-age women, **1**-20*t*
  reproductive-age women, **1**-17*t*
Courvoisier's sign, **7**-4*t*
Cracked tooth syndrome, **9**-19
Cranial nerve testing, **9**-6*t*
Crepitus, **8**-20
Crescent sign, **8**-37
Crohn's disease (CD), **7**-51–59
Cromolyn sodium, **5**-7–8
Cryptococcus neoformans, **5**-37, **11**-30*t*
Cryptosporidium, **7**-25*t*
Cubital tunnel syndrome, **8**-24
Culdocentesis, **12**-45
Cushing's syndrome, **12**-57
Cutaneous candidiasis, **3**-30–31, **12**-189–191
Cyclobenzaprine, **8**-5, **9**-35*t*
Cyclooxygenase-2 (COX) inhibitors, **7**-69, **8**-74
Cyclosporine, **7**-56
Cyproheptadine, **9**-32*t*
Cyproterone acetate, **12**-59
Cyst(s)
  Bartholin's, **12**-211–214
  breast, **4**-16–17
  epidermal, **12**-205–206
  ganglion, **8**-33–34
  marsupialization of, **12**-212, **12**-214*f*

ovarian, **12**-79, **12**-89–94
Cystadenomas, **12**-89
Cystic duct obstruction, **7**-5, **7**-7
Cytolytic vaginitis, **12**-180–181, **12**-186*t*
Cytomegalovirus, **11**-30*t*, **11**-52

D

Dacryocystitis, **2**-10
Danazol, **4**-7, **9**-33*t*, **12**-9, **12**-51
D-dimer assay, **6**-11
Death, leading causes of, **1**-12*t*
Deep vein thrombosis (DVT)
　anticoagulation therapy for, **6**-12–14
　coagulation defects and, **6**-8
　diagnostic tests for, **6**-10–11
　lower-extremity, **6**-12–14
　mortality rates, **6**-8
　physical examination findings, **6**-10
　predisposing factors, **6**-8
　risk factors, **6**-8–9
　sites of, **6**-9
　symptoms of, **6**-9–10
　treatment of, **6**-12–14
Degenerative disk disease, **8**-69–72
Dehydroepiandrosterone sulfate (DHEA), **12**-65
Delavirdine, **11**-35*t*
Demodex folliculorum, **3**-2
Depo-medroxyprogesterone acetate, **12**-104
Depression
　adjustment disorder with, **14**-20–23
　in adolescents, **1**-12
　antidepressants for, **14**-24*t*, **14**-25–27
　description of, **12**-102, **14**-19
　diagnostic tests for, **14**-22
　dysthymia, **14**-20–23
　evaluation of, **14**-21–22
　follow-up for, **14**-28
　major, **14**-19–20, **14**-23
　patient education regarding, **14**-27–28
　selective serotonin reuptake inhibitors for, **14**-23
　treatment of, **14**-22–27
De Quervain's disease, **8**-30–31
Dermatitis
　atopic, **3**-8–10
　contact, **3**-16–18, **12**-191–193
　seborrheic, **3**-51–52
Dermatographism, **3**-8
Dermatological disorders
　acne rosacea, **3**-2–4
　acne vulgaris, **3**-5–7
　atopic dermatitis, **3**-8–10
　burns. *See* Burns
　carbuncles, **3**-32–33
　cellulitis, **3**-14–15
　contact dermatitis, **3**-16–18
　dyshidrotic eczema, **3**-19–20

folliculitis, **3**-21–23
fungal infections. *See* Fungal infections
furuncles, **3**-32–33
impetigo, **3**-34–35
molluscum contagiosum, **3**-36–37
paronychia, **3**-38–39
pediculosis, **3**-40–42
pityriasis rosea, **3**-43–44
psoriasis, **3**-45–47
scabies, **3**-48–50
seborrheic dermatitis, **3**-51–52
warts, **3**-53–54
Dermatophytes, **3**-24
Desipramine, **14**-24*t*
Dexamethasone, **3**-17
Diabetes mellitus
　definition of, **10**-40
　diagnostic criteria, **10**-40*t*
　epidemiology of, **10**-40–41
　gestational, **10**-40
　glycemic control, **10**-41*t*
　resources for, **10**-50
　type 1
　　complications of, **10**-43–44
　　definition of, **10**-40
　　evaluation of, **10**-44–45
　　follow-up for, **10**-48
　　insulin preparations for, **10**-42*t*, **10**-43*f*, **10**-45
　　patient education regarding, **10**-47–48
　　treatment of, **10**-45–47
　type 2
　　complications of, **10**-52, **10**-54
　　definition of, **10**-40, **10**-51
　　evaluation of, **10**-54–55
　　follow-up for, **10**-57–58
　　glycemic control for, **10**-52
　　oral agents for, **10**-53*t*
　　pathogenesis of, **10**-51–52
　　patient education regarding, **10**-56–57
　　treatment of, **10**-55–56
Diabetic ketoacidosis, **7**-6, **7**-8, **10**-43
Diabetic nephropathy, **10**-43
Diabetic retinopathy, **10**-54
Diarrhea
　acute, **7**-23, **7**-26, **11**-5*f*
　characteristics of, **7**-23–28, **7**-62
　chronic, **7**-23, **7**-26
　diagnostic tests for, **11**-4–5
　differential diagnosis, **7**-25*t*
　epidemiology of, **11**-2
　infectious, **11**-2–7
　patient education regarding, **11**-7
　traveler's, **7**-27, **11**-6–7
　treatment of, **7**-26–27, **11**-5–7
Diastolic dysfunction, **6**-15–16
Diazepam, **9**-12*t*, **9**-35*t*
Diclofenac, **8**-76*t*
Dicloxacillin, **5**-35

atopic dermatitis treated with, 3-9
  bacterial folliculitis treated with, 3-22
  cellulitis treated with, 3-15
Didanosine, 11-34*t*
Dietary reference intakes (DRI), **16**-7, **16**-8*t*
Digitalis glycosides, **6**-19*t*, **6**-20
Digoxin, **6**-19*t*
Dihydroergotamine, **9**-31*t*, **9**-34*t*
Dihydrotestosterone (DHT), **12**-53
Dilation and curettage (D&S), **12**-8
Diltiazem, **6**-34*t*
Diltiazem hydrochloride, **9**-33*t*
Dimenhydrinate, **14**-54
Diphenhydramine, 3-9, 3-17, **12**-191–192
Diphenoxylate, 7-26
Dipropionate, **5**-7
Direct fluorescent antibody (DFA), **13**-13*t*
Disease-modifying antirheumatic drugs (DMARDs), **8**-12–14
Disease-specific protocols, 1-5
Disequilibrium, **9**-8–9
Disseminated gonococcal infection (DGI), **13**-18–19, **13**-21–22
Diuretics
  heart failure treated with, **6**-19*t*, **6**-21
  hypertension treated with, **6**-34
  loop, **6**-19*t*, **6**-21
  potassium-sparing, **6**-34*t*
  thiazide, **6**-34*t*
Diverticular disease, 7-29–32
Diverticulitis, 7-29–31
Diverticulosis, 7-29
Dizziness, **9**-8–15
Domestic violence, **14**-30–34
Donovanosis, **13**-4*t*, **13**-25–28
Doxepin, **9**-33*t*, **14**-24*t*
Doxycycline
  chlamydia treated with, **13**-14
  gonorrhea treated with, **13**-21
  granuloma inguinale treated with, **13**-27
  lymphogranuloma venereum treated with, **13**-48
  pelvic inflammatory disease treated with, **12**-84
  pneumonia treated with, **5**-41
  syphilis treated with, **13**-56
  traveler's diarrhea treated with, 7-27
Droperidol, **9**-12*t*
Drug use/abuse
  diagnostic tests for, **14**-5
  epidemiology of, **14**-2
  evaluation of, **14**-4–5
  indicators of, **14**-4*t*
  patient education regarding, **14**-5–6
  psychiatric illness comorbidity with, **14**-8
  recovery from, **14**-9
Dual-energy x-ray absorptiometry (DEXA), **10**-20, **12**-114
Duct ectasia, 4-10–11
Dumping syndrome, 7-24
Duodenal ulcers, 7-64, 7-66
Dysesthetic vulvodynia, **12**-224–226, **12**-230
Dysfunctional uterine bleeding (DUB), **12**-3

Dyshidrotic eczema, 3-19–20
Dysmenorrhea, **12**-37–41
Dyspareunia, **12**-135, **12**-141–142
Dyspepsia, 7-5–6, 7-69
Dysthymia, **14**-20–23

E

Ear disorders
  otitis externa, **5**-29–30
  otitis media, **5**-31–32
Eating disorders
  anorexia nervosa. *See* Anorexia nervosa
  bulimia nervosa. *See* Bulimia nervosa
  treatment of, **14**-41
Ebastine, **5**-46
Ecthyma, 3-34
Ectopic pregnancy, **12**-42–47, **12**-96, **12**-98*t*, **14**-64
Eczema marginatum. *See* Tinea cruris
Efavirenz, **11**-36*t*
Elbow pain, **8**-23–26
Elder abuse, 1-24
Electrocardiogram (EKG)
  angina pectoris evaluations, **6**-4
  deep vein thrombosis evaluations, **6**-11
  heart failure evaluations, **6**-18
  palpitations evaluation, **6**-44
Electronystagmogram, **9**-10*t*
Embolism, pulmonary, **6**-9–11, **6**-13
Emphysema
  definition of, **5**-17
  diagnostic tests, **5**-20
  physical examination findings, **5**-18
  signs and symptoms of, **5**-17
  treatment of, **5**-20–22
Empty sella syndrome, **12**-25, **12**-32
Enalapril, **6**-19*t*, **6**-34*t*
Endocarditis prophylaxis, **6**-38*t*–40*t*
Endometrial biopsy, **12**-114, **12**-116
Endometrial cancer, **12**-111
Endometrial polyps, **12**-121–123
Endometriomas, **12**-89
Endometriosis, **12**-48–52, **12**-64, **12**-100
Endophthalmitis, 2-22
Endoscopic retrograde cholangiopancreatography (ERCP), 7-15
Endoscopy, 7-41, 7-66–67
Enemas, 7-21*t*
Energy requirements, **16**-11–12
Entamoeba histolytica, 7-25*t*, **11**-2, **11**-3*t*, **11**-6
Enterobacteriaceae, 2-19
Enzyme-linked immunosorbent assay (ELISA), **11**-25, **13**-13*t*
Eosinophilic folliculitis, 3-22
Epicondylitis, **8**-23–26
Epidermal cysts, **12**-205–206
Epidural steroid injections, **8**-67
Epilepsy, **9**-37
Epistaxis, **5**-23–24

Epley maneuver, **9**-14*t*

Epstein-Barr virus (EBV), **11**-52

Ergotamine tartrate, **9**-31*t*, **9**-34*t*

Erythema migrans, **11**-43*t*

Erythromycin
    acne vulgaris treated with, **3**-6
    bronchitis treated with, **5**-16
    cellulitis treated with, **3**-15
    chancroid treated with, **13**-6
    chlamydia treated with, **13**-14
    granuloma inguinale treated with, **13**-27
    group A beta-hemolytic streptococcus treated with, **5**-35
    lymphogranuloma venereum treated with, **13**-48
    otitis media treated with, **5**-32

Escherichia coli, **5**-37, **7**-25*t*, **11**-2, **11**-3*t*, **12**-81, **12**-151–152, **12**-211

Essential fatty acids, **4**-7

Estrogen
    amenorrhea treated with, **12**-29
    deep vein thrombosis and, **6**-9
    migraine headache treated with, **9**-33*t*

Estrogen replacement therapy, **10**-21–22, **12**-115*t*

Ethambutol, **11**-65*t*

Ethinyl estradiol, **12**-207, **14**-54

Ethmoid sinusitis, **9**-18

Ethosuximide, **9**-40*t*

Etodolac, **8**-76*t*

Exercise, **16**-11

Exercise-induced bronchospasm, **5**-2, **5**-8

Extracorporeal shock-wave lithotripsy, **7**-16

Exudative diarrhea, **7**-23

Eye
    acne rosacea involvement of, **3**-2
    disorders of. *See* Ophthalmological disorders
    herpes zoster of, **11**-75
    injuries of, **2**-11–13

F

Facial nerve, **9**-2–3

Facial pain
    anatomy of, **9**-16, **9**-17*f*
    musculoskeletal disorders that cause, **9**-19
    neuralgia, **9**-16, **9**-18
    neurological causes of, **9**-16, **9**-18
    otolaryngological causes of, **9**-18–19

Facial paralysis, **9**-4

Factor V Leiden, **6**-8

Famciclovir, **12**-228, **13**-33–34

Famotidine, **7**-37*t*, **7**-68

Fatigue, **10**-14–17

Fat necrosis of breast, **4**-12–13

Fats (dietary), **16**-4–5

Felbamate, **9**-41*t*

Felodipine, **6**-34*t*

Female orgasmic disorder, **12**-134–135

Femoral hernia, **7**-48

Fenofibrate, **6**-27*t*

Fenoprofen, **8**-76*t*

Fexofenadine, **5**-46

Fiber, **16**-6–7, **16**-7*t*

Fibric acid derivatives, **6**-27*t*

Fibroadenoma, **4**-14–15

Fibroids, **12**-87–94, **12**-101

Fibromyalgia, **8**-3–7, **12**-102

Finasteride, **12**-59

Fine-needle aspiration biopsy
    breast cancer evaluations, **4**-4
    cyst evaluations, **4**-16

Finger
    pain in, **8**-27–35
    trigger, **8**-32–33

Finklestein's test, **8**-30

First-degree burns, **3**-11–13

Fluconazole, **12**-190, **12**-228

Fluid cysts of breast, **4**-16–17

Flumadine. *See* Rimantadine

Flunisolide
    asthma treated with, **5**-6–7
    chronic obstructive pulmonary disease treated with, **5**-21

Fluocinolone acetonide, **12**-198

5-Fluorouracil, **13**-42

Fluoxetine, **9**-33*t*, **9**-35*t*, **12**-128, **14**-15, **14**-24*t*, **14**-42

Flurbiprofen, **8**-77*t*

Flutamide, **12**-59

Fluticasone, **5**-6–7

Fluvoxamine, **14**-15, **14**-24*t*

Folate, **10**-13*t*

Folate-deficiency anemia, **10**-6, **10**-10–11

Follicle-stimulating hormone (FSH), **12**-25, **12**-29

Folliculitis, **3**-21–23

Food Guide Pyramid, **16**-2, **16**-2*f*

Foot pain, **8**-52–57

Foreign body, ocular, **2**-11–13

Forensic examination
    request for, **14**-62*f*
    sexual assault, **14**-56*f*–61*f*

Formoterol, **5**-7

Fosinopril, **6**-19*t*, **6**-34*t*

Fothergill's sign, **7**-4*t*

Fox-Fordyce disease, **12**-209–210

Fracture
    ankle, **8**-48–51
    calcaneal, **8**-53–54
    spinal, **8**-60

Free radicals, **16**-9

Frontal sinusitis, **9**-18

Frozen shoulder, **8**-18

Fructose, **16**-3

Fungal infections
    cutaneous candidiasis, **3**-30–31
    description of, **3**-24
    moniliasis, **3**-30–31
    tinea corporis, **3**-25–26
    tinea cruris, **3**-29

tinea pedis, **3**-27–29
tinea versicolor, **3**-24–25
Fungal keratitis, **2**-19–20
Furosemide, **6**-19*t*, **6**-34*t*
Furuncles, **3**-32–33
Furunculosis, **3**-21
Fusobacterium nucleatum, **12**-170

G

Gabapentin, **9**-40*t*, **12**-230
Galactocele, **4**-18–19
Galactorrhea, **4**-20–22, **12**-32, **12**-34
Galactose, **16**-3
Gallstones, **7**-14–17, **12**-112
Ganglion cysts, **8**-33–34
Gardnerella vaginalis, **12**-81, **12**-170, **12**-182
Gastroesophageal reflux, **7**-33–38
Gastrointestinal bleeding, **7**-39–42
Gastrointestinal disorders
    abdominal pain, **7**-2–10
    anal fissures, **7**-43–47
    appendicitis, **7**-11–13
    cholecystitis, **7**-14–17
    constipation, **7**-18–22
    diarrhea. *See* Diarrhea
    diverticular disease, **7**-29–32
    gastroesophageal reflux, **7**-33–38
    gastrointestinal bleeding, **7**-39–42
    heartburn, **7**-33–38
    hemorrhoids, **7**-43–47
    hernia, **7**-48–50
    inflammatory bowel disease, **7**-51–59
    irritable bowel syndrome, **7**-60–63, **12**-101
Gatifloxacin, **13**-22
Gemfibrozil, **6**-27*t*
Generalized anxiety disorder, **14**-11, **14**-13, **14**-16–17
Generalized seizures, **9**-37
Genital ulcers, **13**-4*t*, **13**-5*f*, **13**-42*t*
Genital warts, **13**-42*t*–43*t*
Genitourinary disorders. *See specific disorder*
Geriatric depression scale (GDS), **1**-21
Gestational diabetes mellitus, **10**-40
Giant cell arteritis, **9**-19, **9**-30
Giardia lamblia, **7**-25*t*, **11**-2, **11**-3*t*, **11**-6
Glaucoma, **2**-14–16
Glimepiride, **10**-53*t*
Glipizide, **10**-53*t*
Glomerulations, **12**-101
Glossopharyngeal neuralgia, **9**-18
Glucosamine, **8**-10–11
Glucose, **16**-3
Glucosidase inhibitors, **10**-53*t*
Glyburide, **10**-53*t*
Goiter, **10**-33–34
Gonadotropin-releasing hormone agonists, **4**-7, **12**-104, **12**-106, **12**-129

Gonadotropins, **12**-78
Gonococcal conjunctivitis, **2**-6–8
Gonococcal pharyngitis, **5**-35
Gonorrhea
    anal infection, **13**-21–22
    complications of, **13**-17–18
    diagnostic tests for, **13**-20–21
    disseminated infection, **13**-18–19, **13**-21–22
    epidemiology of, **13**-17
    evaluation of, **13**-18–19
    follow-up for, **13**-23
    genital infection, **13**-21–22
    patient education regarding, **13**-23
    pharyngeal infection, **13**-22
    physical examination findings, **13**-19–20
    in pregnancy, **13**-22
    sites of, **13**-17
Granuloma inguinale, **13**-25–28
Graves' disease, **10**-33–34
Griseofulvin, **12**-190
Group A beta-hemolytic streptococcus, **5**-33–36
Guidelines for Adolescent Preventive Services, **1**-13
Guttate psoriasis, **3**-45–46
Gynecologic cancers, **1**-28

H

Haemophilus ducreyi, **13**-2
Haemophilus influenzae, **5**-12, **5**-37, **5**-48, **5**-51
Hair growth, **12**-53–54
Hallpike-Dix test, **9**-10*t*
Hand pain, **8**-27–35
Harris and Benedict formula, **16**-11
Hashimoto's thyroiditis, **10**-33, **12**-25
Headache
    classification of, **9**-23, **9**-24*t*
    cluster, **9**-28–29, **9**-34*t*
    definition of, **9**-23
    evaluation of, **9**-24–25
    facial pain caused by, **9**-16
    migraine. *See* Migraine headache
    primary, **9**-23, **9**-24*t*
    secondary, **9**-23, **9**-24*t*
    tension-type, **9**-29–30, **9**-35*t*
    treatment of, **9**-25–26
Health care issues
    adolescents, **1**-10–13
    behavioral factors that affect, **1**-9
    lesbians, **1**-27–29
    overview of, **1**-8–10
Health insurance, **1**-9–10
Heartburn, **7**-33–38
Heart failure
    definition of, **6**-15
    diagnostic tests for, **6**-18
    diastolic dysfunction, **6**-15–16
    epidemiology of, **6**-15

etiology of, 6-15
left, 6-16
pathophysiology of, 6-15
patient education regarding, 6-20–21
physical examination findings, 6-17
right, 6-16
symptoms of, 6-16–17
systolic dysfunction, 6-15
treatment of, 6-18–20
Heel fat pad atrophy, 8-53–56
Helicobacter pylori, 3-2, 7-33, 7-64, 7-67–70
Hemangiomas, 12-208–209
Hemiplegic migraine, 9-26
Hemoglobin H disease, 10-3–4
Hemolytic anemia, 10-5–6, 10-10
Hemorrhoids, 7-43–47
Heparin
    deep vein thrombosis treated with, 6-12–14
    low molecular weight, 6-12–13
Hepatitis
    definition of, 11-8
    patient education regarding, 11-18–19
Hepatitis A (HAV)
    antibody to, 11-11–12
    description of, 11-8, 11-11
    diagnostic tests for, 11-11–12
    prophylaxis, 11-29t
    treatment of, 11-15
Hepatitis B (HBV)
    description of, 11-8–9, 11-11
    diagnostic tests for, 11-12–13
    postexposure prophylaxis, 11-16–17, 11-29t
    treatment of, 11-15–17
Hepatitis B core antigen (HBcAg), 11-12
Hepatitis B e antigen (HBeAg), 11-12
Hepatitis B surface antigen (HBsAg), 11-12
Hepatitis C (HCV)
    antibodies to, 11-13
    description of, 11-9, 11-11
    diagnostic tests for, 11-13–14
    RNA, 11-14
    treatment of, 11-17–18
Hepatitis D (HDV)
    description of, 11-10–11
    diagnostic tests for, 11-14
    treatment of, 11-18
Hepatitis E (HEV)
    description of, 11-10–11
    diagnostic tests for, 11-14
    treatment of, 11-18
Hepatitis G, 11-10
Hernia, 7-48–50
Herpes simplex virus (HSV)
    asymptomatic, 13-31
    clinical presentation of, 13-30–31
    diagnostic tests for, 13-33
    incidence of, 13-29
    keratitis caused by, 2-19

nonprimary first-episode, 13-30–31
patient education regarding, 13-34–35
during pregnancy, 13-29–30
prevalence of, 13-29
primary, 13-30, 13-31t, 13-32–33
recurrent, 13-31t, 13-31–34
treatment of, 12-228–229
type 1, 13-29
type 2, 13-29
ulcers associated with, 13-4t
Herpes zoster, 9-18, 11-73–75
Hidradenitis suppurativa, 12-206–208
High-density lipoprotein (HDL), 6-2, 6-22, 16-5
High-grade squamous intraepithelial lesion (HSIL), 12-21f
Highly active antiretroviral therapy (HAART), 11-32, 11-32t–37t
Hip pain, 8-36–38
Hirsutism, 12-53–60
Histamine H2-receptor blockers, 7-37t, 7-68
Histoplasma capsulatum, 5-37, 11-30t
HMG-CoA reductase inhibitors, 6-26, 6-27t
Homosexuality. See Lesbians
Hordeolum, 2-17–18
Hormone replacement therapy (HRT)
    benefits of, 12-110–111
    breast cancer and, 4-3, 12-111
    deep vein thrombosis and, 6-9
    description of, 1-19–20, 12-110
    hormonal preparations for, 12-115t
    osteoporosis treated with, 10-21–22, 12-110–111
    postmenopausal uses, 12-117
    prescribing of, 12-116t
    risks associated with, 12-111–112
    systemic lupus erythematosus and, 10-29
5-HT$_1$ serotonin agonists, 9-27, 9-32t
Beta-human chorionic gonadotropin (hCG), 12-44, 12-78
Human immunodeficiency virus (HIV)
    acute retroviral syndrome, 11-23
    antiretroviral therapy for, 11-32, 11-32t–37t
    classification of, 11-21t
    consultations, 11-38
    diagnostic tests for, 11-22, 11-25–31
    drug resistance assays, 11-28t
    highly active antiretroviral therapy for, 11-32, 11-32t–37t
    latent tuberculosis in, 11-67t
    in lesbians, 1-28
    manifestations of, 11-23–24
    opportunistic infections, 11-27, 11-29t–31t
    Pap smear considerations, 11-27–28
    pathophysiology of, 11-20–22
    patient education regarding, 11-38–39
    physical examination findings, 11-24–25
    plasma RNA testing, 11-26, 11-26t
    pregnancy considerations, 11-39
    prevalence of, 11-20
    progressive, 11-23–24
    risk factors, 11-22–23
    syphilis and, 13-58–59
    transmission of, 11-20

treatment of, **11**-31–38
viral load measurements, **11**-22
Human papillomavirus (HPV)
  biology of, **13**-37
  description of, **1**-28, **3**-53, **12**-229, **13**-37
  diagnostic tests for, **13**-39–40
  evaluation of, **13**-38–39
  incidence of, **13**-37–38
  latent, **13**-39
  patient education regarding, **13**-41
  prevalence of, **13**-37–38
  transmission of, **13**-38
  treatment of, **13**-40–41
  types of, **13**-38*t*
Hyaluronan, **8**-10–11
Hydralazine, **6**-20
Hydrochlorothiazide, **6**-34*t*
Hydrocodone, **8**-75*t*
Hydrocortisone, **3**-17
Hydromorphone, **9**-31*t*
Hydrops fetalis, **10**-3
11ß-hydroxylase deficiency, **12**-54
21-hydroxylase deficiency, **12**-54
3ß-hydroxysteroid dehydrogenase deficiency, **12**-54
Hydroxyzine
  atopic dermatitis treated with, **3**-9
  contact dermatitis treated with, **3**-17, **12**-192
Hyoscyamine sulfate, **7**-62
Hyperhomocysteinemia, **6**-8
Hypericum perforatum, **14**-26
Hyperlipidemia
  coronary heart disease risks and, **6**-22–23
  definition of, **6**-22
  diagnostic tests for, **6**-24
  dietary recommendations for, **6**-26*t*
  HMG-CoA reductase inhibitors for, **6**-26, **6**-27*t*
  lipoproteins, **6**-22
  patient education regarding, **6**-28
  symptoms of, **6**-23–24
  treatment of, **6**-24–26
Hyperosmolar hyperglycemic nonketotic syndrome (HHNS),
    10-52, **10**-54
Hyperprolactinemia, **4**-20, **4**-21*t*, **12**-24–25, **12**-31, **12**-34,
    12-64, **12**-76
Hypertension
  definition of, **6**-29
  diagnostic tests for, **6**-31–32
  epidemiology of, **6**-30
  essential, **6**-29
  isolated systolic, **6**-30
  patient education regarding, **6**-36
  physical examination findings, **6**-31
  risk factors, **6**-29–30, **6**-32
  secondary, **6**-30
  symptoms of, **6**-30–31
  treatment of
    blood pressure goals, **6**-32–33
    lifestyle modification, **6**-33

overview of, **6**-32–33
  pharmacologic, **6**-33–36
  white coat, **6**-30
Hypertriglyceridemia
  coronary heart disease risks, **6**-23
  treatment of, **6**-26
Hypoactive sexual desire, **12**-132–133, **12**-135–136
Hypoglycemia, **10**-43
Hypomenorrhea, **12**-5
Hypothalamus
  amenorrhea, **12**-25, **12**-32–34
  infertility caused by, **12**-64
Hypothyroidism, primary, **10**-33–35, **10**-38–39, **12**-25, **12**-65
Hysterectomy, **12**-10
Hysterosalpingography (HSG), **12**-8, **12**-68

Ibuprofen, **8**-77*t*, **9**-31*t*, **9**-35*t*, **10**-16, **12**-9
Iliopsoas sign, **7**-4*t*
Iliopsoas syndrome, **8**-61, **8**-63
Imipramine, **12**–163, **14**-15, **14**-24*t*
Imiquimod, **13**-42
Immunizations
  description of, **1**-15*t*
  hepatitis A, **11**-15
  influenza, **5**-26
  mumps-measles-rubella, **11**-58
  pneumococcal, **5**-41
  varicella zoster virus, **11**-70
Impedance plethysmography, **6**-11
Impetigo, **3**-34–35
Impingement sign, **8**-19
Indapamide, **6**-34*t*
Indinavir, **11**-36*t*
Indomethacin, **8**-77*t*, **9**-34*t*
Industrial hygienist (IH), **15**-4
Infectious diarrhea, **11**-2–7
Infertility. *See also* Pregnancy
  age-related, **12**-65–66, **12**-71
  clomiphene citrate, **12**-69, **12**-76–80
  definition of, **12**-62
  endocrine-factor, **12**-64–65, **12**-70–71
  evaluations, **12**-66–69
  immunological, **12**-65, **12**-71
  luteal phase defect, **12**-72
  male-factor, **12**-62–63, **12**-69
  pelvic-factor, **12**-63–64, **12**-69–70
  unexplained, **12**-65, **12**-71
Inflammatory acne, **3**-6–7
Inflammatory bowel disease (IBD), **7**-51–59
Infliximab, **7**-56
Influenza, **5**-25–28, **11**-29*t*
Infracalcaneal bursitis, **8**-54
Inguinal hernia, **7**-48
Insoluble fiber, **16**-6
Insulin, **10**-42*t*, **10**-43*f*, **10**-45, **10**-56

Interferons
  genital warts treated with, **13**-43*t*
  hepatitis treated with, **11**-16–18
International Federation of Gynecology and Obstetrics
  staging, **12**-217*t*
Interstitial cystitis (IC), **12**-101, **12**-164–166
Intraductal papilloma, **4**-23–24
Intrauterine adhesions (IUAs), **12**-24
Intrauterine insemination, **12**-74–75
In vitro fertilization (IVF), **12**-65
Ipratropium, **5**-6
Iridocyclitis, **2**-22
Iritis, **2**-22
Iron, dietary, **10**-11, **10**-12*t*, **16**-9
Iron-deficiency anemia, **10**-2–3, **10**-4*t*, **10**-9–11
Irritable bowel syndrome (IBS), **7**-60–63, **12**-101
Isolated systolic hypertension, **6**-30
Isometheptene mucate, **9**-31*t*
Isoniazid, **11**-64, **11**-65*t*–66*t*
Isosorbide dinitrate, **6**-20
Isotretinoin, **3**-6–7
Isradipine, **6**-34*t*
Itraconazole, **12**-190
Ixodes ricinus, **11**-42

K

Kehr's sign, **7**-4*t*
Keratitis, **2**-19–20
Keratoconus, **3**-8
Keratosis pilaris, **3**-8
Ketoconazole, **3**-25, **11**-32, **12**-59, **12**-228
Ketoprofen, **8**-77*t*
Ketorolac, **8**-77*t*
Klebsiella pneumoniae, **5**-37
Knee
  anatomy of, **8**-39
  osteoarthritis of, **8**-43, **8**-45–47
Knee pain
  acute, **8**-39–43
  anatomy of, **8**-39
  chronic, **8**-43–47
Kustner's sign, **7**-4*t*

L

Labyrinthitis, **9**-9
Lachman's test, **8**-41
Lactobacilli-overgrowth syndrome. *See* Cytolytic vaginitis
Lamivudine, **11**-16, **11**-34*t*
Lamotrigine, **9**-40*t*
Lansoprazole, **7**-37*t*, **7**-68–69
Large bowel obstruction, **7**-5, **7**-7, **7**-9
Latent tuberculosis, **11**-66*t*–67*t*
Lateral epicondylitis, **8**-23–26
Laxatives, **7**-20, **7**-21*t*

Learned helplessness, **14**-31
Leflunomide, **8**-13
Legionella pneumophila, **5**-37
Lentigo, **12**-200
Lentigo maligna, **12**-203
Lesbians
  definition of, **1**-27
  gynecologic cancers in, **1**-28
  inadequate utilization of services by, **1**-28–29
  mental health issues, **1**-28
  obesity in, **1**-28
  prevalence of, **1**-27
  sexually transmitted diseases in, **1**-28
  substance use, **1**-27–28
Leukotriene modifiers, **5**-7
Leuprolide acetate, **12**-51
Levetiracetam, **9**-41*t*
Levofloxacin, **5**-40, **11**-6, **12**-84, **12**-154, **13**-14, **13**-21
Liability insurance, **1**-6–7
Lichen sclerosus, **12**-195–197
Lidocaine, **9**-34*t*
Lightheadedness, **9**-9
Lipid-lowering agents, **6**-5
Lipoproteins
  high-density, **6**-2, **6**-22, **16**-5
  low-density, **6**-2, **6**-22, **6**-25, **16**-5
  very-low-density, **6**-22
Lisinopril, **6**-19*t*, **6**-34*t*
Listeria monocytogenes, **2**-19, **7**-25*t*, **11**-3*t*
Lithium carbonate, **9**-34*t*
Locked knee, **8**-42
Lomefloxacin, **13**-22
Longevity, **1**-8
Loop diuretics, **6**-19*t*, **6**-21
Loperamide, **7**-54, **7**-62, **11**-6
Lopinavir, **11**-37*t*
Lovastatin, **6**-27*t*
Low back pain
  acute, **8**-59–69
  causes of, **8**-59
  chronic, **8**-59, **8**-69–72
  conditions associated with, **8**-58
  definition of, **8**-58
  disability risks, **8**-58–59
Low-density lipoprotein (LDL), **6**-2, **6**-22, **6**-25, **16**-5
Low-grade squamous intraepithelial lesion (LSIL), **12**-18*f*–20*f*
Low molecular weight heparin, **6**-12–13
Lumbar corset, **8**-68
Lumbar disk herniation, **8**-60–63
Lupus anticoagulants, **10**-28*t*
Luteinized unruptured follicle, **12**-71
Luteinizing hormone (LH), **12**-25, **12**-29, **12**-53
Lyme disease, **11**-42–48
Lymphadenitis, **3**-14, **13**-47
Lymphangitis, **3**-14
Lymphogranuloma venereum (LGV), **13**-4*t*, **13**-45–49

M

Macroadenoma, **12**-25
Macrocytic anemias, **10**-6–7
Magnetic resonance imaging, **6**-11
Major depression, **14**-19–20
Malic acid, **8**-6
Malocclusion, **9**-43–44
Malpractice, **1**-6–7
Mammography, **4**-4
Mantoux test, **11**-62
Maprotiline, **14**-24*t*
Mastalgia. *See* Breast pain
Mastitis
    nonpuerperal, **4**-25–26
    periductal, **4**-10–11
Maxillary sinusitis, **9**-18
McClintock's sign, **7**-4*t*
McMurray's test, **8**-41
Measles, **11**-49–51
Meclizine, **9**-12*t*
Meclofenamate, **8**-77*t*
Medial cruciate ligament (MCL) tear, **8**-40
Medial epicondylitis, **8**-23–26
Medroxyprogesterone acetate, **12**-29, **12**-58
Mefenamic acid, **8**-77*t*, **12**-9
Megaloblastic anemia, **10**-9
Meglitinide, **10**-53*t*
Melanoma, **12**-202–204
Meloxicam, **8**-74*t*
Ménière's syndrome, **9**-9
Menometrorrhagia, **12**-5
Menopause
    complementary and alternative therapies for, **12**-112
    description of, **12**-109–110
    evaluations, **12**-112–114
    hormone replacement therapy for. *See* Hormone
        replacement therapy (HRT)
Menorrhagia, **12**-5, **12**-9–10
Menstrual cycle, **12**-124
Menstrual migraine (MM), **9**-26
Mental health care
    adolescents, **1**-12
    lesbians, **1**-28
Meperidine, **9**-31*t*
6-Mercaptopurine, **7**-55–56
Mesalamine, **7**-55–57
Metered-dose inhaler, **5**-9–10
Metformin, **10**-53*t*, **12**-33
Methotrexate, **7**-56, **8**-13
Methylprednisolone, **5**-6–7
Methylxanthines, **5**-7
Methysergide maleate, **9**-32*t*, **9**-34*t*
Metoclopramide, **7**-37*t*, **9**-32*t*
Metolazone, **6**-34*t*
Metoprolol succinate, **6**-19*t*, **6**-34*t*
Metoprolol tartrate, **6**-19*t*, **6**-34*t*
Metronidazole
    acne rosacea treated with, **3**-3

bacterial vaginosis treated with, **12**-173
Crohn's disease treated with, **7**-575
diverticulitis treated with, **7**-31
hidradenitis suppurativa treated with, **12**-207
infectious diarrhea treated with, **11**-6
pelvic inflammatory disease treated with, **12**-84
syphilis treated with, **14**-54
Trichomonas vaginalis vaginitis treated with, **12**-184
Metrorrhagia, **12**-5, **12**-9
Miconazole, **12**-177
Microadenoma, **12**-25
Microcytic anemia, **10**-2–5, **10**-4*t*, **10**-8–9
Microsporidia, **7**-25*t*
Middle-age women
    counseling of, **1**-20*t*
    demographics of, **1**-18
    health assessments, **1**-19*t*
    health care issues for, **1**-18–21
    leading causes of death in, **1**-12*t*
    preventive health care, **1**-20*t*
    risk assessments, **1**-20*t*
    screenings, **1**-18–19
Miglitol, **10**-53*t*
Migraine headache
    characteristics of, **9**-26–28
    treatment of, **9**-27–28, **9**-31*t*–33*t*
    vertigo caused by, **9**-10–11
Mind-body therapies (MBTs), **8**-6
Minerals, **16**-7–9
Mini mental status exam (MMSE), **1**-21
Minocycline, **3**-3, **3**-6, **12**-207
Minors, **1**-12–13, **14**-47–48
Mirtazapine, **14**-24*t*
Misoprostol, **7**-68–69, **8**-9
Mitral valve prolapse (MVP), **6**-37–41
Mittelschmerz, **12**-96
Mixed incontinence, **12**-158–159
Mizolastine, **5**-46
Mobiluncus, **12**-170
Moexipril, **6**-34*t*
Molluscum contagiosum, **3**-36–37
Mondor's disease, **4**-31–32
Moniliasis, **3**-30–31
Monoamine oxidase inhibitors (MAOIs), **14**-16, **14**-47
Mononucleosis, **11**-52–54
Monounsaturated fats, **16**-5
Montelukast, **5**-7
Moraxella catarrhalis, **5**-37
Morphine sulfate, **9**-31*t*
Mucopurulent cervicitis, **13**-12
Multidrug-resistant tuberculosis, **11**-60–61
Mumps, **11**-55–56
Mupirocin, **3**-9
Murphy's sign, **7**-4*t*
Muscle relaxants, **8**-66
Musculoskeletal disorders
    ankle pain, **8**-48–51
    bursitis, **8**-15–17

carpal tunnel syndrome, **8**-27–30
elbow pain, **8**-23–26
fibromyalgia, **8**-3–7
foot pain, **8**-52–57
ganglion cysts, **8**-33–34
hip pain, **8**-36–38
knee pain. *See* Knee pain
osteoarthritis, **8**-8–11, **8**-31–32
overview of, **8**-2
rheumatoid arthritis, **8**-12–14
shoulder pain, **8**-18–23
tendinitis, **8**-15–17
trigger finger, **8**-32–33
Mycobacterium africanum, **11**-60
Mycobacterium avium complex, **11**-29t
Mycobacterium tuberculosis, **11**-29t, **11**-60
Mycoplasma hominis, **12**-81, **12**-170, **12**-182
Mycoplasma pneumoniae, **5**-37
Myocardial infarction (MI)
    description of, **6**-2
    risk factors, **6**-3
Myoclonic seizures, **9**-37
Myofascial pain, **9**-19, **12**-102, **12**-107
Myomas, **12**-87

N

Nabumetone, **8**-78t
Nadolol, **6**-34t, **9**-32t
Nafarelin, **12**-51
Naproxen, **8**-78t, **9**-35t, **10**-16
Naproxen sodium, **8**-78t, **9**-31t, **9**-35t, **10**-16
Naratriptan, **9**-32t
Narcotics, **12**-106
National Asthma Education and Prevention Program
    (NAEPP), **5**-2
Nedocromil sodium, **5**-7
Nefazodone, **14**-24t
Neisseria gonorrhoeae, **11**-3t, **12**-63–64, **12**-81, **12**-96,
    12-176, **13**-14, **13**-17
Neisseria meningitidis, **13**-18
Nelfinavir, **11**-37t
Neuralgia, **9**-16, **9**-18, **9**-18t, **9**-21
Neurological disorders
    Bell's palsy, **9**-2–8, **11**-47
    dizziness, **9**-8–15
    facial pain. *See* Facial pain
    headache. *See* Headache
    seizures, **9**-37–42
    temporomandibular disorder, **9**-43–48
Neurosyphilis, **13**-51, **13**-56, **13**-58
Nevi, **12**-200–201
Nevirapine, **11**-35t
Niacin, **6**-27t
Nicardipine, **6**-34t
Nicotine gum, **14**-66–67
Nicotine replacement, **14**-65–66

Nicotinic acid, **6**-27t
Nifedipine, **6**-34t, **9**-32t
Nipple discharge, physiologic, **4**-27–28
Nisoldipine, **6**-34t
Nitric oxide, **6**-5
Nitroglycerin, **6**-5
Nizatidine, **7**-37t, **7**-68
Nodular melanoma, **12**-203–204
Non-nucleotide reverse transcriptase inhibitors
    (NNRTIs), **11**-35t–36t
Nonpuerperal mastitis, **4**-25–26
Nonsteroidal anti-inflammatory drugs (NSAIDs)
    acute knee pain treated with, **8**-42
    bursitis treated with, **8**-16–17
    dysmenorrhea treated with, **12**-39–40
    elbow pain treated with, **8**-24
    low back pain treated with, **8**-66
    menorrhagia treated with, **12**-9
    metrorrhagia treated with, **12**-9
    osteoarthritis treated with, **8**-9
    peptic ulcer disease and, **7**-64–65, **7**-69
    shoulder pain treated with, **8**-20
    tendinitis treated with, **8**-16–17
    types of, **8**-76t–78t
Norfloxacin, **11**-6, **13**-22
Normocytic anemia, **10**-5–6, **10**-9
Nortriptyline, **9**-33t, **14**-24t
Nosebleed. *See* Epistaxis
Nosocomial pneumonia, **5**-37
Nucleic acid amplification tests (NAATs), **13**-20
Nucleotide reverse transcriptase inhibitors (NRTIs), **11**-34t–35t
Nurse Practice Act, **1**-5
Nursing practice
    boundaries of, **1**-5
    standardized procedures for, **1**-5–6
Nutrients
    antioxidants, **16**-9
    carbohydrates, **16**-3–4
    fats, **16**-4–5
    overview of, **16**-2
    protein, **16**-3, **16**-3t
Nutrition
    fiber, **16**-6–7
    Food Guide Pyramid, **16**-2, **16**-2f
    minerals, **16**-7–9
    recommendations for, **16**-12
    reduced meat diet, **16**-5–6
    vegetarian diet, **16**-5–6, **16**-6t
    vitamins, **16**-7–9
    water, **16**-7
Nystatin, **11**-32, **12**-177

O

Obesity
    hypertension risks, **6**-29
    in lesbians, **1**-28

in reproductive-age women, 1-13
Obturator sign, 7-4*t*
Occipital neuralgia, **9**-18, **9**-21
Occupational health
  consultation for, **15**-8–9
  environmental assessments, **15**-2–3
  exposures
    history-taking, **15**-5*f*–7*f*
    treatment of, **15**-8
  overview of, **15**-2–3
  patient education regarding, **15**-9
  resources, **15**-8*t*
  work site evaluations, **15**-4
Occupational Safety and Health Administration (OSHA), **15**-3
Office of Research on Women's Health, 1-8
Ofloxacin, **11**-6, **12**-84, **12**-154, **13**-21
Older women
  abuse of, 1-24
  counseling for, 1-23*t*
  health assessments, 1-22*t*
  health care issues for, 1-21–24
  leading causes of death in, 1-12*t*
  preventive health care, 1-23*t*
  risk assessments, 1-23*t*
  screenings, 1-21–24
Oligomenorrhea, **12**-5
Olsalazine, **7**-55, **7**-57
Omeprazole, **7**-37*t*, **7**-68–69, **8**-9
Open-angle glaucoma, **2**-14–16
Ophthalmological disorders
  blepharitis, **2**-2–3
  cataracts, **2**-4–5
  chalazion, **2**-17–18
  conjunctivitis, **2**-6–9
  dacryocystitis, **2**-10
  eye injury, **2**-11–13
  glaucoma, **2**-14–16
  hordeolum, **2**-17–18
  keratitis, **2**-19–20
  pinguecula, **2**-21
  pterygium, **2**-21
  uveitis, **2**-22–23
Ophthalmoplegic migraine, **9**-26
Opioids, **8**-66
Opportunistic infections, **11**-27, **11**-29*t*–31*t*
Oral contraceptives, **12**-26, **12**-39
Orthostatic syncope, **9**-11
Oseltamivir, **5**-27
Osmotic diarrhea, **7**-23
Osteoarthritis (OA)
  basilar joint of thumb, **8**-31–32
  characteristics of, **8**-8–11
  hip, **8**-36–37
  knee, **8**-43, **8**-45–47
Osteomyelitis, **8**-53
Osteoporosis
  bone mineral density evaluation, **10**-19
  definition of, **10**-18

diagnostic tests for, **10**-20–21
epidemiology of, **10**-18
hormone replacement therapy for, **10**-21–22, **12**-110–111
morbidity and mortality, **10**-18–19
pathophysiology of, **10**-18
physical examination findings, **10**-20
risk factors, **10**-19–20
treatment of, **10**-21–23
Otalgia, **9**-18
Otitis externa, **5**-29–30
Otitis media, **5**-31–32
Otorhinolaryngological disorders
  epistaxis, **5**-23–24
  otitis externa, **5**-29–30
  pharyngitis, **5**-33–36
  rhinitis, **5**-43–47
Ovarian cancer, **12**-89, **12**-112
Ovarian cysts, **12**-79, **12**-89–94
Ovarian masses, **12**-89–94
Ovarian remnant syndrome, **12**-101
Ovarian stromal hyperthecosis, **12**-54
Overactive bladder (OAB), **12**-161–163
Overflow incontinence, **12**-158
Oxaprozin, **8**-78*t*
Oxcarbazepine, **9**-41*t*
Oxybutynin chloride, 12–162, **12**-165
Oxycodone, **8**-75*t*, **9**-31*t*
Oxymetazoline, **5**-49

P

Paget's disease
  of breast, **4**-29–30
  of vulva, **12**-193–194
Pain
  abdominal, **7**-2–10, **7**-62
  ankle, **8**-48–51
  breast, **4**-6–9
  chest wall, **4**-6–9
  elbow, **8**-23–26
  facial. *See* Facial pain
  finger, **8**-27–35
  foot, **8**-52–57
  hand, **8**-27–35
  hip, **8**-36–38
  jaw, **9**-48. *See also* Temporomandibular disorder
  low back. *See* Low back pain
  myofascial, **9**-19, **12**-102, **12**-107
  pelvic, **12**-48, **12**-81
  processing of, **9**-16
  psychogenic, **8**-70
  psychologic, **12**-102
  shoulder, **8**-18–23
  vulvodynia-related. *See* Vulvodynia
  wrist, **8**-27–35
Pain questionnaire, **12**-105*f*
Palpitations, **6**-42–45

Pancreatitis, **7**-5, **7**-7
Panic disorder, **14**-10–12, **14**-14–16
Pantoprazole, **7**-37*t*, **7**-68
Papilloma, intraductal, **4**-23–24
Papillomatosis, **4**-23, **12**-224
Pap smears, **11**-27–28
Parathyroid hormone (PTH), **10**-23
Paronychia, **3**-38–39
Paroxetine, **9**-33*t*, **12**-128, **14**-24*t*
Partial seizures, **9**-37
Patellofemoral pain (PFP) syndromes, **8**-43–45
Patient Health Questionnaire, **14**-22
Pediculosis capitis, **3**-40–42
Pediculosis corporis, **3**-40–42
Pediculosis pubis, **3**-40–42
Pelvic inflammatory disease (PID), **12**-64, **12**-81–86, **12**-98*t*,
    12-100–101, **13**-17
Pelvic masses
    adenomyosis, **12**-87–94
    description of, **12**-87
    fibroids, **12**-87–94
    ovarian masses, **12**-89–94
Pelvic pain
    acute, **12**-96–99
    chronic, **12**-100–108
    description of, **12**-48, **12**-81
Penbutolol, **6**-34*t*
Penicillin V, **5**-35
Peptic ulcer disease (PUD)
    contributing factors, **7**-64–65
    description of, **7**-39, **7**-64
    diagnostic tests for, **7**-66–67
    risk factors, **7**-65
    treatment of, **7**-67–70
Peptostreptococcus, **12**-81, **12**-170
Pergolide, **12**-31
Periductal mastitis, **4**-10–11
Perihepatitis, **13**-10
Perimenopause, **12**-109
Peritonitis, **7**-5, **7**-7
Pernicious anemia, **10**-6
Pessaries, **12**-159
Phalen's test, **8**-28
Pharyngitis, **5**-33–36, **13**-10
Phenobarbital, **9**-41*t*
Phenytoin, **9**-40*t*, **12**-230
Phlebitis, superficial, **4**-31–32
Phonophoresis, **8**-16
Physical therapy, **8**-67
Physiologic nipple discharge, **4**-27–28
Pindolol, **6**-34*t*
Pinguecula, **2**-21
Pink puffer, **5**-18
Pioglitazone, **10**-53*t*, **12**-33
Pirbuterol, **5**-6
Piriformis syndrome, **8**-61
Piroxicam, **8**-78*t*
Pituitary gland disorders, **12**-31–32

Pityriasis alba, **3**-8
Pityriasis rosea, **3**-43–44
Pityriasis versicolor, **3**-24–25
Pityrosporum ovale, **3**-51
Pivot shift, **8**-41
Plantar fascia
    anatomy of, **8**-52
    rupture of, **8**-53–56
Plantar fasciitis, **8**-52–57
Plantar fibromatosis, **8**-53
Plantar wart, **3**-53–54
Plesiomonas, **11**-3*t*
Pneumococcal vaccination, **5**-41
Pneumocystis carinii, **5**-37, **11**-29*t*
Pneumonia
    atypical, **5**-39
    bacterial, **5**-38–39
    community-acquired, **5**-37
    complications of, **5**-37–38
    definition of, **5**-37
    diagnostic tests for, **5**-40
    nosocomial, **5**-37
    pathogens associated with, **5**-37
    physical examination findings, **5**-39–40
    PORT criteria and scoring for, **5**-37–38, **5**-38*t*
    treatment of, **5**-40–41
    viral, **5**-39
Podophyllotoxin, **13**-40, **13**-42*t*
Polycystic ovary syndrome (PCOS), **12**-25–26, **12**-32–34,
    12-54, **12**-65, **12**-70
Polymenorrhea, **12**-5
Polymyalgia rheumatica (PR), **8**-59
Polypharmacy, **1**-23–24
Polyps, **12**-121–123
Polyunsaturated fats, **16**-5
Pompholyx. *See* Dyshidrotic eczema
Porphyria, **7**-6, **7**-8
Posterior blepharitis, **2**-3
Posterior uveitis, **2**-22–23
Postmenopausal bleeding, **12**-5, **12**-10
Post-traumatic stress disorder (PTSD), **14**-52
Potassium-sparing diuretics, **6**-34*t*
Poverty, **1**-9
Pravastatin, **6**-27*t*
Prednisolone, **5**-6–7
Prednisone
    asthma treated with, **5**-6–7
    chronic obstructive pulmonary disease treated with, **5**-21
    cluster headache treated with, **9**-34*t*
    contact dermatitis treated with, **3**-17
    Crohn's disease treated with, **7**-55
Pregnancy. *See also* Infertility
    alcohol use during, **14**-2
    ectopic, **12**-42–47, **12**-96, **12**-98*t*, **14**-64
    gonorrhea treatment during, **13**-22
    herpes simplex virus during, **13**-29–30
    HIV-infected patient, **11**-39
    prenatal care, **1**-16–17

race-based risks, **1**-17–18
recommended dietary allowances during, **16**-8*t*
resources for, **15**-3*t*
syphilis during, **13**-59
systemic lupus erythematosus and, **10**-29–30
teenage, **1**-11–12
varicella zoster virus exposure during, **11**-69
violence during, **1**-18
Premature ovarian failure (POF), **12**-24, **12**-30–31, **12**-34, **12**-65, **12**-71
Premenstrual dysphoric disorder (PMDD), **12**-124–130
Premenstrual syndrome (PMS), **12**-124–130
Prenatal care, **1**-16–17
Prerosacea, **3**-2
Prescriptive authority, **1**-6
Presyncope, **9**-9, **9**-11
Prevotella, **12**-170
Primary care
  chronic illness and, **1**-3
  definition of, **1**-2
  multidisciplinary approach, **1**-3
  providers of, **1**-2–3
Primidone, **9**-41*t*
Prinzmetal's angina, **6**-2
Procedure-specific protocols, **1**-5
Prochlorperazine, **9**-12*t*, **9**-32*t*
Proctitis, **13**-10
Proctocolitis, **13**-47
Professional liability insurance, **1**-6–7
Progesterone, **12**-29, **12**-129
Progestogens, **12**-115*t*
Prokinetic agents, **7**-37*t*
Prolactin, **4**-21, **12**-64
Prolactinoma, **12**-64
Prolactin-secreting adenoma, **12**-25, **12**-64
Prolotherapy, **8**-71
Promethazine, **9**-12*t*, **9**-32*t*
Pronator syndrome, **8**-24
Propionibacterium acnes, **3**-5
Propoxyphene, **8**-75*t*, **9**-31*t*
Propranolol, **6**-34*t*
Protease inhibitors (PIs), **11**-36*t*–37*t*
Protein, **16**-3, **16**-3*t*
Protein C deficiency, **6**-8
Protein S deficiency, **6**-8
Proteus mirabilis, **12**-151
Proton pump inhibitors, **7**-37*t*, **7**-68
Protriptyline, **9**-33*t*, **14**-24*t*
Pruritus, **3**-8–9
Pseudomonas aeruginosa, **2**-19, **3**-21, **3**-38, **5**-12, **5**-29, **5**-37
Psoriasis, **3**-45–47
Psychogenic pain, **8**-70
Psychosocial development, **1**-11*t*
Psychosocial issues and stressors, **1**-9
Psychotherapy, **14**-14
Pterygium, **2**-21
Puddle sign, **7**-4*t*
Pudendal neuralgia, **12**-230

Pulmonary angiogram, **6**-10
Pulmonary embolism (PE), **6**-9–11, **6**-13
Pulmonary function tests, **5**-19
Pyelonephritis, **12**-151–152, **12**-154–155
Pyogenic granuloma, **12**-208–209
Pyospermia, **12**-69
Pyrazinamide, **11**-64, **11**-65*t*–66*t*

Q

Q angle, **8**-44
Quinapril, **6**-19*t*, **6**-34*t*

R

Rabeprazole, **7**-37*t*, **7**-68
Radiation burns, **2**-11–12
Raloxifene, **9**-33*t*
Ramipril, **6**-19*t*, **6**-34*t*
Ramsay Hunt syndrome, **9**-3, **9**-4*t*, **11**-73
Ranitidine, **7**-37*t*, **7**-68
Rape, **14**-51
Rape trauma syndrome, **14**-51
Rapidly destructive hip disease (RDHD), **8**-36
Reactive vulvitis, **12**-191–193
Recommended dietary allowances (RDAs), **16**-7, **16**-8*t*
Reflux esophagitis, **7**-33
Reimbursement, **1**-6
Reiter's syndrome, **13**-10–11
Relaxation exercises, **14**-70*t*
Relenza. *See* Zanamivir
Repaglinide, **10**-53*t*
Reproductive-age women. *See also* Pregnancy
  counseling of, **1**-17*t*
  demographics of, **1**-13
  health care issues, **1**-8, **1**-13–18
  leading causes of death in, **1**-12*t*, **1**-13
  preventive health care, **1**-17*t*
  reproductive health assessments, **1**-14–16
  risk assessments, **1**-17*t*
Respiratory disorders
  acute bronchitis, **5**-15–16
  asthma. *See* Asthma
  bronchiectasis, **5**-12–14
  bronchitis, **5**-15–16
  influenza, **5**-25–28
  pneumonia. *See* Pneumonia
Reticulocytosis, **10**-6
Retinal detachment, **2**-11, **2**-13
Retinoic acid, **3**-6
Retrocalcaneal bursitis, **8**-54
Reye's syndrome, **5**-25
Rheumatoid arthritis (RA), **8**-12–14
Rhinitis, **5**-43–47
Rifabutin, **11**-65*t*
Rifampin, **11**-64, **11**-65*t*–66*t*

Rimantadine, **5**-27
Ringworm. *See* Tinea
Risedronate, **10**-22
Ritonavir, **11**-37*t*
Rizatriptan, **9**-32*t*
Rofecoxib, **8**-10, **8**-74*t*
Rosiglitazone, **10**-53*t*, **12**-33
Rotator cuff arthropathy, **8**-18
Rotator cuff impingement syndrome, **8**-18
Rovsing's sign, **7**-4*t*
Rubella, **11**-57–59
Rubeola. *See* Measles
Rule of nines, **3**-11

S

S-adenosyl-L-methionine (SAMe), **8**-5, **14**-26
Safe sex practices, **13**-6*t*
Salmeterol, **5**-7
Salmonella, **7**-25*t*, **11**-3*t*
Salsalate, **8**-76*t*
Saquinavir, **11**-37*t*
Sarcoptes scabiei, **3**-48. *See also* Scabies
Saturated fats, **16**-4–5
Scabies, **3**-48–50
Sciatica, **8**-60–63
Scopolamine, **9**-12*t*
Screenings
    abuse, **14**-32*t*
    breast cancer, **4**-2–6
    middle-age women, **1**-18–19
    older women, **1**-21–24
Seasonal allergy, **2**-6–8
Seborrheic dermatitis, **3**-51–52
Seborrheic keratosis, **12**-201–202
Secondary amenorrhea, **12**-24–34
Second-degree burns, **3**-11–13
Secretory diarrhea, **7**-23
Seizures, **9**-37–42
Selective estrogen receptor modulators (SERM), **10**-22–23
Selective serotonin reuptake inhibitors (SSRIs)
    anorexia nervosa treated with, **14**-42
    anxiety disorders treated with, **14**-15
    depression treated with, **14**-23
    description of, **9**-33*t*, **9**-35*t*, **12**-128
    side effects of, **14**-25–26
Semen analysis, **12**-63*t*, **12**-74
Semont maneuver, **9**-14*t*
Serotonin agonists, **9**-27, **9**-32*t*
Sertraline, **9**-33*t*, **12**-128, **14**-24*t*
Sexual abuse, **14**-46–50
Sexual activity, **1**-10–11
Sexual arousal disorder, **12**-133–134, **12**-138–140
Sexual assault. *See also* Trauma, Violence
    definition of, **14**-51
    diagnostic tests for, **14**-53
    epidemiology of, **14**-51

    evaluation of, **14**-52–53
    follow-up for, **14**-55
    forensic examination form, **14**-56*f*–61*f*
    patient education regarding, **14**-54–55
    post-traumatic stress disorder caused by, **14**-52
    rape, **14**-51
    treatment for, **14**-53–54
Sexual aversion disorder, **12**-133, **12**-136
Sexual dysfunction
    anorgasmia, **12**-134–135, **12**-140–141
    assessment questions, **12**-145
    in child sexual abuse victims, **14**-47
    definition of, **12**-132
    drug-induced, **14**-25
    dyspareunia, **12**-135, **12**-141–142
    hypoactive sexual desire, **12**-132–133, **12**-135–136
    sexual arousal disorder, **12**-133–134, **12**-138–140
    sexual aversion disorder, **12**-133, **12**-136
    treatment of, **12**-137
    vaginismus, **12**-135, **12**-142–143
Sexually transmitted diseases (STDs)
    adolescents, **1**-11
    bacterial vaginosis, **12**-170
    chancroid, **13**-2–8
    chlamydia. *See* Chlamydia
    gonorrhea. *See* Gonorrhea
    herpes simplex virus. *See* Herpes simplex virus
    human papillomavirus. *See* Human papillomavirus
    incidence of, **1**-9
    in lesbians, **1**-28
    lymphogranuloma venereum, **13**-4*t*, **13**-45–49
    syphilis. *See* Syphilis
Sexual maturity rating, **1**-10*t*, **1**-13
Sexual orientation, **1**-29. *See also* Lesbians
Sheehan's syndrome, **12**-25, **12**-64
Shigella, **7**-25*t*, **11**-2, **11**-3*t*
Shingles. *See* Herpes zoster
Shoulder pain, **8**-18–23
Shoulder sign, **8**-32
Sialadenitis, **9**-18
Simvastatin, **6**-27*t*
Sinusitis
    acute, **5**-48–50
    chronic, **5**-51–52
    facial pain caused by, **9**-18
Small bowel obstruction, **7**-2, **7**-7, **7**-9
Smoking
    cessation of, **14**-64–68
    deep vein thrombosis risks, **6**-9
    description of, **1**-9
Social phobia, **14**-11–13, **14**-16
Socioeconomic issues, **1**-9
Soluble fiber, **16**-6–7
Sonohysteroscopy, **12**-68
Specific phobia, **14**-11–12, **14**-16
Sperm, **12**-62–63
Spinal stenosis, **8**-69–70
Spirometry, **5**-4

Spironolactone, **6**-20, **6**-34*t*, **12**-58
Spondylolisthesis, **8**-59, **8**-61, **8**-63, **8**-69–70
Spondylolysis, **8**-61, **8**-63, **8**-69–70
Sprain
    ankle, **8**-48–51
    lumbosacral, **8**-59
Spurling's sign, **8**-19
Squamous cell carcinoma, **12**-216–220
Squamous cell hyperplasia, **12**-197–199
Squamous intraepithelial lesion
    definition of, **12**-14
    high-grade, **12**-21*f*
    low-grade, **12**-18*f*–20*f*
Stable angina, **6**-2
Standard of care, **1**-6
Staphylococcus aureus, **2**-10, **2**-17, **2**-19, **3**-14, **3**-21, **3**-32,
        3-34, **3**-38, **5**-37, **5**-48, **5**-51, **7**-25*t*, **12**-146–147
Staphylococcus epidermidis, **2**-19, **12**-151
Staphylococcus saprophyticus, **12**-151–152
Stavudine, **11**-34*t*
Strangulated hernia, **7**-48
Streptococcus pneumoniae, **2**-10, **2**-19, **5**-37, **5**-48, **5**-51, **11**-29*t*
Streptococcus pyogenes, **2**-19, **3**-38
Streptomycin, **11**-65*t*
Stress management, **14**-69–72
Stress urinary incontinence (SUI), **12**-157–158
Stroke, **12**-111
Substance abuse/use
    criteria for, **14**-3*t*
    in lesbians, **1**-27–28
    treatment for, **14**-3–5, **14**-9
Substance dependence, **14**-2, **14**-3*t*
Suicide, **14**-20, **14**-27
Sulcus sign, **8**-20
Sulfasalazine, **7**-55, **7**-57
Sulfonylureas, **10**-53*t*
Sulindac, **8**-78*t*
Sumatriptan, **9**-32*t*, **9**-34*t*
Sumner's sign, **7**-4*t*
Superficial phlebitis, **4**-31–32
Superficial spreading melanoma, **12**-203
Superficial thrombophlebitis, **6**-9, **6**-13
Sycosis, **3**-21
Symmetrel. *See* Amantadine
Syncope, **9**-11
Syphilis
    acquired immunodeficiency syndrome and, **13**-50
    definition of, **13**-50
    diagnostic tests for, **13**-53–56
    epidemiology of, **13**-50
    follow-up for, **13**-58–59
    human immunodeficiency virus and, **13**-58–59
    latent, **13**-50–51, **13**-55–58
    patient education regarding, **13**-57–58
    physical examination findings, **13**-52–53
    during pregnancy, **13**-59
    primary, **13**-51–54, **13**-58
    secondary, **13**-51–53, **13**-55, **13**-58
    tertiary, **13**-50–51, **13**-58
    transmission of, **13**-50
    treatment of, **13**-56–58
    ulcers associated with, **13**-4*t*
Systemic lupus erythematosus (SLE)
    complications of, **10**-29
    course of, **10**-28
    description of, **7**-6, **7**-8, **10**-25
    diagnostic criteria for, **10**-26*t*
    differential diagnosis, **10**-29
    epidemiology of, **10**-25
    laboratory tests for, **10**-28*t*, **10**-29, **10**-31
    management of, **10**-29
    manifestations of, **10**-27*t*
    pathogenesis of, **10**-25
    patient education regarding, **10**-31–32
    pregnancy and, **10**-29–30
    screening questionnaire for, **10**-30*t*
    symptoms of, **10**-25–27
Systolic dysfunction, **6**-15

T

Talor tilt test, **8**-49
Tamiflu. *See* Oseltamivir
Tamoxifen, **4**-7, **9**-33*t*
Tanner staging, **1**-10*t*, **1**-13
Tarsal tunnel syndrome, **8**-53–54
Teenage pregnancy, **1**-11–12
Temporal arteritis, **9**-19, **9**-30
Temporomandibular disorder (TMD), **9**-43–48
Temporomandibular dysfunction, **9**-19
Tendinitis, **8**-15–17
Tenofovir, **11**-35*t*
Tension-type headache, **9**-29–30, **9**-35*t*
Terbutaline
    asthma treated with, **5**-6
    bronchitis treated with, **5**-16
Terconazole, **12**-177
Testosterone, **12**-196
Tetracycline, **7**-69
    acne rosacea treated with, **3**-3
    acne vulgaris treated with, **3**-6
    bronchitis treated with, **5**-16
    hidradenitis suppurativa treated with, **12**-207
    syphilis treated with, **13**-56
Thalassemia, **10**-3–5, **10**-4*t*, **10**-10
Theca lutein cysts, **12**-89
Theophylline, **5**-7–8
Thermal burns, **2**-11–12
Thiazide diuretics, **6**-34*t*
Thiazolidinediones, **10**-53*t*
Third-degree burns, **3**-11–13
Thompson test, **8**-49
Thrombophlebitis, superficial, **6**-9, **6**-13
Thrombosis
    deep vein. *See* Deep vein thrombosis

mesenteric venous, 7-8
Thyroid disorders, **10**-33–39
Thyroid nodules, **10**-33–35, **10**-37–39
Thyroid-stimulating hormone, **10**-37*t*
Thyrotoxicosis, **10**-33–35, **10**-37–39
Tiagabine, **9**-41*t*
Tick-borne diseases, **11**-42–48
Tietze's syndrome, **4**-6
Tinea capitis, **3**-26–27
Tinea corporis, **3**-25–26
Tinea cruris, **3**-29
Tinea pedis, **3**-27–29
Tinea versicolor, **3**-24–25
Tinel's sign, **8**-28
Tioconazole, **12**-177
Tissue plasminogen activator (TPA), **6**-13
Tobacco. *See also* Smoking
    cessation of use, **14**-64–68
    history of, **14**-64–65
Tolbutamide, **10**-53*t*
Tolmetin, **8**-78*t*
Toma's sign, **7**-4*t*
Topiramate, **9**-40*t*
Torsemide, **6**-19*t*, **6**-34*t*
Toxic shock syndrome (TSS), **12**-146–150
Toxoplasma gondii, **11**-29*t*
Trandolapril, **6**-34*t*
Tranexamic acid, **12**-10
Transcutaneous electrical nerve stimulation, **12**-40
Trauma. *See also* Sexual assault
    dizziness caused by, **9**-10
    eye, **2**-11–13
    rape, **14**-51
Traveler's diarrhea, **7**-27, **11**-6–7
Trazodone, **9**-35*t*, **14**-24*t*
Treponema pallidum, **13**-2, **13**-5, **13**-50, **13**-53
Triamcinolone acetonide, **12**-198
    asthma treated with, **5**-6–7
    chronic obstructive pulmonary disease treated with, **5**-21
Triamterene, **6**-34*t*
Trichloroacetic acid (TCA), **13**-42
Trichomonas vaginalis, **12**-182–185
Trichomonas vaginalis vaginitis, **12**-182–185, **12**-186*t*
Trichomoniasis, **12**-182–185, **12**-186*t*
Trichopyton rubrum, **3**-25–26
Tricyclic antidepressants, **14**-15, **14**-24*t*, **14**-25, **14**-42. *See also* Antidepressants
Trigeminal neuralgia, **9**-16, **9**-18*t*, **9**-21
Trigger finger, **8**-32–33
Triiodothyronine, **10**-36*t*
Trimethobenzamide hydrochloride, **14**-54
Trimethoprim/sulfamethoxazole
    bronchiectasis treated with, **5**-13
    chronic obstructive pulmonary disease treated with, **5**-21
    granuloma inguinale treated with, **13**-27
    otitis media treated with, **5**-32
    sinusitis treated with, **5**-49, **5**-52
    traveler's diarrhea treated with, **7**-27
    urinary tract infection treated with, **12**-154
Trimipramine, **14**-24*t*
Trochanteric bursitis, **8**-36
Tuberculosis, **11**-29*t*
    definition of, **11**-60
    diagnostic tests for, **11**-62–63
    epidemiology of, **11**-60
    evaluation of, **11**-61–62
    latent, **11**-66*t*–67*t*
    medications for, **11**-65*t*–66*t*
    multidrug-resistant, **11**-60–61
    patient education regarding, **11**-66, **11**-68
    treatment of, **11**-63–64, **11**-65*t*–66*t*
Tumor necrosis factor, **8**-13
Tzanck smear, **11**-71

U

Ulcer(s)
    corneal, **2**-19
    duodenal, **7**-64, **7**-66
    genital, **13**-4*t*, **13**-5*f*
Ulcerative colitis (UC), **7**-51–59
Umbilical hernia, **7**-48
Unstable angina, **6**-2
Ureaplasma urealyticum, **12**-63
Ureteral obstruction, **7**-7
Urethral caruncle, **12**-209
Urethral syndrome, **12**-101, **13**-10
Urinary incontinence (UI), **1**-22–23, **12**-157–160
Urinary tract infection (UTI), **12**-98*t*, **12**-151–156
Urolithiasis, **12**-96
Ursodeoxycholic acids, **7**-16
Uterine bleeding, **12**-3–10, **12**-4*t*
Uveitis, **2**-22–23

V

Vaccinations. *See* Immunizations
Vaginal intraepithelial neoplasia (VAIN), **12**-233–234
Vaginismus, **12**-135, **12**-142–143
Vaginitis
    atrophic, **12**-167–169, **12**-186*t*
    cytolytic, **12**-180–181, **12**-186*t*
    Trichomonas vaginalis, **12**-182–185
Vaginosis, bacterial, **12**-170–173
Valacyclovir, **11**-74, **12**-228, **13**-33–34
Valdecoxib, **8**-74*t*
Valproic acid, **9**-34*t*, **9**-40*t*
Varicella zoster immunoglobulin (VZIG), **11**-71–72, **11**-72*t*
Varicella zoster virus (VZV), **11**-29*t*, **11**-69–73. *See also* Herpes zoster
Varicocele, **12**-62, **12**-69
Vasomotor rhinitis, **5**-43–47
Vasovagal vasopressor syncope, **9**-11
Vegetarian diet, **16**-5–6, **16**-6*t*

Venlafaxine, **14**-24*t*
Venous thromboembolism, **12**-111–112
Verapamil, **6**-34*t*, **9**-32*t*, **9**-34*t*
Verruca plana, **3**-53
Verruca plantaris, **3**-53
Verruca vulgaris, **3**-53–54
Verrucous carcinoma, **12**-214–215
Vertigo
  benign paroxysmal positional, **9**-9
  description of, **9**-8, **9**-12
Very-low-density lipoproteins (VLDL), **6**-22
Vestibular neuronitis, **9**-9
Vestibular suppressants, **9**-12*t*
Vestibulitis, **12**-224, **12**-229
Vibrio cholerae, **7**-25*t*, **11**-3*t*, **11**-6
Vibrio parahaemolyticus, **7**-25*t*
Violence. *See also* Sexual assault
  description of, **1**-18
  domestic, **14**-30–34
Viral conjunctivitis, **2**-6–8
Viral pharyngitis, **5**-33–36
Viral pneumonia, **5**-39
Viral rhinitis, **5**-43–47
Virchow's triad, **6**-8
Virilization, **12**-53
Vitamin(s), **16**-7–9
Vitamin B$_6$, **12**-130
Vitamin B$_{12}$ deficiency anemia, **10**-10–11
Vulva
  acrochordons of, **12**-206
  Bartholin's cyst/abscess, **12**-211–214
  basal cell carcinoma of, **12**-219–220
  caruncle of, **12**-209
  contact dermatitis of, **12**-191–193
  cutaneous candidiasis of, **12**-189–191
  dark lesions of, **12**-200–204
  epidermal cysts of, **12**-205–206
  Fox-Fordyce disease, **12**-209–210
  hemangiomas of, **12**-208–209
  hidradenitis suppurativa of, **12**-206–208
  lentigo of, **12**-200
  lichen sclerosus, **12**-195–197
  melanoma of, **12**-202–204
  nevi of, **12**-200–201
  Paget's disease of, **12**-193–194
  seborrheic keratosis, **12**-201–202
  squamous cell carcinoma of, **12**-216–220
  squamous cell hyperplasia of, **12**-197–199
  verrucous carcinoma of, **12**-214–215
  white lesions of, **12**-195–199
Vulvar intraepithelial neoplasia (VIN), **12**-195, **12**-200, **12**-221–223
Vulvar melanosis, **12**-201
Vulvar vestibulitis, **12**-224, **12**-229
Vulvodynia
  definition of, **12**-224
  diagnostic tests for, **12**-227–228
  differential diagnosis, **12**-225*t*
  dysesthetic, **12**-224–226, **12**-230
  evaluation of, **12**-226–227
  iatrogenic factors, **12**-229
Vulvovaginitis, candidal, **12**-174–179

W

Warts
  dermatological, **3**-53–54
  genital, **13**-42*t*–43*t*
Water, **16**-7
Weight, **16**-11
Whitehead, **3**-5
Wrist pain, **8**-27–35

X

Xylometazoline, **5**-49

Y

Yersinia, **7**-25*t*, **11**-3*t*

Z

Zafirlukast, **5**-7–8
Zalcitabine, **11**-35*t*
Zanamivir, **5**-27
Zidovudine, **11**-35*t*
Zileuton, **5**-7
Zollinger-Ellison syndrome, **7**-65–66, **7**-69
Zolmitriptan, **9**-32*t*, **9**-34*t*
Zonisamide, **9**-41*t*